Gerontological Nursing

Gerontological Nursing

CONCEPTS AND PRACTICE

EDITION 2

Mary Ann Matteson, PhD, RN, CS, FAAN
Thelma and Joe Crow Endowed Professor
University of Texas Health Science Center at San Antonio
School of Nursing
San Antonio, Texas

Eleanor S. McConnell, PhD, RN
Clinical Nurse Specialist
Durham Geriatric Research, Education, and Clinical Center
Department of Veterans Affairs

Research Assistant Professor
Duke University School of Nursing

Senior Fellow
Center for the Study of Aging and Human Development
Duke University
Durham, North Carolina

Adrianne Dill Linton, PhD, RN
Associate Professor
University of Texas Health Science Center at San Antonio
School of Nursing
San Antonio, Texas

W.B. SAUNDERS COMPANY
A Division of Harcourt Brace & Company
PHILADELPHIA LONDON TORONTO
MONTREAL SYDNEY TOKYO

W.B. Saunders Company
A Division of Harcourt Brace & Company

The Curtis Center
Independence Square West
Philadelphia, Pennsylvania 19106

Library of Congress Cataloging-in-Publication Data

Matteson, Mary Ann.
Gerontological nursing: concepts and practice / Mary Ann Matteson,
Eleanor S. McConnell, Adrianne Dill Linton.—2nd ed.

p. cm.

Includes bibliographical references and index.

ISBN 0-7216-3785-X

1. Geriatric nursing.   I. McConnell, Eleanor S.   II. Linton,
  Adrianne Dill.   III. Title.
  [DNLM: 1. Geriatric Nursing.   WY 152 M435g 1996]

RC954.M37 1996   610.73'65—dc20

DNLM/DLC   95-42808

Gerontological Nursing: Concepts and Practice, second edition   ISBN 0-7216-3785-X

Printed in the United States of America

Last digit is the print number: 9   8   7   6   5   4   3   2

To our husbands, Steve, Randy, and Ken

Contributors

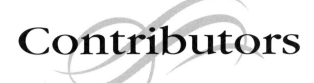

Susan J. Barnes, MSN, RNC, Doctoral Candidate

Associate Faculty, Cochite College, Douglas, Arizona

Context of Services—Network of Care; Gerontological Care in Community Care Settings

Lucille B. Bearon

Assistant Professor and Extensions Specialist, Adult Development/Aging, Department of Family and Consumer Sciences, North Carolina State University, Raleigh, North Carolina; Adjunct Clinical Assistant Professor, School of Nursing, Duke University, Durham, North Carolina

Psychosocial Problems Associated with Aging

Margaret L. Bell, BSN, MPH, PhD

Assistant Professor, University of Texas Health Science Center at San Antonio School of Nursing, San Antonio, Texas

Nutritional Considerations

Dorothy J. Brundage, PhD, RN, FAAN

Associate Professor, Duke University School of Nursing, Durham, North Carolina

Age-Related Changes in the Genitourinary System

Brenda Lewis Cleary, PhD, RN, CS, FAAN

Adjunct faculty, Duke University School of Nursing, Durham; University of North Carolina School of Public Health, Chapel Hill, North Carolina; Texas University HSC School of Nursing, Lubbock, Texas; Executive Director, North Carolina Center for Nursing, Raleigh, North Carolina

Age-Related Changes in the Special Senses

Nancy J. Girard, BSN, MSN, PhD

Chair, Acute Nursing Care Department and Associate Professor, University of Texas Health Science Center, School of Nursing, San Antonio, Texas

Gerontological Nursing in Acute Care Settings

Joseph T. Hanlon, PharmD, MS

Coordinator of Pharmacogeriatrics, Center for the Study of Aging and Human Development, Duke University Medical Center, Durham, North Carolina; Clinical Associate Professor, University of North Carolina School of Pharmacy, Chapel Hill, North Carolina

Pharmacological Considerations

J. Taylor Harden, PhD, RNC

Former Associate Professor, University of Texas Health Science Center School of Nursing, San Antonio, Texas; Nurse Scientist Administrator, National Institutes of Health, National Institute of Nursing Research, Bethesda, Maryland

Nursing Diagnoses Related to Psychosocial Alterations

Joanne S. Harrell, BA, BSN, MN, PhD

Associate Professor, School of Nursing, University of North Carolina at Chapel Hill; Director, Center for Research on Preventing/Managing Chronic Illness in Vulnerable People, School of Nursing, University of North Carolina at Chapel Hill, Chapel Hill, North Carolina

Age-Related Changes in the Cardiovascular System; Age-Related Changes in the Respiratory System

Martha L. Henderson

Clinical Assistant Professor, Department of Community and Mental Health, University of North Carolina School of Nursing, Chapel Hill, North Carolina

Ethical Considerations

Pauline Lee, EdD, MSN, RNC

Assistant Professor/Clinical and Interim Chair, Department of Family Nursing Care, University of Texas Health Science Center at San Antonio School of Nursing, San Antonio, Texas

Age-Related Changes in the Endocrine System

Deborah Lekan-Rutledge, MSN, RNC, CCCN

Adjunct Clinical Assistant Professor, University of North Carolina School of Nursing, Chapel Hill; Clinical Nurse Specialist, Gerontological Nursing, Chapel Hill, North Carolina

Functional Assessment; Gerontological Nursing in Long-Term Care Facilities

Adrianne Dill Linton, PhD, RN

Associate Professor, University of Texas Health Science Center at San Antonio School of Nursing, San Antonio, Texas

Age-Related Changes in the Neurological System; Age-Related Changes in the Gastrointestinal System; Age-Related Changes in the Genitourinary System; Age-Related Changes in the Endocrine System; Pharmacological Considerations

Mary Ann Matteson, PhD, RN, CS, FAAN

Thelma and Joe Crow Endowed Professor, University of Texas Health Science Center at San Antonio School of Nursing, San Antonio, Texas

Biological Theories of Aging; Age-Related Changes in the Integument; Age-Related Changes in the Musculoskeletal System; Age-Related Changes in the Neurological System; Age-Related Changes in the Endocrine System; Psychosocial Aging Changes; Psychosocial Problems Associated with Aging

Eleanor S. McConnell, PhD, RN

Clinical Nurse Specialist, Durham Geriatric Research, Education, and Clinical Center, Department of Veterans Affairs; Research Assistant Professor, Duke University School of Nursing; Senior Fellow, Center for the Study of Aging and Human Development, Duke University, Durham, North Carolina

Conceptual Bases for Gerontological Nursing Practice: Models, Trends, and Issues; Ethical Considerations; Nursing Diagnoses Related to Physiological Alterations; Psychosocial Problems Associated with Aging; Pharmacological Considerations

Ann T. Murphy, RN, MSN

Clinical Nurse Specialist, Adult and Geriatric Health, Durham Veterans Affairs Medical Center; Senior Fellow, Center for the Study of Aging and Human Development, Duke University, Durham, North Carolina

Nursing Diagnoses Related to Physiological Alterations

Susan Ann Ruzicka, BSN, MSN(R)

Doctoral Student, University of Texas Health Science Center, San Antonio, Texas

Nursing Diagnoses Influenced by Setting of Care

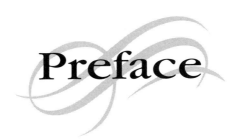

Preface

The first edition of *Gerontological Nursing: Concepts and Practice* was published in 1988. It was written to provide a comprehensive, research-based reference for nurses who cared for and about the elderly. The enthusiastic response to that book and the many suggestions from readers encouraged the authors/ editors to undertake a second edition. Some of the reasons and circumstances that prompted the first edition continue to exist today. The aging population is increasing steadily, creating challenges, opportunities, and a demand for more nurses prepared in this specialty. In addition, generalist nurses must seek sources of information to guide their practice because the populations being seen throughout agencies of care are ever more elderly.

Much nursing literature on gerontology is experiential rather than research based. Research in gerontology is broad based and nurses can draw from biological, social, and medical research literature. The book describes the aging process across the health care continuum from wellness to illness. Physiological and psychological aspects of aging are described in detail, as well as assessment and practice in all settings using the nursing process.

This book is organized into five units. Unit I provides an overview of gerontological nursing with an emphasis on the conceptual bases for practice. Unit II is an exploration of physiological aging changes; a systems approach is employed to describe age-related changes. Special attention is given to research, differentiating between changes related to age and those related to lifestyle or pathology. The nursing process is applied as detailed nursing assessment is presented, followed by common nursing diagnoses, related interventions, and evaluation criteria. Unit III, psychosocial changes, explores sociocultural influences on aging and important psychosocial problems. Pharmacologic and nutritional considerations make up Unit IV. Unit V explores gerontological nursing in a variety of care settings: acute care, long-term care, and the community.

The second edition contains a completely new literature review and updated references. Extensive reference lists reflect a thorough review of the recent literature in nursing, medicine, and social science. In addition, nursing diagnoses are updated from the most recent NANDA conference possible. The general format remains familiar to readers who used the first edition; however, streamlining of content between chapters has minimized overlap and ensured better readability for both students and busy practitioners. Throughout the book, tables are used to summarize theoretical and practice concepts for easy accessibility, and numerous assessment forms are reproduced to provide a comprehensive reference.

Mary Ann Matteson
Eleanor S. McConnell
Adrianne Dill Linton

Acknowledgments

We would like to thank our families, friends, and colleagues who have supported us during the revision process. We especially thank our contributors who have again shared their expertise with us. We are particularly appreciative of Dr. Harvey Cohen and Dr. Patty Hawken for their encouragement and support; Dr. Jo Ann Crow, Stephen Matteson, Jr., Dr. Nancy Maebius, and Dr. Nancy Girard for their help with artwork and photography; and Anna Melinda Bell and Mary K. Wooten, R.N., M.S.N., C.E.T.N, for technical assistance. We are also grateful to Ilze Rader for her professional editorial guidance, support, and patience; Marie Thomas, editorial assistant; David Harvey, copy editor; and Mike Carcel, production manager.

Contents

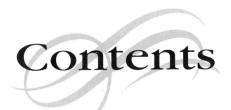

1
Overview of Gerontological Nursing
1

2
Physiological Aging Changes
173

3

Psychosocial Aging Changes
553

4

The Clinical Sciences
737

5

Care Settings
791

Overview of Gerontological Nursing

1

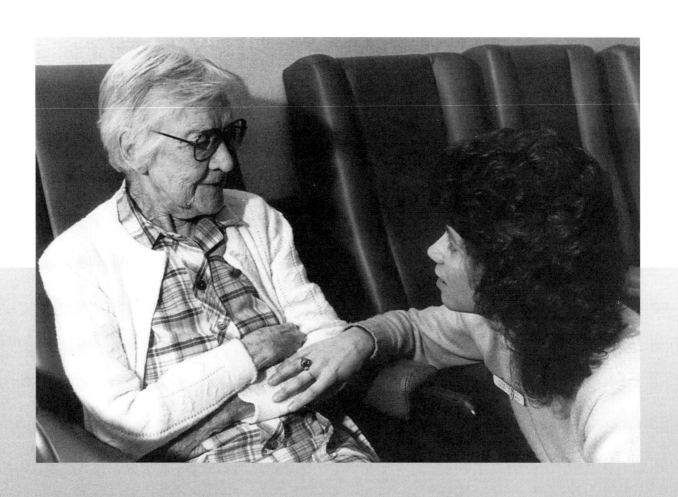

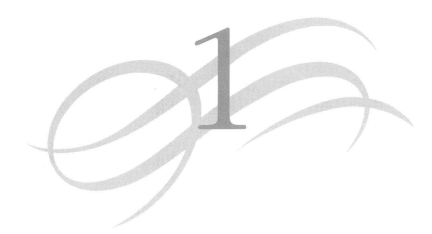

Conceptual Bases for Gerontological Nursing Practice: Models, Trends, and Issues

ELEANOR S. McCONNELL

OBJECTIVES

Describe the purpose of a conceptual framework for nursing care of the elderly.

Discuss the conceptual bases for gerontological nursing practice, including the definitions of aging and old age, health and disease in older age, environmental influences on aging, and nursing and aging clients.

Trace the history of gerontological nursing and its influence on health care of the elderly.

Create a model of gerontological nursing practice within the context of health services to the elderly.

Apply the gerontological nursing model to the nursing care of older clients.

Discuss the need for a research base for clinical practice in gerontological nursing.

Examine the need for formal educational opportunities in gerontological nursing.

Analyze the issues related to standards of gerontological nursing care in the hospital, nursing home, and community.

A conceptual framework is a set of concepts that guides decisions about *what* to assess and diagnose, *how* to intervene, and *what* to evaluate.

Gordon, 1982, p. 21

Elderly people are an extremely diverse group of individuals who possess a broad range of abilities and needs in all domains of function. This reality, along with the varied lifestyles, environmental conditions, and life histories characteristic of old people, creates the need for highly individualized nursing care. Nursing of the elderly is thus a complex specialty—one that must allow for many different perspectives and accommo-date diverse research findings and theoretical approaches.

THE CONCEPTUAL FRAMEWORK

Purpose

A conceptual framework for nursing care of the elderly serves several purposes. First, it specifies the relevant scientific foundations upon which gerontological nursing is practiced. Second, it clarifies the values and assumptions that underlie this type of nursing practice. Finally, it shows how concepts from diverse fields of study come together to guide nursing practice, and suggests nursing research to enhance the scientific and theoretical bases for nursing practice with the aged.

Gerontology has a diversity of conceptual approaches and conflicting research findings; therefore, all models presently guiding clinical nursing practice with older persons will change and evolve. They may eventually meld into a unified nursing model for care of the elderly, although it is doubtful this will happen soon. The current trend in nursing theory development is to focus on the development of midrange theories to guide nursing practice, such as theories of uncertainty (Mishel, 1990) or theories of excess disability in the cognitively impaired (Dawson et al., 1993).

Elements

Nurses should resolve the following questions when developing a conceptual framework for nursing practice with the elderly:

1. What assumptions, beliefs, and values about nursing and the elderly influence my practice?
2. What do nurses offer the elderly in health care?
3. What is the range of expected health outcomes for older persons?
4. What is the nature of the professional nurse's relationship with other health care providers of the elderly?

The answers to these questions influence the type of nursing care delivered to older people. For example, does the nurse believe that old people are capable of growth and attainment of new goals, or does the nurse believe that aging results in decrements in all spheres of function? With the first perspective, the full range of therapeutic options remains open. With the second viewpoint, the goal of nursing older persons is to help the old person give up most responsibilities so that energy can be conserved for maintaining physiological integrity. Support for both viewpoints can be found.

Perspectives of nurses on the scope of practice, definitions of health and illness in the aged, and relationships with other health care providers also influence the nursing care the older person receives. This chapter contains an explicitly formulated conceptual framework for nursing practice with the elderly. It draws from general systems theory, the basic biomedical and behavioral sciences, gerontology, and nursing theory. Other conceptual frameworks for nursing of the aged are used throughout this text. No attempt is made to promote one framework over another. Each nurse must develop and use a framework that provides a useful guide for practice. The only requirements are that it be scientifically grounded and periodically re-evaluated in light of new research or practice findings.

CONCEPTUAL BASES FOR GERONTOLOGICAL NURSING PRACTICE

Gerontology and Geriatrics

Gerontology is the study of the processes of aging and the problems of older people. Although observations about the nature of aging are as old as written history, gerontology is considered a young science. Most significant advances in gerontology have occurred since 1950. Gerontological research is conducted at all levels of living system organization: from the subcellular level through the organ system levels and human organism level to the social-cultural levels of organization.

Gerontology is an applied science; gerontologists use no unique investigative tools. Biochemists, physiologists, pharmacologists, psychologists, sociologists, anthropologists, health care providers, and a host of other professionals are involved in the study of aging. Findings from gerontological research enhance understanding of the nature of aging and old people and help remove stereotypic ideas from clinical practice. Relevant findings from the gerontology literature are summarized throughout the text as they apply to the health care of older people.

Gerontology seeks to understand the processes and effects of normal aging. *Geriatrics*, in contrast, is the study and practice of the medical problems and care of older people

with diseases. Geriatric research seeks to understand the causes, consequences, and factors that modify disease expression in the elderly.

Limitations of Gerontological Research

Controversy exists over which functional changes associated with aging are caused by aging alone, which are caused by lifestyle factors alone, and which by disease processes. In the abstract it is possible to distinguish primary aging changes (those changes that are the result of the aging process only) from secondary aging changes (those resulting from disease, lifestyle, or both) (Rowe and Kahn, 1987). However, in practice it is difficult to distinguish these two types of aging-related changes. Many of the early studies of aging were based on cross-sectional studies of ill and institutionalized old people. Conclusions drawn from these studies tend to portray the elderly and the aging process in a very negative manner. The validity of these conclusions is increasingly being questioned for two reasons: (1) an institutionalized population is not representative of all older people; and (2) in cross-sectional studies, it is difficult to determine whether the differences between young and old are due to aging or to some other factor, such as disease or a cohort effect.

For example, consider the differences in performance ability on the following task between people over the age of 65 years and those under 45: "Describe the importance of Pearl Harbor Day."

The fact that older people perform better on this task than do younger people could be interpreted by a naive investigator as an aging-related phenomenon. However, astute observers know that the difference between groups is due to a difference in the history they have experienced (a cohort factor) and not to an aging process. If the abilities of the younger group in performing a task are measured over time (a longitudinal design), it would eventually be learned that the performance of the group was not affected by age. This is a trivial example, but consider the following more clinically relevant example.

Intelligence is frequently measured by standardized tests. In the past it was concluded on the basis of cross-sectional studies using standardized tests that intelligence declined with age. Critics now question this conclusion for several reasons. How does one know whether the difference between young people and old people in "intelligence" (assuming that intelligence is indeed what is measured by these instruments) is due to aging or to some other factor, such as differences in educational level, differences in nutritional status during their formative years, or cultural bias within the test itself? There is no way of knowing, and therefore the conclusion that intelligence declines with age becomes suspect.

Studies employing a longitudinal design circumvent the problem of a cohort effect leading to erroneous conclusions. However, such studies are expensive and time-consuming to conduct. Additionally, these studies may be biased by a "survivor effect." The survivor effect refers to the problem that results from not knowing whether the individuals who live to *complete* the longitudinal study represent the "average" individual or an especially advantaged subpopulation. This limits the generalizability of study results. Therefore, both longitudinal and cross-sectional studies are useful. It is important to understand the limitations of both research designs, and to be open to revising long-standing opinions or generalizations about the effects of aging as results from newer studies become available. The challenge for gerontological nurses is to remain abreast of the new information being generated about the aging process and older people.

Thus, while the breadth and scope of research in gerontology is impressive, significant gaps exist in the scientific base for clinical practice with old people. The difficulties inherent in generalizing about the nature of aging and old people are exemplified by the problem of arriving at a generally accepted definition of "aging" and "old."

Definitions of Old Age

Common dictionary definitions of old age and related terms reflect the variety of meanings and connotations for the words aged, aging, old, and elderly held by lay people. The term "old" can be used to mean "wise," "familiar," or, in a less positive vein, "declining in vigor and strength" (Webster's, 1991, p. 821). Scientific definitions offer similar variety in tone. Biological definitions often emphasize decline in structure or function of cells and organs, but some are more neutral in tone, defining aging as merely the changes that accrue with the passage of time. Because there is a diversity in definitions of old, clinicians should be alert to the possibility for miscommunication when generalizations are made about "old" people or the "aging process."

In a landmark study, Butler (1975) drew attention to the ambivalent notions of old age held by Americans, which range from the "golden ager" to the "old geezer" or "old biddy" stereotypes. He contended that these conflicting stereotypes combine "wishful thinking and stark terror." The terror is grounded in a natural fear of death and disability; the wishful thinking is based on reluctance to confront the impact of current lifestyle choices on function in later life. Most people do not realize that important factors influencing the quality of life in old age are as numerous as physical health, personality, earlier life experiences, the environment surrounding late life events, and social support, including finances, housing, health care, social roles, recreation, and spiritual pursuits. Butler proposed a more realistic view of aging as "neither inherently miserable nor inherently sublime—like every stage of life it has problems, joys, fears, and potentials" (p. 2). His insights about stereotypes of aging remain salient over 20 years later.

The fact that aging has cultural, social, psychological, and biological meanings makes definitions of descriptive terms difficult to fit all cases. The segment of life referred to as "old age" spans 40 years; it is therefore misleading to try to characterize people in this age group as homogeneous. Terms such as "young-old" are used to describe those aged 55 to 74 years and "old-old" to refer to those 75 years and older.

Caranasos (1993) has proposed a nomenclature for subdividing age cohorts that is likely to develop a widespread following. He suggests using the terms "early old age" to denote those aged 65 to 74, "middle old age" for those aged 75 to 84, and "late old age" for those over 84.

The term "frail elderly," once used to refer to those over 75, is now used to mean something quite specific about vulnerability to disease as the result of decrements in organ system function (Buchner and Wagner, 1992).

Two common approaches to defining people as old are the chronological approach and the functional approach (Schroots and Birren, 1990). The *chronological method* defines a certain age as old—for example, 65 years—and compares the number of years an individual has lived against this standard. It is the most popular approach because it is economical and objective. Use of chronological age to establish who is elderly may be convenient, but it tells little about function or performance.

The *functional approach* to defining "old" evaluates the functional performance of the individual against standard adult performance. This is analogous to the use of developmental screening tests in children, such as the Denver Developmental Screening Test. Those adults who do not meet predetermined criteria for young adult performance are considered "old." For a simple example, one commonly used performance standard for adults is employment. Since it is normal for adults to engage in paid employment, retired adults are thus considered "old."

A practical application of the use of functional age rather than chronological age is in the area of decisions about employment. Since the enactment of the Age Discrimination in Employment Act, mandatory retirement at age 70 is illegal. Chronological age can be used as a reason for dismissal only if it can be shown to be the only valid criterion upon which inferences about the ability to perform the job can be based (Spirduso and MacRae, 1990). Motor performance testing has been proposed as an alternative means for determining ability to perform job tasks. At one time, this approach was criticized because of inadequate information about the work capacity of older adults (Kahn, 1983). Studies are now emerging that help clarify the potential work capacity of older adults. In a study of over 38 million people aged 55 to 74 who had worked at some time since their 45th birthday, 58 per cent of the population had no difficulty with motor performance on tasks associated with job performance. The tasks that were studied included (1) walking one quarter of a mile and ascending 10 stairs without resting; (2) endurance for sitting or standing for 2 hours without resting; (3) lower and upper body strength, such as stooping, crouching, or kneeling, and carrying 25- or 10-pound loads; (4) ability to reach up overhead or out in front of the body; and (5) fine motor skills such as grasping with the fingers (Kovar and LaCroix, 1987). As more data emerge about performance capabilities of older people, it is likely that functional age criteria will be used instead of chronological age criteria.

Although broad application of the functional approach to age grading is expensive, because it requires individualized assessment of many domains of function, society is increasingly less willing to rely on inaccurate categorization of the functional abilities of its elders.

Sometimes the chronological and functional methods are used together. Chronological age criteria are first applied, and then a functional test of age is used. The combined approach is being used increasingly to make decisions about employment of people over 65. It is also used when scarce or expensive resources must be allocated. For example, Medicare uses the concept of "homebound" status (a judgment of functional ability) to determine which Medicare recipients will receive home health benefits. Functional criteria are thus used to subdivide the chronologically defined "elderly" population in order to determine who receives certain costly resources.

For the purposes of this text, terms such as "elderly," "old," and "aged" refer to those aged 65 years and older, unless otherwise specified. When the data are available, characteristics of the young-old and old-old populations are described separately. The semantic difficulties in defining "the elderly" are important, for they reflect the power of labels in defining social opportunities for old people. While this may seem only tangentially related to health, most definitions of health are related to ability to carry out social role expectations.

Impact of Age-Related Changes on the Individual

Aging is a highly individualized process that affects each person in unique ways. Aging is the result of the interaction among genetic endowment, environmental influences, lifestyles, and the effects of disease processes. Therefore, people become increasingly diverse as they age, and it is difficult to predict with certainty a person's health status or functioning level on the basis of chronological age alone. However, certain generalizations discussed below can be culled from the burgeoning research literature in gerontology and geriatrics.

Physiological Changes

As currently understood, biological aging of humans results in progressive, irreversible, decremental changes in the characteristics of organs such as the endocrine glands, myocardium, vasculature, connective tissue, and neurons. The precise mechanism of these changes is unclear, but nearly universal changes in functioning of organ systems in human aging can be discerned. Specific descriptions of age-related changes in structure and function in each body system are contained in Unit II. Biological aging changes have little effect on the functional performance of the individual in the resting state; however, in the stressed state, deficits in function are appreciated because of impairment of homeostatic mechanisms. Examples of common stressors that adversely affect elderly function are drugs, disease, massive life change, and increased physical demand.

Organ systems most commonly and severely affected by age-related changes include the renal, cardiovascular, and neurological systems. Impairment in homeostatic mechanisms implies that clinicians must be particularly alert for signs of body system failure, and must also be aware of the potential for induction of iatrogenic disease because of the reduced margin for error in therapeutics in the aged. Examples of how to exercise such care are discussed in detail throughout the text.

Disease adversely affects function in the elderly. Sophistication in assessment and diagnosis is required to identify the presence of disease as a source of declining function, since disease presentation is often altered in the elderly. Some of the dysfunctions induced by disease in late life are reversible and some are not. The cure of disease is not always feasible in the elderly, and sometimes overaggressive treatment may result in more debility. Judicious treatment of diseases, with consideration of the functional costs as well as benefits, may enhance function in the elderly.

Sensory acuity tends to decline with age, and the threshold for sensory perception increases. Old people are therefore likely to require modification of sensory inputs to perform optimally. Increased lighting intensity, modulation of voice pitch and volume, and modification of the pace of information presentation are useful techniques in enhancing reception of sensory stimuli.

Psychological Changes

Research findings regarding changes in cognition, personality, and affect with aging are conflicting. An extensive body of cross-sectional studies conclude that age-related declines in cognitive abilities exist, but newer, longitudinal studies cast doubt on just how severe the deficits are, and have served to moderate the conclusion that decline is due to aging alone. Additionally, researchers are increasingly interested in identifying what factors are responsible for observed decline, so that potential modifying interventions can be identified and tested (Schaie, 1989). Intelligence is a multidimensional concept, and the effects of age versus disease on the various components of intelligence are not fully understood. Performance on intelligence tests depends on environmental characteristics, sensory ability, time constraints, motivation, educational level, social expectations, and a variety of other variables that cannot always be adequately controlled.

Kogan (1990) reports that research continues to confirm relative stability of personality traits with aging. However, self-concept continues to develop throughout the lifespan and may be affected by aging-related physiological changes and life transitions (Reinke et al., 1985). The self-concept is a product of perceived changes in body structure and function and the reflected appraisal of others in the environment. In late life, self-concept is relatively stable, but self-esteem fluctuates more with the role changes that accompany old age (Atchley, 1969). Self-esteem is composed of the feelings resulting from comparing who one is with the idealized self. Well-regarded past performance contributes to positive self-esteem in later life (Atchley, 1984). Thus, while aging changes and social responses to these changes influence how individuals perceive themselves and others perceive them, lifestyle and past performance are also important.

Multiple losses are a common feature of late life. Changes of any type are associated with some loss; increasing age results in an accumulation of losses. Aging involves processes that both enhance the older person's ability to cope with loss and increase the difficulty of adjustment to losses. Bereavement is most associated with declines in mental health; physical deterioration has also been associated with bereavement. Loss is therefore another stressor that may impair function.

Social Changes

Family structures are altered with age, but family values and relationships follow patterns that are more enduring than the influence of a single member and thus exert greater influence on family functioning than does the impact of aging. Aging-related changes in family structure are not associated with breakdown of extended family networks. Family relationships are governed by family values and norms that are characterized by continuity across generations.

Social responses to aging-related changes in individuals are culturally determined. Some cultures place a high value on the contributions of people of advanced years. Other cultures place a higher value on the contributions of the young. American culture is a mixture of many cultural groups; however, the dominant cultural group currently places its highest values on innovation, newness, independent function, and youth. As a greater proportion of American society becomes old, social values and institutions may evolve to better meet the needs of the aged. More recently, policy analysts have noted the importance of reconsidering the social structures that support the aged, particularly as greater numbers of people live into advanced age. The need is, in the words of one leader, "to broaden the debate about preparing for an aging society in a comprehensive manner. . . ." (Torres-Gil and Puccinelli, 1994, p. 749; Silverstone, 1994).

Current gerontological and geriatric literature emphasizes focusing on functional integrity rather than on structural deficits in defining health. Knowledge of the functional impact of age-related changes helps nurses modify nursing approaches to consider the developmental level when designing and implementing care.

Health and Disease in the Aged

Definitions of Health, Disease, and Illness

Health, disease, and illness are related concepts that apply to people of all ages. For the purposes of this text, disease refers to identifiable pathological processes, whereas illness refers to the human experience of the disease (Suchman, 1963; Wu, 1973). Health is a state of being with multiple determinants (Orem, 1991). It implies continued development and successful adaptation to adverse conditions, including diseases. Physiological as well as psychological, social, and cultural factors influence health status by placing different demands on the human organism, as well as by providing different supports. Health is characterized by "integrated functioning oriented toward maximizing individual potential while maintaining balance and purposeful direction in the environment" (Dunn, 1961).

Determining health status in the elderly is difficult, because few well-defined norms describe health in the aged. Emerging results from large-scale epidemiological studies such as the Establishment of a Population for Epidemiologic Studies of the Elderly (EPESE) studies and the National Health and Nutrition Examination Survey (NHANES), and inclusion of more functionally oriented questions on the National Health Interview Survey, are important first steps in establishing norms regarding functional health for older people. With time, they may allow definitive statements to be made regarding health norms.

Lawton's concept of "The Good Life" is useful for considering the health of the aged in the broadest possible context. According to this model, well-being consists of four intersecting but relatively autonomous sectors of life: psychological well-being, perceived quality of life, objective environment, and behavioral competence. Although psychological well-being is influenced by behavioral competence, it is not wholly dependent upon it, suggesting that the older person may achieve high levels of psychological well-being despite impairments in behavioral competence or deficits in the other determinants of the good life (Lawton, 1983; Lawton, 1991).

Behavioral competence (Fig. 1–1) is "the theoretical upper limit of capacity of the individual to function in the areas of biological health, sensation and perception, motor behavior, and cognition" (Lawton, 1983). Often, concepts of health are restricted to the elements of behavioral competence.

However, if Lawton's concept of well-being as multisectored is correct, all domains of well-being should be included in a concept of health for the elderly, for, with advancing years and diminished functional capacity, aspects of life and well-being other

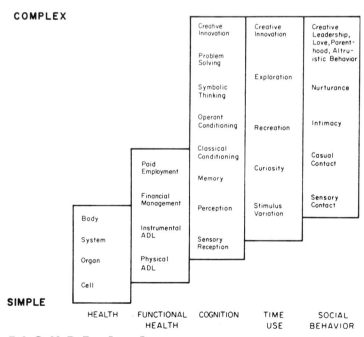

FIGURE 1–1

Lawton's concept of behavioral competence. (ADL: Activities of daily living.) (Redrawn from Lawton, M.P. Environment and other determinants of well-being in older people. *Gerontologist* 23:350, 1983.)

FIGURE 1–2

Self-assessment of health status in community-dwelling older adults by age group. (Redrawn from Van Nostrand, J.F., Furner, S.E. and Suzman, R. (eds.). Health data on older Americans: United States, 1992. *Vital and Health Statistics Series 3, Analytic and Epidemiological Studies,* No. 27. DHHS Publication (PHS) 93-1411, January 1993.)

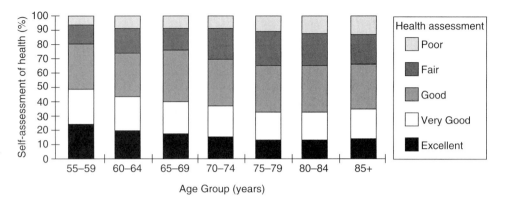

than behavioral competence may assume greater importance.

Patterns of Health and Disease in the Elderly

Health patterns in the aged have not been as comprehensively studied as patterns of disease. Objective measures of function, such as ability to maintain a household and ability to care for self independently, suggest that most of the elderly enjoy good health.

Self-assessment of health status in the elderly correlates highly with objective measures of health status (Maddox, 1962; Engle and Graney, 1985–1986; Gulick, 1986; Cress et al., 1995). Figure 1–2 shows that most old people consider themselves to be in good-to-excellent health, but with increasing age, there is an increasing tendency to rate health as poor or fair (Van Nostrand et al., 1993).

Old people are susceptible to many of the diseases of younger adults. Studies of patterns of disease in the United States reveal that three major categories of disease in the elderly require special consideration (Kohn, 1985): (1) diseases that occur to varying degrees in all aged persons, such as arteriosclerosis or cataracts; (2) diseases with increased incidence in those of advanced age but that do not occur universally, such as neoplastic disease, diabetes mellitus, and some dementing disorders; and (3) diseases that have more serious consequences in the elderly because of their reduced ability to maintain homeostasis compared with the young—for example, pneumonia, influenza, and trauma.

The last category of diseases is particularly important for clinicians, for age-related differences in disease presentation and course are too often overlooked. The subtleties of disease presentation in the elderly frequently pose diagnostic dilemmas for clinicians (Henderson, 1985).

Chronic versus acute disease is another way to characterize disease patterns in the elderly. The incidence of acute conditions declines with age (Fig. 1–3). Eighty-six per cent of the elderly have some chronic disease, and most suffer from more than one. Along with chronic diseases, old people suffer disproportionately from functional disabilities, which consist of the inability to perform a necessary activity of daily living. The need to estimate the prevalence and

FIGURE 1–3

Change in rates of chronic and acute disease with age. (Redrawn from National Health Interview Survey, 1991. NCHS Series 10, No. 24.)

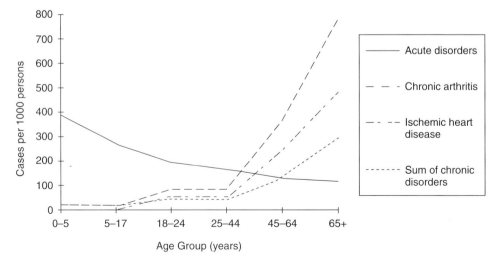

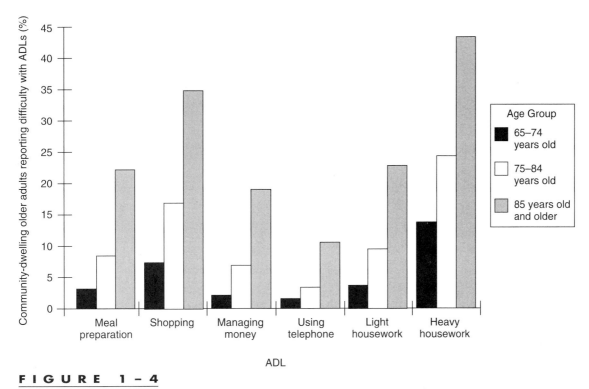

FIGURE 1 – 4

Percentage of community-dwelling older adults who experience difficulty with selected instrumental activities of daily living (ADLs). (Redrawn from Van Nostrand, J.F., Furner, S.E. and Suzman, R. (eds.). Health data on older Americans: United States, 1992. *Vital and Health Statistics Series 3, Analytic and Epidemiological Studies,* No. 27. DHHS Publication (PHS) 93-1411, January 1993.)

incidence of disability has received increasing attention from the National Center for Health Statistics, because of the importance of functional status to health in the elderly, and because of the financial impact of disability.

Estimates of disability are generally obtained by interviewing older people and, if necessary, their caregivers, about difficulties in performing selected activities and the length of time those difficulties are experienced. Self-report has been considered to be the only practical way to obtain functional status information on large numbers of older adults, although there is increasing support for the inclusion of direct observation of physical performance of functional tasks, even in epidemiological studies (Guralnik et al., 1989). It is important to recognize that self-report of function does not always correspond to ratings of function when observed directly (Magaziner and Guralnik, 1992; Cress et al., 1995). Some people tend to underestimate their abilities, while others tend to underreport problems. These estimates of disability should be interpreted with the understanding that they are based on self-report of function.

Figures 1–4 and 1–5 show that functional disability in the community-dwelling elderly advances steadily with increasing age. Difficulty performing basic and instrumental activities of daily living increases with age. Rates of dependency for those aged 65 to 74 are relatively low: 1.5 to 13.5 per cent require assistance with basic activities, and 2 to 13 per cent with instrumental activities. In contrast, those over age 85 have nearly three times as high a rate of dependency as those aged 65 to 74. Rates of functional disabilities in nursing home patients are summarized in Figure 1–6.

Surveys of physicians' office visits show that most encounters for the elderly are due to chronic disease. The most frequent diseases in outpatient medical practice for those aged 65 years and above in the United States are summarized in Table 1–1. Of the top ten diseases listed by age category, only once does an acute illness appear—upper respiratory infection.

Most hospital admissions for those over age 65 years are due to chronic conditions (Table 1–2). Of the acute diseases that result in hospitalization, many can be linked to a chronic disease process, either because they represent adverse sequelae of a chronic disease—for example, hip fracture resulting

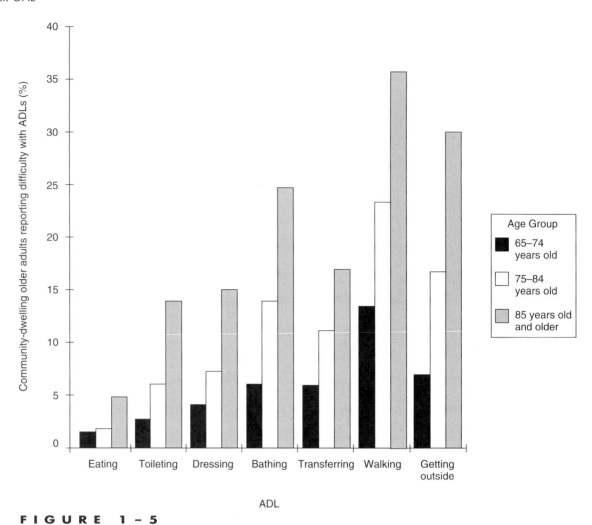

FIGURE   1 – 5

Percentage of community-dwelling older adults with difficulty performing basic activities of daily living (ADLs). (Redrawn from Van Nostrand, J.F., Furner, S.E. and Suzman, R. (eds.). Health data on older Americans: United States, 1992. *Vital and Health Statistics Series 3, Analytic and Epidemiological Studies,* No. 27. DHHS Publication (PHS) 93-1411, January 1993.)

from osteoporosis—or because they are causally related to a chronic disease such as myocardial infarction and atherosclerotic heart disease.

Old people represent a disproportionate share of American hospital costs. Their hospitalizations are significantly longer, the average length of stay increasing with age. Figures from 1987 show average lengths of stay ranging between 2.1 and 11.7 days for men aged 55 to 59 and between 7.1 and 12.9 for men over 85. A similar trend exists for women, with lengths of stay ranging between 6.0 and 10.2 days for women aged 55 to 59 and between 8.0 and 12.9 for women over 85 (Furner and Kozak, 1993).

The prevalence of chronic disease is very high in the 5 per cent of those over age 65 years who live in nursing homes. Data from the National Nursing Home Survey reveal a 99 per cent prevalence of chronic disease among nursing home residents, with an average of 3.9 chronic conditions per resident. Chronic diseases such as arteriosclerosis, stroke, cancer, hip fracture, congestive heart failure, chronic brain syndrome, and diabetes mellitus account for over 50 per cent of the admission diagnoses for these patients. Over half of nursing home patients surveyed were dependent in terms of mobility, continence, or both (Hing and Bloom, 1990).

Impact of Chronic Disease on the Individual

Chronic disease and acute disease differ along four dimensions: causation, duration, identity, and outcomes (Burish and Bradley,

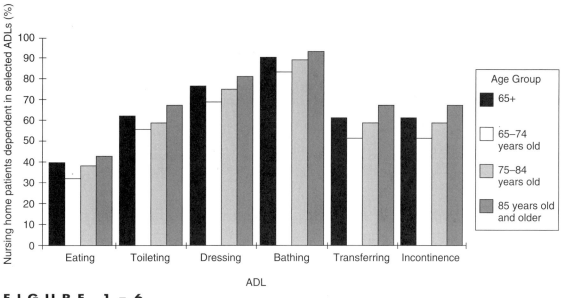

FIGURE 1-6

Percentage of institutionalized older adults dependent in selected activities of daily living (ADLs). (Redrawn from Hing, J.E. and Bloom, B. Long-term care for the functionally dependent elderly. *National Center for Health Statistics Vital Health Stat* 13:104, 1991.)

1983). Chronic diseases usually have multiple causes, many of which are related to lifestyle. They have slow, insidious onsets, with indeterminate duration. It is often difficult for the individual to have a clear understanding of the disease because it is characterized by exacerbations and remissions; there may be periods when the individual has the disease but experiences no symptoms. Moreover, chronic illnesses may affect nearly all aspects of the older person's life. Effects of chronic disease may include impaired functioning, problems with sleep and comfort, changes in mood or affect, and disruptions in family and social life (Funk et al., 1993). Although the ultimate outcomes of chronic disease are often predictable, the course or trajectory of illness is less so. The day-to-day experience of chronic disease may be fraught with uncertainty and unpredictability. Indeed, chronic illness has been described as the experience of living with chronic uncertainty (Mishel, 1993). In contrast, acute diseases usually have specific etiologies, with rapid onset and relatively short duration. Understanding of the disease is simpler, and the symptoms are more overt. Symptoms resolve with cure of the disease, and outcomes are usually favorable. Thus, acute diseases have cures, whereas chronic diseases require ongoing management and lifestyle change.

Strauss (1973) contended that the person with chronic disease must learn to assume control over the management of the disease, rather than relinquishing control to professionals. Successful adaptation to chronic disease requires the following competencies from the individual:

- Preventing and managing medical crises
- Managing therapeutic regimens
- Controlling symptoms
- Organizing time efficiently
- Preventing or living with social isolation
- Adjusting to changes in the course of the disease
- Normalizing interactions with others, and lifestyle, despite the disease
- Managing uncertainty

Individuals obtain help from family, kin, and neighbors, as well as health professionals, but the health professionals are usually not the focal point for coping with the disease. This idea counters traditional American notions of health care, which emphasize professional intervention for the cure of disease (Schmidt, 1985). This conflict between the needs of those with chronic disease and the acute-care orientation of the American medical care system may underlie some of the widespread dissatisfaction with health care for the elderly.

Wu (1973) and Gordon (1966) defined a model for developing behavior norms for

T A B L E   1 – 1

Number of Mentions of Most Frequent All-listed Diagnoses for Ambulatory Patients 55 Years of Age and Over and Rank for Males and Females, by Age: United States, 1985 (data based on reporting by a sample of office-based physicians)

RANK	AGE, MOST FREQUENT ALL-LISTED[1] DIAGNOSES, AND ICD-9-CM CODE[2]	NUMBER OF MENTIONS PER 1,000 VISITS	RANK Male	RANK Female
	55–59 years			
1	Essential hypertension 401	143	1	1
2	Diabetes mellitus 250	61	2	2
3	Chronic ischemic heart disease 414	28	3	17
4	Neurotic disorders 300	26	9	4
5	Disorders of refraction and accommodation 367	26	6	5
6	Osteoarthritis and allied disorders 715	25	4	9
7	Arthropathies, other and unspecified 716	19	10	11
8	Obesity 278	16	27	10
9	Bronchitis 490	16	16	13
10	Acute upper respiratory infections 465	16	47	6
	60–64 years			
1	Essential hypertension 401	159	1	1
2	Diabetes mellitus 250	83	2	2
3	Chronic ischemic heart disease 414	46	3	3
4	Osteoarthritis and allied disorders 715	28	5	5
5	Disorders of refraction and accommodation 367	26	8	4
6	Arthropathies, other and unspecified 716	21	10	9
7	Chronic airway obstruction, not elsewhere classified 496	19	4	38
8	Neurotic disorders 300	19	19	7
9	Angina pectoris 413	19	6	22
10	Cardiac dysrhythmias 427	17	16	11
	65–69 years			
1	Essential hypertension 401	157	1	1
2	Diabetes mellitus 250	78	2	2
3	Chronic ischemic heart disease 414	47	3	5
4	Osteoarthritis and allied disorders 715	43	10	3
5	Cataract 366	30	8	4
6	Cardiac dysrhythmias 427	26	5	6
7	Angina pectoris 413	24	6	11
8	Chronic airway obstruction, not elsewhere classified 496	23	4	17
9	Arthropathies, other and unspecified 716	23	9	9
10	Disorders of refraction and accommodation 367	22	11	8
	70–74 years			
1	Essential hypertension 401	145	1	1
2	Diabetes mellitus 250	81	2	2
3	Chronic ischemic heart disease 414	53	3	4
4	Cataract 366	48	5	3
5	Osteoarthritis and allied disorders 715	35	8	5
6	Cardiac dysrhythmias 427	27	6	10
7	Chronic airway obstruction, not elsewhere classified 496	27	4	12
8	Heart failure 428	25	9	8
9	Arthropathies, other and unspecified 716	24	18	6
10	Glaucoma 365	24	14	7

those with chronic diseases as the impaired role:

any activity undertaken by a disabled person who no longer views himself as ill, but is restricted physically and/or psychosocially, for the purposes of maintaining control of his impaired condition, prevention of complications attending such conditions, and reserving role responsibilities commensurate with his controlled or convalescent state. (Wu, p. 188)

Aspects of impaired role expectations that foster adaptation to chronic disease include

- Encouragement of resumption of normal behaviors and responsibilities within the limits of disability.
- Expectation that the individual retain control over management of disease.
- Encouragement of acceptance of impairment, while capitalizing on remaining capacities.
- Integration of the impaired person into the society at large.

According to Wu, adoption of the im-

TABLE 1–1

Number of Mentions of Most Frequent All-listed Diagnoses for Ambulatory Patients 55 Years of Age and Over and Rank for Males and Females, by Age: United States, 1985 (data based on reporting by a sample of office-based physicians) *Continued*

RANK	AGE, MOST FREQUENT ALL-LISTED[1] DIAGNOSES, AND ICD-9-CM CODE[2]	NUMBER OF MENTIONS PER 1,000 VISITS	RANK Male	RANK Female
	75–79 years			
1	Essential hypertension 401	170	1	1
2	Diabetes mellitus 250	91	2	2
3	Chronic ischemic heart disease 414	67	3	4
4	Cataract 366	61	5	3
5	Osteoarthritis and allied disorders 715	48	7	5
6	Heart failure 428	37	6	7
7	Cardiac dysrhythmias 427	34	4	9
8	Glaucoma 365	32	8	6
9	Arthropathies, other and unspecified 716	27	12	8
10	Neurotic disorders 300	21	15	11
	80–84 years			
1	Essential hypertension 401	133	1	1
2	Cataract 366	74	5	2
3	Chronic ischemic heart disease 414	72	2	3
4	Diabetes mellitus 250	56	8	4
5	Heart failure 428	54	3	6
6	Osteoarthritis and allied disorders 715	54	6	5
7	Glaucoma 365	32	9	7
8	Cardiac dysrhythmias 427	30	7	11
9	Other eye disorders 379	27	14	8
10	Chronic airway obstruction, not elsewhere classified 496	27	4	26
	85 years and over			
1	Essential hypertension 401	122	4	1
2	Chronic ischemic heart disease 414	77	1	3
3	Cataract 366	74	3	2
4	Heart failure 428	66	2	4
5	Diabetes mellitus 250	44	5	5
6	Osteoarthritis and allied disorders 715	37	9	6
7	Glaucoma 365	35	8	8
8	Cardiac dysrhythmias 427	*33	6	12
9	Other disorders of urethra and urinary tract 599	*31	16	9
10	Other skin cancer 173	*31	7	11

[1]"All-listed" means listed as first, second, or third diagnosis.
[2]Coded according to the *International Classification of Diseases, Ninth Revision, Clinical Modification.*
SOURCE: National Center for Health Statistics: Data from the National Ambulatory Medical Care Survey.
From Furner, S.E. and Kozak, L.J. Acute care. *In* Van Nostrand, J.F., Furner, S.E. and Suzman, R. (eds.). Health Data on Older Americans: United States, 1992. *Vital and Health Statistics Series 3: Analytic and Epidemiological Studies* No. 27. DHHS Publication No. (PHS) 93-1411, 1993.

paired role is facilitated by the following conditions:

- Congruence between old behaviors and the new behaviors the disabled person is expected to learn.

- Capacity to learn new behaviors.

- Motivation to adopt the impaired role.

- Preparation for the role, through rehearsal of the new behaviors.

- Gradual transition from the well or sick role.

Not all individuals with chronic diseases are able to master the competencies described by Strauss or assume the impaired role. However, those who do not assume this role experience a lower health status, because they fail to reintegrate themselves into society to the fullest extent possible, and they are more vulnerable to the adverse effects of chronic disease exacerbations.

Mastering chronic disease is by no means a trivial or simple task. The work and care involved in chronic disease management can pervade the affected individual's life (Corbin and Strauss, 1988). The complexities of disease management while the person continues to lead a "normal" life can be enormous. Astute clinicians, when assisting those with chronic disease, will be aware of the phase of the chronic illness, the individual's trajec-

TABLE 1 - 2

Number of Patients Discharged, Rate of Discharges, Days of Care, and Average Length of Stay for Males 55 Years of Age and Over, by Age and Selected First-listed Diagnoses: United States, 1981 and 1987 (discharges from non-Federal short-stay hospitals)

AGE, FIRST-LISTED DIAGNOSIS, AND ICD-9-CM CODE[1]	DISCHARGES				DAYS OF CARE		AVERAGE LENGTH OF STAY	
	Number in Thousands		Number Per 1,000 Population		Number in Thousands		Stay in Days	
	1981	1987	1981	1987	1981	1987	1981	1987
55–59 years								
Diseases of heart ... 391–392.0,393–398,402,404,410–416,420–429	227	238	41.5	44.8	1,846	1,407	8.1	5.9
Malignant neoplasms ...140–208,230–234	91	76	16.6	14.3	954	704	10.5	9.3
Cerebrovascular disease ...430–438	30	31	5.5	5.9	292	366	9.6	11.7
Inguinal hernia ...550	37	25	6.8	4.6	179	52	4.8	2.1
Fractures, all sites ...800–829	23	23	4.2	4.0	192	154	8.3	7.4
Hyperplasia of prostate ...600	24	21	4.4	3.9	154	93	6.4	4.5
60–64 years								
Diseases of heart ... 391–392.0,393–398,402,404,410–416,420–429	224	270	46.9	53.1	1,864	1,681	8.3	6.2
Malignant neoplasms ...140–208,230–234	117	118	24.4	23.3	1,207	1,036	10.3	8.8
Cerebrovascular disease ...430–438	36	42	7.5	8.3	419	376	11.7	8.9
Hyperplasia of prostate ...600	40	39	8.3	7.6	288	186	7.2	4.8
Inguinal hernia ...550	39	31	8.2	6.1	190	66	4.8	2.2
Pneumonia, all forms ...480–486	19	26	4.0	5.1	206	215	10.8	8.4
65–69 years								
Diseases of heart ... 391–392.0,393–398,402,404,410–416,420–429	271	285	68.6	63.3	2,506	1,992	9.3	7.0
Malignant neoplasms ...140–208,230–234	153	131	38.8	29.0	1,959	1,186	12.8	9.1
Cerebrovascular disease ...430–438	56	60	14.2	13.4	628	537	11.2	8.9
Hyperplasia of prostate ...600	53	59	13.6	13.2	454	294	8.5	5.0
Pneumonia, all forms ...480–486	26	35	6.7	7.7	260	334	9.9	9.6
Inguinal hernia ...550	38	24	9.7	5.4	205	64	5.4	2.6
70–74 years								
Diseases of heart ... 391–392.0,393–398,402,404,410–416,420–429	221	294	75.0	88.2	2,169	2,128	9.8	7.2
Malignant neoplasms ...140–208,230–234	145	145	49.3	43.4	1,815	1,228	12.5	8.5
Cerebrovascular disease ...430–438	62	67	20.9	20.1	674	607	10.9	9.1
Hyperplasia of prostate ...600	58	54	19.5	16.2	513	283	8.9	5.3
Pneumonia, all forms ...480–486	34	48	11.7	14.4	417	479	12.1	10.0
Inguinal hernia ...550	31	21	10.7	6.4	193	74	6.1	3.5

16

75–79 years

Condition	ICD code[1]								
Diseases of heart	391–392.0,393–398,402,404,410–416,420–429	166	223	87.6	98.3	1,683	1,748	10.1	7.9
Malignant neoplasms	140–208,230–234	106	111	55.9	49.0	1,366	1,092	12.9	9.8
Cerebrovascular disease	430–438	57	63	30.0	27.7	834	587	14.7	9.4
Pneumonia, all forms	480–486	27	47	14.4	20.9	326	470	11.9	9.9
Hyperplasia of prostate	600	35	46	18.7	20.5	314	263	8.9	5.7
Fractures, all sizes	800–829	14	20	7.3	9.0	226	237	16.5	11.7

80–84 years

Condition	ICD code[1]								
Diseases of heart	391–392.0,393–398,402,404,410–416,420–429	118	157	110.4	128.3	1,215	1,163	10.3	7.4
Malignant neoplasms	140–208,230–234	62	61	57.9	49.7	780	639	12.7	10.5
Cerebrovascular disease	430–438	45	48	42.1	39.4	580	466	12.9	9.7
Pneumonia, all forms	480–486	20	47	19.2	38.5	259	472	12.7	10.0
Hyperplasia of prostate	600	22	29	20.5	23.9	224	182	10.3	6.2
Fractures, all sites	800–829	14	21	13.2	17.2	328	275	23.4	13.0

65 years and older

Condition	ICD code[1]								
Diseases of heart	391–392.0,393–398,402,404,410–416,420–429	868	1,054	82.2	87.0	8,563	7,714	9.9	7.3
Malignant neoplasms	140–208,230–234	506	485	47.9	40.0	6,449	4,522	12.8	9.3
Cerebrovascular disease	430–438	252	273	23.8	22.5	3,090	2,498	12.2	9.1
Pneumonia, all forms	480–486	141	222	13.4	18.4	1,652	2,190	11.7	9.8
Hyperplasia of prostate	600	181	206	17.1	17.0	1,690	1,166	9.3	5.7
Fractures, all sites	800–829	80	97	7.6	8.0	1,280	1,168	16.0	12.0

75 years and over

Condition	ICD code[1]								
Diseases of heart	391–392.0,393–398,402,404,410–416,420–429	376	476	102.6	110.8	3,888	3,595	10.3	7.7
Malignant neoplasms	140–208,230–234	207	210	56.5	48.8	2,675	2,109	12.9	10.1
Cerebrovascular disease	430–438	134	146	36.5	34.0	1,788	1,354	13.4	9.3
Pneumonia, all forms	480–486	81	140	22.0	32.5	976	1,377	12.1	9.9
Hyperplasia of prostate	600	70	93	19.1	21.7	724	588	10.4	6.3
Fractures, all sites	800–829	49	61	13.3	14.2	891	766	18.2	12.5

85 years and over

Condition	ICD code[1]								
Diseases of heart	391–392.0,393–398,402,404,410–416,420–429	98	96	131.1	119.4	991	683	10.7	7.1
Pneumonia, all forms	480–486	33	45	46.4	56.0	391	435	11.9	9.6
Malignant neoplasms	140–208,230–234	40	38	56.7	43.6	530	377	13.4	10.0
Cerebrovascular disease	430–438	32	35	45.7	47.0	374	301	11.6	8.6
Fractures, all sites	800–829	21	20	30.0	24.4	337	254	15.9	12.9
Hyperplasia of prostate	600	13	17	18.0	21.5	185	143	14.6	8.2

[1]Coded according to the *International Classification of Diseases, Ninth Revision, Clinical Modification.*
SOURCE: National Center for Health Statistics: Data from the National Hospital Discharge Survey.
From Furner, S.E. and Kozak, L.J. Acute care. *In* Van Nostrand, J.F., Furner, S.E. and Suzman, R. (eds.). Health Data on Older Americans: United States, 1992. *Vital and Health Statistics Series 3: Analytic and Epidemiological Studies* No. 27. DHHS Publication No. (PHS) 93-1411,1993.

tory of illness, the work involved in managing the illness, and the contingencies that affect the conduct of illness-related work.

Since chronic diseases cannot be cured, clinicians must shift their emphasis from cure of disease to fostering the individual's adaptation to disease effects. This is achieved through the processes of care and coordination. It is important to consider the impact of a disease on the patient's functional abilities, psychoemotional status, social support network, and quality of life. These data are essential for helping the individual to adapt to the chronic disease. The challenge of chronic disease for health care professionals is summarized as follows:

Helping those afflicted with chronic disease means far more than simply displaying compassion or having medical competence. Only through knowledge of and sensitivity to the social aspects of symptom control, regimen management, crisis prevention, handling dying and death itself, can one develop truly beneficial strategies for dealing with specific diseases and chronic illnesses in general. (Strauss, 1973, p. 39)

Broad definitions of health used for younger adults apply to the elderly. With advanced age, however, operational definitions of health focus on maintenance of social functioning and prevention of adverse consequences from chronic diseases. Achievement of these two goals allows for maximum individual autonomy, a characteristic valued highly by adults in Western society (Evans, 1984). Individual autonomy must be supported before interdependence can be achieved. The ability to achieve interdependence offers the highest potential for continued interpersonal, cognitive, and spiritual development in old age.

Environmental Influences

Concepts of Environment

Nurses have been concerned about the impact of environmental conditions on the health of individuals since the time of Nightingale. The concept of environment is regarded as an essential element in any model of nursing. Orem (1991) considers the environment to have interrelated physical and psychosocial aspects. She believes that a suitable environment is essential in promoting continued development and regards environmental modification as a key nursing method.

Study of the environment has profited from the research of many different disciplines, such as geographers, architects, psychologists, sociologists, nurses, occupational therapists, social workers, and urban planners. Unfortunately, no universally accepted theory of the environment exists to guide practice. Indeed, there is considerable disagreement on the attributes of the environment that most influence behavior.

Components of the Environment

The first step in developing a concept of the environment is defining its geographical boundaries. The environment under consideration may be as large as a community, a neighborhood, or an institution or as small as a ward, a home, or an individual room. The next step is to characterize the objective and transactional attributes of the environment.

Objective attributes of the environment include the quantity and qualities of various objects and people within the geographical boundary. These attributes can be reliably measured. Examples include population density, sex, racial mix, frequency of interaction, lighting intensity, noise level, colors, temperature, spatial arrangements, and size and type of specific objects, such as furniture, assistive devices, and personal items.

The environment also has transactional attributes, resulting from a person's interaction with it. Transactional attributes of the environment are the symbolic meaning of objects within it; its familiarity; the task demands of certain activities; and the role expectations, norms, and values within it.

Ittleson et al. (1976) described four different forms of environmental experience:

1. The environment is experienced as an *external physical place*, which is perceived with the sense organs.
2. The environment is experienced as an *extension of self*. A poignant example is describing an elderly hospital patient as "a 74-year-old nursing home resident," as if that is sufficient to characterize the individual socially. Conversely, others may define the environment by the individual, in comments such as "This room is just not the same without him."
3. The environment is experienced as a *social system*, with a complex set of roles, expectations, norms, rules, and processes. Homes, clinics, stores, nursing homes, churches, and hospitals all differ sharply in this respect.
4. Many have had the experience of associating a certain place or environmental attribute with specific *emotions*, such as sadness, anxiety, fear, joy, or relief.

All behavior takes place within some environment. The characteristics of the environment have tremendous impact on the performance of tasks, from simple to complex.

Environmental Layers

Barris et al. (1985) proposed a model for structural analysis of the environment based on a concept that describes the environment as a series of interacting layers: objects, tasks, social groups, and culture/values. Each layer of the environment, alone or in combination with other layers, influences the behavior of the individual.

Models of Person-Environment Interaction

To understand the impact of the environment on the individual, static descriptions of the environment alone are not enough. Several models have been developed to explain the impact of person-environment interactions over time, including the stress and adaptation framework, the press-competence model, and person-environment congruence. These models overlap, but each provides unique insights into person-environment interactions.

Stress and Adaptation Framework

The field of stress research as it relates to health outcomes has a long tradition, dating back to the 1940s research on catastrophic events, and Selye's work on the General Adaptation Syndrome in the 1950s. Although stress research has been criticized on methodological grounds (see Wykle et al., 1992 for an excellent review), and because it has a tendency to promote an overly simplistic focus on negative outcomes of life stressors, rather than on the potential for positive outcomes from stressful events (Lieberman, 1992), stress research continues to provide a useful heuristic framework that can organize diverse research findings and inform clinical care of the elderly.

According to Byrne and Thompson (1978), the human organism is composed of a set of open systems. Human beings can thus be conceived of as energy units that must achieve a balance of energy utilization and conservation. To survive, humans must be able to regulate their internal environment despite extreme variations in external environmental conditions. The tendency to maintain this consistent internal environment is called *homeokinesis*. It depends on the system's ability to *adapt* to varying levels of inputs from the environment. Humans achieve this through complex interactions among the neuroendocrine, cardiovascular,

and psychological subsystems, which result in self-regulation. Successful adaptation results in achievement and maintenance of a steady state of function. In humans, the steady state is a condition of load balanced with capability (Kahn et al., 1964; McGrath, 1970).

Humans thrive when environmental demands match the individual's capabilities, *not* in a demand-free environment (Clarke, 1984). Thus, for humans, stress is

a state that is always present in man, but . . . is intensified when there is a change or threat with which the individual must cope. The term stressor . . . refer(s) to the factor or agent that causes an intensification of the stress state. (Byrne and Thompson, 1978, p. 42)

Increased demands on the individual may precipitate what Selye (1956) termed the *general adaptation syndrome* (GAS). Three phases in human response to stressors are described: alarm, resistance, and exhaustion (Selye, 1956). During the first phase, the stressor is perceived and the organism prepares to respond. This is known as the "fight or flight" phase and typically lasts a short time. The second phase is when adaptation usually occurs. Some behavioral change usually accompanies the physiological response to the stressor. Finally, if adaptation does not occur and the intensified stress state continues, exhaustion occurs because the individual's adaptive reserves are depleted. These individuals require external intervention to support physiological function until the stressor is removed or adaptation occurs.

Although stress cannot be observed directly, intensification of stress levels can be observed by changes in the pattern of the individual's behaviors and observation of responses mediated by the autonomic nervous system, such as changes in vital signs and pupil size and diaphoresis. Assisting individuals to maintain physiological integrity as they respond to stressful situations is a part of nursing practice (Byrne and Thompson, 1978). To promote adaptation, nurses must be alert for signs of intensifying stress states. Scott et al. (1982) emphasized that interactions between individuals and the *environment* may intensify the stress response, meaning that modification of environmental variables is an important nursing function.

Since the elderly have diminished adaptive capabilities because of their diminished functional reserves in all organ systems, nurses should be particularly alert for signs of intensified stress states in older persons. Additionally, the patterns of illness characteristic in the elderly result in the average older person experiencing a disproportionately large number of simultaneously occurring stressors compared with younger adults. Older people are therefore likely to have high demands on their compensatory reserves. However, they are also likely to have previous experience with a variety of stressors and therefore have well-developed coping resources.

Stress and adaptation concepts for nursing of the elderly include the following:

- Stress arises from transactions between the individual and the environment. Stress is intensified when there is awareness of demands that strain or exceed available resources (Scott et al., 1982; Kahana, 1992).

- Humans experience both physiological and psychological stress. The ability to adapt to these stressors is one measure of health (Murray and Zetner, 1985).

- The stress response is a psychophysiological phenomenon, mediated by both cognitive processes and neuroendocrine processes within the organism (Kasl, 1992).

- Adaptation to stressors is mediated by cognitive appraisal of the stressor, the extent of social support, personality and internal coping resources, the number of simultaneously occurring stressors, previous experience with the stressor, and the duration of exposure to the stressor (Lazarus and Folkman, 1984).

- Maladaptive responses to stressors and overexposure to stress have been linked to certain chronic diseases prevalent in older persons, such as diabetes mellitus, hypertension, and depression (Eisdorfer and Wilkie, 1977).

- Environmental characteristics are sources of both stressors and supports for older persons (Lawton and Nahemow, 1973). Environmental variables should therefore be modified to match the behavioral competence of the individual.

Ecological Psychology Framework

A primary tenet of environmental psychology is that behavior is a function of personal and environmental characteristics. Many researchers have elaborated on this proposition. Two models that have influenced practitioners in gerontology include the environmental press-competence model (Lawton and Nahemow, 1973) and Kahana's (1982) person-environment congruency model.

In the press-competence model, both the objective and transactional attributes of the environment combine to produce a set of demands or expectations. The demands may be physical—for example, the ability to walk up a flight of stairs to get to the bathroom—or they may be interpersonal, such as a demand for daily conversation with a visitor or housemate. The combination of physical and interpersonal demands is known as *environmental press*. The press-competence model of behavior shows that adaptive behavior and positive affect are the result of environmental demands balanced by the individual's biological and behavioral competence (Lawton et al., 1984). Thus, when environmental demands exceed individual competence, maladaptation and negative emotional affect occur. Similarly, an environment characterized by minimal demands will result in maladaptation for the highly competent individual.

A concept derived from this model is the environmental docility hypothesis: as an individual's competence decreases, behavior is increasingly influenced by environmental factors. For example, as an individual's mobility decreases, the ability to maintain urinary continence more and more depends on the distance to the toilet and the ease of finding it.

The person-environment congruence model agrees with the press-competence model (Kahana, 1975). Psychological well-being is viewed as the result of congruence between personal needs and perceived attributes of the environment, such as privacy, order, or affiliation. An oversupply or undersupply of these qualities will result in incongruence. The concepts of sensory deprivation and sensory overload (Wohlwill, 1974) are consistent with this model.

Temporal Influences on Person-Environment Interactions

The effects of activity within an environment over time must be considered before the full impact of individual-environment interaction can be understood.

Social Breakdown Hypothesis

The social breakdown model proposed by Bengtson (1973) is one way of explaining how individuals and environments influence each other over time. Figure 1–7 summarizes the process of social breakdown. Individuals who are in an environment appropriate to their level of competence and needs perform optimally and receive messages from the environment reinforcing their mastery of various tasks. If environmental demands and individual capabil-

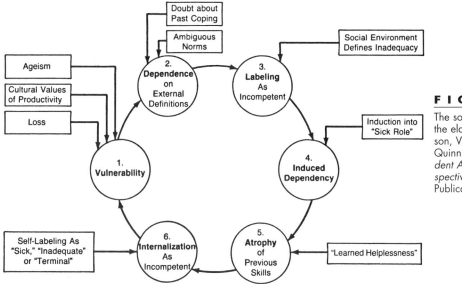

FIGURE 1 – 7

The social breakdown hypothesis applied to the elderly. (From Kuypers, J.A. and Bengtson, V.L. Perspectives on the older family. *In* Quinn, W.H. and Hughston, G.A. *Independent Aging: Family and Social Systems Perspectives.* Rockville, MD: Aspen Publications, 1985.)

ity are mismatched, a negative cycle of ever-diminishing opportunity results, unless some event occurs to interrupt this cycle.

CASE EXAMPLE
Impact of Environmental Change

Mr. P. has been admitted to the hospital for tests after a series of falls. He lives alone and has no family in the immediate area. He is put in a room with another patient. Floor space is limited, with technical equipment, gauges, buzzers, no control over heating/cooling systems, and shared access to bathrooms (or he must use a bedpan, urinal, or bedside commode). The novelty of the objects surrounding him makes even routine task performance more difficult. Thus, he seems more tentative and dependent in the hospital setting than in a familiar environment.

He has been told not to perform tasks without assistance, but he does not remember how the nurse said to operate the intercom system. He is embarrassed to ask to be taken to the toilet. The hospital schedule is different from his own. Acquiring new knowledge about diagnostic procedures, diseases, or postdischarge care is also a complex task.

Mr. P., a "loner," now has interaction with many different health care providers on the hospital staff who often use medical jargon and acronyms that need to be explained. Visiting hours are restricted and he must share the room's only phone. Most conversations with staff are about the technical aspects of care and diagnosis rather than his adjustment to the hospital, care regimen, or changes in his functioning level.

In the cultural layer of the environment, the old person truly is in a foreign world. In addition to language differences, customs regarding privacy, communication, and requests for assistance differ markedly from those in the home environment. Treatment success is measured by resolution of acute illness rather than a return to the previous functioning level, which is likely to be the criterion used by the older person. Misunderstandings about rituals and goals may result in miscommunications between patients and care providers, which at the very least may heighten the patient's anxiety and at worst may lead to serious misunderstandings about posthospital care and prognosis, which in turn may foster unnecessary dependency.

Add to this structural analysis of the environment the concepts of the social breakdown hypothesis. The hospitalized old person encounters difficulty in mastering the new communications system, resulting in increased difficulty performing basic tasks like toileting. The individual has an "accident" and wets the bed, and the staff unthinkingly provides incontinence pads. While this step may present little difficulty for the short-stay patient or for the patient with a secure self-image as a continent individual, to the long-stay patient this may represent the first step in a long spiral of functional decline.

Given the substantial differences in all levels of the environment from one location to another, and the relative dependence of old persons on environmental characteristics, nurses should become particularly adept at analyzing environmental attributes and the degree to which they enhance or detract from the older person's ability to function independently.

Although no unitary theory of the effects of person-environment interaction exists, useful conceptual models can be applied to the analysis of clinical situations and home environments of older persons.

Influences of Environmental Attributes on Function

Considering the effects of environmental attributes is a useful way to organize a wide variety of observations and generalizations about disparate influences on the health status of community-dwelling older adults.

Physical Environment

Aspects of the physical environment that may impinge upon the older person's health include housing, neighborhood, and the microenvironment. These interact with the social and task aspects of the old person's environment. For example, some neighborhoods encourage more social interaction than others. Some housing arrangements are more physically challenging than others: for example, the fifth-story walk-up apartment versus the ground-level garden apartment.

A demographic study showed that disability rates among community-dwelling older adults were reduced during the 1980s (Manton et al., 1993); the older population increased 14.7 per cent, while the number of people defined as chronically disabled increased by only 9.2 per cent. One possible explanation advanced for the decrease is the increased use of adaptive devices, such as raised toilet seats, shower seats, and tub stools.

The objective qualities of the environment, through the individual's perceptions of it and interactions with it over time, may result in memories, long-standing friendships, and feelings.

Some nurses are involved in community planning decisions and in assisting individuals with decisions about relocation to a new environment, but more often nurses are involved in manipulating elements in the environment that immediately surrounds the aged individual. Varying such aspects as lighting intensity, glare, and background noise to compensate for age-related changes in sensory capacity are interventions familiar to most nurses. Similarly, the use of adaptive equipment, such as eating utensils with oversized handles or raised toilet seats to assist those with musculoskeletal disabilities, is also within the scope of nursing practice. Nurses also teach older persons and their friends and relatives about environmental modifications to enhance function.

Interpersonal Environment

Family, religious groups, and neighborhood groups are all potentially important environmental considerations influencing function in old age. The best-studied group is the family, but in the absence of family ties, neighborhood friendships and religious ties shape older persons' responses to illness.

FAMILY. Research has shown repeatedly that old people are well connected to their family groups (Shanas, 1979; Bengtson et al., 1990). Cultural norms and values are transmitted and reinforced primarily within the family. Beliefs about health, illness, aging, and dying are forged within the family unit; therefore, knowledge of the cultural background of the individual is important if these factors are to be considered in providing care.

Independence is highly valued in American society. The importance of independence as a characteristic of adulthood should be assessed in each family. The meanings attached to independence and dependence in a given family unit have important consequences for the adjustment to chronic disease and age-related decrements in function. In some families, becoming dependent means giving up the rights and responsibilities of adulthood. Other families are more accepting of dependency in some spheres of function, allowing adults to engage in help-seeking behavior without insisting on role reversal.

Another cultural consideration that may influence the health of the old person is the manner in which death and dying are viewed. Some cultures view death as a normal part of life, whereas others are extremely fearful about it. Religiosity, ethnicity, and individual life experience shape these attitudes and beliefs. Extreme anxiety related to the threat of death may be manifested in multiple somatic complaints, in excessive preoccupation with body functions, or through less specific symptoms of anxiety. Unresolved conflicts between family members regarding the dying process may make fulfilling older individuals' wishes about their dying process difficult to carry out.

Old people are both providers and recipients of assistance within family networks.

Many patterns of mutual aid exist; these are usually shaped more by cultural norms and long-standing family-life patterns, such as household arrangements and norms, than by the chronological age of family members (Bengtson et al., 1990). When asked whom they would turn to in times of crisis, 90 per cent of the elderly identify family members, although the degree to which that family member would actually respond is variable (Tobin and Kulys, 1980). Thus, family may represent either a source of objective resources or a source of demand for the older person. Indeed, there is increasing concern about the burdens of caregiving on family members (see Wright et al., 1993 for an extensive review). Patterns of caregiving described by Chappell (1990) suggest that in most instances (70 per cent) there is one "primary" informal caregiver for a disabled older person, and one third of caregivers, usually spouses, describe themselves as sole caregivers.

The integrity of the family network into advanced age has implications for the health of older people, for it has been shown that social support is strongly correlated with health and well-being in people of all ages, including the elderly (Antonucci, 1990). Assistance among family members may take the form of emotional support, financial assistance, help with day-to-day chores, and provision of personal care for those with self-care impairments. Additionally, involvement in a family group is an important source of role fulfillment and therefore contributes to an evolving self-concept for the older person. Finally, families serve as mediating agents between the older person and bureaucratic institutions.

The family is not always an effective or completely self-sufficient support for older persons. The burden of caregiving can be great, and tensions generated by long-standing familial conflict may lead to abuse. Recent demographic studies show a trend toward a smaller, younger population to care for the aged and an increasing prevalence of "blended" families, i.e., families with complex structures as a result of remarriage following death or divorce. In addition, women, the traditional caregivers of dependent family members, are entering the paid work force in unprecedented numbers. The family aspect of the social environment of the aged will continue to be difficult to characterize.

NONFAMILY SOCIAL GROUPS. Other sources of social support, values, and norms include friendships, religious groups, and the neighborhood. The friendship role is important to older persons and relates to patterns of earlier life. For those living alone, neighborhood friends are an important source of assistance, particularly in times of illness. Participation in religious activities may influence access to support services. Religious activity may also be associated with reduced anxiety regarding death, although this is not a universal finding (Kalish, 1985). Finally, religious activity influences an individual's beliefs about the meaning of illness and the use of life-extending technologies.

Societal and Cultural Influences

Societal and community variables are viewed both as influences on environment and as an integral part of the environment. According to Howell (1980), physical attributes of communities are the result of conscious planning. They thus have the potential for being engineered to facilitate function for people of all ages. Locations of Social Security offices, shops, and medical facilities attending to the needs of special populations reflect social values. For example, suburban shopping centers reflect our orientation toward the automobile and a class value that shoppers have cars.

Certain societal values have an impact on the health and well-being of the aged in the United States (Achenbaum, 1985): the American fascination with newness, simple answers to complex problems, and emphasis on self-reliance. Community and societal values thus shape the physical and social environments in which the elderly live.

American society is young compared with other Western cultures, and values new ideas over traditions and youth over the aged. The political system runs in four-year cycles, meaning that success is measured in a relatively short time frame rather than over decades.

Twentieth-century Americans excel at the development of technological answers to problems and have had the luxury of nearly limitless resources to apply to problems identified as high national priorities. The space program and the war on cancer are two recent examples. Unfortunately, Americans have less experience with providing ongoing assistance under conditions of scarce resources, particularly in health care. Greater attention has been paid to curing and treating disease than to disease prevention. The attitude that no money should be spared to cure disease prevails, but when people must live with the effects of incurable diseases, a commitment to addressing the problems in care for these people is less impressive.

T A B L E 1 – 3
Generic Nursing Methods

ASSESSMENT	DIAGNOSIS	PLANNING	INTERVENTION	EVALUATION
Inspection	Analysis of data	Goal setting	Further assessment	Establishing outcome
Auscultation	Testing diagnostic	Choosing methods to	Referral	criteria
Palpation	hypotheses	achieve goal	Doing for another	Comparing reassessment
Percussion	Stating diagnoses	Setting priorities	Caring	data with outcome
Listening			Administration of prescribed	criteria
Selecting appropriate tests			medicines and treatments	
Communicating			Creating a milieu or modifying	
			the environment	
			Exercising	
			Teaching	
			Counseling	
			Coordinating	
			Advocating	
			Setting limits	
			Lobbying	
			Supervising	
			Documenting care given	
			Monitoring health status in-	
			dices	

The predominant model in Western health care for approaching the problem of disease is to isolate a unitary cause and develop a drug or vaccine to address the etiological agent. This often leads to depersonalization, which in turn fosters dehumanization of care (Leventhal et al., 1982). This approach is singularly unsuited to the multidetermined problems of the elderly.

The high value placed on independent function in adults has the effect of making those in need of assistance or special consideration seem inferior. The common result of this attitude is dehumanization of those who seek assistance, through negative stereotyping or through token programs of assistance. Only in recent years has the issue of removing barriers to those with physical handicaps (regardless of age) been addressed seriously. The mainstream of public life was for many years off limits to those with physical dependencies.

Many of the dominant American values are at variance with the values that would provide humane conditions for those with infirmities. Although most old people at any one time are probably not adversely affected by these values, people with significant impairments are negatively influenced. This in turn influences the concerns of nurses who care for those with infirmities, as well as those who hope to avoid such infirmities.

Now that we have described some key influences on gerontological health care—the aged, the environment, and patterns of health and illness—it is time to focus on the nursing profession and its special role in addressing the health needs of older adults.

Nursing and the Elderly

Definitions of Nursing

Nursing is the diagnosis and treatment of human responses to actual or potential health problems. (ANA, 1995, p. 6)

Nursing is a deliberative problem-solving process, grounded in the biomedical, behavioral, and social sciences, that aims to restore and promote health or, for dying persons, achieve a dignified death. The aims of nursing are achieved through the activities of caring, counseling, teaching, referring, doing for, coordinating, and implementing prescribed treatments for individuals, as well as through supervising, teaching, and evaluating those who perform or who are preparing to perform these functions. The activities of nursing are carried out within the framework of nursing process: assessing, diagnosing, planning, intervening, and evaluating. This process applies to clients at several levels of organization: the individual, the family, and the community.

Nursing process is a systematic approach to designing and implementing care appropriate to the needs of nursing clients. This approach uses methods common to other professional groups. The generic subprocesses and methods used by all nurses in caring for clients are summarized in Table

1–3. Some of these methods may require modification for use with elderly clients, but they are all applicable to this population.

Contributions of Nursing to Health of the Aged

Nurses, by virtue of their training and perspective, have much to contribute to promotion of health in the elderly. Nursing's tradition emphasizes health and illness care, coordination of services as well as provision of service directly, and a whole-person approach. These perspectives counter the trends in the medical model toward fragmentation and emphasis on disease states rather than on individual function (McBride, 1993).

Nursing practice centers on compensation, treatment, and prevention of self-care deficits, with promotion of maximal biopsychosocial function within a specific environment as its primary goal. The elderly can obtain from nurses comprehensive assistance in ways of preventing self-care deficits, compensating for self-care deficits, and adjusting to developmental changes.

Nursing Models

Nursing models are diverse, but all are concerned with the concepts of human nature, health, environment, and nursing actions. Nurses regard human beings as integrated biopsychosocial organisms, in dynamic interaction with their environment, capable of continued growth and development until death.

Health is a state of the human organism judged by comparing the observable signs and behavior of the individual with previously defined criteria of functioning. Health is characterized by purposeful integrated functioning in the environment, and includes biological, psychological, and social well-being, not merely the absence of disease.

The environment is a complex entity, consisting of physical, chemical, interactional, and cultural characteristics. Two important systems in the environment that influence individual health and behavior are the family and complex organizations in the community.

Nurses are a professional group in society who work to promote the health of individuals, families, and communities, both independently and collaboratively with other professionals, by diagnosing and treating human responses to illness. Professional nursing practice is based on scientific knowledge and experience of nursing situations. It is conducted according to a systematic process of assessment, diagnosis, planning, intervention, and evaluation.

Self-Care Model of Nursing

Orem's (1991) self-care model, one of many well-accepted frameworks for nursing practice, demonstrates that nursing care results from interaction between a patient who has a deficit in the need for self-care and the ability to provide it independently, and a nurse trained in design and implementation of nursing systems to compensate for deficits.

Orem's concept of self-care nursing is grounded in the work of Henderson (1955), Orlando (1961), and Wiedenbach (1964). Hill and Smith (1985) noted that many nursing models use the concept of self-care, although they may not use the term explicitly. Examples given include Hall's "care-core-cure" model (Hall, 1966; George, 1980), Roy's adaptation model (Roy and Roberts, 1981), and Blattner's concept of holistic nursing (Blattner, 1981).

Orem believes that the ability to nurse requires knowledge of such diverse disciplines as science, the humanities, and the arts; experiential knowledge of nursing cases; a complex skill repertoire; and motivations that allow for prudence and a willingness to provide nursing. The self-care framework has particular relevance for nursing practice with the aged because of its emphasis on self-care and individual functioning—two central concerns of older people and their families.

KEY CONCEPTS. The key elements of Orem's self-care model are defined in Table 1–4. The relationships between these concepts are depicted in Figures 1–8 to 1–10.

In Orem's self-care model, the purpose of nursing is to assist individuals whose self-care capabilities are unequal to their needs. Ideally, this assistance helps the individual regain or attain the needed capability. For some people this is not an attainable goal. In such cases the nurse is responsible for assisting the individual to compensate for the inability in self-care through identification of appropriate dependent-care agents—often family or friends. Figure 1–8 depicts Orem's typology of nursing care systems in which the degree of initiative from the nurse and patient varies in accord with the patient's dependence. Nurses practicing within a self-care framework utilize the nursing process described in the next section.

Assessment determines whether the individual is a legitimate nursing client, by calculating the therapeutic self-care demand

TABLE 1-4
Definition of Concepts in Orem's Self-Care Model

Self-Care. Activities that individuals usually initiate and perform on their own behalf to maintain life, health, and well-being.
Dependent Care. Activities taken on behalf of individuals to maintain life, health, and well-being who are unable to perform self-care either because of developmental level or disabling conditions.
Self-Care Requisites. Human needs that are met through the practice of self-care. Three types exist: universal, developmental, and health deviation.
Universal Self-Care Requisites. Those needs of all humans to sustain life, including the need to

- take in sufficient air, fluid, and food
- eliminate waste
- balance activity and rest, solitude and social interaction
- prevent injury
- achieve normality

Developmental Self-Care Requisites. Those needs that occur during various stages of the life cycle, which must be met for appropriate continued growth and development. In the elderly, this includes an environment that allows for reminiscing and one that supports

- adaptation to age-related changes, such as sensory deficits, and
- the effects of environmental change and loss of possessions, roles, friends, and functional capacity

Health Deviation Self-Care Requisites. Those needs that must be met if diseases are to be managed or cured. Specific categories include

- seeking appropriate medical assistance for pathological conditions
- developing awareness of and attending to effects of pathological conditions
- carrying out medically prescribed diagnostic, therapeutic, and rehabilitative measures for the treatment or prevention of diseases to maintain integrated functioning, to compensate for disabilities, and to prevent further disease-related disability
- developing awareness of adverse effects of medical care measures
- modifying self-concept in light of special needs for care or lifestyle modification
- learning to live with the effects of diseases and treatment in a lifestyle that promotes growth

Self-Care Agency. The ability for engaging in self-care, which depends on a set of human abilities for deliberate action: the ability to attend to specific things, to understand the nature of things, to understand the need to change or regulate things, to acquire knowledge. These abilities develop through learning and practice of self-care activities.
Therapeutic Self-Care Demand. Specific self-care activities that must be performed for an individual for some duration, which is determined by assessing an individual's self-care requisites and determining what needs to be done to meet them.
Self-Care Deficit. State in which a person's abilities are less than those required for meeting a therapeutic self-care demand. The lack of ability may be due to decreased motivation, skill, or knowledge.
Nursing Agency. Complex capabilities needed to assist others in the exercise of self-care, acquired through specialized education in the nursing disciplines.
Nursing System. All the actions and interactions that take place between nurses and patients in nursing practice situations. Nursing systems are supportive educative, partly compensatory, or wholly compensatory.

(From Orem, D. *Nursing Concepts of Practice.* 4th ed. St. Louis: Mosby-Year Book, 1991.)

based on comparison of the person's self-care requisites and self-care capacities (or self-care agency). When self-care agency is exceeded by demand, a need for nursing care exists. The relevant nursing diagnoses should be formulated, providing the basis for choice of the type of nursing care (Fig. 1-9) and design of the nursing system. Assessment culminates in an initial choice of nursing care system, providing a framework for planning and implementation.

The nurse assists individuals by planning and implementing a system of nursing care appropriate to their unique situation. In the supportive-educative system, the nurse acts primarily as a consultant to the client, at the individual's request. Clients perform their own self-care and seek out the needed resources to meet their goals. In the partly compensatory system, the nurse assists with those self-care skills that the client is unable to perform independently, but goal setting is collaborative. In the wholly compensatory system, the nurse performs all self-care activities for the client and identifies needs and goals for the client. This does not preclude involvement of the patient and family members regarding preferences, but the major responsibility for directing the care rests with a dependent-care agent, either family or nurse.

Figure 1-10 shows the relationship between patient dependency, self-care deficits, and need for support. As patient dependency increases, the need for support increases. The balance between the amount of support provided by formal and informal support systems is determined by two factors: (1) the capabilities, interests, and values of informal support system members; and (2) the degree of technical nursing expertise required by the patient. For example, an individual with newly diagnosed diabetes mellitus requires a high amount of technical expertise to learn to meet new self-care demands. The same patient requires relatively small amounts of assistance with activities of daily living. Thus, this patient requires increased support from formal sources and decreased help from the informal support network. In contrast, the individual with hemiplegia requires skillful support persons to provide dependent care on a daily basis; however, once the caregivers have been taught the requisite skills, only minimal support from formal organizations is required.

The self-care framework provides a useful means for consideration of family involvement in the life of the older adult. When self-care demands exceed self-care agency, three major possibilities emerge. The older person either (1) has unmet needs for self-care, (2) receives assistance from profes-

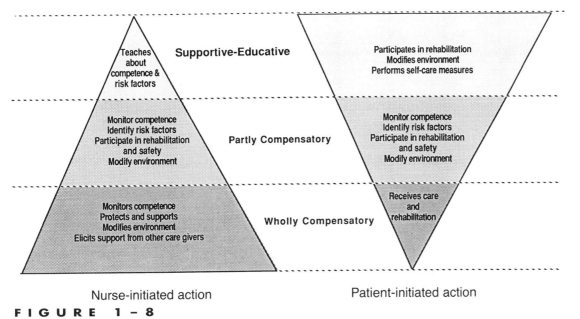

FIGURE 1 – 8

Typology of nursing systems within a self-care framework.

sional caregivers, or (3) receives assistance from family caregivers. In most cases, the older adult experiences some combination of the three possibilities, as depicted in Figure 1–10. If an individual without any self-care deficits receives tremendous amounts of help from family or formal organizations, it is likely that something is amiss. Similarly, if an individual has many unmet self-care de-

mands and there is no support from family or professionals, intervention is warranted.

The self-care model for nursing practice has stood the tests of time and validation by nurses in practice and education. The framework, first proposed in 1959, has undergone considerable refinement and testing since then. It serves as the conceptual framework in some schools of nursing and for nursing

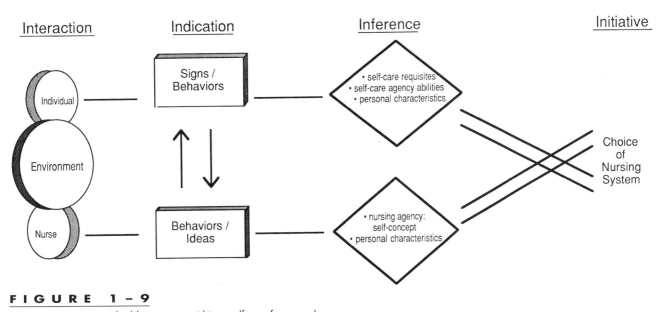

FIGURE 1 – 9

Nursing assessment with older persons within a self-care framework.

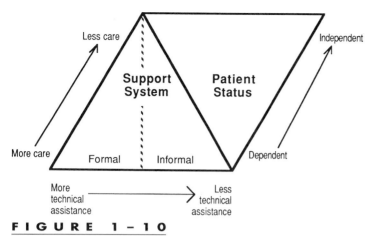

FIGURE 1 – 10

Specification of support and technical assistance by patient status.

services in both acute-care and long-term-care settings. In addition, an active, formalized network of nurses interested in the self-care model is currently working toward further development and refinement.

Critics of the self-care model charge that it introduces unusual terminology and does not sufficiently include family and community as recipients of care. Other critics describe the theory as merely descriptive rather than prescriptive. Other equally well accepted nursing models are in use.

Orem's framework has been used successfully by a number of gerontological nurses. Contributions of other nursing practitioners and theorists are integrated into this framework as they apply to various patient care situations.

Nursing Process and the Elderly

Knowledge of age-related changes and the societal responses to the aging population calls for a modification in generic nursing approaches when working with the aged. Modifications are discussed according to the steps of the nursing process. Although the nursing process is divided into discrete steps for the purposes of discussion, in practice these steps are a cyclical process that is carried on many, many times in each patient encounter. Thus, in conducting the assessment, the nurse can begin to achieve some of the goals of gerontological nursing with a client. For example, as the nurse assesses activity patterns in the elderly patient, the very act of inquiring about this domain of function may "raise the consciousness" in the elderly person that activity is important regardless of age. This small intervention may enhance the effectiveness of subsequent

health teaching, for the person's "teachable moment" may occur at an earlier time than would have been the case without the timely intervention during the assessment encounter. Giduz and Snow (1987) further suggest that the act of intervening as one assesses is essential to obtaining accurate information about the capacity of the older person. Because the performance level of those with functional impairments is sensitive to environmental factors, it is important to measure performance not only under the conditions in which the nurse finds the older person but also under more favorable conditions. For example, biomechanical studies of the requirements for getting out of a chair independently show that chair height is of critical importance, with less force (strength) required for getting out of chairs that are above knee height (Alexander et al., 1991). Elderly individuals may have considerable difficulty getting out of many so-called standard-height chairs because their sitting surface is below knee height. The likelihood of success in rising from a chair is increased by raising the seat level to above knee height (Weiner et al., 1993; Finlay et al., 1983). Therefore, before concluding that an older person is unable to transfer from a sitting to a standing position, the nurse should observe the person's performance while attempting to arise from chairs of different heights.

Another example of the interplay among steps in the nursing process is a nurse who assesses a depressed elderly person. By valuing that individual sufficiently to spend time listening to the concerns, the nurse helps improve that person's self-esteem. Since assessment is a form of nursing intervention, it is important for the nurse to evaluate the impact of the assessment on the individual. Such evaluation will be discussed in detail in a later chapter.

Assessment

Assessment of an older person is a complex, time-consuming process. It is impossible to perform a comprehensive assessment of an older person at one encounter because of the wealth of information to be gathered, the tendency of older persons to reminisce, and the reality that at first it may be difficult to establish trust with an older person. The many frameworks and tools to guide the process of assessment are discussed in detail in later chapters. Key aspects of assessment that should be kept in mind by the gerontological nurse include pace, multidimensionality, emphasis on functional changes rather than structural changes, and the relationship between assessment and intervention.

With advancing age, information processing is slowed (Gilmore, 1989). To obtain accurate measures of an individual's abilities, the time allowed for assessment should be sufficient for the older person to interpret questions or directives and to rest in between. This generally requires that nurses use a slower pace than that used with younger adults. The precise timing should be individualized, as no two people age in precisely the same manner.

Each problem an older person encounters is likely to have several contributing factors. Additionally, each problem is apt to influence other aspects of life. Therefore, it is important to assess a problem or symptom from each dimension of an individual's being. For example, an older person who has urinary incontinence has a genitourinary system problem. Such a problem may be affected or possibly caused by infectious disease, pharmacological agents used to treat other diseases, neurological dysfunction, musculoskeletal problems, or psychological or social factors. The impact of urinary incontinence is experienced by multiple systems, including but not limited to the integument, the family, and the community in which the person resides.

Thus, gerontological nurses should consider many potential contributors to a problem and the multiple ramifications of a problem upon the client's life. This is most readily accomplished by using a multidimensional framework for assessment. Lawton's concept of "the good life" is an example of a multidimensional framework for assessment. Others have been proposed by Pfeiffer et al. (1978), Orem (1991), and Becker and Cohen (1984).

Aging results in many changes in body structures and in functional capacity. Research has shown that there is often no one-to-one correlation between altered structure and impaired function. Therefore, it is insufficient to simply catalogue the structural changes seen in an individual to have an adequate database for nursing care. It is critical to determine the older individual's *functional abilities* in conjunction with structural assessment. For example, in an elderly diabetic individual it is insufficient to note that the client has an above-the-knee amputation of the left leg. It is important to note the person's ability to perform the functions of ambulation, dressing, bathing, social activities, and ability to maintain a household. It

is also important to consider the function of the peripheral vascular system in the remaining limb.

As all nurses must work within time constraints, it is often most efficient to focus the assessment process on function, and note structural abnormalities and strengths as function is assessed.

Diagnosis

The act of diagnosing, or specifying the problems or needs for nursing intervention from assessment data, is the next step in nursing process. A nursing diagnosis is defined by the North American Nursing Diagnosis Association (NANDA) as "a clinical judgment about individual, family or community responses to actual and potential health problems/life processes. Nursing diagnoses provide the basis for selection of nursing interventions to achieve outcomes for which the nurse is accountable" (NANDA, 1994, p. 7). The standard format for communicating nursing diagnoses includes a diagnostic label, an etiological statement, and defining characteristics that support the diagnostic statement.

Nurses have diagnosed patient problems since the time of Nightingale, but only in recent years has attention been directed toward achieving consistency in terminology. NANDA was first convened in 1973 as a broad constituency of practicing nurses and nursing theorists who believed in the importance of the classifying phenomena that nurses assess and treat. NANDA remains the driving force behind establishing a broadly accepted classification of nursing diagnoses that can be used to support a variety of key clinical, administrative, and research activities: an ideal that has not yet been realized. Disagreements persist over whether the taxonomic structure is useful, and the approval process for new diagnostic labels, although more deliberative than in the past, does not require a strong body of evidence (see NANDA, 1994, pp. 105–107, for an overview of requirements). An alphabetized list of NANDA-approved nursing diagnoses as of the eleventh conference (NANDA, 1994) is reproduced on page 30. The newest categories accepted for testing are marked with an asterisk. Given the controversies over the nursing diagnosis taxonomy and classification process, the approach taken in this textbook is to discuss broad clusters of diagnostic categories throughout the text, especially in Chapters 14, 17, and 21, emphasizing more specific labels when the conceptual or empirical gerontological

---

BOX 1 – 1

Diagnoses Currently Accepted for Testing and Use by the North American Nursing Diagnosis Association (NANDA), 1994

Activity Intolerance
Activity Intolerance, Risk for
Adaptive Capacity: Intracranial, Decreased
Adjustment, Impaired
Airway Clearance, Ineffective
Anticipatory Grieving
Anxiety
Aspiration, Risk for
Body Image Disturbance
Body Temperature, Risk for Altered
Bowel Incontinence
Breastfeeding, Effective
Breastfeeding, Ineffective
Breastfeeding, Interrupted
Breathing Pattern, Ineffective
Caregiver Role Strain
Caregiver Role Strain, Risk for
Chronic Low Self-Esteem
Chronic Pain
Colonic Constipation
Communication, Impaired Verbal
Community Coping, Ineffective
Community Coping, Potential for Enhanced
Confusion, Acute
Confusion, Chronic
Constipation
Constipation, Colonic
Constipation, Perceived
Decisional Conflict (specify)
Decreased Cardiac Output
Defensive Coping
Denial, Ineffective
Diarrhea
Disorganized Infant Behavior
Disorganized Infant Behavior, Risk for
Disuse Syndrome, Risk for
Diversional Activity Deficit
Dysfunctional Grieving

Dysfunctional Ventilatory Weaning Response
Dysreflexia
Energy Field Disturbance
Environmental Interpretation Syndrome, Impaired
Family Coping: Compromised, Ineffective
Family Coping: Disabling, Ineffective
Family Coping: Potential for Growth
Family Process: Alcoholism, Altered
Family Processes, Altered
Fatigue
Fear
Fluid Volume Deficit
Fluid Volume Deficit, Risk for
Fluid Volume Excess
Functional Incontinence
Gas Exchange, Impaired
Grieving, Anticipatory
Grieving, Dysfunctional
Growth and Development, Altered
Health Maintenance, Altered
Health Seeking Behaviors (specify)
Home Maintenance Management, Impaired
Hopelessness
Hyperthermia
Hypothermia
Incontinence, Bowel
Incontinence, Functional
Incontinence, Reflex
Incontinence, Stress
Incontinence, Total
Incontinence, Urge
Individual Coping, Ineffective
Infant Feeding Pattern, Ineffective
Infection, Risk for
Injury, Risk for
Knowledge Deficit (specify)
Loneliness, Risk for

---

nursing literature warrants greater specificity. For example, it is our belief that it is unwise to distinguish an entity such as "impaired environmental interpretation syndrome" from "altered thought processes" until more work has been done delineating the advantages of such a fine-grained classification. The more specific label has considerable overlap with the broader, older label, as individuals with altered thought processes generally have difficulty interpreting environmental cues. Thus, it is unclear what benefit the new, more specific category confers in clinical care. Nursing research is

needed to determine whether the more specific, concrete labels represent an improvement over the more established labels.

Despite the problems with nursing diagnosis classification development described above, several aspects of NANDA's efforts are helpful to the profession and justify the use of NANDA labels when possible. First, use of NANDA labels contributes to increased consistency in use of language, facilitating communication between nurses across the functional areas of practice, administration, teaching, and research. Second, a nursing diagnosis taxonomy facilitates the

---

BOX 1–1

Diagnoses Currently Accepted for Testing and Use by the North American Nursing Diagnosis Association (NANDA), 1994 *Continued*

Management of Therapeutic Regimen: Community, Ineffective

Management of Therapeutic Regimen: Families, Ineffective

Management of Therapeutic Regimen: Individual, Effective

Management of Therapeutic Regimen: Individual, Ineffective, Noncompliance (specify)

Memory, Impaired

Nutrition: Less than Body Requirements, Altered

Nutrition: More than Body Requirements, Altered

Nutrition: Potential for More than Body Requirements, Altered

Oral Mucous Membrane, Altered

Organized Infant Behavior, Potential for Enhanced

Pain

Pain, Chronic

Parent/Infant/Child Attachment, Risk for Altered

Parental Role Conflict

Parenting, Altered

Parenting, Risk for Altered

Perceived Constipation

Perioperative Positioning Injury, Risk for

Peripheral Neurovascular Dysfunction, Risk for

Personal Identity Disturbance

Physical Mobility, Impaired

Poisoning, Risk for

Post-Trauma Response

Powerlessness

Protection, Altered

Rape-Trauma Syndrome

Rape-Trauma Syndrome: Compound Reaction

Rape-Trauma Syndrome: Silent Reaction

Reflex Incontinence

Relocation Stress Syndrome

Role Performance, Altered

Self-Care Deficit:
  Bathing/Hygiene
  Dressing/Grooming
  Feeding
  Toileting

Self-Esteem, Chronic Low

Self-Esteem, Situational Low

Self-Esteem Disturbance

Self-Mutilation, Risk for

Sensory/Perceptual Alterations (specify) (visual, auditory, kinesthetic, gustatory, tactile, olfactory)

Sexual Dysfunction

Sexuality Patterns, Altered

Situational Low Self-Esteem

Skin Integrity, Impaired

Skin Integrity, Risk for Impaired

Sleep Pattern Disturbance

Social Interaction, Impaired

Social Isolation

Spiritual Distress

Spiritual Well-Being, Potential for Enhanced

Spontaneous Ventilation, Inability to Sustain

Suffocation, Risk for

Swallowing, Impaired

Thermoregulation, Ineffective

Thought Processes, Altered

Tissue Integrity, Impaired

Tissue Perfusion, Altered (specify type) (renal, cerebral, cardiopulmonary, gastrointestinal, peripheral)

Total Incontinence

Trauma, Risk for

Unilateral Neglect

Urge Incontinence

Urinary Elimination, Altered

Urinary Retention

Violence, Risk for: Self-Directed or Directed at Others

---

statistical reporting of patient problems in various settings of care. Without a systematic means of classifying nursing phenomena, it is impossible to develop general information about the frequency with which these problems are encountered. The World Health Organization's 10th Revision of the International Classification of Diseases (ICD-10) will include nursing diagnoses jointly proposed by NANDA and the American Nurses' Association (ANA) in addition to the traditional medical diagnoses and procedures (Fitzpatrick et al., 1989; NANDA, 1994, pp. 110–114).

Not all aspects of nursing practice fall into the domain of problems that nurses are licensed to treat *independently*. Although nurse theorists continue to discuss independent versus dependent nursing functions, it is generally acknowledged that health care in our society is a complex endeavor, involving interdependent practice by many health and illness care providers. This is particularly true in the case of older persons who suffer from multiple chronic diseases, because their treatment often requires the expertise of several disciplines. Nurses must be able to contribute skillful nursing care to the efforts of other providers in a collaborative manner if the health care needs of individuals are to be best served.

Carpenito (1983) uses the term *clinical problem* for those patient problems that nurses treat collaboratively with other professionals. An example of a clinical problem is diabetes mellitus. Nurses often monitor the patient's serum glucose and teach patients and families about disease management, yet they do not diagnose or prescribe drug treatment for this disease. Nurses do assess and treat independently certain patient responses to diabetes mellitus, for example, knowledge deficit: symptoms of hypo/hyperglycemia. It is, however, too limiting to confine discussion of elderly patient problems to those within the domain of independent nursing practice. Therefore, in this text, clinical problems of old people that are treated collaboratively, as well as nursing diagnoses, are discussed.

Accurate diagnosis depends on careful assessment and understanding of developmental influences on behavior. The scarcity of normative data on health responses in the aged is an important limitation to nursing diagnoses for the elderly. However, gerontological nursing should be practiced within the larger framework of currently accepted nursing practice. Therefore, where possible throughout this book the latest nursing diagnosis nomenclature is used. Older people frequently present diagnostic dilemmas because of the complex interaction between aging process, disease process, and the environment. The existing nursing diagnosis taxonomy at times does not reflect the nature of gerontological nursing problems. Conditions for which no appropriate nursing diagnostic category is specified in the nationally accepted taxonomy are treated as clinical problems. New nursing diagnostic categories undoubtedly will be developed as gerontological nursing phenomena are better understood.

Most gerontological nurses practice within a multidisciplinary environment. It is therefore important to be aware of diagnoses or problems identified by other disciplines, keeping in mind that only nurses are prepared to diagnose patient problems within the scope of nursing practice.

Planning

The nurse planning care for the older person should be aware of environmental influences on the patient's life situation and on the nurse's practice world. Two important types of environmental influences are the health care system and the social system.

These may affect the nurse's priorities, or focus, in caring for a patient, the resources available to the patient and nurse for goal attainment, and the time available for goal achievement.

For example, individuals cared for in the Department of Veterans' Affairs health care system have resources available to them different from those available to indigent patients in a rest home. The nurse working with either type of individual must consider what goals are appropriate for that person, given the options and resources available. Healthful outcomes are possible in both situations, but the specific goals and strategies are likely to be quite different.

Similarly, individuals from large, healthy families in which the long-standing cultural norm is to "take care of your own" have different potentials and a wider range of options than do those without family or friends and with limited finances. These influences may dramatically affect judgments about what goals are attainable, which in turn helps shape nursing activities with that person.

Mutual goal setting is emphasized in working with the aged. Most older persons have developed an extensive repertoire of coping skills and adaptations that form a delicately balanced system for maintaining equilibrium. Unthinking interference with this system may create disaster for the older person with diminished compensatory reserve. Older persons who suffer from dependency remain entitled to the privileges accorded adults. Basic civil rights are sometimes abridged by well-meaning helpers, who assume that disability renders the older person incapable of setting goals. While this may be true for a very small minority of extremely impaired older persons, it is vital to respect the adult status of the older person, and mutual goal setting is a fundamental way to accomplish this. As is the case for other forms of assessment, there are promising methods emerging for helping older adults to articulate their goals that allow clinicians to quantitate progress toward those goals (Bearon et al., 1994).

Involvement of family members in the planning of nursing care is important for old people with self-care deficits, because 60 to 80 per cent of long-term care received by older persons is given by family members. It is not always a simple matter to determine which family members are appropriate to include, but defining the functional family unit is essential in assessment of those in need of long-term care.

A final aspect of planning nursing care for

the elderly that warrants discussion is the increased likelihood of multidisciplinary team involvement. There is an emerging body of research on the effects of team care and team functioning on patient outcomes (e.g., see Wood-Dauphinee et al., 1984). Greater numbers of health care providers increase the complexity of the planning process but result in the expertise of a wide variety of specialists. There is a risk that without careful joint planning of care, disciplines may work at cross-purposes, resulting in suboptimal care for the client. Face-to-face communication with workers in other disciplines is often needed, as well as written communication to facilitate joint planning. The issue of leadership for the multidisciplinary team has historically been problematic because of interprofessional struggles for power and autonomy. Nurses should be knowledgeable about behaviors that facilitate positive team interaction and be prepared to support the patient or family member who becomes the leader in firmly establishing goals for health care.

Intervention

The range of nursing interventions available to nurses who work with the elderly is as broad as with any other age group. The full complement of generic nursing skills identified in Table 1–3 applies to care of the aged. Implementation of such interventions is affected by the aging process in two ways: some interventions are used more frequently, and the manner of implementing a given activity may vary. For example, the fragmented nature of the health care system for the aged requires nurses to be involved in coordination of services more often than in nursing practice with younger adults. The high prevalence of functional disability in the aged results in more use of rehabilitation nursing techniques and assistance with self-care activities than in younger adult groups.

A good example of modifying accustomed nursing activities is health teaching, an intervention commonly used with patients of all ages. Many health education materials have been developed with a younger population in mind; examples of modifications for the elderly include use of larger print for those with presbyopia (aging-related decreased visual acuity) and slowing the pace of a slide-tape presentation because it presents too much material too quickly for an elderly individual's processing abilities (Pierce, 1980). Another example includes the use of older people as models in health promotional literature and audio-visual materials.

Evaluation

Evaluation of nursing practice includes setting criteria and comparing patient progress with those criteria. The process is the same in gerontological nursing; however, the generally accepted criteria for "success" and the frequency by which progress is measured may vary. Also, setting priorities of goals may be different in the elderly as compared with the young. Some examples of these principles follow.

In the nursing care of a young adult with diabetes mellitus, lifestyle modification regarding medication, diet, and exercise is a critical goal, because habits fostered early in the course of the disease may prevent diabetic complications, and better control of the diabetes contributes positively to health status. In the older diabetic, other factors must be considered. It may be more important for older diabetics to socialize at a congregate meal, even though they may suffer the effects of higher blood glucose levels because it is more difficult to follow their prescribed diet away from home than to have better-controlled diabetes but no opportunities for social interaction. The goal of optimal social function may take precedence over euglycemia for the older adult, but this would rarely be the case for a younger adult. The difference in priorities is the result of developmental level as well as the different social opportunities available to these individuals.

Timing of evaluation may also vary in the case of the aged person. Many of the problems that confront younger people require interventions that have effects measurable in a relatively short time. In an aged person with chronic illness, the time needed to see results may be greatly extended. Even in acute illness, the time period for evaluation of results may be prolonged in the elderly. For example, a 35-year-old who sustains a hip fracture in an automobile accident is likely to begin ambulating sooner than an 80-year-old with the same type of fracture because the old person is apt to have complicating medical problems, which will prolong the healing process. It is self-defeating for both patient and nurse to use the same standards for progress in both patients.

Much of gerontological nursing consists of the application of nursing processes and methods with special attention to the unique influences of the aging process on health and illness. It is important to keep in mind the similarities and differences between gerontological nursing practice and generalist nursing practice.

Elements of nursing practice that remain the same, regardless of the age of the client group, include

- Goals of nursing
- Generic nursing process and methods
- Professional practice norms: (1) following standards of practice and code of ethics and (2) accountability to clients

Modifications in nursing practice because clients are of advanced age include

- Slowed pace of the nursing process
- Emphasis on functional abilities
- Expanded nursing diagnosis taxonomy to include phenomena specific to the elderly
- Attention to the social, economic, and political influences on health care to the elderly
- Attention to the effects of the aging process on disease presentation and responses to disease and treatments
- Increased alertness for signs of an intensified stress state
- Increased attention to environmental modifications as an intervention or as a source of problems for the old person

Modifications because of the location of care at the time of the nurse-patient encounter include

- Financial resources available to implement a plan of care
- Health care professionals available to implement a plan of care
- Priority setting
- The old person's goals

Modifications necessary because of developmental level include

- Goal and priority setting
- Increased attention to concerns about dying process
- Increased attention to coping with chronic diseases

Before presenting a specific model of gerontological nursing practice, it is worthwhile to reflect on the history of the specialty of gerontological nursing and on emerging trends in clinical practice.

HISTORY OF GERONTOLOGICAL NURSING

The history of gerontological nursing is influenced by the development of nursing as a profession. Although the need for a gerontological nursing specialty was identified as early as 1900, formalization of the specialty occurred only in 1966, as other specialties in nursing were being formally recognized.

The first gerontological nursing text was published in 1950 by Newton. Like many nursing texts of the day, the material was long on aphorism and short on scientific rationale. During this period in nursing's history, nursing research began to grow, and some of the earliest published nursing research concerned chronic disease and the elderly (Mack, 1952). Norton et al. (1962) conducted a landmark study describing the problems of hospitalized older people and the conditions under which nurses cared for them in the United Kingdom. At approximately the same time, Schwartz et al. (1964) published their study of the psychosocial needs of elderly ambulatory patients. These nursing activities, along with political action being generated to establish governmental health insurance for the aged, set the stage for the establishment of gerontological nursing as a specialty. In 1962 the ANA convened the first meeting of a Conference Group on Geriatric Nursing Practice. Four years later a Division of Geriatric Nursing Practice was established, giving nursing of the aged specialty status along with maternal child health, medical-surgical nursing, psychiatric nursing, and community health nursing.

1965–1981

The period following the enactment of Medicare and Medicaid was one of rapid growth in health care generally. Federal funding for nursing training stimulated growth in nursing practice and education in the form of "expanded roles" for nurses, rapid increases in the numbers of nurses prepared at the master's and doctoral levels, and an increased interest in theory building in nursing science.

Medicare and Medicaid spawned tremendous growth in the nursing home and hospital industries. Medicare legislation provided payment for medical care for older persons, with physicians as the gatekeepers of the system, but excluded most preventive and long-term care. Reimbursement was calculated on a "cost-plus" basis, providing an incentive for expansion of services. Tremendous problems were encountered in obtaining reasonable standards of care in nursing homes. Lax regulations and liberal funding levels led to flagrant abuses of infirm older people. Although Medicare and Medicaid regulations initially stimulated reforms in both hospitals and nursing homes, Medicare reimbursement regulations were slow to keep pace with the increasing support in health policy research for preventive care, community-based long-term care, and expanded nursing roles.

Large-scale longitudinal studies of the aging process began to mature during the 1960s and 1970s, providing the scientific base for much of the modern perspectives on aging. Increased government funding for education, service, and research expanded university-based research and teaching efforts in gerontology and geriatrics. During this era, social policy for care of the aged evolved in the form of the Older Americans' Act and amendments to the Social Security Act. Limited funding spawned a variety of services for the elderly in communities ranging from senior centers to home-based care providers.

1981–1990

A watershed year in gerontological nursing, 1981 marked the beginning of major public policy shifts away from Federal involvement in social programs of all types, including health care financing. The Omnibus Reconciliation Act (OBRA) of 1981 liberalized Medicare home health benefits by removing the limit on the number of visits allowed and the requirement for prior hospitalization. This led to the rapid growth in home health and dramatically changed the acuity level of patients being cared for in the home. The Tax Equity and Fiscal Responsibility Act of 1983 changed Medicare reimbursement for hospitals from a cost-based system to a prospective payment system, creating, for the first time since 1965, an incentive for hospitals to contain costs rather than expand services and costs.

Concern about the high cost of health care led to experiments in financing health care for the aged in the late 1970s, which resulted in more widespread implementation of new models for care provision, such as reimbursement for care coordination, or "case-management" services, increased use of nonphysicians as gatekeepers for care, increased centralization of diverse community-based services, and prepaid care.

The 1980s were characterized by an increased interest in health promotion and fitness, and a slowly growing understanding of the limitations of technology to cure all ills. During this same period, increased interest in the ethical aspects of long-term care was evident, fueled both by clinical dilemmas such as the Cruzan case and by economic concerns that the elderly were consuming more than their fair share of health care resources (Callahan, 1987).

Fundamental changes also occurred during this period in delivery of health care services. The number of hospital beds decreased, and new institutions for the delivery of medical care emerged, including "urgent care" centers, ambulatory surgery facilities, and outpatient rehabilitation centers. These innovations have the potential to benefit older people by containing costs through decreased overhead and hospitalization and by fostering the development of new care models, but they may also further fragment care, increasing the potential for those with complex care needs to have difficulties. For example, ambulatory surgery for cataract removal is frequently performed on older people. Some older adults undergoing this procedure are at high risk for developing acute delirium as a result of exposure to the sedative medications used intraoperatively, and may have difficulty learning new skills required during the recovery phase, such as eyedrop instillation. These innovations in technology and health service delivery call for increased vigilance on the part of nurses to ensure that patients have adequate information and skill to perform self-care.

1991 to the Present

During the late 1980s, and into the present, we are experiencing some of the benefits of gerontological educational and research initiatives. With attention to health care reform, there is a greater willingness to examine expanded roles of nurses in care of the aged, particularly if they can substitute for more costly services, such as physician or hospital services (DeAngelis, 1994).

It is no longer a rarity to find health care providers from many disciplines with specialized training in gerontology or geriatrics. The Geriatric Research, Education, and Clinical Centers (GRECCs) of the US Department of Veterans Affairs provide substantial leadership in training geriatric physicians and dentists, as well as facilitating training of other gerontological health care providers, including nurses. In addition to their training mission, the GRECCs have served as focal points for the development of new knowledge in geriatric care through the establishment of both basic and applied research programs. The GRECCs have been instrumental in developing novel approaches to care of the elderly, such as Geriatric Evaluation and Management Units (GEMUs) and in training a new cadre of clinical investigators in geriatrics. Geriatric Education Centers (GECs) are now widespread throughout the country in academic health sciences centers, providing multidisciplinary continuing education for health care providers.

In research, several developments have fostered improvements in care of the aged, including increased emphasis on the outcomes of health care, the maturation of the National Institute on Aging and its extramural funding program, and the establishment of the National Institute for Nursing Research (NINR).

The medical outcomes movement has focused increased attention on whether care received by older adults is appropriate and effective (Lawlor, 1992). Outcomes research is currently spearheaded by the US Agency for Health Care Policy and Research (AHCPR), under its Medical Treatment Effectiveness Program. One goal of this approach is to examine variability in treatment approaches for common conditions, and determine (if a suitable scientific basis exists) a recommended set of approaches to assessment and treatment of these conditions that can reduce treatment variability and cost, improve quality, and enhance patient outcomes (Kravitz et al., 1992). A highly visible outcome of the AHCPR's work on outcomes research has been the promulgation of guidelines for assessment and treatment of common problems of older people, such as pain, urinary incontinence, and pressure sores. Other practice areas receiving attention from the AHCPR include care of those with benign prostatic hyperplasia, stroke, ischemic heart disease, low back pain, cataracts, joint replacement surgery, diabetes, and pneumonia (Lawlor, 1992).

Maturation of the extramural research program of the National Institute on Aging (NIA) means that the scientific basis for clinical care of the aged is growing. Large-scale epidemiological studies of the aged (Established Populations for Study of the Elderly [EPESE]) are now ongoing in several parts of the country; centers for the study of Alzheimer's disease have been established; and major funding initiatives to determine how best to prevent disability have also been launched, including the Frailty and Injuries:

Cooperative Studies of Intervention Techniques (FICSIT) trials (jointly sponsored by the NIA and NINR [see below]), and most recently with the establishment of several Older Americans' Independence Centers (OAICs) throughout the country, named in honor of the late Claude D. Pepper (a long-time political advocate for needs of the elderly).

Finally, establishment of a National Institute for Nursing Research (NINR) further helps to expand the knowledge base for gerontological nursing practice. In addition to funding individual and cooperative studies of common clinical problems affecting the elderly, the NINR funds original research projects and provides limited funding for nurse scientist training. Thus, a cadre of well-prepared nurse scientists to study nursing care problems of the aged is now emerging.

OPPORTUNITIES FOR GERONTOLOGICAL NURSES: A LOOK INTO THE FUTURE

Opportunities for gerontological nurses are better than ever, because there is greater demand for services and better preparation of practitioners owing to an enhanced research base. The tremendous variety of human situations and needs that confront the gerontological nurse is striking. There is ample opportunity for direct care, counseling, teaching, and advocacy in most positions. Research and policy contributions of gerontological nurses are receiving increasing recognition. Futrell and associates (1980) listed the following roles open to gerontological nurses:

- Direct provider of health services
- Independent practitioner
- Educator of patients, families, other health care professionals, and communities
- Researcher
- Consultant to community agencies and long-term care facilities
- Collaborator with other disciplines
- Advocate
- Health planner
- Health and social policy maker
- Administrator
- Counselor

The frontiers of gerontological nursing lie in *how* these roles are enacted: in what settings of care, with what creativity, and with what rewards or sacrifices.

The ongoing transition from institution-based care to community-based care is likely to continue into the next century. Gerontological nurses are therefore likely to be found in greater numbers in home health agencies, day hospital or day care programs, hospices, primary care settings, and wellness programs than ever before. Gerontological nurses can expect to practice with relative autonomy in these settings, assuming ever-increasing responsibility for independent nursing assessment and initiating referrals to other disciplines as indicated by the patient's functional status. The role of nurse as coordinator of care, perhaps with the title of "case manager," is likely to increase in prominence.

For example, University of Pennsylvania School of Nursing has been a leader in development of model nurse-managed clinics, such as nurse-run clinics for assessment and treatment of urinary incontinence, that have spawned similar models of care in non–university-affiliated private practice settings (Mooney et al., 1993). More recently, this school has established a nurse-managed geriatric rehabilitation center (Evans et al., 1995). Heine and Bahr (1993) reviewed a series of newer gerontological nursing practice models, including health maintenance organization (HMO) services in long-term care facilities and gerontological nurse practitioner services in congregate housing sites, and predicted that nursing practice will continue to relocate to be closer to where the older people themselves are customarily found, rather than in traditional health care settings. The cost effectiveness of using advanced practice nurses in discharge planning for the frail elderly has been established (Naylor et al., 1994). Studies documenting the cost effectiveness of nurse practitioners are being reported (Buchanan et al., 1990), as are more explicit practice descriptions (Sullivan, 1992).

The expansion of prospective payment systems such as HMOs in ambulatory and long-term care is likely to enhance the role of nurses as primary care providers. Thus, nurse practitioners may become more prominent as direct service providers, and an even greater blurring of the boundaries between medicine and nursing in primary care may result. Legislation to allow direct reimbursement to community nursing centers would pave the way for multispecialty nursing practices, in which the gerontological nurse could obtain help with the specialized needs of an older person and family from an enterostomal therapist, a nurse psychotherapist, and a nutrition support team, among other specialists.

A smaller proportion of the care of the aged will be given in nursing homes and hospitals, although there is likely to be a demand for increased sophistication of nursing care for the aged in these settings. As pressures continue to mount for cost containment in health care generally, nurses will be forced to think critically about how to achieve therapeutic end points efficiently. Systems such as care maps (Thompson et al., 1991; Bejciy-Spring, 1991) to chart a predicted course of care are likely to become more commonplace. Practicing nurses should be aware that such care innovations can be misused, as when care maps substitute for individualized patient assessment and care (Wells, 1994).

The history of gerontological nursing and current trends in the specialty underscore the importance of maintaining an approach to practice based on a strong nursing tradition, influenced by knowledge from gerontology and geriatrics. What follows is specification of an approach to gerontological nursing, along with case examples of its application.

MODEL OF GERONTOLOGICAL NURSING PRACTICE

Definitions

Gerontological nursing is " . . . a health service that incorporates generic nursing methods [see Table 1–3] and specialized knowledge about the aged to establish conditions within the client and within the environment that will do the following:

1. Increase health conducive behaviors in the aged
2. Minimize and compensate for health-related losses and impairments of aging
3. Provide comfort and sustenance through the distressing and debilitating events of aging, including dying and death
4. Facilitate the diagnosis, palliation, and treatment of disease in the aged" (Gunter and Estes, 1979b, pp. 91–92)

In Table 1–5 the definition proposed by Gunter and Estes reflects the evolution of gerontological nursing over the past 40 years. We believe this is the most comprehensive definition of gerontological nursing available, and it is not restricted to any one theoretical perspective for nursing.

To complete the framework for geronto-

T A B L E   1 – 5
Evolution of a Definition of Gerontological Nursing

THEORIST	DEFINITION	CONTRIBUTION
Newton, 1950	"Geriatrics is, then, that branch of medical and nursing science that deals with the treatment and care of disease conditions in old people, including also constructive health practice and prevention of disease" (Newton, 1950, p. 18). "Nursing as a companion science complementing medicine has a responsibility in making these later years healthful, happy, and economically productive." "One concept of geriatrics is basic; it is that old age can be satisfying, that it need not be a period of idle sitting and waiting for the inevitable death. . . . It is not a matter of making him young again. It is, on the contrary, an adjustment of health commensurate with his years; helping him to use what normal capacities he possesses with the firm conviction that each interval of life has its own particular satisfactions and potentialities, provided that health for the age level is maintained and opportunity for the utilization of one's potentialities is granted by society" (Newton, 1950, p. 21).	First definition of geriatric nursing
Norton, 1965	Geriatrics is "the positive approach to preserve and to restore human ability in old age," and geriatric nursing practice is divided into two categories, "the rehabilitation category, for patients who have a potential to regain the ability of basic self-care, and the irremediable category—geriatric long-stay or chronic—for patients who have gone beyond medical reclaim and need some degree of nursing care for the remainder of their lives" (Norton, 1965, paraphrased in Gunter and Miller, 1977).	Geriatric nursing researcher; differentiates supportive nursing from rehabilitative nursing care
American Nurses Association, Division of Geriatric Nursing Practice, 1970	"Geriatric nursing is concerned with the assessment of nursing needs of older people; planning and implementing nursing care to meet those needs; and evaluating the effectiveness of such care to achieve and maintain a level of wellness consistent with the limitations imposed by the aging process." Identified primary factors that make nursing of older persons different, including effects of aging process, multiplicity of losses, atypical presentation and response to disease, multiple chronic illnesses, and cultural and societal values and attitudes toward old people.	First nationally recognized definition
Baker, 1976	Adds to ANA definition: "The aim of any nursing intervention . . . should be to help the elderly maintain independent lives in their own homes for as long as possible" (Baker, 1976).	Focus on independence and home care
Gunter and Estes, 1979a	"Gerontic nursing is proposed to be a health service that incorporates generic nursing methods and specialized knowledge about the aged to establish conditions within the client and within the environment that will do the following: 1. Increase health conducive behaviors in the aged, 2. Minimize and compensate for health-related losses and impairments of aging, 3. Provide comfort and sustenance through the distressing and debilitating events of aging, including dying and death, 4. Facilitate the diagnosis, palliation, and treatment of disease in the aged" (Gunter and Estes, 1979b, pp. 91–92).	Explicitly addresses care of the dying
Eliopoulos, 1979	"The focus of gerontological and geriatric nursing is to take action in a planned, organized and therapeutic manner: 1. To strengthen the individual's self-care capacities, 2. To eliminate or minimize self-care limitations, 3. To provide direct care services by acting for, doing for, or partially assisting the individual when universal self-care or therapeutic demands cannot be independently fulfilled" (Eliopoulos, 1979, p. 70).	Applies a major nursing theory to care of the elderly
Wells, 1980	"Modern nursing care of the elderly should be about mobilization, not bedcare; it should be about regaining and maintaining skills and abilities, not acceptance of less than the older individual's maximum functional level. Underlying such dynamic nursing care of the old is comfort and support" (Wells, 1980, p. 7).	Blends rehabilitative nursing with supportive nursing care
Bahr, 1981	"The goal of gerontological nursing care is to help elderly clients function as fully as possible by realizing their highest potential" (Bahr, 1981, p. 24).	Introduces notion of highest potential (a developmental concept) into gerontological nursing definitions

logical nursing practice, the various environments in which gerontological nursing is practiced must be considered, along with how they influence the process and outcomes of gerontological nursing. Additionally, the following structural elements of gerontological nursing are specified:

1. Characteristics of the recipients of gerontological nursing
2. Assumptions that underpin the practice model
3. Essential knowledge and competencies of gerontological nurses
4. Standards for care

The process of care is then described, using illustrative case examples, and criteria for evaluation of gerontological nursing are proposed.

Context of Health Services to the Aged

Nursing care of the aged takes place within the environment of a complex health care delivery system. Since gerontological nursing typically is practiced in a team context, it is essential that clinicians understand the problems of the current health care system and how they influence opportunities for practice by nurses and other health care providers.

There is widespread acknowledgment that serious problems exist with the way the American health care system addresses the problems of the aged. Key problems include

- Preferential reimbursement under Medicare for acute illness rather than for chronic disease care, health promotion, or disease prevention
- Emphasis on institutional care rather than community-based care
- Physician control of access to reimbursement for long-term care services, leading to underutilization of nonphysician and noninstitutional providers of care
- Lack of specialized training in geriatrics/ gerontology for most health care providers
- Many providers of services with few formal linkages or systematic care coordination, leading to serious fragmentation of services
- Reimbursement, eligibility, and availability of service considerations taking precedence over patient and family goals for health in determining access to services
- Poor mechanisms for ensuring high quality care, as measured by maintaining functional ability

The roots of these problems are discussed in more detail in Chapter 20. Each of the problems outlined above influences the practice of gerontological nursing.

Influence of Health Care System for the Elderly on Nursing Practice

A fragmented and medically oriented system of health care has predictable effects on the practice of nursing, including demands for greater clinical nursing sophistication, and an ability to see the nursing role quite broadly, including providing advocacy for elderly patients. Tremendous tension exists between the imperatives just listed and the fact that many nurses caring for old people have little formalized training in care of the aged. Numerous studies and authoritative bodies have documented and decried the lack of gerontological nursing content in basic nursing curricula at both the baccalaureate and associate degree levels (Small, 1993; Carignan, 1991, citing Johnson and Connelly, 1990; Kuehn, 1991). The National League for Nursing has tried to provide leadership in building a consensus for strengthening requirements for gerontological nursing content. However, as noted by Waters (1993, p. xiv), nursing curricula in general have been slow to amend their content from an acute disease treatment perspective to one that emphasizes "the chronic degenerative diseases of lifestyle and aging." Small (1993) notes that faculty give lip service to teaching nursing across the lifespan, but often fail in the gerontological nursing arena because of their own lack of preparation.

The result of poor preparation in nursing care of the aged is nurses who are frustrated when the care provided is perceived by patients and their families to be inadequate or unrewarding. These frustrations may be at the root of the negative attitudes toward the aged observed in experienced nurses (Haight et al., 1994).

The nursing profession has a well-conceived and long-standing commitment to considering both the wellness and illness needs of patients. Despite this, nurses are frequently in the position of having to focus on only a narrow portion of an individual patient's problems, because of the goals of the systems in which they work. This adds to the frustration of working with older people, because there is a gap between what should be and what is feasible in many practice settings.

For example, in acute care hospitals the major focus of the institution is on diagnosis and treatment of acute medical problems. Once those goals have been accomplished, the patient is considered healed and is expected to leave that subunit of the health care system. Nurses who work with older patients in the hospital must be alert to prevent functional losses, for such losses have considerable impact on a patient's health and self-care status. Once function is lost in the acute care setting, there is little opportunity to assist patients to regain self-care abilities, because the emphasis in most hospitals is on diagnosis and cure rather than rehabilitation.

The nurse in the hospital who works with the elderly should be concerned with preventing functional loss for two reasons. First, a nurse is in the best position to assess and monitor changes in a patient's functional status and to intervene to promote maintenance of functional independence. Second, if functional ability is lost during a hospitalization, the nurse will probably have lost the opportunity to participate in assisting the patient to regain function, because of the environmental emphasis on resolution of acute medical or surgical problems. The one opportunity available to assist in this aspect of the patient's care is participating in discharge planning. However, despite careful discharge planning, inadequate reimbursement for nonhospital services, the uneven distribution of services, and the unpredictable quality of gerontological care in various long-term care settings may conspire to deny old people the opportunity to receive assistance in regaining self-care abilities, or in adjusting to their loss.

The need for gerontological nurses to focus broadly on patient needs pervades every component of the health care system. The nursing home nurse must be knowledgeable about acute health problems, despite the institution's focus on rehabilitation and chronic care, because failure to have such knowledge further fragments care and may have serious consequences for the patient. Likewise, acute care nurses must be knowledgeable about the long-term impact of prolonged immobility and should take steps to prevent complications such as contractures and malnutrition and to recognize coping difficulties early in the patient's stay. One example of an organized approach to accomplishing these goals is reported by Kresevic et al. (1993), who have developed a specialized acute care unit for elderly hospitalized patients. A literature concerning practical strategies to bridge gaps between settings of care is starting to emerge (e.g., see Trella, 1994).

Nurses who work with the aged should be knowledgeable about the nuances of local service options for the elderly and use that information to guide their planning for optimal care. Gerontological nurses have a responsibility for developing a working knowledge of the services available to the elderly in a given community. This responsibility is analogous to their responsibility for obtaining adequate orientation to a new nursing unit in an institutional setting.

Nurses may find themselves frustrated by conflicts between their work settings' emphasis on efficiency and cost containment and the awareness that older individuals generally require careful care coordination that is often time-consuming and therefore expensive.

Multidisciplinary Nature of Gerontological Nursing Practice

Complexities in describing the nature and influence of professional nursing practice in health care of the aged arise from the relationships between nursing and the other health care professionals and institutions affecting it. Since much of health care today is multidisciplinary in nature, members of the other health care professions are keenly interested in activities of the nursing profession and vice versa. Changes in the role definition of one set of health care providers affect the roles and functions of other providers. These complex relationships affect the scope of practice, as well as the availability of services to old people.

While the number of disciplines needed for each patient varies with the individual patient's needs, the concepts of shared data gathering and management techniques, along with advanced expertise and accountability for specialty practice, are characteristic of every patient care situation. Some of the regulatory bodies and professional organizations that influence gerontological nursing practice are listed in Table 1–6. Diagramming the complex interrelationships among these organizations would be impossible.

The organization of nursing personnel to care for older persons is also complex and may be confusing to non-nurses. A diverse group provides nursing care to the elderly in America. At least 11 different levels of preparation exist for those providing nursing care to the aged (Table 1–7), and the only consistent credentialing mechanism throughout the United States for these various providers of nursing care is the state licensing mechanism for registered nurses and licensed practical nurses. Additional credentialing mechanisms that help differentiate practitioners of different levels are earned degrees (in the case of advanced practitioners) and the certification program sponsored by the American Nurses Association for specialist practitioners.

Additionally, nurses may function in a variety of capacities, such as direct caregivers, physician extenders, managers, teachers, consultants, and researchers; they may practice in many different settings, including hospitals, rehabilitation centers, ambulatory care clinics, mental health centers, long-stay institutions, and the home. This results in some confusion as to what precisely nurses are prepared to do in health care, and at what level. This situation is particularly difficult for consumers of nursing services who reached maturity in the era before the proliferation of roles and responsibilities that characterize modern nursing.

Five levels of nursing personnel are involved in care of the elderly:

Level I: Nursing Assistants

Level II: Licensed practical nurses

Level III: Professional nurses

Level IV: Advanced level practitioners (clinical specialists, nurse practitioners, administrators of nursing services for the aged)

Level V: Nurse scientists/gerontologists

Several factors influence the need for this broad range of providers. Demographic trends in the United States show that a rapidly increasing proportion of the recipients of health care are elderly. This makes it important that every professional nurse practicing in an adult health setting have some gerontological nursing skill. The current system of health care financing for the elderly in the United States dictates the involvement of paraprofessionals in care of the elderly. There is a great need for further development of the scientific basis of gerontological nursing practice, and most practicing professional nurses do not have sufficient educational preparation to conduct nursing research independently.

Although the need for the involvement of diverse levels of caregivers in the care of the elderly is recognized, under the definition of gerontological nursing used in this text, only Levels III to V practitioners qualify for definition as gerontological nurses. The other two levels of providers assist professional nurses in the conduct of gerontological nursing but are not gerontological nurses. Practitioners at the first two levels carry out selected aspects of care of the elderly under the supervision of the professional nurse.

TABLE 1 – 6
Organizations Affecting Gerontological Nursing Practice

PUBLIC SECTOR	PRIVATE SECTOR
Federal	
Department of Health and Human Services	Professional Organizations
Health Care Financing Administration	American Nurses Association (ANA)
National Institutes of Health	National League for Nursing (NLN)
Institute of Medicine	National Practical Nurses Association
Division of Nursing	American Academy of Nursing
Public Health Service	American Academy of Colleges of Nursing
Department of Labor	American Medical Association
National Labor Relations Board	American Health Care Association
Occupational Health and Safety Office	National Homecaring Council
Department of Defense	American Geriatrics Society
Department of Veterans Affairs	Gerontological Society of America
Armed Services Nurse Corps	American Hospital Association
Department of Agriculture	AARP
Food and Drug Administration	National Council on Aging (NCoA)
State*	
State Board of Nursing	State Nurses Association
State Board of Medical Examiners	State Medical Society
State Board of Pharmacy	Schools of Nursing
Medical Care Commission	Universities (public and private)
Department of Human Resources	State Hospital Association
Division of Health Services	State Nursing Home Association
Division of Mental Health	State Visiting Nurse Association
Division of Facility Services	
Division of Aging	
Division of Medical Assistance	
Local	
County Commissioners	District Nurses Association
Local Health Board	County Medical Society
Local Nursing Home Ombudsman Program	
Local School Board	
Community Mental Health Center Board	
Area Agency on Aging	

* North Carolina serves as the example.

Elements of a Gerontological Nursing Model

Recipients of Gerontological Nursing

Recipients of gerontological nursing include those who seek assistance in adjusting to age-related changes in their postadulthood health status or in that of a family member, and any individual over the age of 65 years who receives nursing care from a professional nurse who practices according to the definition listed earlier. According to Orem (1991), any aged individual whose self-care demands exceed the ability to meet

T A B L E   1 – 7

Levels of Nursing Practitioners Involved in Care of the Aged

PRACTITIONER	FUNCTION	EDUCATION PREPARATION
Nursing assistant, also known as patient care assistant (PCA), nurses' aide (NA)	Assists professional nurse in patient care tasks	Certified through taking short courses at technical colleges or through inservice training. Competency-based evaluation must be passed.
Licensed practical nurse (LPN) or licensed vocational nurse (LVN)	Assists professional nurse in patient care tasks	Technical college or vocational high school preparation, must pass licensure exam and maintain licensure to practice
Registered nurse (RN)	Practices professional nursing with patients/clients in any health care setting	Multiple levels of entry including Associate degree (ADN) in 2-year program Diploma (3-year hospital-based program) Baccalaureate degree (BSN), 4-year university-based program Nursing doctorate (ND), 4-year program after college degree in another field State licensure required for all levels of entry
Nurse practitioner (NP) (sometimes also qualified by specialty area such as pediatric nurse practitioner (PNP) or family nurse practitioner (FNP)	Performs "medical" acts such as management of chronic disease, prescription of medicines, diagnosis of disease	Multiple levels of entry including Certificate programs open to any RN regardless of level of preparation and Master's level programs; all are RNs certified jointly by state boards of nursing and medicine
Clinical specialist	Advanced practitioner of nursing, clinical teacher	Master's degree (MSN, MN), also are RNs
Nurse scientist	Nurse research and/or nurse educator	Doctor of Nursing Science (DNSc) or Doctor of Philosophy (PhD) in nursing or other field (psychology, sociology, physiology, anthropology), public health, epidemiology

those demands is an appropriate recipient of gerontological nursing care.

Although chronological age is a poor indicator of the impact of aging on an individual, and an even poorer indicator of needs, it is used to mark the target population for this text for two reasons. First, there are no universally accepted markers of an individual's place on the continuum of aging. Second, aging is a social phenomenon as well as a physiological and psychological one, and the chronological age of 65 years has significant meaning in our society. It is the age of retirement, when society begins to allow individuals, as a normal course of events, to begin to relinquish younger adult roles. It is also the age at which most Americans become eligible to benefit from the major health care financing system for the elderly, Medicare.

It is regrettable that a more satisfactory marker for gerontological nursing clients does not exist. However, as gerontology and gerontological nursing research progress, more accurate markers of this target population may emerge, based on better delineation of the altered responses that accompany aging.

Assumptions

The elderly have specific, although diverse, responses to the interplay among age-related biological changes, developmental tasks, and social environment. They are capable of attaining the full range of health statuses, despite the increased incidence of chronic disease in late life and the increased vulnerability to illness. The context in which older persons currently receive health care is disease oriented, fragmented, and institutionally based. Nurses, regardless of their theoretical framework for practice, are concerned with preserving health and function as well as preventing and curing disease, from a biopsychosocial perspective. For these reasons, nurses are important health care providers for the elderly.

Other assumptions that undergird our model of gerontological nursing are as follows:

1. Older individuals and their families can be viewed as open systems, capable of change, growth, and mutual interaction.

2. Human beings have the potential to develop their intellectual and practical skills and the motivation essential for self-care and care of dependent family members.

3. Human development requires the formation and maintenance of specific environmental conditions that promote known developmental processes at each period of the life cycle.

4. Older individuals are affected in unique ways by the combined effects of the aging process, the disease process, lifestyle, and environment.

5. Old people are capable of making independent decisions, unless some well-documented pathological process interferes with this ability. This capability is presumed to be intact unless demonstrated otherwise.

6. Elderly people are interested in learning more about health and aging.

7. Health status and developmental status are two separate but related concepts. Health is a multidimensional concept that allows for the presence of well-being despite the presence of pathological processes in body subsystems.

8. Nursing is one of several health services, all of which are helping services designed to assist individuals experiencing states of social dependency.

9. Old people have the potential to benefit from a wide variety of health services, if appropriately targeted. Nurses are not and should not be the sole providers of care but should function within a multidisciplinary team context.

10. Given the necessary information, older people can reduce their dependence on medical and institutional services.

11. Health teaching can help older people maintain and protect their health and prevent disease or complications and disabilities.

12. Gerontological nursing is practiced within the framework of professional nursing and therefore is subject to professional norms and the code of ethics.

Essential Competencies for Practice of Gerontological Nursing

The necessary competencies for gerontological nursing practice are influenced by the level at which the nurse will function and the role expectations of the nurse. For example, gerontological nurses in a clinical role require an expertise different from that of a gerontological nurse scientist. However, a common body of knowledge, skills, and attitudes essential for good clinical nursing practice with the aged has developed. This knowledge and its relationship to other related fields are depicted in Figure 1–11. We will describe the specific competencies needed by the clinical gerontological nurse in addition to generic professional nursing preparation.

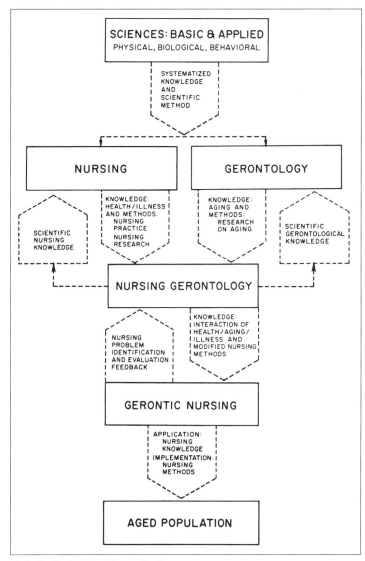

FIGURE 1 – 1 1

Knowledge base of gerontological nursing. (From Gunter, L. and Estes, C. *Education for Gerontic Nursing.* New York: Springer Publishing Company © 1979, p. 38, used by permission.)

Knowledge

A gerontological nurse should be knowledgeable about basic professional nursing practices and theories, *and also*

- The physical, psychological, and social aspects of aging throughout the lifespan, and the resultant impact on the individual and family

- The pathophysiology, epidemiology, and treatment of chronic diseases commonly encountered by older people, and the impact of these disease processes and associated therapeutic regimens on elderly individuals and their families

- The spectrum of health services available to the elderly in the community, and how that relates to the national spectrum of health services
- The signs and symptoms of atypical presentation of disease in the elderly
- The altered pharmacology of drugs in the elderly
- The influence of environmental factors on human performance and health status in the aged
- The impact of ethnicity on responses to aging-related changes, disease, and developmental events
- Specific standards of nursing care for older individuals
- Approaches to health promotion and disease prevention in late life
- The range of ethical reasoning frameworks that apply to care of the aged

Skills

Gerontological nurses should be skillful in applying generic nursing methods to care of the aged, and be able to

- Utilize research findings from gerontology as well as nursing and the biomedical and behavioral sciences to inform nursing practice
- Interact effectively with individuals who have sensory loss
- Perform multidimensional assessment of the elderly person using existing standardized tools and individualized approaches
- Function as members of a coordinated multidisciplinary or interdisciplinary team in providing care to the aged
- Implement rehabilitative nursing techniques
- Help clients integrate past life with present
- Include the older person and family members in developing goals for nursing care, even if the individual has significant communication or cognitive impairments
- Modify the environment to maximize the older person's ability to function independently
- Provide excellent palliative, supportive, and spiritual care for those who are dying
- Counsel the grieving
- Consider ethical dilemmas encountered by old people, their kin, and their health care providers

- Help families and communities overcome hostilities toward the elderly
- Participate in professional activities designed to improve health care for the elderly
- Supervise the efforts of paraprofessional and lay caregivers in providing nursing care to the aged
- Teach paraprofessional and lay caregivers and old people about the impact of the aging process and the disease process on self-care abilities and requisites of older persons
- Teach paraprofessional and lay caregivers and old people about techniques to achieve self-care objectives
- Establish developmentally appropriate criteria for evaluation of nursing care

Attitudes

Most gerontological experts and clinicians would agree that nurses need to be able to free themselves of biases toward aging and older people, but specifying the attitudes desirable for the gerontological nurse is considerably more difficult. The attitudes of nurses and nursing students toward the elderly have been studied extensively (see Treharne, 1990 and Haight et al., 1994 for reviews), but little is known of the impact of such attitudes on patient outcomes. Anecdotal data suggest that negative attitudes toward the elderly, based on stereotypical thinking, have negative effects on health outcomes.

Obtaining the necessary attitudes, skills, and knowledge for the successful practice of gerontological nursing is not a simple process. Ideally, generic nursing programs should provide adequate preparation for professional nurses in gerontological nursing; however, the curricula of most schools of nursing historically have lacked adequate gerontological nursing content. Another avenue for developing the needed competencies lies in continuing education programs. These vary in depth of content and in opportunities for precepted clinical practice. Many continuing education providers offer courses that cover some of the competencies needed by gerontological nurses. The federally funded, multidisciplinary Geriatric Education centers are increasing the availability of high-quality continuing education in gerontological nursing. Journals, textbooks, and audiovisual aids may be used by nurses for self-study. Advanced training at the Master's degree level is available in a number of nursing schools for preparation of gerontological nurse specialists. Those who cannot pursue graduate study yet who practice primarily with older adults are left to design their own programs to arrive at the proper mix of didactic instruction and precepted clinical practice. Carefully planned exposure to gerontology, either in basic nursing curricula or in continuing education settings, enhances attitudes of nursing personnel toward the elderly (Haight et al., 1994).

Standards

Gerontological nursing should be practiced in accordance with standards developed by the nursing profession. The American Nurses Association Division of Gerontological Nursing Practice has developed and refined standards for practice (ANA, 1970, 1976, 1987, 1995), which provide an excellent guide for evaluation of nursing practice.

The current ANA standards for gerontological nursing practice address organization of gerontological nursing services, make specific recommendations for the process of nursing care of the aged, and describe the context for gerontological nursing as one where interdisciplinary teamwork is practiced; where nursing theory and research are used to inform clinical practice; where the cost-effectiveness of care options is considered; where nurses participate in quality improvement activities, professional development, and research activities; and where nurses practice according to the ANA Code for Nurses. The standards for implementation of nursing process emphasize the importance of systematic and comprehensive data collection, the use of nursing diagnosis, and the development and evaluation of interventions based on nursing diagnoses and goals mutually established with the patient and family. Walker and Knapp (1990) have developed examples of implementing the ANA standards for gerontological nursing practice using a quality improvement approach.

Scope of Practice

The nature and scope of nursing practice is influenced by the *needs of the patients* in a given *setting*. The range of health and illness needs that old people experience is extremely broad. There is a place for nursing action at nearly any point along the health-illness continuum. Likewise, there is potential for nursing practice in every location in which old people are found.

The *focus* of nursing care in the many settings where nursing of the elderly is practiced may be as broad as the range of needs

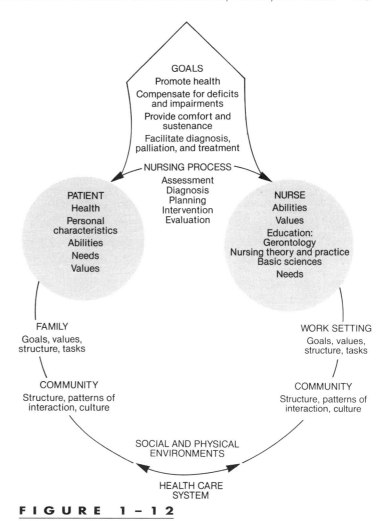

F I G U R E   1 – 1 2

Schematic view of gerontological nursing practice.

encountered. For example, in a congregate housing project for the elderly, nurses may be responsible for organizing and teaching an exercise class (a wellness activity) and, in the same day, be responsible for initiating advanced emergency care to an elderly person who has suffered a cardiopulmonary arrest. The nurse caring for an aged person in an intensive care unit is responsible for administering highly technological interventions to patients with multiple organ system dysfunction. That nurse is also responsible for monitoring the patient's psychoemotional response to illness and the intensive care environment, as failure to do so may result in a technical success in controlling organ system pathology without concomitant restoration of the individual's functional ability.

Process

Figure 1–12 diagrams the elements of gerontological nursing practice. The goal of each gerontological nurse-patient interaction is to establish conditions within client and environment that will promote healthy behaviors; compensate for disease-related losses and impairments; prevent further disease-related losses; promote comfort; and facilitate the diagnosis, palliation, and treatment of disease. These goals are achieved through interactions between patient and nurse, which are guided by the nursing process activities of assessment, diagnosis, planning, intervention, and evaluation. Three examples showing application of this model to practice with selected elderly individuals are given next.

Application of Gerontological Nursing Models

Case Examples

These case studies demonstrate the influences of dependency level, environment, and life stage on the process of gerontological nursing. The elderly people discussed here demonstrate the rich variability in the types of nursing encounters that are possible.

Text continued on p. 62

CASE 1. Supportive-Educative Nursing System

Mr. Green's environment was his home, and the nurse's environment was a general medical clinic with a geriatric evaluation team. The initial request for assistance came from the patient's physician, to help reduce the burden of caregiving for a demented wife, which was adversely affecting his health. The nursing system developed was in the *supportive-educative mode*; thus, the client established the priorities. The approaches used by the nurse over the 6-month period are summarized in the case feature, along with client outcomes.

Key issues in providing care for Mr. Green were his need to unburden and to explore the function that his burdens served, in helping him avoid considering his own life stage. The nurse's role was to provide active listening and counseling regarding his death anxiety and his specific concerns about adequate care for his wife if he should predecease her. He was also in conflict about providing the best possible physical care without violating her religious beliefs.

Important strengths in this client's environment included adequate finances and a small but very active and devoted extended family. The Greens had a 30-year relationship with their domestic help, and Mr. Green's sister-in-law lived nearby and assisted with the daily meal preparation. This case is an excellent example of how finances can be used in partial supplement of relatively scarce family resources. It also highlights the importance of working with a flexible definition of family, for the hired helpers in many ways functioned as family.

IDENTIFYING INFORMATION: 83-year-old white retired university faculty member seen in general medical clinic. Primary medical problems include mitral regurgitation w/ congestive heart failure (CHF) (compensated) and stress of caregiving for demented wife.

CONDITIONING FACTORS
AGE: 83
SEX: Male
EDUCATIONAL LEVEL: Postcollegiate

ENVIRONMENTAL FACTORS
HOUSEHOLD STATUS: Lives with wife and has three housekeepers
MARITAL STATUS: Married

FAMILY SUPPORT: No children, many friends and neighbors
ETHNICITY: Caucasian, Protestant religion
FORMAL ORGANIZATION INVOLVEMENT: None

UNIVERSAL SELF-CARE REQUISITES
Air*
HISTORY/HABITS: No smoking
SYMPTOMS: Dyspnea on exertion, paroxysmal nocturnal dyspnea
PERCEPTIONS: Feels air intake adequate except during episodes of dyspnea
PHYSICAL EXAMINATION/INSPECTION: Respiratory rate = 20 at rest; ↑ to 26 w/moderate activity. No deformities of chest wall.
AUSCULTATION: Breath sounds: Clear, all lobes

CASE 1.   Supportive-Educative Nursing System

continued

PERCUSSION: Normal resonance

PALPATION: Fremitus: No increase in any lobe

ENVIRONMENTAL FACTORS: No respiratory irritants. Client has to climb one flight of stairs to bedroom.

PERFORMANCE: Ability to deep breathe: Intact. Dyspnea on performance of activities of daily living (ADLs) or independent ADLs (IADLs): not if adequately paced.

Fluid

HISTORY/HABITS: 6 glasses of fluid per day. Takes furosemide, 40 mg q day.

SYMPTOMS: Dizziness on changing position rapidly

PERCEPTIONS: Thirst seldom present

PHYSICAL EXAMINATION: Skin turgor: Loose; mucous membranes moist

INSPECTION: No edema, neck veins flat. No abdominal distention.

AUSCULTATION: No orthostatic changes in blood pressure. BP = 160/85 sitting.

ENVIRONMENTAL FACTORS: Able to access water/other fluids ad lib

PERFORMANCE: Able to pour and drink fluids without difficulty

Food

HISTORY/HABITS: Usual meal patterns: Three meals per day, with major meal at midday. No snacks in between.

SYMPTOMS: No symptoms related to food intake

PERCEPTIONS: Feels food intake is adequate. Body image: Perceives self as normal-thin. Meaning of food to individual: social activity and you have to eat to live.

ENVIRONMENTAL FACTORS: Nearest grocery store approx. 2 miles away. Housekeepers do shopping. Kitchen on ground floor, readily accessible. Paid help and sister-in-law (78 years old) assist with meal preparation. No health hazards in kitchen.

PHYSICAL EXAMINATION: Weight = 130 lbs. Height = 5'3".

INSPECTION: Appearance of mucous membranes: Moist, red. Muscle mass = small. Biochemical measures: No abnormalities: Hgb, TP, B_{12}. Oral-motor reflexes: Intact.

PERFORMANCE: Does not prepare meals independently but can afford and obtain necessary assistance. Able to feed self. Able to swallow without difficulty.

Elimination*

HISTORY/HABITS: Frequency of elimination: Urinates approximately every 2 hours; fears being incontinent. Sometimes has difficulty starting and stopping stream. Uses milk of magnesia approx. once a month. Usually has BM q day. Does not use pads, catheters or other devices to control elimination.

SYMPTOMS/URINARY: Admits frequency but denies burning, incontinence

FECAL: Denies constipation, pain on elimination

PERCEPTIONS: Believes that a monthly purgative is necessary to prevent constipation

PHYSICAL EXAMINATION/INSPECTION: No odor of urine or feces; no evidence of soiling

AUSCULTATION: Bowel sounds normal

PALPATION: No abdominal masses or distended bladder. Rectal examination shows no fecal impaction; prostate moderately enlarged, regular, nontender.

ENVIRONMENTAL FACTORS: Toilets on both floors of house with unrestricted access. No assistive devices used.

PERFORMANCE: Urination or defecation not observed

Activity/Rest*

HISTORY/HABITS: Sedentary lifestyle except for walking

DRUGS: Takes no sedatives or analgesics. Uses long-acting nitrate for control of CHF.

SLEEP PATTERNS: Approx. 6 hours of sleep at night, sometimes interrupted by wife awakening to toilet

SYMPTOMS: No chest pain or dyspnea on exertion. No musculoskeletal pain. Complains of falling asleep in the middle of tasks without realizing it.

PERCEPTIONS: Believes in the value of walking as a health-promoting activity.

PHYSICAL EXAMINATION/INSPECTION: Muscle mass within normal limits (WNL), range of motion in all joints WNL

AUSCULTATION: Resting heart rate = 78/min, regular

ENVIRONMENTAL FACTORS: Shares bedroom with wife who has severe dementia and is attended by a nursing assistant at night. House is in quiet, safe neighborhood with little traffic, which allows for safe walking. No assistive devices used.

Solitude/Social Interaction*

HISTORY: Many long-time friends in area. Goes out to dinner once a week. Reports

continued on following page

CASE 1. Supportive-Educative Nursing System

continued

social activity slightly restricted since wife's illness but is able to get out when paid caregivers are present. Hearing impairment impedes conversation. He does not feel secure in operation of hearing aid. Denies visual impairment if he wears his glasses.

EXAMINATION: Has difficulty manipulating hearing aid and does not know how to check for dead batteries. Communication otherwise unimpaired.

ENVIRONMENT: Has lived in the same house and community for over 50 years. Has ready access to public transportation, which he is able to use without difficulty.

Injury Prevention

HISTORY: No report of falls or accidental injury in past year. Not concerned about personal safety. Walks 1 mile three times a week, weather permitting.

EXAMINATION: Skin intact without evidence of bruising or other trauma. Musculoskeletal and neurological examination within normal limits except for hearing loss. No orthostatic hypotension. Vision intact with glasses on. Mental status examination shows judgment intact, no other cognitive deficits.

ENVIRONMENT: Must climb stairs to bedroom. Bathrooms on both floors in house, without grab rails; transfers are cautious but secure. Lighting adequate throughout house.

Normality

HISTORY: Denies recent major departures from lifestyle. Health care practices such as medication taking, trips to outpatient clinic are normal for age group. Household management is done per his usual lifestyle. Caregivers have been a part of the household for over 30 years. Manages his own finances.

EXAMINATION: No evidence of deviant behavior or appearance

DEVELOPMENTAL SELF-CARE REQUISITES
Care of Dependent Family Members*

HISTORY: Expresses considerable concern about the adequacy of care provided for his wife who has a dementing illness. She is a Christian Scientist and would not seek medical treatment. He is not a Christian Scientist and is in conflict about his duty to her: He believes in the value of medical care but does not want to compromise her religious beliefs. He worries about providing the best possible care for her urinary incontinence and tendency to fall.

PERFORMANCE: Wife receives excellent custodial care from paid caregivers the patient arranged. He also provides her with excellent emotional support and diversional activity.

Acceptance of Own Mortality

HISTORY: Is concerned about making proper arrangements for care of his wife if he should predecease her. Has no other immediate family living, yet has many friends who visit regularly and allow him opportunity to reminisce.

PERFORMANCE: Initiates discussion about aging, being closer to death, with appropriate sadness and without nonverbal cues of anxiety.

Acceptance of Age-Related Limitations

HISTORY: Accepted retirement without undue hardship. Perceives he can do most things he wants to do if paced properly but is annoyed by sleep pattern disturbance.

PERFORMANCE: Paces self well, is realistic about activities undertaken, and allows housekeepers to take on more strenuous caregiving tasks. Retains exercise habit to retain fitness within limits of cardiovascular disease.

HEALTH DEVIATION SELF-CARE REQUISITES*

HISTORY: Has medical diagnoses of mitral regurgitation with CHF, benign prostatic hypertrophy, and presbycusis. Medications include Lanoxin, 0.25 mg daily; Nitro-Dur patch, 1 daily; Lasix, 40 mg daily; and KCl elixir, 40 mEq daily. Reports no adverse side effects from medications. Physician wants patient to begin using low-flow oxygen at night. Patient has been fitted with a hearing aid.

PERFORMANCE: Demonstrates medication dosing accurately but cannot describe purposes of each medicine, symptoms of toxicity, or impact of not taking medications. Calls physician if he becomes severely short of breath. Cannot manipulate hearing aid skillfully. Cannot demonstrate simple maintenance maneuvers.

---

*Indicates deficit relationship: need for nursing care.

OVERALL GOALS
1. Client will experience less worry over adequacy of care for wife.
2. Client will have normal sleep pattern.

SELF-CARE DEFICIT AND NURSING DIAGNOSIS	GOAL	NURSING INTERVENTIONS	OUTCOMES
Air Impaired gas exchange, related to pulmonary congestion secondary to congestive heart failure, manifested by paroxysmal nocturnal dyspnea	No episodes of paroxysmal nocturnal dyspnea	Guide in obtaining home oxygen apparatus. Teach how to use oxygen and rationale for use of oxygen.	Episodes of paroxysmal nocturnal dyspnea resolved with use of night-time oxygen
Activity-Rest Alteration in sleep pattern, related to concerns about obtaining proper care for wife and paroxysmal nocturnal dyspnea, manifested by unexpectedly falling asleep at unwanted times	Have normal sleep pattern, 6 hours per night with one planned 1-hour nap	Guide patient in performing in-depth assessment of sleep/wake patterns. See interventions under impaired gas exchange and ineffective individual coping.	Sleep disturbance spontaneously resolved during assessment phase
Solitude/Social Interaction Altered sensory perception: hearing related to knowledge deficit re use and care of hearing aid, manifested by inability to hear clearly despite hearing aid, and client's statements regarding insecurity about use of hearing aid	Be able to engage in conversation with others at normal volume. Be knowledgeable about hearing aid care and use.	Teach care of hearing aid: To remove impacted cerumen, how to check for batteries working, how to replace battery	Performed satisfactory return demonstration of battery check, cerumen check, and battery replacement
Developmental Self-Care Requisites Providing care for dependent spouse: Ineffective individual coping related to: 1. Knowledge deficit re care requirements of wife 2. Spiritual distress re value conflict in obtaining medical care for wife against her religious beliefs 3. Loss of confidante	Resolve feelings of conflict regarding care for wife. Understand supportive care needs of wife.	Teach specific care needs of wife to paid caregivers regarding exercise, toileting, and environmental modification Explain and demonstrate to paid caregivers prompted voiding techniques, environmental modification, ways of integrating exercise with her existing routines	Feelings of conflict regarding wife's care remained unresolved. Expressed relief at obtaining high-quality custodial care for her. Client established more permanent arrangements for management of finances, allowing for increased time with wife and decreased task burden

continued on following page

OVERALL GOALS

1. Client will experience less worry over adequacy of care for wife.
2. Client will have normal sleep pattern.

continued

SELF-CARE DEFICIT AND NURSING DIAGNOSIS	GOAL	NURSING INTERVENTIONS	OUTCOMES
4. Burden of caregiving for severely impaired spouse, manifested by difficulty in making decisions about family finances, ambivalence about securing medical care for wife		*Support* client by engaging in active listening to reminiscences, concerns regarding feelings of accomplishment, review of options regarding continuing care for wife. Help client clarify sense of duty to wife.	
Health Deviation Self-Care Requisite			
Knowledge deficits regarding treatment for congestive heart failure, benign prostatic hypertrophy–induced altered urination pattern, and bowel management, related to preoccupation with wife's care, and lack of exposure to information on these problems	Will be knowledgeable about (1) purposes of medications, side effects, and risks of noncompliance; (2) reasons for altered urinary elimination pattern and indications for seeking medical advice; and (3) alternative means of preventing constipation	Interventions deferred until first four diagnoses resolved, then: Spaced teaching regarding medications, prostatic hypertrophy, and prevention of constipation	Able to describe symptoms of digitalis toxicity and adverse effects of overdose of diuretic and need to call physician Expressed relief regarding urinary tract symptoms. Chose to continue managing bowels as previously.

CASE 2. Partly Compensatory Nursing System

The second case demonstrates the implementation of a *partly compensatory system* in a 72-year-old retired African-American laborer, who was referred to a community-based long-term care project because of frequent hospital admissions for exacerbations of angina and congestive heart failure. The nurse was a case manager in the community long-term care project. Factors that complicated Mr. Gray's care included establishing trust and his limited financial resources.

Mr. Gray had negative feelings about the existing community agencies because they had frequently terminated services to him for reasons he did not understand. According to the home health nurse, his care had been terminated because he no longer met the homebound criteria of Medicare, as he had been seen at the local fast-food restaurant having breakfast. Further exploration revealed that Mr. Gray believed that breakfast was the most important meal of the day. When receiving Medicare home health services, his home health aide did not arrive until noon, and he had been instructed not to cook for himself. In solving the problem of obtaining a hot breakfast, he removed himself from

CASE 2. Partly Compensatory Nursing System

continued

eligibility for home health services. This left him without any assistance in the home, and these circumstances had precipitated several hospital admissions. He was reluctant to trust another nurse from another community agency; however, in time sufficient trust was established to achieve the goals of the relationship. Mr. Gray's goals were to stay out of the hospital and to have some help doing household chores. The goals of the nursing system were mutually derived, with the nurse having considerable input into what accomplishments would help keep him out of the hospital.

The second barrier to achievement of goals for Mr. Gray was financial. He was eligible for Medicaid but had a deductible, which meant that he had to be able to keep track of receipts for his medical bills and submit them to his eligibility worker on a regular basis. This simple record-keeping task was beyond his abilities, but with the collaboration of his case manager and his daughter, his eligibility was maintained. Although Mr. Gray had family willing to assist him, he was reluctant to ask for help because he felt he was being a burden.

IDENTIFYING INFORMATION: 72-year-old black man referred to community-based long-term care project because of frequent readmissions to the hospital due to poorly controlled coronary artery disease.

CONDITIONING FACTORS
AGE: 72
SEX: Male
ETHNICITY: Southern, African-American, Protestant background
EDUCATIONAL LEVEL: 4th grade
MARITAL STATUS: Widowed 10 years
HOUSEHOLD STATUS: Subsidized apartment for the handicapped, lives alone
FAMILY SUPPORT: Two daughters, five grandchildren

UNIVERSAL SELF-CARE REQUISITES
Air
HISTORY/HABITS: Smokes 1 pack per day; 40 pack-year history
SYMPTOMS: Morning cough productive of white sputum. No dyspnea at rest but becomes dyspneic with minor exertion (e.g., preparing meals, walking less than 100 feet).
PERCEPTIONS: Understands adverse effects of smoking but does not want to quit. Does not believe that pulmonary symptoms adversely affect his quality of life.
EXAMINATION: Barrel-chested, hyperresonant to percussion. Bibasilar rales, clear with coughing. Respiratory rate = 22 per min at rest, increases to 30 per min with minor exertion.
ENVIRONMENT: Lives in apartment equipped

for the physically handicapped. No steps to climb.

Fluid
HISTORY/HABITS: Drinks water throughout the day, in addition to coffee and tea with meals. Total in excess of 1800 ml per day.
SYMPTOMS: Denies thirst, weakness.
PERCEPTIONS: Drinks water because he's heard it's good for you. Doesn't believe in sodium restriction.
EXAMINATION: Oral mucosa moist, no orthostatic hypotension. 2+ peripheral edema in lower extremities bilaterally.
ENVIRONMENT: Indoor plumbing, easy access to water.

Food*
HISTORY/HABITS: Breakfast is favorite meal of the day. Does not like to cook for himself for fear of injuring self. Has been going to local fast-food restaurant for ham on biscuit every morning, which violates the 2-gm sodium restriction prescribed by MD (see Health Deviation Self-Care Requisites).
PERCEPTION: Does not think sodium restriction is important in managing his hypertension and CHF
EXAMINATION: Weight = 145, height = 5'8". No evidence of nutritional deficiency except for mild lower extremity muscle atrophy. Biochemical indices all within normal limits.
ENVIRONMENT: Kitchen adequately equipped. Homemaker from local Council on Aging comes 3 days a week to assist with meal preparation and grocery shopping.

continued on following page

CASE 2. Partly Compensatory Nursing System

continued

Activity/Rest*
HISTORY/HABITS: Sleeps approximately 7 hours a night with only one interruption to urinate. Has no difficulty getting back to sleep. Naps off and on during the day.
SYMPTOMS: Chest pain, claudication, and dyspnea if activities are too strenuous or not paced slowly
PERCEPTIONS: Frustrated by slowness, inability to keep up with family and friends. Does not want to be a burden to family.
PERFORMANCE: Independent in basic ADLs if allowed to go at slow pace. Maximum activity level during day is walk to apartment manager's office, approximately 100 level meters from apartment, which he can do in about 10 minutes. Does not do housekeeping. Only sedentary activities.
ENVIRONMENT: Home well-adapted to limitations
Solitude/Social Interaction
HISTORY/HABITS: Daughter calls daily. Homemaker visits three times a week. Visits with apartment manager approx. three times a week. Visits with neighborhood children daily, which he enjoys.
SYMPTOMS: Expresses frustration at inability to participate in family activities as in the past, because of decreased endurance
EXAMINATION: Mental status examination without evidence of cognitive impairment. Auditory and visual examinations within normal limits. No communication deficits.
ENVIRONMENT: Apartment building provides many satisfying opportunities for social interaction
Injury Prevention
HISTORY/HABITS: Does not cook in oven or on stove. Cautious when walking outside apartment. Always wears socks and slippers. Does not inspect feet daily. Daily telephone check with daughter.
SYMPTOMS: No history of recent falls, burns, or drug overdosage. Complains of decreased sensation in hands and feet.
PERCEPTIONS: Feels secure with current injury prevention program
EXAMINATION: Mental status: judgment, memory, and problem-solving abilities intact. Sensory: Diminished sensation to pinprick, hands and lower extremities to midcalf. Visual acuity sufficient to allow ready identification of obstacles; can read print on medication bottles.

ENVIRONMENT: Apartment uncluttered. Has appliances such as toaster oven, which he could be taught to use safely.
Normality*
HISTORY/PERCEPTIONS: Describes self as crippled from heart disease
PERFORMANCE: Does not perform meal preparation, transportation, grocery shopping independently. Has difficulty with complex financial management. Socially appropriate adult male without obvious deformity or disability. Limited in normal adult activities by dyspnea, pain, and fear of injury.

DEVELOPMENTAL SELF-CARE REQUISITES
Acceptance of Mortality
HISTORY: Has survived several myocardial infarctions—feels he is ready to die "whenever the Lord is ready for me." Is able to visit with family regularly, has opportunity to reminisce with family and neighborhood children.
PERFORMANCE: Does not appear anxious when discussing death
Care of Dependent Family Members
HISTORY: Wife has been deceased 15 years. Shows no signs of unresolved grief. Not responsible for care of other family members.
Adjustment to Age-Related Limitations*
HISTORY: Expresses regret about decreased ability to keep up with family socially
PERFORMANCE: Does not attempt unrealistic tasks

HEALTH DEVIATION SELF-CARE REQUISITES*
Chronic Diseases

1. **Coronary artery disease with angina pectoris, S/P acute myocardial infarction ×3**
   Requires ability to

- Take nitrates as prescribed
- Modify activity within limits of pain and dyspnea
- Know when to seek medical care for unrelieved chest pain or increasing frequency of chest pain

2. **Hypertension and congestive heart failure**
   Requires ability to

- Take diuretic as prescribed
- Adhere to 2-gm sodium-restricted diet

CASE 2. Partly Compensatory Nursing System

continued

3. **Peripheral vascular disease**
   Requires ability to

- Pace activity
- Inspect lower extremities daily for evidence of trauma
- Seek medical care for foot lesions

4. **Chronic obstructive pulmonary disease**
   Requires ability to

- Pace activities
- Seek medical care for changes in sputum production, increasing dyspnea

HISTORY: Patient unable to describe purposes of medications or implications of noncompliance. Says he would seek medical care if chest pain became intolerable.
PERFORMANCE: Noncompliant with medications, diet. Repeated hospitalizations over the past year for decompensated CHF, uncontrolled angina. Financial resources insufficient to pay for medications each month.

_____

* Indicates deficit relationship: need for nursing care.

OVERALL GOALS

1. Client will reside in an environment that prevents injury, allows for continued growth.
2. Client will demonstrate enhanced skills for coping with chronic disease.

SELF-CARE DEFICIT AND NURSING DIAGNOSIS	GOAL	NURSING INTERVENTIONS	OUTCOMES
Air			
Potential ineffective gas exchange related to decreased lung surface area for ventilation secondary to chronic lung disease, congestive heart failure; manifested by dyspnea on exertion	Will not experience periods of dyspnea during routine activities	Do for: Monitor congestive heart failure and chronic lung disease for signs of decompensation Support: Home health aide to encourage reduced smoking, compliance with diet, medications, and activity restrictions Teach: Impact of noncompliance on dyspnea	No episodes of severe dyspnea reported or observed
Food			
Potential alteration in nutrition less than body requirements related to inability to prepare meals safely according to therapeutic diet	Will eat three nutritionally balanced meals per day within limits of 2-gm sodium diet Will maintain body weight of 145 lbs Will not manifest signs of nutritional deficiency	Do for: Obtain home health aide 5 days a week to assist with meal preparation, grocery shopping, and encourage dietary compliance. Family to provide meals on weekends. Teach: Client and family re diet restrictions, impact of noncompliance	No evidence of nutritional deficiency Weight maintained

continued on following page

OVERALL GOALS

1. Client will reside in an environment that prevents injury, allows for continued growth.
2. Client will demonstrate enhanced skills for coping with chronic disease.

continued

SELF-CARE DEFICIT AND NURSING DIAGNOSIS	GOAL	NURSING INTERVENTIONS	OUTCOMES
Fluid			
Potential fluid greater than body requirements related to dietary sodium indiscretion, or noncompliance with medications, manifested by decompensation of congestive heart failure	Will exhibit optimal fluid and electrolyte balance, as demonstrated by normal blood pressure, absence of peripheral edema or persistent rales	Do for: Monitor blood pressure, edema, orthostasis	Maintained blood pressure and edema within acceptable range
Potential fluid less than body requirements related to diuretic overdose, manifested by orthostatic hypotension, weakness, mental status changes		Support: Home health aide to encourage compliance with medications	Maintained Medicaid eligibility
		Teach: Regarding medications, rationale, and impact of under- and overdosage	
		Guide: Family regarding Medicaid application process and record-keeping requirements	
Activity/Rest			
Activity intolerance related to decreased tissue perfusion and impaired ventilation secondary to coronary artery disease, chronic obstructive lung disease, and sedentary lifestyle, manifested by inability to perform housekeeping, grocery shopping, extensive ambulation without dyspnea and claudication	Will demonstrate independence in basic activities of daily living without dyspnea or claudication	Teach: Daily exercise regimen to increase strength and endurance; effects of noncompliance. Impact of pacing and work simplification techniques on endurance.	Independent in basic activities of daily living without dyspnea or claudication
		Support: Home health aide to encourage compliance with exercise regimen	
Solitude/Social Interaction			
Altered role relationships related to reduced activity tolerance and claudication, manifested by verbalization of inability to maintain accustomed social relationships	Express satisfaction with level of social activity	Teach: Exercise regimen. Use of calendar to facilitate pacing of activities.	Remains frustrated with inability to keep up with younger members of family
		Support: Active listening to establish meaning of lost social activity, counseling to help client integrate loss	

OVERALL GOALS
1. Client will reside in an environment that prevents injury, allows for continued growth.
2. Client will demonstrate enhanced skills for coping with chronic disease.

continued

SELF-CARE DEFICIT AND NURSING DIAGNOSIS	GOAL	NURSING INTERVENTIONS	OUTCOMES
Protection from Injury Potential for injury: Burn related to peripheral neuropathy, hands and feet, manifested by decreased sensation, strength, and coordination in hands, and reduced sensation in feet	Will not experience burn or traumatic injury	Do for: Home health aide to assist with housekeeping, cooking Teach: Daily inspection of feet for evidence of small trauma Need to refrain from certain types of cooking, such as placing heavy objects in oven, and test temperature of bath water with thermometer rather than relying on hands or feet	No injury sustained
Normality Alteration in comfort: Pain in legs related to reduced peripheral vascular circulation, manifested by patient report of pain on ambulation, relieved by rest and leg elevation	Reduced frequency of episodes of pain. Enhanced feelings of control over pain.	Teach: Influences of smoking on claudication. Exercise program to promote development of collateral circulation. Impact of pacing of activities on pain. Relaxation exercises to help alleviate pain. Do for: Home health aide 5 days a week to assist with housekeeping activities Support: Instruct home health aide to allow time to listen to client's frustrations re pain	Pain largely alleviated by femoral-popliteal bypass surgery
Health Deviation Self-Care Requisites Self-care deficit: Money management related to mismatch between educational level and demands of Medicaid system for careful record keeping, manifested by inability to keep receipts and demonstrate meeting deductible each month	Will remain on Medicaid and have bills paid on timely basis	Do for: Arrange for client's daughter to serve as financial recordkeeper. Client retains decision-making authority regarding how to spend money. Teach: Explain rudiments of recordkeeping system to client's daughter and refer her to social	Patient remained on Medicaid, had no problems getting prescriptions filled. Voiced no concerns about daughter's increased involvement. Family satisfied with arrangement. Only hospital admission was elective for bypass

continued on following page

OVERALL GOALS

1. Client will reside in an environment that prevents injury, allows for continued growth.
2. Client will demonstrate enhanced skills for coping with chronic disease.

continued

SELF-CARE DEFICIT AND NURSING DIAGNOSIS	GOAL	NURSING INTERVENTIONS	OUTCOMES
Ineffective coping with chronic diseases, related to poor financial situation, poor understanding of diseases, manifested by noncompliance with diet and medications, frequent readmission to hospital for control of coronary heart failure, noncompliance with therapeutic regimen related to knowledge deficits, financial status, educational level, manifested by failure to take medications, diet, and exercise as prescribed	Reduced numbers of hospital admissions for control of chronic diseases Increased understanding of diseases and impact of noncompliance	worker for more detailed instructions Support: Home health aide 5 days a week to encourage compliance with treatment regimen and provide emotional support Guide: Counseling from registered nurse regarding adjustments to chronic diseases: Diet, activity, social relationships, medications, pain control Teach: Purposes of therapeutic regimen, impact of noncompliance Do for: Securing family member to serve as recordkeeper to maintain Medicaid eligibility and reduce financial burden of disease	surgery on lower extremity Compliance with diet, medications, and exercise greatly improved

CASE 3. Wholly Compensatory Nursing System

Mrs. Brown, a 74-year-old widowed white woman with severe dementia and cardiopulmonary disease, demonstrates someone who requires a *wholly compensatory nursing system.*

Mrs. Brown was referred by her daughter to a community-based long-term care project to obtain additional assistance. She had lived in a nursing home for 1 year until 2 months before the referral. When the patient was hospitalized because of an exacerbation of chronic obstructive pulmonary disease (COPD), the family decided to care for her at home because they felt the nursing home care was inadequate for her needs.

Initially, the family was close to being in crisis. The patient's nocturnal behavioral disturbances were creating heightened stress levels in the household. The daughter reported inability to concentrate at work because of inadequate sleep, and she feared that continued caregiving would adversely affect her marriage. Despite these strong feelings of burden, the daughter refused to consider nursing home placement as an option.

The nurse's role was formally defined as that of health assessor and case manager. The nursing technologies used in this case included counseling, teaching, and coordinating. The nurse arranged for additional help in the home through the long-term care program, which stabilized the family situation temporarily. Additionally, the nurse arranged for occupational therapy consultation. The occupational therapist was able to demonstrate to the caregivers the untapped performance capacity of the client. The fact that the client was living in an environment that was less demanding than her capabilities contributed to her nocturnal restlessness, for on the days when her activity level was higher and she was engaged in more complex activities (for example, helping with specific tasks in meal preparation, such as vegetable paring), the nocturnal restlessness diminished.

Despite these interventions, the family again experienced a crisis when one of the paid helpers threatened to quit. Once again, the daughter exhibited symptoms of high stress and made statements like "I know I just cannot go on like this, but I will not put mother in a nursing home. I'll just have to leave things to the Lord." The nurse was concerned about the potential for neglect or even abuse of the patient if no intervention was taken. Just as an impasse seemed inevitable, an apartment in a newly constructed subsidized housing project in the family's neighborhood became available. Buoyed by this unexpected resource, and the prospect of being able to care for the patient outside her home, the daughter redoubled her efforts to find a replacement live-in helper, and was successful. The daughter was able to marshal the emotional resources to move the mother and monitor a cadre of paid caregivers, once the stressors of the continual presence of her mother and nocturnal disturbances were removed.

This care arrangement made demands of a different sort on the daughter, as she had to visit daily and respond to illnesses and vacations of caregivers. However, the alternative living arrangement proved to be a much more stable arrangement than when Mrs. Brown lived with her daughter. An additional bonus was that the paid helpers received well the teaching regarding increasing the patient's activity level; her activity level increased and her nocturnal restlessness abated.

IDENTIFYING INFORMATION: Mrs. Brown is a 74-year-old white woman referred to a community-based long-term care program by daughter because family was unable to care for client alone. Client had formerly resided in an intermediate-care facility, but daughter took her back home because of dissatisfaction with the care.

CONDITIONING FACTORS
AGE: 74
SEX: Female
EDUCATIONAL LEVEL: Grade school

ENVIRONMENTAL FACTORS
HOUSEHOLD STATUS: Lives with daughter, son-in-law, and grandchildren
MARITAL STATUS: Widowed
FAMILY SUPPORT: Has five living children; only one daughter is active in client's care
ETHNICITY: White, southern, fundamentalist Christian
FORMAL ORGANIZATION INVOLVEMENT: Department of Social Services: Provides chore service 30 hours per week. Community mental health center: Is seen by geropsychiatrist monthly for medication adjustment.

UNIVERSAL SELF-CARE REQUISITES
Air
HISTORY/HABITS: No history of smoking
SYMPTOMS: No cough, dyspnea
PERCEPTIONS: Client unable/unwilling to answer questions re this
PHYSICAL EXAMINATION/INSPECTION: Respiratory rate = 24/minute, mild kyphosis
AUSCULTATION: Breath sounds clear
PERCUSSION: No hypo/hyperresonance
PALPATION: No increased fremitus
ENVIRONMENTAL FACTORS: No respiratory irritants in home
PERFORMANCE: Able to deep breathe on command; no dyspnea on performance of ADLs or IADLs
Fluid
HISTORY/HABITS: Usual fluid intake unknown; no diuretics
SYMPTOMS: Denies dizziness
PERCEPTIONS: Never asks for water or fluid according to daughter
PHYSICAL EXAMINATION/INSPECTION: Skin turgor adequate, mucous membranes moist; no edema, neck veins flat
AUSCULTATION: No orthostatic changes in blood pressure

continued on following page

CASE 3. Wholly Compensatory Nursing System

continued

ENVIRONMENTAL FACTORS: Water and fluids readily accessible

PERFORMANCE: Client drinks when beverage is served but does not initiate drinking on her own

Food

HISTORY/HABITS: Ate three meals a day, snacked in between, major meal at noontime

SYMPTOMS: Does not enjoy food yet denies nausea

PERCEPTIONS: Client feels she eats adequately; body image: "Normal"

ENVIRONMENTAL FACTORS: Grocery stores not within walking distance; client does not have mental capacity to grocery shop independently. Kitchen accessible at all times. Client does not have capacity to prepare meals independently. Daughter and hired caregivers assist with meal preparation. No health hazards in kitchen.

PHYSICAL EXAMINATION/INSPECTION: Height = 5 ft. Weight = 108 lbs, no change in 6 mos; mucous membranes moist; muscle mass adequate for ambulation; oral-motor reflexes intact. No pathological reflexes.

PERFORMANCE: Able to assist in food preparation if given small, simple tasks. Is able to feed self. Is able to swallow without difficulty.

Elimination*

HISTORY/HABITS: Has bowel movement daily. Uses milk of magnesia q wk. Uses incontinence pads to protect furniture but is continent if toileted regularly.

SYMPTOMS: No report of urinary frequency, burning. Has night-time incontinence. Chronic constipation but no pain on elimination.

PERCEPTIONS: Believes bowels must move every day. Lifelong laxative user.

PHYSICAL EXAMINATION/INSPECTION: No odor of urine or feces on clothes in room. No evidence of soiling of clothes.

AUSCULTATION: Bowel sounds active

PALPATION: No abdominal masses or distended bladder. Rectal examination: Moderate amount of putty-like feces.

PERCUSSION: Bladder not distended

ENVIRONMENTAL FACTORS: Toilet approximately 20 feet from living room. Unrestricted access to toilet most of the day. Incontinence pads in evidence in bedroom and living room.

PERFORMANCE: Patient able to void on command. No difficulties with transfer or positioning. Able to complete all tasks required in elimination with reminders.

Activity/Rest*

HISTORY/HABITS: Sedentary lifestyle: Housewife. Drugs: Takes low-dose Haldol. *Sleep patterns are erratic. Does not sleep well at night, keeps other members of household awake moaning for attention. Naps during the day.

SYMPTOMS: No musculoskeletal or cardiac pain that limits mobility. Psychiatric illness does limit activity, as client perceives that she "cannot" move or do for herself.

PERCEPTIONS: Believes she cannot be very active. Her nerves are too bad, she is too weak.

PHYSICAL EXAMINATION/INSPECTION: Muscle mass adequate in lower extremities. Range of motion in all joints.

AUSCULTATION: Resting heart rate = 82, regular

ENVIRONMENTAL FACTORS: Client has own room, but it is right next door to other family members' bedrooms. Family supplements Title XX chore worker's salary so that she is available to attend to client at night. House is in suburban neighborhood, conducive to moderate outdoor physical activity. Other household members are sedentary, do not value physical activity.

PERFORMANCE: Client engages only in ADL activity, except for occasional trips to fast-food restaurant (in car) to buy a milkshake. Client rests throughout day, except when engaged in ADLs or asking for attention.

Solitude/Social Interaction*

HISTORY/HABITS: Prior to illness, interacted within family unit and at church. Since illness, only interacts with family and hired helper, around symptoms and ADLs.

SYMPTOMS: Does not verbalize loneliness or fears of interacting with others.

PERCEPTIONS: No recent changes in availability of social contacts.

PHYSICAL EXAMINATION/INSPECTION: Body language is withdrawn: Keeps eyes closed even when being asked questions directly. No functional sensory deficits.

ENVIRONMENTAL FACTORS: Has lived with daughter's family for past 2 months. Before this, lived in nursing home. No recent losses. No age peers immediately available.

PERFORMANCE: Initiates conversation only regarding her symptoms of "dry eyes" or moans to request repositioning. Is not able

CASE 3. Wholly Compensatory Nursing System

continued

to converse on a variety of topics. Socially inappropriate behaviors include lack of eye contact during conversation, continuous moaning about eyes or need to be repositioned. No evidence of persecutory, delusional, or hallucinatory ideation.

Injury Prevention

HISTORY/HABITS: Family does not allow client to be left unattended. Caregivers administer medications.

SYMPTOMS: No history of recent falls or other accidents

PERCEPTIONS: Neither client nor family expresses concern about safety measures

PHYSICAL EXAMINATION/INSPECTION: No evidence of burns, other trauma. Muscle mass and strength adequate for activity level. Sensory status intact. No orthostatic blood pressure changes.

ENVIRONMENTAL FACTORS: Lighting, stair and floor repair adequate. Little clutter in house. Emergency medical assistance readily available.

PERFORMANCE: Able to perform ADLs with assistance without injury. Mental status examination: Shows deficits in memory, judgment, and problem-solving ability. Can follow two-stage command.

Normality*

HISTORY/HABITS: Lifelong role-relationships: Work: Homemaker and mother. Family roles: See above. Leisure pursuits: Church.

SYMPTOMS: Does not pursue any previously enjoyed social activities

PERCEPTIONS: Victim stance with regard to illness

PHYSICAL EXAMINATION: Has "dry eyes" syndrome, symptoms consistent with senile dementia of Alzheimer's type. Has history of hip fracture, myocardial infarction.

ENVIRONMENTAL FACTORS: Children are geographically close, but most do not visit; closest daughter is in role-reversal situation, as dependent care agent. Others in household regard chronic diseases as very disabling but remain frustrated by nocturnal anxiety and symptoms. They do not view client as capable of purposeful activity.

PERFORMANCE: Client does not contribute to community. Client is clothed in pajamas unless there is a special occasion for going outside. Uses incontinence pads routinely. Client does not have roles other than self-care, and recipient of dependent care.

DEVELOPMENTAL SELF-CARE REQUISITES

1. **Provision of needed care for client without sacrificing other family goals***
   Client's daughter expresses concerns about husband and children's tolerance for nighttime disturbances. These interfere with daytime functioning and, in daughter's words: "There is no peace in our house with mother there, yet I cannot send her to a nursing home."

2. **Ego integrity versus despair**

3. **Death anxiety**
   Unable to obtain adequate assessment information secondary to patient's cognitive impairment

HEALTH DEVIATION SELF-CARE REQUISITES

1. **Senile dementia of Alzheimer's type (SDAT):* Need for assistance with self-monitoring, self-care activities (see Universal Self-Care Requisites above), or independent goal setting**
   Necessary assistance provided for ADLs, but attention was given to maximizing client's strengths and activity level

2. **Antipsychotic medications: Need for supplemental eyedrops, increased likelihood of elimination problems, knowledge of side effects of medications**
   Family has obtained necessary assistance for monitoring adverse effects of medications but does not have optimal bowel regimen in place

---

* Indicates deficit relationship: need for nursing care.

OVERALL GOALS

1. Client will experience function at highest possible level of independence.
2. Family relationships of client will be normalized.

SELF-CARE DEFICIT AND NURSING DIAGNOSIS	GOAL	NURSING INTERVENTIONS	OUTCOMES
1. Alteration in thought process related to senile dementia, Alzheimer's type, manifested by impairments in memory, judgment, and problem-solving ability	Will function at highest possible cognitive level	*Teaching and guidance* of caregivers regarding techniques to enhance patient's ability to process information despite disease, e.g., use of simple patterns of communication; reducing environmental stimulation; use of habits and routines	Caregivers began including patient more in decision making appropriate to her cognitive level, instead of making decisions for her or frustrating her with decisions that were too difficult
2. Alteration in patterns of urinary elimination, related to cognitive impairments, manifested by inability to remain continent without assistance	Achieve urinary continence in daytime	*Taught* caregivers about toileting schedules, use of habit training in achieving continence	Daytime continence achieved. Incontinence pads removed from living room.
3. Alterations in bowel elimination: Constipation, related to chronic laxative use, anticholinergic medications, manifested by routine use of milk of magnesia and presence of stool in rectal vault	Every-other-day bowel movement without laxative	*Taught* caregivers alternative methods of bowel management: Increasing fluid and fiber intake, exercises	Family uninterested in attempting to modify this behavior
4. Alterations in role relationships, secondary to extreme dependency needs, nocturnal restlessness, manifested by daughter's feelings of crisis	Daughter's sense of crisis will be resolved. Family role relationships will more nearly approximate baseline (before patient's dementing illness began).	*Supported and guided* daughter in her attempts to find alternative living arrangements for patient, to reduce the burden of dependent care	Patient settled in own apartment, with paid helpers providing the majority of care and daughter able to "visit" more socially
5. Self-care deficit: Total; related to cognitive deficits and helplessness, manifested by nonperformance of activities of daily living without assistance	Will have basic needs for hygiene, nutrition, elimination, and exercise met, without inducing excess dependency	*Taught* caregivers how to provide care while maximizing patient's abilities to do for herself	See No. 3. Patient's hygiene adequate, hydration and nutrition adequate, medications taken as prescribed.

OVERALL GOALS

1. Client will experience function at highest possible level of independence.
2. Family relationships of client will be normalized.

continued

SELF-CARE DEFICIT AND NURSING DIAGNOSIS	GOAL	NURSING INTERVENTIONS	OUTCOMES
6. Alterations in family process, related to extreme dependency, nocturnal restlessness, and live-in help within household, manifested by family's complaints of change in habits, ability to function normally	Family restored to usual habits, mode of operation	*Counseled* daughter and son-in-law regarding care options. *Guided* through bureaucratic procedures to assist in obtaining additional assistance	Caregiver's stress level reduced gradually. Reported marriage less strained and job performance no longer affected.
7. Diversional activity deficit, related to cognitive deficits, and caregiver's perception of client as unable to pursue meaningful activity, manifested by long periods of inactivity except for ADL performance	Will engage in at least one purposeful activity during day consistent with previous lifestyle	*Arranged for* occupational therapy evaluation and treatment, and *taught* caregivers different options for occupying patient's time in purposeful manner	Had monthly "special" interaction with therapist, and caregivers began including her in simple meal preparation tasks
8. Sleep pattern disturbance, related to inactivity and cognitive impairments, manifested by nocturnal restlessness	Will sleep minimum of 6 hours uninterrupted between midnight and 6:00 A.M.	*Taught* caregivers about relationship between activity and sleep patterns, anxiety and restlessness. *Offered* concrete suggestions about structuring time so that patient would become fatigued at night	Instances of nocturnal restlessness declined from nightly to weekly or less often
9. Anxiety, related to senile dementia, Alzheimer's type; manifested by short attention span, agitation when attempts are made to engage client in typical adult activities, and nocturnal restlessness	Will have reduced intensity of anxious behaviors, such as crying out for help, nocturnal restlessness. Will not experience adverse side effects of anxiolytic medications	*Taught* caregivers about relationship between communication problems and performance deficits in dementia and anxiety, manifested by restlessness, and techniques of modifying tasks to match patient's capabilities (see No. 1)	Still on low-dose anxiolytic agent. Nocturnal restlessness decreased, and restlessness diminished during familiar special tasks. No evidence of somnolence or decreased function because of anxiolytic use.

ISSUES IN GERONTOLOGICAL NURSING

Enhancing the Scientific Basis for Clinical Practice

Gerontological nursing continues to suffer from an inadequate scientific basis for practice, although prospects for its enhancement are good (Wells, 1993). The scientific base for gerontological nursing practice has grown considerably since 1950. Larger numbers of nurse researchers, coupled with an increased interest in gerontology and geriatrics at academic centers worldwide, have supported the expansion of the knowledge base in gerontological nursing.

With the establishment of the NINR in 1986, a growing number of federal research dollars have been allocated to the study of physical as well as psychosocial problems in the aged. In addition, nurse scientists have continued to serve as valued collaborators in multidisciplinary research. For example, Hoch has made important contributions to the understanding of sleep disorders in the elderly (Hoch et al., 1992a, 1992b, 1994). Similarly, a variety of nurse scientists have contributed to the study of urinary incontinence (Brink et al., 1994; Wells et al., 1991; Wyman et al., 1990, 1993; Bump et al., 1991); acute cognitive impairment (Pompei et al., 1994; Neelon et al., 1992); chronic cognitive impairment (Beck et al., 1991, 1993; Berg et al., 1991; Kolanowski et al., 1994); and dysmobility (Hogue et al., 1993; Evans and Strumpf, 1988). Lang et al. (1990) summarized a wide body of research demonstrating the contribution that nursing research has made to development of newer and more effective models of care for the aged.

In addition to the more applied research cited above, there is a growing cadre of nurse scientists who are doing more basic research that is also pertinent to development of a scientific basis for gerontological nursing practice. For example, Clipp and colleagues examined the long-term effects of combat experience on the late life development and health of older veterans (Elder et al., 1994; Elder and Clipp, 1989). The fact that nurse scientists participate in both clinical and basic research augurs well for the development of a basic and applied science base for gerontological nursing practice. Another positive trend in gerontological nursing research is the emergence of programs of gerontological nursing research as the dominant model, rather than the "one-shot" study, to address key gerontological nursing concerns. Finally, the increased numbers of doctorally prepared gerontological nurses,

and the greater availability of funding for research on topics that are salient to gerontological nursing practice, bode well for continued development of gerontological nursing science.

Although problems persist in disseminating research findings to gerontological nurses, a variety of mechanisms are being developed to enhance research utilization in nursing generally. For example, Sigma Theta Tau, the international nursing honorary society, has developed sophisticated information resources for research dissemination, including an "on-line" journal of nursing knowledge, available only through computer access. In addition, Sigma Theta Tau sponsors research utilization awards for individuals or teams of nurses who demonstrate successful application of new research findings to practice. Kilpack et al. (1991) received such an award for their work using research-based interventions to reduce falls in elderly hospitalized patients. Other approaches to research utilization include larger-scale projects based at major university nursing centers. The University of North Carolina at Chapel Hill for a number of years sponsored a series of conferences and publications that emphasized writing research findings with an eye toward helping clinicians identify applications of research to practice (Funk et al., 1989). All the monographs from this project have papers with direct applicability to gerontological nursing. More recently, at the University of Iowa an exemplary model for research dissemination in nursing has been developed and implemented (Titler et al., 1994).

Two areas of research in which gerontological nurses can make important contributions are understanding the patterns of causation of common self-care problems of the elderly, and validation of effective nursing technologies for care of the aged and their families. Common self-care problems of older persons include prevention of injury, promotion of continence, promotion of high self-esteem, compensation for cognitive impairment, and compensation for altered physical mobility. Members of other disciplines have shown considerable research interest in these topics. There is a great need for systematic investigation into the prevalent self-care problems of older people from a nursing perspective, with nurses as both principal investigators and collaborators with members of other disciplines.

Another essential area for gerontological nursing research concerns staffing patterns in long-term care (Institute of Medicine, 1986). There is widespread agreement among professional nurses that current minimum standards for nurse staffing in institutions are inadequate, despite the fact that standards have improved marginally since the passage of the nursing hom regulation reforms associated with the OBRA of 1987. We continue to lack data that are adequate to support specific ratios of professional nurses to paraprofessional staff or number of staff needed for patients with various levels of dependency. As a greater body of knowledge about the relationship between nursing staff levels and patient outcomes emerges from studies based on resident data such as that provided by the nursing home minimum data set (e.g., see Spector and Drugovich, 1989), the nursing profession will be in a better position to prescribe needed improvements in staffing.

Improving the Educational Preparation for Gerontological Nursing

A 1975 American Nurses Association survey revealed that 85 per cent of the schools with basic nursing education programs did *not* offer courses in gerontological nursing. The following progress has since been reported. First, a survey of 454 nursing programs at all levels (associate degree, diploma, baccalaureate, master's, and doctoral) showed that half of the topic areas in a questionnaire listing key gerontological nursing content were endorsed as taught in 90 per cent of respondents. The amount of gerontological nursing content increased with length of the program; associate degree programs generally reported less gerontological content than baccalaureate and master's programs (ANA, 1986). Over one half of the nursing master's programs responding reported having a gerontological nursing major or specialty, but the specific content taught in these programs can vary widely (Wells, 1993).

Specific problems contributing to inadequate educational preparation in gerontological nursing include: (1) the fact that many nursing faculty responsible for teaching gerontological content have little or no formal preparation in gerontological nursing; (2) underutilization of community-based practice sites, and (3) persistent low enrollment in gerontological nursing advanced practice programs (NLN, 1991).

There are encouraging signs that national nursing leaders are taking steps to address the problems of adequate educational preparation for gerontological nursing at all levels

of professional practice. The NLN has supported publication of a series of papers reporting the results of deliberations among gerontological nursing leaders as they contemplate new approaches to gerontological nursing education. Heine (1993) emphasizes the need for partnerships between a variety of clinical practice sites and schools of nursing in training gerontological nurses of the future.

The primary mode for improving gerontological nursing expertise of practicing nurses and nurse faculty has been through continuing education programs. Many schools of nursing offer ongoing continuing education programs in gerontological nursing. The federal government has funded multidisciplinary Geriatric Education Centers, which have been successful in providing a stable base of continuing education for providers who lack geriatric training (Waters, 1994). In addition, specific gerontological specialty tracts are now commonplace in most health sciences schools.

Developing and Promoting Suitable Models of Care

Many models, including the professional rehabilitation team and primary nursing models have been developed to foster continuity, accountability, and maintenance or restoration of function, yet these models are seldom applied to older persons. The benefits of the rehabilitation team for individuals who experience traumatic disability have long been recognized. However, older persons are often excluded from rehabilitation programs, either on the basis of age alone or because the rehabilitation team is not knowledgeable about the effects of the aging process and its interaction with chronic disease. Older people with the potential for regaining function or learning compensatory responses are relegated to custodial care because they do not measure up to norms developed with younger people in mind. Yet there is ample evidence that older persons are able to benefit from rehabilitative and multidisciplinary team approaches (Applegate et al., 1991; Rubenstein et al., 1991).

Primary nursing is another model of care well suited to the needs of older people that is seldom seen in long-term care. It is an excellent model for the care of older people because it emphasizes continuity, coordination, and accountability. Unfortunately, the prevailing administrative opinion regarding older people and primary nursing is that older people require considerable physical care, and there is little professional skill in providing such care. Budgets are limited, particularly in long-term care, and quality is sacrificed for quantity to meet the required amount of body power needed to transfer and position dependent patients. Some long-term care settings have instituted modified primary nursing systems to take advantage of the continuity and accountability features of a primary nursing system, and have the primary nurse responsible for supervising a stable group of nursing assistants who care for a group of elderly patients (Patterson, 1985; Campbell, 1985).

The institutional model of care has been extensively criticized on the grounds of both its expense and its long history of abuses and generally unsatisfactory response to the needs of individuals. Despite the plethora of projects that successfully demonstrate the effectiveness of noninstitutional models in meeting the needs of the elderly, institutions remain the cornerstone of acute and long-term care for the aged.

Nurses must continue to be in the forefront of advocacy for models of care that are cost effective in meeting the needs of older people and their families in a consistent, co-ordinated, continuous, accountable, and ethical manner. To effectively participate in policy formation, gerontological nurses must be knowledgeable consumers of health policy research, particularly those studies concerned with the cost effectiveness of alternative models of care. As concern about the cost of care has grown, cost effectiveness studies have proliferated. However, not all of these are well designed, and the reader must pay careful attention to the limitations of the study design.

Many cost effectiveness studies consider the question of cost effectiveness from only one perspective, such as that of Medicare or Medicaid. Although this tactic simplifies research methods, it tends to oversimplify the question of cost effectiveness by failing to account for all social costs and benefits. A second limitation of the cost effectiveness literature is the short duration of most studies. Measurement of costs over a 1- to 2-year period fails to capture adequately the long-range impact of functional disability. The cumulative costs of custodial care contrasted with those of rehabilitative care have yet to be studied.

Many of the cost effectiveness studies currently available in long-term care do not ask the questions that are of most interest to nurses. Non-nurse investigators may not research new clinical management ideas because they lack the insights generated from clinical experience and personal observation.

Nurses need to be proactive in the health policy arena, conducting cost effectiveness research along with other types of research.

Specifying and Enforcing Standards of Care

The existing ANA standards for gerontological nursing care provide useful guidance but are insufficient to guide the development and evaluation of larger programs. Also, the ANA standards lack any enforcement mechanism, and they have not been included systematically in standards of care for hospitals, nursing homes, or home care. The gerontological nursing literature does not identify the numbers and types of personnel necessary to bring about desired patient outcomes in a specific patient population. Nurses in acute care complain about inadequate time to promote self-care or address the emotional needs of elderly patients, and there is general consensus that the nurse staffing minimums enforced by most states for nursing homes are woefully inadequate. Yet millions of Americans are cared for in these institutions each year.

Home care has received less scrutiny than institutional settings from regulatory agencies (Zimmerman, 1991), although this is changing with the greater influx of third-party reimbursement dollars. According to Mundinger (1983), monitoring of quality in home care has been extremely limited and has focused on process criteria and record keeping rather than on patient outcomes.

Hospitals: Issues and Ideas

The impact of prospective reimbursement for Medicare patients in hospitals has been profound. Although there are well-publicized concerns about the dangers of premature discharge of dependent older people from the hospital (Champlin, 1985), there is evidence to suggest that shorter lengths of stay may lead to better functional outcomes for some older patients (McConnell et al., 1986). The most humane, and perhaps most cost-effective, arrangement is to have ample rehabilitative and supportive services available outside the acute care setting for the elderly who require care following hospitalization. Some hospitals are diversifying so that they provide not only acute care but rehabilitative and long-term care services as well.

The contribution of professional nursing to the well-being of patients and the economic health of the hospital is achieving new recognition. It is possible that the new respect accorded nurses under the prospective payment system can be parlayed into a potent force for upgrading standards of care for the hospitalized elderly. For example, as hospitals become more interested in diversifying services, gerontological nurses should be prepared to identify the gaps in community-based services and encourage the hospital administration to develop the needed missing services.

The standards of nursing care established by the Joint Commission on Accreditation of Health Care Organizations (JCAHO) do not acknowledge that gerontological nursing is a specialty or that older patients require special attention. There is a great need to upgrade the standards of care for the elderly in hospitals, as the potential for adverse outcomes exists if nurses are inadequately prepared. Another problem with JCAHO standards is that they focus primarily on process measures rather than patient outcome measures. As more and more attention is focused on reducing length of stay to contain hospital costs, it will be important to develop outcome measures to use as discharge parameters as well as for evaluation of the quality of care.

Nursing Homes: Issues and Ideas

Serious problems regarding the standards for institutional long-term care are well documented (Institute of Medicine, 1986; Vladek, 1980; Moss and Halamandaris, 1977). Resolution of the substandard care that currently predominates in the field will require a combination of strategies.

The work of the American Nurses' Foundation (ANF) and the American College of Nursing Home Administrators (ACNHA) to upgrade the preparation of nurse administrators in long-term care is an essential step toward improving the competence of nurse administrators in long-term care, so that there will be a stronger voice for clinical issues in the administrative decision-making process. The development of several models of teaching nursing homes provides a broad base from which to attack the various problems in providing basic services for the elderly in long-term care. Further discussion of the ANF/ACNHA and teaching nursing home projects is contained in Chapter 24.

The Institute of Medicine (IOM) committee on reform of nursing home regulation will remain a classic that documents the history of the widespread problems in nursing home regulation and care.

The nursing home regulation changes initiated by the IOM report, and enacted through the OBRA of 1987, are resulting in slow changes in practice. Some of the key changes in nursing home care that have resulted from the reform include dramatic reduction in restraint usage, mandatory pre-service training, more specific requirements for in-service training, and certification of nursing assistants. In addition, the requirement that each resident have a uniform, functionally oriented assessment on admission that must be updated on a routine basis has laid the foundation for outcome-based quality monitoring. Establishment of the minimum resident assessment (also known as the Minimum Data Set or MDS) is likely to foster the conduct of research into important, but heretofore unanswerable questions about the natural history of functional decline in nursing home patients, and other key clinical questions (George, 1994).

Despite the substantial gains that have been made through legislative reforms, there remains a need for nurses to be vigilant in advocating a higher standard of care for nursing home residents. Burger (1993) points out that some of the compromises, such as allowing individual nursing facilities to obtain waivers of staffing requirements if they can demonstrate a nursing shortage, have not been followed up according to the original agreement. Thus, there is potential for erosion of the hard-won gains in basic standards of care.

Gerontological nurses should participate in nursing home ombudsman advisory committees, where there is a unique opportunity to provide consumer education regarding the issue of inadequate standards of care and possible remedies.

Community and Home Care: Issues and Ideas

Community-based care for the elderly has not been well scrutinized. The assumption that an individual in his or her own home is more autonomous and therefore less vulnerable is not always well founded. According to Spiegel (1983, p. 419), "In this setting a peculiar opportunity exists for the provision of poor services, overutilization and for totally inadequate observation of the quality of care." There is concern among some observers (Spiegel, 1983; Hall et al., 1977) that the difficulties in achieving and maintaining a reasonable standard of nursing care in home care may exceed those encountered in the institutional setting with the current movement toward deprofessionalization of home care. Concerns about quality are based on the fact that home care is more decentralized than institutional care, and therefore supervision and quality assessment are more costly and difficult to achieve. The problem is compounded by inconsistencies in standards for home care used by the various accrediting and licensing bodies (Trager, 1980). Historically, little attention has been paid to monitoring the quality of care in the home or clinic setting (Mundinger, 1983). Unless the standards for training and supervision of paraprofessionals in home health care are strengthened to exceed the standards in institutional care, there is nothing to prevent home health care from suffering the same inadequacies documented in institutional care. Fortunately, home health care has a history of proactively developing standards for training and care and engaging in a peer-review system. There is also a long history of high-quality professional nursing involvement and autonomy in home care, dating to the early twentieth century (Mundinger, 1983). However, nurses should remain vigilant against dilution of the quality of professional services in home care. As the individuals who require highly technological care leave the hospital setting for the home, there is a great risk of fragmentation and repetition of organizational problems experienced in the acute care setting.

Nurses have a tremendous challenge ahead as new forms of community-based care for the elderly emerge. Increased utilization of adult day care and day hospitals will require new role development by gerontological nurses. However, some of the new models for community-based care seem specifically designed to exclude participation by professional nurses, emphasizing the use of paraprofessionals. Reforms in Medicare reimbursement practices, although now allowing direct third-party reimbursement to nurse practitioners and nurse anesthetists (Towers, 1992), continue to value nursing services less than physician services (Sullivan, 1992). Moreover, other studies have shown that enabling legislation does not always ensure implementation of third-party reimbursement for nurses in advanced practice (Scott and Harrison, 1990). Nurses should strive to become active in policy-making positions on local boards of health, councils on aging, and hospitals so that the full potential of gerontological nursing is considered in program development.

Developing and Validating Adequate Quality Assurance Mechanisms

Medicare and Medicaid have emphasized process criteria in evaluation of nursing services to the aged (Zimmerman, 1991). Dur-ing the 1990s the emphasis has shifted to outcome-based assessment, in part as the result of the implementation of the Nursing Home MDS, which allows for systematic recording of changes in resident status over time. Although this represents a welcome shift from the paperwork-oriented surveys many nurses have experienced, there are problems associated with outcome-based quality assurance as well. Nurses should be concerned that the pendulum does not swing too far in the other direction, to the extent that process criteria are ignored. A nurse or facility should not be penalized when caring for patients who make "unhealthy" choices if such choices are truly informed and if the patient's judgment or comprehension is not severely impaired. For example, if "number of patient falls" is chosen as a key indicator of quality, a good facility may be unfairly penalized. The facility may have a low rate of restraint use because patients and families have made an informed choice to accept the risk of falling rather than accept the loss of dignity associated with restraint use. The potential for inadequacies exists if the wrong outcomes are chosen as tracer conditions. The outcome of interest in facilities should be episodes of fall-related injury rather than the number of patient falls. Facility A may have a higher rate of falls than Facility B but a lower rate of fall-related injury. If number of falls alone is chosen as the tracer condition, the facility has an incentive to err on the side of physical safety, thus restraining patients more than is necessary.

The outcomes chosen as tracer conditions will probably represent a compromise between what is easily and objectively measured (e.g., skin integrity and presence/absence of contractures) and those outcomes of most importance to nursing home residents (e.g., degree of autonomy, freedom to make choices about self-care practices). Reasonable "middle ground" alternatives, such as changes in functional status, are expensive to assess and are influenced by variables other than the nursing care delivered.

Ensuring Adequate Reimbursement for Gerontological Nursing Care

Obtaining adequate reimbursement for gerontological nursing is an essential step toward improving the quality of health care for older persons. The salaries of nurses in home-based and institutional long-term care are depressed relative to acute care settings, making recruitment of the best nurses difficult.

The reasons for the underfunding of long-term care are complex. Undervaluing of nursing care in general is part of the problem. See Lynaugh and Fagin (1988) for a historical perspective of the problem nursing faces generically, and the authors' view of the prospects for change. Additional factors include the low status of the elderly in U.S. society and the fact that most older people have health problems that do not lend themselves to either simple or highly technological solutions. It is far more difficult to capture a community's imagination with stories of heroic consistency in caring for someone with Alzheimer's disease than to excite them with stories about the latest microsurgical techniques.

Nursing care in hospitals and nursing homes traditionally has been priced as a part of the room rate, along with housekeeping, food service, maintenance, and the mortgage. There is therefore little understanding on the part of policy makers or the public of the true cost of high-quality gerontological nursing care. It is assumed that high-quality care would be prohibitively expensive without adequate investigation into the matter. Dissimilar facilities are considered comparable if the daily rate is comparable, yet facilities differ substantially in the amount of the budget they allocate to professional nursing care. As has been argued for hospitals, it is necessary in nursing homes to separate charges for nursing care from the "bed and board" or "hotel" services, so that there is a better understanding of what the nursing care dollar is buying. Community and home care organizations usually have more clearly defined prices for nursing services, although in some organizations the charge per visit may exceed the cost of providing the nursing service, so that less profitable services are subsidized.

Another obstacle to adequate reimbursement for nursing services is that direct reimbursement to nurses for nursing practice traditionally has not been allowed by most third-party reimbursors. This practice leads to further inflation of cost of care by inserting overhead expenses or requirements for physician services that may not be needed by the older person. Until the "excess charges" attached to nursing care are removed, it will be difficult to obtain adequate reimbursement for gerontological nursing care. Fortunately, barriers to direct reimbursement to nurses in advanced practice roles (NPs and CNSs) are starting to come down.

The case of attempting to obtain direct reimbursement for gerontological nurse practitioners is a prime example of policymakers ignoring the existing research data. Numerous studies document the cost effectiveness of nurse practitioners in general and gerontological nurse practitioners in particular (Naylor et al., 1994; Romeis et al., 1985; Schultz and McGlone, 1977; Sox, 1979; Linn, 1976; Freund, 1981). Despite the wealth of literature, Medicare for many years persisted in not allowing direct reimbursement to nurses, even when it would save the system money.

Specific changes in federal rules and some state legislation bode well for the future of widespread direct third-party reimbursement for nurses in advanced practice. O'Connor (1993) notes that for selected nurses in advanced practice, direct reimbursement can be realized under the four major federal health programs: Medicare, Medicaid, Civilian Health and Medical Program of the Uniformed Health Services (CHAMPUS), and Federal Employee Health Benefits Program (FEHBP). As part of the OBRA legislation, there was a provision for reimbursement for Medicaid certification visits made in nursing homes. Additionally, Medicare now allows direct third-party reimbursement to nurse practitioners practicing in medically underserved areas. Finally, some states (e.g., North Carolina) have enacted legislation that provides for direct reimbursement for nurse practitioners and psychiatric/mental health clinical nurse specialists. There is sufficient activity in this arena that manuals now exist (e.g., see Mittelstadt, 1993) on how to obtain up-to-date information on rules governing reimbursement, procedures, and ways to access additional information. In summary, the future looks promising for direct reimbursement for nurses. However, it is important to remember that issues regarding adequate reimbursement for nurses are political as well as administrative. Although there is great need for nurse administrators to specify the cost of high-quality gerontological nursing care, obtaining adequate reimbursement levels is inherently a political process. Nurses must become active lobbyists with legislators and health policymakers to ensure an adequate funding base for care. Nurses will also need to be aggressive in demonstrating their effectiveness under new systems of reimbursement, such as prepaid systems, to other health care professionals and the public at large. As consumers become more aware of the benefits of gerontological nursing, demand for the services and reimbursement may follow.

Increasing the Availability of Interdisciplinary Team Care for the Elderly

The complexity of care for many older persons makes a persuasive argument for the usefulness of teams in geriatric care. Unfortunately, review of current geriatrics journals shows tremendous diversity in the composition of the geriatric treatment team. Research findings about conditions under which teams thrive are limited.

As nurses gain increasing recognition of their abilities to provide and coordinate care for complex patients, their authority and status may rise accordingly. The critical question will then become: Can nurses perform better than physicians have often done in facilitating older people's access to high-quality interdisciplinary team care? The risk is that nurses, given the authority, will not make the effort to work collaboratively with members of other disciplines. If nurses use their skill and new status wisely, resisting the temptation to be all-knowing and all-skillful in the guise of protecting the patient from too many providers, elderly people and their caregivers will be the beneficiaries. Nurses who have well-developed communications skills and who are knowledgeable about group dynamics have a great deal to offer any team.

SUMMARY

Gerontological nursing practice builds upon the theories and methods of nursing practice generally. The nurse must consider the developmental issues unique to those of advanced years and be particularly astute in addressing environmental demands in providing care. These traits, in addition to skillful assessment and use of nursing interventions, are likely to result in enhanced health outcomes for the older person and more rewarding practice for the nurse.

Gerontological nursing remains at a crossroads. Increased public awareness and interest in the problems of the aged place gerontological nursing in the spotlight. The influence of nurses in health care is on the upswing. The challenge before us is clear: Can we lead health care of the aged into a more enlightened era, where well-prepared, rehabilitation-oriented teams of motivated professionals provide individualized, goal-oriented, cost-effective care for older people? Or will gerontological nurses become guardians of the status quo—where need for care is equated with the potential for reimbursement, where custodial care predominates in the name of cost containment, where nurses base their practice on myth and custom rather than on scientific reasoning and ethical principles—and follow the medical profession's lead into a fragmented system of care? The choice is ours to make.

REFERENCES

Achenbaum, W.A. Societal perceptions of aging and the aged. *In* Binstock, R. and Shanas, E. *Handbook of Aging and the Social Sciences.* New York: Van Nostrand Reinhold, 1985, pp. 129–148.

Alexander, N.B., Schultz, A.B. and Warwick, D.N. Rising from a chair: Effects of age and functional ability on performance biomechanics. *J Gerontol Med Sci* 46: M91–M98, 1991.

American Nurses Association. *Standards of Geriatric Nursing Practice.* Kansas City, MO: Division of Geriatric Nursing Practice, American Nurses Association, 1970.

American Nurses Association. *Nursing and Long-Term Care: Toward Quality Care for the Aging.* Publication No. GE4-3m. Kansas City, MO: American Nurses Association, 1975.

American Nurses Association. *Standards of Gerontological Nursing Practice.* Kansas City, MO: Division of Gerontological Nursing Practice, American Nurses Association, 1976.

American Nurses Association, *Nursing's Social Policy Statement.* Publ #NP-107. Washington, DC: American Nurses Publishing, 1995.

American Nurses Association. *A Statement on the Scope of Gerontological Nursing Practice.* Kansas City: MO: Division of Gerontological Nursing Practice, American Nurses Association, 1981.

American Nurses Association. *A Challenge for Change. The Role of the Gerontological Nurse.* Kansas City, MO: Division of Gerontological Nursing Practice, American Nurses Association, 1982.

American Nurses Association. *Professional Practice for Nurse Administrators in Long-Term Care Facilities.* Kansas City, MO: American Nurses Foundation, 1984.

American Nurses Association. *Gerontological Nursing Curriculum: Survey Analysis and Recommendations.* Kansas City, MO: American Nurses Association, 1986.

American Nurses Association. *Standards and Scope of Gerontological Nursing Practice.* Kansas City, MO.: Council on Gerontological Nursing. ANA, 1987.

American Nurses Association. *Scope and Standards of Gerontological Nursing Practice.* Publ. #GE-14. Washington, DC: American Nurses Publishing, 1995.

Antonucci, T.C. Social supports and social relationships. *In* Binstock, R.H. and George, L.K. (eds.). *Handbook of Aging and the Social Sciences.* 3rd ed. San Diego: Academic Press, 1990, pp. 205–227.

Applegate, W.B., Graney, M.J., Miller, S.T. and Elam, J.T. Impact of a geriatric assessment unit on subsequent health care charges. *Am J Pub Health* 81:1302–1306, 1991.

Atchley, R.C. Respondents v. refusers in an interview study of retired women. *J Gerontol* 24:424–427, 1969.

Atchley, R.C. *The Social Forces in Later Life.* Belmont, CA: Wadsworth, 1984.

Bahr, S.R.T. Overview of gerontological nursing. *In* Hogstel, M.O. (ed.). *Nursing Care of the Older Adult.* New York: John Wiley & Sons, 1981, Chapter 1.

Baker, D. *The Role of Nursing in Care of the Elderly in Health, Sickness and Terminal Care.* Geneva: World Health Organization, 1976.

Barris, R., Kielhofner, G., Levine, R. and Neville, A.M.

Occupation as interaction with the environment. *In* Kielhofner, G. (ed.). *A Model of Human Occupation.* Baltimore: Williams & Wilkins, 1985, Chapter 4.

Bearon, L., Crowley, G.M., Chandler, J. et al. Personal functional goals: A new approach to assessing patient-relevant outcomes. *Gerontologist* 34 (Special Issue):239, 1994.

Beck, C., Rossby, L. and Baldwin, B. Correlates of disruptive behavior in cognitive impaired elderly nursing home residents. *Arch Psychiatr Nurs* 5(5):281–291, 1991.

Beck, C.K., Heacock, P., Rapp, C.G. and Shue, V. Cognitive impairment in the elderly. *Nurs Clin North Am* 28(2):335–347, 1993.

Becker, P. and Cohen, J.H. The functional approach to the care of the elderly: A conceptual framework. *J Am Geriatr Soc* 32(1):923–929, 1984.

Bejciy-Spring, S.M. Nursing case management: Application to neuroscience nursing. *J Neurosci Nurs* 23:390–397, 1991.

Bengtson, V. *The Social Psychology of Aging.* New York: Bobbs-Merrill, 1973.

Bengtson, V., Rosenthal, C. and Burton, L. Families and aging: Diversity and heterogeneity. *In* Binstock, R. and George, L. (eds.). *Handbook of Aging and the Social Sciences.* 3rd ed. San Diego: Academic Press, 1990, Chapter 14.

Berg, L., Buckwalter, K., Chafetz, P.K. et al. Special care units for persons with dementia. *J Am Geriatr Soc* 39(12):1229–1236, 1991.

Birren, J.E. A contribution to the theory of aging: As a counterpart of development. *In* Birren, J.E. and Bengtson, V.L. (eds.). *Emergent Theories of Aging.* New York: Springer, 1988.

Birren, J. and Renner, V.J. Research on the psychology of aging: Principles and experimentation. *In* Birren, J.E. and Schaie, K.W. (eds.). *Handbook of the Psychology of Aging.* New York: Van Nostrand Reinhold, 1977, pp. 3–38.

Blattner, B. *Holistic Nursing.* Englewood Cliffs, NJ: Prentice-Hall, 1981.

Bortz, W. The physics of frailty. *J Am Geriatr Soc* 41:1004–1008, 1993.

Brimmer, P.F. Past, present and future in gerontological nursing research. *J Gerontol Nurs* 5:27–34, 1979.

Brink, C., Wells, T.J., Sampselle, C.M. et al. A digital test for pelvic muscle strength in women with urinary incontinence. *Nurs Res* 43(6):352–356, 1994.

Brody, S.J., Cole, L., Storey, P. and Wink, N.J. The geriatric nurse practitioner: A new medical resource in the skilled nursing home. *J Chronic Dis* 29:537–543, 1976.

Buchanan, J.L., Bell, R.M., Arnold, S.B. et al. Assessing cost effects of nursing home based geriatric nurse practitioners. *Health Care Financing Rev* 11(3):67–78, 1990.

Buchner, D.M. and Wagner, E. Preventing frail health. *Clin Geriatr Med* 8(1):1–17, 1992.

Bump, R.C., Hurt, W.G., Fantl, J.A. and Wyman, J.F. Assessment of Kegel pelvic muscle exercise performance after brief verbal instruction. *Am J Obstet Gynecol* 165(2):322–327, 1991.

Burger, S.G. Nurses, stand up for nursing home reform. Editorial. The American Nurse, July/August 1993, pp. 5–6.

Burish, T.G. and Bradley, L.A. *Coping with Chronic Disease: Research and Applications.* New York: Academic Press, 1983.

Burke, M. and Sherman, S. *Gerontological Nursing: Issues and Opportunities for the 21st Century.* New York: National League for Nursing, 1993.

Butler, R. *Why Survive? Growing Old in America.* New York: Harper & Row, 1975.

Byrne, M.L. and Thompson, L.F. *Key Concepts for the Study and Practice of Nursing.* 2nd ed. St. Louis: C.V. Mosby, 1978.

Callahan, D. *Setting Limits: Medical Goals for an Aging Society.* New York: Simon & Schuster, 1987.

Campbell, S.O. Primary nursing: It works in long-term care. *J Gerontol Nurs* 11(12):12–16, 1985.

Campion, E.W., Jette, A. and Berkman, B. An interdisciplinary geriatric consultation service: A controlled trial. *J Am Geriatr Soc* 31:792, 1983.

Caranasos, G.J. A more opportune description of the stages of aging. Letter to the Editor. *J Am Geriatr Soc* 41:888, 1993.

Carignan, A.M. The content domain. *In* Waters, V. (ed.). *Teaching Gerontology.* New York: National League for Nursing, 1991, pp. 35–54.

Carpenito, L.J. *Nursing Diagnosis: Application to Clinical Practice.* Philadelphia: J.B. Lippincott, 1983.

Carroll-Johnson, R.M. (ed.). *Classification of Nursing Diagnoses: Proceedings of the Ninth Conference.* Philadelphia: J.B. Lippincott, 1990.

Carroll-Johnson, R.M. and Paquette, M. (eds.). *Classification of Nursing Diagnoses: Proceedings of the Tenth Conference.* Philadelphia: J.B. Lippincott, 1994.

Champlin, L. DRGs: Putting the squeeze on your older patients. *Geriatrics* 40(7):77–81, 1985.

Chappell, N.L. Aging and social care. *In* Binstock, R. and George, L. (eds.). *Handbook of Aging and the Social Sciences.* 3rd ed. San Diego: Academic Press, 1990, Chapter 23.

Clarke, M. Stress and coping: Constructs for nursing. *J Adv Nurs* 9:3–13, 1984.

Comfort, A. *The Biology of Senescence.* London: Routledge & Paul, 1956.

Corbin, J. and Strauss, A. *Unending Work and Care: Managing Chronic Illness at Home.* San Francisco: Jossey-Bass, 1988.

Cress, M.E., Schechtman, K.B., Mulrow, C. et al. Relationship between physical performance and self-perceived physical function. *J Am Geriatr Soc* 43:93–101, 1995.

Daly, J.M., McCloskey, J.C. and Bulecheck, G.B. Nursing interventions classification use in long-term care. *Geriatr Nurs* 15(1):41–46, 1994.

Dawson, P., Wells, D. and Kline, K. *Enhancing the Abilities of Persons with Alzheimer's and Related Dementias: A Nursing Perspective.* New York: Springer, 1993.

DeAngelis, C. Nurse practitioner redux. *JAMA* 271:868–871, 1994.

Dunn, H. *High Level Wellness.* Arlington, VA: W.R. Beatty, 1961.

Eisdorfer, C. and Wilkie, F. Stress, disease, aging and behavior. *In* Birren, J.E. and Schaie, K.W. (eds.). *Handbook of the Psychology of Aging.* New York: Van Nostrand Reinhold, 1977, Chapter 12.

Elder, G.H., Jr. and Clipp, E.C. Combat experience and emotional health: Impairment and resilience in later life. *J Pers* 57(2):311–341, 1989.

Elder, G.H., Jr., Shanahan, M.J. and Clipp, E.C. When war comes to men's lives: Life-course patterns in family, work and health. *Psychol Aging* 9(1):5–16, 1994.

Engle, V.F. and Graney, M.J. Self-assessed and functional health of older women. *Int J Aging Hum Dev* 22(4):301, 1985–1986.

Evans, J.G. Prevention of age-associated loss of autonomy: Epidemiologic approaches. *J Chronic Dis* 37:353–363, 1984.

Evans, L.K. and Strumpf, N. Physical restraint of the hospitalized elderly: Perceptions of patients and nurses. *Nursing Research* 37:132–137.

Evans, L.K., Yurkow, J. and Siegler, E.L. The *CARE* Program: A nurse-managed collaborative outpatient program to improve function of frail older people. *J Amer Geriatr Soc* 43:1155–1160, 1995.

Finlay, O.E., Balyes, T.B., Rosen, C. and Milling, J. Effects of chair design, age and cognitive status on mobility. *Age Ageing* 12:329–335, 1983.

Fitzpatrick, J.J., Kerr, M.E., Saba, V.K. et al. Translating nursing diagnosis into ICD Code. *Am J Nurs* 89:493–495, 1989.

Foreman, M.D. Confusion in the hospitalized elderly: Incidence, onset and associated factors. *Res Nurs Health* 12:21–29, 1989.

Freund, C.M. *The Economic Impact of Nurse Practitioner–Patient Delegation Patterns.* Springfield, VA: National Technical Information Service, 1981.

Funk, S.G., Tornquist, E.M. and Champagne, M.T. A model for improving the dissemination of nursing research. *West J Nurs Res* 11:359–365, 1989.

Funk, S.G., Tornquist, E.M., Champagne, M.T. and Wiese, R.A. Caring for the chronically ill: From research to practice. *In* Funk, S.G., Tornquist, E.M., Champagne, M.T. and Wiese, R.A. (eds.). *Key Aspects of Caring for the Chronically Ill: Hospital and Home.* New York: Springer, 1993, pp. 3–7.

Furner, S.E. and Kozak, L.J. Acute care. *In* Van Nostrand, J.F., Furner, S.E. and Suzman, R. (eds.). *Health Data on Older Americans: United States, 1992. Vital and Health Statistics Series 3: Analytic and Epidemiological Studies,* No. 27. DHHS Publication No. (PHS) 93-1411, 1993, Chapter 5.

Futrell, M., Brovender, S., McKinnon-Mullett, E. and Brower, H.T. (eds.). *Primary Health Care of the Older Adult.* North Scituate, MA: Duxbury Press, 1980.

Gallagher, E.B. Lines of reconstruction and extensions in the parsonian sociology of illness. *In* Jaco, E. (ed.). *Patients, Physicians and Illness.* New York: Free Press, 1979, pp. 162–183.

George, J. (ed.). *Nursing Theories: The Base for Professional Nursing Practice.* Englewood Cliffs, NJ: Prentice-Hall, 1980.

George, L.K. Multidimensional assessment instruments. *In* Lawton, M.P. and Teresi, J. (eds.). *Ann. Rev. Geriatrics and Gerontology,* Vol. 14. New York: Springer, 1994, pp. 353–376.

Giduz, B. and Snow, T. (eds.). *Essentials of Geriatric Care.* Rockville, MD: Aspen Systems, 1987.

Gilmore, G.C. Memory and aging: Theory and assessment. *In* Gilmore, G.C., Whitehouse, P.J. and Wykle, M.L. (eds.). *Memory, Aging and Dementia: Theory Assessment and Treatment.* New York: Springer, pp. 1–3, 1989.

Gioella, E.C. (ed.). *Gerontology in the Professional Nursing Curriculum.* New York: National League for Nursing, Pub. 15–2151, 1986.

Goosen, G.M. and Bush, H.A. Adaptation: A feedback process. *In* Sutterley, D. and Donnelly, G. (eds.). *Coping with Stress: A Nursing Perspective.* Rockville, MD: Aspen Systems, 1982, pp. 19–34.

Gordon, G. *Role Theory and Illness.* New Haven, CT: College & University Press, 1966.

Gordon, M. *Nursing Diagnosis.* New York: McGraw-Hill, 1982.

Gulick, E.E. The self-assessment of health among the chronically ill. *Top Clin Nurs* 8(1):74–82, 1986.

Gunter, L. and Estes, C. *Education for Gerontic Nursing.* New York: Springer, 1979a.

Gunter, L. and Estes, C. Tomorrow's aged: Impact of transgenerational trends on nursing education. Presented at ANA 51st Convention, June 1978. *In American Nurses Association: Power: Nursing: Challenge for Change.* Kansas City, MO: American Nurses Association, 1979b.

Gunter, L. and Miller, J. Toward a nursing gerontology. *Nurs Res* 26:208–221, 1977.

Guralnik, J.M., Branch, L.G., Cummings, S.R. and Curb, J.D. Physical performance measures in aging research. *J Gerontol Med Sci* 44:M141–M146, 1989.

Haight, B.K., Christ, M.A. and Dias, J.K. Does nursing education promote ageism? *J Adv Nurs* 20:382–390, 1994.

Hall, H.D., Tufts, J.A. and Ricer-Smith, K. Formulation of a national policy for in-home health and supportive services. Paper presented at a meeting of the American Public Health Association, Washington DC, 1977 (cited in Spiegel, 1983).

Hall, L. Another view of nursing care and quality. *In* Straub, K.M. and Parker, K.S. (eds.). *Continuity of Patient Care: The Role of Nursing.* Washington DC: Catholic University of America Press, 1966.

Heine, C. Enhancing gerontological nursing knowledge through curriculum and collaboration. *In* Heine, C. (ed.). *Determining the Future of Gerontological Nursing Education.* New York: National League for Nursing, Pub. No. 14-2508, 1993.

Heine, C. and Bahr, S.R.T. New practice models in long-term care. *In* Burke, M. and Sherman, S. New York: National League for Nursing, 1993, pp. 27–36.

Henderson, V. *Textbook of the Principles and Practice of Nursing.* 5th ed. New York: Macmillan, 1955.

Hill, L. and Smith, N. *Self-Care Nursing: Promotion of Health.* Englewood Cliffs, NJ: Prentice-Hall, 1985.

Hing, J.E. and Bloom, B. Long term care for the functionally dependent elderly. *National Center for Health Statistics Vital Health Stat* 13(104), 1990.

Hoch, C.C., Dew, M.A., Reynolds, C.F., 3rd et al. A longitudinal study of laboratory and diary-based sleep measures in healthy "old-old" and "young-old" volunteers. *Sleep* 17(6):489–496, 1994.

Hoch, C.C., Reynolds, C.F., 3rd, Buysse, D.J. et al. Sleep disordered breathing in healthy and spousally bereaved elderly: A one-year follow-up. *Neurobiol Aging* 13(6):741–746, 1992a.

Hoch, C.C., Reynolds, C.F., 3rd, Jennings, J.R. et al. Daytime sleepiness and performance among healthy 80 and 20 year olds. *Neurobiol Aging* 13(2):353–356, 1992b.

Hogue, C.C., Cullinan, S. and McConnell, E.S. Exercise interventions for the chronically ill: Review and prospects. *In* Funk, S.G., Tornquist, E.M., Champagne, M.T. and Wiese, R.A. (eds.). *Key Aspects of Caring for the Chronically Ill: Hospital and Home.* New York: Springer, 1993, pp. 59–78.

Howell, S.C. Environments and aging. *In* Eisdorfer, C., Besdine, R.W., Birren, J.E. et al. (eds.). *Annual Review of Gerontology and Geriatrics.* Vol. 1. New York: Springer, 1980, pp. 237–260.

Hultsch, D.F. and Dixon, R.A. Learning and memory in aging. *In* Birren, J.E. and Schaie, K.W. (eds.). *Handbook of the Psychology of Aging.* 3rd ed. San Diego: Academic Press, 1990, pp. 171–200.

Institute of Medicine, National Academy of Sciences. *Report of Committee on Nursing Home Regulation Reform.* Washington DC: National Academy of Sciences, 1986.

Isaacs, B. Rehabilitation for the elderly. *Int Rehab Med* 6: v–viii, 1984.

Ittleson, W.H., Franck, K.A. and O'Hanlon, T.J. The nature of environmental experience. *In* Wapner, S., Cohen, S.B. and Kaplan, B. (eds.). *Experiencing the Environment.* New York: Plenum Press, 1976, pp. 187–206.

Jackson, J. and Antonucci, T.C. Social support processes in health and effective functioning of the elderly. *In* Wykle, M.L., Kahana, E. and Kowal, J. (eds.). *Stress and Health Among the Elderly.* New York: Springer, 1992, pp. 72–95.

Johnson, H.A. (ed.). *Relations Between Normal Aging and Disease.* New York: Raven Press, 1985, p. vi.

Johnson, M.A. and Connelly, J.R. *Nursing and Gerontology: Status Report.* Washington DC: Association for Gerontology in Higher Education, 1990.

Kahana, E. A congruence model of person-environment interaction. *In* Lawton, M.P., Windley, P.G. and Byers,

T.O. (eds.). *Aging and the Environment.* New York: Springer, 1982, pp. 97–121.

Kahana, E. Epilogue: Stress research and aging: Complexities, ambiguities, paradoxes, and promise. *In* Wykle, M.L., Kahana, E. and Kowal, J. (eds.). *Stress and Health Among the Elderly.* New York: Springer, 1992, pp. 239–256.

Kahn, R. Productive behavior: Assessment, determinants, and effects. *J Am Geriatr Soc* 31:750–757, 1983.

Kahn, R., Wolfe, D., Quinn, R.P. and Snoek, J.D. *Organizational Stress: Studies in Role Conflict and Ambiguity.* New York: John Wiley & Sons, 1964.

Kalish, R.A. The social context of death and dying. *In* Binstock, R. and Shanas, E. *Handbook of Aging and the Social Sciences.* New York: Van Nostrand-Reinhold, 1985.

Kasl, S.V. Stress and health among the elderly: Overview of issues. *In* Wykle, M.L., Kahana, E. and Kowal, J. (eds.). *Stress and Health Among the Elderly.* New York: Springer, 1992, pp. 5–34.

Kayser-Jones, J. *Old, Alone and Neglected.* Berkeley: University of California Press, 1981a.

Kayser-Jones, J. Gerontological nursing research revisited. *J Gerontol Nurs* 7:217–223, 1981b.

Kilpack, V., Boehm, J., Smith, N. and Mudge, B. Using research-based interventions to decrease patient falls. *Appl Nurs Res* 4(2):50–55, 1991.

Kingsdale, J. Marrying regulatory and competitive approaches to health care cost containment. *J Health Polit Policy Law* 4(1):20–42, 1978.

Kogan, N. Personality and aging. *In* Birren, J. and Schaie, K. W. (eds.). *Handbook of the Psychology of Aging.* New York: Academic Press, 1990, pp. 330–346.

Kohn, R.R. Aging and age-related diseases. Normal processes. *In* Johnson, H.A. (ed.). *Relations Between Normal Aging and Disease.* New York: Raven Press, 1985, pp. 1–44.

Kolanowski, A., Hurwitz, S., Taylor, L.A. et al. Contextual factors associated with disturbing behaviors in institutionalized elders. *Nurs Res* 43(2):73–79, 1994.

Kovar, M.G. and LaCroix, A.Z. Aging the eighties: Ability to perform work related activities. *National Center for Health Statistics Advance Data* 136:1–12, 1987.

Kravitz, R.L. and Greenfield, S. Differences in the mix of patients among medical specialties and systems of care: Results from the Medical Outcomes Study. *JAMA* 267:1617–1623, 1992.

Kresevic, D.M., Landefeld, C.S., Palmer, R. and Kowal, J. Managing acute exacerbations of chronic illness in the elderly. *In* Funk, S.G., Tornquist, E.M., Champagne, M.T. and Wiese, R.A. (eds.). *Key Aspects of Caring for the Chronically Ill: Hospital and Home.* New York: Springer, 1993, Chapter 11.

Kuehn, A. Essential gerontological content for the associate degree nursing curriculum: A national study. *Geriatr Nurs* 17:20–27, 1991.

Laforge, R.G., Spector, W.D. and Sternberg, J. The relationship of vision and hearing impairment to one-year mortality and functional decline. *J Aging Health* 4(1):126–148, 1992.

Lang, N.M., Kraegel, J.M., Rantz, M.J. and Krejci, J.W. *Quality of Health Care for Older People in America: A Review of Nursing Studies.* New York: American Nurses Association, 1990.

Lawlor, E.F. The medical outcomes movement. *Public Policy and Aging Report* 4(6):1–3, 9, University of Chicago, 1992.

Lawton, M.P. Environment and other determinants of well-being in the aged. *Gerontologist* 24:350–354, 1983.

Lawton, M.P. A multidimensional view of quality of life in frail elders. *In* Birren, J.E., Lubben, J.E., Rowe, J.C. and Deutchman, D.E. (eds.). *The Concept and Measurement of Quality of Life in the Frail Elderly.* San Diego: Academic Press, 1991, pp. 3–27.

Lawton, M.P., Altman, I. and Wohlwill, J.F. Dimensions of environment-behavior research: Orientations to place, design, process and policy. *In* Altman, I., Lawton, M.P. and Wohlwill, J.F. (eds.). *Elderly People and the Environment.* New York: Plenum Press, 1984, pp. 1–16.

Lawton, M.P. and Nahemow, L. Ecology and the aging process. *In* Eisdorfer, C. and Lawton, M.P. (eds.). *Psychology of Adult Development and Aging.* Washington, DC: American Psychological Association, 1973, pp. 619–674.

Lazarus, R.S. and Folkman, S. *Stress, Appraisal and Coping.* New York: Springer, 1984.

Leventhal, H., Nerenz, D.R. and Leventhal, E. Feelings of threat and private views of illness: Factors in dehumanization in the medical care system. *In* Baum, A. and Singer, J.E. (eds.). *Advances in Environmental Psychology.* Vol. 4. *Environment and Health.* Hillsdale, NJ: Lawrence Erlbaum Associates, 1982, pp. 85–114.

Lieberman, M. Limitations of psychological stress model: Studies of widowhood. *In* Wykle, M.L., Kahana, E. and Kowal, J. (eds.). *Stress and Health Among the Elderly.* New York: Springer, 1992, pp. 133–150.

Linn, L.S. Patient acceptance of the family nurse practitioners. *Med Care* 24:357, 1976.

Lipsitz, L. and Goldberger, E. A loss of complexity and aging. Potential application of fractal and chaos theory to senescence. *JAMA* 267:1806–1809, 1992.

Lynaugh, J. and Fagin, C. Nursing comes of age. *Image J Nurs Sch* 20:184–190, 1988.

Mack, M. Personal adjustment of chronically ill people under home care. *Nurs Res* 1:9–30, 1952.

Maddox, G.L. Some correlates of differences in self-assessments of health status among the elderly. *J Gerontol* 17:180–185, 1962.

Magaziner, J. and Guralnik, J. The utility of performance measures of physical functioning: Insights from ongoing studies. *Gerontologist* 32 (Special Issue II):101, 1992.

Manton, K.G., Corder, L. and Stallard, E. Changes in use of personal assistance and special equipment from 1982 to 1989: Results from the 1982 and 1989 NLTCS. *Gerontologist* 33:168–176, 1993.

Martin, D.C., Morycz, R., McDowell, B.J. et al. Community-based geriatric assessment. *J Am Geriatr Soc* 33:602, 1985.

McBride, A. Managing chronicity: The heart of nursing care. *In* Funk, S.G., Tornquist, E.M., Champagne, M.T. and Wiese, R.A. (eds.). *Key Aspects of Caring for the Chronically Ill: Hospital and Home.* New York: Springer, 1993, Chapter 2.

McConnell, E.S., Wildman, D.S. and Harrell, J.S. Functional changes in the hospitalized elderly on a general medical unit. Presented at International Nursing Research Congress, University of Alberta, Calgary, May 1986.

McGrath, J.E. (ed.). *Social and Psychological Factors in Stress.* New York: Holt, Rinehart and Winston, 1970.

Mendelson, M.A. *Tender Loving Greed.* New York: Alfred A. Knopf, 1974.

Mikulencak, M. Aging population in US to affect delivery of care. *American Nurse* July/August, 1993, p. 12.

Mishel, M.H. Reconceptualization of the uncertainty in illness theory. *Image J Nurs Sch* 22:256–262, 1990.

Mishel, M.H. Living with chronic illness: Living with uncertainty. *In* Funk, S.G., Tornquist, E.M., Champagne, M.T. and Wiese, R.A. (eds.). *Key Aspects of Caring for the Chronically Ill: Hospital and Home.* New York: Springer, 1993, pp. 46–58.

Mittelstadt, P. (ed.). *The Reimbursement Manual: How to Get Paid for Your Advanced Practice Nursing Services.* Washington, DC: American Nurses Publishing, 1993.

Mooney, R.A., Newman, D.K., Smith, D.A. and Grey,

M. Establishing a continence service using AHCPR guidelines. *Ostomy Wound Management* 39(34):38–30, 1993.

Moos, R. and Lemke, S. *Group Residences for Older Adults.* New York: Oxford University Press, 1994.

Moss, F. and Halamandaris, V. *Too Old, Too Sick, Too Bad.* Rockville, MD: Aspen Systems, 1977.

Mundinger, M.O. *Home Care Controversy: Too Little, Too Late, Too Costly.* Rockville, MD: Aspen Systems, 1983.

Murray, R. and Zetner, J. *Nursing Concepts for Health Promotion.* 3rd ed. Englewood Cliffs, N.J.: Prentice-Hall, 1985.

NANDA. *Nursing Diagnoses: Definitions and Classification: 1995–1996.* Philadelphia, PA: NANDA, 1994.

NANDA. Nursing Diagnosis Submission Guidelines and Diagnostic Review Cycle. *In* Carroll-Johnson, R.M. (ed.). *Classification of Nursing Diagnoses: Proceedings of the Ninth Conference.* Philadelphia: J.B. Lippincott, 1991, Appendix A.

National League for Nursing. *Gerontology in the Nursing Curriculum.* New York: National League for Nursing, 1992.

National League for Nursing. *Nursing Data Review.* New York: National League for Nursing, 1991.

Naylor, M., Brooten, D., Jones, R. et al. Comprehensive discharge planning for the hospitalized elderly: A randomized clinical trial. *Ann Intern Med* 120:999–1006, 1994.

Neelon, V.J., Champagne, M.T., McConnell, E.S. et al. Use of the Neechan Scale to assess acute confusional states of hospitalized older adults. *In* Funk, S.G., Tornquist, E.M., Champagne, M.T. and Wiesen, R.M. (eds.). *Key Aspects of Elder Care.* New York: Springer, 1992.

Neugarten, B.L. Personality and aging. *In* Birren, J.E. and Schaie, K.W. (eds.). *Handbook of the Psychology of Aging.* New York: Van Nostrand Reinhold, 1977, pp. 626–649.

Newton, K. *Geriatric Nursing.* St. Louis, C.V. Mosby, 1950.

Norton, D., McLaren, R. and Exton-Smith, N. *An Investigation of Geriatric Nursing Problems in Hospital.* National Corporation for the Care of Old People, 1962. Edinburgh: Churchill Livingstone, 1975 (reprinted).

Odenheimer, G.S., Beaudet, M., Jette, A.M. et al. Performance-based driving evaluation of the elderly driver: Safety, reliability and validity. *J Gerontol Med Sci* 49:M153–M159, 1994.

Orem, D. *Nursing: Concepts of Practice.* 4th ed. St. Louis: Mosby-Year Book, 1991.

Orlando, I.J. *The Dynamic Nurse-Patient Relationship.* New York: G.P. Putnam's Sons, 1961.

Palmore, E. and Manton, K. Modernization and the status of the aged. *J Gerontol* 16:504–507, 1974.

Patterson, J. Development of the registered nurse who selects nursing home practice. Unpublished paper presented at the Teaching Nursing Home Program annual meeting, Robert Wood Johnson Foundation, Cincinnati, November 13–15, 1985.

Pfeiffer, E. (ed.). *Multidimensional Functional Assessment: The OARS Methodology.* 2nd ed. Durham, NC: Duke University Press, 1978.

Pierce, P.M. Intelligence and learning in the aged. *J Gerontol Nurs* 6:267–270, 1980.

Pompei, P., Foreman, M., Rudberg, M.A. et al. Delirium in hospitalized older persons: Outcomes and predictors. *J Am Geriatr Soc* 42(8):809–815, 1994.

Reff, M.E. and Schneider, E.L. *Biological Markers of Aging.* Washington, DC: United States Department of Health & Human Services, N.I.H. Publ. No. 82-2221, 1982.

Reinke, B.J., Homes, D.S. and Harris, R.L. The timing of psychosocial changes in women's lives: The years 25–45. *J Pers Soc Psychol* 48:1353–1364, 1985.

Renner, V.J. and Birren, J.E. Stress: Physiological and psychological manifestations. *In* Birren, J.E. and Sloane, R.B. (eds.). *Handbook of Mental Health and Aging.* Englewood Cliffs, NJ: Prentice-Hall, 1980, pp. 310–336.

Riley, M.W. Age strata in social systems. *In* Binstock, R. and Shanas, E. (eds.). *Handbook of Aging and the Social Sciences.* New York: Van Nostrand Reinhold, 1976, Chapter 13.

Riley, M.W. Introduction: Life course perspectives. *In* Riley, M.W. (ed.). *Aging from Birth to Death: Interdisciplinary Perspectives.* Boulder, CO: Westview Press, 1979, pp. 3–13.

Rockstein, M., Chesky, J.A. and Sussman, M.L. Comparative biology and evolution of aging. *In* Finch, C.E. and Hayflick L. (eds.). *Handbook of the Biology of Aging.* New York: Van Nostrand Reinhold, 1977, p. 4.

Rogers, M. Change through environmental interaction makes aging exciting: Interview. *J Gerontol Nurs* 11(2):35–36, 1985.

Romeis, J.C., Schey, H.M., Marion, G.S. and Keith, F.F. Extending the extenders: Compromise for the geriatric specialization-manpower debate. *J Am Geriatr Soc* 33:339, 1985.

Rowe, J. and Kahn, R.L. Human aging: Usual and successful. *Science* 237:143–149, 1987.

Rowe, J., Wang, S.Y. and Elahi, D. Design, conduct and analysis of human aging research. *In* Schneider, E.L. and Rowe, J. (eds.). *Handbook of the Biology of Aging.* 3rd ed. New York: Academic Press, 1990, pp. 63–71.

Roy, C. and Roberts, S. *Theory Construction in Nursing: An Adaptation Model.* Englewood Cliffs, NJ: Prentice-Hall, 1981.

Rubenstein, L.Z., Stuck, A.E., Siu, A.L. and Wieland, D. Impacts of geriatric evaluation and management programs on defined outcomes: Overview of the evidence. *J Am Geriatr Soc* (Suppl): 39:8S–16S, 1991.

Salthouse, T.A. Cognitive competence and expertise in aging. *In* Birren, J.E. and Schaie, K.W. (eds.). *Handbook of the Psychology of Aging.* 3rd ed. San Diego: Academic Press, 1990, Chapter 18.

Schaie, K.W. The hazards of cognitive aging. *Gerontologist* 29:484–493, 1989.

Schmidt, M.D. Meet the health care needs of older adults by using a chronic care model. *J Gerontol Nurs* 11(9):30–34, 1985.

Schroots, J.J.F. and Birren, J.E. Concepts of time and aging in science. *In* Birren, J.E. and Schaie, K.W. (eds.). *Handbook of the Psychology of Aging.* 3rd ed. San Diego: Academic Press, 1990, pp. 45–64.

Schultz, P.R. and McGlone, F.B. Primary health care provided to the elderly by a nurse practitioner/physician team: Analysis of cost effectiveness. *J Am Geriatr Soc* 25:443–446, 1977.

Schwartz, D., Henley, B. and Zeitz, L. *The Elderly Ambulatory Patient: Nursing and Psychosocial Needs.* New York: Macmillan, 1964.

Scott, C.L. and Harrison, O.A. Direct reimbursement of nurse practitioners in health insurance plans of research universities. *J Prof Nurs* 6(1):21–32, 1990.

Scott, D.W., Oberst, M.T. and Dropkin, M.J. A stress-coping model. *In* Sutterley, D. and Donnelly, G. (eds.). *Coping with Stress: A Nursing Perspective.* Rockville, MD: Aspen Systems, 1982, pp. 3–18.

Selye, H. *The Stress of Life.* New York: McGraw-Hill, 1956.

Shanas, E. The family as a social support system in old age. *Gerontologist* 19:169–174, 1979.

Shanas, E. and Sussman, M. The family in later life: Social structure and social policy. *In* Fogel, R., Hatfield, E., Kessler, S.B. and Shanas, E. (eds.). *Aging: Stability and Change in the Family.* New York: Academic Press, 1981, pp. 211–232.

Shock, N.W. Physiological aspects of aging in man. *Annu Rev Physiol* 23:97–122, 1961.

Shock, N.W. Systems integration. *In* Finch, C.E. and

Hayflick L. (eds.). *Handbook of the Biology of Aging.* New York: Van Nostrand Reinhold, 1977, p. 661.

Silverstone, B. Public policies on aging: Reconsidering old-age eligibility. *Gerontologist* 34:724–725, 1994.

Small, N.R. National consensus conference on gerontological nursing competencies. *In* Heine, C. (ed.). *Determining the Future of Gerontological Nursing Education.* New York: National League for Nursing, 1993, pp. 27–31.

Southern Council on Collegiate Education for Nursing and Southern Regional Educational Board. *Gerontological Nursing Issues and Demands Beyond the Year 2005: A Position Paper.* Atlanta, GA: SREB, 1993.

Sox, H.C. Quality of patient care by nurse practitioners and physician assistants: A ten year perspective. *Ann Intern Med* 91:459, 1979.

Spector, W.D. and Drugovich, M.L. Reforming nursing home quality regulation: Impact on cited deficiencies and nursing home outcomes. *Med Care* 27:789–801, 1989.

Spiegel, A.D. *Home Health Care.* Owings Mills, MD: National Health Publishing, 1983.

Spirduso, W.W. and MacRae, P.G. Motor performance and aging. *In* Birren, J.E. and Schaie, K.W. *Handbook of the Psychology of Aging.* 3rd ed. San Diego: Academic Press, 1990, pp. 171–200.

Strauss, A. America: In sickness and in health: Chronic illness. *Society* 10(6):33–39, 1973.

Strauss, A. *Chronic Illness and the Quality of Life.* St. Louis: C.V. Mosby, 1975.

Strumpf, N. and Evans, L. Physical restraint of the hospitalized elderly: Perceptions of patients and nurses. *Nurs Res* 37(3):132–137, 1988.

Suchman, E.A. *Sociology and the Field of Public Health.* New York: Russell Sage Foundation, 1963, p. 65.

Sullivan, E.M. Nurse practitioners and reimbursement. *Nurs Health Care* 13(5):236–241, 1992.

Thompson, K.S., Caddick, K., Mathie, J. et al. Building a critical path for ventilator dependency. *Am J Nurs* 91:28–31, 1991.

Titler, M.G., Kleiber, C., Steelman, V. et al. Infusing research into practice to promote quality care. *Nurs Res* 43(5):307–313, 1994.

Tobin, S.S. and Kulys, R. The family and services. *In* Eisdorfer, C., Besdine, R.W., Birren, J.E. et al. (eds.). *Annual Review of Gerontology and Geriatrics.* Vol. 1. New York: Springer, 1980, pp. 370–399.

Topf, M. Theoretical considerations for research on environmental stress and health. *Image* 26:289–293, 1994.

Torres-Gil, F.M. and Puccinelli, M.A. Mainstreaming gerontology in the policy arena. *Gerontologist* 34:749–752, 1994.

Towers, J. The status of Medicare reimbursement for nurse practitioners. *J Am Acad Nurse Pract* 4(3):129–130, 1992.

Trager, B. Home health care and national health policy. *Home Health Care Services Q* 1(2):1–103, 1980.

Treharne, G. Attitudes toward care of elderly people: Are they getting better? *J Adv Nursing* 15:777–781, 1990.

Trella, R. From hospital to nursing home: Bridging the gaps in care. *Geriatr Nurs* 15(6):313–316, 1994.

United States Senate Committee on Human Resources. Age Discrimination in Employment Amendments. Hearings before the Subcommittee on Labor, July 26–27, 1977. Washington, DC: U.S. Government Printing Office, 1977.

Van Nostrand, J.F., Furner, S.E. and Suzman, R. (eds.). Health Data on Older Americans: United States, 1992. *Vital and Health Statistics Series 3: Analytic and Epidemiological Studies,* No. 27. DHHS Publication No. (PHS) 93-1411, 1993.

Vladeck, B.C. *Unloving Care: The Nursing Home Tragedy.* New York: Basic Books, 1980.

Walker, S.N. and Knapp, M.T. Development and use of the ANA standards of gerontological nursing practice. *J Nurs Qual Assur* 4(3):1–14, 1990.

Waters, V. Introduction: Convening the Conference. *In* Burke, M. and Sherman, S. (eds.). *Gerontological Nursing: Issues and Opportunities for the 21st Century.* New York: National League for Nursing, 1993, pp. xiii–xiv.

Waters, V. Other resources: People and organizations. *In* Waters, V. (ed.). *Resources for Teaching Gerontology.* New York: National League for Nursing Publ. No. 14-2608, 1994.

Webster's New World Dictionary. Springfield, MA: G&C Merriam, 1991, p. 821.

Weindruch, R., Hadley, E.C. and Ory, M. Overview: Reducing frailty and falls in older persons. *In* Weindruch, R., Hadley, E.C. and Ory, M. (eds.). *Reducing Frailty and Falls in Older Persons.* Springfield, IL: Charles C Thomas, 1991, pp. 5–12.

Weiner, D.K., Long, R., Hughes, M.A. et al. When older adults face the chair-rise challenge. *J Am Geriatr Soc* 41:6–10, 1993.

Wells, D.L. Discharge decision making as a pragmatic and moral activity: An empirical and theoretical analysis. *Gerontologist* (Special Issue) 34:376–377, 1994.

Wells, T. Setting the agenda for gerontological education. *In* Heine, C. (ed.). *Determining the Future of Gerontological Nursing Education.* New York: National League for Nursing, Publ. No. 14-2508, 1993.

Wells, T., Brink, C.A., Diokno, A.C. et al. Pelvic muscle exercise for stress urinary incontinence in elderly women. *J Am Geriatr Soc* 39(8):785–791, 1991.

Wells, T. Nursing committed to the elderly. *In* Reinhardt, A.M. and Quinn, M.D. (eds.). *Current Practice in Gerontological Nursing.* St. Louis: C.V. Mosby, 1979, pp. 187–196.

Wells, T.J. *Problems in Geriatric Nursing Care: A Study of Nurses' Problems in Care of Old People in Hospitals.* New York: Churchill Livingstone, 1980.

Wiedenbach, E. *Clinical Nursing: A Helping Art.* New York: Springer, 1964.

Wohlwill, J.F. The physical environment. *In* Moos, R.H. and Insels, P.M. (eds.). *Issues in Social Ecology.* Palo Alto, CA: National Press Books, 1974, pp. 180–188.

Wohlwill, J.F. and Kohn, I. Dimensionalizing the environment mainfold. *In* Wapner, S., Cohen, S.B. and Kaplan, B. (eds.). *Experiencing the Environment.* New York: Plenum Press, 1976, pp. 19–53.

Wolanin, M.O. Nursing intervention. *In* Burnside I. (ed.). *Nursing and the Aged.* New York: McGraw-Hill, 1981, pp. 421–430 (1st ed); 404–408, (2nd ed).

Wood-Dauphinee, S.L., Shapiro, S., Bass, E. et al. A randomized trial of team care following stroke. *Stroke* 15:864–872, 1984.

Wright, L.K., Clipp, E.C. and George, L.K. Health consequences of caregiver stress. *Med Exerc Nutr Health* 2:181–195, 1993.

Wu, R. *Behavior and Illness.* Englewood Cliffs, NJ: Prentice-Hall, 1973.

Wykle, M.L., Kahana, E. and Kowal, J. (eds.). *Stress and Health Among the Elderly.* New York: Springer, 1992.

Wyman, J.F., Elswick, R.K., Jr., Ory, M.G. et al. Influence of functional, urological and environmental characteristics on urinary incontinence in community-dwelling older women. *Nurs Res* 42(5):270–275, 1993.

Wyman, J.F., Harkins, S.W. and Fantl, J.A. Psychosocial impact of urinary incontinence in the community-dwelling population. *J Am Geriatr Soc* 38(3):282–288, 1990.

Zimmerman, D.R. Impact of new regulations and data sources on nursing home quality of care. *In* National League for Nursing (ed.). *Mechanisms of Quality in Long-Term Care.* New York: National League for Nursing Publ No. 41-2382, 1991, pp. 29–42.

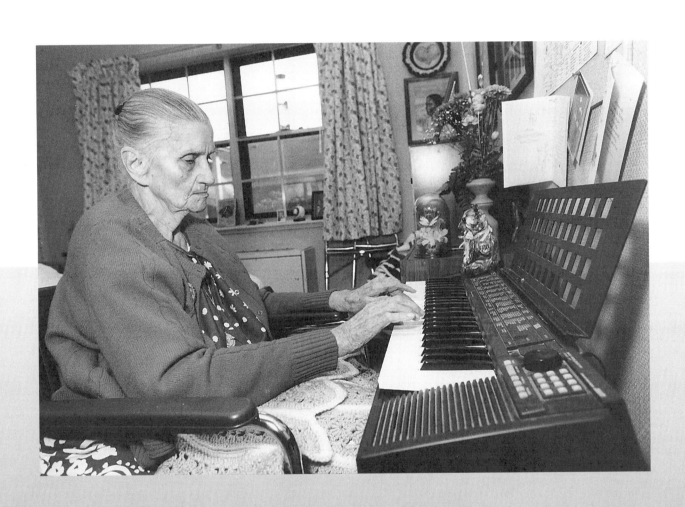

Functional Assessment

DEBORAH LEKAN-RUTLEDGE

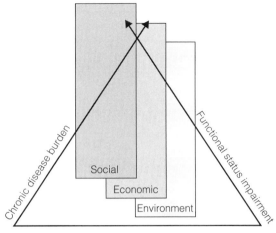

FIGURE 2-1

Interrelationship of chronic disease burden and functional status impairment.

COMPREHENSIVE FUNCTIONAL ASSESSMENT

Background

Although the significance of function in health and illness has been long appreciated, it was not until the 1950s that its importance was recognized as the numbers of older and disabled persons grew and the prevalence of chronic disease increased (Katz and Stround, 1989). The importance of function was affirmed by the U.S. Commission on Chronic Illness and the World Health Organization, which fostered the development of a scientific base for measurement. Further theoretical research and instrument development examined key constructs of functional health: activities of daily living (ADL) and instrumental activities of daily living (IADL) and psychological and social variables.

Definition

Functional status is defined as a person's ability to perform the activities necessary to ensure well-being, and it is conceptualized as the integration of three domains of function: biological, psychological (cognitive and affective), and social. Functional assessment is derived from a systems model, which observes that the interrelationship of these domains contributes to overall behavior and function. In older persons, adaptive responses to stressors in each of these domains assume increasing importance. Although developmental and aging processes cause wide variations in clinical profiles, broadening assessment procedures of the biological domain to include those from the psychosocial domains makes the impact of health problems clearer. Assessment of each of these domains provides a critical estimation of the person's overall health, need for care and services, and prognosis.

The interrelationships of the biopsychosocial domains that are mediated by chronic disease burden and functional status are illustrated in Figure 2–1. Quality of life is influenced by each of these factors when deficits exist. As the chronic disease burden increases, the risk for functional impairments also increases, and the quality of life is threatened.

Nursing assessment historically has been grounded in addressing the wholeness of the individual and the interrelationships of biopsychosocial domains. Nursing and other disciplines have also addressed measurement issues for screening and comprehensive assessment, program development, service delivery, and evaluation in older populations. Standardized measures not only provide a mechanism for systematic evaluation but also a language for interdisciplinary communication.

Comprehensive Geriatric Assessment

The prevalence of chronic disease and risk for functional disability introduces special considerations in nursing assessment. Key points are described by Gurland and Wilder (1984).

1. Most elderly people have more than one health or social problem.
2. The assessment of one problem often involves its distinction from other problems that it may resemble (e.g., the separation of depression from dementia).

3. The etiology or sustaining mechanisms of one problem may be best understood by reference to concomitant problems that occur with advancing age.

4. The prognosis of the primary problem may vary with associated problems (e.g., the chronicity of depression in elderly persons varies with the presence of physical illness).

5. The appropriate treatment depends on the combination of problems encountered and may require ongoing monitoring of all problems to prioritize treatments and later to make treatment adjustments.

6. Judgments of progress must take into account the possibility that one problem may get better while another gets worse. The treatment that improves one problem may aggravate another.

7. The consequences of deterioration in one problem area (e.g., intellectual deterioration) may be most evident in the emergence of another problem (e.g., functional impairment).

Comprehensive geriatric assessment (CGA) is the multidisciplinary evaluation of the older person in the following domains: physical health and mental, social, and economic function. The purpose of CGA is to uncover, describe, and explain the multiple problems of the older person and to identify the person's strengths and resources. The hallmark of CGA is the role of the multidisciplinary team. The "core team" consists of a physician, nurse, and social worker. Other professionals may include a pharmacist, psychiatrist, audiologist, speech pathologist, dentist, nutritionist, podiatrist, clinical psychologist, optometrist, occupational or physical therapist, and a member of the clergy. Support from other medical specialties may also be needed (Solomon, 1988). The role of the interdisciplinary team is to tackle problems systematically and organize a coordinated plan of care to facilitate better outcomes. CGA is a diagnostic rather than a therapeutic process in that outcomes depend on the implementation of the care plan. Just as important, the team is responsible for monitoring progress and making changes as needed (Solomon, 1988).

The rationale for CGA is grounded in the understanding that older persons typically present with clinically complex, interrelated problems that require more complex evaluation and intervention than can realistically be provided by a single discipline. This is particularly true for the older, more frail patient.

The National Institutes of Health Consensus Development Conference in 1987 reviewed the scientific base for CGA and concluded that CGA is effective in improving important health outcomes in older persons in various health settings. It must be noted that for CGA to be considered efficacious, in light of the amount of time and effort various disciplines contribute, the interdisiplinary care plan must be implemented. CGA has been conducted in both inpatient or outpatient settings; however, its effectiveness appears to be most favorable in inpatient geriatric medical and geriatric rehabilitation units, in which systematic follow-up care and treatment is possible (Solomon, 1988).

Formal programs that link CGA with treatment are called GEM (Geriatric Evaluation and Management) programs. GEM programs endeavor to improve care outcomes and quality of life for older patients, including decreasing morbidity and disability, and to improve survival. Although GEM programs vary greatly in how they are organized and the services they may deliver, the common element is the performance of CGA (Rubenstein et al., 1991). Additional activities may include outreach and casefinding, professional consultation, provision of extensive treatment and rehabilitation, and implementation of primary care or case management (Rubenstein et al., 1991). A number of controlled studies have demonstrated improved diagnostic accuracy, use of long-term care service (both community-based and institution-based), improved functional status, drug management, and hospital or acute care utilization (Rubenstein et al., 1991). The cost benefits have not been well documented; however, with improved early recognition of problems, preventive or rehabilitative treatment, better management of chronic disease, and reduced use of inpatient hospital and nursing home services, the costs associated with the program are focused on keeping the individual highly functional with the best quality of life rather than focusing exclusively on managing acute episodic illness.

The role of CGA in early detection of disease and dysfunction provides a quantifiable way of measuring and describing changes in function. One study comparing the clinical judgment of physicians and nurses with specific instruments to measure mental status, nutritional status, visual acuity, gait, and activities of daily living in geriatric medical inpatients found that severe impairments were recognized, but clinicians missed detecting moderate impairment in mental status, nutrition, vision, and continence (Pinholt et al., 1987). In another report, nonphysician clinic personnel administered formal geriatric assessment tools to medical outpatients. Overall, 56 per cent had at least one meaningful impairment, but few of these problems had been recognized before the survey (Miller et al., 1990). The use of systematic assessment tools is particularly important to detect early signs of impairment, which may be remediable through early intervention (Pinholt et al., 1987).

In the early 1970s, there was growing awareness of the increasing numbers of older people and their needs for long-term care services. As the numbers of nursing homes burgeoned, concern about community-based alternatives for long-term care also grew. Research in screening and comprehensive assessment procedures led to the development of instruments that were used to provide longitudinal data about aging adults, to describe their characteristics and functional capacity, and to predict the service needs of older persons. One of the best-known instruments is the Duke OARS methodology (Duke University Center for The Study of Aging and Human Development, 1978).

The Duke OARS (Older Adults Resources and Services) instrument describes the characteristics of older persons using five dimensions: social, economic, mental health, physical health, and activities of daily living. Various measures for each of these dimensions formed the Multidimensional Functional Assessment Questionnaire (MFAQ). Services are grouped into 24 categories and described in terms of the kinds of services provided and the costs associated with these services. The questionnaire requires about 45 minutes to 1 hour to complete, and some training is necessary to use the instrument accurately (Maddox, 1989).

Community-based screening and assessment initiatives are being used in a number of state governments in providing long-term care services. In Oregon, the Client Assessment Planning System (CAPS) performs three functions: (1) pre-admission screening to assist in placement decisions, (2) estimate of functional capacities for use by case managers, and (3) program planning and evaluation (Maddox, 1989). In Connecticut, screening procedures are utilized to establish eligibility for long-term care services and for nursing home placement. The screening procedure is conducted in approximately 20 minutes, then it is Faxed to the Department of Income Maintenance for review by a registered nurse (Maddox, 1989). The central role of standardized screening and assessment is clear, yet barriers remain in paying for the cost of assessment and in coordinating services that are fragmented with regard to eligibility, the amount of service that can be made available, and payment structure.

In rehabilitation settings, instruments have been developed to document the severity of disability and the benefits of treatment. In 1983, when prospective payment was mandated for Medicare patients in acute care hospitals, rehabilitation facilities were exempted, since diagnosis-related groups (DRGs) did not appropriately document rehabilitation outcomes. At that time, the American Congress of Rehabilitation Medicine and the American Academy of Physical Medicine and Rehabilitation established a task force to develop a uniform data system for medical rehabilitation (Laughlin et al., 1992; Granger and Hamilton, 1992). With federal funding, the Center for Functional Assessment Research at the State University of New York at Buffalo developed the Uniform Data System (UDS) for Medical Rehabilitation. The UDS provides a formal method to assess, collect, and communicate information regarding the patient's disability and the outcome of rehabilitation programs from admission to discharge (Laughlin et al., 1992; Center for Functional Assessment Research, 1990).

The UDS has several components: the functional independence measure (FIM), demographic data, and financial and diagnostic information. The FIM is an 18-item, 7-level, Likert-type scale representing items that commonly occur in patients with neurologic or musculoskeletal disorders (Fig. 2–2). The categories, which include mobility, self-care, communication, and others, reflect the burden of care and cost of disability. One category, transfer, is shown in Figure 2–2. The FIM is designed to be brief, simple to use, discipline-free, and sensitive to change over the course of a comprehensive rehabilitation program (Laughlin et al., 1992).

The UDS Data Management Service analyzes and reports on patients discharged from rehabilitation hospitals that subscribe to the system. The UDS is used in 35 states in 139 medical rehabilitation hospitals. Recent reports indicate that across impairment groups there is significant, timely, and measurable functional improvement of patients undergoing rehabilitation (Granger and Hamilton, 1992; Granger and Hamilton, 1993). Good interrater reliability and validity have been established.

In long-term care, the development of a comprehensive instrument for resident assessment was mandated by Congress as one

LEVELS		NO HELPER
	7 Complete Independence (Timely, Safely) 6 Modified Independence (Device)	

	Modified Dependence
	  5 Supervision
	  4 Minimal Assist (Subject = 75%+)
	  3 Moderate Assist (Subject = 50%+)
	Complete Dependence
	  2 Maximal Assist (Subject = 25%+)
	  1 Total Assist (Subject = 0%+)
		HELPER

	ADMIT	DISCHG	FOL-UP
Self Care A. Eating B. Grooming C. Bathing D. Dressing—Upper Body E. Dressing—Lower Body F. Toileting			
Sphincter Control G. Bladder Management H. Bowel Management			
Mobility Transfer: I. Bed, Chair, Wheelchair J. Toilet K. Tub, Shower			
Locomotion L. Walk/wheel Chair M. Stairs	w c	w c	w c
Communication N. Comprehension O. Expression	a v v n	a v v n	a v v n
Social Cognition P. Social Interaction Q. Problem Solving R. Memory			
Total FIM			

NOTE: Leave no blanks; enter 1 if patient not testable due to risk.

Amplification of FIM Item I and Levels of Dependence

I. Transfer: Bed, Chair, Wheelchair   Includes all aspects of transferring to and from bed, chair, and wheelchair, and coming to a standing position, if walking is the typical mode of locomotion.

FIGURE 2–2

Functional independence measure (FIM). (From Research Foundation, State University of New York, copyright 1990.)

No Helper

7. Complete Independence

If walking: approaches, sits down and gets up to a standing position from a regular chair; transfers from bed to chair. Performs safely.

If in a wheelchair: approaches a bed or chair, locks brakes, lifts foot rests, removes arm rest if necessary, and performs either a standing pivot or sliding transfer and returns. Performs safely.

6. Modified Independence

Requires adaptive or assistive device (including a prosthesis or orthosis) such as a sliding board, a lift, grab bars, or special seat or chair or brace or crutches; takes more than reasonable time or there are safety considerations.

Helper

5. Supervision or Setup

Requires supervision (e.g., standing by, cuing, or coaxing) or setup (positioning sliding board, moving foot rests, and so on)

4. Minimal Contact Assistance

Subject performs 75% or more of transferring tasks.

3. Moderate Assistance

Performs 50% to 74% of transferring tasks.

2. Maximal Assistance

Performs 25% to 49% of transferring tasks.

1. Total Assistance

Performs less than 25% of transferring tasks.

Comment: When assessing bed to chair transfer, the subject begins and ends in the supine position.

F I G U R E   2 – 2   *Continued*

---

part of the Omnibus Budget Reconciliation Act of 1987. A national resident assessment system was developed under contract by the Health Care Financing Administration to provide a structure and language in which to understand the needs of long-term care residents, design care plans, evaluate quality of care, and describe the national long-term care population for planning and policy efforts (Morris et al., 1990). Proposed regulations addressed the need for uniform resident assessment that would include data on the nursing home resident's functional, medical, mental, and psychosocial status upon admission and on a periodic basis.

The uniform resident assessment marked a dramatic shift in nursing facility survey for certification. Prior to this initiative, the survey process focused on a nursing home's written policies and structural procedures, such as staffing levels, as indicators of adequate or inadequate care. Years of research demonstrated the inadequacy of this approach. A shift toward a more outcome-based approach would redirect the focus to observing the actual care provided to the resident and resident outcomes over time (Morris et al., 1990).

The Resident Assessment Instrument en-compasses two interrelated components: the Minimum Data Set (MDS) (see Appendix) and the Resident Assessment Protocols (RAPS). The MDS is a four-page assessment tool that contains core items necessary for comprehensive assessment of nursing facility residents. It has 16 different sections, or "screens," for assessing specific functions. It also provides triggers, which are individual items or groups of items that identify specific issues or problems to be further assessed and addressed in careplanning. When the triggers are identified, the RAP must be completed. Trigger questions address problems such as incontinence, restraints, disruptive behavior, and skin ulcers. The RAP targets a potential problem and provides recommendations for further assessment and careplanning. The RAP can be helpful to guide nurses and other team members in further systematic assessment, problem-solving, and careplanning, particularly when staff lack a gerontological background (Haight, 1992). Both the MDS and the RAPS strongly link resident assessment with careplanning on a continuing basis, providing a structure for responsiveness to changes in a resident's functional status (Fig. 2–3).

The Resident Assessment Instrument is used widely in nursing facilities, since a mechanism for comprehensive standardized assessment of resident function is a condition for participation for facility reimbursement under Medicare and Medicaid. However, states have the option of developing their own assessment systems, provided the Health Care Financing Administration deems that the alternative instruments conform with the MDS (Morris et al., 1990).

Unidimensional Instruments for Functional Assessment

Instruments and scales have been developed for specific domains of function. Use of standardized measures can improve clinical decision making, since important aspects of that domain are less likely to be missed and can facilitate communication among disciplines when summary scores of recognized and accepted measures give brief, meaningful information about a person's function.

Physical Health

Measures of physical health attempt to derive a global determination of overall health and fitness. Some measures inquire about the presence of illness or disease, whereas others may cover items related to activities of daily living and instrumental activities of daily living (Kane and Kane, 1981). Commonly used indicators of physical health include diagnoses and conditions present, symptoms, handicaps, categories of drugs taken, severity of illness indicators, and quantification of medical services utilized—for example, number of hospital days per year, bed days per year, or days unable to perform usual activities per year (Kane, 1984). Self-ratings of health and disability may also be included in such measures.

The Cumulative Illness Rating Scale is an instrument designed to measure overall health and burden of disease in the elderly based on the degree of impairment in 13 organ systems (Linn et al., 1968; Parmalee et al., 1995). Each of these systems is rated and scored on a 5-point scale according to severity of impairment (from none to extremely severe). The score obtained reflects the accumulation of impairment and disease and may be a more accurate predictor of life expectancy than chronological age. Psychological aspects that may affect physical function are not identified in this scale, although it is known that mental functioning does affect physical functioning (Granick, 1983).

The Health Index is a scale that measures

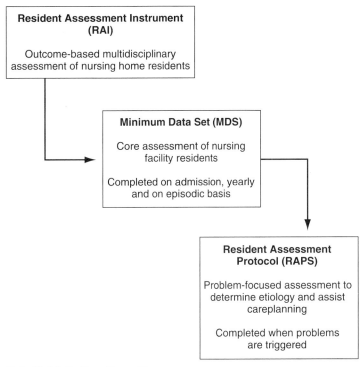

FIGURE 2 – 3

Comprehensive resident assessment in the nursing facility: The resident assessment instrument (RAI), minimum data set (MDS), and resident assessment protocols (RAPS).

the presence, extent, and duration of 40 common ailments (heart trouble, high blood pressure, stroke, tumor, and so on). Four points are given for each major illness and two points for minor illness (Rosencranz and Pihlblad, 1970). Additional points are given for episodes of confinement to the house, bed, or hospital during the preceding month. Based on the total number of points, the individual is classified into one of five categories indicating the severity of illness and confinement.

The Sickness Impact Profile (SIP) is a measure of health status that is used to detect changes over time (Bergner et al., 1976; Bergner et al., 1981). It was designed to be used generically in different populations (such as hip fracture patients), in individuals and in groups of patients, and across geographical and cultural groups. SIP is an interviewer-administered questionnaire with statements describing sickness-related behavioral dysfunction in 14 categories—for example, social interaction, ambulation, nutrition, sleep and rest, daily work, household management, mobility and confinement, and leisure pastimes. For instance, the social interaction section includes such statements as, "I make many demands, for example, insist that people do things for me, tell them how

T A B L E   2 – 1
Katz Index of Activities of Daily Living (ADL)

Independence means without supervision, direction, or active personal assistance, except as specifically noted below. This is based on actual status and not ability. A patient who refuses to perform a function is considered as not performing the function, even though he or she is deemed able.

Bathing (Sponge, shower, or tub)
Independent: assistance only in bathing a single part (back or disabled extremity) or bathes self completely
Dependent: Assistance in bathing more than one part of body; assistance in getting in or out of tub; does not bathe self

Dressing
Independent: gets clothes from closets and drawers; puts on clothes, outer garments, braces; manages fasteners; act of tying shoes is excluded.
Dependent: does not dress self or remains partly undressed

Going to Toilet
Independent: gets to toilet; gets on and off toilet; arranges clothes, cleans organs of excretion (may manage own bedpan used at night only and may or may not be using mechanical supports)
Dependent: uses bedpan or commode or receives assistance in getting to and using toilet

Transfer
Independent: moves in and out of bed and in and out of chair independently (may or may not be using mechanical supports)
Dependent: assistance in moving in or out of bed and/or chair; does not perform one or more transfers

Continence
Independent: urination and defecation entirely self-controlled
Dependent: partial or total incontinence in urination or defecation; partial or total control by enemas, catheters, or regulated use of urinals and/or bedpans

Feeding
Independent: gets food from plate or its equivalent into mouth (precutting of meat and preparation of food, as buttering bread, are excluded from evaluation)
Dependent: assistance in act of feeding (see above); does not eat at all or parenteral feeding

Evaluation Form

Name _____ Date of Evaluation _____

For each area of functioning listed below, circle description that applies (the word "assistance" means supervision, direction, or personal assistance).

Bathing—either sponge bath, tub bath, or shower

Receives no assistance (gets in and out of tub by self if tub is usual means of bathing)	Receives assistance in bathing only one part of body (such as back or a leg)	Receives assistance in bathing more than one part of body (or does not bathe self)

Dressing—gets clothes from closets and drawers; puts on clothes, including underclothes, outer garments; manages fasteners (including braces, if worn)

Gets clothes and gets completely dressed without assistance	Gets clothes and gets dressed without assistance except for tying shoes	Receives assistance in getting clothes or in getting dressed or stays partly or completely undressed

Toileting—going to the "toilet room" for bowel and urine elimination; cleaning self after elimination and arranging clothes

Goes to "toilet room," cleans self, and arranges clothes without assistance (may use object for support such as cane, walker, or wheelchair and may manage night bedpan or commode, emptying same in morning)	Receives assistance in going to "toilet room" or in cleansing self or in arranging clothes after elimination or in use of night bedpan or commode	Does not go to room termed "toilet" for the elimination process

Transfer

Moves in and out of bed and in and out of chair without assistance (may use object for support such as cane or walker)	Moves in or out of bed or chair with assistance	Does not get out of bed

Continence

Controls urination and bowel movement completely by self	Has occasional "accidents"	Supervision helps keep urine or bowel control; catheter is used or is incontinent

Feeding

Feeds self without assistance	Feeds self except for getting assistance in cutting meat or buttering bread	Receives assistance in feeding or is fed partly or completely by tubes or intravenous fluids

From Katz, S., Ford, A.B., Moskowitz, R.S., et al. Studies of illness in the aged. The index of ADL: A standardized measure of biological and psychosocial function. *JAMA* 185:94–98, 1963. Copyright 1963, American Medical Association.

to do things" and "I am going out less to visit people."

The SIP is being used to examine the impact of chronic illness, such as back pain and chronic lung disease, on functioning, to determine whether a profile exists unique to populations with different chronic diseases, and to evaluate the efficacy of treatment programs. Reliability and validity are satisfactory, and the SIP "is feasible to administer even to the very sick, is relevant to their needs, and adds information beyond that provided by other data" (Bergner et al., 1981, p. 805). The SIP has also been shown to be a useful outcome measure in studies of the effects of interventions to reduce frailty, in a variety of settings (Cress et al., 1995).

Functional Status

Scales of functional status address activities of daily living (bathing, dressing, feeding, transfers, continence, and ambulation) and instrumental activities of daily living (housekeeping, shopping, taking medicines, using transportation, using the telephone, cooking, and managing money) that are usually necessary for independent living (Kane, 1984). Measurement of functional status can reveal the physical abilities of patients and the kinds of assistance they may need (Doyle et al., 1986). Direct observation is considered more reliable and sensitive to change as it is freer from bias, although it can be time consuming.

"Environmental artifacts," however, may influence performance of activities of daily living (Katz et al., 1963). For example, most hospitals and nursing homes require nurses to supervise and/or assist patients during bathing (getting into showers or tubs) and transfers. Care may be provided by the nurse for the sake of safety and convenience and to economize on time, instead of encouraging the individual to do as much as possible. This can result in functional status ratings that are lower than they might be in the absence of such restrictions (Katz et al., 1963).

The Katz Index of ADL (Katz et al., 1963) is a well-known scale used extensively in assessing the treatment outcomes of the elderly and chronically ill (Table 2–1). Six different functions are measured and scored according to the individual's actual performance of these functions, not the individual's ability to perform them. The rating is dichotomous, with one point awarded for each dependent item, although an intermediate description identifies skills the individual can perform with some help. The intermediate

descriptions are classified as dependent for certain functions (e.g., continence) and independent for others (e.g., bathing, dressing). The six functions of bathing, dressing, toileting, transfer, continence, and feeding are conceived as being hierarchically ordered, with the pattern of recovery from a disabling illness in later life similar to the order of development of primary functions in children. Conversely, loss of function begins with complex activities, and the most basic and least complex activities are retained the longest. Recovery proceeds through three stages: early independence in feeding and continence; subsequent recovery of transfer and going to the toilet; and complete independence in bathing and dressing (Katz et al., 1963). A combined measure of all six ADL functions can be used to gauge change over time. The Katz Index is strongly related to the nursing time required by patients (Lyden and Lau, 1991).

An expanded version of the Katz Index adds items that address IADL activities. The Spector-Katz ADL Scale includes items such as housework, shopping, and strenuous physical activity, which encompass a wider range of physical function as encountered in ambulatory elderly (Spector et al., 1987). The scale also has hierarchical properties so that failure to perform a moderately or minimally difficult task would imply inability to perform a more complex task.

The PULSES profile (Table 2–2) provides a measure of general functional performance in mobility and self-care, medical status, and psychosocial factors (Granger et al., 1979). PULSES is an acronym for Physical condition, Upper limbs (self-care), Lower limbs (mobility), Sensory components, Excretory functions, and Support factors. Each item is scored on a 4-point scale from independent to dependent. Scores range from 6/6 for intact functioning to 6/24 for complete dependence. A score of 16 or more describes the very severely disabled. The PULSES profile has been used in rehabilitation settings to predict response to intensive rehabilitation and to monitor changes in function.

The Barthel Index (Table 2–3) rates specific self-care abilities (such as drinking from a cup and dressing upper and lower body) and mobility functions (such as walking 50 yards, using stairs, propelling wheelchair) (Mahoney and Barthel, 1965; Granger et al., 1979). The total scores are graded for different degrees of independence, and items are individually weighted. The maximum score of 100 indicates independence in all items but may not reflect the individual's ability to live alone (Kane and Kane, 1981). A score of

TABLE 2-2
PULSES Profile*

P—Physical condition: Includes diseases of the viscera (cardiovascular, gastrointestinal, urological, and endocrine) and neurological disorders:
1. Medical problems sufficiently stable that medical or nursing monitoring is not required more often than 3-month intervals.
2. Medical or nurse monitoring is needed more often than 3-month intervals but not each week.
3. Medical problems are sufficiently unstable as to require regular medical and/or nursing attention at least weekly.
4. Medical problems require intensive medical and/or nursing attention at least daily (excluding personal care assistance only).

U—Upper limb functions: Self-care activities (drink/feed, dress upper/lower, brace/prosthesis, groom, wash, perineal care) dependent mainly upon upper limb function:
1. Independent in self-care without impairment of upper limbs.
2. Independent in self-care with some impairment of upper limbs.
3. Dependent upon assistance or supervision in self-care with or without impairment of upper limbs.
4. Dependent totally in self-care with marked impairment of upper limbs.

L—Lower limb functions: Mobility (transfer chair/toilet/tub or shower, walk, stairs, wheelchair) dependent mainly upon lower limb function:
1. Independent in mobility without impairment of lower limbs.
2. Independent in mobility with some impairment in lower limbs, such as needing ambulatory aids, a brace, or prosthesis, or else fully independent in a wheelchair without significant architectural or environmental barriers.
3. Dependent upon assistance or supervision in mobility with or without impairment of lower limbs, or partly independent in a wheelchair or when there are significant architectural or environmental barriers.
4. Dependent totally in mobility with marked impairment of lower limbs.

S—Sensory components: Relating to communication (speech and hearing) and vision:
1. Independent in communication and vision without impairment.
2. Independent in communication and vision with some impairment such as mild dysarthria, mild aphasia, or need for eyeglasses or hearing aid, or regular eye medication.
3. Dependent upon assistance, an interpreter, or supervision in communication or vision.
4. Dependent totally in communication or vision.

E—Excretory functions (bladder and bowel):
1. Complete voluntary control of bladder and bowel sphincters.
2. Control of sphincters allows normal social activities despite urgency or need for catheter, appliance, suppositories, etc. Able to care for needs without assistance.
3. Dependent upon assistance in sphincter management or else has accidents occasionally.
4. Frequent wetting or soiling from incontinence of bladder or bowel sphincters.

S—Support factors: Consider intellectual and emotional adaptability, support from family unit, and financial ability
1. Able to fulfill usual roles and perform customary tasks.
2. Must make some modification in usual roles and performance of customary tasks.
3. Dependent upon assistance, supervision, encouragement, or assistance from a public or private agency owing to any of the above considerations.
4. Dependent upon long-term institutional care (chronic hospitalization, nursing home, etc.) excluding time-limited hospital for specific evaluation, treatment, or active rehabilitation.

* PULSES total: best score is 6, worst score is 24.
From Granger, C.V., Albrecht, G.L., and Hamilton, B.B. Outcome of comprehensive medical rehabilitation: Measures of PULSES profile and the Barthel index. *Arch Phys Med Rehab* 60:145–154, 1979.

40 or less describes the very dependent individual. Barthel scores of less than 60 have resulted in an individual being placed in a long-term care facility 90 per cent of the time (Clark, 1984). The Barthel Index, like the PULSES profile, is a useful complement to clinical judgment when predicting rehabilitation potential and outcomes, disposition, and care requirements.

Instrumental activities of daily living (IADL) constitute a range of activities more complex than those needed for personal self-care. Included are being able to cook, shop, telephone, and manage finances (Kane and Kane, 1981; Katz, 1983). Table 2–4 illustrates the categories of IADL (Lawton and Brody, 1969). IADL scales tend to emphasize tasks commonly performed by women and may put men at a disadvantage because of social roles. For example, men may have been excluded during married life from food preparation or doing laundry, tasks considered essential IADL functions. Items that tap social role performance in older men (such as "fixing things around the house" or gardening) have not been included in IADL scales (Kane and Kane, 1981).

It is particularly important to measure IADL in individuals living in the community. Impairment in IADL may precede other impairments and may be a detriment to independent living. However, knowing the existing needs allows for the appropriate matching of services and family support to enable the individual to live independently for as long as possible.

The Rapid Disability Rating Scale–2 (Table 2–5) is an 18-item questionnaire with a

TABLE 2 - 3

Barthel Index with Corresponding Values for Independent Performance of Tasks*

INDEX	"CAN DO BY MYSELF"	"CAN DO WITH HELP OF SOMEONE ELSE"	"CANNOT DO AT ALL"
SELF-CARE INDEX			
1. Drinking from a cup	4	0	0
2. Eating	6	0	0
3. Dressing upper body	5	3	0
4. Dressing lower body	7	4	0
5. Putting on brace or artificial limb	0	−2	0 (not applicable)
6. Grooming	5	0	0
7. Washing or bathing	6	0	0
8. Controlling urination	10	5 (accidents)	0 (incontinent)
9. Controlling bowel movements	10	5 (accidents)	0 (incontinent)
MOBILITY INDEX			
10. Getting in and out of chair	15	7	0
11. Getting on and off toilet	6	3	0
12. Getting in and out of tub or shower	1	0	0
13. Walking 50 yards on the level	15	10	0
14. Walking up/down one flight of stairs	10	5	0
15. IF NOT WALKING: Propelling or pushing wheelchair	5	0	0 (not applicable)

* Barthel total: best score is 100; worst score is 0.
From Granger, C.V., Albrecht, G.L., and Hamilton, B.B. Outcome of comprehensive medical rehabilitation: Measures of PULSES profile and the Barthel index. *Arch Phys Med Rehab* 60:145–154, 1979.

4-point rating scale that incorporates ADL, IADL, degree of disabilities (e.g., sensory impairments, communication, and diet), and degree of special problems such as depression and mental confusion (Linn and Linn, 1982). This scale attempts to account for some of the functional disability related to the presence of confusion or depression. As with other functional status scales, rating what the individual actually does, not what the individual can potentially do, is emphasized. The items on the scale are used to predict mortality, with the best predictors being the need for assistance with eating, incontinence, time in bed, diet, and depression (Linn and Linn, 1982). The scale is useful for patient monitoring and determining changes in level of care.

The Physical Performance Test (PPT) combines validated items from several scales that evaluate multiple dimensions of physical function at various levels of difficulty (Reuben and Siu, 1990). The PPT is a 9-item test requiring direct observation and timed measurement of performance of various ADL and IADL activities (Table 2–6). The variables assessed include fine motor function, upper coarse motor function, balance, mobility, coordination, and endurance. Specific observed ADL activities include eating, transferring, dressing, and locomotion. Degree of difficulty ranges from minimal difficulty, such as eating, or writing a sentence; to

moderate difficulty, such as lifting a book; to very difficult, such as climbing stairs. Items are scored on a 5-point scale (ranging from "capable or fastest" to "0") and summed for a maximum of 36 points for the 9-point scale. The 7-item scale omits stair climbing for a maximum of 28 points. Reliability and validity tests were satisfactory, and there is high agreement between self-reported ability to complete the PPT items and the patient's actual ability as observed by the tester.

The PPT is a brief and easily administered and scored test for screening for functional impairments. It holds practical appeal since it addresses a wide range of function but is not cumbersome, as are some more detailed comprehensive evaluations. The PPT has been shown to be both reliable and valid (Reuben and Siu, 1990).

Psychological Function: Cognitive and Affective Status

Psychological impairment, most notably depression and dementia, is strongly correlated with decreased quality of life and functional impairments. Screening assessment of both cognitive and affective function should be a part of any geriatric assessment approach, keeping in mind that screening alone is insufficient to confirm a diagnosis.

It is recommended that cognitive and af-

TABLE 2-4
Scale for Instrumental Activities of Daily Living (IADL)

MALE SCORE		FEMALE SCORE
	A. Ability to use telephone	
1	1. Operates telephone on own initiative; looks up and dials numbers, etc.	1
1	2. Dials a few well-known numbers	1
1	3. Answers telephone but does not dial	1
0	4. Does not use telephone at all	0
	B. Shopping	
1	1. Takes care of all shopping needs independently	1
0	2. Shops independently for small purchases	0
0	3. Needs to be accompanied on any shopping trip	0
0	4. Completely unable to shop	0
	C. Food preparation	
	1. Plans, prepares, and serves adequate meals independently	1
	2. Prepares adequate meals if supplied with ingredients	0
	3. Heats and serves prepared meals, or prepares meals but does not maintain adequate diet	0
	4. Needs to have meals prepared and served	0
	D. Housekeeping	
	1. Maintains house alone or with occasional assistance (e.g., heavy-work domestic help)	1
	2. Performs light daily tasks such as dish washing and bed making	1
	3. Performs light daily tasks but cannot maintain acceptable level of cleanliness	1
	4. Needs help with all home maintenance tasks	1
	5. Does not participate in any housekeeping tasks	0

MALE SCORE		FEMALE SCORE
	E. Laundry	
	1. Does personal laundry completely	1
	2. Launders small items; rinses socks, stockings, etc.	1
	3. All laundry must be done by others	0
	F. Mode of transportation	
1	1. Travels independently on public transportation or drives own car	1
1	2. Arranges own travel via taxi, but does not otherwise use public transportation	1
0	3. Travels on public transportation when assisted or accompanied by another	1
0	4. Travel limited to taxi or automobile, with assistance of another	0
0	5. Does not travel at all	0
	G. Responsibility for own medication	
1	1. Is responsible for taking medication in correct dosages at correct time	1
0	2. Takes responsibility if medication is prepared in advance in separate dosages	0
0	3. Is not capable of dispensing own medication	0
	H. Ability to handle finances	
1	1. Manages financial matters independently (budgets, writes checks, pays rent and bills, goes to bank); collects and keeps track of income	1
1	2. Manages day-to-day purchases, but needs help with bank for major purchases, etc.	1
0	3. Incapable of handling money	0

From Lawton, H.P., and Brody, E.M. Assessment of older people: Self-maintaining and instrumental activities of daily living. *Gerontologist* 9:179, 1969.

fective functions be measured independently of one another, as impairments in both areas may coexist in the same individual and may be difficult to differentiate (Kane and Kane, 1981). The social environment may adversely affect the emotional state, leading to symptoms such as sadness, loneliness, anxiety, and "paranoia," which may result in poor performance on tests of cognitive function although no organic dementing process may exist.

Cognitive status measurements identify a number of areas for evaluation: attention, memory, orientation, calculation, language, visual-spatial ability, concentration, and abstraction and judgment. Because full-scale psychological testing is often impractical in elderly people, shorter tests have been developed to measure different attributes of cognitive function. There is variation in the cognitive functions evaluated and the questions included in different mental status examinations (Kane and Kane, 1981).

Kittner and associates (1986) note that mental status screening tests may introduce bias, particularly with variables such as educational level. They underscore that the gold standard against which screening tests are measured is a clinical evaluation that incorporates a detailed history and comprehensive mental status evaluation.

The Folstein Mini-Mental State Examination (MMSE) (Table 2–7) tests orientation, registration, attention and calculation, recall, language, and ability to follow a three-part command (Folstein et al., 1975). The highest possible score is 30, and a score of 23 or less may be found in individuals with dementia, schizophrenia, delirium, or an affective disorder. The severity of cognitive impairment

TABLE 2 - 5
Rapid Disability Rating Scale-2 (RDRS-2)

Directions: Rate what the person *does* to reflect current behavior. Circle one of the four choices for each item. Consider rating with any aids or prostheses normally used. None = completely independent or normal behavior. Total = that person cannot, will not, or may not (because of medical restriction) perform a behavior or has the most severe form of disability or problem.

ASSISTANCE WITH ACTIVITIES OF DAILY LIVING

Eating	None	A little	A lot	Spoon-feed; intravenous tube
Walking (with cane or walker if used)	None	A little	A lot	Does not walk
Mobility (going outside and getting about with wheelchair, etc., if used)	None	A little	A lot	Is housebound
Bathing (include getting supplies, supervising)	None	A little	A lot	Must be bathed
Dressing (include help in selecting clothes)	None	A little	A lot	Must be dressed
Toileting (include help with clothes, cleaning, or help with ostomy/catheter)	None	A little	A lot	Uses bedpan or unable to care for ostomy/catheter
Grooming (shaving for men, hairdressing for women, nails, teeth)	None	A little	A lot	Must be groomed
Adaptive tasks (managing money/possessions; telephoning; buying newspaper, toilet articles, snacks)	None	A little	A lot	Cannot manage

DEGREE OF DISABILITY

Communication (expressing self)	None	A little	A lot	Does not communicate
Hearing (with aid if used)	None	A little	A lot	Does not seem to hear
Sight (with glasses, if used)	None	A little	A lot	Does not see
Diet (deviation from normal)	None	A little	A lot	Fed by intravenous tube
In bed during day (ordered or self-initiated)	None	A little (<3 hr)	A lot	Most/all of time
Incontinence (urine/feces, with catheter or prosthesis, if used)	None	Sometimes	Frequently (weekly +)	Does not control
Medication	None	Sometimes	Daily, taken orally	Daily; injection (+ oral if used)

DEGREE OF SPECIAL PROBLEMS

Mental confusion	None	A little	A lot	Extreme
Uncooperativeness (combats efforts to help with care)	None	A little	A lot	Extreme
Depression	None	A little	A lot	Extreme

From Linn, M.W., and Linn, B.S. The rapid disability rating scale-2. *J Am Geriatr Soc* 30:378-382, 1982.

can be classified into three levels, with 24 to 30 indicating no cognitive impairment, 18 to 23 mild impairment, and 0 to 17 severe cognitive impairment. Following an extensive review of the literature, the MMSE was determined to have satisfactory reliability and construct validity. The test is highly sensitive for moderate to severe cognitive impairment and less sensitive for mild degrees of impairment (Tombaugh and McIntyre, 1992).

The MMSE may produce false-positive results; up to a third of patients assessed were incorrectly identified as cognitively impaired (Folstein et al., 1985). This may be attributed partly to the fact that MMSE scores may be significantly affected by age, education, and cultural background (Tombaugh and McIntyre, 1992). Educational attainment below the eighth grade level may be associated with lower test performance and possible misclassification of dementia. Furthermore, the reading and writing part of the test may be difficult for those with visual impairment or physical limitations such as arthritis or hemiplegia (Tombaugh and McIntyre, 1992).

Certain items may be biased against elders with less than 9 years of education—for example, the design-copying item and mathematical calculations. The MMSE should not be used for persons with less than a ninth grade education or those who are not fluent in English.

Notwithstanding the MMSE's wide acceptability in clinical and research applications and its documented high level of reliability, there have been attempts to increase the test's sensitivity and specificity. One alternative has been to modify the content of the MMSE to exclude particular questions or to add questions that would be more independent of education, age, and cultural variables. One revision modifies content, adds four new test items, and expands the range of scoring, which is 0 to 30, to 0 to 100 (Teng et al., 1987).

The Short Portable Mental Status Questionnaire (SPMSQ) (Table 2-8) consists of 10 questions testing remote memory, awareness of current events, and mathematical ability (Pfeiffer, 1975). This test is part of the multi-

T A B L E   2 - 6
The Physical Performance Test (PPT) Scoring Sheet

	TIME	SCORING	SCORE
1. Write a sentence (Whales live in the blue ocean)	_____sec*	≤10 sec = 4 10.5–15 sec = 3 15.5–20 sec = 2 >20 sec = 1 unable = 0	_____
2. Simulated eating	_____sec	≤10 sec = 4 10.5–15 sec = 3 15.5–20 sec = 2 >20 sec = 1 unable = 0	_____
3. Lift a book and put it on a shelf	_____sec	≤2 sec = 4 2.5–4 sec = 3 4.5–6 sec = 2 >6 sec = 1 unable = 0	_____
4. Put on and remove a jacket	_____sec	≤10 sec = 4 10.5–15 sec = 3 15.5–20 sec = 2 >20 sec = 1 unable = 0	_____
5. Pick up penny from floor	_____sec	≤2 sec = 4 2.5–4 sec = 3 4.5–6 sec = 1 >6 sec = 1 unable = 0	_____
6. Turn 360 degrees	discontinuous steps 0 continuous steps 2 unsteady (grabs, staggers) 0 steady 2		_____
7. 50-foot walk test	_____sec	≤15 sec = 4 15.5–20 sec = 3 20.5–25 sec = 2 >25 sec = 1 unable = 0	_____
8. Climb one flight of stairs†	_____sec	≤5 sec = 4 5.5–10 sec = 3 10.5–15 sec = 2 >15 sec = 1 unable = 0	_____
9. Climb stairs†	Number of flights of stairs up and down (maximum 4)		_____
TOTAL SCORE (maximum 36 for 9-item, 28 for 7-item)			_____ 9-item _____ 7-item

* For timed measurements, round to nearest 0.5 second.
† Omit for 7-item scoring.
From Reuben, D.B., and Siu, A.L. An objective measure of physical function of elderly outpatients: The Physical Performance Test. *J Am Geriatr Soc* 38:1105–1112, 1990.

dimensional OARS (Older Adults Resources and Services) instrument and has been used extensively in elderly people. Each error is scored as 1 point, with intact mental function indicated by less than two errors and severe impairment indicated by eight to ten errors. The scoring is adjusted for educational level, because it was found that this variable introduced bias (Pfeiffer, 1975).

The Neurobehavioral Cognitive Status Examination (NCSE) is a screening test to detect and characterize cognitive dysfunction for geriatric medicine patients (Kiernan et al., 1987; Schwamm et al., 1987). The first part of the test rates a patient's consciousness, attention, and orientation. Then a graded series of questions is asked in each of five areas: language, constructional ability, memory, calculation, and verbal reasoning. Each of the sections begins with a difficult item (called the screen); if the patient answers this item correctly, the particular skill is considered intact and no other questions in this category are asked. If the patient fails the

TABLE 2-7
The Mini-Mental State Examination

Patient _____ Examiner _____ Date _____

Maximum Score	Score	
		ORIENTATION
5	( )	What is the (year) (season) (date) (day) (month)?
5	( )	Where are we (state) (county or neighborhood) (town) (hospital) (floor)?
		REGISTRATION
3	( )	Name 3 objects: 1 second to say each. Then ask the patient all 3 after you have said them. Give 1 point for each correct answer. Then repeat them until he/she learns all 3. Count trials and record.
		Trials _____
		ATTENTION AND CALCULATION
5	( )	Serial 7s. 1 point for each correct answer. Stop after 5 answers. If the patient refuses to *attempt* serial 7s, spell "world" backward.
		RECALL
3	( )	Ask for the 3 objects repeated above. Give 1 point for each correct answer.
		LANGUAGE
2	( )	Name a pencil and watch. (2 points)
1	( )	Repeat the following "No ifs, ands, or buts." (1 point)
3	( )	Follow a 3-stage command: "Take a paper in your hand, fold it in half, and put it on the floor." (3 points)
1	( )	Read and obey the following: CLOSE YOUR EYES. (1 point)
1	( )	Write a sentence. (1 point)
1	( )	Copy design. (1 point)
_____		Total Score
		ASSESS level of consciousness along a continuum _____
		Alert Drowsy Stupor Coma

screen, then a series of questions of graded difficulty are asked. Patients who fail the screen may still demonstrate abilities in the normal range through their performance on these additional items. Test administration is between 5 minutes (in normal patients who answer the screens correctly) to 10 to 20 minutes for patients with impairments. Results are summarized in a profile format rather than a single summary score.

In a geropsychiatric sample, the NCSE was found more effective than the MMSE in distinguishing individuals with organic brain disorders from those with affective disorders, based on the number of clinical subscales yielding scores indicating impairment (La Rue, 1992). In depressed patients with no indication of neurological disorder, only a small proportion scored completely within normal limits; therefore, La Rue recommends using this test in conjunction with additional mental status measures.

In nursing practice in hospital settings, early recognition and intervention for acute confusion and delirium syndromes is recognized as critical in the recovery process. Nurses may rely more on assessment of level of alertness and orientation but overlook reporting other signs of fluctuations in mental status and deterioration in cognitive function (Neelon et al., 1989; Champagne et al., 1987). Delirium may be difficult to recognize because of its fluctuating pattern, presenting symptoms may be mild and difficult to recognize, and symptoms vary significantly from patient to patient. The negative consequences of acute confusion, which are manifested as serious functional impairment, are well established. The use of an assessment tool in clinical practice ensures that early cognitive impairment is detected, findings are communicated among team members, and interventions directed at optimizing cognitive function are implemented.

A clinical nursing instrument for rapid bedside assessment of cognitive and behavioral performance has been developed for primary application in hospitalized elderly

T A B L E 2 - 8
Short Portable Mental Status Questionnaire (SPMSQ)

Instructions: Ask questions 1 through 10 in this list and record all answers. Ask question 4A only if patient does not have a telephone. Record total number of errors based on ten questions.

+	−

1. What is the date today? _____

   Month   Day   Year

2. What day of the week is it? _____
3. What is the name of this place? _____
4. What is your telephone number? _____
4A. What is your street address? _____
   (Ask only if patient does not have a telephone.)
5. How old are you? _____
6. When were you born? _____
7. Who is the President of the U.S. now? _____
8. Who was President just before him? _____
9. What was your mother's maiden name? _____
10. Subtract 3 from 20 and keep subtracting 3 from each new number, all the way down.

_____ Total Number of Errors

Scoring: 0–2 errors = intact mental function
3–4 errors = mild intellectual impairment
5–7 errors = moderate intellectual impairment
8–10 errors = severe intellectual impairment
Allow one more error if subject had only grade school education.
Allow one fewer error if subject has had education beyond high school.

From Pfeiffer, E. A short portable mental status questionnaire for the assessment of organic brain deficit in elderly patients. *J Am Geriatr Soc* 23:433–441, 1975.

patients. The NEECHAM Confusion Scale is a structured database that is derived during routine nursing assessments (Neelon et al., 1989). The NEECHAM evaluates nine information-processing, performance, and vital function items, which are each divided into three levels of assessment (Fig. 2–4). Level 1 evaluates responsiveness to meaningful information: attentiveness, ability to follow complex commands, and orientation and memory. Level 2 evaluates the integrity of sensory-motor behavior and speech. Level 3 evaluates physiological control and stability, including vital functions, oxygenation, and continence (see Box 2–1).

The NEECHAM total score is calculated by adding the scores for the three levels. The range of scores is from 0 (minimal responsiveness) to 30 (normal function). Scores of 0 to 19 indicate moderate to severe confusion, scores of 20 to 24 indicate mild or early development of confusion, and scores above 24 are classified as "not confused." Sensitivity is reported to be 95 per cent, specificity 78 per cent, and predictive value 57 per cent. In another study, sensitivity and specificity were reported at 30 per cent and

92 per cent and the predictive value at 81 per cent (Siemsen, 1992). The overall reliability of the NEECHAM for determining level of confusion is good.

Using the NEECHAM in a study of hospitalized elderly patients, 39.2 per cent demonstrated some level of confusion. In comparison, the Folstein Mini-Mental State Examination detected cognitive impairment in 60 per cent in this sample. This difference could be explained by education level attained by the patients, since education attainment below the eighth grade level is known to influence lower scoring on the MMSE. The NEECHAM is both feasible and clinically useful in the acute care setting.

The Clinical Assessment of Confusion Scale was developed from observations described by nurses about acute confusion in hospitalized older persons (Vermeersch, 1992). The Scale comes in two versions: CAC-A, a 25-item screening instrument, and CAC-B, a 58-item comprehensive assessment with one screening item and seven subscales. The CAC-A addresses five underlying dimensions of confusion: cognition, general behavior, motor activity, orientation, and

NEECHAM CONFUSION SCALE

NAME/ID: _____

DATE: _____ TIME: _____

SCORED BY: _____

LEVEL 1–PROCESSING

PROCESSING–ATTENTION: (Attention–Alertness–Responsiveness)

__4__ Full attentiveness/alertness: responds immediately and appropriately to calling of name or touch—eyes, head turn; fully aware of surroundings, attends to environmental events appropriately.

__3__ Short or hyper attention/alertness: either shortened attention to calling, touch, or environmental events or hyper alert, over-attentive to cues/objects in environment.

__2__ Attention/alertness inconsistent or inappropriate: slow in responding, repeated calling or touch required to elicit/maintain eye contact/attention; able to recognize objects/stimuli, though may drop into sleep between stimuli.

__1__ Attention/alertness disturbed: eyes open to sound or touch; may appear fearful, unable to attend/recognize contact, or may show withdrawal/combative behavior.

__0__ Arousal/responsiveness depressed: eyes may/may not open; only minimal arousal possible with repeated stimuli; unable to recognize contact.

PROCESSING–COMMAND: (Recognition–Interpretation–Action)

__5__ Able to follow a complex command: "Turn on nurse's call light". (Must search for object, recognize object, perform command.)

__4__ Slowed complex command response: requires prompting or repeated directions to follow/complete a complex command. Performs complex command in "slow"/over-attending manner.

__3__ Able to follow a simple command: "Lift your hand or foot, Mr . . . ". (Only use 1 object)

__2__ Unable to follow direct command: follows command prompted by touch or visual cue—drinks from glass placed near mouth. Responds with calming affect to nursing contact and reassurance or hand holding.

__1__ Unable to follow visually guided command: responds with dazed or frightened facial features, and/or withdrawal-resistive response to stimuli, hyper/hypoactive behavior; does not respond to nurse gripping hand lightly.

__0__ Hypoactive, lethargic: minimal motor/responses to environmental stimuli.

PROCESSING–ORIENTATION: (Orientation, Short-term Memory, Thought/Speech Content)

__5__ Oriented to time, place, and person: thought processes, content of conversation or questions appropriate. Short-term memory intact.

__4__ Oriented to person and place: minimal memory/recall disturbance, content and response to questions generally appropriate; may be repetitive, requires prompting to continue contact. Generally cooperates with requests.

__3__ Orientation inconsistent: oriented to self, recognizes family but time and place orientation fluctuates. Uses visual cues to orient. Thought/memory disturbance common, may have hallucinations or illusions. Passive cooperation with requests (cooperative cognitive protecting behaviors).

__2__ Disoriented and memory/recall disturbed: oriented to self/recognizes family. May question actions of nurse or refuse requests, procedures (resistive cognitive protecting behaviors). Conversation content/thought disturbed. Illusions and/or hallucinations common.

__1__ Disoriented, disturbed recognition: inconsistently recognizes familiar people, family, objects. Inappropriate speech/sounds.

__0__ Processing of stimuli depressed: minimal response to verbal stimuli.

LEVEL 2–BEHAVIOR

BEHAVIOR–APPEARANCE:

__2__ Controls posture, maintains appearance, hygiene: appropriately gowned or dressed, personally tidy, clean. Posture in bed/chair normal.

__1__ Either posture or appearance disturbed: some disarray of clothing/bed or personal appearance, or some loss of control of posture, position.

__0__ Both posture and appearance abnormal: disarrayed, poor hygiene, unable to maintain posture in bed.

F I G U R E   2 – 4

The NEECHAM Confusion Scale. (Copyright 1985/1989, Virginia J. Neelon.)

Illustration continued on following page

BEHAVIOR—MOTOR:

_4_ Normal motor behavior: appropriate movement, coordination and activity, able to rest quietly in bed. Normal hand movement.

_3_ Motor behavior slowed or hyperactive: overly quiet or little spontaneous movement (hands/arms across chest or at sides) or hyperactive (up/down, "jumpy"). May show hand tremor.

_2_ Motor movement disturbed: restless or quick movements. Hand movements appear abnormal—picking at bed objects or bed covers, etc. May require assistance with purposeful movements.

_1_ Inappropriate, disruptive movements: pulling at tubes, trying to climb over rails, frequent purposeless actions.

_0_ Motor movement depressed: Limited movement unless stimulated; resistive movements.

BEHAVIOR—VERBAL:

_4_ Initiates speech appropriately: able to converse, can initiate and maintain conversation. Normal speech for diagnostic condition, normal tone.

_3_ Limited speech initiation: responses to verbal stimuli are brief and uncomplex. Speech clear for diagnostic condition, tone may be abnormal, rate may be slow.

_2_ Inappropriate speech: may talk to self or not make sense. Speech not clear for diagnostic condition.

_1_ Speech/sound disturbed: altered sound/tone. Mumbles, yells, swears or is inappropriately silent.

_0_ Abnormal sounds: groaning or other disturbed sounds. No clear speech.

LEVEL 3—PHYSIOLOGIC CONTROL

PHYSIOLOGIC MEASUREMENTS:

Recorded Values: Normals:

_____ Temperature   (36–37°)   _____ Periods of apnea/hypopnea present? 1 = yes, 0 = no

_____ Systolic BP   (100–160)   _____ Oxygen therapy prescribed?

_____ Diastolic BP   (50–90)   0 = no, 1 = yes, but not on, 2 = yes, on now.

_____ Heart Rate [HR]   (60–100)
Regular/Irregular   (circle one)

_____ Respirations   (14–22)   (Count for one full minute)

_____ O_2 sat   (93 or above)

VITAL FUNCTION STABILITY: (Count abnormal SBP and/or DBP as one value; count abnormal and/or irregular HR as one; count apnea and/or abnormal resp. as one; and abnormal temp. as one.)

_2_ BP, HR, TEMP, RESPIRATION within normal range with regular pulse

_1_ Any one of the above in abnormal range

_0_ Two or more in abnormal range

OXYGEN SATURATION STABILITY:

_2_ O_2 sat in normal range (93 or above)

_1_ O_2 sat 90 to 92 or is receiving oxygen

_0_ O_2 sat below 90

URINARY CONTINENCE CONTROL:

_2_ Maintains bladder control

_1_ Incontinent of urine in last 24 hours or has condom cath

_0_ Incontinent now or has indwelling or intermittent catheter or is anuric

_____ LEVEL 1 Score: Processing
(0–14 points)

_____ LEVEL 2 Score: Behavior
(0–10 points)

_____ LEVEL 3 Score: Integrative Physiological Control
(0–6 points)

_____ TOTAL NEECHAM (0–30 points)

Total Score of:	Indicates:
0–19	Moderate to severe confusion
20–24	Mild or early development of confusion
25–26	"Not confused," but at high risk for confusion
27–30	"Not confused," or normal function

F I G U R E   2 – 4   *Continued*

BOX 2-1
Instructions for Scoring the NEECHAM Confusion Scale

The NEECHAM total score range runs from 0 (minimal responsiveness) to 30 (normal function). The NEECHAM has nine scaled items divided into three domains (subscales) of assessment: Cognitive–Information Processing, Behavior and Performance, and Physiological Control. Subscale 1 measures key cognitive functions and is given the greatest weight (0–14). Subscale 2 (0–10) measures behavioral manifestations. Subscale 3 (0–6) is given the least weight, because hospitalized patients in general are likely to have abnormal values on one or more of these items.

Points are assigned for the item level description that represents the patient's response or behavior during the rater's interaction. Accurate scoring of the NEECHAM requires sensitivity to cultural differences and awareness of physical disabilities (visual, hearing, motor, etc.) that may affect the subject's response. The patient need not exhibit every behavior in the item description level to score at that point level, but behavior(s) should be representative. Although some training is required, interrater reliability of professional nurses is good. Data needed to score the NEECHAM can be collected during 10 minutes of routine patient observations and vital sign assessment.

COGNITIVE–INFORMATION PROCESSING

Note patient's level of responsiveness on entering the room—eye contact, recognition, etc.

Note whether patient can maintain attentiveness and understand both verbal and visual information. Does the patient require repeated contact to stay focused or aroused? Do verbal or facial cues suggest understanding of interaction: example: patient anticipates required action by visual cues (open mouth to visual thermometer cue).

Observe for complex or cued command responses. Is patient able to initiate or complete a telephone call or nurse "call" procedure? Depending on the type of system and after initial orientation to procedure, the subject's ability to "call" the nurse can be used as a measure of complex command processing. Observe how the patient would "find and activate call system" (a complex system requires locating the "call instrument," picking it up from bedside table, activating nurse signal among several possible choices, and responding to call-back). Is the task completed with normal speed and without prompting? Can the patient respond only to cued commands (visual or touch cues)?

Orientation and short-term memory can be tapped without typical "Do you know what day/date this is." What part of the day, what meal he/she has eaten, what place this is are examples of information obtained in routine care interaction.

BEHAVIOR AND PERFORMANCE

Score patient's awareness and actions in managing appearance, posture, and position (do not rate routine nursing hygiene care, only patient function).

Are there "hyperactive" movements or purposeless movements? Does the subject show abnormal hand/finger movements—"picking" at sheets?

Differentiate between culturally grounded slow speech and difficulty in speaking, initiating speech, appropriate speech, etc.

PHYSIOLOGICAL CONTROL

The vital signs are scored as defined in the scale. Observe the patient's response and awareness. Does he/she anticipate the procedure and assist or require repeated prompting or cueing?

Oxygen stability is scored by a noninvasive measure of oxygen saturation (pulse oximetry). Note subject's position and whether oxygen is being administered (flow-rate). In place of oximeter measurements, scoring can be done by scoring one point loss for required oxygen therapy and one point loss for the presence of apnea (greater than 15-sec period during a 1-minute observation and more than one observation).

Scoring continence is confounded by clinical care factors as well as by interactive effects of deteriorating cognitive and physical function in those who develop acute confusion. Score as defined in item, but note whether subject needs assistance to toilet, requested help, and whether help was delayed.

Box continued on following page

B O X   2 – 1 *Continued*
Instructions for Scoring the NEECHAM Confusion Scale

SCORING

			Points
Items 1–3	Processing-Attention		= 0–4
	Processing-Command		= 0–5
	Orientation-Memory		= 0–5
			0–14
Items 4–6	Behavior-Appearance		= 0–2
	Behavior-Motor		= 0–4
	Behavior-Verbal		= 0–4
			0–10

27–30 = "Not confused," or normal processing
25–26 = "Not confused," but at risk for confusion
20–24 = Mild or early developing confusional state
0–19 = Moderate to severe confusion

Scores for subjects with severe chronic cognitive impairment may differ from the above ranges (with or without superimposed acute confusional state).

HELPFUL HINTS FOR SCORING THE NEECHAM CONFUSION SCALE

- Score the NEECHAM at the completion of the interaction. Read all scoring options for each item before selecting item score.
- In scoring a patient, it is not uncommon for a 1- or 2-point difference to occur between ratings—a change of more than 2 points is considered clinically significant and warrants a more complete assessment.
- Be creative, develop an approach that is comfortable and gets the necessary information. The key is to be consistent in assessment and scoring.
- Cognitive ability may fluctuate even in a short 15-minute period. Should this occur, score the lowest level observed during the entire interaction.
- Record only what you observe during the present interaction, not what was seen previously.
- Pay attention to the patient's awareness or reaction to surroundings as well as what occurs in your interaction.
- Avoid asking "yes" and "no" questions as the basis for scoring.

Clinician guidelines for the use of the NEECHAM Confusion Scale can be obtained from Virginia J. Neelon, Ph.D., R.N. CB# 7460, University of North Carolina at Chapel Hill, Chapel Hill, NC 27599.

psychotic/neurotic behavior. Items are scored on a weighted scale and summed for a total score. The higher the score, the greater the confusion. The CAC-B Scale includes an item to rate level of consciousness and seven subscales which are rated and summed: cognition, general behavior, motor activity/speech-motor ability/sensory acuity, orientation, behaviors that threaten the safety of the patient, psychotic/neurotic behavior, and ability to interact/perform ADL/speech content. Subscales are summed, and the higher the score, the greater the degree of confusion. Reliability, sensitivity, and validity testing results are not conclusive. Both scales offer a 4-level scoring system to determine the severity of the acute confusion, ranging from possible confusion to severe confusion.

Affective status measurements attempt to differentiate the severe and sustained depression that puts individuals at risk for deteriorating function, self-destructive behavior, and high mortality rates from the saddened mood states common in the whole population (Kane, 1984). Older persons who are depressed may mistakenly be judged to be demented. As a result, inappropriate treatment or lack of treatment may ensue.

Individuals who are depressed may respond to items on mental status examinations by saying "I don't know" and therefore perform poorly. Since many mental status examinations do not differentiate between dementia and depression, "I don't know" responses should be a clue that further assessment is necessary. In addition, inconsistent performance on mental examinations suggests the influence of depression.

A number of screening tools for depression have been validated in older persons, although none have been validated in the "old-old." In older persons with multiple chronic illnesses and functional impairments, the meaning of poor scores can often be uncertain. Nevertheless, depression screening tools can be helpful to detect major depression in older persons, thus opening opportunities for treatment.

The Geriatric Depression Scale (GDS) is a self-rated scale that is frequently used to assist in the diagnosis of depression in medical and geriatric patients. The GDS consists of 30 yes-no items that take approximately 5 minutes to complete (Table 2–9). The GDS has been validated in elderly community and inpatient populations (Yesavage et al., 1983; Koenig et al., 1988) and in community elderly with mild to moderate dementia (Feher et al., 1992). The questions on the GDS focus on the psychological aspects of depression, in contrast to other tools that may also address somatic variables. The accuracy of the GEDS in patients with dementia has been questioned for the reason that memory-impaired patients would not accurately recall depressive symptoms over the recent past. However, it seems that only minimal memory ability is needed for accurate self-report as is required in the GDS, although validity in severely demented patients has not been established (Feher et al., 1992). In patients with dementia who tend to deny deficits in cognitive function, results should be interpreted with caution as depressive symptoms may also be denied (Feher et al., 1992).

The GDS has been found to be feasible, accurate, and acceptable for use in clinical practice (Koenig et al., 1988). At a cut-off score of 11, the 95 per cent confidence intervals for sensitivity and specificity were high, at 84 to 93 per cent. Since the tool is completed by the older person, it might be necessary in some cases to provide further explanation about instructions or to read items from the test.

The Brief Carroll Depression Rating Scale (BCDRS) is a self-administered test that consists of 12 items requiring a yes-no response and takes about 2 minutes to complete (Duke University Center for the Study of Depression in Later Life, 1986). In a comparison study with the GDS, the BCDRS demonstrated the highest sensitivity and specificity at a cut-off score of 6. At this score, a diagnosis of major depression is excluded (Koenig et al., 1988). In comparison with the GDS, Koenig and colleagues determined that

TABLE 2–9
The Geriatric Depression Scale

Instructions to patient: Choose the best answer (yes or no) to each question about how you felt the past week.

1. Are you basically satisfied with your life?
2. Have you dropped many of your activities and interests?
3. Do you feel that your life is empty?
4. Do you often get bored?
5. Are you hopeful about the future?
6. Are you bothered by thoughts you can't get out of your head?
7. Are you in good spirits most of the time?
8. Are you afraid that something bad is going to happen to you?
9. Do you feel happy most of the time?
10. Do you often feel helpless?
11. Do you often get restless and fidgety?
12. Do you prefer to stay at home, rather than going out and doing new things?
13. Do you frequently worry about the future?
14. Do you feel you have more problems with memory than most?
15. Do you think it is wonderful to be alive now?
16. Do you often feel downhearted and blue?
17. Do you feel pretty worthless the way you are now?
18. Do you worry a lot about the past?
19. Do you find life very exciting?
20. Is it hard for you to get started on new projects?
21. Do you feel full of energy?
22. Do you feel that your situation is hopeless?
23. Do you think that most people are better off than you are?
24. Do you frequently get upset over little things?
25. Do you frequently feel like crying?
26. Do you have trouble concentrating?
27. Do you enjoy getting up in the morning?
28. Do you prefer to avoid social gatherings?
29. Is it easy for you to make decisions?
30. Is your mind as clear as it used to be?

Scoring: Score 0 for each item that is "nondepressive" and 1 point for each "depressive" answer ("depressive" answers are no for questions 1, 5, 7, 9, 15, 19, 21, 27, 29, and 30 and yes for all others). Normal score for the aged is 0–10.

From Yesavage, J.A., Brink, T.L., Rose, T.L., et al. Development and validation of a geriatric depression screening scale: A preliminary report. *J Psychiatr Res* 17:37–49, 1983.

this test performed equally as well in ruling out major depression.

The Beck Depression Inventory (Table 2–10) consists of 13 items related to mood, self-image, and somatic complaints that are scored on a 4-point scale according to the degree of severity for each item (Beck and Beck, 1972). The questionnaire is a shortened version of the original 21-item form and can be self-administered or administered by the clinician in about 5 minutes. A score of greater than 16 indicates severe depression, whereas a score of less than 4 represents minimal or no depression. The Beck Depression Inventory has been shown to permit effective discrimination among groups of patients with varying degrees of depression. It also reflects changes in the in-

TABLE 2-10
Beck Depression Inventory, Short Form

Instructions: This is a questionnaire. On the questionnaire are groups of statements. Please read the entire group of statements in each category. Then pick out the one statement in that group that best describes the way you feel today, that is, *right now!* Circle the number beside the statement you have chosen. If several statements in the group seem to apply equally well, circle each one.

Be sure to read all the statements in each group before making your choice.

A. (Sadness)
3 I am so sad or unhappy that I can't stand it.
2 I am blue or sad all the time and I can't snap out of it.
1 I feel sad or blue.
0 I do not feel sad.

B. (Pessimism)
3 I feel that the future is hopeless and that things cannot improve.
2 I feel I have nothing to look forward to.
1 I feel discouraged about the future.
0 I am not particularly pessimistic or discouraged about the future.

C. (Sense of failure)
3 I feel I am a complete failure as a person (parent, husband, wife).
2 As I look back on my life, all I can see is a lot of failures.
1 I feel I have failed more than the average person.
0 I do not feel like a failure.

D. (Dissatisfaction)
3 I am dissatisfied with everything.
2 I don't get satisfaction out of anything anymore.
1 I don't enjoy things the way I used to.
0 I am not particularly dissatisfied.

E. (Guilt)
3 I feel as though I am very bad or worthless.
2 I feel quite guilty.
1 I feel bad or unworthy a good part of the time.
0 I don't feel particularly guilty.

F. (Self-dislike)
3 I hate myself.
2 I am disgusted with myself.
1 I am disappointed in myself.
0 I don't feel disappointed in myself.

G. (Self-harm)
3 I would kill myself if I had the chance.
2 I have definite plans about committing suicide.
1 I feel I would be better off dead.
0 I don't have any thought of harming myself.

H. (Social withdrawal)
3 I have lost all of my interest in other people and don't care about them at all.
2 I have lost most of my interest in other people and have little feeling for them.
1 I am less interested in other people than I used to be.
0 I have not lost interest in other people.

I. (Indecisiveness)
3 I can't make any decisions at all anymore.
2 I have great difficulty in making decisions.
1 I try to put off making decisions.
0 I make decisions about as well as ever.

J. (Self-image change)
3 I feel that I am ugly or repulsive-looking.
2 I feel that there are permanent changes in my appearance and they make me look unattractive.
1 I am worried that I am looking old or unattractive.
0 I don't feel that I look any worse than I used to.

K. (Work difficulty)
3 I can't do any work at all.
2 I have to push myself very hard to do anything.
1 It takes extra effort to get started at doing something.
0 I can work about as well as before.

L. (Fatigability)
3 I get too tired to do anything.
2 I get tired from doing anything.
1 I get tired more easily than I used to.
0 I don't get any more tired than usual.

M. (Anorexia)
3 I have no appetite at all anymore.
2 My appetite is much worse now.
1 My appetite is not as good as it used to be.
0 My appetite is no worse than usual.

Scoring: 0–4 = None or minimal depression
8–15 = Moderate depression
5–7 = Mild depression
16+ = Severe depression

From Beck, A.T., Ward, C.H., Mendelson, M., et al. An inventory for measuring depression. *Arch Gen Psychiatr* 4:561–571, 1961. Copyright 1961, American Medical Association.

Now I'd like to ask you some questions about your family and friends.

Are you single, married, widowed, divorced, or separated?
1 Single 3 Widowed 5 Separated
2 Married 4 Divorced — Not answered

If "2" ask following

Does your spouse live here also?
1 *Yes*
2 *No*
— *Not answered*

Who lives with you?
(Check "yes" or "no" for each of the following.)

Yes	No	
_____	_____	No one
_____	_____	Husband or wife
_____	_____	Children
_____	_____	Grandchildren
_____	_____	Parents
_____	_____	Grandparents
_____	_____	Brothers and sisters
_____	_____	Other relatives (does not include in-laws covered in the above categories)
_____	_____	Friends
_____	_____	Nonrelated paid help (includes free room)
_____	_____	Others (specify) _____

In the past year how often did you leave here to visit your family and/or friends for weekends or holidays or to go on shopping trips or outings?
1 *Once a week or more*
2 *1–3 times a month*
3 *Less than once a month or only on holidays*
4 *Never*
— *Not answered*

How many people do you know well enough to visit with in their homes?
3 Five or more
2 Three to four
1 One to two
0 None
— Not answered

About how many times did you talk to someone—friends, relatives or others—on the telephone in the past week (either you called them or they called you)? (If subject has no phone, question still applies.)
3 Once a day or more
2 Twice
1 Once
0 Not at all
— Not answered

How many times during the past week did you spend some time with someone who does not live with you, that is, you went to see them, or they came to visit you, or you went out to do things together?

How many times in the past week did you visit with someone, either with people who live here or people who visited you here?
3 *Once a day or more*
2 *Two to six*
1 *Once*
0 *Not at all*
— *Not answered*

Do you have someone you can trust and confide in?
2 Yes
0 No
— Not answered

Do you find yourself feeling lonely quite often, sometimes, or almost never?
0 Quite often
1 Sometimes
2 Almost never
— Not answered

Do you see your relatives and friends as often as you want to, or are you somewhat unhappy about how little you see them?
1 As often as wants to
2 Somewhat unhappy about how little
— Not answered

Is there someone *(outside this place)* who would give you any help at all if you were sick or disabled, for example, your husband/wife, a member of your family, or a friend?
1 Yes
0 No one willing and able to help
— Not answered

  If "yes" ask a and b.

a. Is there someone *(outside this place)* who would take care of you as long as needed, or only for a short time, or only someone who would help you now and then (for example, taking you to the doctor, or fixing lunch occasionally, etc.)?

1 Someone who would take care of subject indefinitely (as long as needed)

2 Someone who would take care of subject for a short time (a few weeks to 6 months)

3 Someone who would help subject now and then (taking to the doctor or fixing lunch, etc.)

— Not answered

b. Who is this person?
  Name _____
  Relationship _____

RATING SCALE
Rate the current social resources of the person being evaluated along the 6-point scale presented below. Circle the *one* number that best describes the person's present circumstances.

1. Excellent Social Resources: Social relationships are very satisfying and extensive; at least one person would take care of him (her) indefinitely.

2. Good Social Resources: Social relationships are fairly satisfying and adequate and at least one person would take care of him (her) indefinitely, *or*
Social relationships are very satisfying and extensive, and only short-term help is available.

3. Mildly Socially Impaired: Social relationships are unsatisfactory, of poor quality, few; but at least one person would take care of him (her) indefinitely, *or*
Social relationships are fairly satisfactory and adequate, and only short-term help is available

4. Moderately Socially Impaired: Social relationships are unsatisfactory, of poor quality, few; and only short-term care is available, *or*
Social relationships are at least adequate or satisfactory, but help would only be available now and then.

5. Severely Socially Impaired: Social relationships are unsatisfactory, of poor quality, few; and help would be available only now and then, *or*
Social relationships are at least satisfactory or adequate, but help is not available even now and then.

6. Totally Socially Impaired: Social relationships are unsatisfactory, of poor quality, few; and help is not available even now and then.

Note: Italicized questions apply to those living in institutions.
From Duke University Center for the Study of Aging and Human Development. *Multidimensional Functional Assessment: The OARS Methodology.* Durham, NC: Duke University Press, 1978.

T A B L E   2 – 1 2
Social Dysfunction Rating Scale

Directions: Score each of the items as follows:
1. Not present   3. Mild   5. Severe
2. Very Mild   4. Moderate   6. Very severe

SELF-ESTEEM

1. _____ Low self-concept (feelings of inadequacy, not measuring up to self-ideal)
2. _____ Goallessness (lack of inner motivation and sense of future orientation)
3. _____ Lack of a satisfying philosophy or meaning of life (a conceptual framework for integrating past and present experiences)
4. _____ Self-health concern (preoccupation with physical health, somatic concerns)

INTERPERSONAL SYSTEM

5. _____ Emotional withdrawal (degree of deficiency in relating to others)
6. _____ Hostility (degree of aggression toward others)
7. _____ Manipulation (exploiting of environment, controlling at other's expense)
8. _____ Overdependency (degree of parasitic attachment to others)
9. _____ Anxiety (degree of feeling of uneasiness, impending doom)
10. _____ Suspiciousness (degree of distrust or paranoid ideation)

PERFORMANCE SYSTEM

11. _____ Lack of satisfying relationships with significant persons (spouse, children, kin, significant persons serving in a family role)
12. _____ Lack of friends, social contacts
13. _____ Expressed need for more friends, social contacts
14. _____ Lack of work (remunerative or nonremunerative, productive work activities that normally give a sense of usefulness, status, confidence
15. _____ Lack of satisfaction from work
16. _____ Lack of leisure time activities
17. _____ Expressed need for more leisure, self-enhancing and satisfying activities
18. _____ Lack of participation in community activities
19. _____ Lack of interest in community affairs and activities that influence others
20. _____ Financial insecurity
21. _____ Adaptive rigidity (lack of complex coping patterns to stress)

Patient: _____   Rater: _____   Date: _____

*From Linn, M.W., Sculthorpe, W.B., Evje, M., et al. A social dysfunction rating scale. *J Psychiatr Res* 6:299–306, 1969. Reprinted with permission from Elsevier Science Ltd., Pergamon Imprint, Oxford, England.

tensity of depression over time (Beck and Beck, 1972).

Social Functioning

Measures of social functioning take into consideration two distinctly different dimensions: the social network and social support. Berkman (1983) notes that the social network is defined as the web of social relationships that surrounds a person, including the number and frequency of contacts, the presence of a confidant, the durability of the network, geographical proximity, and reciprocity (mu-

tual helping). Social support is defined as the emotional, instrumental, or financial aid that is obtained from the social network. All social networks do not provide the same degree of support and assistance; therefore some measurement of perceived social support is usually included in social functioning instruments (Blazer, 1982). Social networks tend to be very dynamic, especially so in the elderly who confront many significant life changes. Therefore, repeated assessment is necessary, particularly during stressful circumstances.

Adequate social resources may act as a "buffer" against adverse effects and facilitate independence and functional ability (Cole, 1985), whereas their absence may play a role in disease causation (Berkman, 1983). Luke and associates (1982) found that a low level of social interaction was associated with poor mental functioning and health problems. Findings from a large community-based longitudinal study indicate that people lacking many social and community ties were 2.5 times as likely to die during the follow-up period as those with many ties (Berkman, 1983). Maintaining some level of social contact seems to be an important determinant of health.

The Social Resource Scale (Table 2–11) is a well-known measure of social function. This scale is a part of the Older Adults Resources and Services (OARS) community survey questionnaire. It obtains information about family structure (marital status, living-in companions, frequency of family visits), contact with friends, availability of a confidant, satisfaction with the social interaction pattern, and availability of someone to help if the individual becomes sick or disabled. When the scale is administered to persons in institutions, different questions (noted in italics) are substitued for the standard items that may not apply.

In a study in which data from the OARS survey were used to control for variables, Blazer (1982) found that three parameters in the Social Resources Scale predicted mortality in an elderly community population 30 months after the initial assessment. The three parameters included perceived support, frequency of social contact, and available attachments. Ten potentially confounding variables that could influence mortality, such as physical health status, cognitive functioning, cigarette smoking, stressful life events, and so forth, were controlled in the analysis. By accounting for variables within the physical and social context, possible causes of mortality were statistically controlled. Blazer notes that the influence of emotional status at the time of measurement may contribute to the perception of social support.

The Social Dysfunction Rating Scale (Table 2–12) measures the dysfunctional aspects of adjustment (Linn et al., 1969). Effective coping, problem solving, and adaptive behavior are integral to healthy social functioning. The scale emphasizes the individual's personal and interpersonal behavior pattern by measuring the presences of negative attributes or coping approaches that affect social functioning. The scale assesses social dysfunction within five factors: apathetic detachment, dissatisfaction, hostility, health-finance, and manipulative-dependency and is useful in evaluating treatment outcomes.

Standardized assessment instruments should be used with a specific goal in mind and in accordance with their guidelines for use. Before using instruments, permission from the author may be necessary. Many instruments have detailed instruction manuals to assist practitioners in their use. The strengths, weaknesses, and accuracy of the test being used should be considered, and its use should complement clinical practice (Applegate et al., 1990). Results should be interpreted within the context of other information about the individual. Although much remains to be learned, careful use of instruments that are appropriate to the setting and population being served can result in improved clinical decision making, outcomes, and service delivery.

NURSING ASSESSMENT OF ELDERLY PEOPLE

Nursing Foundations

The purpose of nursing assessment of elderly people is to identify patterns of functioning that deviate from baseline or from accepted standards (norms). A systematic approach is advocated to ensure comprehensiveness and efficiency. Nurses should develop an approach that accommodates their nursing framework, the objectives of the work setting, and the needs of the clients being served. Approaches to comprehensive assessment may vary depending upon the practice setting.

Conducting the Nursing Assessment

Several processes occur simultaneously during an assessment encounter. For example, while discussing with the older person the reason for seeking medical or nursing assistance, the nurse assessor will be using all the senses to evaluate the older person's response to the questions, the ability to articulate concerns, affective mood, sensory-perceptual function, comfort level, overall body integrity, and grooming. At the same time the nurse will modify the interaction style to accommodate sensory-perceptual deficits (through voice modulation and attention to body language), provide support and instill confidence and trust, provide information about health concerns, and provide reinforcement for positive health behaviors. Tentative nursing diagnoses are formulated and areas of further data collection are determined.

Much assessment information is directly accessible to the nurse during patient care encounters. Whenever possible, the nurse should be taking advantage of natural opportunities for gathering data (during the bath, at meals, during transfers), since actual performance is an important assessment finding. In nursing facility and nursing home settings there can be many opportunities, often over a period of days, to collect data.

The assessment encounter also provides the opportunity for the nurse and older person to identify or establish mutual expectations. The nurse can clarify his or her role and responsibilities with regard to the older person's needs and concerns. The older person can be encouraged to discuss strategies for meeting identified needs. The mutual interaction and collaboration between the nurse and the older person fosters the expectation that the client will participate in decision making and care. The client will be in control to the greatest extent possible, with the nurse serving a supportive role. For clients who are not able to articulate their needs or concerns, the nurse serves a supportive and advocacy role, compensating for the client's limitations and, whenever possible, engaging family and friends to assist in assessment. This approach is the beginning of a therapeutic milieu in which client needs are central.

Life review can facilitate the identification of unresolved developmental issues, concerns about role transitions and new living situations, altered social networks, altered health status, and expectations for the future. Life review is adaptive and healing in elderly people, contrary to the negative stereotype that reminiscing is an indication of "living too much in the past" or of being "out of touch with reality." Some guidance from the nurse will keep the life review from dominating the assessment.

Special Considerations

Prior to assessing the older person it is helpful to keep in mind the following points.

COORDINATE. Plan the focus of the assessment, what will be covered, and how the assessment will be conducted. Unless there is an emergency, begin with the person's concerns. Plan for enough time to attain your goals, and match your pace with the older person. Do not expect to cover everything in one encounter; instead, plan for several encounters if possible. Be relaxed and patient. It is helpful to be aware of any special communication barriers (visual decrements, hearing loss, aphasia, impaired cognition) in advance or very early in the interview so that adjustments in communication techniques can be made.

ANTICIPATE. Be alert to signs and symptoms of medical illness presenting in atypical fashion. Plan to screen for problems that have high prevalence in the aged with an impact on functional ability (e.g., dysmobility, cataracts, urinary incontinence, falls, polypharmacy, acute confusion). To compensate for anxiety that may interfere with formal testing (for example, in the mental status examination), establish rapport by recognizing the person's concerns. Introduce testing techniques by explaining how the information will help individualize the person's care.

MANIPULATE. Modify the environment to match the older person's needs. In the surrounding physical environment, reduce noise levels (especially "white noise" generated from activity in hallways, other people in the room, television, radio, outdoor noise, intercoms). Ensure a comfortable temperature, adequate space and lighting, and privacy.

To enhance the person's ability to engage fully in the encounter, consider the personal factors involved such as comfort and communication. Enhance comfort by positioning the older person comfortably or assisting him or her to sit in an upright position if in bed to promote vision and eye contact, hearing, and alertness. Inquire about pain, thirst, and the need to use the toilet (and intervene beforehand or reschedule the interview if possible). Face the client to allow for lip reading. Make sure assistive devices, including hearing aids and glasses, are on (and in good working order). Hand-held voice amplifiers can be valuable equipment for the nurse to use with hearing-impaired persons. They are easily obtained and are relatively inexpensive. Proceed in a relaxed pace, and do not rush the interaction. Be patient! Maximize the use of silence to allow the person to collect his or her thoughts in order to formulate and answer questions or verbalize concerns.

DEMONSTRATE. Have the older person demonstrate skills such as activities of daily living and instrumental activities of daily living when indicated. For example, watch the person drink a glass of water, eat, get dressed, and walk. Observe communication patterns with others. Direct observation is the most reliable method of data collection.

VALIDATE. Check information obtained from the older person with other persons such as family members, nursing staff, physician, to elicit their perception of the older person's health problems, concerns, and

TABLE 2–13

First-Level Approach: Introduction and Client/Nurse Appraisal of Problems and Concerns

APPROACH	PROCESS COMMENTS
Approach the client: note appearance, posture, spontaneous activity, grooming, hygiene, comfort, presence of others, facial expression, attentiveness, interest	Cues gathered about musculoskeletal, neurological, GU, GI, cardiovascular, and pulmonary systems, cognitive and emotional function, senses, social support
Address the client by name. Introduce self: "My name is . . . I prefer to be called . . . What do you like to be called?"	Hearing. Ability to respond to social situation, cues about cognitive and effective function
Offer to shake hands or grasp client by the hand	Neuromuscular function, strength, skin temperature, texture
Establish eye contact, ask about visual ability and use of glasses. Position self in full view of client. Adjust lighting for brightness but avoid glare	Vision
Ask about any hearing difficulties and if client can hear you clearly. Ask about use of hearing aid, lip reading, better hearing in one ear over the other	Cues about hearing and cognitive function
"How are you feeling today?" If a clinic visit, "What brings you here today?" or "Is anything troubling you lately?" Probe specifically with open-ended questions, e.g., "Oh, you're hurting, tell me more about that."	Self-assessment of health, symptoms assessment, cognitive and verbal function, communication skills, optimism, emotional response
"What would you like help with today?" Note the issues identified and the order of concerns	Cues about client's priorities, expectations, response to health or social problems or concerns
Summarize the interaction so far. "Mrs. J., we have approximately 45 minutes together to address your concerns. I think that will give us time to deal with the concerns you have voiced. I would like to proceed now by asking you a few more questions and then do the following examination procedures for these reasons."	Establish trust, contract for and set mutual expectations for the encounter, prioritize concerns, validate inferences with the client

functional status. Also, validation with an objective data source such as the medical record is helpful. This helps increase the accuracy of the data.

REPEAT. Assess at more than one encounter and at different times of the day. Older persons have "good" days and "bad" days, and in some cases assessing at different times of the day can yield different results. For example, early morning stiffness or pain or late afternoon and evening fatigue can negatively affect performance of activities of daily living in a way that is not characteristic of the person's usual functioning and manner of compensation. Also, the older person may not feel wholly cooperative in the assessment encounter if not feeling at his or her best.

Four-Level Nursing Assessment

Although traditional methods of assessment tend to include the history, physical examination, and laboratory and diagnostic data, "examining room" assessments rarely include the kinds of information that give the nurse clues to the actual client situation (Wolanin, 1980). Examinations can produce anxiety in the elderly, and since examinations are often conducted in unfamiliar environments, the situation can even be threatening. Direct observation of performance of activities of daily living is imperative. Each level of the assessment progressively focuses on the impact of aging, health issues, and developmental alterations in the biological, social, and psychological domains of the individual. Nursing assessment guides the determination of nursing diagnosis and appropriate nursing intervention.

First-Level Assessment

The first level of assessment is the introductory, or "first impression," phase of the encounter. The nurse observes the older person's overall appearance and physical function, sensory function, and the ability to communicate. General signs and symptoms are observed. Key issues and concerns are elicited from the client, and mutual expectations concerning the conduct of the assessment and the solution of problems are outlined. As a result, the assessment may become targeted in certain areas, stemming from the "chief complaint." At this point, problem areas for which careful attention is warranted may become evident, serving as a focal point in future assessment. Table 2–13 describes some of the approaches the nurse can use in the first-level

assessment. This introductory encounter provides cues about potential sensory and cognitive deficits, general health status and concerns or problems, social support, and expectations for care.

Second-Level Assessment

The second level of assessment involves the use of screening techniques to detect functional impairments. Screening is based on the principle that most human functioning can be described hierarchically. It is possible to infer integrity of some body systems by observing intact function in tasks that require the integration of several systems. For example, intact neuromuscular functioning is necessary in order to feed oneself. The ability to perform this task without difficulty indicates integrity of several cranial nerves (specifically II, IX, X) and the peripheral nerves innervating the upper extremity, good range of motion of upper extremity, hand-eye coordination, fine motor coordination, vision, judgment, and the ability to follow simple commands.

Those who are "screened in" are subject to further assessment to determine whether the diagnosis is valid. The sensitivity of a test refers to the percentage of persons with the problem or risk factor who are correctly identified by the test. A test that is extremely sensitive will identify both those persons who have the diagnosis and some who do not. The specificity of a test measures the degree to which the noncases score as negative. Ideally, a screening test correctly identifies most of the patients who have the diagnosis (high sensitivity) with a minimum of false-positives (high specificity). It is important to note that the sensitivity and specificity of a screening test may vary according to the conditions under which the test is administered.

Screening techniques serve to uncover problems that are not already diagnosed or that place an individual at high risk because of the high prevalence and morbidity associated with the problem. Screening is a parsimonious task. Screening measures tend to be brief, containing only essential diagnostic information. Further diagnostic evaluation is necessary, however, to confirm the problem and etiology. The techniques in Table 2–14 address general function in a natural environment, emphasizing the integration of systems. Table 2–15 identifies screening techniques targeting significant impairments associated with functional health patterns. Rationale and implications of screening for

T A B L E   2 – 1 4
Screening Techniques Useful in Various Settings

TECHNIQUE	PURPOSE
"Take off your shoes"	Mobility, agility, vision, fine motor coordination, support network, complex task
"Show me your medicines"	Vision, over-the-counter and prescription medications, memory, literacy, compliance
Set test	Cognition, alternate thought process
Remember three objects	Cognition, alternate thought process
Face-hand test	Describe brain pathology
Genogram	Describe support network, altered family process
Orthostatic BPs	Potential for injury, fall
"What do you do for enjoyment?"	Anhedonia, depression
"Describe a typical day"	Diversional activities deficit, self-care deficit

physical health problems are listed in Table 2–16.

Screening for medical problems for which available and effective interventions exist is advocated in elderly people as a health promotion and health maintenance strategy (Sloane, 1984). Recommended screening procedures are listed in Table 2–17. Screening for psychosocial impairments may be more difficult. Kane and Kane (1981) suggest that periodic detailed assessment may be more appropriate. Screening for risk factors, such as bereavement, living alone, absence of a confidant or someone to turn to in an emergency, substance abuse, or caregiver stress can be followed by in-depth assessment.

Third-Level Assessment

The third level of assessment involves using a comprehensive nursing assessment framework to collect specific data systematically in the biological, social, and psychological domains. Comprehensive nursing assessment assures that baseline data in each area of function are collected. The comprehensive assessment may also serve to rule in or rule out potential problems hypothesized earlier in the encounter. Data are organized into 11 categories, or functional health patterns (Gordon, 1982).

This level of assessment helps validate the objective and subjective findings to determine the nursing diagnoses. For example, the cue (the objective or subjective finding or observation) collected about mobility, such as not being able to bend down to take off shoes, leads to the inference (the nurse's interpretation of the meaning of the cue)

that activities of daily living and self-care may be impaired. Inferences and cues are validated during the comprehensive third-level assessment to determine the causes of and contributing factors to functional impairments.

Health Perception–Health Management
HISTORY/INTERVIEW

1. "How would you describe your health?"
2. "Describe the health problems you are having now and how they are being managed (diet, medications, exercise or activity limitations, therapy, and so on)." Consider the overall degree of disability observed in the client relative to the health problems and medical diagnoses identified by the client or obtained from the health record.
3. Elicit understanding of health problems and rationale for management.
4. Elicit information about medication usage, reason for use, side and toxic effects, and monitoring tasks.
5. Ask about management of health problems and any difficulty carrying out regimen. If treatment plan is not consistently carried out, does client understand risks?
6. "Are there things you would like to do but can't because of your health or medical problems?" Elicit the impact of health problems and treatment modalities on functioning. Is client satisfied with health outcomes?
7. If the individual lives at home, is he or she able to maintain the home and perform instrumental activities of daily living? Is assistance available to perform those things the individual is unable to accomplish?

OBJECTIVE ASSESSMENT

1. Observe for indicators of effective management related to special care measures (e.g., diet, skin care, glucose monitoring, toxic drug effects, smoking cessation, exercise, weight control, and so on).
2. Observe the environment for potentially hazardous conditions. Note floor surfaces, clutter, lighting, condition of appliances, heating system, presence of vermin, food storage, cleanliness, steps and uneven surfaces, and location and condition of bathroom.

Nutritional–Metabolic Pattern
HISTORY/INTERVIEW

1. Obtain food intake profile: 24-hour or 3-day diary to determine RDA equivalents;

TABLE 2-15
Functional Health Patterns Screening Assessment

FUNCTIONAL PATTERN	ASSESSMENT SCREEN	ABNORMAL TRIGGER	TARGETED ASSESSMENT
Health Perception–Health Management Pattern	"Have you experienced a major illness in the past year?"	Yes	Further assessment on impact and management of health condition.
	"Have you had a fall in the past?"	History of a fall	Administer fall risk assessment.
	"Do you smoke or drink alcohol?"	Yes	Assess health habits and identify health promotion opportunities.
	"Do you take more than 3 medications?"	Yes	Review medication list for polypharmacy, polyprovider, adverse effects
Nutritional Pattern	Height, weight, body mass index (BMI) measurement	BMI above or below normal range	Nutritional assessment
	"What did you have to eat and drink yesterday? Do you eat fewer than two meals per day or find you don't always have money to buy food?"	Oral intake and nutritional resources inadequate	
Elimination Pattern	"Do you ever lose urine or wet on yourself?" "Do you ever wear pads for protection?"	Responds yes to questions, or observation suggests incontinence may be a problem	Bowel and bladder elimination assessment
	"Do you use a laxative or enema more than once per month?"		
Activity–Exercise Pattern	Lower extremities: "Rise from a chair, walk 10 feet, turn around, walk back, sit down."	Gait, balance, pace postural stability abnormal	Administer Katz Index of ADL Scale, Short-FIM
	Upper extremities: "Comb your hair; reach for the book off the bookshelf and hand it to me."	Inability to walk or transfer or perform simple maneuvers	
	"Do you have trouble with making meals, shopping, housekeeping, transportation?"	Yes	Full IADL assessment
	"Do you have trouble with stairs inside or outside your home?"	Yes	Home environment assessment
Cognitive–Perceptual Pattern	Depression: "Do you feel sad or depressed? If yes, have you felt this way for longer than 2 weeks?"	Yes	Administer Geriatric Depression Scale
	Cognitive impairment: "I am going to name three objects. I will ask you to remember these names now, and repeat them in a few minutes."	Failure to name objects	Administer Folstein Mini-Mental State Exam
	Vision: Test vision using eye chart.	Vision less than 20/70 with corrective lenses	Referral to ophthalmologist
	Hearing: Whisper test: From behind, whisper a word or short sentence in each ear and have patient repeat.	Incorrect response	Check ears for cerumen, irrigate if necessary, retest. Referral to audiologist
Sleep–Rest Pattern	"Do you have trouble falling asleep, sleeping well, or feeling rested when you wake up?"	Yes	In-depth sleep assessment
Self-perception–Self-concept Pattern	"Do you ever experience pain?" "If yes, are you able to manage the pain so you can meet your needs?"	Yes; pain not well managed	Administer Visual Analogue Pain Scale
Role–Relationship Pattern	"Who would help you in case you became ill, or in an emergency?"	Lack of social resource and friend or confidant	Initiate in-depth assessment of social network, Social Resource Scale
	"Who do you talk to on a regular basis?"		
Sexuality–Reproductive Pattern	"Are you having any difficulty with intimacy or sexuality?"	Yes	Initiate in-depth assessment
Coping–Stress Tolerance Pattern	"Have you experienced a crisis in the past 2 years? If yes, was it resolved to your satisfaction? Is there unresolved conflict?"	Yes	Initiate further assessment of coping patterns
Value–Belief Pattern	"Are you experiencing conflict with regard to spirituality or your beliefs?"	Yes	Further assessment of spirituality and life meaning

T A B L E   2 – 1 6
Screening for Physical Health Problems

PARAMETER	RATIONALE	IMPLICATIONS
Number of medications	Incidence of adverse drug reactions increases with number of medications taken	Can be used as a criterion for in-depth review of patient Consult with pharmacist, nurse, or physician
Falls	Falls can be an early indicator of a variety of physical problems Falls can indicate that the person is having problems with changing physical, sensory, and mental abilities Falls can lead to serious health problems and death	People with history of recurrent falls are good candidates for in-depth review If facility has large number of falls or fall-related injuries: Examine potential environmental contributors more closely, e.g., restraint use, mobility programs, lighting, physical barriers, etc. Examine records for evidence of in-depth assessment for intrinsic factors contributing to falls, e.g., drugs, muscle weakness, vision impairment
Sleep disturbance	Insomnia may signal major physical or mental illnesses Nighttime wakefulness can be a problem for caregivers and can precipitate early institutionalization Bad sleep habits may lead to overuse and abuse of sleeping medications	Recent changes in sleep habits should be evaluated
Visual disturbance	Visual changes often have gradual onset Vision should be checked every 2 years or when new symptoms of visual disturbance are identified Some visual disorders can be controlled IF they are identified early Problems with depth perception can result in falls	Patients who complain of visual disturbance should have some evidence in their records of more in-depth evaluation of the problem Observe staff or family interacting with visually impaired patients. Their verbal and nonverbal behavior should indicate that they are aware that the individual has a disturbance and that they know how to help the individual compensate
Hearing difficulty	Over 60 per cent of those over the age of 70 years have some impairment in hearing ability Hearing loss is not usually identified by the older person Information is generally MISheard not UNheard. Consonants are the first sounds to be lost Changes in behaviors can be an early signal of hearing impairment	During the course of the interview, vary the level and pitch of your voice; note any changes in ability to comprehend your questions Early in the interview, make sure you ask an open-ended question to determine whether the person is following the conversation If you note problems with hearing, determine whether efforts have been made to obtain a hearing evaluation, using staff interview or record review
Fatigue	Tiredness or weakness may be the only symptom of a major illness for some older people Dietary deficiencies and adverse drug effects can cause tiredness Many chronic and acute illnesses cause disturbances in sleep patterns	Complaints of excessive tiredness, weakness, or fatigue should be evaluated for their etiology; consult with physician, nurse, dietitian, and/or pharmacist
Forgetfulness	Complaints of forgetfulness are more indicative of depression but may signal the onset of delirium or dementia Forgetfulness and problems with memory or planning daily activities can escalate and result in major physical or emotional health problems Problems with remembering important information are NOT a normal part of aging	Try to determine the nature of the memory impairment and seek validation If memory deficits are clearly identifiable, then historical data may not be accurate; try to validate information with impartial observer, when possible Look for documentation of baseline mental function; if the staff or family does not know baseline mental function, it is not possible to detect changes in cognitive function, often the first (or only) sign of serious underlying disease
Pain	Complaints of pain are NOT common for the elderly Complaints of pain often signal the onset of a new disease or worsening of an existing problem Many new medications are now available to manage chronic pain New pain is usually symptomatic of a new health problem Pain limits functional abilities and causes excessive dependence	A plan for chronic pain management should be in evidence for all patients who complain of such Acute pain should be evaluated carefully for etiology. This should be reflected in the record Observe how PRN medications are used. Does the patient always have to ask? Needs for medication (particularly in cognitively impaired patients) should be anticipated by caregivers and pain medication or other comfort techniques offered, particularly after an acutely painful episode

T A B L E   2 – 1 6 *Continued*
Screening for Physical Health Problems

PARAMETER	RATIONALE	IMPLICATIONS
Extremes in weight	Rapid weight loss can be an indicator of cancer Rapid weight changes may signal the onset of depression Weight changes may signal the onset of worsening chronic illnesses or an acute episode of disease Weight changes also may indicate a change in ability to eat, or in the availability of helpers to assist in or supervise eating	Extremes in weight should be noted and information on whether or not weight has changed over the last 3 months should be obtained If there have been weight gains or losses of more than 5 pounds per month, THEN refer to dietitian or RN for evaluation of adequacy of assessment and treatment plan
Extreme difficulty getting about (walking, transferring)	Inability to move about poses a safety hazard. It also places the older person at risk for the many hazards associated with immobility Inability to walk is often remediable, sometimes the result of deconditioning, chronic disease, lack of equipment or helpers, or fear of falling after one fall Use of a wheelchair is NOT necessarily an indicator of nonambulatory status	Observe transfer or patient being ambulated Interview staff regarding current exercise regimen Obtain consultation from RN about adequacy of assessment and treatment plan and presence of hazards of immobility
Smell of urine or feces	Incontinence is *not* a part of normal aging. There are *many* remediable causes of incontinence, both psychological and physical All patients deserve evaluation and treatment for this problem	Try to determine length of problem and whether or not the problem has been evaluated in-depth, through interview or record review. THEN Consult with RN to determine whether the evaluation and treatment program are adequate
Observation of wetness	The inability to control urine may be a result of inaccessible toilet areas or discomfort about asking for assistance OR it may signal a problem with mental ability to anticipate the need to go or to sense voiding is occurring. Incontinence is *not* a part of normal aging. There are *many* remediable causes of incontinence, both psychological and physical All patients deserve evaluation and treatment for this problem	Note the general reaction or response of the older person and the caregiver to the incident. This is needed in further assessment of the nature of the problem Determine duration of problem and whether it has been evaluated in-depth previously, through use of interview and record review. THEN Consult with nurse relative to the adequacy of evaluation and management plan
Dried stool or soiling	The ability to toilet oneself is a marker of general self-care abilities Slovenly appearance or stool on clothing can be a strong indicator of depression, dementia, abuse, poor home environment, or a variety of other problems that require intervention	Evaluate the mental abilities of the person. If they are intact, then begin to ascertain the nature and duration of incontinence Consult with RN regarding adequacy of evaluation and management plan
Extreme shortness of breath	Difficulty with breathing with conversation is not normal and is indicative of a major medical problem Shortness of breath can be one of the few symptoms of infection or acute illness in the elderly	Anyone experiencing shortness of breath during the course of an interview should be assessed to evaluate the adequacy of the current treatment regimen
Bruises	Many older people bruise easily Many older people cannot identify how they got bruised Bruises CAN indicate rough handling and signal early signs of abuse Bruises can also indicate repeated falls or problems with mobility Bruises can additionally indicate the need for environmental modifications to improve safety Extensive bruising can also result from medication side effects and may require readjustment of regimens	If bruises are noted on the extremities, try to determine how the bruising occurred If the older person cannot tell you, ask family members, if available, or staff If there are other markers of possible abuse or neglect, investigate this possibility more thoroughly Consult another team member for further assessment and validation of findings
Burns	Scalds and blisters are often the result of water heaters that are too hot, or cooking accidents	Should lead to evaluation of water temperature, bathing procedures

From Snow, T.L., and McConnell, E.S. *Program on Aging,* School of Medicine, Chapel Hill, NC: University of North Carolina, 1986.

TABLE 2-17
Screening in the Elderly

HISTORY AND PHYSICAL EXAMINATION
Cancer-related check-up: yearly after age 40, includes physical examination for cancer of the thyroid, breasts, testicles, prostate, lymph nodes, skin and oral cavity; digital rectal exam; pelvic examination of all women; and health counseling
Assessment of physical, social, and psychological function: every 2 years until age 75, then annually

TESTS AND PROCEDURES
Mammography: yearly at least through age 75 years
Pap smears: regularly until age 65 years, then every 3 to 5 years
Stools for occult blood: yearly; flexible sigmoidoscopy every 3 to 5 years for average-risk individuals, barium enema every 3 to 5 years for those at high risk
Blood pressure: at every visit to provider, at least yearly
Vision examination and tonometry for glaucoma: every 2 years
Hearing examination: at every visit to provider
Thyroid assay: every 2 years
Measurement of height, weight: every visit to provider, at least yearly

DISCRETIONARY STUDIES
Blood hemoglobin
Serum protein and albumin
Tuberculin test
Urine cytology
Audiometry
Dental examination

From Eddy, D.M. Screening the "well elderly" (letter). CA 36: 318-339, 1986; and Sloane, P.D. How to maintain the health of independent elderly. *J Am Geriatr Soc* 39:93-104, 1984.

determine food preferences, cultural traditions, and knowledge of dietary needs.

2. Does client have difficulty ingesting food: chewing, salivating, altered taste sensation, swallowing, regurgitation, stomach fullness, bloating, impaired manual dexterity (paresis, weakness, joint pain or deformity, tremors), impaired cognition, fatigue?

3. Are there any foods the client is unable to eat (dairy products, food allergies, salted food) or must eat (potassium- or calcium-rich food)?

4. Has client experienced a recent (past 6 months) weight gain or loss? Is body mass index abnormal—above 27 or below 22?

5. Does fluid intake approximate 1 cup of liquid per 20 pounds of weight (include between-meal beverages and foods with high water content)?

6. Does any aspect of underlying illnesses, medical treatment, or environmental factors affect intake?

OBJECTIVE ASSESSMENT

1. Note general appearance: observe for dry skin, muscle weakness, pale conjunctiva, agitation or confusion, lethargy. Note condition of mouth, tongue, mucous membranes, gums, and teeth.

2. Note weight above or below 10 to 20 per cent of ideal weight for height and body frame. Is nutritional intake adequate to meet metabolic needs?

3. Observe client eating a meal: note actual intake, food preferences, ability to feed self and swallow food, enjoyment in eating, position and comfort, time needed to finish the meal, any encouragement needed.

4. Assess skin color, temperature, and sensation. Note skin turgor, dryness or excessive oiliness, flaking, bruises, lacerations, moles, lesions, rashes, discolorations.

5. Note alterations such as a stoma, incision, fistula, skin graft, or pressure sores. Note skin integrity, evidence of poor healing or infection, tissue granulation, circulation, and odor.

6. Observe oral mucous membranes for dryness, cracking, bleeding, ulcers, infection.

Elimination
HISTORY/INTERVIEW (URINARY)

1. Inquire about recent pattern of urinary elimination. Is there a recent change or problem in frequency, amount, dysuria, urgency, nocturia, urinary incontinence?

2. Elicit beliefs about relationship between fluid intake or medication (particularly diuretic and anticholinergic) and urinary frequency.

3. Has urinary dysfunction affected socialization and quality of life?

OBJECTIVE ASSESSMENT

1. Palpate for distended bladder, observe urine character, amounts, color, specific gravity, sedimentation, blood, protein, glucose, leukocytes, nitrite.

2. Note evidence of renal or urinary tract problem: check for fever, abdominal pain, chills, dysuria, constipation/fecal impaction, hematuria, heavy sedimentation in urine, anuria, strong odor to urine. Obtain urine specimen for culture and sensitivity if UTI is suspected.

3. In men, rectal examination to palpate for enlarged prostate, rectal tone. Note force of urine stream, hesitancy, volume, postvoid dribbling. In women, rectal examination to note rectal tone. Examine external genitalia. In women, observe for vaginal prolapse, urethritis, atrophic vaginitis, vaginal discharge.

4. Initiate voiding record for several days, documenting voiding times, amounts, whether continent or incontinent, and assistance and/or equipment needed when using the toilet. Do problem-focused assessment to differentiate further the type of incontinence. Check postvoid residual when bladder emptying problem is suspected.

5. Identify contributing factors to incontinence: medications, impaired mobility, fecal impaction, dehydration, urinary tract infection, unfamiliar environment, cognitive impairment, lack of timely assistance, pain, depression, psychological reaction, new medical problem resulting in weakness.

HISTORY/INTERVIEW (BOWEL)

1. Describe bowel function: frequency, amount, consistency, diameter and size of bowel movements, fecal incontinence, and any pain or discomfort when passing stools. Obtain laxative use history.

2. Is fluid and dietary fiber intake adequate?

3. Inquire about past and current bowel problems: constipation, impaction, hemorrhoids, anal fissures, diarrhea, fecal incontinence, flatus. What are expectations for bowel habits?

OBJECTIVE ASSESSMENT

1. Rectal examination: presence/absence of stool, consistency, guaiac testing, presence of hemorrhoids, fissure, sphincter tone, fecal incontinence.

2. Abdominal examination: palpate for masses, tenderness; auscultate for bowel sounds; percuss for dullness or tympany.

3. Observe, when possible, actual intake of food and fluid and compare with reported intake and calculated need of client.

Activity–Exercise
HISTORY/INTERVIEW

1. Ask the individual to recall a "typical" day's activities and a recent day's activities within the past week to determine alterations in habits or activities. Ask about activity patterns, meals, out-of-house activities, sleep adequacy and rest periods, socialization, interests, hobbies. Inquire about instrumental activities of daily living: telephoning, housekeeping, grocery shopping, meal preparation, doing laundry.

2. Inquire about the client's usual exercise/activity pattern and any limitations or changes.

3. Ascertain history of altered tissue perfusion: high blood pressure, heart trouble, angina, dizziness, edema, numbness or tingling in extremities, coldness in extremities, claudication.

4. Obtain respiratory history of symptoms: cough, dyspnea, sputum, orthopnea, previous infection, smoking history, allergies, environmental pollution.

5. Elicit client's beliefs about value of activity/exercise.

6. Has the individual had a fall(s) in the past year? Did injury result? Does fear of falling interfere with mobility pattern? Has previous fall(s) resulted in a higher degree of functional impairment due to pain, injury, weakness, and so on?

7. Does client have outside interests or hobbies that provide enjoyment and diversion? Any recent changes in diversional activities? If new health problems limit continuing participation in hobbies, can client identify other areas of interest to pursue?

OBJECTIVE ASSESSMENT

1. Vital signs at rest, after moderate activity (such as dressing or bathing), and vigorous activity (such as walking a long distance or after exercising). Check the blood pressure in three positions: supine, sitting, and standing. A greater than 20 mm Hg drop in systolic pressure is significant for orthostasis. Check apical-radial and peripheral pulses.

2. Observe respiratory pattern (rate, depth, rhythm, type), nasal flaring, cyanosis, asymmetrical chest expansion. Auscultate lungs and note crackles, wheezes, diminished sounds. Assess coughing pattern and sputum.

3. Assess range of motion: active or passive, in all joints. Note stiffness, pain, limited range, contractures, or deformities.

4. Inspect muscles for symmetry, mass, tremor, spasm, strength.

5. Assess balance (sitting and standing), standing and transfer ability, and gait. Have individual walk 15 feet and note stability, posture, endurance, and pace. Note safe use of adaptive equipment or whether equipment may be indicated.

6. Assess self-care in feeding, dressing, bathing, toileting, transferring, and instrumental activities (such as telephoning, housekeeping, grocery shopping). Determine level of independence and types of assistance needed. Also elicit the kind of direct care needed.

7. Are there mechanical restrictions of movement: casts, splints, traction, incisions, restraints, IV lines, catheters, ventilators? Does client maneuver safely within the confines of the mechanical restriction?

Sleep–Rest Pattern
HISTORY/INTERVIEW

1. Inquire about usual bedtime, arousal time, and nap frequency and duration. Ask about any difficulty getting to sleep, staying asleep, nightmares, quality of sleep. Ask about pain as an inhibitor of restful sleep. Any recent change in sleep pattern?

2. Ask about sleeping aids and bedtime rituals: television, music, warm bath, food, drugs, alcohol, and so on. Inquire about the qualities of the environment.

3. Inquire about client's expectations regarding sleep and understanding about altered sleep patterns with aging.

OBJECTIVE ASSESSMENT

1. Keep a sleep/wake diary to record naps, bedtime, nighttime sleeping duration, how rested person feels when awakening, daytime lethargy, dreams or nightmares, nighttime awakenings (nocturia, pain, dreams, worries, noise), effectiveness of bedtime aids. Does environment (noise, lights, restraints, roommate, and so on) affect sleep?

2. For sleep difficulties, observe the individual (or ask family member to observe) while sleeping, noting positioning, movement, restlessness, periods of wakefulness, snoring, apnea, talking, and efforts to get out of bed.

3. Observe for adverse impact of sleeping patterns or sleep medication functioning (daytime naps, lethargy, irritability).

Cognitive–Perceptual Pattern
HISTORY/INTERVIEW

1. Inquire about any difficulties with communication: articulating words, forming ideas, sensory deficits, language barriers, memory impairment, information processing and comprehension.

2. Ask about adequacy of sensory function and any recent changes: vision, hearing, tactile (temperature, sensitivity), smell, taste.

3. Have drugs and other therapies interfered with communication pattern, senses, memory and/or cognition?

4. Have there been any recent changes in cognitive abilities? Does cognitive impairment affect client's ability to manage obligations such as managing money or keeping track of personal belongings? Is there risk for injury when left alone (fire, wandering)?

5. Does individual exhibit an understanding of own aging, health issues, medications and treatments, and self-care requirements for health promotion? Has a new health problem evolved requiring new information for self-care?

OBJECTIVE ASSESSMENT

1. Note the usual pattern of communication: verbosity, content, quality of speech (tone, pitch, pace, dialect, slurring, stuttering, and so on), language barrier, aphasia, eye contact.

2. Note client's comprehension (ability to follow commands or content of speech of others) and spontaneity in responding to verbal interaction.

3. Administer mental status screening examination to evaluate cognitive function.

4. Note situational factors that affect communication and cognition: pain, environment (sensory deprivation or overload, relocation), impaired mobility, metabolic alterations (fluid and electrolyte imbalance), surgery, sensory deficits, drugs, anxiety and fear, sleep deprivation, grief, psychological disorder.

5. Assess sensory function.

Vision. Can individual read large and small print in the newspaper? See the numbers on a clock 20 feet away? Use a hand-held Snellen chart (Fig. 2–5)? Can the client identify numbers, with or without glasses or contact lenses, to 20/70 at least? When was individual's last eye examination? Any visual field defects, change in central or peripheral vision, hemianopia, decreased acuity, poor night vision? Can individual distinguish between blue-green and red-yellow?

Olfaction. Can individual smell the scent of a flower as she or he used to? Differentiate smells such as lemon, menthol, coffee, vinegar?

Auditory. Can individual hear low-pitched and high-pitched voices equally well? Have individual repeat three numbers or objects after first whispering them and then repeating them in a normal tone of voice (using two different sets of numbers or objects). Any complaint of ringing in the ears? When was the last hearing test? Does individual use a hearing aid? Is it kept in good working order? When is it used?

Tactile. Can individual distinguish between heat and cold, dull and sharp? Any numbness, tingling, or paresthesia in the extremities?

Gustatory. Does individual need to season food liberally? Have food preferences changed related to changes in taste? Can in-

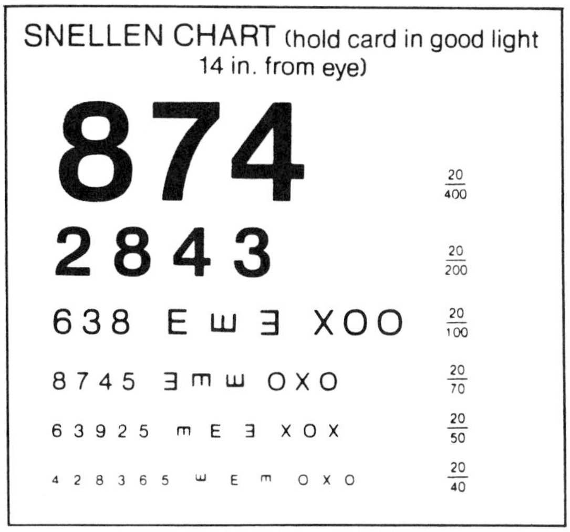

FIGURE 2-5

Vision assessment guide.

dividual distinguish between salty, sweet, and bitter flavors?

Kinesthetic. Does individual experience one-sided neglect related to hemiparesis? Have individual close eyes, then place person's extremities in different positions, asking him or her to describe the location and position of the extremity.

Observe effectiveness of pain-coping measures on behavior, verbalization of comfort, participation in self-care and activities, and social interaction pattern.

Emotional Reactions

HISTORY/INTERVIEW

1. Is the client's affect appropriate to the situation? Does client display a range of emotional behaviors? Does client experience feelings of prolonged sadness, worthlessness, sense of loss, inability to cope, thoughts of suicide? If so, assess emotional state further by screening for depression.

2. Does client admit to inability to concentrate, forgetfulness, worry about the past, rumination, apprehension, nervousness, lack of self-confidence?

3. What are client's goals for the future?

OBJECTIVE ASSESSMENT

1. Do client's facial expressions and nonverbal cues coincide with verbal content?

2. Does client's perception of social and emotional status match information received from other sources?

Self-Perception–Self-Concept Pattern

HISTORY/INTERVIEW

1. Does the client indicate increased sadness or identify a recent loss (relationship,

health, status, role, financial, and so on) that has been traumatic? Has client had difficulty concentrating?

2. How has client adjusted to aging effects on body system structure and function? How would individual describe the self? Has body image been altered? Have the effects of aging and illness affected the individual's self-concept?

3. Has individual achieved self-acceptance and recognition of self-worth? Ask the individual: "Would you change any part of your life? Live any part over? Can you describe what your life has meant to you?"

Role–Relationship Pattern

HISTORY/INTERVIEW

1. Inquire about social status: marital status, educational level, work history, retirement, living arrangement and number in household, transportation, and ability to meet financial obligations.

2. Ask client to identify family members, their age, sex, health status, and where they live. How many family members does client feel close to? Ask about non-kin "family" members on whom client may rely for support.

3. Describe how family members relate to one another, get and make decisions? Would client like family relationships to be different? Is there a family crisis or stressor that is currently taxing the family?

4. Inquire about socialization pattern: number of persons seen in the past week, whom client confides in (confidant), quality of relationships (whom does client keep in contact with, how often), any conflicts. Who helps client in times of need or when things be-

come difficult (hospitalization, illness, crisis)?

5. Does individual express fear or ambivalent feelings about any family members or friends? Does individual understand difference between physical and verbal/psychological abuse?

6. Has individual ever been a victim of a crime or interpersonal violence? What were the circumstances? How was it resolved? How did individual cope? Does the individual still feel vulnerable?

7. Has client experienced relocation, either temporary or permanent? What impact has relocation had on social interaction patterns?

8. Does individual have a telephone? Can the individual dial the appropriate telephone numbers to obtain assistance when needed (neighbor, relative, emergency 911)? Is the telephone emergency system available to the individual? Is there a local telephone visitation service if the individual is isolated socially or geographically?

OBJECTIVE ASSESSMENT

1. If family members become involved in the individual's care, note the frequency and pattern of interactions and type of assistance provided (psychological support and visits, financial assistance, direct care, telephone calls, transportation, gifts). Observe how decision making proceeds, if conflicts arise, and how conflict is dealt with.

2. Assess for bodily injury: bruises, lacerations, and inquire about the surrounding circumstances. Observe family interaction patterns within the family unit (particularly caregivers who provide direct care to the individual) for potential for mistreatment.

Sexuality–Reproductive Pattern
HISTORY/INTERVIEW

1. Have patterns of sexual contact changed recently? Are there problems with discomfort or pain during intercourse, male impotence, decreased opportunity, decreased satisfaction? Any concerns about current intimacy needs?

2. Does individual recognize intimacy (warm, close, nonsexual relationships) as a form of sensuality?

3. Does the individual express a desire for improvement in sexual relationships through counseling, gynecological or urological evaluation, or referral to self-help groups for older persons?

OBJECTIVE ASSESSMENT

1. Does the verbal content and enthusiasm

with which the individual describes sexuality and intimacy indicate satisfaction? Does individual articulate wishes that things could be different and therefore better?

2. Have there been recent or past experiences that have demonstrated the responsiveness of the social network (hospitalization, illness, transition)?

Coping–Stress Tolerance Pattern
HISTORY/INTERVIEW

1. How has client managed crises in the past? Ask client to identify examples of effective and ineffective ways of coping (confrontation, avoidance, discussion, praying, meditation, humor, activity increase or decrease, seek presence of others, crying, indulgence in food, cigarettes, alcohol, drugs, and so on).

2. Has client experienced recent loss (actual or perceived): status, prestige, valued possessions, divorce, independence, death of loved one, change in environment, financial, health status/disease or effects of aging, peer relationship, lack of recognition from others?

OBJECTIVE ASSESSMENT

1. Assess the range of coping skills being employed and their effectiveness. Does client engage in stress-reducing activities such as socializing, gardening, crafts, cooking, hobbies, caring for a pet, exercise?

Value–Belief Pattern
HISTORY/INTERVIEW

1. What are client's values and beliefs about spirituality? Does client identify a religious preference? Does client actively practice religious faith? Does the client seek religious guidance?

2. Are there barriers to participation in religious rituals, such as lack of transportation, impaired mobility, poor hearing and vision, urinary incontinence, pain, feeling of hopelessness, depression, questioning of faith?

3. Does client verbalize doubts or inner conflict about religion and own faith?

OBJECTIVE ASSESSMENT

1. Note content of speech references to religious affiliation or relationship with spiritual being. Follow up on references to death and dying.

2. Assess verbal content of despair or loss of faith or lack of meaningfulness in life. Help individual articulate values and beliefs.

Fourth-Level Assessment

The fourth level of assessment, the problem-focused assessment, elicits more detailed, in-depth information in a diagnostic category to rule in or rule out a nursing diagnosis. The specific etiology of the nursing diagnosis is identified at this level. In addition, referral to other health professionals may be necessary. For example, in-depth assessment of the contributing factors to urinary incontinence, pain, ineffective coping, or social isolation may be necessary if the problems are not clearly represented. Further history and physical information and laboratory or diagnostic evaluation may be in order. Problem-focused assessment strategies can be found in the related chapters throughout the text.

Minimum Data Set (MDS) for Nursing Facility Resident Assessment and Care Screening*

*See discussion on pages 2 to 6.

Appendix

FACE SHEET FOR NURSING FACILITY RESIDENT ASSESSMENT AND CARE SCREENING (MDS)
BACKGROUND INFORMATION/INTAKE AT ADMISSION

[ ] = Code the appropriate response | b. | = Check (✓) if response is applicable

I. IDENTIFICATION INFORMATION

1. RESIDENT NAME _____
(First)　　　(Middle Initial)　　　(Last)

ID# _____

2. DATE OF CURRENT ADMISSION [ ][ ] — [ ][ ] — [ ][ ][ ][ ]
Month　　Day　　Year

3. MEDICARE No. (SOC. SEC. or Comparable No. if no Medicare No.)

4. FACILITY PROVIDER NO.
Federal No.

5. GENDER　1. Male　　2. Female

6. RACE/ETHNICITY
1. American Indian/Alaskan Native　4. Hispanic
2. Asian/Pacific Islander　5. White, not of
3. Black, not of Hispanic origin　　Hispanic origin

7. BIRTHDATE [ ][ ] — [ ][ ] — [ ][ ][ ][ ]
Month　　Day　　Year

8. LIFETIME OCCUPATION _____

9. PRIMARY LANGUAGE
Resident's primary language is a language other than English.　0. No　　1. Yes _____
(Specify)

10. RESIDENTIAL HISTORY PAST 5 YEARS
(Check all settings resident lived in during 5 years prior to admission)
a. Prior stay at this nursing home | a.
b. Other nursing home/residential facility | b.
c. MH/psychiatric setting | c.
d. MR/DD setting | d.
e. NONE OF ABOVE | e.

11. MENTAL HEALTH HISTORY
Does resident's RECORD indicate any history of mental retardation, mental illness, or any other mental health problem?　0. No　　1. Yes

12. CONDITIONS RELATED TO MR/DD STATUS
Check all conditions that are related to MR/DD Status, that were manifested before age 22, and are likely to continue indefinitely.
a. Not Applicable—no MR/DD (Skip to Item 13) | a.
　MR/DD with Organic Condition
b. Cerebral palsy | b.
c. Down's syndrome | c.
d. Autism | d.
e. Epilepsy | e.
f. Other organic condition related to MR/DD | f.
g. MR/DD with no organic condition | g.
h. Unknown | h.

13. MARITAL STATUS
1. Never Married　3. Widowed　5. Divorced
2. Married　　4. Separated

14. ADMITTED FROM
1. Private home or apt.　3. Acute care hospital
2. Nursing facility　　4. Other

15. LIVED ALONE　0. No　1. Yes　2. In other facility

16. ADMISSION INFORMATION AMENDED
(Check all that apply)
a. Accurate information unavailable earlier | a.
b. Observation revealed additional information | b.
c. Resident unstable at admission | c.

II. BACKGROUND INFORMATION AT RETURN/READMISSION

1. DATE OF CURRENT READMISSION [ ][ ] — [ ][ ] — [ ][ ][ ][ ]
Month　　Day　　Year

2. MARITAL STATUS
1. Never Married　3. Widowed　5. Divorced
2. Married　　4. Separated

3. ADMITTED FROM
1. Private home or apt.　3. Acute care hospital
2. Nursing facility　　4. Other

4. LIVED ALONE　0. No　1. Yes　2. In other facility

5. ADMISSION INFORMATION AMENDED
(Check all that apply)
a. Accurate information unavailable earlier | a.
b. Observation revealed additional information | b.
c. Resident unstable at admission | c.

III. CUSTOMARY ROUTINE (ONLY AT FIRST ADMISSION)

1. CUSTOMARY ROUTINE (Year prior to first admission to a nursing home)
(Check all that apply. If all information UNKNOWN, check last box only.)

CYCLE OF DAILY EVENTS
a. Stays up late at night (e.g., after 9 pm) | a.
b. Naps regularly during day (at least 1 hour) | b.
c. Goes out 1+ days a week | c.
d. Stays busy with hobbies, reading, or fixed daily routine | d.
e. Spends most time alone or watching TV | e.
f. Moves independently indoors (with appliances, if used) | f.
g. NONE OF ABOVE | g.

EATING PATTERNS
h. Distinct food preferences | h.
i. Eats between meals all or most days | i.
j. Use of alcoholic beverage(s) at least weekly | j.
k. NONE OF ABOVE | k.

ADL PATTERNS
l. In bedclothes much of day | l.
m. Wakens to toilet all or most nights | m.
n. Has irregular bowel movement pattern | n.
o. Prefers showers for bathing | o.
p. NONE OF ABOVE | p.

INVOLVEMENT PATTERNS
q. Daily contact with relatives/close friends | q.
r. Usually attends church, temple, synagogue (etc.) | r.
s. Finds strength in faith | s.
t. Daily animal companion/presence | t.
u. Involved in group activities | u.
v. NONE OF ABOVE | v.
w. UNKNOWN—Resident/family unable to provide information | w.

Signature and Date of RN Assessment Coordinator: _____
Signatures and Dates of Others Who Completed Part of the Assessment:

_____　_____

_____　_____

END

Form 1827HH　　BRIGGS, Des Moines, IA 50306　(800) 247-2343　PRINTED IN U.S.A.　　　　　(9-90)

MINIMUM DATA SET
FOR NURSING FACILITY RESIDENT ASSESSMENT AND CARE SCREENING (MDS)
(Status in last 7 days, unless other time frame indicated)

Code "NA" or (—) = Information unavailable or untrustworthy

☐ = Write in the appropriate alpha or numeric response

☐ = Check (✓) if response is applicable

UPON COMPLETION OF THIS FORM, GO TO RAP TRIGGER LEGEND.

SECTION A. IDENTIFICATION AND BACKGROUND INFORMATION

1. ASSESSMENT DATE
☐☐ — ☐☐ — ☐☐☐☐
Month   Day   Year

2. RESIDENT NAME
(First)   (Middle Initial)   (Last)

3. SOCIAL SECURITY NO.

4. MEDICAID NO. (If applicable)

5. MEDICAL RECORD NO.

6. REASON FOR ASSESSMENT
1. Initial admission assess.   4. Annual assessment
2. Hosp/Medicare reassess.   5. Significant change in status
3. Readmission assessment   6. Other (e.g., UR)

7. CURRENT PAYMENT SOURCE(S) FOR N.H. STAY
(Billing Office to indicate; *check all that apply*)
a. Medicaid ☐ a.   d. VA ☐ d.
b. Medicare ☐ b.   e. Self pay/Private insurance ☐ e.
c. CHAMPUS ☐ c.   f. Other ☐ f.

8. RESPONSIBILITY/LEGAL GUARDIAN
(*Check all that apply*)
a. Legal guardian ☐ a.   d. Family member responsible ☐ d.
b. Other legal oversight ☐ b.   e. Resident responsible ☐ e.
c. Durable power attrny./health care proxy ☐ c.   f. NONE OF ABOVE ☐ f.

9. ADVANCED DIRECTIVES
(*For those items with supporting documentation in the medical record, check all that apply*)
a. Living will ☐ a.   f. Feeding restrictions ☐ f.
b. Do not resuscitate ☐ b.   g. Medication restrictions ☐ g.
c. Do not hospitalize ☐ c.   h. Other treatment restrictions ☐ h.
d. Organ donation ☐ d.   i. NONE OF ABOVE ☐ i.
e. Autopsy request ☐ e.

10. DISCHARGE PLANNED WITHIN 3 MOS.
(*Does not include discharge due to death*)
0. No   1. Yes   2. Unknown/uncertain

11. PARTICIPATE IN ASSESSMENT
a. Resident   b. Family
0. No   0. No
1. Yes   1. Yes
2. No family
a. ☐   b. ☐

12. SIGNATURES (Indicate section(s) completed next to name)
Signature & Date of RN Assessment Coordinator
_____
Signatures, Titles & Dates of Others Who Completed Part of the Assessment
_____
_____
_____
_____

SECTION B. COGNITIVE PATTERNS

1. COMATOSE
(*Persistent vegetative state/no discernible consciousness*)
0. No   1. Yes (Skip to SECTION E)

2. MEMORY
(*Recall of what was learned or known*)
a. Short-term memory OK—seems/appears to recall after 5 minutes
0. Memory OK   1. Memory problem ▲²   a. ☐
b. Long-term memory OK—seems/appears to recall long past
0. Memory OK   1. Memory problem ▲²   b. ☐

3. MEMORY/RECALL ABILITY
(*Check all that resident normally able to recall during last 7 days*)   Fewer than 3 ✓ = ▲²
a. Current season ☐ a.   d. That he/she is in a nursing home ☐ d.
b. Location of own room ☐ b.   e. NONE OF ABOVE are recalled ☐ e.
c. Staff names/faces ☐ c.

4. COGNITIVE SKILLS FOR DAILY DECISION-MAKING
(*Made decisions regarding tasks of daily life*)
0. Independent—decisions consistent/reasonable ▲⁴
1. Modified independence—some difficulty in new situations only ▲⁴ ▲²
2. Moderately impaired—decisions poor; cues/supervision required ▲⁴ ▲²
3. Severely impaired—never/rarely made decisions ▲²

5. INDICATORS OF DELIRIUM—PERIODIC DISORDERED THINKING/AWARENESS
(*Check if condition over last 7 days appears different from usual functioning*)
a. Less alert, easily distracted ●¹   a. ☐
b. Changing awareness of environment ●¹   b. ☐
c. Episodes of incoherent speech ●¹   c. ☐
d. Periods of motor restlessness or lethargy ●¹   d. ☐
e. Cognitive ability varies over course of day ●¹   e. ☐
f. NONE OF ABOVE   f. ☐

6. CHANGE IN COGNITIVE STATUS
Change in resident's cognitive status, skills, or abilities in last 90 days
0. No change   1. Improved   2. Deteriorated ●¹ ▲¹⁴

SECTION C. COMMUNICATION/HEARING PATTERNS

1. HEARING
(*With hearing appliance, if used*)
0. Hears adequately—normal talk, TV, phone
1. Minimal difficulty when not in quiet setting
2. Hears in special situation only—speaker has to adjust tonal quality and speak distinctly
3. Highly impaired/absence of useful hearing

2. COMMUNICATION DEVICES/TECHNIQUES
(*Check all that apply during last 7 days*)
a. Hearing aid, present and used   a. ☐
b. Hearing aid, present and not used   b. ☐
c. Other receptive comm. technique used (e.g., lip read)   c. ☐
d. NONE OF ABOVE   d. ☐

3. MODES OF EXPRESSION
(*Check all used by resident to make needs known*)
a. Speech ☐ a.   c. Signs/gestures/sounds ☐ c.
b. Writing messages to express or clarify needs ☐ b.   d. Communication board ☐ d.
       e. Other ☐ e.
       f. NONE OF ABOVE ☐ f.

4. MAKING SELF UNDERSTOOD
(*Express information content—however able*)
0. Understood
1. Usually Understood-difficulty finding words or finishing thoughts
2. Sometimes Understood-ability is limited to making concrete requests ▲⁴
3. Rarely/Never Understood ▲⁴

5. ABILITY TO UNDERSTAND OTHERS
(*Understanding verbal information content-however able*)
0. Understands
1. Usually Understands-may miss some part/intent of message ▲²
2. Sometimes Understands-responds adequately to simple, direct communication ▲² ▲⁴ ▲⁵
3. Rarely/Never Understands ▲² ▲⁴ ▲⁵

6. CHANGE IN COMMUNICATION/HEARING
Resident's ability to express, understand or hear information has changed over last 90 days
0. No change   1. Improved   2. Deteriorated ●¹

SECTION D. VISION PATTERNS

1. VISION
(*Ability to see in adequate light and with glasses if used*)
0. Adequate—sees fine detail, including regular print in newspapers/books
1. Impaired—sees large print, but not regular print in newspapers/books ●³
2. Highly Impaired—limited vision, not able to see newspaper headlines, appears to follow objects with eyes ●³
3. Severely Impaired—no vision or appears to see only light, colors, or shapes ●³

●= Automatic Trigger   ▲ = Potential Trigger

1 - Delirium   5 - ADL Functional/Rehabilitation Potential   9 - Behavior Problems   13 - Feeding Tubes   17 - Psychotropic Drug Use
2 - Cognitive Loss/Dementia   6 - Urinary Incontinence and Indwelling Catheter   10 - Activities   14 - Dehydration/Fluid Maintenance   18 - Physical Restraints
3 - Visual Function   7 - Psychosocial Well-Being   11 - Falls   15 - Dental Care
4 - Communication   8 - Mood State   12 - Nutritional Status   16 - Pressure Ulcers

Form 1828HH   © 1990 Briggs Corporation, Des Moines, IA 50306 (800) 247-2343   PRINTED IN U.S.A.
Copyright limited to addition of trigger system.

1 of 4   Rev. 3/91

Resident Name _____ I.D. Number _____

2.	VISUAL LIMITATIONS/ DIFFICULTIES	a. Side vision problems—decreased peripheral vision; (e.g., leaves food on one side of tray, difficulty traveling, bumps into people and objects, misjudges placement of chair when seating self) ●[3]	a.
		b. Experiences any of the following: sees halos or rings around lights, sees flashes of light; sees "curtains" over eyes	b.
		c. NONE OF ABOVE	c.
3.	VISUAL APPLIANCES	Glasses; contact lenses; lens implant; magnifying glass 0. No 1. Yes	

SECTION E. PHYSICAL FUNCTIONING AND STRUCTURAL PROBLEMS

1. ADL SELF-PERFORMANCE *(Code for resident's PERFORMANCE OVER ALL SHIFTS during last 7 days*—Not including setup)

0. **INDEPENDENT**—No help or oversight—OR—Help/oversight provided only 1 or 2 times during last 7 days.

1. **SUPERVISION**—Oversight encouragement or cueing provided 3+ times during last 7 days—OR—Supervision plus physical assistance provided only 1 or 2 times during last 7 days.

2. **LIMITED ASSISTANCE**—Resident highly involved in activity, received physical help in guided maneuvering of limbs, or other nonweight bearing assistance 3+ times—OR—More help provided only 1 or 2 times during last 7 days.

3. **EXTENSIVE ASSISTANCE**—While resident performed part of activity, over last 7-day period, help of following type(s) provided 3 or more times:
   — Weight-bearing support
   — Full staff performance during part (but not all) of last 7 days.

4. **TOTAL DEPENDENCE**—Full staff performance of activity during entire 7 days.

2. ADL SUPPORT PROVIDED—*(Code for MOST SUPPORT PROVIDED OVER ALL SHIFTS during last 7 days; code regardless of resident's self-performance classification)*

0. No setup or physical help from staff   2. One-person physical assist
1. Setup help only   3. Two+ person physical assist

			1 SELF-PERFORMANCE	2 SUPPORT
a.	BED MOBILITY	How resident moves to and from lying position, turns side to side, and positions body while in bed 3 or 4 for self-perf = ▲[5]		
b.	TRANSFER	How resident moves between surfaces—to/from: bed, chair, wheelchair, standing position (EXCLUDE to/from bath/toilet) 3 or 4 for self-perf = ▲[5]		
c.	LOCO-MOTION	How resident moves between locations in his/her room and adjacent corridor on same floor. If in wheelchair, self-sufficiency once in chair 3 or 4 for self-perf = ▲[5]		
d.	DRESSING	How resident puts on, fastens, and takes off all items of street clothing, including donning/removing prosthesis 3 or 4 for self-perf = ▲[5]		
e.	EATING	How resident eats and drinks (regardless of skill) 3 or 4 for self-perf = ▲[6]		
f.	TOILET USE	How resident uses the toilet room (or commode, bedpan, urinal); transfers on/off toilet, cleanses, changes pad, manages ostomy or catheter, adjusts clothes 3 or 4 for self-perf = ▲[5]		
g.	PERSONAL HYGIENE	How resident maintains personal hygiene, including combing hair, brushing teeth, shaving, applying makeup, washing/drying face, hands, and perineum (EXCLUDE baths and showers)		

3. BATHING How resident takes full-body bath, sponge bath, and transfers in/out of tub/shower (EXCLUDE washing of back and hair. Code for most dependent in self-performance and support. Bathing Self-Performance codes appear below.) 3 or 4 for (a) = ▲[5]

0. Independent—No help provided
1. Supervision—Oversight help only
2. Physical help limited to transfer only
3. Physical help in part of bathing activity
4. Total dependence

| | | a. | b. |

4. BODY CONTROL PROBLEMS *(Check all that apply during last 7 days)*

a. Balance—partial or total loss of ability to balance self while standing ▲[11]	a.	g. Hand—lack of dexterity (e.g., problem using toothbrush or adjusting hearing aid)	g.
b. Bedfast all or most of the time ▲[11]	b.	h. Leg—partial or total loss of voluntary movement ▲[11]	h.
c. Contracture to arms, legs, shoulders, or hands	c.	i. Leg—unsteady gait	i.
d. Hemiplegia/hemiparesis ▲[11]	d.	j. Trunk—partial or total loss of ability to position, balance, or turn body ▲[11]	j.
e. Quadriplegia ▲[11]	e.	k. Amputation	k.
f. Arm—partial or total loss of voluntary movement	f.	l. NONE OF ABOVE	l.

5.	MOBILITY APPLIANCES/ DEVICES	*(Check all that apply during last 7 days)*	
		a. Cane/walker [a.]	d. Other person wheeled	d.
		b. Brace/prosthesis [b.]	e. Lifted (manually/mechanically)	e.
		c. Wheeled self [c.]	f. NONE OF ABOVE	f.
6.	TASK SEG-MENTATION	Resident requires that some or all of ADL activities be broken into a series of subtasks so that resident can perform them. 0. No 1. Yes	▲
7.	ADL FUNC-TIONAL REHAB. POTENTIAL	a. Resident believes he/she capable of increased independence in at least some ADLs ▲[5]	a.
		b. Direct care staff believe resident capable of increased independence in at least some ADLs ▲[5]	b.
		c. Resident able to perform tasks/activity but is very slow	c.
		d. Major difference in ADL Self-Performance or ADL Support in mornings and evenings (at least a one category change in Self-Performance or Support in any ADL)	d.
		e. NONE OF ABOVE	e.
8.	CHANGE IN ADL FUNCTION	Change in ADL self-performance in last 90 days 0. No change 1. Improved 2. Deteriorated ▲[14]	

SECTION F. CONTINENCE IN LAST 14 DAYS

1. CONTINENCE SELF-CONTROL CATEGORIES *(Code for resident performance over all shifts.)*

0. **CONTINENT**—Complete control

1. **USUALLY CONTINENT**—BLADDER, incontinent episodes once a week or less; BOWEL, less than weekly

2. **OCCASIONALLY INCONTINENT**—BLADDER, 2+ times a week but not daily; BOWEL, once a week

3. **FREQUENTLY INCONTINENT**—BLADDER, tended to be incontinent daily, but some control present (e.g., on day shift); BOWEL, 2-3 times a week

4. **INCONTINENT**—Had inadequate control. BLADDER, multiple daily episodes; BOWEL, all (or almost all) of the time.

| a. | BOWEL CON-TINENCE | Control of bowel movement, with appliance or bowel continence programs if employed | |
| b. | BLADDER CONTI-NENCE | Control of urinary bladder function (if dribbles, volume insufficient to soak through underpants), with appliances (e.g., foley) or continence programs, if employed 2, 3 or 4 = ▲[6] | |

2.	INCONTI-NENCE RELATED TESTING	*(Skip if resident's bladder continence code equals 0 or 1 AND no catheter is used)*	
		a. Resident has been tested for a urinary tract infection	a.
		b. Resident has been checked for presence of a fecal impaction, or there is adequate bowel elimination	b.
		c. NONE OF ABOVE	c.

3.	APPLIANCES AND PROGRAMS	a. Any scheduled toileting plan [a.]	e. Did not use toilet room/commode/urinal	e.
		b. External (condom) catheter ▲[6] [b.]	f. Pads/briefs used ▲[6]	f.
		c. Indwelling catheter ▲[6] [c.]	g. Enemas/irrigation	g.
		d. Intermittent catheter ▲[6] [d.]	h. Ostomy	h.
			i. NONE OF ABOVE	i.

| 4. | CHANGE IN URINARY CONTINENCE | Change in urinary continence or programs in last 90 days 0. No change   1. Improved   2. Deteriorated | |

SKIP TO SECTION J IF COMATOSE

SECTION G. PSYCHOSOCIAL WELL-BEING

1.	SENSE OF INITIATIVE/ INVOLVE-MENT	a. At ease interacting with others	a.
		b. At ease doing planned or structured activities	b.
		c. At ease doing self-initiated activities	c.
		d. Establishes own goals	d.
		e. Pursues involvement in life of facility (i.e., makes/keeps friends; involved in group activities; responds positively to new activities; assists at religious services)	e.
		f. Accepts invitations into most group activities	f.
		g. NONE OF ABOVE	g.
2.	UNSETTLED RELATION-SHIPS	a. Covert/open conflict with and/or repeated criticism of staff ●[7]	a.
		b. Unhappy with roommate ●[7]	b.
		c. Unhappy with residents other than roommate ●[7]	c.
		d. Openly expresses conflict/anger with family or friends ●[7]	d.
		e. Absence of personal contact with family/friends	e.
		f. Recent loss of close family member/friend	f.
		g. NONE OF ABOVE	g.

●= Automatic Trigger   ▲ = Potential Trigger

1 - Delirium	5 - ADL Functional/Rehabilitation Potential	9 - Behavior Problems	13 - Feeding Tubes	17 - Psychotropic Drug Use
2 - Cognitive Loss/Dementia	6 - Urinary Incontinence and Indwelling Catheter	10 - Activities	14 - Dehydration/Fluid Maintenance	18 - Physical Restraints
3 - Visual Function	7 - Psychosocial Well-Being	11 - Falls	15 - Dental Care	
4 - Communication	8 - Mood State	12 - Nutritional Status	16 - Pressure Ulcers	2 of 4 Rev. 3/91

Resident Name _____ I.D. Number _____

3.	PAST ROLES	a. Strong identification with past roles and life status	a.
		b. Expresses sadness/anger/empty feeling over lost roles/status ●7	b.
		c. *NONE OF ABOVE*	c.

SECTION H. MOOD AND BEHAVIOR PATTERNS

1.	SAD OR ANXIOUS MOOD	*(Check all that apply during last 30 days)*	
		a. **VERBAL EXPRESSIONS of DISTRESS** by resident (sadness, sense that nothing matters, hopelessness, worthlessness, unrealistic fears, vocal expressions of anxiety or grief) ●9	a.
		DEMONSTRATED (OBSERVABLE) SIGNS of mental DISTRESS	
		b. Tearfulness, emotional groaning, sighing, breathlessness ●8	b.
		c. Motor agitation such as pacing, handwringing or picking ●6	c.
		d. Failure to eat or take medications, withdrawal from self-care or leisure activities ●8 ▲14	d.
		e. Pervasive concern with health ●8	e.
		f. Recurrent thoughts of death—e.g., believes he/she is about to die, have a heart attack ●8	f.
		g. Suicidal thoughts/actions ●8	g.
		h. *NONE OF ABOVE*	h.
2.	MOOD PERSISTENCE	**Sad or anxious** mood intrudes on daily life over last 7 days—not easily altered, doesn't "cheer up" 0. No 1. Yes ●8	
3.	PROBLEM BEHAVIOR	*(Code for behavior in last 7 days)* 0. Behavior **not exhibited** in last 7 days 1. Behavior of this type occurred **less than daily** 2. Behavior of this type occurred **daily or more frequently**	
		a. **WANDERING** (moved with no rational purpose; seemingly oblivious to needs or safety) 1 or 2 = ●9	a.
		b. **VERBALLY ABUSIVE** (others were threatened, screamed at, cursed at) 1 or 2 = ●9	b.
		c. **PHYSICALLY ABUSIVE** (others were hit, shoved, scratched, sexually abused) 1 or 2 = ●9	c.
		d. **SOCIALLY INAPPROPRIATE/DISRUPTIVE BEHAVIOR** (made disrupting sounds, noisy, screams, self-abusive acts, sexual behavior or disrobing in public, smeared/threw food/feces, hoarding, rummaged through others' belongings) 1 or 2 = ●9	d.
4.	RESIDENT RESISTS CARE	*(Check all types of resistance that occurred in the last 7 days)* a. Resisted taking medications/injection	a.
		b. Resisted ADL assistance	b.
		c. *NONE OF ABOVE*	c.
5.	BEHAVIOR MANAGEMENT PROGRAM	**Behavior problem has been addressed by clinically developed behavior management program.** (Note: Do not include programs that involve only physical restraints or psychotropic medications in this category.) 0. No behavior problem 1. Yes, addressed 2. No, not addressed	
6.	CHANGE IN MOOD	Change in mood in last 90 days 0. No change 1. Improved 2. Deteriorated ▲1	
7.	CHANGE IN PROBLEM BEHAVIOR	Change in problem behavioral signs in last 90 days 0. No change 1. Improved 2. Deteriorated ●1	

SECTION I. ACTIVITY PURSUIT PATTERNS

1.	TIME AWAKE	*(Check appropriate time periods—last 7 days)* Resident awake all or most of time (i.e., naps no more than one hour per time period) in the:	
		a. Morning 7a.m.–Noon (or when resident wakes up)	a.
		b. Afternoon Noon–5p.m.	b.
		c. Evening 5p.m.–10p.m. (or bedtime)	c.
		d. *NONE OF ABOVE*	d.
2.	AVERAGE TIME INVOLVED IN ACTIVITIES	0. Most—(more than 2/3 of time) ▲10 2. Little—(less than 1/3 of time) ▲10 1. Some—(1/3 to 2/3 time) ▲10 3. None ▲10	
3.	PREFERRED ACTIVITY SETTINGS	*(Check all settings in which activities are preferred)*	
		a. Own room	a.
		b. Day/activity room	b.
		c. Inside NH/off unit	c.
		d. Outside facility	d.
		e. *NONE OF ABOVE*	e.

4.	GENERAL ACTIVITIES PREFERENCES (adapted to resident's current abilities)	*(Check all specific preferences whether or not activity is currently available to resident)*			
		a. Cards/other games	a.	f. Spiritual/religious activ.	f.
		b. Crafts/arts	b.	g. Trips/shopping	g.
		c. Exercise/sports	c.	h. Walking/wheeling outdoors	h.
		d. Music	d.	i. Watch TV	i.
		e. Read/write	e.	j. *NONE OF ABOVE*	j.
5.	PREFERS MORE OR DIFFERENT ACTIVITIES	Resident expresses/indicates preference for other activities/choices. 0. No 1. Yes ●10			

SECTION J. DISEASE DIAGNOSES

Check only those diseases present that have a relationship to current ADL status, cognitive status, behavior status, medical treatments, or risk of death. (Do not list old/inactive diagnoses.) (If none apply, check the NONE OF ABOVE box)

1.	DISEASES	**HEART/CIRCULATION**			
		a. Arteriosclerotic heart disease (ASHD)	a.	r. Manic depressive (bipolar disease)	r.
		b. Cardiac dysrhythmias	b.	**SENSORY**	
		c. Congestive heart failure	c.	s. Cataracts	s.
		d. Hypertension	d.	t. Glaucoma	t.
		e. Hypotension	e.	**OTHER**	
		f. Peripheral vascular disease	f.	u. Allergies	u.
		g. Other cardiovascular disease	g.	v. Anemia	v.
		NEUROLOGICAL		w. Arthritis	w.
		h. Alzheimer's	h.	x. Cancer	x.
		i. Dementia other than Alzheimer's	i.	y. Diabetes mellitus	y.
		j. Aphasia	j.	z. Explicit terminal prognosis	z.
		k. Cerebrovascular accident (stroke)	k.	aa. Hypothyroidism	aa.
		l. Multiple sclerosis	l.	bb. Osteoporosis	bb.
		m. Parkinson's disease	m.	cc. Seizure disorder	cc.
		PULMONARY		dd. Septicemia	dd.
		n. Emphysema/asthma/COPD	n.	ee. Urinary tract infection- in last 30 days ▲14	ee.
		o. Pneumonia	o.	ff. *NONE OF ABOVE*	ff.
		PSYCHIATRIC/MOOD			
		p. Anxiety disorder	p.		
		q. Depression	q.		
2.	OTHER CURRENT DIAGNOSES AND ICD-9 CODES	260–263.9=●12 276.5=▲14 291.0, 292.81, 293.0, 293.1=●1	
		a.	
		b.	
		c.	
		d.	
		e.	
		f.	

SECTION K. HEALTH CONDITIONS

1.	PROBLEM CONDITIONS	*(Check all problems that are present in last 7 days unless other time frame indicated)*			
		a. Constipation	a.	j. Pain—resident complains or shows evidence of pain daily or almost daily	j.
		b. Diarrhea ▲14	b.		
		c. Dizziness/vertigo ▲14	c.		
		d. Edema	d.	k. Recurrent lung aspirations in **last 90 days**	k.
		e. Fecal impaction	e.		
		f. Fever ▲14	f.		
		g. Hallucinations/delusions	g.	l. Shortness of breath	l.
		h. Internal bleeding ▲14	h.	m. Syncope (fainting)	m.
		i. Joint pain	i.	n. Vomiting ▲14	n.
				o. *NONE OF ABOVE*	o.
2.	ACCIDENTS	a. Fell—past 30 days ●11	a.	c. Hip fracture in **last 180 days**	c.
		b. Fell—past 31-180 days ●11	b.	d. *NONE OF ABOVE*	d.

Resident Name _____   I.D. Number _____

3.	STABILITY OF CONDITIONS	a. Conditions/diseases make resident's cognitive, ADL, or behavior status unstable—fluctuating, precarious, or deteriorating.	a.
		b. Resident experiencing an acute episode or a flare-up of a recurrent/chronic problem.	b.
		c. *NONE OF THE ABOVE*	c.

SECTION L. ORAL/NUTRITIONAL STATUS

1.	ORAL PROBLEMS	a. Chewing problem [a.]	c. Mouth pain ●[15]	c.
		b. Swallowing problem [b.]	d. *NONE OF ABOVE*	d.
2.	HEIGHT AND WEIGHT	*Record height (a) in inches and weight (b) in pounds.* Weight based on most recent status in **last 30 days**; measure weight consistently **in accord with standard facility** practice—e.g., in a.m. after voiding, before meal, with shoes off, and in nightclothes. HT (in.) [a.] WT (lb.) [b.]	
		c. **Weight loss** (i.e., 5% + **in last 30 days**; or 10% in **last 180 days**) 0. No 1. Yes ●[12] ▲[14]	c.
3.	NUTRITIONAL PROBLEMS	a. Complains about the taste of many foods ●[12] [a.]	d. Regular complaint of hunger ●[12]	d.
		b. Insufficient fluid; dehydrated ●[14] [b.]	e. Leaves 25%+ food uneaten at most meals ●[12] ▲[14]	e.
		c. Did **NOT** consume all/almost all liquids provided **during last 3 days** ▲[14] [c.]	f. *NONE OF ABOVE*	f.
4.	NUTRITIONAL APPROACHES	a. Parenteral/IV ▲[14] ●[12] [a.]	e. Therapeutic diet ●[12]	e.
		b. Feeding tube ▲[14] ●[13] [b.]	f. Dietary supplement between meals	f.
		c. Mechanically altered diet ●[12] [c.]	g. Plate guard, stabilized built-up utensil, etc.	g.
		d. Syringe (oral feeding) ●[12] [d.]	h. *NONE OF ABOVE*	h.

SECTION M. ORAL/DENTAL STATUS

1.	ORAL STATUS AND DISEASE PREVENTION	a. Debris (soft, easily movable substances) present in mouth prior to going to bed at night ●[15]	a.
		b. Has dentures and/or removable bridge	b.
		c. Some/all natural teeth lost—does not have or does not use dentures (or partial plates) ●[15]	c.
		d. Broken, loose, or carious teeth ●[15]	d.
		e. Inflamed gums (gingiva), oral abscesses, swollen or bleeding gums, ulcers, or rashes ●[15]	e.
		f. Daily cleaning of teeth/dentures If not checked = ●[15]	f.
		g. *NONE OF ABOVE*	g.

SECTION N. SKIN CONDITION

1.	STASIS ULCER	(i.e., open lesion caused by poor venous circulation to lower extremities) 0. No 1. Yes	
2.	PRESSURE ULCERS	*(Code for highest stage of pressure ulcer)* 0. No pressure ulcers 1. Stage 1 A persistent area of skin redness (without a break in the skin) that does not disappear when pressure is relieved ●[12] ●[16] 2. Stage 2 A partial thickness loss of skin layers that presents clinically as an abrasion, blister, or shallow crater ●[12] ●[16] 3. Stage 3 A full thickness of skin is lost, exposing the subcutaneous tissues—presents as a deep crater with or without undermining adjacent tissue ●[12] ●[16] 4. Stage 4 A full thickness of skin and subcutaneous tissue is lost, exposing muscle and/or bone ●[12] ●[16]	
3.	HISTORY OF RESOLVED/CURED PRESSURE ULCERS	Resident has had a pressure ulcer that was resolved/cured in **last 90 days** 0. No 1. Yes	

4.	SKIN PROBLEMS/CARE	a. Open lesions other than stasis or pressure ulcers (e.g., cuts)	a.
		b. Skin desensitized to pain/pressure/discomfort	b.
	If None Checked From C Thru G = ▲[16]	c. Protective/preventive skin care	c.
		d. Turning/repositioning program	d.
		e. Pressure-relieving beds, bed/chair pads (e.g., egg crate pads)	e.
		f. Wound care/treatment (e.g., pressure ulcer care, surgical wound)	f.
		g. Other skin care/treatment	g.
		h. *NONE OF ABOVE*	h.

SECTION O. MEDICATION USE

1.	NUMBER OF MEDI-CATIONS	**(Record the number of *different medications* used in the last 7 days; enter "0" if none used.)**	
2.	NEW MEDI-CATIONS	Resident has received new medications during the **last 90 days** 0. No 1. Yes	
3.	INJECTIONS	*(Record the number of days injections of any type received during the last 7 days.)*	
4.	DAYS RECEIVED THE FOLLOWING MEDICATION	(Record the number of days during last 7 days; *Enter "0" if not used; enter "1" if long-acting meds. used less than weekly)*	
		a. Antipsychotics 1-7 = ▲[9] ▲[11] ▲[17]	a.
		b. Antianxiety/hypnotics 1-7 = ▲[9] ▲[11] ▲[17]	b.
		c. Antidepressants 1-7 = ▲[9] ▲[11] ▲[17]	c.
5.	PREVIOUS MEDICATION RESULTS	*(SKIP this question if resident currently receiving antipsychotics, antidepressants, or antianxiety/hypnotics—otherwise code correct response for last 90 days)* Resident has previously received psychoactive medications for a mood or behavior problem, and these medications were effective (without undue adverse consequences). 0. No, drugs not used 1. Drugs were effective 2. Drugs were not effective 3. Drug effectiveness unknown	

SECTION P. SPECIAL TREATMENTS AND PROCEDURES

1.	SPECIAL TREAT-MENTS AND PROCE-DURES	SPECIAL CARE—*Check treatments received during the last 14 days.*			
		a. Chemotherapy [a.]	f. IV meds	f.
		b. Radiation [b.]	g. Transfusions	g.
		c. Dialysis [c.]	h. O₂	h.
		d. Suctioning [d.]	i. Other _____	i.
		e. Trach. care [e.]	j. *NONE OF ABOVE*	j.
		THERAPIES—*Record the number of days each of the following therapies was administered (for at least 10 minutes during a day) in the last 7 days:*	
		k. Speech—language pathology and audiology services	k.
		l. Occupational therapy	l.
		m. Physical therapy	m.
		n. Psychological therapy (any licensed professional)	n.
		o. Respiratory Therapy	o.
2.	ABNORMAL LAB VALUES	Has the resident had any **abnormal lab values during the last 90-day period**? 0. No 1. Yes 2. No tests performed	
3.	DEVICES AND RESTRAINTS	*Use the following code for last 7 days:* 0 Not used 1 Used less than daily 2 Used daily	
		a. Bed rails	a.
		b. Trunk restraint 1 or 2 = ▲[9] ●[18]	b.
		c. Limb restraint 1 or 2 = ▲[9] ●[18]	c.
		d. Chair prevents rising 1 or 2 = ▲[9] ●[18]	d.

● = **Automatic Trigger**   ▲ = **Potential Trigger**

1 - Delirium	5 - ADL Functional/Rehabilitation Potential	9 - Behavior Problems 13 - Feeding Tubes 17 - Psychotropic Drug Use
2 - Cognitive Loss/Dementia	6 - Urinary Incontinence and Indwelling Catheter	10 - Activities 14 - Dehydration/Fluid Maintenance 18 - Physical Restraints
3 - Visual Function	7 - Psychosocial Well-Being	11 - Falls 15 - Dental Care
4 - Communication	8 - Mood State	12 - Nutritional Status 16 - Pressure Ulcers

QUARTERLY REVIEW FOR NURSING FACILITY RESIDENT ASSESSMENT AND CARE SCREENING (MDS)

(Sequence of questions on this Quarterly Review have been numbered to coincide with the Minimum Data Set.)

RESIDENT NAME _____

RESIDENT SOC. SEC. NO. ☐☐☐ – ☐☐ – ☐☐☐☐

☐ = Write in the appropriate alpha or numeric response.

☐ = Check (✓) if response is applicable

UPON COMPLETION OF THIS FORM, GO TO RAP TRIGGER LEGEND

IF COMATOSE, SKIP TO SECTION E

			DAYS 90	180	270
		SECTION B. COGNITIVE PATTERNS			
2.	MEMORY	*(Recall of what was learned or known)*			
		a. Short-term memory OK—seems/appears to recall after 5 minutes 0. Memory OK 1. Memory problem ▲²	a.		
		b. Long-term memory OK—seems/appears to recall long past 0. Memory OK 1. Memory problem ▲²	b.		
4.	COGNITIVE SKILLS FOR DAILY DECISION-MAKING	Made decisions regarding tasks of daily life *(Code response)* 0. **Independent**—decisions consistent/reasonable ▲⁴ 1. **Modified independence**—some difficulty in new situations only ▲⁴ ▲² 2. **Moderately impaired**—decisions poor; cues/supervision required ▲⁴ ▲² 3. **Severely impaired**—never/rarely made decisions ▲²			

		SECTION C. COMMUNICATION/HEARING PATTERNS			
4.	A. MAKING SELF UNDERSTOOD	*(Express information content—however able)* 0. Understood 1. Usually Understood—difficulty finding words or finishing thoughts 2. Sometimes Understood—ability is limited to making concrete requests ▲⁴ 3. Rarely/Never Understood ▲⁴			
5.	B. ABILITY TO UNDERSTAND OTHERS	*(Understanding verbal information content—however able.)* 0. Understands 1. Usually Understands—may miss some part/intent of message ▲² 2. Sometimes Understands—responds adequately to simple, direct communication ▲² ▲⁴ ▲⁵ 3. Rarely/Never Understands ▲² ▲⁴ ▲⁵			

		SECTION E. PHYSICAL FUNCTIONING AND STRUCTURAL PROBLEMS			
1.	ADL SELF-PERFORMANCE	*(Code for resident's PERFORMANCE OVER ALL SHIFTS during last 7days—Not including setup)* 0. **INDEPENDENT**—No help or oversight OR—Help/oversight provided only 1 or 2 times during last 7 days. 1. **SUPERVISION**—Oversight encouragement or cueing provided 3+ times during last 7 days —OR—Supervision plus physical assistance provided only 1 or 2 times during last 7 days. 2. **LIMITED ASSISTANCE**—Resident highly involved in activity, received physical help in guided maneuvering of limbs, or other nonweight bearing assistance 3+ times—OR—More help provided only 1 or 2 times during last 7 days. 3. **EXTENSIVE ASSISTANCE**—While resident performed part of activity, over last 7day period, help of following type(s) provided 3 or more times: – Weight-bearing support – Full staff performance during part (but not all) of last 7 days. 4. **TOTAL DEPENDENCE**—Full staff performance of activity during entire 7 days.			
b.	TRANSFER	How resident moves between surfaces—to/from: bed, chair, wheelchair, standing position (EXCLUDE to/from bath/toilet) 3 or 4 = ▲⁵			
c.	LOCO-MOTION	How resident moves between locations in his/her room and adjacent corridor on same floor. If in wheelchair, self-sufficiency once in chair. 3 or 4 = ▲⁵			
d.	DRESSING	How resident puts on, fastens, and takes off all items of street clothing, including donning/removing prosthesis. 3 or 4 = ▲⁵			
e.	EATING	How resident eats and drinks (regardless of skill) 3 or 4 = ▲⁶			
f.	TOILET USE	How resident uses the toilet room (or commode, bedpan, urinal); transfers on/off toilet, cleanses, changes pad, manages ostomy or catheter, adjusts clothes 3 or 4 = ▲⁵			
3a.	BATHING	How resident takes full-body bath/shower, sponge bath, and transfers in/out of tub/shower (EXCLUDE washing of back and hair. *Code for most dependent in self-performance and support.* Bathing Self-Performance codes appear below.) 0. Independent—No help provided 1. Supervision—Oversight help only 2. Physical help limited to transfer only 3. Physical help in part of bathing activity ▲⁵ 4. Total dependence ▲⁵			

UPON COMPLETION OF THIS FORM, GO TO RAP TRIGGER LEGEND — DAYS 90 | 180 | 270

		SECTION F. CONTINENCE IN LAST 14 DAYS	90	180	270
1.		CONTINENCE SELF-CONTROL CATEGORIES *(Code for resident's PERFORMANCE over all shifts)* 0. **CONTINENT**—Complete control 1. **USUALLY CONTINENT**—BLADDER, incontinent episodes once a week or less; BOWEL, less than weekly. 2. **OCCASIONALLY INCONTINENT**—BLADDER, 2+ times a week but not daily; BOWEL, once a week. 3. **FREQUENTLY INCONTINENT**—BLADDER, tended to be incontinent daily, but some control present (e.g., on day shift); BOWEL, 2-3 times a week. 4. **INCONTINENT**—Had inadequate control. For BLADDER, multiple daily episodes; for BOWEL, all (or almost all) of the time.			
a.	BOWEL CONTINENCE	Control of bowel movement, with appliance or bowel continence programs, if employed.			
b.	BLADDER CONTI-NENCE	Control of urinary bladder function (if dribbles, volume insufficient to soak through underpants), with appliances (e.g., foley) or continence programs, if employed. 2,3 or 4 = ▲⁶			

IF COMATOSE, SKIP TO SECTION J

		SECTION H. MOOD AND BEHAVIOR PATTERNS	90	180	270
2.	MOOD PER-SISTENCE	**Sad or anxious** mood intrudes on daily life over last 7 days—not easily altered, doesn't "cheer up." 0. No 1. Yes ●⁸			
3.	PROBLEM BEHAVIOR	*(Code for behavior in last 7 days)* 0. Behavior **not exhibited** in last 7 days 1. Behavior of this type occurred **less than daily** 2. Behavior of this type occurred **daily or more frequently**			
		a. **WANDERING** (moved with no rational purpose; seemingly oblivious to needs or safety) 1 or 2 = ●⁹	a.		
		b. **VERBALLY ABUSIVE** (others were threatened, screamed at, cursed at) 1 or 2 = ●⁹	b.		
		c. **PHYSICALLY ABUSIVE** (others were hit, shoved, scratched, sexually abused) 1 or 2 = ●⁹	c.		
		d. **SOCIALLY INAPPROPRIATE BEHAVIOR** (made disrupting sounds, noisy, screams, self-abusive acts, sexual behavior or disrobing in public, smeared/threw food/feces, hoarding, rummaged through others' belongings) 1 or 2 = ●⁹	d.		

		SECTION J. DISEASE DIAGNOSES	260-263.9 = ●¹²	276.5 = ▲¹⁴	291.0-293.1 = ●¹
	*Include **ONLY THOSE DISEASES DIAGNOSED IN THE LAST 90 DAYS THAT HAVE A RELATIONSHIP** to current ADL status, behavior status, medical treatments, or risk of death.*				
2.	OTHER CURRENT DIAGNOSES AND ICD-9 CODES				

		SECTION L. ORAL/NUTRITIONAL STATUS	90	180	270
2.	HEIGHT/ WEIGHT	c. Weight Loss (i.e., 5%+ in last 30 days; or 10% in last 180 days) 0. No 1. Yes ●¹² ▲¹⁴	c.		

		SECTION O. MEDICATION USE	90	180	270
4.	DAYS RECEIVED THE FOLLOWING MEDICATION	*(Record the number of days during the last 7 days; enter "0" if not used; enter "1" if long-acting meds. used less than weekly)* a. Antipsychotics 1-7 = ▲⁹ ▲¹¹ ▲¹⁷	a.		
		b. Antianxiety/hypnotics 1-7 = ▲⁹ ▲¹¹ ▲¹⁷	b.		
		c. Antidepressants 1-7 = ▲⁹ ▲¹¹ ▲¹⁷	c.		

		SECTION P. SPECIAL TREATMENTS AND PROCEDURES	90	180	270
3.	DEVICES AND RESTRAINTS	*Use the following code for last 7 days:* 0. Not used 1. Used less than daily 2. Used daily			
		b. Trunk restraint 1 or 2 = ▲⁹ ●¹⁸	b.		
		d. Chair prevents rising 1 or 2 = ▲⁹ ●¹⁸	d.		

SIGNATURES REQUIRED ON REVERSE SIDE ➤

● = Automatic Trigger
▲ = Potential Trigger
1 - Delirium
2 - Cognitive Loss/Dementia
3 - Visual Function
4 - Communication
5 - ADL Functional/Rehab. Potential
6 - Urinary Incont. and Indwelling Cath.
7 - Psychosocial Well-Being
8 - Mood State
9 - Behavior Problems
10 - Activities
11 - Falls
12 - Nutritional Status
13 - Feeding Tubes
14 - Dehydration/Fluid Maint.
15 - Dental Care
16 - Pressure Ulcers
17 - Psychotropic Drug Use
18 - Physical Restraints

MDS QUARTERLY REVIEW — Signature, Title and Date of Staff Completing the Assessment
NOTE: Indicate sections completed next to Signature and Title.

90-Day Assessment - FIRST QUARTER

Signature of RN
Assessment Coordinator _____

Others Who Completed Part of the Assessment

Signature/Title   Date

_____

_____

_____

_____

_____

Date of Assessment:

Month	Day	Year

Review indicates change necessary to plan of care?

❏ Yes   ❏ No

_____

_____

_____

_____

_____

_____

_____

_____

180-Day Assessment - SECOND QUARTER

Signature of RN
Assessment Coordinator _____

Others Who Completed Part of the Assessment

Signature/Title   Date

_____

_____

_____

_____

_____

Date of Assessment:

Month	Day	Year

Review indicates change necessary to plan of care?

❏ Yes   ❏ No

_____

_____

_____

_____

_____

_____

_____

270-Day Assessment - THIRD QUARTER

Signature of RN
Assessment Coordinator _____

Others Who Completed Part of the Assessment

Signature/Title   Date

_____

_____

_____

_____

_____

Date of Assessment:

Month	Day	Year

Review indicates change necessary to plan of care?

❏ Yes   ❏ No

_____

_____

_____

_____

_____

_____

_____

REFERENCES

Anthony, J.C., et al. Limits of the Mini-Mental State as a screening test for dementia and delirium among hospital patients. *Psychol Med* 12:397–408, 1982.

Applegate, W.B., Blass, J.P., and Williams, T.F. Instruments for the functional assessment of older patients. *N Engl J Med* 322(17):1207–1213, 1990.

Beck, A.T., and Beck, R.W. Screening depressed patients in family practice: A rapid technique. *Postgrad Med* 52(6):81–85, 1972.

Bender, P. Deceptive distress in the elderly. *Am J Nurs* 10:29–33, 1992.

Bergner, M., Bobbitt, R.A., Carter, W.B., and Gilson, B.S. The sickness impact profile: Development and final revision of a health status measure. *Med Care* 19(8):787–805, 1981.

Bergner, M., Bobbitt, R.A., Pollard, W.E., et al. The sickness impact profile: A validation of a health status measure. *Med Care* 14(1):57–67, 1976.

Berkman, L.F. The assessment of social networks and social support in the elderly. *J Am Geriatr Soc* 31(12):743–749, 1983.

Blazer, D.G. Social support and mortality in an elderly community population. *Am J Epidemiol* 115(5):684–693, 1982.

Brody, J.A., and Foley, D.J. Epidemiologic considerations. *In* Schneider, E.L. (ed.). *The Teaching Nursing Home*. The Beverly Foundation. New York: Raven Press, 1985, pp. 9–25.

Carnevali, D.L. The diagnostic reasoning process. *In* Carnevali, D.L., Mitchell, P.H., Woods, N.F., and Tanner, C.A. *Diagnostic Reasoning in Nursing*. Philadelphia: J.B. Lippincott, 1984, pp. 25–56.

Carpenito, L.J. *Nursing Diagnosis: Application to Clinical Practice*. Philadelphia: J.B. Lippincott, 1983.

Carpenito, L.J. *Nursing Diagnosis: Application to Clinical Practice*. 4th ed. Philadelphia: J.B. Lippincott, 1992.

Center for Functional Assessment Research. *Guide for the Use of the Uniform Data Set for Medical Rehabilitation*. Version 3.1. Buffalo, NY: State University of New York at Buffalo, March, 1990.

Champagne, M.T., Neelon, V.J., McConnell, E.S., and Funk, S. The NEECHAM Confusion Scale: Assessing acute confusion in the hospitalized and nursing home elderly. *The Gerontologist* 27(October, special), 4A:1989.

Clark, G.S. Functional assessment in the elderly. *In* Williams, T.F. (ed.). *Rehabilitation in the Aging*. New York: Raven Press, 1984, pp. 111–124.

Cole, E. Assessing needs for elders' networks. *JOGN Nursing* 11(7):31–34, 1985.

Cress, M.E., Schechtman, K.B., Mulrow, C., et al. Relationship between physical performance and self-perceived physical function. *J Am Geriatr Soc* 43:93–101, 1995.

Doyle, G.E., Dunn, S.I., Thadani, I., and Lenihan, P. Investigating tools to aid in restorative care for Alzheimer's patients. *J Gerontol Nurs* 12:19–24, 1986.

Duke University Center for the Study of Aging and Human Development. *Multidimensional Functional Assessment: The OARS Methodology*. Durham, NC: Duke University Press, 1978.

Duke University Center for the Study of Depression in Later Life. *Depression Evaluation Schedule for the Elderly*. Durham, NC: Department of Psychiatry, Duke University Medical Center, 1986.

Falcone, A.R. Comprehensive functional assessment as an administrative tool. *J Am Geriatr Soc* 31(11):642–650, 1983.

Farina, A., Arenberg, D., and Guskins, S. A scale for measuring minimal social behavior. *J Consult Psychol* 21:265–268, 1957.

Feher, E.P., Larrabee, G.J., and Crook, T.H. Factors at-

tenuating the validity of the geriatric depression scale in a dementia population. *J Am Geriatr Soc* 40:906–909, 1992.

Folstein, M.F., Anthony, J.C., and Parhad, L. The meaning of cognitive impairment in the elderly. *J Am Geriatr Soc* 33(4):228–235, 1985.

Folstein, M.F., Folstein, S.E., and McHugh, P.R. Mini-mental state: A practical method for grading the cognitive state of patients for the clinician. *J Psychiatr Res* 12:189–198, 1975.

Fried, L.P., Storer, D.J., King, D.E., and Lodder, F. Diagnosis of illness presentation in the elderly. *J Am Geriatr Soc* 39(2):117–123, 1991.

Giduz, B.H., Snow, T.L., Sanchez, C.J., et al. *Geriatric First Aid Kit*. Chapel Hill, NC: University of North Carolina, Program on Aging, 1986.

Gordon, M. *Nursing Diagnosis: Process and Application*. New York: McGraw-Hill, 1982.

Gordon, M. *Nursing Diagnosis: Process and Application*. 2nd ed. New York: McGraw-Hill, 1987.

Granger, C.V., Albrecht, G.L., and Hamilton, B.B. Outcome of comprehensive medical rehabilitation: Measures of PULSES profile and the Barthel index. *Arch Phys Med Rehab* 60:145–154, 1979.

Granger, C.V., and Hamilton, B.B. UDS Report: The uniform data system for medical rehabilitation report of first admissions for 1990. *Am J Phys Med Rehab* 71(2):108–113, 1992.

Granger, C.V., and Hamilton, B.B. The uniform data system for medical rehabilitation report of first admissions for 1991. *Am J Phys Med Rehab* 72(1):33–38, 1993.

Granick, S. Psychologic assessment technology for geriatric practice. *J Am Geriatr Soc* 31(12):728–742, 1983.

Guralnik, J.M., LaCroix, A.Z., Everett, D.F., and Kovar, M.G. *Aging in the eighties: The prevalence of comorbidity and its association with disability*. Advance data from vital and health statistics. No. 170. Hyattsville, MD: National Center for Health Statistics, 1989.

Gurland, B.J., and Wilder, D.E. The CARE interview revisited: Development of an efficient, systematic clinical assessment. *J Gerontol* 39(2):129–137, 1984.

Haight, B.K. Putting OBRA into practice. *J Gerontol Nurs* 18:43–45, 1992.

Henderson, M.L. Altered presentations. *Am J Nurs* 85(10):1104–1106, 1985.

Institute of Medicine (Berg, R.L., and Cassells, J.S.). *The Second Fifty Years; Promoting Health and Preventing Disability*. Washington, D.C.: National Academy Press, 1992.

Kane, R.A. Instruments to assess functional status. *In* Cassel, C., and Walsh, J. (eds.). *Geriatric Medicine*. Vol 11. New York: Springer-Verlag, 1984, pp. 132–140.

Kane, R.A., and Kane, R.L. *Assessing the Elderly: A Practical Guide to Measurement*. Lexington, MA: Lexington Books, 1981.

Katz, S. Assessing self-maintenance: Activities of daily living, mobility, and instrumental activities of daily living. *J Am Geriatr Soc* 31(12):721–726, 1983.

Katz, S., Ford, A.B., Moskowitz, R.S., et al. Studies of illness in the aged. The Index of ADL: A standardized measure of biological and psychosocial function. *JAMA* 185:94–98, 1963.

Katz, S., and Stroud, M.W. Functional assessment in geriatrics: A review of progress and directions. *J Am Geriatr Soc* 37:267–271, 1989.

Kiernan, R.J., Mueller, J., Langston, J.W., and Van Dyke, C. The neurobehavioral cognitive status examination: A brief but differentiated approach to cognitive assessment. *Ann Intern Med* 107:481–485, 1987.

Kittner, S.J., et al. Methodological issues in screening for dementia; The problem of education and adjustment. *J Chron Dis* 39(3):163–170, 1986.

Koenig, H.G., Meador, K.G., Cohen, H.J., and Blazer,

D.G. Self-rated depression scales and screening for major depression in the older hospitalized patient with medical illness. *J Am Geriatr Soc* 36(8):699–706, 1988.

La Rue, A. Neuropsychological assessment. *In Aging and Neuropsychological Assessment.* New York: Plenum Press, 1992.

Laughlin, J.A., Granger, C.V., and Hamilton, B.B. Outcomes measurement in medical rehabilitation. *Rehab Mgt* Dec/Jan: 57–58, 1992.

Lawton, H.P. and Brody, E.M. Assessment of older people: Self-maintaining and instrumental activities of daily living. *Gerontologist* 9:179, 1969.

Lawton, M.P. The functional assessment of elderly people. *J Am Geriatr Soc* 19(6):465–481, 1971.

Lawton, M.P. Dimensions of morale. *In* Kent, D., Kastenbaum, R., and Sherwood, S. (eds.). *Research Planning and Action for the Elderly.* New York: Behavioral Publications, 1972.

Linn, B.S., Linn, M.W., and Gurel, L. Cumulative illness rating scale. *J Am Geriatr Soc* 16(9):622–626, 1968.

Linn, M.W., and Linn, B.S. The rapid disability rating scale–2. *J Am Geriatr Soc* 30(6):378–382, 1982.

Linn, M.W., Sculthorpe, W.B., Evje, M., et al. A social dysfunction rating scale. *J Psychiatr Res* 6:299–306, 1969.

Luke, E., Norton, W., and Denbigh, K. Prevalence of psychologic impairment in an advanced age population. *J Am Geriatr Soc* 30(2):114–122, 1982.

Lyden, P.D., and Lau, G.T. A critical appraisal of stroke evaluation and rating scales. *Stroke* 22:1345–1352, 1991.

Maddox, G.L. Functional screening and assessment. *Long-Term Care Adv* 1(2):1–9, 1989.

Mahoney, F.I., and Barthel, D.W. Functional evaluation: The Barthel Index. *Maryland State Med J* 14:61–65, 1965.

Miller, D.K., Morley, J.E., Rubenstein, L.Z., et al. Formal geriatric assessment instruments and the care of older general medical outpatients. *J Am Geriatr Soc* 38(6):645–651, 1990.

Molde, S. Understanding patients' agendas. *Image* 18(4):145–147, 1986.

Morris, J.N., Hawes, C., Fries, B.E., et al. Designing the national resident assessment instrument for nursing homes. *Gerontologist* 30:293–307, 1990.

Neelon, V.J., Funk, S.F., Carlson, J.T., and Champagne, M.T. The NEECHAM Confusion Scale: Relationship to clinical indicators of acute confusion in hospitalized elders. *The Gerontologist* 29(October, special), 65A:1989.

Parmalee, P.A., Thuras, P.D., Katz, I.R., and Lawton, M.P. Validation of the cumulative illness rating scale in a geriatric residential population. *J Am Geriatr Soc* 43:130–137, 1995.

Pendleton, S.H. Clarification or obfuscation? *Am J Nurs* 86(8):944, 1986.

Pfeiffer, E. A short, portable mental status questionnaire for the assessment of organic brain deficit in elderly patients. *J Am Geriatr Soc* 23(10):433–441, 1975.

Pfeiffer, E., Johnson, T., and Chiofolo, F. Functional assessment of elderly subjects in four service settings. *J Am Geriatr Soc* 29(10):433–436, 1981.

Pinholt, E.M., Kroenke, M.C., Hanley, M.C., et al. Functional assessment of the elderly: A comparison of standard instruments with clinical judgment. *Arch Intern Med* 147:484–488, 1987.

Reuben, D.B., and Siu, A.L. An objective measure of physical function of elderly outpatients: The Physical Performance Test. *J Am Geriar Soc* 38:1105–1112, 1990.

Rice, D.P., and LaPlante, M. Chronic illness, disability, and increasing longevity. *In* Sullivan, S., and Lewin, M.E. (eds.). *The Economics and Ethics of Long-Term Care and Disability.* Washington, D.C.: The American Enterprise Institute for Public Policy Research, 1988.

Robinson, B.E., Lund, C.A., Keller, D., et al. Validation of the functional assessment inventory against a multidisciplinary home care team. *J Am Geriatr Soc* 34(12):851–854, 1986.

Rosencranz, H.A., and Pihlblad, C.T. Measuring the health of the elderly. *J Gerontol* 25(1):129–133, 1970.

Rubenstein, L.A., Stuck, A.E., Siu, A.L., and Wieland, D. Impacts of geriatric evaluation and management programs on defined outcomes: Overview of the evidence. *J Am Geriatr Soc* 39(Suppl):9S–16S, 1991.

Rubenstein, L.V., Calkins, D.R., Greenfield, S., et al. Health status assessment for elderly patients: Report of the society of general internal medicine task force on health assessment. *J Am Geriatr Soc* 37:562–569, 1989.

Schouten, J. Important factors in the examination and care of old patients. *J Am Geriatr Soc* 23(4):180–183, 1975.

Schwamm, L.H., Van Dyke, C., Kiernan, R.J., et al. The neurobehavioral cognitive status examination: Comparison with the cognitive capacity screening examination and the mini-mental state examination in a neurosurgical population. *Ann Intern Med* 107:486–491, 1987.

Siemsen, G.C., Miller, J., Neumann, A.H., and Lucas, C.M. The predictive value of the NEECHAM Scale. *In* Funk, S.G., Tornqvist, E.M., Champagne, M.T., and Weise, R.A. (eds.). *Key Aspects of Eldercare: Managing Falls, Incontinence, and Cognitive Impairment.* New York: Springer, 1992, pp. 289–299.

Siu, A.L., Beers, M.H., and Morgenstern, H. The geriatric "medical and public health" imperative revisited. *J Am Geriatr Soc* 41:78–84, 1993.

Sloane, P.D. How to maintain the health of independent elderly. *J Am Geriatr Soc* 39:93–104, 1984.

Sokolovsky, J., and Cohen, C.L. Measuring social interaction of the urban elderly: A methodological synthesis. *Int J Aging Hum Devel* 13(3):233–243, 1981.

Solomon, P.H. Geriatric assessment: Methods for clinical decision-making. *JAMA* 259(16):2450–2452, 1988.

Spector, W.D., Katz, S., and Murphy, J.B. The hierarchical relationship between activities of daily living and instrumental activities of daily living. *J Chron Dis* 40:481–485, 1987.

Stewart, A.L., Greenfield, S., Hays, R.D., et al. Functional status and well-being of patients with chronic conditions. Results from the medical outcomes study. *JAMA* 262(7):907–913, 1989.

Tanner, C.A. Factors influencing the diagnostic process. *In* Carnevali, D.L., Mitchell, P.H., Woods, N.F., and Tanner, C.A. (eds.). *Diagnostic Reasoning in Nursing.* Philadelphia: J.B. Lippincott, 1984a, pp. 61–82.

Tanner, C.A. Diagnostic problem-solving strategies. *In* Carnevali, D.L., Mitchell, P.H., Woods, N.F., and Tanner, C.A. (eds.) *Diagnostic Reasoning in Nursing.* Philadelphia: J.B. Lippincott, 1984b, pp. 83–104.

Teng, E.L., Chiu, H.C., Schneider, L.S., et al. Alzheimer's dementia: Performance on the mini-mental state examination. *J Consult Clin Psychol* 55:96–100, 1987.

Tombaugh, T.N., and McIntyre, N.J. The mini-mental state examination: a comprehensive review. *J Am Geriatr Soc* 40:922–935, 1992.

Vermeersch, P.E.H. Clinical assessment of confusion. *In* Funk, S.G., Tornquist, E.M., Champagne, M.T., and Wiese, R.A. (eds.): *Key Aspects of Eldercare: Managing Falls, Incontinence, and Cognitive Impairment.* New York: Springer, 1992, pp. 251–261.

Wolanin, M.O. Mental health assessment as a part of the physiological status of the elderly. *In* American Nurses Association (eds.). *New Directions for Nursing in the 80's.* Kansas City, MO: ANA, 1980, pp. 91–97.

Yesavage, J.A., Brink, T.L., Rose, T.L., et al. Development and validation of a geriatric depression screening scale: A preliminary report. *J Psychiatr Res* 17(1):37–49, 1983.

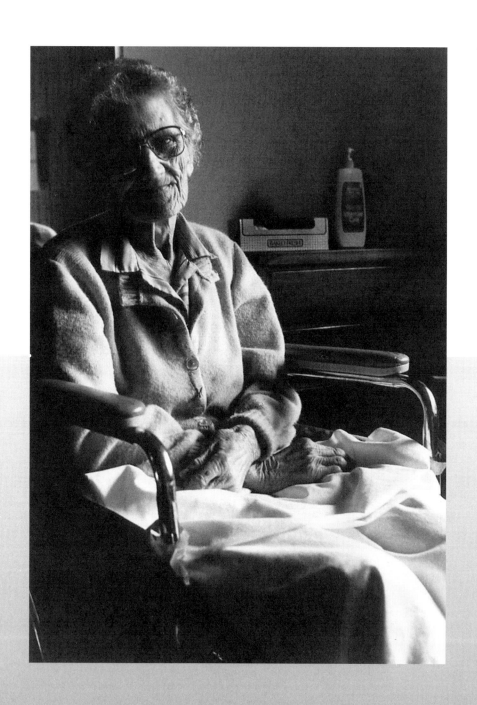

Ethical Considerations

MARTHA L. HENDERSON
ELEANOR S. McCONNELL

OBJECTIVES

Define and describe professional ethics and ethical dilemmas related to nursing care of the elderly.

❖

Employ ethical models and principles as frameworks for ethical decision making in gerontological nursing.

❖

Utilize specific processes and techniques to promote ethical decision making in the care of older clients.

❖

Relate community and societal ethical problems, such as rationing of services, euthanasia, and rights of institutionalized patients, to standards of nursing care of the elderly.

❖

Analyze individual and family ethical dilemmas and formulate appropriate nursing care measures.

THE NURSE'S RESPONSIBILITY FOR ETHICAL ACTION
Ethics Defined
Traditional Ethical Theories
Nursing Ethics
Nature of Ethical Dilemmas in Caring for the Elderly
ETHICAL DECISION-MAKING FRAMEWORKS FOR GERONTOLOGICAL NURSES
Ethical Decision-Making Processes
Moral Principles Applicable to Care of the Aged
Specific Techniques to Promote Ethical Decision Making in Care of the Elderly
COMMUNITY AND SOCIETAL ETHICAL PROBLEMS
Standards of Care
Rationing of Services
Euthanasia
Rights of Institutionalized Patients
Research and the Aged
INDIVIDUAL AND FAMILY ETHICAL DILEMMAS

To be a nurse requires the willing assumption of ethical responsibility in every dimension of practice.

M.E. Levine (1977)

THE NURSE'S RESPONSIBILITY FOR ETHICAL ACTION

Nurses have great potential to help solve problems encountered in the health care of elderly people. Many of these problems are ethical, requiring nurses to see themselves as appropriate problem solvers of ethical issues. Whether or not they exercise this responsibility consciously or knowledgeably, nurses make ethical decisions quite frequently.

The field of nursing ethics, especially related to care of elderly people, has expanded greatly in recent years. First has come the development of an ethic of care. This new theory of moral reasoning has contributed significantly to the knowledge base of ethical inquiry and the process of ethical analysis. The second area of expansion relates to the Cruzan case, and, in turn, to the passage of the Patient Self-Determination Act, a Federal law passed in 1990 (described and discussed later). The increased awareness and use of advance directives at the end of life has brought ethical considerations into the forefront of gerontological practice.

Ethics Defined

Ethics is a systematic, thoughtful process to determine right or best decisions. For nurses, this means deciding the best course of action for those in their care.

Ethics illuminates our understanding of human problems and is concerned with the "distinction between what is and what ought to be" (May, 1983, p. 13). Ethics provides a clearer picture of the world as it is and as it might become, thus offering deeper insight into problems and liberating thoughtful choices as solutions to problems. Ethics can help define the ideal in both the individual nurse and the nursing profession, and it focuses on the quality of the decisions made and actions taken.

Ethics is closely related to values and to legal guidelines for right behavior. Values are accepted beliefs about what is right, usually shaped by tradition, society, respected others, and institutions of respect, such as churches or synagogues. One's personal values may influence how one perceives and evaluates a situation. It is important for nurses to acknowledge their own value systems and to realize that these are subjectively held sets of beliefs that may differ significantly from the patient's value system. This acknowledgement will help nurses take care not to impose unconsciously their values onto the patient. As clinicians gain greater understanding of diverse cultural influences on the experience of health and illness, awareness of one's values and how they may differ from a particular patient's values becomes ever more important (Caralis et al., 1993; Pawlson, 1995).

The law sets parameters that determine what decisions and actions are permissible. Institutional regulations further delineate how the law will be implemented. Although values and laws always have an influence on decision making, they are obviously not sufficient in terms of ethical considerations. To practice ethics means to go beyond one's personal values and society's legal constraints and thoughtfully discern what is right.

Traditional Ethical Theories

The discipline of ethics is historically rooted in philosophy and theology. As Western thought developed, there was interest in discerning right thought and conduct to guide society and individuals. Two major theories developed to guide the process of decision making about what is right or best: deontology and utilitarianism. Now added to these is an ethics of care.

DEONTOLOGY, OR FORMALISM. Deontology is based on the work of Immanuel Kant. It proposes that right decisions are made by following certain rules or principles (Fig. 3–1). Decisions are based on rational and logical thought processes. Deontology is also called an ethic of duty or obligation. Adherents feel bound to follow the principles they think guide persons on a moral path. Examples of moral principles that are well accepted today include beneficence (do good), nonmaleficence (do no harm), autonomy (self-determination), respect for personhood, alleviation of suffering, death with dignity, and preservation of life. These principles are general and only point the way to ethical decisions.

Sometimes principles conflict, and the moral agent must decide which principle is more important in a particular situation. For example, a terminally ill patient may be suffering and want to cease all aggressive treatment so that she may die. The nurse may consider very important both the principle to preserve life and the principle to support the autonomy of a patient. The nurse may decide that the principle of autonomy has higher priority than the principle of preserving life, and thus support the patient in her decision to forego life-sustaining treatment.

UTILITARIANISM. Utilitarianism, or consequentialist ethics, is based on a process of weighing the consequences of one's proposed decision. In this theory, the right decision is the one in which the benefits outweigh the burdens. Thus, for any decision, the pros and cons are carefully predicted and considered before any decision is made (Fig. 3–2).

In a societal context, utilitarianism calls for the greatest good for the greatest number. It is often used in discussions of the allocation of scarce resources. Utilitarian theory conflicts with the traditional medical value of doing all one can and mobilizing all available resources for a single individual. Utilitarian theory is sometimes applied to undervalued older clients who have lived a long life and have begun to experience chronic physical and mental health problems.

ETHIC OF CARE. In the last 10 years, women theorists have begun questioning the traditional models of ethical inquiry, primarily because they reflect a society that has not

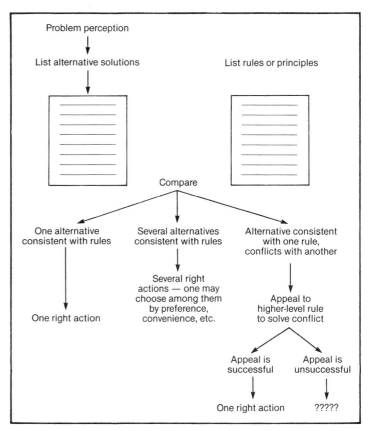

F I G U R E 3 – 1

Formalism, or the deontological ethical method. (From Brody, H. *Ethical Decisions in Medicine.* 2nd ed. Boston: Little, Brown, 1981.)

included the thought and experience of women (Gilligan, 1982; Noddings, 1984; Ahronheim et al., 1994).

Gilligan notes that the work of Kohlberg (1969) on the development of moral reasoning included research only on boys and showed a predominance of concern for individual human rights. Gilligan concludes from studying girls that they judge what is right and wrong within the context of relationships. Kohlberg's subjects worried about people interfering with each other's rights, whereas Gilligan's subjects were concerned about not hurting others when they could help. "To admit the truth of the women's perspective to the conception of moral development is to recognize for both sexes the importance throughout life of the connection between self and other, the universality of the need for compassion and care" (Gilligan, 1982, p. 98).

Traditionally, ethics has focused on moral reasoning based on principles and propositions. The language has been that of masculine concepts of justice, duty, rules. Noddings asserts that a more natural approach to ethics is through feminine concepts of re-

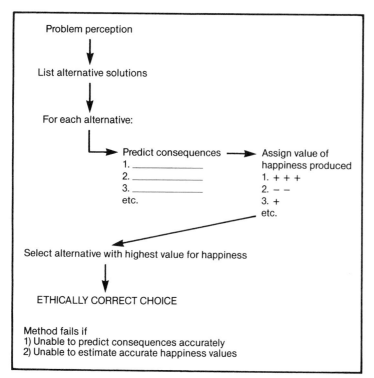

Problem perception

List alternative solutions

For each alternative:

Predict consequences ———→ Assign value of
1. _____   happiness produced
2. _____   1. + + +
3. _____   2. − −
etc.   3. +
                          etc.

Select alternative with highest value for happiness

ETHICALLY CORRECT CHOICE

Method fails if
1) Unable to predict consequences accurately
2) Unable to estimate accurate happiness values

FIGURE 3 – 2

Utilitarianism, or the act-utilitarian ethical method, which proposes the greatest good for the greatest number. (From Brody, H. *Ethical Decisions in Medicine*. 2nd ed. Boston: Little, Brown, 1981.)

latedness, receptivity, and responsiveness. Moral decisions are made in real situations and begin with a "longing for goodness and not with moral reasoning" (Noddings, 1984, p. 2). The caring relationship is ethically basic and includes reciprocity, although there is a "one-caring" and "one cared-for." She proposes that an ethic of caring must "be directed to the maintenance of conditions that will permit caring to flourish" (pp. 1–5).

It is interesting that the shift in emphasis from a principle-based approach to ethical reasoning to an ethic of care may be helpful in working with individuals from some ethnic minority groups. Review of a series of papers concerning ethical considerations with nonwhite minority groups, including African-Americans, Hispanic-Americans, Native Americans, Asians, and Pacific Islanders, suggests that some well-accepted procedures for practicing "preventive ethics," such as obtaining advance directives, may work in a manner that is contrary to cultural norms of these groups (Bedolla, 1995; Hepburn and Reed, 1995; Mouton et al., 1995; Yeo, 1995). The ethic of care, with its emphasis on considering contextual factors, may provide some

more satisfactory approaches than is true for principle-based ethics.

Nursing Ethics

As a field, nursing ethics has developed over the last 15 years. During this period, nursing ethics started with traditional approaches and recently has begun defining more specifically what nursing has to bring to the issue of determining what is best for patients.

Nursing Ideal

A professional assumes certain ethical standards and ideals of practice. An ethical professional must have several qualities: (1) maximal competence in the prescribed area of service, (2) contribution of a service that has significant social value; (3) ability to practice with a high degree of autonomy, and (4) competent decision making in his or her area of expertise and work setting.

Historically, nursing ethics has strongly emphasized the value of a holistic perspective, which is shared by the humanities. Nightingale insisted that nursing address all needs of patients: physical, spiritual, emotional, social, and intellectual. She also contended that nursing was an art as well as a science. Sward comments on shared values of nursing and the humanities and suggests that health care be concerned with a broad understanding of the human situation involving psychological, social, economic, and environmental factors, not just narrowly defined scientific factors. The nursing profession is interested in the quality of life, not just the quantity of life (i.e., the duration of one's life). Nurses see the practitioner-patient relationship as a potentially creative and therapeutic force in healing. Nurses are also interested in broad ethical issues such as resource allocation and desire for personal meaning in patient encounters. In short, they have a strong interest in humanizing health care (Sward, 1980).

There is a tradition in ethics, called virtue ethics, that looks at the character of the moral agent to determine the quality of the decisions made. The moral agent with the highest of ethical standards and ideals will be able to make the best decisions. Nightingale alluded to the moral nature of the profession of nursing by noting that it should be considered a "calling" (Jameton, 1984). According to Henderson (1982, p. 30), "Ethics involves clarifying one's own idea: Who I ought to be, as a nurse: What is my commitment to my patient? The fundamental issue of who the nurse is precedes the issue of what the nurse does."

The concept of advocacy has been used to describe the ideal role of the nurse in relationship to the patient (Winslow, 1984; Copp, 1986, Gadow, 1980b, Henderson, 1990b). The nurse as advocate supports the principle of autonomy and is instrumental in helping patients maximize their freedom of informed choice about their care.

According to Copp (1986, p. 259):

Among health care professionals who attend the patient, nurses are in a privileged position if they are willing to recognize and accept advocacy opportunities. Not only do nurses attend patients when distress is immediate, but they attend them for sustained periods of time, often providing those intimate details of physical and emotional care that lead to a deepened knowledge of a person as a distinct and unique human being.

Nurses can enable patients to "authentically exercise their freedom of self-determination" as they help patients clarify what they want to do in a specific situation, based on their beliefs and values (Gadow, 1980a).

Principle-Based Ethics in Nursing

Despite the limitations of principle-based ethics, nurses still find principles that guide their practice useful. In addition to the general ethical principles as they apply to geriatric populations that will be discussed later in this chapter, nurses have a professional code of ethics, which states principles that apply to all nurses as they fulfill their specific roles. Codes of ethics often exceed the legal standards for practice. Violation of a code of ethics is not punishable by law, but the American Nurses' Association may impose sanctions, such as reprimands, censure, suspension, or expulsion, for violation of the Code for Nurses (Thompson and Thompson, 1981). The code of ethics with interpretive statements (American Nurses' Association, 1976) is worthy of every nurse's attention, study, and adherence.

A Nursing Ethic of Care

Based on the work of Noddings and Gilligan cited earlier, some nursing theorists have adapted the ethic of care to nursing as a necessary complement to traditional principle-based ethics (Benner and Wrubel, 1989; Watson, 1985; Cooper, 1989, 1991). The essential elements of an ethic of care are that moral choices are made in particular situations, by unique human beings who are in relationships with others. The nurse, as the professional person who is the "one-caring," is able to facilitate the patient working through a morally demanding situation, by virtue of a caring, reciprocal relationship in which patient and nurse get to know, trust, and appreciate each other. The nurse can help the patient discern what is best in accordance with the patient's values, feelings, and goals at this particular time. According to Benner and Wrubel (1989), embodiment, or making tangible the human situation that seeks understanding, is necessary in detail to define the worthwhile and the good. Disembodied reasoning is critically limited in relevant ethical understanding.

Nursing theory and knowledge assume concepts of person, health, environment, and nursing. An emerging concept in the metaparadigm of nursing is the element of caring. Caring is the foundational substance of nursing and must be explicitly incorporated into practice (Watson, 1985). In a study of critical care nurses, Cooper (1991) found that they used with patients both principle-based ethical reasoning and an ethic of care to discern what was best. The contextual and relational nature of the ethics of care allowed the patient and nurse to struggle with the full complexity of the situation and find a solution that uniquely fit that individual in that circumstance.

Nature of Ethical Dilemmas in Caring for the Elderly

Health care of elderly people offers the nurse as ethicist a particularly challenging arena. Ethical dilemmas in the care of older people can be identified on many levels, including societal, family, and individual.

COMMUNITY AND SOCIETAL ISSUES. At the societal level, several types of dilemmas predominate: (1) the prevailing *standard of care* for older people as contrasted with that for younger people; (2) the issue of *rationing of scarce or costly health care resources,* such as surgical procedures, rehabilitation, health promotion, and disease prevention; (3) the issue of *euthanasia;* (4) the *rights of institutionalized patients* or other recipients of health care; and (5) *balancing the need for research* into the problems of the aged *with the rights of aged persons to participate or refuse to participate* as research subjects.

INDIVIDUAL AND FAMILY ISSUES. For individuals and their families, other types of concerns prevail, including: (1)

when to limit aggressive care, (2) how to handle mental incompetence while preserving personhood, (3) how to preserve autonomy in decision making about health care, and (4) conflicts of interest among family members, care providers, and the individual in making individual placement or treatment decisions.

Nurses and their patients feel the effects of unresolved ethical dilemmas in their practice almost daily. The result of many poorly resolved dilemmas is frustration about the quality of care given and the quality of life left to the older person (Hirschfeld, 1985).

In the last few years, the increased availability of technology in long-term care settings has served to heighten levels of confusion and ambiguity about moral choices. Long-term care nurses in institutions and in home care are very sensitive to this, because they are often present when patients' conditions require a decision about whether to use a life-sustaining intervention, and because of their long associations with residents and their families. Confusion about the nurses' role in moral decision making and conflicts over how the decisions are made create stress for family members and professional caregivers alike (Paier and Miller, 1991).

Explicit consideration of the issues underlying moral dilemmas in health care of the aged helps the gerontological nurse achieve greater understanding of the forces that shape the practice world and may also provide direction for a new, more satisfying, course of action.

ETHICAL DECISION-MAKING FRAMEWORKS FOR GERONTOLOGICAL NURSES

A formalized framework for ethical decision making is extremely useful in guiding the consideration of the various ethical problems encountered by older people and their caregivers. Before specifying an ethical decision-making framework, the nurse must be aware of pitfalls in ethical reasoning. Ethical decision making in health care is informed by a variety of conflicting, but equally valid, concepts of morality, and these different theoretical frameworks influence outcomes. Four fallacies in ethical reasoning are described by Hynes (1980):

- **Reductionistic thinking,** in which the individuals involved in the dilemma insist that there is only one moral dilemma in each case, when generally several moral problems coexist.

- **"Ethical dominoes,"** in which the contention is made that bad, but not necessarily related, consequences will result from an action; for example, if children with severe birth defects are allowed to die, then adult children will be given permission to kill unwanted elderly parents. The conclusion does not logically follow from the first statement.

- **"Ethical quagmires"** that result when all the ethical problems in one situation are considered simultaneously, overwhelming the individuals in the situation. It is more productive to consider each issue in turn.

- **"Exception arguments,"** for example, discussion of the "miracle case," rather than the usual outcomes of a certain set of health care circumstances. "Everyone said she was going to die, but she proved them wrong . . ."

Hynes recommends constructing an individualized ethical decision-making system based upon an understanding of the common fallacies in ethical reasoning previously listed as well as an appreciation for the traditional approaches to ethical decision making and the varied value systems held by individuals.

Ethical Decision-Making Processes

In this era of increasing moral complexity, choices are often unclear. The "right" or "best" decision is not readily apparent, and ethical dilemmas can be disturbing for patients, families, and professional caregivers.

Ethical dilemmas, choices between equally unsatisfactory alternatives, offer no "clearly best" solution; they usually involve interrelationships characterized by conflicts and tension (Davis and Aroskar, 1978). The ethical dilemmas frequently facing health professionals who work with older clients concern the following topics: (1) death and suicide, (2) competency, (3) disclosure of health information, and (4) distribution of health care resources.

The essential elements to be considered when approaching an ethical dilemma are (1) the specific ethical problem, (2) the facts of the situation, (3) the decision-making questions, (4) who the decision makers are, (5) the moral principles involved, (6) the options and consequences that pertain to the situation, and (7) an ethic of care that includes compassionate discernment of the patient's wishes and best interest.

In working with families of older persons, those family members who have been the most intensely involved should have more influence in the decision-making process than those who have had little contact with the client. Decision-making questions identify the decision maker (patient, physician, family, nurse, client, therapist), the criteria by which the decision is made (social, legal, physiological, economic), the degree of informed consent needed by the client, and moral principles involved. Underlying ethical theories are considered when looking at alternatives for actions and identifying a framework for decision making.

Hynes (1980) cites a useful approach to ethical decision making based on a model first described by Brody (1976). The model suggests that the following questions be asked to identify, clarify, and resolve ethical dilemmas:

1. What is the health problem, and what is the corresponding ethical question? For example, terminal illness is a health problem that often raises the ethical question of aggressiveness of care.

2. Who is involved in the health/ethical dilemma? All individuals who have an interest in the decision are likely to be affected. In addition to the patient, caregivers of all types often have an interest in the decision. Family, professional, and paraprofessional caregivers may experience conflicts with personal or professional values when decisions to limit aggressiveness of care are made.

3. What is the role of each person involved? Technical expert is one important role in making decisions about aggressiveness of care. Other equally important roles include that of the patient, advocate for the patient's values if the patient is unable to speak, and advocate for the rights of others, such as family caregivers.

4. Am I the decision maker for either the health problem or ethical problem? Hynes contends that often either no one wants to claim responsibility for making the decision or everyone involved feels responsible for the decision. In the first case, the patient may suffer unnecessarily, because life is prolonged or because adequate symptom control is not achieved. When everyone involved feels responsible, conflicts among personal value preferences of the caregivers may override the patient's right to self-determination.

5. What are the implications of the possible decisions for myself and for the others involved? According to Hynes, the more al-

ternative solutions are generated, the more likely it is that many values and viewpoints can be accommodated.

6. Does the decision reinforce my general value orientation? The final step is an attempt to get the decision maker to respond consistently. It also helps the professional to confront conflicts between personal and professional ethics. When professionals repeatedly find themselves in personal conflict with decisions made in accordance with professional or workplace ethics, it may be time to re-evaluate personal ethics or reconsider the wisdom of working in a setting where conflicts between personal and professional ethics are frequent.

Another quite useful framework for identifying and analyzing ethical problems in nursing practice is outlined by Thompson and Thompson (1981). Here are their guidelines, modified slightly:

1. Review the situation.
   a. Determine what health problems exist.
   b. Identify what decisions need to be made.
   c. Separate the ethical components of the decisions from those that can be based solely on a scientific knowledge base.
   d. Identify all the individuals or groups affected by the decision(s).
2. Gather additional information needed to decide a course of action.
3. Identify the relevant ethical principles.
   a. Discuss the historical, philosophical, and religious bases for each of the principles.
4. Identify your own values and beliefs:
   a. From family and other personal experience.
   b. From obligations specified in the Code for Nurses.
5. Identify values and beliefs of others involved in the situation.
   a. Consider historical, philosophical, and religious bases for the values and beliefs of others to enhance understanding.
6. Identify the value conflicts in the situation.
7. Discuss who is best able to make the decision(s).
8. Identify the fullest possible range of possible decisions and actions.
   a. Identify implications/consequences of the possible decisions and actions.
   b. Identify the congruence between possible decisions and actions and the Code for Nurses.

9. Decide on a course of action as the nurse in the situation and implement.
10. Evaluate the outcomes of the decision and use this information in the future when confronted with similar situations.

Nurses should be conversant with the various ethical decision-making frameworks available for use. Which model is chosen is less important than that the gerontological nurse be able to apply a valid framework to the ethical dilemmas that will inevitably arise in practice situations.

Moral Principles Applicable to Care of the Aged

Some moral principles that undergird standards of care for elderly people include the following: (1) the right to quality health care, (2) respect for the personhood of the aged, (3) the principle of beneficence, (4) the principle of autonomy or self-determination, and (5) the principle of distributive justice. Application of each principle to care of the elderly is discussed next.

THE RIGHT TO QUALITY HEALTH CARE. Elderly persons in the United States share in a general right of all to quality health care. According to Farley and Powers (1975),

This nation has long recognized from its founding the fundamental rights of all persons to life, liberty, and the pursuit of happiness. These rights are essentially related to the physical and psychological well-being of persons. From them derives directly, then, a right to the maintenance of health. This in turn implies a right to the availability of comprehensive health care services . . . which meet current professional standards.

The right to quality health care for elderly people means that they have adequate access to the best care available. Practically speaking, this means that older citizens have a right to the same high standards of health care as those in any other age group. The same standard should apply in terms of quality of care, although the same type of care may not be appropriate. For example, older individuals have a right to complete evaluation of a problem, information on treatment options, and participation in the decision making about the best course of treatment. If a terminally ill patient develops a new problem, the health care team, including the patient, may elect not to assess the problem using invasive techniques. However, the election of a less aggressive course of assessment and treatment should not mean that the standard for complete, high quality care should be sacrificed with older people.

Astute observers note that advance directives not to undertake advanced life support are sometimes overinterpreted by clinicians to mean that all curative therapies should be abandoned. Such a stance oversimplifies the issues at stake. Haber (1986) discusses a range of technology available in health care for the aged and suggests that high-quality care can often be provided to the aged with low technology services. The issue of rationing certain technologies using chronological age as the criterion is extremely controversial, partly because of the serious limitations of using chronological age as a predictor of functional status or quality of life. Since age alone is a poor predictor of functional status and well-being, older people should receive care in consideration of their unique life situations as suggested by the ANA Code for Nurses.

RESPECT FOR THE INDIVIDUAL. Elderly people deserve respect for their personhood. Inherently they are worthy and valuable, especially in ways that make them unique individuals. They are not merely a means to some other end. Kant (1964, p. 96) explicates this fundamental principle in ethics as follows:

So act that you treat humanity in your own person and in the person of everyone else . . . as an end and never merely as a means.

Although it has been argued that the elderly person is "an irrepeatable amalgam of experience and hope, a center of freedom and love" (Jonsen, 1976, p. 98), older people are often treated stereotypically and thus are depersonalized. One way in which the elderly are depersonalized is in the derogatory generalizations that are made about them, an example of ageism. Proclamations that all old people are set in their ways and not open to change indicate disrespect for the elderly as persons. In contrast, respect for older persons involves appreciation of the special characteristics and needs that are more common in the elderly population. For example, as a group, older people have less income and increasing health care needs. A respectful response to this dilemma would be for society adequately to subsidize the health costs of the elderly. Respect for personhood in the aged means treating them with the best health care available that is specifically designed to meet their particular needs. It means respecting the elderly as decision makers who deserve to be informed and allowed to make decisions about their living and dying, including participation or nonparticipation in research and teaching efforts.

May (1982) contends that the aged should not be excluded from expectations of moral responsibility. He provides a novel description of virtues called for by advanced age, including courage, humility, patience, simplicity, benignity, and hilarity. Although not all would agree with these virtues, the point that respect for the individual includes consideration of the older person's moral responsibilities to others is valid and sometimes overlooked.

BENEFICENCE. The principle of beneficence, or "doing good," means that the highest good will be done for elderly people in a particular situation. Obviously, use of this principle must involve providing an interpretation of what is "good." According to Gadow (1980b), in medicine, the criteria for defining benefit relate to the alleviation of suffering and the preservation of life. Although these are generally accepted benefits of care, they are still subject to interpretation and weighing of benefits to define the highest value. The best thing to do in the case of a terminally ill patient who wants to die may be to alleviate suffering by withholding antibiotic therapy rather than prolonging life. Some ethicists claim that this action would violate the principle of doing no harm (nonmaleficence), whereas others would contend that inappropriately aggressive treatment of this person in this situation would be harmful. Deciding with the patient and/or family what is most beneficial given the particular circumstances and then facilitating that action is an example of "doing good" in the care of the aged.

The establishment of programs to enable elderly persons to stay as healthy, functional, and independent as possible could be regarded as beneficent. Beneficence relies on the sensitivity of the provider to detect and interpret the needs of a patient and then to respond in a caring and helpful way. Beneficence also requires looking at the long-term benefits or harms of treatment. In certain situations, immediate beneficial results are realized for the patient and family when lives are saved. However, the years of disability that sometimes ensue may not be judged beneficial. It can be argued that society has an obligation to provide long-term quality of life for those aged who "benefit" from aggressive treatment in acute situations. Ethical decisions thus have long-term implications however difficult it may be to predict certain outcomes.

AUTONOMY OR SELF-DETERMINA-TION. The principle of autonomy or self-determination is critical in caring for the aged. Respecting the principle of autonomy means that elderly patients will be respected as decision makers about their own care. All competent older persons have a perspective on their own best interests, shaped by their values and beliefs developed over a lifetime, that defines each individual as a unique person. Based on this unique set of values and beliefs, individuals assess alternatives, arrive at preferences, and try to implement that preference, either individually or with the assistance of others.

In health care situations, frail older persons have varying abilities to exercise autonomy, and therefore clinicians have specific responsibilities to an older patient in order to respect autonomy. These include (1) recognizing and acknowledging the validity of the values and beliefs of the older person, especially when the clinician differs with those values and beliefs; (2) assisting the older person to identify relevant values and beliefs; (3) assisting the older person to express a value-based preference; and (4) refraining from interfering with the implementation of that preference by the older person, or assisting with its implementation as necessary, given the limitations on the older person's ability (McCullough, 1990). Although autonomy is a complex, multidimensional concept that has eluded simple definitions, an underlying theme among all definitions is the presumption that individuals are the best judges of what is in their interest (Caplan, 1990).

Nursing home patients experience particular difficulties in exercising autonomy. Inherent in satisfactory nursing home life is resolution of the "dialectic between autonomy and security needs," a dialectic that requires continual renegotiation for satisfactory function (Parmalee and Lawton, 1990). Recognition of this difficult reality has spawned a thought-provoking study of "everyday ethics" in nursing homes that raises the startling prospect that for some individuals, the "morality of the mundane" may be a determining factor in quality of life for frail nursing home patients (Kane and Caplan, 1990). Realizing the importance of the potential for violations of autonomy in everyday living is a particularly important function for nurses, as they are frequently in a position to enforce decisions about everyday routines. They often decide whether or not an individual's choice, even one that may be contrary to conventional wisdom or one that may disrupt ward routine, should be upheld.

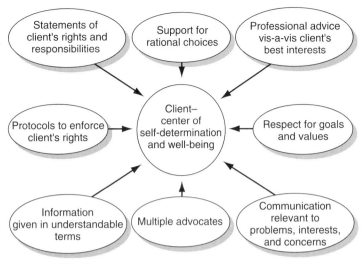

FIGURE 3 – 3

Factors that foster patient participation in health care decision making. (Redrawn from Bandman, E.L., and Bandman, B. Ethical decision making in nursing: Values and guidelines. *In* Bandman, E.L., and Bandman, B. (Eds.). *Nursing Ethics in the Lifespan.* Norwalk, CT: Appleton-Century-Crofts, 1985.)

Ironically, it is in the care of people with questionable capacity to make decisions that autonomy becomes such a predominant issue. Gadow (1980b, p. 684) suggests that if a patient is not self-determining, the principle of autonomy requires action that will most likely facilitate or restore autonomy or that has "the least possibility of permanently precluding it." For those patients who wish to waive their autonomy in deference to their care provider's advice, it must be clear that this decision was consciously and freely

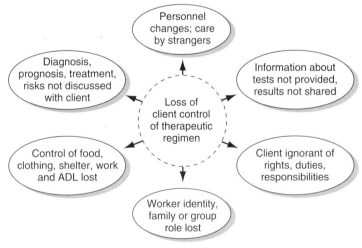

FIGURE 3 – 4

Constraints on the patient's participation in health care decisions. (Redrawn from Bandman, E.L., and Bandman, B. Ethical decision making in nursing: Values and guidelines. *In* Bandman, E.L., and Bandman, B. (Eds.). *Nursing Ethics in the Lifespan.* Norwalk, CT: Appleton-Century-Crofts, 1985.)

made. When there is a possible clash between what the health care professionals feel is most beneficial and what the patient wants, the principle of autonomy dictates that the patient's wishes should supersede the care provider's recommendation.

Legally, all adults are presumed to be competent to make their own decisions unless a court of law has been convinced that an individual is unable to make rational decisions or to care for self or property adequately, usually as the result of old age, mental illness, or mental retardation (Kapp, 1981; Regan, 1983). However, health care professionals cannot consider a consent or refusal of treatment valid if they have reason to believe that the individual is incapable of making a rational decision.

Ethicists and clinicians recognize that individuals may have varying capacity to make different types of decisions. For example, although a person in the early stages of a dementing illness may not be able to handle all business affairs, he or she may be quite capable of voicing values and opinions about treatment decisions, and preferences about daily routines and activities. The principle of autonomy requires that an elderly client be allowed, and in fact encouraged, to function at the highest level of decision making possible. Often, if a person is given the pertinent information at a time when thinking ability is clearest and patiently allowed the time necessary to process the information and make a decision, he or she can express helpful advice to caregivers regarding a treatment plan. Drane (1985) has incorporated these ideas into a "sliding scale" model of competency, in which the standards for determining competence are based on the type of decision required regarding health care. The greater the potential for harm from the decision, the more rigorous the standard for competency.

As basic as the principle of autonomy is to our freedom as human beings, it is often subtly undermined in the care of elderly individuals. Figure 3–3 diagrams the factors that promote patient autonomy. Figure 3–4 diagrams constraints on patient involvement in decision making. Clearly nurses have tremendous power to foster or constrain patient autonomy.

Adult children often put pressure on health care professionals to tell them their parent's diagnosis and prognosis and options for treatment before sharing the information with the elder patient. The temptation is for the clinicians and adult children to make decisions, supposedly in the best interest of the patient, instead of respecting the patient's autonomous decision-making ability.

When older individuals are unable to make decisions for themselves, surrogate decision makers, usually family members, can respect the patient's wishes by making decisions in accordance with the patient's general values and past choices. This practice is based on the principle of "substituted judgment," which means trying to decide as the patient would decide if he or she were capable. "Best interest" is another principle of decision making that directs the surrogate to decide what seems optimal for the patient's good, since specific wishes may be unknown, and perhaps includes factors such as the relief of suffering, the quality of life presently and in the future, and the return of function (President's Commission, 1983).

DISTRIBUTIVE JUSTICE. Distributive justice deals with problems of allocation and equitable distribution of scarce resources. Although there are several bases for claims in distributive justice, the two that apply most aptly to the elderly are contribution and need. Jonsen (1976, p. 102) interprets Hobhouse's rule for distribution as follows:

Distributive justice is the equal satisfaction of equal need, subject to the adequate maintenance of useful functions.

Avorn (1984) warns that methods of distributing medical resources, such as measuring the worth of an individual in terms of present earning capability or absence of disability, have a built-in bias against elderly persons. Many people think of the elderly as unproductive parasites that drain societal resources. They forget that most older people have been contributing to our society all their lives in various ways, including working in paying jobs and birthing and raising children who are now productive. The nature of their contribution may be different now from when they were younger, but they continue to contribute their knowledge, wisdom, and experiences to others as grandparents, volunteers, consultants, and church members. They are therefore due their share of societal goods and services. Some societies expect productivity according to one's abilities, and then share goods and services according to the needs of the people. In such a system, the elderly are due whatever they need to maintain their health and autonomy. Since health care resources are finite, how will priorities be determined? Jonsen (1976 p. 102) contends that

. . . if, in fact, it could be shown that the provision of health services to the elderly becomes so costly, in money and energy, that the health of those by whose taxable productivity the health system exists is compromised, it would not be unjust to reduce care for the elderly until equity is restored. But . . . only if this is the case would such a policy be just.

"Life boat ethics," or making decisions based on who will be sacrificed for the greater good, should be a last resort, used only after all other measures to meet existing needs have been exhausted. It is possible that if all decisions to use (or not use) costly, high technology measures were judiciously made, sufficient funds would be added to the health care resource pool to pay for some chronic disease needs that are currently neglected. The implication of distributive justice is that all health care needs of elderly individuals would receive attention, not just those acute needs that are amenable at certain times to inpatient medical manipulation. Distributive justice would not allow curtailment of services using chronological age alone as a criterion.

In this age of anticipated rationing because of high costs and the necessity for cost-containment, Eddy (1991) suggests that "essential" care be defined for all citizens to set minimum standards of care. This would entail identifying specific interventions, patient indications, estimation and evaluation of benefits, harms, and costs, and a comparison with alternative treatments. Using outcome criteria to justify costly interventions will become increasingly commonplace in all age groups. It may become evident through proper research into effectiveness of interventions that some high-technology procedures and treatments in the acute care setting are less beneficial than some less costly outpatient rehabilitative and maintenance interventions that would apply to many of the chronically ill at home. A related basic ethical question is whether a society is obligated to provide the appropriate long-term maintenance therapies to patients whose lives have been prolonged through aggressive interventions in the hospital.

Specific Techniques to Promote Ethical Decision Making in Care of the Elderly

Many techniques have been advocated to facilitate the ethical decision-making process in health care. The use and limitations of selected techniques are analyzed next.

The Value History

McCullough (1984) discusses the usefulness of the patient's "value history" in preserving patient autonomy and respect for personhood when faced with dilemmas involving impaired competence. The value history is defined as a summary of the patient's values and beliefs prior to the onset of a cognitive impairment that impedes exercising autonomous judgment. Ideally, the value history is obtained when the individual is fully competent, but remember that some cultural groups may not understand the need for discussing end-of-life decisions well in advance of their occurrence (Hepburn and Reed, 1995; Mouton et al., 1995). A sophisticated values history would allow the patient to rank values—for example, "(1) I want to maintain my capacity to think clearly; (2) I want to avoid unnecessary pain and suffering; (3) I want to be treated in accord with my religious beliefs and traditions." Then the patient could give specific advance directives regarding treatment preferences.

If a patient is not able to give a value history, the next best option is to construct a value history with the help of family members or significant others. The contention is made that a value history can inform the practitioner's decisions about agressiveness of care when the older individual is no longer able to reason.

There are two major limitations to this technique. First, most clinicians are not trained in eliciting information about patient's values. Second, if they are able to elicit such information, often the patient is not questioned about values until there is some crisis, when it may be too late for patients to express themselves and significant others may not be sure about the specifics of the patient's value history.

Patient Self-Determination Legislation

With the advancement of technology that enables prolongation of life, the increased interest in autonomy and self-determination by consumers, and the increased consciousness of the high cost of technological aggressiveness at the end of life, special attention is now being paid to end-of-life decisions. Specifically, there is increased interest in having older adults prepare advance directives declaring what kind of care they want at the end of life. Advance directives often are used to limit the amount of aggressive treatment in terminal illness, although they can serve the broader purpose of clearly indicating care wishes, to remove the burden of decision making from a family member.

The Nancy Cruzan case in Missouri, ultimately decided by the United States Supreme Court, is a pivotal case in the matter of limiting treatment. Nancy Cruzan was injured in a motor vehicle accident in January, 1983, and she laid in a persistent vegetative state until she died in December, 1990. In 1988, Ms. Cruzan's parents decided that she would not want to continue to live in her existing state, and they petitioned a trial court for permission to remove her feeding tube. The favorable decision was overturned by the Missouri Supreme Court in November, 1988. In Missouri, an initial consent for treatment of an unconscious patient cannot be changed by the family or doctor. The only way treatment can be withdrawn is if the treatment causes pain to the patient, or if the patient left clear and convincing evidence that she did not want treatment before she became incompetent. Although Ms. Cruzan had communicated generally that she would not want to continue to live if she were "a vegetable" and could not live "halfway normal" (Wolf, 1990, p. 38), the state judged that she had not been sufficiently explicit to convince the state that its right to preserve life should be superseded. When the United States Supreme Court heard the case, they could not find any constitutional reason for overturning the state's decision. The impact of the Supreme Court decision was that states would be free to rule in this area. Although most states now have laws that uphold living wills, each state's statutes differ. Some states, such as Missouri, are very restrictive and protective of life, requiring a high standard of proof that an individual does not want to continue to live in a compromised state of existence. The implication is that written patient-initiated advance directives will be increasingly important in limiting treatment (Cranford, 1990; Lynn and Glover, 1990).

Another landmark event in this area of end-of-life decisions, undoubtedly growing out of the Cruzan case, was the passage of the Patient Self-Determination Act by the Federal government in 1990, which became effective in December, 1991. The Act was passed as part of the Omnibus Reconciliation Act of 1990. According to one of the architects of the legislation,

It is the purpose of this act to ensure that a patient's right to self-determination in health care decisions be communicated and protected . . . The traditional right to accept or reject medical or surgical treatment should be available to an adult while competent, so that in the event that such adult becomes unconscious or otherwise incompetent to make decisions, such adult would more easily continue to control decisions affecting their (sic) health care.

The act requires that any health care institution accepting Medicare or Medicaid monies must inform all clients of their right to make decisions about their care, including the right to accept or reject medical or surgical treatment. Clients must be given written information about their right to have advance directives according to state law. Institutions must have written policies about patients' rights and document on their charts whether or not they have executed an advance directive.

Living Wills

Most institutions have developed policies and forms that allow patients several kinds of advance directives. The living will, or patient's right to a natural death, is the oldest and most common form of advance directive. A living will generally stipulates that in the event of a terminal illness, the client does not desire any life-prolonging treatment. In most states, this document must be witnessed by two disinterested witnesses, that is, people who will not benefit from the patient's estate and who do not work for the institution providing care. It must also be notarized.

Durable Power of Attorney for Health Care Decisions

Another form of advance directive is the durable power of attorney for health care decisions. This document allows the patient to appoint a legal surrogate for health care decisions. The surrogate serves as a spokesperson for the patient when he or she becomes incapable of making the necessary choices about treatment. The surrogate should know the patient well, having paid particular attention to understanding the patient's values, philosophy, and preferences regarding end-of-life treatment decisions.

Even though the option for appointment of a durable power of attorney is now available, patients often do not take advantage of this. In a study of 43 competent hospitalized elders who participated in a discussion about advance directives, only 35 per cent showed an interest in appointing a durable power of attorney, versus 10 per cent who showed an interest in completing a living will. In general, these patients showed no urgency to appoint surrogates and did not

anticipate decisional incapacity. Patients who were more highly educated showed less suspicion about completing advance directives (Shawler, 1992).

In a study of 103 nursing home residents who were offered the opportunity to appoint a durable power of attorney, 25 per cent wished to execute this document. Of those patients, 90 per cent chose a relative, with 64 per cent choosing a son or daughter. Sixty per cent had never discussed their wishes for future medical care with anyone, although over 90 per cent had certain preferences about accepting or refusing care. Interest in life-sustaining treatment declined significantly as cognitive function was perceived as declining in the future, and as the treatment became permanent instead of temporary. Over one half of the residents in the nursing home were too cognitively impaired to participate in the study or to execute a durable power of attorney (Cohen-Mansfield, 1991).

Treatment Preferences

Although the living will is gaining in popularity and use, a limitation in the use of this document is the generality of its directive. Although such a will states that the patient does not want "extraordinary measures" in the face of terminal illness, it does not explicitly address what the individual considers extraordinary. It is increasingly commonplace for individuals to document types of treatment to be avoided more specifically, for example, cardiopulmonary resuscitation (CPR), ventilator, tube feedings, intravenous feedings, and antibiotics. In a study of 63 residents of a retirement community who had living wills, Henderson (1990a) found a significant decrease in death anxiety associated with the opportunity for residents to express their specific preferences about treatment options.

Although specific identification of patient preferences may be desired by providers and family members, when these preferences are expressed they are not always followed. Danis and colleagues (1991) documented nursing home cases in which patient wishes were not followed, although in most cases patient's preferences were heeded.

Despite the increased attention to the need for more formalized approaches to decision making about aggressiveness of care for seriously ill patients, initiating, documenting, and implementing a coordinated team effort in this area can be challenging. The first step is to give the patient and family the information and opportunity to discuss advance directives in the context of an individual's particular situation. Wanzer (1984) points out the paramount role of the patient in decision making when aggressive treatment is considered to be death prolonging and there is a medical indication to diminish aggressiveness. However, in a study of Do Not Resuscitate (DNR) decisions in seriously ill patients in three teaching hospitals in Texas, the resuscitation issue had not been settled in 13 per cent of the first survey (174 patients) and 7 per cent of the second survey (162 patients). In the total of 72 decisions not to resuscitate, the physician had made the decision with the family in 13 of the cases and had not discussed it with the patient, although the patient was competent.

How to increase the frequency of patients executing advanced directives has been investigated (Ouslander et al., 1993; High, 1993; Luptak, 1994). A number of different approaches have been developed to help elderly persons and their family members understand the concept, to consider carefully the issues involved in making advance directives, and to create possible end-of-life scenarios, all in the hope of "developing an understanding of the authentic wishes of the patient concerning treatment" (Hepburn and Reed, 1995). Counseling models and written materials have been used. Educational materials are widely available through organizations such as the American Association of Retired Persons (AARP, 1994) and through bioethics centers, which often are located in universities.

Few studies have examined beliefs cross-culturally. Caralis and colleagues (1993) compared views concerning end-of-life decisions of African-Americans, Hispanic-Americans and non-Hispanic whites. Fifty-five per cent of Hispanic-Americans said they would want to be admitted to an intensive care unit if they had dementia, compared with only 19 per cent of whites given the same scenario. Cultural differences may influence not only the specific decision made but also a patient's or family's willingness to formalize these arrangements (Hepburn and Reed, 1995).

It is difficult to get patient and family preferences discussed and documented, but also there is often disagreement among staff members as to the best decision for patients. Some nursing staff may disagree with the physician (Wilson, 1992), and house officers may disagree with the attending physicians (Winkenwerder, 1985). Team consensus about ethical decisions can be facilitated if differing value systems of providers are recognized, disagreements are openly aired, there

is an increase in formal ethics teaching, ethics consultants are used to help resolve difference, and a plan is formulated and re-evaluated periodically (Winkenwerder, 1985).

Once decisions are made, they must be communicated. For example, the information that a patient has DNR orders in effect must be available to all caregivers at all times. In a pilot study in a Milwaukee hospital, DNR patients were designated by blue armbands and the notation "DNR" beside their names. In this way, patients would have less likelihood of being resuscitated inappropriately (Centala, 1990).

Medical Futility

Discussion is growing about the ethics of offering what may be considered futile treatment because of increasing information about the ineffectiveness of CPR in many seriously ill patients (Gray, 1991) and increased attention to the benefits and burdens of treatments with questionable value (Callahan, 1991). The Council on Ethical and Judicial Affairs of the American Medical Association has concluded that physicians have no obligation to obtain consent for DNR orders when CPR is deemed to be futile. Tomlinson and Brody (1990) also argue that patients should not be offered futile treatment and given a "false choice" but that end-of-life decisions should be discussed so that patients begin to face the lack of viable options and the inevitability of their death.

Truog and colleagues (1992) question "futility" as a rationale to deny patients the option of CPR or other treatment, because some patients may beat the statistical odds against survival, and some may be willing to live with a compromised quality of life. Truog also disagrees with precluding aggressive treatment options unless the outcomes are undeniably futile, because the patient's lack of readiness to die may provide motivation to fight harder to live, and may in fact, enable the patient to survive despite the odds.

The nurse should be ready to give the patient relevant information and support him or her in making as clear a decision as possible.

Ethics Committees

Interdisciplinary ethics committees have grown in number in the last 20 years. A number of factors have led to increased interest in their use in health care, including (1) the growing sophistication of medical technology, (2) an increasing recognition that there is usually a range of acceptable options in patient care rather than just one best way, (3) a desire to be protected from litigation in controversial situations, (4) a growing awareness that factors other than medical criteria influence clinical decisions, (5) an increasing need for arbitration between patient desires and health care institutions, (6) an increasing likelihood that certain technologies or services will be rationed, (7) a need for religious groups to have a forum for discussing the conflicts between religious beliefs and health care practices, and (8) a need for a forum where the conflicting values of various parties with a stake in the outcome of clinical decisions can be aired (McCormick, 1984).

The functions of ethics committees are generally three: education, policy development, and consultation or case review. Newly formed ethics committees often spend the first several months of their meetings educating their members regarding their purpose, ethical principles, and process, and deciding upon how they would like to function. They then broaden their educational efforts to include workshops for staff and conducting ethics conferences.

Policy development is an important function of ethics committees because it fills a void between the macrolevel of policy dictated by the government and other third party-payers and the microlevel of individual decisions. Singer (1990) calls this the mesolevel, where policies help define the moral mission of the institution, promote fair treatment by explicating criteria that pertain to similar clinical situations—for example, admission criteria for intensive care units—and foster institutional discussions when management is unclear.

Consultation is usually the last and most difficult function that ethics committees provide. There are several models for consultation on individual cases, where providers usually seek advice: (1) full committee review of a case, (2) a consultant reviewing the case and presenting it to the committee for input (3) a consultant reviewing and advising on the case, and bringing it back to the committee for post-hoc discussion, and (4) a consultant reviewing and advising on the case alone (Singer, 1990). There is no consensus as to which is the most effective method for case consultation; this area needs more study and evaluation.

A variety of obstacles to the effective functioning of institutional ethics committees have been identified, including physician resistance, safeguarding patient confidentiality, and conflicts between the ethics committee's activities and the institution's self-interest. Experts in the field advise consideration of these potential problems early in the establishment of the committee to facilitate its proper functioning (McCormick, 1984; Craig et al., 1986).

Membership of institutional ethics committees varies from one institution to another and often is dictated by the express purposes of the committee. The President's Commission for the Study of Ethical Problems (1983) advocates a diverse membership. Craig and associates (1986) contend that particular attention should be paid to the roles of lawyers and community representatives on the committee. They caution that if lawyers are included, conflict of interest may arise between the attorney's role as member versus counsel to the committee. Some voice concern that including members of the community on the committee will increase the risk of breaches in confidentiality of patient information, although one could argue that the benefits of diversifying the committee with public representation far outweigh the risks.

The issue of the appropriateness of patient and family participation in their case review within the ethics committee is controversial. Agich and Younger (1991) suggest that the committee's responsibility for balancing conflicts and seeking the best decision is helpful in considering whether to allow committee access to the patient/family. Patient and family input are essential to any case discussion, but this might most easily and comfortably be obtained in a one-to-one discussion with a consultant or committee member and shared with the group later. Obviously, if a patient or family insist on attending the meeting, they should be welcomed.

Hospital ethics committees generally include nurses. A survey in Illinois polled acute care institutions about nurse participation in ethics committees in that state (Oddi and Cassidy, 1990). There was an average of 2.19 nurses on the 115 committees that responded. Forty-six per cent of the nurses were master's degree prepared, 69 per cent of which were in nursing administration. Most of the nurses had taken a course in ethics on an undergraduate or graduate level. Oddi and Cassidy found that a nurse's contribution to the committee was enhanced if the nurse had some formal ethics training, years of clinical experience, master's degree level of education, and tenure on the committee beyond 1 year.

Ethics committees are just beginning to be formed in nursing homes. In 1988, a national survey of 4504 nursing home administrators was conducted to learn about the use of ethics committees. Twenty-nine per cent of the administrators responded. Only 2 per cent (nine facilities) of those responding reported having an ethics committee. The existence of a committee depended in part on large size and religious affiliation. The most frequent cases reviewed by the committee concerned treatment decisions, capacity for decision making, and formulating a professional code of ethics. Facilities without ethics committees often used institutional policies or legal advice to help in ethical dilemmas. Nine per cent sought the advice of a philosopher or ethics expert (Glasser et al., 1988).

The increase in technology and the complexity of care in nursing homes, as well as the lack of guidelines regarding appropriateness of certain treatments such as resuscitation and tube feedings, make ethical decision making increasingly difficult. Ethics committees or policies regarding treatment are needed. A pilot study in a 300-bed long-term care facility in Alberta, Canada, pointed out the ethical problems associated with tube feedings (Wilson, 1992). Ten patients were studied, and the following questions emerged as the data were examined:

1. Who should decide to initiate tube feeding?
2. How should the decision be made?
3. What are valid reasons for initiating and continuing tube feeding?
4. Is it permissible to withdraw tube feeding?
5. Is tube feeding an appropriate and effective life support?

Nurses must be involved in such ethical decisions for nursing home patients since they know these patients and their families well. More widespread establishment of ethics committees in nursing homes would help to ensure that an ethical reasoning approach is applied to these difficult decisions.

A final consideration in the development of an institutional ethics committee is the degree to which the institution expects its providers to consult with and abide by the decisions of the committee. Three models generally prevail. In the first, the decision to consult the committee is optional, and compliance with the committee's recommendations is left to the discretion of the professional(s) involved. A second model involves mandatory review of certain decisions, for example, review of "do not rescuscitate" orders in incompetent patients, but the professionals retain the authority for the final decision. A third model calls for mandatory review and compliance with the committee's recommendations. The first model risks that the decisions of the committee will be ignored. Craig and associates (1986) strongly recommend against the third model, because of the dilution of responsibility for decisions and the potential negative legal ramifications of using the ethics committee as a decision-making body.

Although not all health care institutions have formalized ethics committees, the plethora of ethical dilemmas in the care of the aged make them a worthwhile consideration for any institution or agency caring for large numbers of older people.

Legal Remedies

A variety of legal remedies exist to prevent or redress unethical practices in health care. Such remedies range from incompetence proceedings, to identification of a surrogate to act for an individual who is incapable of autonomous decision making, to lawsuits against negligent or incompetent practitioners. The primary purpose of such legal remedies is to keep professionals from applying different standards of care simply because of age.

GUARDIANSHIP. *Legal guardianship* is a mechanism that allows a surrogate to exercise individual rights for an older person who is no longer mentally competent. However, guardianship can also have the effect of denying people exercise of their rights. According to Regan (1983, p. 283), the typical statutory definition

. . . describes an incompetent as one who, by reason of mental illness, drunkenness, drug addiction, or old age, is incapable of caring for himself and/or providing for his family or is liable to dissipate his property or become the victim of designing persons. Thus, in declaring a person incompetent, a court is making two findings: (1) that the person suffers from a condition affecting mental capacity; and (2) that certain functional disabilities result from this condition, such as inability to do business, manage property, or make personal care decisions.

It should be emphasized that mental illness and incompetence are not the same; incompetence is one possible outcome of mental illness. Considerable confusion is generated by imprecise use of the term "incompetence" in professional and lay circles. Although specific criteria do not exist for the functional determination of incompetence, the following questions are often used (Kapp, 1981, p. 366):

- Can the person make choices concerning his or her life?

- Are the outcomes of these choices reasonable?

- Are these choices based on "rational" reasons?

- Is the person able to understand the implications of the choices she or he makes?

- Does the person actually understand the implications of the choices?

When incompetence is established through court proceedings, a guardian is appointed by the court to be responsible for the care of the incompetent person and his or her estate. Other terms used for guardian include conservator, committee, and curator. The guardian may be an individual or a corporation. Limited or full guardianship may be granted. In *limited guardianship,* the court specifies the particular types of decisions the individual is incapable of making, and the guardian is empowered to act as surrogate only in those areas (Kapp, 1981). When limited guardianship is not available, the guardian is called a plenary guardian. Plenary guardians are empowered to make decisions about the incompetent person's financial assets, where and with whom the incompetent person will live, and consent or refusal of medical treatment. Individuals who have involuntarily appointed plenary guardians lose many rights often taken for granted, including the rights to vote, marry, make a will, and sue others. Performance of the guardian is monitored by the court, and the guardian may be held liable for failing to act in the incompetent person's best interests.

Understanding the various motivations for pursuing guardianship, the different forms guardianship may take, and the implications of the various forms is important when advising older people, their families, and caregivers. Kapp (1981) contends that court-appointed guardianship arises out of one of two motives: (1) altruism, or a sincere desire to help another individual, and (2) administrative convenience, such as when a service provider benefits from a patient having a guardian to ensure payment of bills. The latter motive for guardianship proceedings has been criticized as unduly compromising individual autonomy. This is particularly true in states where there is no provision for limited guardianship. Kapp (1981) contends that such severe restrictions of civil rights under plenary guardianship argues for more widespread use of limited guardianship.

Although the foregoing are examples of legal transfer of decision-making power, in practice, care providers often consult competent adult children when making decisions for incompetent elderly people without going through any legal processes. Although this practice may at times be appropriate, it should be viewed with caution. Occasionally, adult children may make decisions for their parents based largely on convenience to them rather than in the "best interest" of the older person or according to patient preferences. Also, "incompetent" elderly people may be unable to perform some cognitively demanding tasks but may still retain an understanding of choices about treatment or aggressiveness of care. Long-standing values may persist and may be available to a failing older adult when mental faculties have become limited.

POWER OF ATTORNEY. This is a form of voluntary guardianship in which a competent individual freely appoints a surrogate decision maker. In most states voluntary guardianships are automatically invalidated if the individual becomes incompetent, although a *durable power of attorney,* which does not expire if the individual becomes incompetent, is recognized in some states. A durable power of attorney's authority can be specified to cover health care decisions.

PAYEE STATUS. The Social Security Administration recognizes a *"payee" status* for relatives of elderly individuals who are unable to manage their financial affairs because of physical or mental infirmity. This procedure does not require court proceedings and has no impact on the rights of the individual to make decisions in other domains. It merely allows another individual to cash the older person's social security check and, by implication, manage a major source of income. Some elderly people establish joint checking accounts to allow a friend or family member to assist in financial management. These are examples of options for assisting older people in financial management when their abilities are limited, without going through court proceedings.

Team Conferences

The notion of team decision making as a means of ensuring that ethical decisions are made is gaining increasing popularity (Thompson and Thompson, 1981). One advantage of this approach is that a wider variety of alternative actions may be identified because of the diversity of the group. Membership on the decision-making team is an important consideration. For patient autonomy to be respected, it is critical that the patient, and often family members, be included as a part of the team. Another advantage of team decision making is that when the major parties involved or affected by a decision are included in a decision, there is less likelihood that the course of action chosen will later be sabotaged by one or more members of the team (e.g., conflicts over a "do not resuscitate" order).

A limitation of this approach is that decision making becomes more cumbersome, and there is not always time to involve a large team. However, many decisions affecting the elderly do not require immediate resolutions, and there is ample time for team involvement. Another potential limitation of team conferences for the resolution of ethical problems is the "risky shift" phenomenon observed in small group process. This refers to the situation in which individuals behave less conservatively when in a group than when alone because of external pressure of the group (Lieberman et al., 1973). The concern is that patient autonomy or individual professional standards will be sacrificed for the sake of compromise or group harmony. In some instances this is a positive outcome, particularly when an impasse has been reached and a family member needs emotional and moral support for choosing the only feasible alternative.

COMMUNITY AND SOCIETAL ETHICAL PROBLEMS

There is widespread agreement in the United States that there are serious problems with the way in which the health care issues of older people are addressed. The roots of these problems are discussed in other chapters and include ageism, poverty, low status, fear of growing old, changing demography, changing role of women in society, fear of disability, and competing social priorities. The discussion to follow centers on specific problems in health care for the aged that prevail in most communities. Each set of problems is considered within an ethical decision-making framework.

Standards of Care

The prevailing standard of health care for older people in the United States is based on an inadequate understanding of the aging process and the care needs of the elderly. Current inadequacies of the United States health care system for the aged are described in Chapters 1 and 20. Problems regarding high-quality health care for the elderly pervade acute, long-term, and community care, although the nature of the problem in each setting is somewhat different. In acute care, the primary problem is expense and subspecialization: the difficulties of obtaining individualized care despite great expense and retaining personal autonomy in the hospital (Panicucci, 1983). Abuses as well as the poor standard of care in nursing homes have been well documented for many years (Mendelson, 1974; Moss and Halmandaris, 1977; Vladeck, 1980; Institute of Medicine, 1986). The problems of quality of care in the community are more difficult to document because so much happens behind closed doors. However, problems of long waiting lists for in-home services, inadequate intensity of rehabilitative services, and inadequate reimbursement for in-home services have been described (Sheehan, 1984).

Many older people receive care that is less than adequate for their needs in a country that some believe provides the best health care in the world. Reasons cited for the current inadequacy of care include cost, insufficient numbers of adequately trained personnel in geriatrics and gerontology, and inadequate knowledge base in gerontology/ geriatrics. Supporters of the current system of health care for older adults contend that suggested changes, such as expansion of community-based long-term care services or tighter control on application of unproved medical technologies, are too costly or impractical (Weissert, 1985). Specific remedies suggested to resolve the problems of poor quality care for the elderly should be considered in light of applicable ethical principles. This process should assist individual nurses in deciding which course of action to support. The following discussion illustrates the use of an ethical decision-making framework to analyze the issues that undergrid the dilemma of expansion of community-based long-term care services.

Deciding Whether to Support Expansion of Community-Based Long-Term Care Options

Development of more sophisticated in-home services to provide a better alternative to nursing home care for those with severe dependencies has been proposed as a response to the widespread dissatisfaction with institutional long-term care. Some factors that press for more serious consideration of expansion of community-based long-term care services include the following:

- Most older people say they would prefer to stay in their own homes rather than go to an institution.

- The quality of care for elderly persons in most nursing homes is substandard (Institute of Medicine, 1986).

- The quality of care in proposed community settings is poorly described.

- In most communities, community-based services are underdeveloped or inadequately reimbursed so that a majority of the care burden falls upon family members.

- Governmental reports suggest that expansion of in-home services is too costly to be supported by the government unless they truly substitute for institutional care.

- Traditional caregivers are becoming less available to provide services at no cost as more women enter the paid work force.

National demonstration projects have been conducted to evaluate the feasibility and cost impact of some programs, and therefore there is a sizable data base from which to project the impact of such activity. To evaluate the public policy alternative of controlling the growth of nursing home beds while expanding community-based services, an ethical decision-making framework is applied.

The Problem

Should the government be encouraged to expand reimbursement for community-based long-term care services while limiting use of institutional services?

The Actors

- Old people, whose care options are directly affected by such policies.

- Family members of old people, who currently provide an estimated 80 per cent of community-based long-term care services.

- Health care professionals, who prescribe and deliver care to patients, set standards of care, and evaluate quality of care.

- Insurers, who pay for the majority of health care in the United States.

- Home care industry, which is increasing its profits from providing long-term care services.

- Nursing home industry, which has tradi-

tionally profited from providing long-term care services.

- Federal and state governments (indirectly, the public), which traditionally have funded the majority of reimbursed long-term care services.

Analysis

The problem can be analyzed by using the table on the following page.

Options for Nursing Action

After careful analysis of the problem, at least three options for nursing action are possible.

1. Do nothing. This would violate the elderly person's rights of access to quality health care and self-determination; it shows disrespect to the client's individuality and rejects the principles of beneficence and distributive justice.

2. Lobby for increased reimbursement of community-based long-term care services. This time- and energy-consuming option respects individuality, the principle of beneficence, and the rights of access to quality health care and self-determination. It may also violate the principle of distributive justice and risks alienating those who want to maintain an institutional model of long-term care.

3. Support the prevailing institutionally based model of long-term care services. This option violates the rights to quality health care (unless most institutions are significantly improved) and self-determination (unless the individual so chooses). It may also show disrespect for individuality and violate the principles of beneficence and distributive justice.

After considering the ethical principles involved, it is difficult for the authors to rationalize the continued restrictions on expanded in-home services for the aged using ethical reasoning, primarily because it limits the options for high quality care. The next step for nurses who accept this argument is to decide what courses of action are available.

Interventions at the public policy level to change the limits on home-care services may seem a bit far removed from day-to-day nursing practice. The following discussion shows how such dilemmas affect the nurse at a patient care level.

It is worth noting that the current situation presents two types of problems for nurses. First, nurses must decide the extent

Expansion of Community-Based Long-Term Care Options

MORAL PRINCIPLE	RELEVANCE TO CASE	CONCLUSION
The right of everyone to have equal access to quality care.	For younger adults, the prevailing standard of care is to obtain the greatest rehabilitation in the least restrictive environment. Younger people with chronic disabilities have access to group homes and half-way houses designed to assist with their reintegration into the community.	An argument for the development of home care options.
Respect for individuality. Older people deserve respect for their own lifestyle and preferred living site.	Due consideration should be given to the often documented desire of older people to remain in their homes for as long as possible without unduly burdening their children. Callahan (1985) argues that there is little support in the US for forcing children to provide financially for their elders.	An argument for expansion of in-home services.
Beneficence demands that the health care system provide for the highest good for the elderly.	Mortality after admittance to a nursing home is high. Patient morale in nursing homes is lower than that of elderly of similar functional level in the community. In-home services, as currently organized, place tremendous burdens on families. If the service provider does not appear for work, the family must usually serve as replacement or the older person does without. Increasing the availability of in-home services may increase the societal expectation that adult children care for their parents at home, without recognizing the attendant difficulties on family members if institutional services are reduced.	If what is good for the older person is the main consideration, expanded home care services are indicated. If what is good for the family members is the main consideration, expanded in-home services may or may not be indicated.
The right of self-determination means that older people should make their own decisions.	Expanding in-home services should enhance the ability of most older people to choose what is the most attractive option for the majority—continuing to live in their own home with supportive services as needed. There is a risk that the reduced availability of institutional services will influence an individual's choice to enter a facility.	Since most older people want to remain in their homes, a social policy of expanded in-home services is supported by this principle.
The principle of distributive justice mandates that health services be distributed fairly. This means that there must be "equal satisfaction of equal need, subject to the maintenance of useful function" (Jonsen, 1976).	Studies on the cost effectiveness of community-based alternatives to long-term care suggest that the former may be more costly than nursing home care over the long term, in part because older people live longer in home care settings (Weissert, 1985). Contributing to the expense is the variability among the programs being evaluated, such as the different types of personnel used (Capitman et al., 1986). The associated costs of caring for older people in acute care settings owing to the unavailability of acceptable long-term care options and the actual cost of expanded in-home care options have not been reported.	Without specific cost data, it is difficult to argue that expanded in-home services will be so expensive that "the health of those by whose taxable productivity the health system exists" will be compromised (Jonsen, 1976).

to which they should support a suggested system reform. Second, nurses should evaluate their current work practices to determine the degree to which they support the status quo through their daily practice.

Conflict Between Nursing Standards and Reimbursement Policies

A nurse works for a home health agency in a rural setting. She routinely assesses pa-

tients' needs for in-home services. Her agency cannot afford to see many patients without a source of reimbursement. Most of the patients cared for by this agency are unable to afford in-home services privately. The nurse in question has a number of patients who meet the requirement for skilled nursing observation because they have indwelling catheters. The only way for these patients to receive home health aide services and regular nursing visits in this community is if a "skilled nursing need" is documented and the care can be reimbursed under Medicare.

Some of the patients on the nurse's caseload could potentially do without an indwelling catheter; however, someone would need to evaluate the patient's ability to void completely and be present to implement a toileting schedule. If the catheter is removed, within a short period of time the patient would no longer qualify for skilled nursing care and aide service funded by Medicare would be discontinued.

The Problem

A nurse's responsibility is to promote maximum functional independence and minimize the risk of disease. Which course of action, removing the indwelling catheter or maintaining the catheter and the home health aides, is the correct decision?

The Actors

- Patient, who has the right to refuse or accept treatment.
- Nurse, who is responsible for assessing need for care, making recommendations for care to the physician, implementing plan of care, coordinating other in-home service providers, and monitoring the patient's response to care and diseases.
- Physician, who is responsible for writing orders for home health care.
- Family of the patient, who are expected to provide "unskilled" personal services.
- Home health agency, which has the right to refuse or accept clients and the responsibility to remain fiscally solvent.

Analysis

The decision technically belongs to the patient and the physician. If a competent adult, the patient has the right to refuse treatment. The physician is the director of the patient's home care plan in the eyes of Medicare and is the individual entitled to write the order for continuing or discontinuing the indwelling catheter.

However, the decision should be influenced by a variety of considerations, including patient functional status, availability of other support services in the community including family, and prognosis of the patient without home health aide support. The nurse is in the best position to make many of these judgments and therefore should be involved in the decision-making process. Exclusion of the nurse from this process is likely to lead to a decision based on incomplete data and incorrect assumptions. The problem can be analyzed by using the table on the following page.

Options for Nursing Action

After careful analysis, at least five options for nursing action are possible.

1. The catheter remains in place; home-care providers continue as before. This would place the patient at greater risk for urinary tract infection and body image disturbance. The patient's autonomy may be violated if his or her wishes are not clarified. The right to high-quality care is violated if the incontinence is not thoroughly evaluated.

2. The nurse finds aides to assist with the toileting schedule, and the catheter is removed. The principle of beneficence, the right to high-quality care, and respect for personhood are maintained as long as the patient approves of the new aides. The principle of distributive justice may be infringed upon if excessive amounts of time or money are needed to identify and pay for the aides.

3. The nurse arranges for a thorough evaluation of the incontinence problem. There is decreased likelihood of violating the patient's right to high-quality care unless the third-party reimburser denies services because the catheter is considered medically unnecessary. Autonomy and respect for personhood are violated if the patient does not want to be evaluated.

4. The nurse clarifies the patient's preference for managing incontinence and other needs for assistance with ADLs. This reduces the risks of violating autonomy and disrespecting personhood but may infringe upon the principle of distributive justice if increased nursing time is expended. The right to high quality of care is abridged if evaluation is not offered.

5. The nurse discusses the problem with the supervisor and urges that their agency join others in seeking regulatory reform to permit restorative care without loss of benefits. This risks annoying the supervisor, resulting in closer scrutiny of the nurse's actions and of third-party payers in reviewing claims, but the principles of beneficence and the right to quality care are maintained if the regulations are changed.

A decision for action should be made after considering all the data. After a decision is implemented, it should be evaluated for ethical consistency; that is, can the rationale based on ethical principles be shown to uphold the decision?

Nursing Standards and Reimbursement Policies

MORAL PRINCIPLE	RELEVANCE TO CASE	CONCLUSION
Beneficence requires doing the highest good in a health care situation, such as eliminating preventable health problems and maximizing independence.	Preventable problems include urinary tract infection, delirium, body image disturbance from long-term catheter usage, reduced mobility, and excess dependency on tubes, all of which would be facilitated by removal of the catheter. However, removal would mean that "skilled nursing" services would not be required and subsequent lack of reimbursement would interfere with obtaining adequate helpers to implement a toileting schedule. Removal of the catheter may also increase the likelihood of skin irritation from urine, fungal skin infections from chronic wetness, altered self-image from chronic incontinence, and social isolation secondary to urine odor.	The principle of beneficence is violated regardless of the choice, unless conditions for obtaining assistance are somehow changed.
Autonomy mandates self-determination or free choice by the client.	No information is given about the patient's wishes. If the patient prefers to retain the catheter rather than give up home assistance, then the choice is made more clear. However, if the patient wants the catheter removed but the necessary continence management program is unaffordable, it is unlikely that the patient would choose to remain wet most of the time.	The system needs to be changed so that true options for obtaining necessary care are possible.
Individual respect means human needs for dignity (including hygiene and continence) must be met.	A program for maintaining continence under the present system requires a demeaning appliance or is prohibitively expensive for most individuals.	If the client wants no catheter, funding for aide help must be sought.
Right to quality health care means that the elderly have a right to thorough evaluation and management of their health problems according to the same standard as others.	No information is given about how the incontinence problem was evaluated. A thorough evaluation may reveal remediable causes.	Respecting the individual's right to high-quality health care would ensure that the individual has had the benefit of (and has agreed to) a complete evaluation of the incontinence.
Distributive justice means that the elderly deserve their fair share of resources.	Hiring adequate help to assist patient to manage without a catheter may be prohibitively expensive for the patient.	Volunteer help or funding may be sought to provide home aides.

Rationing of Services

Another societal problem regarding health care for the aged concerns the possibility of rationing of certain services and resources. This prospect becomes more likely as insurance programs such as Medicare begin to institute drastic cost-containment measures. Now that hospitals are reimbursed at a fixed fee, there is incentive to withhold expensive procedures as the individual's care becomes increasingly costly.

Haber (1986) contends that rationing of health care services on the basis of age already has occurred in the United States. He discusses the limitations to the various generic approaches to health care rationing. The approaches described include (1) the market approach, (2) the selection committee approach, (3) the lottery approach, and (4) the customary approach (patients selected according to clinical suitability). The first approach discriminates against the socially and economically disadvantaged, whereas the second and fourth approaches depend substantially on professional judgment and may be perceived as arbitrary.

Most gerontologists contend that chronological age is not an appropriate criterion for the rationing of health services. However, functional incapacity may well become the criterion applied to expensive technologies. In some cases it can be argued that advanced age decreases the individual's ability to benefit from a complex medical therapy because of age-associated decrements in homeostatic reserve. Although the justice of such decisions will be debated for years to come, it is important to recognize that rationing is already a feature of care of the elderly.

Any discussion of rationing of services should therefore incorporate an awareness that some services are already being rationed for the elderly. The basis for rationing certain types of health care may not be prohibitive cost or limited benefit but regulatory custom. For example, because Medicare reimbursement for chronic disease care is highly restricted, the services of such valuable practitioners as geriatric nurse practitioners and some rehabilitative therapies are, in effect, available only to those who can afford to pay for the services out of private funds. Home health care, although beneficial to many with chronic diseases, is "rationed" by only allowing reimbursement during unstable episodes of the disease.

Nurses should be prepared to discuss rationing of health care services to the aged from at least two viewpoints: (1) the rationing of new technologies, and (2) the need for opening debate on the wisdom of the current system of rationing low-technology services, such as home health services.

Euthanasia

Euthanasia is another controversial topic concerning the aged. The debate is complicated by imprecise use of terminology. Some individuals consider euthanasia to be when a health care provider acts in ways to promote comfort and not prolong a life of suffering, whereas others consider euthanasia to be a more active process of hastening death (Rachels, 1975).

Volicer (1986) contends that the need for euthanasia is due to inappropriate use of medical technologies and failure of the courts and philosophers to reach a consensus regarding the acceptability of limiting medical care for those in persistent vegetative states or those with advanced dementia. Some controversy exists over whether or not a true distinction exists between active euthanasia, in which action is taken to terminate someone's life, and passive euthanasia, in which measures that would prolong life are avoided (Rachels, 1975). However, in one survey, 23 religious groups refused to condone active euthanasia, whereas only 3 condemned passive euthanasia (Volicer, 1986).

Proponents of euthanasia contend that individuals with chronic, progressive, incurable illnesses should have access to an easy and painless death without prolonged suffering. The concept of foregoing extraordinary measures to promote a comfortable death is not new. Watts and Cassel (1984, p. 239) quote a Catholic theologian named Banez, who in 1595 stated that

. . . a person is bound only "to preserve his life by nourishment and clothing common to all, by medicine common to all, and even through some ordinary and common anguish, but not through any extraordinary or horrible pain, or anguish, nor by any undertakings extraordinarily disproportionate to one's state in life."

Opponents of euthanasia object to the concept from two major standpoints. First, some have religious beliefs that consider human intervention that influences an individual's death to be immoral (Volicer, 1986). These individuals revere the sanctity of continued living, regardless of the circumstances. A second major challenge to euthanasia comes from those who fear that indiscriminate criteria will be used to denote suffering, and rather than being a right, an early death will become an obligation of the elderly in our society. Hirschfeld (1985) offers a grim reminder that this is far from a remote possibility in western society. She notes that, in 1939, Nazi Germany instituted a "Euthanasia Program," in which

. . . persons who, according to human judgment, are incurably ill may, upon the most serious evaluation of their medical condition, be accorded a mercy death. (Nuremburg, 1949–1953)

She states that the killings began with infirm individuals and spread to ethnic groups and social deviants.

The goal of a comfortable death for individuals with terminal diseases is an integral part of nursing practice. However, nurses should be alert for ways in which individual autonomy is compromised by well-meaning interventions. There is an ever-present risk of paternalistic practice in health care. As eloquently stated by Hirschfeld (1985, p. 322),

Acceptable proxy assessment [of quality of life] assumes that a second person has the knowledge upon which to base quality of life judgments for another. A crucial question becomes: To what degree is such proxy judgment on a demented person's quality of life based upon such knowledge and *to what degree does it reflect projections of often unreflected and deep-seated fears and value judgments* (emphasis added)?

Recently there has been controversy over the discontinuation of life-sustaining treatments in the terminally ill (Annas, 1985; Volicer, 1986). The controversy centers on the conflict between the individual's right to refuse medical treatment and the professional's obligation to preserve health and safety. The concerns that exist about the misinterpretation of a patient's "refusal" of treatment are evidenced by the New Jersey

Supreme Court's decision to distinguish between nursing homes and other care settings in such matters, by establishing an elaborate procedure involving an ombudsman when withdrawal of life-sustaining treatment is considered in incompetent nursing home patients. However, this decision does not specify a procedure for patients who are hospitalized or in the home (Annas, 1985).

It is unlikely that anything approaching a national consensus on the appropriateness of euthanasia in care of elderly people will emerge soon. In a society characterized by pluralism in religious belief and cultural background, such an expectation is unrealistic. Most state laws currently support consideration of advance directives from the individual in determining aggressiveness of care. When caring for the elderly, nurses should be alert for instances in which advance directives are not being honored as well as cases in which the older person may be coerced into a less aggressive mode of care than is warranted by the individual's functional status or previously expressed desires.

Rights of Institutionalized Patients

Individuals in institutions are particularly vulnerable to infringements on their rights to self-determination. There is an inherent tension between the need for protection because of impaired functional status and the protection of the individual's autonomy. In long-term care institutions, the problem has been partially addressed by the enactment of the Nursing Home Patient's Bill of Rights as a part of the Medicare/Medicaid certification procedure. Similar bills of rights also have been enacted as law in some states.

Codification of the rights of institutionalized patients is a step in the right direction toward preserving patient autonomy. However, nurses must remain vigilant if the spirit as well as the letter of the law is to be honored. For example, people in nursing homes have the right to make private phone calls or to receive visitors in private. However, actually achieving privacy in an institutional environment can be extremely difficult. It requires staff who truly believe that privacy is an important part of supporting someone's personhood. In practice, it is easier to pretend that the patient does not really mind who overhears a telephone conversation or who intrudes on a visit with a friend.

Other rights of institutionalized patients may be extremely difficult to exercise. For example, a patient may have the right to complain about care and to select another care provider, but, in reality, the numbers and types of care providers in long-term care are extremely limited. When this is the case, the patient or family will be understandably fearful of reprisal if care is criticized too sharply.

Protecting the rights of institutionalized patients requires great sensitivity to the vulnerability of this population and a willingness to be honest with oneself about when patient's rights are abridged in the name of efficiency or beneficence. Without such sensitivities, all the codification of "rights" will be virtually meaningless.

Research and the Aged

Ethical dilemmas abound when considering research and the aged. On one hand, there are legitimate concerns about the potential for exploitation of elderly individuals as research subjects. When elderly persons are concentrated in settings such as nursing homes or retirement communities, it may be tempting for a researcher to see a "captive audience" and barrage these residents with requests to do research. Some advocate treating elderly people as a particularly vulnerable group that should be excluded from research populations unless their participation is absolutely essential for answering the research question. For many years this approach was taken by the National Cancer Institute when conducting clinical trials on cancer chemotherapy protocols (Kerr and Chabner, 1983).

However, the need for geriatric health care to have a scientific basis has led to criticism of excluding elderly patients from research protocols merely on the basis of chronological age (Dubler, 1993). Although it may be more time-consuming to explain the purposes of research to individuals who are hard of hearing or unaccustomed to considering themselves as potential subjects in research endeavors, for the quality of gerontological health care to advance, carefully planned research efforts must include the elderly as subjects.

As with many dilemmas in health care of the aged, using chronological age alone as in inclusion or exclusion criterion for research is inappropriate. It is extremely important to consider the following steps:

- Provide information about the purposes and methods of the study in a manner that is comprehensible to the potential subjects.

- Decide when written consent versus assent is acceptable in research procedures.

- Decide when an individual is competent to give informed consent to a research protocol.

- Decide what type of proxy consent is appropriate if the individual is unable to give informed consent.

A detailed discussion of these issues is beyond the scope of this text. For further study, the reader is referred to Wolanin (1980), Hoffman and associates (1983), Ratzan (1984), Cassel (1988), Cohen-Mansfield et al. (1988), and the American College of Physicians (1989).

INDIVIDUAL AND FAMILY ETHICAL DILEMMAS

Numerous ethical dilemmas are involved in providing care to elderly patients and their families. The following examples present familiar problems that consider possible actions based on an ethical reasoning framework. These examples show only some of the ways to approach ethically difficult situations. The reader is encouraged to attempt other systematic evaluations of similar situations to arrive at ethically sound decisions.

A Nurse's Conflict with a "Do Not Resuscitate" Order

Mr. C. is a patient in an intermediate care facility with moderately advanced Alzheimer's disease. He is functionally independent with supervision and spends the majority of his day wandering around the facility, talking to himself. It is rare that anyone carries on a meaningful conversation with him, as the majority of the time he hallucinates or talks about subjects, usually with a high level of sexual content, that have no apparent relationship to current reality. He had a cardiac arrest one morning and was resuscitated by the nursing staff. The physicians are upset because the patient had a "do not resuscitate" order in effect. The nurse's response was that the nursing assistant had begun the resuscitation effort, and besides, she could not, in good conscience, *not* resuscitate the patient, as he was so viable.

The Problem

A nurse feels in conflict with a "do not resuscitate" order for a severely demented patient because he seems "too viable."

The Actors

- Patient, who is directly affected by the outcomes of the order and nursing actions.

- Family, who are asked to serve as surrogate decision makers.

- Nursing staff, who must carry out the order and often serve as surrogate family to demented, institutionalized patients.

- Physician, who must decide whether or not to write the order.

- Other patients and staff in the facility who may serve as significant others.

Analysis

Legally, the decision must be made by the physician, although it should be formulated in consultation with patient and family, using data about the patient's functional level from all caregivers. Ethically, it should involve anyone who has an interest in the patient.

The problem can be analyzed by using the table on the following page.

Options for Nursing Action

After careful analysis, the options for nursing action can be summarized as in Figure 3–5.

1. Do not carry out the DNR order. The autonomy principle is violated because the patient's surrogates agreed to DNR status. The refusal permits adherence to the nurse's interpretation of respecting the patient's personhood and his right to the highest-quality care available. The nurse risks being terminated for failure to adhere to agency policies and may violate the distributive justice principle.

2. Follow the DNR order. The autonomy principle is honored, but respect for personhood may be violated if the wrong surrogate has been chosen or if no surrogate exists. One interpretation of the principle of distributive justice is also upheld.

3. Contact the physician and ask for reconsideration of the DNR order. The physician or family may be angered at the "intrusion" into the patient-physician relationship and the questioning of a difficult decision. There is a decreased likelihood of unwitting disrespect for personhood, an increased understanding of the reasons for the decision, and more information upon which nurses can base their actions.

4. Contact the family members and ask for reconsideration of the DNR order. The physician or family may be angered at the

Conflict with a "Do Not Resuscitate" Order

MORAL PRINCIPLE	RELEVANCE TO CASE	CONCLUSION
Beneficence in this case may mean honoring life by preserving it or allowing death to come. Doing "good" may be defined by the patient's or family's wishes or by the quality of life and amount of suffering.	If the patient has expressed strong feelings about not prolonging life or suffering and is suffering, then his wishes should be honored and his suffering alleviated. If the patient has not expressed these wishes, then doing good can be equated with preserving life. The "good" may be defined differently by the nurse, patient, or family; conflicts are generated if the patient's wishes are not known.	It is helpful for nurses to clarify their own values in such a situation and discuss with others on the team. Recording data that supports the DNR decision (such as expression of patient wishes) may decrease the nurse's conflicting feelings about carrying out the order.
Preserving autonomy means respecting patients' wishes about the aggressiveness of treatment and communicating these wishes to caregivers verbally or through a living will.	In this instance, the patient is not capable of expressing himself logically or of considering treatment alternatives. If no living will exists, then the principles of "substituted judgment" or "best interest" apply (see page 133). Mr. C's family told the physician they did not want him resuscitated. The nursing staff questioned the adequacy of the family to decide this, since they seldom visited. Nurses have often functioned as surrogate family for institutionalized individuals.	Family members or close friends with whom the patient may have discussed his wishes should be consulted as potential surrogates. Professional caregivers should also participate in decision making, as they are able to contribute information.
Respecting someone's personhood means doing what is consistent with that person's lifestyle and values, including not clinging to life when what made that person uniquely human has largely disappeared.	The nurse involved viewed the patient as a viable human. Respect for personhood may now mean he is given every advantage that any other, less handicapped, person would be given, unless he has expressed a wish to not be resuscitated. The family may be greatly aware of the change in the identity of this person now in comparison with whom they knew him to be most of his life. They view respecting his personhood to mean not clinging to a person whose unique characteristics have diminished considerably.	The facility and care team need to outline a philosophy and discuss a procedure to deal with any conflictual feelings.
Distributive justice demands that health care resources be given fairly to the elderly.	It is often argued that caring for dependent, cognitively impaired older patients is expensive, particularly since their quality of life appears so poor. Denying them life-sustaining care frees resources that can be spent on those with greater potential for a higher quality of life. On the other hand, to be fair, distribution is often based on need rather than the perceived quality of life. Thus, an individual with a life-threatening condition (cardiac arrest) is perceived to be more needy than someone who needs long-term rehabilitative services.	Social ethics, or the public good, needs to contribute to social policy involving equitable use of resources. In individual situations, economics may be considered if continued expenses threaten to drain a family's resources to the point that a family's health is compromised.

"intrusion" into the patient-physician relationship and the questioning of a difficult decision. There is a decreased likelihood of unwitting disrespect for personhood, an increased understanding of the reasons for the decision, and more information upon which nurses can base their actions. There is less likelihood that the physician's values will distort family wishes and prevent the family from reconsidering the decision.

5. Contact the local ombudsman program and charge physician and family with patient neglect. The physician or family is likely to be angered by charges of neglect, making the issue of aggressiveness of care more difficult to discuss. There is a decreased likelihood of unwitting disrespect for personhood. Increased discussion of the reasons for the decision will yield more information upon which nurses can base their actions. There is less likelihood that the physician's values will distort family wishes and prevent the family from reconsidering the decision. The nurse risks disciplinary action for involving "outsiders" in discussion. However, one judge ruled that the

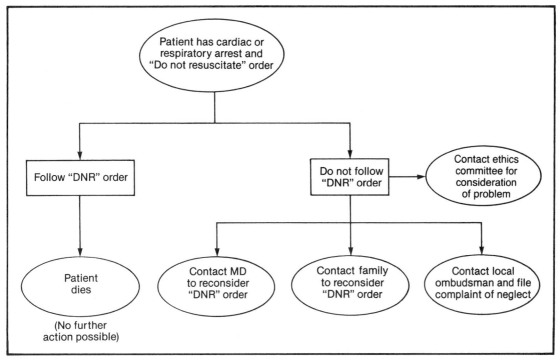

F I G U R E   3 - 5

Decision sequence for conflict with a "Do Not Resuscitate" order (Case Study: Mr. C).

nursing home ombudsman group was the preferred group for making the decisions about withholding or discontinuing life-sustaining treatment in the mentally incompetent (Annas, 1985).

6. Take the problem to the ethics committee of the facility, assuming this is an interdisciplinary, broadly representative group. Responsibility for decision making is "diluted," so the physician feels less personally involved and less accountable for his or her actions. The decision is viewed more objectively with the opportunity for relevant information from several sources to be considered; thus a decision more consistent with the patient's best interest is likely. Discussion, team building, and trust are generated, so the decision can be finally accepted and supported by all, and the individual's values are heard and respected. If the institutional hierarchy and physician's authority seem threatened, team members may feel intimidated and become alienated.

7. Convene a team conference with family and physician and other interested caregivers and significant others, e.g., clergy. Practice "preventive ethics" by discussing a possible DNR order, if the family seems ready, before a crisis arises. Principles of beneficence, autonomy, and respect for personhood can be honored by thoughtful consideration of what the patient wants as

discerned by others who know him or her well. All those involved with the patient have an opportunity to come to a consensus and support each other in providing the highest quality of care as defined by them.

Options 3 to 7 would need to be exercised before the acute situation (cardiac arrest). Options 3 to 6 may be prompted by the Do Not Resuscitate order.

Conflict of Questioning a Patient's Competence

Ms. B. is referred to a community-based long-term care program by her neighbor to obtain in-home services. Ms. B. has early dementia and has received Meals on Wheels and extensive support from her neighbor. She has no children, and her nearest relative, an elderly sister, lives 150 miles away. To receive needed in-home services, Ms. B. must keep careful financial records to qualify for Medicaid. Until now, the neighbor handled Ms. B's finances for her and provided numerous other services, such as visiting, phoning, daily checking, and assistance with meal preparation. Now that the financial record-keeping is becoming more complex, the neighbor is reluctant to remain involved.

Ms. B. has repeatedly stated that she

wants to stay at home. Her neighbor feels that a rest home would be the best place for Ms. B. The local Adult Protective Services unit has a history of routinely institutionalizing incompetent elderly clients with functional impairments.

The nurse case manager sees two options available: (1) to suggest that the neighbor obtain power of attorney so that she has legal authority to act for Ms. B., or (2) to pursue an incompetency proceeding, which involves petitioning the court and removing all rights of self-determination from Ms. B. The dilemma is which course of action to pursue, because Ms. B.'s cognitive capabilities may be such that she cannot be found incompetent, yet she has difficulty understanding complex matters (such as power of attorney).

The Problem

Should power of attorney be obtained or an incompetency procedure be pursued? The first option, although technically less restrictive, will result in immediate rest home placement by the neighbor, whereas the second option will result in withdrawal of formal services and eventual rest home placement through the action of Adult Protective Services, with less family involvement.

The Actors

- Patient, who must agree to power of attorney or experience the consequences of a guardianship procedure.

- Neighbor, who has been the primary support person and is the likely person to manage the patient's financial affairs.

- Sister, next of kin, who cares about the patient but is unable or unwilling to take day-to-day responsibility for the patient's affairs.

- Nurse, who is the patient's care manager and is in the position to make judgments about the need for and arrangement of services.

- Physician, who is responsible for the patient's medical care and perceives that the patient needs some form of supportive care, either rest home or in-home services.

- Lawyer, who is responsible for making a judgment about whether or not a power of attorney is the proper procedure or whether a guardianship procedure is indicated.

- Three local agencies: Adult Protective Services, responsible for guardianship if there are no family members to serve in that capacity. The Case Management Agency, responsible for providing services according to need but restricted by Medicaid eligibility. The Home Health Agency, responsible for providing services if there is an adequate source of reimbursement.

Analysis

A lawyer must make this decision, although he or she is likely to be influenced by information given by the nurse and family.

The problem can be analyzed by using the table on the following page.

Options for Nursing Action

After careful analysis, at least three options for nursing action are possible, as diagrammed in Figure 3–6.

1. Work toward obtaining power of attorney for neighbor. The principle of beneficence is respected, as patient would be able to obtain proper supervision and needed health services. The right to quality of care will be preserved, as bills will be paid while a more supervised environment is sought. Respect for the individual will be preserved, as living conditions will be more suitable than remaining alone at home in an unsafe environment. Autonomy is partially violated, as once power of attorney is obtained, steps will be taken to look for rest home placement. Although not Ms. B's choice, this will enable her to maintain some independence in function. If the neighbor could find someone to help with the bills, Ms. B. might stay independent a while longer, which further preserves her autonomy.

2. Petition court for incompetence proceeding. If Ms. B. is found competent, her autonomy is respected. Although right to quality of care and the principle of beneficence are respected in principle, care will be impossible to maintain since Ms. B. cannot keep the necessary records. If Ms. B. is found incompetent, the court-appointed guardian (probably a public agency official) will look after her affairs. Institutionalization is probable, and input from family and friends will be less readily sought. Her autonomy may not be respected since she can no longer exercise her rights independently. Institutionalization will honor certain rights, as codified in the nursing home patient's bill of rights (part of the conditions for participation for nursing homes under Medicare/Medicaid). The principle of beneficence is probably respected, although the guardian may have difficulty defining "the good" if there is little contact with family and neighbors. Inadvertent disrespect for personhood

Questioning a Patient's Competence

MORAL PRINCIPLE	RELEVANCE TO CASE	CONCLUSION
Beneficence means providing needed services to prevent injury and further functional decline.	In the nurse's judgment, Ms. B. is incapable of meeting basic nutritional and safety needs unassisted. Obtaining power of attorney would stabilize the situation and provide a consistent source of assistance from both informal and formal support systems. Without this help, Ms. B. is likely to decline both functionally and mentally. Some people interpret beneficence as respecting the elderly person's wishes even if health deteriorates.	Beneficence in this situation must be defined functionally.
All persons have the right to high-quality health care.	Ms. B.'s cognitive deficits make it impossible for her to exercise this right unassisted. To be eligible for home-care services under Medicaid, she must be capable and willing to spend a certain proportion of her monthly income on home-care services, but she cannot perform the necessary record-keeping without assistance.	Involved parties should present all options for helping Ms. B. obtain the quality care to which she is entitled.
Respect for personhood entails preserving as many human rights for Ms. B. as possible, including an appreciation of her lifestyle and values.	Respect for personhood includes the need for protection and safety as well as autonomy when a person is cognitively impaired. It also implies that the patient will be involved in discussions regarding placement.	The least restrictive alternative that addresses her needs without unnecessarily taking away any of her rights is indicated.
The principle of autonomy may mean not only self-determination but provision of an environment that encourages maximum autonomy and decision making. This is especially relevant for a cognitively impaired person. Also, the "right" to autonomy carries the responsibility of competent performance.	Ms. B. has repeatedly said that she wants to stay at home. Her neighbor is equally convinced that a rest home is the best place for her. Regardless of whether the neighbor or Adult Protective Services has guardianship or power of attorney, the outcome in this locality is likely to be institutionalization. Ms. B. is more likely to have her wishes respected if an interested friend or neighbor remains involved rather than only a social worker who does not know her well.	Ms. B.'s wish for autonomy must be heard and the limitations on her independence acknowledged as she participates in discussions about her placement. Her neighbor must also be an integral part of the process, and the implications of her role must be considered.

is less likely, as guardians are well supervised. Exploitation of the patient under this system is less likely, but individuals who know the patient personally must be involved in the decision making and care. The choice of an excellent rest home would help ensure that principles of beneficence, respect for personhood, and autonomy would be preserved.

3. Do nothing. The principle of beneficence and respect for the individual and right to quality care are violated, because the patient requires supportive care. However, autonomy is respected.

Conflict over Aggressiveness of Care for a Depressed Elderly Woman

Ms. W. is an 83-year-old woman living in an intermediate care facility with chronic pain secondary to nonunion of a clavicular fracture, heart block, depression, and mild dementia. She has lost 17 pounds in the past month. During two previous hospitalizations, her family has elected not to have a pacemaker put in to treat her heart block. It is not clear whether the patient has been consulted about the pacemaker. The patient, when approached by anyone, keeps repeating "Just leave me alone!"

She is currently being treated with antidepressants prescribed by the consulting geropsychiatrist and has shown some small increase in interaction with others, but she continues to lose weight. The nurse caring for Ms. W. is aware of the following limitations of the care environment:

1. The nursing home has limited volunteer resources.
2. Ongoing outpatient psychotherapy is not an option because the patient has no source of transportation for regular appointments, and no psychotherapist in the community is willing to visit patients in nursing homes.
3. A nurse psychotherapist is willing to come, but because Medicare will not reimburse nurses and the patient is too

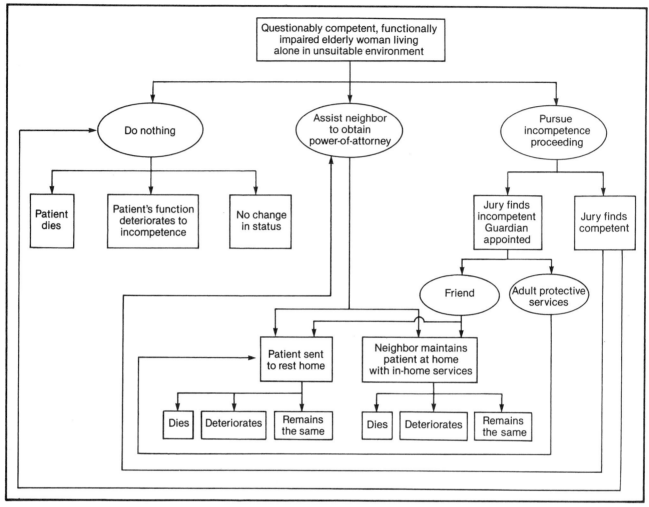

FIGURE 3 - 6

Decision sequence for conflict of questioning a patient's competence (Case Study: Ms. B).

poor to pay privately, psychotherapy is still unavailable to this patient.

The Problem

Given the family's unwillingness to pursue aggressive treatment of her heart block and her recent 10 per cent weight loss, should the patient's depression and refusal to eat be treated aggressively?

The Actors

- Patient, who has the right to accept or refuse treatment and who is the object of the beneficence or neglect.
- Daughter, who will be considered the surrogate decision maker for the patient and has filial obligations to the patient.
- Psychiatrist, who, if the patient is referred, must make the recommendations about treatment options and make judgments about the degree of danger the pa-

tient presents to herself, as well as the patient's ability to reason through treatment options.

- Nurse, who must care for the patient and who is obligated by a professional code of ethics to provide services "with respect for human dignity and the uniqueness of the client . . ." and be accountable for nursing actions and judgments.
- Family physician, who must make decisions about referral to a psychiatrist as well as nutritional supplementation.

Analysis

The patient or family would have to consent to a pacemaker procedure, as they would to psychiatric treatment. Anyone can petition to have the patient committed for psychiatric treatment.

The problem can be analyzed by using the following table.

Aggressiveness of Care

MORAL PRINCIPLE	RELEVANCE TO CASE	CONCLUSION
The principle of beneficence involves a definition of "doing good" in a particular situation. Whenever possible, clues to "doing good" must be obtained from the patient.	To do good would first mean facilitating treatment to return patient to a state in which she was capable of deciding what is "good." The patient's beliefs about undergoing psychiatric care are not known. Depression is a curable disease that can be treated by such modalities as psychotherapy, medications, and electroconvulsive therapy. Malnutrition can result from untreated depression and predisposes the patient to many other problems, including dementia. The patient has only voiced "Just leave me alone," which could indicate clinical depression or a withdrawal from life.	Without knowing the patient's value history, the health team is obligated to act in a conservative (i.e., life-sustaining) manner. An attempt to establish the patient's trust and discuss her desire for continued treatment could be made, but she sounds close-minded.
The right to high-quality health care for everyone involves complete diagnosis, appropriate treatments, and the promotion of comfort within the context of the patient's values.	The characteristics of high-quality care are aggressive evaluation and treatment tempered by respect for the individual's values, not by considerations of age, or economics. Without knowing the patient's values or expressed wishes, in an undepressed state, the health care team can only estimate the quality of care by using the criteria of patient comfort and the completeness of their evaluation and treatment.	Determine with the physician the need for an inpatient work-up of the depression and try to persuade the physician and family to permit a full diagnosis of the problem.
Respect for autonomy or self-determination assumes that the patient is competent, i.e., cognitively intact and able to act in his or her own best interest. Depression would undermine this assumption.	The patient is currently asking to be left alone. Treatment involves violating this request and thus violates her right to self-determination. In order to exercise autonomy the patient must be capable of deciding among the alternatives. This implies that patients must be able to understand the consequences of their actions, which is not true for someone seriously depressed.	If the patient refuses hospitalization, psychiatric evaluation to determine competency and level of depression should be sought.

Options for Nursing Action

After careful analysis, at least three options for nursing action are possible, as diagrammed in Figure 3–7, with consequences outlined here:

1. Encourage referral for inpatient medical or psychiatric evaluation.
   a. The depression may be treatable. The principle of beneficence and the right to quality care are upheld.
   b. The patient or family refuses treatment and suffers the discomfort from evaluation and stigma of mental illness. Although autonomy is upheld, her right to quality care and the principle of beneficence are not upheld.
   c. The patient or family refuses treatment, but the physician successfully petitions for involuntary commitment to treatment. The principle of beneficence and the right to quality care are upheld, although autonomy is violated.

2. Encourage insertion of nasogastric tube.
   a. The patient refuses NG tube. The team is now presented with the problem of whether or not to restrain patient's hands to keep tube in. Autonomy is violated, one interpretation of beneficence is respected, and the right to high-quality care is possibly respected, if incompetency demands overriding the patient's wishes.
   b. The patient accepts NG tube, her weight stabilizes, and her affect remains the same. As the patient is spared further adverse effects from malnutrition, the principles of autonomy and beneficence and the right to quality care are respected as long as the care provider does not overlook a curable cause for the weight loss.

3. Do nothing.
   a. The patient dies. Her autonomy is respected, although the integrity of this principle is weakened if the patient is incompetent. The principle of benefi-

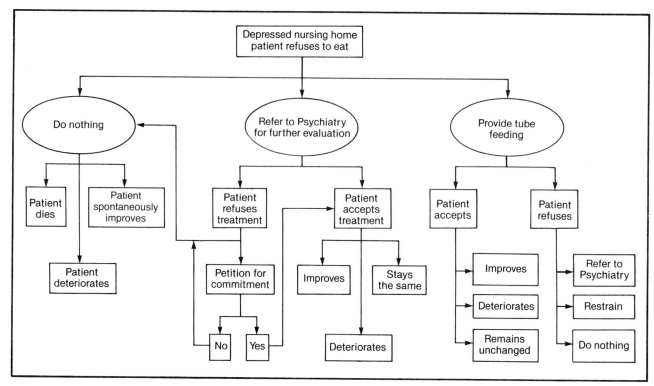

FIGURE 3 – 7

Decision sequence for conflict over aggressiveness of care (Case Study: Ms. W).

cence and the right to high-quality care are violated.

b. The patient lives. Her depression spontaneously remits. The principles of autonomy and beneficence are respected.

SUMMARY

Ethical dilemmas pose challenges that are not easily solved, whether they are on a social policy level or an individual level. The first step in solving them is to recognize the issues and bring them out for discussion and systematic scrutiny against a background of values and principles that can be tested. Several principles to guide ethical decision making for the elderly have been proposed, but there are many more. Contemporary nursing ethical theory suggests that thorough knowledge of the individual patient's situation is an essential, but sometimes overlooked, element of moral reasoning.

Ethical dilemmas call for a process of ethical decision making. This process includes defining the dilemma, gathering all relevant data and principles, considering all possible alternatives with attendant consequences, weighing the options, and making a decision

that can be justified. Health professionals should be educated to understand ethics, think ethically, and involve patients, families and colleagues in discussion. The courts should *not* become the center of ethical decision making. They often assume this responsibility in retrospect because of the failure of health care professionals to anticipate ethical ambiguities and difficulties and to involve all interested and responsible parties in the decision-making process.

Nurses are in an excellent position to help society and individual health professionals think of the ethical ramifications for elderly people in social programs and individual decisions. Yarling (1977, pp. 44–46) challenges the nursing profession to become a social conscience and a prophetic voice demanding better care for the elderly. Not only do nurses have the greatest numbers of any health professional involved in care of the aged, but they have an obligation to work to improve conditions of care:

Professions are created and sustained by a society for the purpose of serving society, and their social and political responsibility should be broadly conceived.

The elderly are growing in number and

needs. The great majority of their health needs concern teaching, counseling, rehabilitation, ongoing evaluation and management of chronic illness, coordination of services, and terminal care, all needs that gerontological nurses are specifically prepared to meet. Because of the intimate connection between needs of the elderly and resources for nursing care, nurses should become spokespersons, alongside the elderly themselves, for better care for this population. Resolution of the issues of adequate reimbursement for efficacious but nontraditional long-term care services, preservation of autonomy, respect for personhood, careful interpretation of beneficence, and thoughtful consideration of distributive justice should be the goal as nurses remind themselves and their colleagues that care of older people is an ethical problem for all in western society to face now.

REFERENCES

Agich, G.J., and Younger, S.J. For experts only? Access to hospital ethics committees. *Hastings Center Report* September/October, 1991, pp. 17–24.

Ahronheim, J.C., Moreno, J., and Zuckerman, C. Assessing the standard theory. Chapter 5 *In Ethics in Clinical Practice.* Boston: Little, Brown, 1994, pp. 65–73.

American Association of Retired Persons (AARP). Advance directives: An important aspect of self-care. *Perspect Health Promotion Aging* 9(2):1, 1994.

American Bar Association Commission on the Mentally Disabled, Developmental Disabilities State Legislative Project. *Guardianship and Conservatorship* (Discussion ed). Chicago: The American Bar Association, 1979, pp. 18–21.

American College of Physicians. Cognitive impaired subjects: Position paper. *Ann Intern Med* 111:843–848, 1989.

American Nurses' Association. *Code for Nurses with Interpretive Statements.* Kansas City, MO: ANA, 1976.

Annas, G.J. When procedures limit rights: From Quinlan to Conroy. *Hastings Center Report,* April, 1985, pp. 24–26.

Applebaum, P.S., and Grisso, T. Assessing patients' capacities to consent to treatment. *N Engl J Med* 319: 1635–1638, 1988.

Aroskar, M. Anatomy of an ethical dilemma's theory and practice. *Am J Nurs* 80 (Apr):658–663, 1980.

Avorn, J. Benefit and cost analysis in geriatric care: Turning age discrimination into health policy. *N Engl J Med* 310:1294–1301, 1984.

Bandman, E.L., and Bandman, B. *Nursing Ethics in the Life Span.* Norwalk, CT: Appleton-Century-Crofts, 1985.

Barritt, E. Florence Nightingale's values and modern nursing education. *Nurs Forum* 12(1):14, 1973.

Bedolla, M.A. The principles of medical ethics and their application to Mexican-American elderly patients. *Clin Geriatr Med* 11(1):131–138, 1995.

Benner, P., and Wrubel, J. *The Primacy of Caring.* Reading, MA: Addison-Wesley, 1989.

Brody, H. *Ethical Decisions in Medicine.* Boston: Little, Brown, 1976.

Callahan, D. Medical futility, medical necessity: The problem without a name. *Hastings Center Report,* July/August, 1991, pp. 30–35.

Callahan, D. What do children owe elderly parents? *Hastings Center Report,* April, 1985, pp. 32–37.

Capitman, J.A., Haskins, B., and Bernstein, J. Case management approaches in coordinated community-oriented long-term care demonstrations. *Gerontologist* 26: 398–404, 1986.

Caplan, A. The morality of the mundane: Ethical issues arising in the daily lives of nursing home residents. *In* Kane, R.A., and Caplan,. A.L. (eds). *Everyday Ethics: Resolving Dilemmas in Nursing Home Life.* New York: Springer Publishing Company, 1990.

Caralis, P.V., Davis, B., Wright, K., et al. The influence of ethnicity and race on attitudes toward advance directives, life-prolonging treatments, and euthanasia. *J Clin Ethics* 4:155, 1993.

Cassel, C.K. Ethical issues in the conduct of research in long-term care. *Gerontologist* 28(Suppl):90–96, 1988.

Centala, M., et al. One way to avoid resuscitation roulette. *Am J Nurs* 6:29–30, 1990.

Cohen-Mansfield, J., et al. Informed consent for research in a nursing home: Process and issues. *Gerontologist* 28(3):355–359, 1988.

Cohen-Mansfield, J., et al. The decision to execute a durable power of attorney for health care and preferences regarding the utilization of life-sustaining treatments in nursing home residents. *Arch Intern Med* 15: 289–294, 1991.

Cooper, M.C. Gilligan's different voice: A perspective for nursing. *J Prof Nurs* 5(1):10–16, 1989.

Cooper, M.C. Principle-oriented ethics and the ethic of care. A creative tension. *Adv Nurs Sci* 14(2):22–31, 1991.

Copp, L.A. The nurse as advocate for vulnerable persons. *J Adv Nurs* 11:255–263, 1986.

Craig, R.P., Middleton, C.L., and O'Donnell, L.J. *Ethics Committees: A Practical Approach.* St. Louis: The Catholic Health Association, 1986.

Cranford, R.E. A Hostage to technology. *Hastings Center Report,* September/October, 1990, pp. 9–10.

Danis, M., et al. A prospective study of advance directives for life-sustaining care. *N Engl J Med* 324:882–888, 1991.

Davis, A., and Aroskar, M. *Ethical Dilemmas in Nursing Practice.* New York: Appleton-Century-Crofts, 1978, pp. 1–18.

Drane, J.F. The many faces of competency. *Hastings Center Report,* April, 1985, pp. 17–21.

Dubler, N.N. Inclusion of elderly individuals in clinical trials: Ethical Issues. In Wegner, N.K. (ed.). *Inclusion of Elderly Individuals in Clinical Trials: Cardiovascular Disease & Cardiovascular Therapy as a Model.* Kansas City, Mo.: Marion-Merrell-Dow, 1993.

Eddy, D.M. What care is essential: What services are basic? *JAMA* 265(6):782–788, 1991.

Evans, L.K., and Strumpf, N.E. Tying down the elderly: A review of the literature on physical restraint. *J Am Geriatr Soc* 36:65–74, 1989.

Farley, M., and Powers, C. Basic statement regarding rights of the elderly to health care and corresponding duties of persons in the medical profession. Working paper prepared for Connecticut State Medical Society, 1975.

Fuchs, V. The rationing of medical care. *N Engl J Med* 311:1572, 1984.

Gadow, S. Existential advocacy: Philosophical foundations of nursing. *In Nursing Images and Ideals.* New York: Springer Publishing Company, 1980a.

Gadow, S. Medicine, ethics and the elderly. *Gerontologist* 20:682–684, 1980b.

Gillick, M. Is the care of the chronically ill a medical prerogative? *N Engl J Med* 310(3):190–193, 1984.

Gilligan, C. *In a Different Voice*. Cambridge, MA: Harvard University Press, 1982.

Gilligan, C., Ward, J.V., Taylor, J.M., and Baridge, B. *Mapping the Moral Domain: A Contribution of Women's Thinking to Psychological Theory and Education*. Boston: Harvard University Press, 1988.

Glasser, G., et al. The ethics committee in the nursing home: Results of a national survey. *J Am Geriatr Soc* 36:150–156, 1988.

Gray, W.A., et al. Unsuccessful emergency medical resuscitation—Are continued efforts in the emergency department justified? *N Engl J Med* 325:1393–1398, 1991.

Haber, P.A.L. Rationing is a reality. *J Am Geriatr Soc* 34:761–763, 1986.

Henderson, M. Ethical considerations for the nurse as primary provider. *In* Lynch, M.L. (ed.). *On Your Own: Professional Growth Through Independent Nursing Practice*. Monterey, CA: Wadsworth Health Sciences Division, 1982.

Henderson, M. Beyond the living will. *Gerontologist* 30(4):480–485, 1990a.

Henderson, M. The nurse as moral agent. *Nursing RSA Verpleging* 5(3):10–16, 1990b.

Hepburn, K., and Reed, R. Ethical and clinical issues with Native-American elders. Clin Geriatr Med 11(1): 97–111, 1995.

High, D.M. Advance directives and the elderly: A study of intervention strategies to increase use. *Gerontologist* 33:342–349, 1993.

Hirschfeld, M.J. Ethics and care for the elderly. *Intern J Nurs Stud* 22:319–328, 1985.

Hobhouse, L.T. *Elements of Social Justice*. New York: Henry Holt, 1922.

Hoffman, P.B., et al. Obtaining informed consent in the teaching nursing home. *J Am Geriatr Soc* 31:565, 1983.

Hynes, K.M. An ethical decision system. In Davis, A.J., and Krueger, J.C. (eds.). *Patients, Nurses, Ethics*. New York: American Journal of Nursing Co., Educational Services Division, 1980.

Institute of Medicine, Committee on Nursing Home Regulation. *Improving the Quality of Care in Nursing Homes*. Washington, D.C.: National Academy Press, 1986.

Jameton, A. *Nursing Practice: The Ethical Issues*. Englewood Cliffs, N.J.: Prentice-Hall, 1984, pp. 19–23.

Jonsen, A.R. Principles for an ethics of health services. *In* Neugarten, B. (ed.). *Social Ethics and the Aging Society*. Chicago: Committee on Human Development, University of Chicago, 1976.

Kane, R.A., and Caplan, A.L. *Everyday Ethics: Resolving Dilemmas in Nursing Home Life*. New York: Springer Publishing Company, 1990.

Kant, I. *In* Paton, H.J. (ed.). *Groundwork of the Metaphysics of Morals*. New York: Harper and Row, 1964, p. 96.

Kapp, M.B. Legal guardianship. *Geriatric Nursing*, Sept/ Oct, 1981, pp. 366–369.

Kerr, I.G., and Chabner, B.A. The effect of age on the clinical pharmacology of anticancer drugs. *In* Yancik, R., et al. (eds.). *Perspectives on Prevention and Treatment of Cancer in the Elderly* (Vol 24 of Aging Services). New York: Raven Press, 1983, pp. 203–213.

Kohlberg, L. Stage and sequence: The cognitive developmental approach to socialization. *In* Goslin, D. (ed.). *The Handbook of Socialization Theory and Research*. Chicago: Rand McNally, 1969, pp. 347–480.

Levine, M.E. Nursing ethics and the ethical nurse. *Am J Nurs* 77:895, 1977.

Lieberman, M.A., Yalom, I., and Miles, M. *Encounter Groups: First Facts*. New York: Basic Books, 1973.

Luptak, B. A method for increasing elder's use of advance directives. *Gerontologist*, 34:409–412, 1994.

Lynn, J., and Glover, J. Cruzan and caring for others. *Hastings Center Report*, September/October, 1990, pp. 10–11.

May, W.F. Who cares for the elderly? *Hastings Center Report*, December, 1982, pp. 31–37.

May, W.F. *The Physician's Covenant: Images of the Healer in Medical Ethics*. Philadelphia: The Westminster Press, 1983, p. 13.

McCormick, R.A. Ethics committees: Promise or peril? *Law Med Healthcare*, September, 1984, pp. 150–152.

McCullough, L.B. Medical care for elderly patients with diminished competence: An ethical analysis. *J Am Geriatr Soc* 32:15–153, 1984.

McCullough, L.B. Phone privileges: Commentary. *In* Kane, R.A., and Caplan, A.L. *Everyday Ethics: Resolving Dilemmas in Nursing Home Life*. New York: Springer Publishing Company, 1990.

Mendelson, M.A. *Tender Loving Greed*. New York: Alfred A. Knopf, 1974.

Moss, F., and Halmandaris, V.J. *Too Old, Too Sick, Too Bad: Nursing Homes In America*. Germantown, MD: Aspen Systems Corporation, 1977.

Moss, R.J., and LaPuma, J. The Ethics of Mechanical Restraint. *Hastings Center Report*, January/February, 1991, pp. 22–24.

Mouton, C.P., Johnson, M.S., and Cole, D.R. Ethical considerations with African-Americans. *Clin Geriatr Med* 11(1):113–130, 1995.

Noddings, N. *Caring: A Feminist Approach to Ethics and Moral Education*. Berkeley, CA: University of California Press, 1984.

Oddi, L.F., and Cassidy, V.R. Participation and perception of nurse members in the hospital ethics committee. *West J Nurs Res* 12(3):307–317, 1990.

Ouslander, J.G., Tymchuk, A.J., and Krynski, M.D. Decisions about enteral feeding among the elderly. *J Am Geriatr Soc* 41:70–77, 1993.

Paier, G., and Miller, P. The development of ethical thought. *J Gerontol Nurs* 17(10):28–31, 1991.

Panicucci, C. Nursing assessment of the hospitalized older adult. *Nurs Clin North Am* 18(2):355–363, 1983.

Parmalee, P.A., and Lawton, M.P. The Design of special environments for the aged. *In* Birren, J.E., and Schaie, K.W. (eds.). *Handbook of the Psychology of Aging*. NY: Academic Press, Inc., 1990, pp. 464–488.

Pawlson, L.G. Ethnogeriatrics: Preface. *Clin Geriatr Med* 11(1):ix–x, 1995.

President's Commission for the Study of Ethical Problems in Medicine and Biomedical and Behavioral Research. *Deciding to Forego Life-Sustaining Treatment: A Report on the Ethical, Medical, and Legal Issues in Treatment Decisions*. Washington, D.C.: U.S. Government Printing Office, March, 1983.

Rachels, J. Active and passive euthanasia. *N Engl J Med* 292:78, 1975.

Ratzan, R.M. Informed consent in clinical geriatrics. *J Am Geriatr Soc* 32:175–176, 1984.

Regan, J.J. Protective services for the elderly: Benefit or threat? *In* Kosberg, J.I. (ed.). *Abuse and Maltreatment of the Elderly: Causes and Interventions*. Boston, John Wright PSG Inc., 1983.

Schwartz, D.A., and Reilly, P. The choice not to be resuscitated. *J Am Geriatr Soc* 34:807–811, 1986.

Shawler, C., et al. Clinical considerations: Surrogate decision-making for hospitalized elders. *J Gerontol Nurs* 18(6):5–11, 1992.

Sheehan, S. *Kate Quinton's Days*. Boston: Houghton Mifflin, 1984.

Siegler, M. Should age be a criterion in health care? *Hastings Center Report* 14:24–27, 1984.

Singer, P.A., et al. Ethics committees and consultants. *J Clin Ethics* 1(4):263–267, 1990.

Steinberg, A., Fitten, L.J., and Kackhuck, N. Patient participation in treatment decision-making in the nursing home: The issue of competence. *Gerontologist* 26:362–366, 1986.

Strumpf, N.E., and Evans, L.K. The ethical problems of prolonged physical restraint. *J Gerontol Nurs* 17(2):27–30, 1991.

Sulmassy, D.P., et al. The quality of mercy: Caring for patients with do not resuscitate orders. *JAMA* 267(5):682–686, 1992.

Sward, K.M. Precedents and prospects for the humanities in nursing. *In* Spicker, S.F., and Gaden, S. (eds.). *Nursing Images and Ideals.* New York: Springer Publishing Company, 1980, pp. 3–33.

Thompson, J.B., and Thompson, H.O. *Ethics in Nursing.* New York: Macmillan Publishing Company, 1981.

Thompson, J.B., and Thompson, H.O. *Bioethical Decision Making for Nurses.* Norwalk, CT: Appleton-Century-Crofts, 1985.

Tomlinson, T., and Brody, H. Futility and the ethics of resuscitation. *JAMA* 264(10):1276–1280, 1990.

Troug, R.D., et al. Sounding board, the problem with futility. *N Engl J Med* 326(23):1560–1564, 1992.

Vladeck, B. *Unloving Care.* New York: Basic Books, 1980.

Volicer, L. Need for hospice approach to treatment of patients with advanced progressive dementia. *J Am Geriatr Soc* 34:655–658, 1986.

Von Preyss-Friedman, S.M., et al. Physician attitude toward tube feeding chronically ill nursing home patients. *J Gen Intern Med* 7:46–51, 1992.

Wanzer, S.H., et al. The physician's responsibility toward hopelessly ill patients. *N Engl J Med* 310(15):955–959, 1984.

Watson, J. *Nursing: Human Science and Human Care.* Norwalk, CT: Appleton-Century-Crofts, 1985.

Watson, J. Caring knowledge and informed moral passion. *Adv Nurs Sci* 13(1):15–24, 1990.

Watts, D., and Cassel, C. Extraordinary nutritional support: A case study and ethical analysis. *J Am Geriatr Soc* 32:237–242, 1984.

Weisensee, M.G., and Kjervik, D.K. Dilemmas in decision making for caregivers of cognitively impaired elderly persons. *J Prof Nurs* 5(4):186–191, 1989.

Weissert, W.G. Seven reasons why it is so difficult to make community-based long-term care cost effective. *Health Serv Res* 20:423–433, 1985.

Wilson, D.M. Ethical concerns in long-term tube feeding. *Image J Nurs Sch* 249:195–199, 1992.

Winkenwerder, W. Ethical dilemmas for house staff physicians. *JAMA* 254(24):3454–3457, 1985.

Winslow, G.R. From loyalty to advocacy: A new metaphor for nursing. *Hastings Center Report,* June, 1984, pp. 32–40.

Wolanin, M.O. Research and the aged. *In* Davis, A.J., and Krueger, J.C. (eds.). *Patients, Nurses, Ethics.* New York: American Journal of Nursing Company, Educational Services Division, 1980.

Wolf, S.M. Nancy Beth Cruzan: In no voice at all. *Hastings Center Report,* January/February, 1990, pp. 18–41.

Yarling, R. The sick aged, the nursing profession and the large society. *J Gerontol Nurs* 3:42–51, 1977.

Yeo, G. Ethical considerations in Asian and Pacific Island elders. *Clin Geriatr Med* 11(1):139–152, 1995.

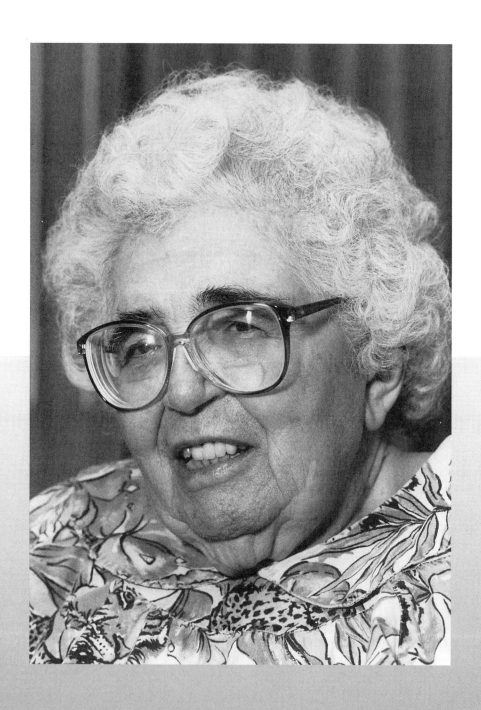

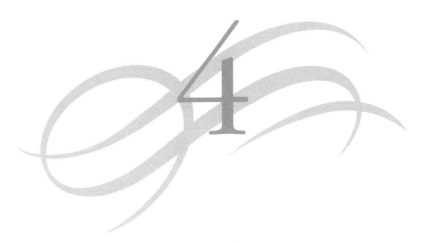

Biological Theories of Aging

MARY ANN MATTESON

For centuries, humankind has been fascinated with the concept of aging, not only from the biological and psychological perspectives but also from the philosophical perspective of aging and death. Theorists have attempted to define aging, to postulate causes of aging, and to develop measures and cures to postpone the aging process. Thus far, attempts to unlock the secrets of the causes of aging have been futile, and results of investigative efforts have been rather speculative. Also, few data suggest that particular preventive and curative measures such as megadoses of vitamins, physical exercise, or youth potions significantly extend the lifespan. This chapter focuses on definitions and concepts of aging and the lifespan with emphasis on early and recent biological theories of aging.

AGING AND THE LIFESPAN

Lifespan is defined as the maximum survival potential for a particular species (*Encyclopedia Britannica*, 1969). In human beings, the lifespan is thought to be about 110 to 115 years, in spite of reports, which have tended to be inaccurate, of groups living well beyond those years. *Life expectancy* is defined as the average observed years of life from birth or any stated age. The present life expectancy at birth in the United States is 71.5 years in men and 78.4 years in women (National Center for Health Statistics, 1987).

The human lifespan can be divided into three stages: (1) embryonic development, which occurs from conception to birth, (2) growth and maturity, which occur from birth through adulthood, and (3) senescence, which occurs at the last stages of adulthood through death. The terms "aging" and "senescence" are frequently used interchangeably, and both are considered to be fundamental and intrinsic properties of most living organisms. Aging can be defined as "the sum of all the changes that normally occur in an organism with the passage of time," whereas senescence is defined as "the last stage of a lifelong process of aging." The aging process has three distinct characteristics:

1. The process is common to all members of a given species,
2. The process is progressive with time, and
3. The process is deleterious, ultimately leading to death (Rockstein and Sussman, 1979).

Aging is a complex and variable phenomenon, for not only do organisms of the same species age at different rates, but the rate of aging varies within a single organism of a given species. Reasons for this variability are not fully known. Some theorists claim that individuals are born with a particular amount of vitality—the ability to sustain life—which continually diminishes with advancing age. The amount of vitality with which individuals begin life and the rate at which that vitality is lost throughout life differ among individuals. Environmental factors also mediate the length of lifespan and time of death (Dychtwald, 1986).

Although medical science has made great strides in conquering infections and acute disease processes, little has been achieved in terms of extinction of chronic disease and extension of the lifespan. In fact, from age 40 years, life expectancy has increased relatively little (Fig. 4–1). In 1900, a man reaching his sixty-fifth birthday could expect to live another 11.5 years, whereas in 1987 he could expect to live another 14.8 years, for a gain of 3.3 years. Women could expect to live another 12.2 years in 1900 and 18.7 years in 1987, for a gain of 6.5 years (National Center for Health Statistics, 1990).

Although life expectancies have changed little for those presently over age 70 years, the elimination of premature death has resulted in a sharp downslope in the natural

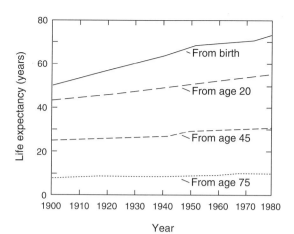

FIGURE 4-1

Change in life expectancy in the United States during the 20th century. From birth, life expectancy has risen from 47 years to 73 years. In contrast, from age 75, the increase has been only from 8 years to 11 years. The greater the age from which life expectancy is calculated, the less has been the improvement. (From Fries, J.F. and Crapo, L.M. The elimination of premature disease. *In* Dychtwald, K. [ed.]. *Wellness and Health Promotion for the Elderly.* Rockville, MD: Aspen, 1986.)

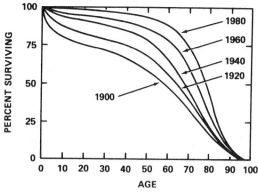

FIGURE 4-2

The rectangularization of survival curves in the United States. (From Fries, J.F. and Crapo, L.M. The elimination of premature disease. *In* Dychtwald, K. [ed.]. *Wellness and Health Promotion for the Elderly.* Rockville, MD: Aspen, 1986.)

lifespan. This phenomenon is known as the "rectangularization of the survival curve" (Fig. 4–2). The curve, which has a rectangular shape, shows that fewer people are dying "prematurely" and more people are living into older age and closer to the natural lifespan (Fries and Crapo, 1986).

The elimination of premature deaths is generally attributed to the conquest of infectious diseases. At the turn of the century, mortality patterns were dominated by acute diseases such as tuberculosis, acute rheumatic fever, smallpox, diphtheria, tetanus, poliomyelitis, and pneumococcal pneumonia. Now they account for only 2 per cent of the health problems that they caused in 1900, whereas chronic illness has become the cause of more than 80 per cent of all deaths and an even higher percentage of disability (Department of Health and Human Services, 1991).

The lengthening life expectancy and increased incidence of chronic illness raise concerns over the possibility of greater numbers of chronically ill, disabled elderly in the population. The prospect of higher health care and societal costs to support dependent elderly people is distasteful to people of all ages. Fortunately, the concept of "compressed morbidity" has been raised by gerontologists as an alternative. The definition of compressed morbidity states that "the average age of onset of a significant permanent infirmity may increase more rapidly than does life expectancy, thus shorten-

ing both the proportion of life spent infirm and the absolute length of the infirm period." In other words, people may live longer, healthier lives and have shorter periods of disability at the end of their lives. In effect, the rectangularization of the survival curve may be followed by the rectangularization of the morbidity curve and compression of morbidity (Fig. 4–3) (Fries and Crapo, 1986).

The strategy for postponing infirmity involves preventive approaches to premature

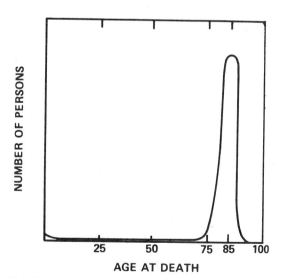

FIGURE 4-3

Mortality according to age, in the absence of premature death. The morbidity curve is made rectangular, and the period of morbidity is compressed between the point of the end of adult vigor and the point of natural death. (From Fries, J.F. and Crapo, L.M. The elimination of premature disease. *In* Dychtwald, K. [ed.]. *Wellness and Health Promotion for the Elderly.* Rockville, MD: Aspen, 1986.)

chronic disease through increased physical, social, and psychological exercise and establishment of formal preventive programs. The focus on health improvement is on chronic rather than acute disease, on morbidity rather than mortality, and on postponement rather than cure (Department of Health and Human Services, 1990).

EARLY BIOLOGICAL THEORIES

The earliest theories of aging were highly speculative and frequently had a philosophical basis. The Greeks were the first people to speculate on the cause of aging. Several hundred years before the birth of Christ, Hippocrates characterized aging as an irreversible and natural event caused by a decrease in body heat. Later, Galen elaborated on this idea by saying that aging was caused primarily by changes in the body's "humors" that produced increased dryness and coldness. He also stated that aging was a lifetime process rather than an event occurring at the end of the lifespan.

Late in the 12th century, Maimonides, a Jewish philosopher, postulated that life was predetermined and unalterable but that the lifespan could be prolonged by taking suitable precautions. Early in the 13th century, Roger Bacon, a European, wrote prolifically about the aging process, so much so that he was imprisoned for his philosophical views. He adhered to the Greek model of decreased heat and dryness related to aging, but added that aging was a pathological process that could be halted by good hygiene. He further postulated that aging was a result of the wear and tear of living; however, the Catholic Church ultimately determined one's lifespan.

Leonardo da Vinci (1452–1519) was the first person to attempt to identify physiological changes associated with aging by performing autopsies on old men and young children. Later, Santorio theorized that aging was manifested through a hardening of fibers and a progressive consolidation of earthy material within one's body. However, it was not until the 18th and 19th centuries that scientists began to investigate seriously the physiological and anatomical processes of aging. According to Darwin, aging was due to a decrease in irritability of nervous and muscular tissues resulting in a failure of the body to respond to stimuli. Other theorists claimed that life was a vital force or intrinsic energy that gradually decreased over time and diminished to the point of death.

After 1900 few scientists and researchers studied aging as a primary interest. In the early 1900s, C. S. Minot studied mortality rates with the use of statistical analysis. The "auto intoxication" theory, which stated that age was attributed to particular physiological systems or conditions, and the "wear and tear" theory, which claimed that organisms had fixed amounts of energy available to them, were predominant at that time. Not until the past several decades did science begin to display a renewed interest in researching biological theories of the aging process, which now include immunity, crosslinkage, free radicals, stress, nutrition restriction, error, and biological programming.

RECENT THEORIES OF AGING

Immunity Theory

The immune system protects the body by seeking out and destroying foreign agents such as viruses, bacteria, fungi, and possibly one's own somatic cells that undergo neoplastic changes. The major organs of the immune system are the bone marrow, the thymus, the spleen, and the lymph nodes. The bone marrow and thymus are considered primary organs; the spleen and lymph nodes are considered secondary or peripheral organs responsible for initiating immunity.

Immune responses depend on a number of different cells and tissues and the complex interactions among them. When an antigen, such as a virus or bacteria, enters the body, two types of immunological reactions may occur. First, the antigen may induce the formation of lymphocytics, which stimulate the synthesis and release of *humoral* antibodies principally involved in the neutralization of bacterial toxins and the destruction of bacteria. Second, the antigen may induce lymphocytes to produce *cell-mediated* reactions such as delayed hypersensitivity or destruction of foreign tissue grafts and tumors. Lymphocytes responsible for the production of effector cells for *humoral* responses are known as B cells because in birds they are processed in a structure known as the bursa of Fabricius. It is speculated that in humans, the B cells are processed in similar lymphoid tissue found in the liver and spleen. T cells, which are processed in the thymus gland in humans, are responsible for the production of effector cells for *cell-mediated* responses (Fig. 4–4).

The primary organs of the immune system (bone marrow and thymus) are thought to be most affected by the aging process. The immune response declines steadily after young adulthood when the thymus begins to decrease both in weight and in its ability to produce T cell differentiation. The effect of aging is most apparent in the T cells, as evidenced by a decline in the humoral immune response, a delay in the skin allograft rejection time, a decrease in the intensity of delayed hypersensitivity, and a decline in the resistance to tumor cell challenge. The bone marrow stem cells may also show reduced efficiency in performing certain functions with older age. As these normal immunological functions decrease, there is an increase in the incidence of infections, autoimmunity, and cancer (Volk and Ershler, 1991; Ben-Yehuda and Weksler, 1992a, 1992b; Cordopatri et al., 1992; Hartwig, 1992; Hirokawa, 1992). Some studies have found that poor nutrition can lead to decreased immune responses; improving nutrition with micronutrients and vitamins, particularly vitamin E, can improve immunity and decrease the risk of infection in old age (Lesourd, 1990; Meydani et al., 1990; Chandra, 1992).

Autoimmunity

According to some scientists, the decrease in immunological functions may result in an increase in the body's autoimmune response. With aging, the body becomes less able to recognize or tolerate "self" antigens, so that the immune system produces antibodies that act against itself. This is evidenced by an increased level of autoantibodies and an increased accumulation of lymphocytes and plasma cells in various tissues of normal, healthy older people. In addition, the graft-versus-host reaction in laboratory animals produces changes similar to those seen in the aging process, such as skin and hair changes, weight loss, increased levels of autoantibodies, and renal changes (Weksler et al., 1990; Huang et al., 1992; Perez et al., 1992).

Crosslinkage Theory

Crosslinking is a chemical reaction that produces irreparable, spontaneous damage to DNA and consequent cell death. This reaction occurs when a crosslinking agent attaches itself to one strand of a DNA molecule. Usually, defense mechanisms excise the agent—together with the piece of the affected DNA—and the damage to the strand is repaired using the unaffected strand as

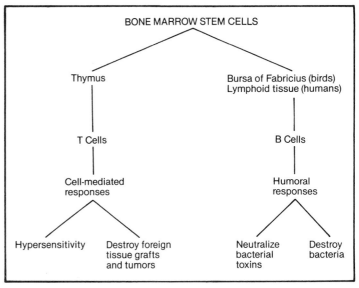

F I G U R E   4 – 4

The immunological process.

the template (Fig. 4–5). When cell division occurs, the DNA strand is then able to part normally. However, with aging, defense mechanisms are not able to excise the cross-

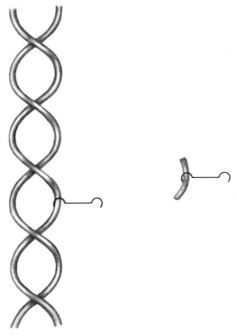

F I G U R E   4 – 5

A crosslinking agent attaches itself at one point on a DNA molecule, involving one strand only. Right, the agent, along with a piece of the DNA affected, is excised by defense mechanisms. The damage is then repaired; the unaffected strand is the template. (From Bjorksten, J. Cross-linkage and the aging process. *In* Rockstein, M., et al. [eds.]. *Theoretical Aspects of Aging*. New York: Academic Press, 1974.)

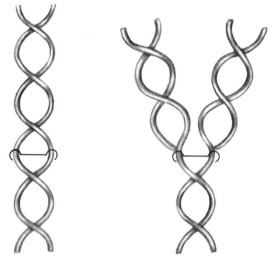

FIGURE 4 - 6

Here the crosslinking agent has become attached to the second strand of DNA before the defense mechanism could excise it. When this has happened the cell is doomed. If the crosslinker is excised, there will be no template for repair as both strands are involved at the same point. If the crosslinker remains, it will block the normal parting of strands in mitosis at a stage where the resultant DNA can neither return to normal nor complete the division. (From Bjorksten, J. Cross-linkage and the aging process. *In* Rockstein, M., et al. [eds.]. *Theoretical Aspects of Aging.* New York: Academic Press, 1974.)

linking agent before it attaches itself to the second DNA strand. The result is an abnormal parting of the strands in mitosis, leading to an incomplete division and cell death (Fig. 4–6) (Bjorksten, 1974).

An accumulation of crosslinking compounds over a lifetime produces the random, irreparable binding together of essential molecules in the cells (Fig. 4–7). These range from DNA within the nucleus to macromolecules such as protein. The crosslinked network interferes with normal cell functioning and impedes intracellular transport. It is thought that the irreversible aging of proteins such as *collagen* is responsible for the ultimate failure of tissues and organs. Collagen is an important connective tissue support for the lungs, heart, muscle, and lining of the vessel walls. Age-related changes in the structure of collagen are partially responsible for arteriosclerosis and the concomitant loss of elasticity in the tissues (Rose, 1991).

Free Radical Theory

Free radicals are "highly reactive cellular components derived from atoms or molecules in which an electron pair has been transiently separated into two electrons that exhibit independence of motion" (Mehlhorn,

1988). The separated electrons have a large amount of free energy and oxidatively attack adjacent molecules. The O_2 molecule most commonly generates free radicals, and the most vulnerable sites are the mitochondrial and microsomal membranes rich in unsaturated lipids. Lipid molecules are especially vulnerable to attack by free radicals, resulting in structural changes and malfunctions. Chemical and structural changes are progressive, with a potential for a chain reaction in which free radicals generate other free radicals. Free radicals do not contain useful biological information and replace genetic order with randomness; thus faulty molecules and cellular debris accumulate in the nucleus and cytoplasm over a lifetime.

Lipofuscin is a pigmented material rich in lipids and proteins that accumulates in many organs with aging. The pigments originate from a peroxidation of components of polyunsaturated acids located in mitochondrial membranes. Lipofuscin appears to have some relationship to free radicals and the process of aging, because the substance is associated with oxidation of unsaturated lipids. The accumulation of lipofuscin interferes with the diffusion and transport of essential metabolites and information-bearing molecules in the cells and may play an im-

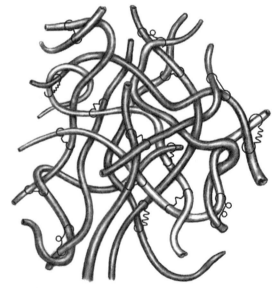

FIGURE 4 - 7

Over a lifetime, dense aggregates are formed intracellularly, by random accidental crosslinkage of any available large molecules with any available crosslinking agents. These aggregates are too dense to be touched by available enzymes. As they accumulate, they may contribute to age-dependent deterioration even more than the genetic molecules. (From Bjorksten, J. Cross-linkage and the aging process. *In* Rockstein, M., et al. [eds.]. *Theoretical Aspects of Aging.* New York: Academic Press, 1974.)

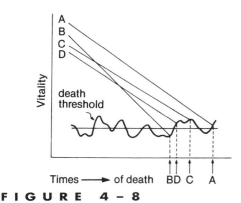

F I G U R E   4 - 8

Diagram of aging. The environmental challenges that an individual has to cope with are never completely constant, so the death threshold fluctuates around a mean value. Individual A ages more rapidly than individual C, yet has a longer lifespan than C. Individual D lives longer than B; yet had these two individuals been challenged by a severe stress at the beginning of their lives, B (the individual with the shorter lifespan), would have had a greater chance of surviving than D. The length of life does not depend simply on the rate at which aging processes are occurring, but on a combination of aging processes and environmental stressors. (From Lamb, M. *Biology of Aging*. New York: John Wiley & Sons, 1977.)

portant part in the aging process (Beregi et al., 1991; Arnheim and Cortopassi, 1992; Wei, 1992).

Wear and Tear Theory

According to the wear and tear theory of aging, chronological age does not determine whether or not one is old; rather, age is a physiological process determined by the amount of stress and damage to which one has been exposed. The process is similar to the mechanical breakdown that is inevitable with an automobile or piece of machinery.

The theory also states that life is essentially a process that gradually spends a given amount of inherited adaptation energy, and stressful activities cause an individual to use up reserves of adaptability that cannot be replaced. Figure 4–8 illustrates the relationship between vitality (adaptation energy), the threshold (environmental stress), and the time of death. Individuals A, B, C, and D are born with given amounts of adaptation energy or vitality and must cope with varying levels of environmental stressors that affect the levels of the death thresholds. Thus individuals A, B, C, and D age at different rates and die at different times because either they were endowed with different levels of vitality or they experienced different levels of stress (Rose, 1991).

Attempts have been made to refute this theory, because it is argued that physical stress and activity such as exercise increase the body's level of functioning rather than use it up. At this point, the stress theory is receiving little support from theorists on aging.

Nutrition Restriction Theory

A number of recent animal studies using rats, mice, and hamsters have concentrated on the premise that restricted nutrition can prolong the lifespan (Yu, 1990; Rose, 1991). The studies are conducted on older rodents in order to explore age-specific mortality rates—that is, mortality associated with advancing age.

Researchers have postulated that the antiaging action related to food restriction occurs through a reduction of energy intake per animal rather than decreased body fat content or decreased metabolic rate. Additionally, there appears to be endocrine and/or nervous system involvement, resulting in metabolic changes that modulate the aging processes in the tissues of the body. Food restriction research has demonstrated links with other physiological aging mechanisms, such as declines in protein synthesis and reductions in reactive oxygen molecules (Goodrick et al., 1990; Tacconi et al., 1991; Masoro, 1992).

Error Theory

According to the error theory of aging, inappropriate information is emitted from the cell nucleus, which interferes with normal cell functioning. It is thought that this process may occur through changes in the base pairing or coding of DNA or through increased levels of error in RNA transcription or protein synthesis (Prunieras, 1991). Information may be lost from the DNA as a result of an accumulation of a certain number of somatic mutations, macromolecular damage, or chromosomal abnormalities. Recently, several reports have focused on an accumulation of mutations in the mitochondrial gene (mt DNA) with age (Bodenteich et al., 1991). Cell mutations are self-perpetuating, for once a mutation is formed subsequent cell divisions develop more mutations until a large fraction of the cells are mutated. Cells are then less able to perform normal functions, and organs become inefficient and senescent.

Cellular mutations are thought to result from extracellular influences, specifically, *radiation*. Major proponents of this theory claim that radiation provokes chromosomal damage, induces or accelerates the development of degenerative diseases, and mimics

TABLE 4-1

Possible Correlation Between Population Doubling Potential and Mean Maximum Species Lifespan

	DOUBLINGS	LIFESPAN (yr)
Galapagos tortoise	90–125	175
Human being	40–60	110
Mink	30–34	10
Chicken	15–35	30
Mouse	14–28	3.5

From Finch, C.E. and Hayflick, L. *Handbook of the Biology of Aging.* New York: Van Nostrand–Reinhold, 1977, p. 171.

the aging process (Lohman et al., 1990; Wallace, 1992).

Biological Programming

Some theorists claim that there appears to be a hereditary basis for aging in man as evidenced by similarities in life expectancies of particular family members. Genealogical studies have shown that the average life expectancy of children whose parents had both died before the age of 60 years was almost 20 years less than the average life expectancy of children of parents who lived more than 80 years. In addition, it has been found that monozygotic twins have more similar life expectancies than dizygotic twins of either the same or opposite sex. It has also been found that monozygotic twins have two times the rate of similarity in causes of death as dizygotic twins of the same or opposite sex (Lints, 1978).

Further evidence supporting the concept of biological programming has come from studies of in vitro cell proliferation in both humans and animals. Cultured normal human fibroblasts were observed to determine the number of divisions in the cell population. It was found that *normal* cells underwent a finite number of population doublings and died; however, cells that had *abnormal* properties were capable of indefinite proliferation in vitro. Fibroblasts derived from human *embryonic* tissue generally undergo 50 population doublings before losing their ability to divide, and fibroblasts isolated from human *adult* tissue undergo about 20 population doublings in vitro. These phenomena seem to indicate that senescence occurs at the cellular level and that cell reproduction is a programmed event under genetic control. Age of the tissue donor also appears to influence and limit cell proliferation in vitro (Norwood and Pendergrass, 1992; Pereira-Smith and Ning, 1992; Wang, 1992).

An interesting comparison was made among various animal species, including humans, in terms of correlations between in vitro cell population doubling potential and the mean maximum lifespan (Table 4–1). It can be noted that the Galapagos tortoise, which has the longest animal lifespan, has the greatest number of cell divisions, whereas the mouse, which lives only about 3 years, has the fewest.

AGING AT THE CELL AND TISSUE LEVELS

Aging changes have been observed by scientists in the cells, tissues, organs, and organ systems that tend to have an effect on body functioning. Generally there is a slowing down of functioning at all levels, beginning at the cellular level. This section discusses biological aging of the cells and tissues, specifically connective tissues. Aging of other types of tissues, organs, and organ systems is discussed in detail in later chapters.

Cells

A cell is defined as a minute protoplasmic mass that, together with other cells, makes up organized tissue. All living matter is composed of cells, all cells arise from other cells, and all metabolic reactions of a living organism take place within cells. There are many different kinds of cells, more than 100 types in the human body; however, all cells have basically the same structure.

Cell Structure

A typical cell is made up of two parts, the nucleus and the cytoplasm. The nucleus controls the chemical reactions and reproduction of the cell and contains chromosomes, which are composed of *deoxyribonucleic acid (DNA)* and protein. The nucleus also contains the *nucleolus,* composed of DNA and protein, which is the principal site of RNA formation. The *nuclear envelope* surrounds the nucleus; it is a porous membrane that separates the nucleus from the cytoplasm.

The cytoplasm contains organelles important to cell functioning, including the *endoplasmic reticulum, ribosomes, mitochondria, microsomes, lysosomes,* and *Golgi bodies.* The cytoplasm is surrounded by the *cell membrane,* separating it from the surrounding fluids (Fig. 4–9). Substances that make up the cell are collectively called *protoplasm;* it is composed mainly of water, electrolytes, proteins, lipids, and carbohydrates.

The Aging Cell

Several age-related changes have been noted in both the nucleus and cytoplasm of aging cells. The nucleus appears to enlarge with aging, although there is no noticeable increase in the amount of DNA. The nucleolus also increases in size and number, and, whereas there is an increase in RNA content, there seems to be a decrease in RNA synthesis and protein metabolism. Chromosomal changes have been observed in the nucleus, with clumping, shrinkage, fragmentation, and dissolution of the chromatin (nondividing chromosomes). The nuclear membrane tends to invaginate with aging, and there is an appearance of intranuclear inclusions (Griffiths and Meechan, 1990).

In the cytoplasm there is fragmentation of the Golgi apparatus, and the mitochondria show alterations in shape and number. Vacuole formation increases with an accumulation of lysosomes. It is thought that lysosomes, which are associated with diges-

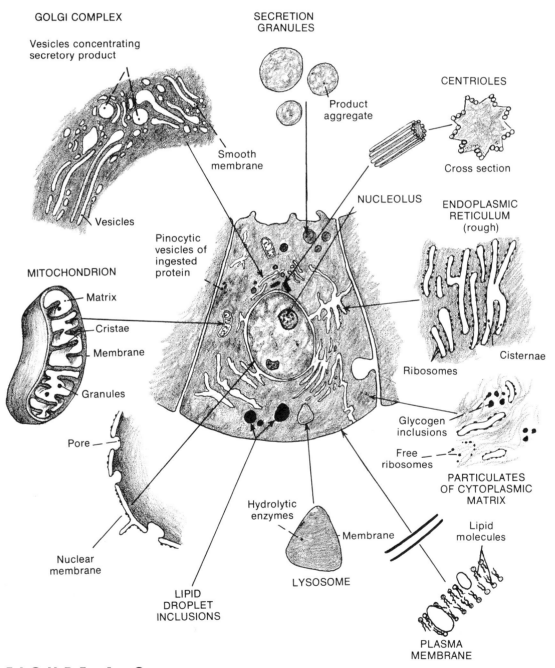

FIGURE 4–9

Parts of a cell as seen through the electron microscope. (After Fawcett, D.W. *Bloom & Fawcett: A Textbook of Histology*, 11th ed. Philadelphia: W.B. Saunders, 1986.)

tion and the breakdown of cell products, may accumulate owing to alterations in the rates of protein turnover or deficiencies in the protein disposal process. Protoplasmic changes associated with cellular aging include an increase in protein content, but a decrease in protein synthesis; an increase in cellular lipids; an accumulation of pigments or lipofuscin, especially in the fixed, postmitotic cells of the nervous tissue and muscle; and a depletion of glycogen (Timiris, 1988; Macieira-Coelho, 1991; Miquel, 1992).

Although the body contains many different cell populations, *all* types of cells show age changes. Not only are cells from older populations larger, but they also tend to decrease in the capacity to divide and repro-

duce. Observers of cells in cultured media report that individual cells proceed through a series of proliferative states, beginning with rapid proliferation, followed by a slowing down, which culminates in a total arrest of DNA synthesis and cell division. As a larger proportion of cells reaches a state of arrest, more and more cells become senescent, resulting in the inability of the remaining cells to repopulate sufficiently. This decrease in the ability of the cell to proliferate with aging is thought to be a major factor in senescence (Warner et al., 1992).

Tissues

Tissues are defined as groups or layers of similarly specialized cells that together perform certain special functions. Various kinds of tissues unite structurally and coordinate activities to form organs, which in turn make up organ systems. There are four basic types of tissues in the body: (1) epithelial tissue, (2) connective tissue, (3) muscle tissue, and (4) nervous tissue. Epithelial tissue forms the covering and lining membranes of the entire body, internal organs, cavities, and passageways. Connective tissue binds together and supports other tissues and includes bone, blood, and lymph tissues. Muscle tissue is divided into two types: striated and smooth. Striated, or voluntary, muscle moves the skeleton, usually at will; smooth, or involuntary, muscle surrounds the walls of the internal organs, such as the heart and stomach. Nerve cells and tissues carry nerve impulses from one part of the body to another.

Aging in the Tissues

As noted earlier, one of the most noticeable changes in aging tissue is the accumulation of the pigmented material *lipofuscin*, especially in the postmitotic tissue of the muscle and nervous tissues. There is also an accumulation of lipids and fat in the tissues. In men, there is a gradual increase in tissue lipids and fat until age 60 years, after which there is a gradual decrease. In women, fat and lipids accumulate in the tissues continuously with no drop-off. Many lipids are stored in the endothelial tissues of artery walls, as well as extracellularly between the elastic lamella and collagen fibers.

Connective tissues are widely distributed throughout the body and are diverse in composition. They contain an *extracellular matrix* made up of ground substance and fibrous proteins, such as *collagen* and *elastin*. Age changes in the tissues are best observed

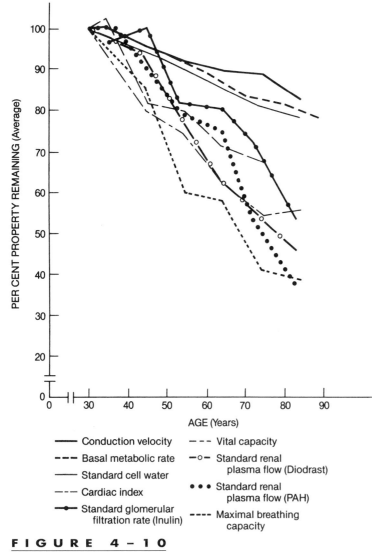

Legend:
— Conduction velocity
--- Basal metabolic rate
— Standard cell water
--- Cardiac index
—•— Standard glomerular filtration rate (Inulin)
--- Vital capacity
—○— Standard renal plasma flow (Diodrast)
••• Standard renal plasma flow (PAH)
---- Maximal breathing capacity

FIGURE 4-10

Efficiency of human physiological mechanisms as a function of age. Levels at 30 years are assigned values of 100 per cent. (From Kohn, R.J. *Aging.* Kalamazoo, MI: The Upjohn Company, 1973.)

in the extracellular matrix, although changes result from alterations in the cells, which synthesize most of the extracellular material.

Collagen is found in all connective tissues and shows the changes in structure with aging described earlier. Elastin is found only in tissues associated with body movement, such as the walls of major blood vessels, heart, lungs, and skin. The elastin content of the tissue decreases with aging but is replaced by *pseudoelastin,* which is either a degradation product or a faulty form of elastin (Hall, 1985). Because of the altered structure and degradation of elastin and collagen, the tissues become stiffer, less elastic and pliable, and less efficient in their functioning (Coni et al., 1992).

AGING AT THE ORGAN LEVEL

As with cells and tissues, the organs experience a decrease in functional capacity with older age. Physiological reserves show a linear decline beginning at age 30 years, especially in the cardiac, respiratory, and renal organs (Fig. 4–10), so that maintenance of homeostasis becomes increasingly difficult (Fries, 1980). Although these changes appear

slowly and over a long period of time, moderate or severe stressors can precipitate unexpected problems or failures of bodily functions as a result of compromised reserve capacity and homeostatic mechanisms (Medalie, 1986). Age-related changes at the organ level are discussed in greater detail in Chapters 7 through 13.

THE AGING PROCESS

The aging process is complex and varied, involving changes in cells, tissues, and organs. It is thought that the aging process is engineered by internal processes, such as genetic programming, and influenced by external sources, such as environmental hazards. Other factors influential in the process of aging are life stressors, lifestyles, and social support systems. The complex interaction of these elements is illustrated in the model in Figure 4–11.

SUMMARY

Aging and senescence are fundamental and intrinsic properties of most living orga-

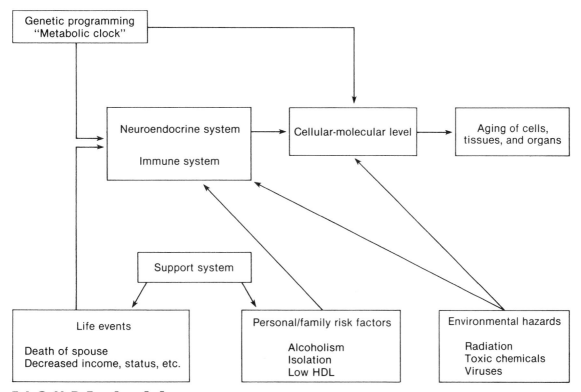

F I G U R E   4 – 1 1

A proposed integrated model of the processes involved in aging. (From Medalie, J.H. An approach to common problems in the elderly. *In* Calkins, E., Ford, A.B. and Katz, P.R. *The Practice of Geriatrics,* 2nd ed. Philadelphia: W.B. Saunders, 1992.)

nisms. Since the beginning of time, humans have attempted to unlock the secrets of aging and prolonging life. Some recent theories of aging are related to immune responses, crosslinkage of DNA, free radicals, stress, error in DNA and RNA coding, and biological programming. Research is continuing to explore and test these theories.

Aging changes have been observed by scientists in the cells, tissues, organs, and organ systems that tend to have an effect on body functioning. Although the body contains many different cell populations, all types of cells show age changes. Not only are cells from the aged larger, but also their capacity to divide and reproduce tends to decline with age. This decline in the ability of the cell to proliferate with aging is thought to be a major factor in senescence.

In the tissues, there is an accumulation of lipofuscin, lipids, and fat. There are also changes in the structure of collagen and a degradation of elastin, so that the tissues become stiffer, less elastic and pliable, and less efficient in their functioning. The organs undergo a decline in functional capacity and ability to maintain homeostasis with aging. Aging occurs slowly and is a complex and dynamic process involving many internal and external influences, including genetic programming and the physical and social environment.

REFERENCES

Arnheim, N. and Cortopassi, G. Deleterious mitochondrial DNA mutations accumulate in aging human tissues. *Mutat Res* 275:157–167, 1992.

Ben-Yehuda, A. and Weksler, M.E. Host resistance and the immune system. *Clin Geriatr Med* 8:701–711, 1992a.

Ben-Yehuda, A. and Weksler, M.E. Immune senescence: Mechanisms and clinical implications. *Cancer Invest* 10: 525–531, 1992b.

Beregi, E., Regius, O. and Rajczy, K. Comparative study of the morphological changes in lymphocytes of elderly individuals and centenarians. *Age Ageing* 20:55–59, 1991.

Bjorksten, J. Crosslinkage and the aging process. *In* Rockstein, M.M., Sussman, M., and Chesky, J. (eds.). *Theoretical Aspects of Aging.* New York: Academic Press, 1974, pp. 43–59.

Bodenteich, A., Mitchell, L.G. and Merril, C.R. A lifetime of retinal light exposure does not appear to increase mitochondrial mutations. *Gene* 108:305–309, 1991.

Chandra, R.K. Effect of vitamin and trace-element supplementation on immune responses and infection in elderly subjects. *Lancet* 340:1127, 1992.

Coni, N., Davison, W. and Webster S. *Ageing: The Facts*, 2nd ed. New York: Oxford University Press, 1992.

Cordopatri, F., Magaraci, F., Iacona, G. et al. Different behavior of phagocytes in young and old subjects. *Boll Soc Ital Biol Sper* 68:337–342, 1992.

Department of Health and Human Services (DHHS). *Healthy People 2000.* Washington, D.C., 1990.

Department of Health and Human Services (DHHS). *Aging America: Trends and Projections.* Washington, D.C., 1991.

Dychtwald, K. (ed.). *Wellness and Health Promotion for the Elderly.* Rockville, MD: Aspen Publications, 1986.

Fries, J.F. Aging, natural death, and the compression of morbidity. *N Engl J Med* 303:130–135, 1980.

Fries, J.F. and Crapo, L.M. The elimination of premature disease. *In* Dychtwald, K. (ed.). *Wellness and Health Promotion for the Elderly.* Rockville, MD: Aspen Publications, 1986, pp. 19–37.

Goodrick, C.L., Ingram, D.K., Reynolds, M.A. et al. Effects of intermittent feeding upon body weight and lifespan in inbred mice: interaction of genotype and age. *Mech Age Develop* 55:69–87, 1990.

Griffiths, T.D. and Meechan, P.J. Biology of aging. *In* Ferraro, K.F. *Gerontology: Perspectives and Issues.* New York: Springer Publishing Company, 1990, pp. 45–57.

Hall, D. Biology of aging—metabolic and structural aspects. *In* Brocklehurst, J.C. (ed.). *Textbook of Geriatric Medicine and Gerontology*, 2nd ed. New York: Churchill-Livingstone, 1985, pp. 46–61.

Hartwig, M. Immune control of mammalian aging: A T-cell model. *Mech Age Develop* 63:207–213, 1992.

Hirokawa, K., Utsuyama, M., Kasai, M. and Kurashima, C. Aging and immunity. *Acta Pathol Jap* 42:537–548, 1992.

Huang, Y.P., Gauthey, L., Michel, M. et al. The relationship between influenza vaccine-induced specific antibody responses and vaccine-induced nonspecific autoantibody responses in healthy older women. *J Gerontol* 47:M50–M55, 1992.

Lesourd, B.M. Immunologic aging. Effect of denutrition. *Ann Biol Clin* 48:309–318, 1990.

Lints, F.A. *Genetics and Aging.* Basel, Switzerland: S. Karger, 1978.

Lohman, P.H., Berends, F. and Vijg, J. DNA damage, metabolism and aging. *Mutat Res* 237:189–210, 1990.

Macieira-Coelho, A. Chromatin reorganization during senescence of proliferating cells. *Mutat Res* 256:81–104, 1991.

Masoro, E.J. Retardation of aging processes by food restriction: an experimental tool. *Am J Clin Nutr* 55: 1250S–1252S, 1992.

Medalie, J.H. An approach to common problems in the elderly. *In* Calkins, E., et al. (eds.). *The Practice of Geriatric Medicine.* Philadelphia: W.B. Saunders, 1986, pp. 47–59.

Mehlhorn, R.J. Oxygen radical generation and protective system: Assessment of their involvement in aging. *In* Timiris, P.S. (ed.). *Physiological Basis of Geriatrics.* New York: Macmillan Publishing Company, 1988, pp. 87–102.

Meydani, S.N., Barklund, M.P., Liu, S. et al. Vitamin E supplementation–enhanced cell-mediated immunity in healthy elderly subjects. *Am J Clin Nutr* 52:557–563, 1990.

Miquel, J. An update on the mitochondrial-DNA mutation hypothesis of cell aging. *Mutat Res* 275:209–216, 1992.

National Center for Health Statistics. *Life Tables.* Vital Statistics of the United States. Washington, D.C., 1987.

National Center for Health Statistics. *Life Tables.* Vital Statistics of the United States. Washington, D.C., 1990.

Norwood, T.H. and Pendergrass, W.R. The cultured diploid fibroblast as a model for the study of cellular aging. *Crit Rev Oral Biol Med* 3:353–370, 1992.

Pereira-Smith, O.M. and Ning, Y. Molecular genetic studies of cellular senescence. *Exp Gerontol* 27:519–522, 1992.

Perez, L., Rodriguez, C., Sepulveda, J.A. and Silva, M.C. Autoimmune phenomena in the elderly. *Rev Med Chil* 119:287–292, 1992.

Prunieras, M. General process of aging. *Rev Franc Gynecol Obstet* 86:421–423, 1991.

Rockstein, M. and Sussman, M. *Biology of Aging.* Belmont, CA: Wadsworth Publishing Company, 1979.

Rose, M.R. *Evolutionary Biology of Aging.* New York: Oxford University Press, 1991.

Tacconi, M.T., Lligona, L., Salmona, M. et al. Aging and food restriction: effect on lipids of cerebral cortex. *Neurobiol Aging* 12:55–59, 1991.

Timiris, P.S. *Physiological Basis of Geriatrics.* New York: Macmillan Publishing Company, 1988.

Volk, M.J. and Ershler, W.B. The influence of immunosenescence on tumor growth and spread: Lessons from animal models. *Cancer Cells* 3:13–18, 1991.

Wallace, D.C. Mitochondrial genetics: A paradigm for aging and degenerative diseases? *Science* 256:628–632, 1992.

Wang, E. Characterization of the absence of a unique DNA-binding protein in senescence but not in their young growing and nongrowing counterparts provides the means to mark the final stage of the cellular aging process. *Exp Gerontol* 27:503–517, 1992.

Warner, H.R., Campisi, J., Cristofalo, V.J. et al. Control of cell proliferation in senescent cells. *J Gerontol* 47:B185–189, 1992.

Wei, Y.H. Mitochondrial DNA alterations as ageing-associated molecular events. *Mutat Res* 275:145–155, 1992.

Weksler, M.E., Schwab, R., Huetz, F. et al. Cellular basis for the age-associated increase in autoimmune reactions. *Int Immunol* 2:329–335, 1990.

Yu, B.P. Food restriction research: Past and present status. *In* Rothstein, M. (ed.). *Review of Biological Research in Aging.* Vol. 4. New York: John Wiley & Sons, 1990, pp. 349–371.

Physiological Aging Changes

2

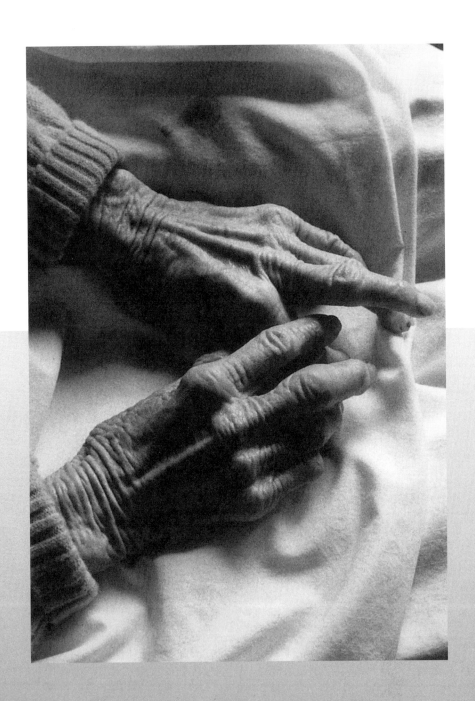

Age-Related Changes in the Integument

MARY ANN MATTESON

OBJECTIVES

List and describe normal skin, hair, and nail changes associated with aging.

❖

Discuss causes of normal skin changes in older persons.

❖

Identify common skin disorders, their causes, and their treatment.

❖

Assess aging persons and their skin and develop nursing diagnoses based on that assessment.

❖

Develop management plans for older persons with skin problems (actual or potential).

The changes in the appearance and function of the skin, perhaps more than any other organ system, reflect the continuous aging process. The primary functions of the skin are protection from environmental stresses, regulation of temperature, mainte-nance of fluid and electrolyte balance, excretion of metabolic wastes, and sensory reception (touch, pain, pressure). Aging changes impinge on these functions, causing a reduction in their effectiveness.

The skin is composed of three layers: the epidermis, or outer layer; the dermis, or middle layer; and subcutaneous tissue that lies beneath the dermis. The epidermis receives its nourishment from the underlying dermis and is divided into four strata (in order from the outer to the inner layer): (1) keratin layer or stratum corneum; (2) granular layer; (3) spinous layer or prickle layer; and (4) basal layer. The outer horny layer contains dead keratinized cells; the inner cellular layers produce melanin (pigment) and keratin (protein). Essentially, the epidermis grows from the basal layer, structures itself in the spinous or prickle layer, establishes the permeability barrier in the granular layer, and sheds itself in the outer cornified layer. The dermis contains blood vessels, nerves, hair follicles, and sebaceous glands. The subcutaneous tissue contains eccrine or sweat glands, some hair follicles, blood vessels, and fat (Fig. 5–1). The three layers are supported by an underlying network of collagen fibers and associated elastin fibers. The collagen fibers attach the skin to the under-

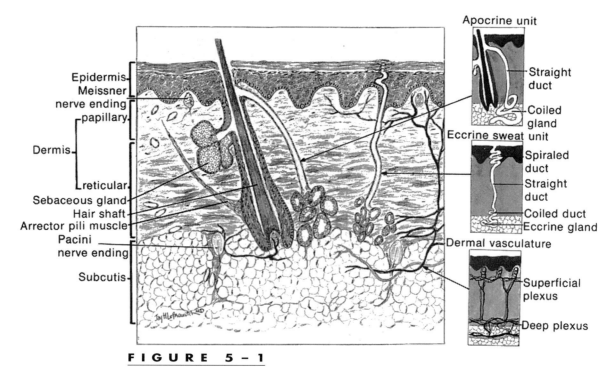

FIGURE 5 – 1

Diagrammatic cross-section of the skin and panniculus. (From Arnold, H.L., Jr., Odom, R.B. and James, W.D. *Andrews' Diseases of the Skin: Clinical Dermatology.* 8th ed. Philadelphia: WB Saunders, 1990, p. 1.)

lying tissues, and the elastin fibers give the skin flexibility, elasticity, and strength. Hair, nails, and sweat glands are considered to be appendages of the skin (Farmer and Hood, 1990).

NORMAL CHANGES

One needs only to look at a person to determine an approximate age. Evidence of advancing age includes wrinkles, sagging skin, gray hair, and baldness. Aging changes are categorized as either intrinsic or extrinsic (Table 5–1). Intrinsic factors are related to aging processes, such as genetic make-up and other bodily changes. Extrinsic factors are primarily due to exposure to sunlight, referred to as "photoaging." Habitual exposure to sunlight can accentuate the changes of chronological aging (Gilchrest, 1990; Kurban and Bhawan, 1990; Lober and Fenske, 1990; Taylor et al., 1990; Kurban and Kurban, 1993). Photoaging can be seen in people who work outdoors and are exposed to sunlight and is evident in the differences in age-related changes in exposed and nonexposed skin. Skin that is usually covered shows little change with age. Blue-eyed, fair-skinned individuals are more susceptible to solar skin damage than are people with darker, more heavily pigmented skin who seem to be well protected (Fitzpatrick and Mellette, 1990; Leyden, 1990; Beylot, 1991; Holzle, 1992; Grady and Ernster, 1992; Green and Drake, 1993). Bhawan et al. (1992) found that facial skin showed more age-related changes than did forearm skin in persons with mild-to-moderate photoaging.

T A B L E   5 – 1
Aging Versus Photoaging: Clinical Changes in Skin

Aging (intrinsic)	Thinning of the skin
	Loss of elasticity
	Deepening of expression lines
	Smooth, unblemished surface
Photoaging (extrinsic)	Fine and coarse wrinkling
	Yellow, lax, leathery texture
	Blotchiness and pigmentary changes
	Telangiectasia
	Actinic keratoses
	Elastotic skin with giant comedones

From Kurban, R.K. and Kurban, A.K. Common skin disorders of aging: Diagnosis and treatment. *Geriatrics* 48:35, 1993.

Epidermis

The *epidermis* shows a generalized thinning with advancing age, although there may be some thickening in sun-exposed areas. Although there is an increased variation in epidermal thickness, the average number of cell layers remains unchanged. The prickle cells of the inner layer of the epidermis show greater variation in nuclear and cytoplasmic size and a less orderly arrangement of cells than in younger people. Cells reproduce more slowly and are larger and more irregular; however, exposed epidermal cells may divide more frequently than unexposed cells. Melanocytes, the cells in the basal layer of the epidermis responsible for the production of melanin, may decrease in number, but the remaining melanocytes increase in size. Sunlight causes activation and proliferation of melanocytes (Ortonne, 1990). Because of these changes, aging skin appears thinner, paler, and more translucent (Montagna and Carlisle, 1990; Branchet et al., 1990).

Dermis and Subcutaneous Tissue

The *dermis* contains blood vessels, nerves, hair follicles, and sebaceous glands, but the major portion (79 per cent) is made up of collagen. The strength and elasticity of the skin are largely due to dermal collagen, and decreased skin strength and elasticity with aging are attributed to collagen changes. Collagen fibers appear to rearrange into thicker bundles, and there is an alteration in their cross-linkage configuration, as described in the previous chapter. Additionally, the number of fibroblasts, which are the cells responsible for the synthesis of protein and collagen, tends to decrease (Kulozik and Krieg, 1989; Lapiere, 1990). This condition is referred to as *elastosis* and is closely associated with exposure to sunlight. It produces a weather beaten or tanned appearance and is most frequently seen in farmers, sailors, white-skinned people living near the equator, and people with fair complexions who sun tan with difficulty (Warren et al., 1991; Kim and Su, 1992; Moloney et al., 1992).

Aging also produces a decrease in the vascularity of the dermal skin, as evidenced by decreasing numbers of epithelial cells and blood vessels. There is greater vascular fragility, leading to the frequent appearance of hemorrhages (senile purpura), cherry angiomas, venous stasis, and venous lakes on the ears, face, lips, and neck. The thinning cells and vessels have a slower rate of repair with aging, resulting in a higher and more severe incidence of decubitus ulcers and slower healing of damaged skin (Fenske and Lober, 1990; Jones and Millman, 1990; Lober and Fenske, 1990). Delayed healing may also be due to other factors, such as circulatory changes, poor nutritional state, sun-induced damage, and lowered resistance to infection (Lober and Fenske, 1991).

The decreased vascularity and circulation in the dermis and the underlying *subcutaneous tissue* also have an effect on drug absorption. Drugs administered subcutaneously are absorbed more slowly, thus prolonging the half-life of the drug. The amount of subcutaneous fat tissue also decreases, especially in the extremities, so that arms and legs appear to be thinner (Goldman, 1979). The skin becomes folded, lined, and wrinkled and has a diminished ability to maintain body temperature and homeostasis (Fenske and Lober, 1990).

Skin Glands

The two major types of skin glands are *sebaceous glands* and *sweat glands*. Sebaceous glands originate in the dermis and secrete *sebum*, an oily, colorless, odorless fluid, through hair follicles. Sweat glands originate in the subcutaneous tissue and are of two major types: *eccrine* and *apocrine*. Eccrine sweat glands are unbranched, coiled, tubular glands that are widely distributed and open directly onto the skin surface. They promote body cooling by allowing the sweat secretions to evaporate from the skin surface. The apocrine sweat glands are large, branched, specialized glands located chiefly in the axillary and genital regions that empty into hair follicles. They are responsible for body odor through bacterial decomposition of the sweat secretions.

Sebaceous glands show increased size with age; however, their function tends to diminish, as seen by a decrease in sebum secretion. In men, the decrease is minimal and does not begin until after the age of 70 years, but in women, there is a gradual diminution in sebum secretion after menopause, and no significant changes occur after the seventh decade. The decrease in sebum secretion and in the number of sebaceous glands results in the dryer, coarser skin associated with aging (Marks, 1987; Young et al., 1993).

Sweat glands generally decrease in size, number, and function with age. In the eccrine glands, the secretory epithelial cells become uneven in size, ranging from normal to small, and there is a progressive accumu-

lation of lipofuscin in the cytoplasm. In the very old, the secretory coils of many eccrine glands are replaced by fibrous tissue, which drastically diminishes their capacity to produce sweat. However, recent studies have found that there is little decrease in sweat production in persons younger than 70 years. The thermal threshold for sweating is raised, so that the amount of sweat output at a body temperature of 38°C decreases. This may be due to the fact that there are fewer blood vessels and nerve cells around the glands that enable the body to respond to temperature changes. Apocrine glands do not decrease in number or size, but they do decrease in function. An accumulation of lipofuscin has also been noted in apocrine glands. The diminished functioning of sweat glands in the elderly greatly impairs the ability to maintain body temperature homeostasis (Downing et al., 1988; Sato and Timm, 1988; Kligman and Balin, 1989; Fenske and Lober, 1990).

Hair

The most obvious change in aging hair is hair color. Half of the population older than 50 years has at least 50 per cent gray body hair, regardless of sex or hair color. Gray hair is determined by an autosomal dominant gene and results from a decreased rate of melanin production by the hair follicle. Hair color generally darkens with age, but this process is reversed with the onset of graying. Graying usually begins at the temples of the head and extends to the vertex of the scalp. It may not occur in the axilla, especially in women, and occurs to a lesser extent in the presternum or pubis.

Changes in hair growth and distribution are also associated with aging. The amount and distribution of hair are determined by racial, genetic, and sex-linked factors; however, almost all older people have a diminution of body hair except on the face. Adults develop a full terminal hair pattern by the age of 40, and this is followed by a progressive loss of hair in reverse order of development. Postmenopausal white women lose trunk hair first, then pubic and axillary hair. Unopposed adrenal androgens produce coarse facial hair in 50 per cent of white women older than 60 years of age, especially on the chin and around the lips (Coni et al., 1980).

Although men also show a general thinning of hair distribution, the hairs of the eyebrows, ears, and nose become longer and coarser. Baldness is often a cause for con-

TABLE 5-2
Common Aging Skin Changes and Selected Treatment Options

COSMETIC SKIN CHANGE	TREATMENT
Wrinkles	Photoprotection
	Tretinoin (Retin-A)
	Collagen injection (Zyderm)
	Chemical peel
	Dermabrasion
	Blepharoplasty
	Face lift
	Fat transplant
Hair loss	Minoxidil (Rogaine)
	Antiandrogens
	Hair transplantation
Gray hair	Hair coloring
Unwanted facial hair	Facial bleaches
	Tweezing
	Depilatories
	Shaving
	Waxing
	Electrolysis
Skin tags	Scissor excision
	Electrodesiccation and curettage
Cherry angiomas	Electrodesiccation and curettage
	Cryosurgery
	Shave excision
Seborrheic keratoses	Cryosurgery
	Electrodesiccation and curettage
	Alpha hydroxy acids
	Glycolic acid
Sebaceous hyperplasia	Photoprotection
	Electrodesiccation and curettage
	Cryosurgery
Solar lentigines	Photoprotection
	3% hydroquinone (Melanex)
	Cryosurgery
Telangiectasia	Photoprotection
	Electrodesiccation

From Fenske, N.A. and Albers, S.E. Cosmetic modalities for aging skin: What to tell patients. *Geriatrics* 45:60, 1990.

cern, particularly in aging men, although women also tend to show some thinning of scalp hair. Frontal recession of the hairline occurs in 80 per cent of older women and 100 per cent of older men. Baldness in men is inherited from the mother and occurs only in the presence of testosterone. Onset is variable and is manifested by an M-shaped pattern of hair loss on either side of the midline or by a thinning patch over the vertex (Kligman and Balin, 1989; Dalziel and Bickers, 1992).

In general, both men and women change from darker, thicker, more numerous hairs to lighter, thinner, and less numerous hairs with aging. Hair changes begin in midlife and become highly noticeable in later life, especially after the age of 60. Women seem to manifest more hair loss on the trunk and extremities, whereas men have greater hair loss on the head.

Aging changes in the skin and hair can have cosmetic effects that are troublesome for older persons. The impact of these changes on physical well-being may not be life threatening, but self-perception and self-esteem can be profoundly affected. Many older adults seek treatment to help them look and feel better. Table 5-2 describes skin changes and treatments currently in use (Fenske and Albers, 1990).

Nails

With aging, nails become dull, brittle, hard, and thick. Most nail changes are due to a diminished vascular supply to the nailbed. Thickening of the nail also results from nutritional disturbances, repeated trauma, inflammation, and local infection. There is approximately a 30 to 50 per cent decrease in the growth rate of nails, from 0.83 mm per week in 30-year-olds to 0.52 mm per week in 90-year-olds. Aging nails show an increase in longitudinal striations, which can cause splitting of the nail surface. This phenomenon can lead to infections and should be treated by bandaging around the distal portion of the finger or toe (Gilchrest, 1986; Orentreich and Durr, 1989; Fenske and Lober, 1990).

Toenails are particularly prone to thickening, perhaps as a result of constant trauma and pressure from shoe coverings. Along with thickening, the toenails may become discolored and grooved and may accumulate debris under the nail. This condition may be exacerbated as the distal portion of the nail works free from the underlying nailbed, accumulating more debris; fungal infections may also follow. Treatment usually consists of periodic debridement of the nail-

TABLE 5-3
Morphological Features of Aging Human Skin

EPIDERMIS	DERMIS	APPENDAGES
Flat dermoepidermal junction	Atrophy	Graying of hair
Variable thickness	Fewer fibroblasts	Loss of hair
Variable cell size and shape	Fewer blood vessels	Conversion of terminal to vellus hair
Occasional nuclear atypia	Shortened capillary loops	Abnormal nail plates
Loss of melanocytes	Abnormal nerve endings	Fewer glands

From Gilchrest, B.A. Skin. In Rowe, J.W. and Besdine, R.W. (eds.). *Health and Disease in Old Age*. Boston: Little, Brown, 1982, p. 383.

YOUNG ADULT

OLD ADULT

FIGURE 5 - 2

Histological changes associated with aging in normal human skin. (From Gilchrest, B.A. Skin. *In* Rowe, J.W. and Besdine, R.W. [eds.]. *Health and Disease in Old Age.* Boston: Little, Brown, 1982.)

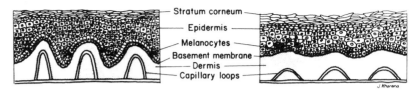

YOUNG ADULT · OLD ADULT — Stratum corneum · Epidermis · Melanocytes · Basement membrane · Dermis · Capillary loops

plate; however, return to normal nail structure rarely occurs after thickening (Helfand, 1983).

Table 5–3 summarizes the morphological features of aging human skin, and Figure 5–2 illustrates the histological changes associated with aging in normal human skin (Gilchrest, 1986).

COMMON DISORDERS

Skin disorders are so common among the elderly that it is difficult to distinguish normal from pathological changes. More than 90 per cent of all older people have some kind of skin disorder. These disorders may result from internal causes, such as diabetes, gout, malignancies, heredity, stress, neurological diseases, liver disease, muscle weakness, vascular and metabolic disorders, toxic reactions to drugs, and obesity. They may also be caused by external sources, such as sunlight, climate, industrial contamination, indoor heating systems, clothing, plant life, and allergic reactions to drugs and cosmetics

(Fenske and Lober, 1990; Fitzpatrick and Mellette, 1990).

The major cause of pathological skin changes is sunlight, which produces the short ultraviolet wavelength that is responsible for sunburning, thickening of the stratum corneum, sun tanning, and increased melanin production. Sunlight produces direct local effects on the skin in the form of elastotic syndromes, keratoacanthomas, premalignant diseases, basal cell epitheliomas, and squamous cell epitheliomas; indirect and direct effects can produce malignant melanomas (Griffiths, 1992).

Skin lesions may be divided into two types—primary and secondary. *Primary lesions* arise from intrinsic (internal) disorders

TABLE 5 - 4

Dermatological Terms

Macule	Flat, nonpalpable lesion differing in color from the surrounding skin
Papule	Small, raised, solid, superficial lesion, usually less than 0.5 cm in diameter
Plaque	Raised, solid, plateau-like lesion, usually more than 0.5 cm in diameter, greater in its diameter than in its depth
Nodule	Raised, solid lesion greater than 0.5 cm in both width and depth
Vesicle	Small (less than 0.5 cm), fluid-filled lesion
Bulla	Large (greater than 0.5 cm), fluid-filled lesion
Pustule	Fluid-filled sack containing cloudy or purulent material
Erosion	Loss of superficial surface epidermis often occurring after the natural breakage of a vesicle, bulla, or papule
Ulcer	Loss of epidermis extending into the dermis or subcutaneous tissue, usually as broad as it is deep
Fissure	Crack in the skin that is usually narrow but deep
Crust	Dried serum or purulent material overlying an erosion or ulcer
Wheal (hive)	Papule or plaque caused by dermal edema
Neoplasm (tumor)	New growth
Excoriation	Scratch marks indicating pruritis
Scale	Thickened stratum corneum
Lichenification	Thickening of the epidermis

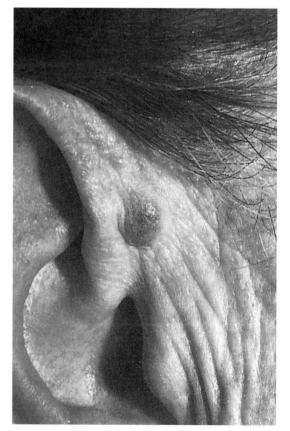

FIGURE 5 - 3

Venous lake. (From Callen, J.P., Greer, K.E., Hood, A.F., et al. *Color Atlas of Dermatology.* Philadelphia: WB Saunders, 1993, p. 98.)

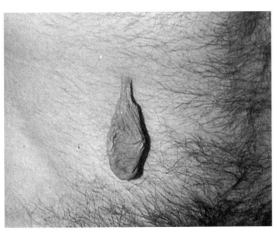

FIGURE 5 – 4

Acrochordon (skin tag). (From Callen, J.P., Greer, K.E., Hood, A.F., et al. *Color Atlas of Dermatology*. Philadelphia: WB Saunders, 1993, p. 130.)

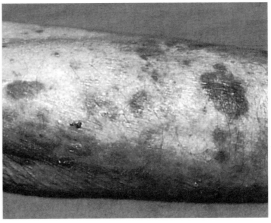

FIGURE 5 – 6

Purpura. (From Callen, J.P., Greer, K.E., Hood, A.F., et al. *Color Atlas of Dermatology*. Philadelphia: WB Saunders, 1993, p. 212.)

or extrinsic (external) irritants. Examples of primary lesions include macules, papules, plaques, nodules, tumors, vesicles, bullae, wheals, pustules, and cysts. *Secondary lesions* arise from primary lesions and include scales, crusts, fissures, erosions, ulcers, and scars (Lombardo, 1979) (Table 5–4).

The most commonly found skin disorders in the elderly are keratoses and skin cancers, followed by fungal infections, dermatitis, pigmentary disturbances, psoriasis, and urticaria. Other lesions frequently seen in the elderly are comedones (blackheads), asteatosis (scaling), cherry angiomas (small, red benign tumors), nevi (moles), skin tags (pedunculated fleshy growths), and lentigos ("liver spots"). In addition, the incidence of senile purpura and senile warts (papillomata) significantly increases, especially in the very old (Kaplan, 1991; Ries et al., 1990). Senile purpura is related to the loss of subcutaneous tissue, which supports the skin

capillaries. Minor trauma can cause small bruises or ecchymotic lesions that are largely found on the extensor surface of the forearms. Forty per cent of older men and 77 per cent of older women show evidence of senile purpura. Senile papillomata are small yellow, brown, or black warts located on the trunk, limbs, and face. Sixty-three per cent of all older people have some senile papillomata (Cape, 1978; Porth and Kapke, 1983; Shelley and Shelley, 1982). Figures 5–3 to 5–6 illustrate several of the common skin lesions associated with aging.

Most of these lesions are considered normal concomitants of aging and cause little discomfort. The greatest concern is the appearance of the skin, which tends to look mottled and spotty. Disorders of the skin that cause the most discomfort are pruritus, keratoses, epitheliomas, malignant melanomas, herpes zoster, psoriasis, and pressure sores.

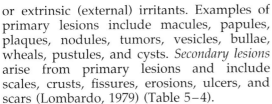

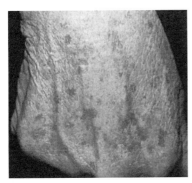

FIGURE 5 – 5

Senile actinic lentigo, or "liver spots." (From Lookingbill, D.P. and Marks, J.G., Jr. *Principles of Dermatology*, 2nd ed. Philadelphia: WB Saunders, 1993, p. 89.)

Pruritus

Idiopathic Pruritus

Pruritus, or generalized itching, is an extremely common geriatric disorder. It may occur with or without a rash and may be caused by internal, external, or psychological factors. When there is no rash, one should look for internal causes, such as hepatic disorders (itching may precede jaundice), uremia, malignancies, anemia, polycythemia, lymphomas, or drug reactions (Table 5–5) (Gilchrest, 1982; Duncan and Fenske, 1990; Phillips, 1992).

Xerosis, excessive dryness, is the most common cause of itching in older persons

TABLE 5-5
Systemic Disorders Sometimes Associated with Pruritus in the Elderly

Renal	Chronic renal failure
Hepatic	Extrahepatic biliary obstruction
	Hepatitis
	Drug ingestion
Hematopoietic	Polycythemia vera
	Hodgkin's disease
	Other lymphomas and leukemias
	Multiple myeloma
	Iron deficiency anemia
Endocrine	Hyperthyroidism
	Diabetes mellitus
Miscellaneous	Visceral malignancies
	Opiate ingestion
	Drug ingestion
	Psychosis

From Gilchrest, B.A. Skin diseases in the elderly. *In* Calkins, E., Ford, A.B. and Katz, P.R. (eds.). *The Practice of Geriatrics.* 2nd ed. Philadelphia: W.B. Saunders, 1992, p. 517.

and is almost inevitable in persons older than 70 years. Decreased sebaceous activity associated with aging promotes dry skin, which is exacerbated by cold, dry weather and excessive washing with soaps and detergents. Dry, scaly, itchy skin most often occurs on the lower legs, hands, and forearms, but itching may occur also in skin folds and in the genital and anal regions. Helfand (1973) found that 85 per cent of 1366 subjects over 65 studied suffered severe xerosis of the feet. The skin may be mildly inflamed with fine scaling, dryness, flakiness, and slight fissuring. Dryness and itching are often relieved by restricting the amount of bathing, by applying lubricants such as bath oils, vegetable shortening, glycerine, and rosewater with either menthol or camphor, or by administering medications such as antihistamines or steroids. The effectiveness of emollients and ointments lies in their ability to coat the skin surface, thereby reducing evaporation and building up the underlying moisture content (Banov et al., 1992; Duncan and Fenske, 1990). Figure 5–7 illustrates dry, flaky skin before and after the application of lubricants. Monk (1993) found a favorable therapeutic effect from transcutaneous electronic nerve stimulation for older persons with severe, chronic, generalized pruritus. Antihistamines, especially those such as terfenadine (Seldane) and astemizole (Hismanal) that can be taken for long periods and full dosages without causing sedation, also may be used for pruritus (Phillips, 1992; Banov et al., 1992).

Other conditions associated with pruritus

are eczema, allergic reactions, and stasis dermatitis with leg ulcers.

Eczema/Dermatitis

Excessive scratching associated with pruritus can lead to *dermatitis* (skin inflammation), which may be acute or chronic. In

---

BOX 5-1
Measures for Treatment and Prevention of Dry Skin

1. Artificial humidification can be done with a home humidifier.

2. The patient may bathe less frequently, using warm rather than hot water.

3. The use of a mild superfatted soap or cleansing cream is helpful, especially in the elderly (e.g., Aveenobar for dry skin, oilated Aveeno bath powder, Oilatum, Basis, Dove soap).

4. The patient should wear protective clothing in cold weather.

5. Moisturizers can be used for restoration of the epidermal water barrier. Occlusive moisturizers coat the surface of the skin, reducing the evaporative loss of moisture from the surface. Vaseline is an excellent moisturizer. A petrolatum-glycerin combination is especially effective in the treatment of dry skin.

6. The use of bath oils for bathing can be extremely hazardous for the elderly because of the increased possibility of slipping in the tub. Creams and moisturizers should be applied after getting out of the bathtub or shower. At that time, the body should be patted dry with a towel and the moisturizing preparation applied. Under these conditions, the skin is fully hydrated, and the moisturizing preparation is more effective in preventing epidermal water loss.

From Callen, J.P., Greer, K.E., Hood, A.F., et al. Color Atlas of Dermatology. Philadelphia: W.B. Saunders, 1993, pp. 100–101.

acute dermatitis, all four signs of acute inflammation are present: erythema (redness), edema, heat, and pain (which may result from the itching and scratching). *Chronic dermatitis* is less obviously inflammatory, and the skin is scalier, darker, thickened, and leathery with exaggerated normal skin markings.

Eczema is a term often used interchangeably with the term dermatitis. In the elderly, dermatitis is not only more difficult to treat, but it also causes more distress. Eczema is characterized by round patches of inflammation that are reddened, scaly, and extremely itchy. The patches are usually located on the fingers, the dorsa of the hands, the forearms, and the anterior tibial area (Fig. 5–8). Drying agents, such as soap and water, are the main causes of eczema, so treatment consists of (1) avoidance of the drying agent and (2) use of a steroid cream for inflammation and antihistamines for itching (Lombardo, 1979; Berliner, 1986). In several clinical trials, 0.05 per cent halobetasol propionate (Ultravate) cream was an effective treatment for atopic dermatitis and other eczematous dermatoses (Guzzo et al., 1991; Kantor et al., 1991).

Seborrheic Dermatitis

This eczematous condition is often bothersome to older people, not only because it causes itching and discomfort but also because of the appearance of the yellowish, greasy scaling of the skin known as dandruff (Fig. 5–9). Overactive sebaceous glands produce the scaly skin, which may be oily or dry. There also may be redness and scaling of the eyebrows, sides of the nose, hairline, sternum, and axilla. Antiseborrheic shampoos are the most effective treatment, along with the twice-daily application of a low-potency topical glucocorticosteroid, such as 1 per cent hydrocortisone cream (Kurban and Kurban, 1993; Segal et al., 1992). Additionally, recent studies have demonstrated the effectiveness of topical lithium succinate for the treatment of seborrheic dermatitis (Cuelenaere et al., 1992; Efalith Multicenter Trial Group, 1992).

Intertrigo

Intertrigo is a form of seborrheic eczema in which inflammation and itching are found in skin folds under the breasts, in the groin, in the transverse abdominal folds, and in the axilla. It is more common in obese elderly persons who do not maintain an appropriate level of cleanliness. Inflammation

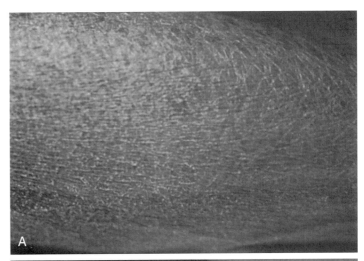

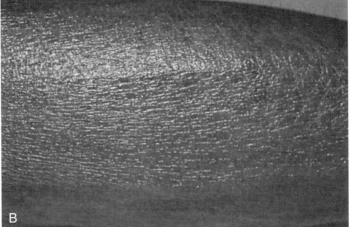

FIGURE 5–7

A and *B,* Dry skin evidenced by flaking scales and roughness. (From Dotz, W.E. and Berman, B. The facts about treatment of dry skin. *Geriatrics* 38: 93–100, 1983.)

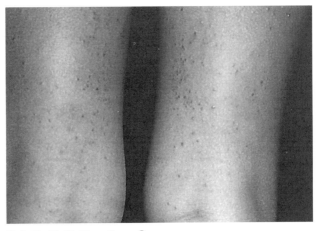

FIGURE 5–8

Papular eczema. (From Callen, J.P., Greer, K.E., Hood, A.F., et al. *Color Atlas of Dermatology.* Philadelphia: W.B. Saunders, 1993, p. 192.)

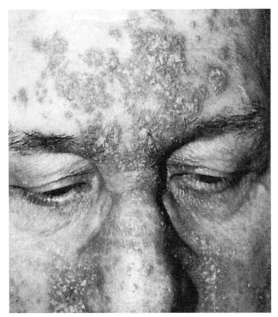

FIGURE 5-9

Severe seborrheic dermatitis of forehead, glabella, wings of the nose, and nasolabial folds. (From Domonkos, A.N., Arnold, H.L., Jr., and Odom, R.B. *Andrews' Diseases of the Skin,* 7th ed. Philadelphia: W.B. Saunders, 1982, p. 219.)

is due to a combination of friction, sweating, and bacterial or monilial infection. Cleanliness is essential for prevention and treatment. The folds should be separated with linen strips, washed with hexachlorophene, and dried thoroughly. Afterwards, 1 per cent topical hydrocortisone cream is applied. Monilial infections are treated locally with nystatin, and bacterial infections are treated with neomycin or fucidic acid (Coni et al., 1980; Elkowitz, 1981; Itin, 1989; McMahon, 1991).

Neurodermatitis

Neurodermatitis (lichen simplex chronicus) is caused by the excessive scratching and rubbing of dry, itchy eczematous skin. The condition can be localized, especially on the dorsal forearms, lateral tibial areas, and posterior neck, or it may be generalized over the entire body. When the condition is localized, the constant scratching and rubbing of a particular area produces *lichenification*—a thickening of the skin. This leads to chronic inflammation and itching, which in turn produce further scratching and rubbing. The result is thickened patches of skin in varying sizes that appear scaly, leathery, and darker than normal (Fig. 5–10). The condition is treated with steroid creams and antihista-

mines for the itch; however, frequent relapses may occur unless the scratching habit is broken. Generalized lichenified lesions often arise in older persons who are agitated and depressed. Treatment for these lesions consists of steroid creams, antihistamines, tranquilizers, and systemic steroids (Marks, 1987; Graham-Brown and Monk, 1988).

Pruritus Ani and Vulvae

These types of dermatitis are found in the perianal area and are due to irritation from heat, swelling, hemorrhoids, or fissures. The resulting rubbing and scratching leads to thickening of the vulvar and perianal skin. Itching frequently occurs at night, causing the appearance of scratch marks in the morning. The condition is complicated by urinary or fecal incontinence and is especially troublesome for chronically ill or confused elderly persons. The major treatment goal is to alleviate the irritation by avoiding irritating medications, using warm compresses or baths, applying mild steroid creams, and administering oral antipruritic medications (Bornstein et al., 1993; Origoni et al., 1990; Ensebio, 1990; Silverman et al., 1989).

Allergic Reactions

The most common allergic reactions after age 50 are (1) allergic eczematous contact dermatitis; (2) allergic drug eruptions; and (3) allergic urticaria (hives). Drugs are the most common cause of allergic reactions in older persons. A maculopapular rash is the most common type of reaction, and it is

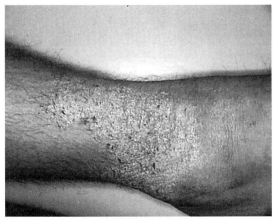

FIGURE 5-10

Lichen simplex chronicus. (From Callen, J.P., Greer, K.E., Hood, A.F., et al. *Color Atlas of Dermatology.* Philadelphia: W.B. Saunders, 1993, p. 194.)

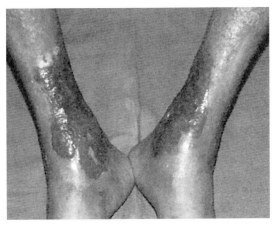

FIGURE 5 – 11

Stasis dermatitis. (From Callen, J.P., Greer, K.E., Hood, A.F., et al. *Color Atlas of Dermatology*. Philadelphia: W.B. Saunders, 1993, p. 231.)

both generalized and itchy. Hives may also result, with severe swelling and itching. Withdrawal of the drug is the primary treatment, along with an antipruritic agent, such as an antihistamine, to relieve the itching (Monroe, 1981; Berliner, 1986).

Stasis Dermatitis with Leg Ulcers

Leg ulcers are the most common chronic wound in the United States, and the incidence increases with age. The prevalence rises from 1 per cent in people aged 70 years to 5 per cent in those aged 90 years, with women outnumbering men 2.8:1. The ulcers are caused by venous insufficiency, arterial insufficiency, neuropathic diabetes, or a combination of these factors; however, venous ulcers are by far the most common, representing 80 to 90 per cent of all cases.

In this condition, the legs, especially the distal portions, become swollen and edematous, interfering with the distribution of nutrients in the skin. There is an eczematous reaction that may be aggravated by scratching or by topical ointments used to alleviate the discomfort. The resulting scratching and inflammation produce infection and skin breakdown, ending in a venous or varicose leg ulcer. Ulceration frequently occurs around the ankle; a bluish-red discoloration surrounds the area (Fig. 5–11). Chronic infection, cellulitis, and crusting occur (Levine, 1990; Burton, 1993; Phillips and Dover, 1991; Stacey et al., 1992).

Treatment of leg ulcers has become increasingly successful when a multidisciplinary, holistic approach has been used. Bed-

rest is no longer necessary, and many outpatient clinics (some that are run by nurses) are devoted exclusively to leg ulcer care. The goals of treatment are to alleviate swelling, eliminate infection, and promote healing. The first step is to determine the cause of the ulcer. Peripheral pulse and sensation should be assessed to rule out arterial disease and neuropathy, respectively. Compression bandages reduce edema, and occlusive dressings provide a moist environment for promoting debridement (Bourne, 1992; Riordan, 1991; Awenat, 1992; Russell and Bowles, 1992).

The leg ulcer clinic at Duke University has had impressive success using the "Duke" boot, which is a combination of elastic self-adherent outer wrap (Coban) and an Unna wrap (Dome-Paste) that provides ambulatory hemodynamic support and patient comfort. Occlusive dressings, topical ointments, corticosteroid therapy, and occasionally antibiotics are used for associated problems,

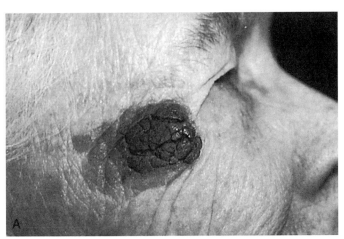

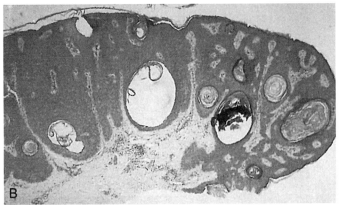

FIGURE 5 – 12

A, Seborrheic keratosis. *B*, Histopathological appearance of a typical case of seborrheic keratosis. (From Callen, J.P., Greer, K.E., Hood, A.F., et al. *Color Atlas of Dermatology*. Philadelphia: W.B. Saunders, 1993, p. 146.)

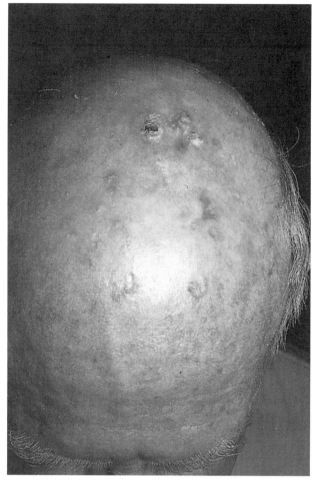

FIGURE 5-13

Actinic keratoses. (From Callen, J.P., Greer, K.E., Hood, A.F., et al. *Color Atlas of Dermatology*. Philadelphia: W.B. Saunders, 1993, p. 311.)

such as venous dermatitis, mild inflammatory changes, and cellulitis (Burton, 1993).

Neoplastic Disorders

Keratoses

SEBORRHEIC KERATOSES. Seborrheic keratoses have been found in up to 88 per cent of persons over 65; in about 50 per cent of the cases, 10 or more lesions were present (Tindall and Smith, 1963). They originate from the horny layer of the epidermis, usually on the unexposed skin of older white persons, or, in some cases, from solar lentigines. The lesions are raised, brownish-gray patches with a surface sheen that lacks roughness or fine granularity. Sometimes the lesions appear on exposed skin, especially around the hairline (Fig. 5–12). The size of the exposed lesions rarely changes; however,

the lesions on covered skin may enlarge and appear darker and more crumbly. Seborrheic keratoses are noninvasive, benign, warty lesions, and they can be removed with chemical peeling agents, such as trichloroacetic acid or tretinoin (Retin-A); delicate electrocautery; carbon dioxide laser vaporization; and cryotherapy if they cause discomfort or embarrassment (Young, 1993).

ACTINIC KERATOSES. These lesions are also known as *senile* or *solar keratoses*. Because actinic keratoses are associated with excessive exposure to sun, they usually appear on the forehead, cheeks, dorsa of the hands and forearms, and on the ears and balding scalp of older men. The keratotic patches begin as small, reddened areas of light-damaged skin (Fig. 5–13). They become well demarcated, gradually losing normal skin surface markings. They appear yellow to brown in color with a rough surface; the patches are often most easily identified by touch.

Fewer than 20 per cent of actinic keratoses develop into squamous cell carcinomas, and even fewer metastasize (Marks, 1987, 1993; Prawer, 1991). Decreased exposure to sunlight may cause the lesions to regress, but because they are potentially malignant, they should be removed. Removal is accomplished through the use of chemical peel, freezing, cautery, and topical creams (Curaderm; masoprocol) (*Oncology*, 1992; Chaum et al., 1991; Olsen et al., 1991).

Epitheliomas

Epitheliomas are tumors derived from the epithelium and are usually found on hair-bearing skin. Two major types of carcinogenic skin epitheliomas frequently seen in the elderly are *basal cell epitheliomas* and *squamous cell epitheliomas*. Although the diagnosis of any form of cancer is frightening to many people, epitheliomas are highly treatable when found early. Basal cell carcinoma occurs three times as often as squamous cell carcinoma. The rate of growth is usually diagnostic of the disease. There is a slow, relentless enlargement of basal cell epitheliomas (approximately 0.1 to 0.4 mm per month), whereas the growth rate of squamous cell epitheliomas is much faster (10 to 20 mm per month) (Robinson, 1983). Studies have found that persons with prior basal cell or squamous cell epitheliomas have a substantial risk of developing another tumor of the same histological type (Marghoob et al., 1993; Karagas et al., 1992).

BASAL CELL EPITHELIOMA. The basal

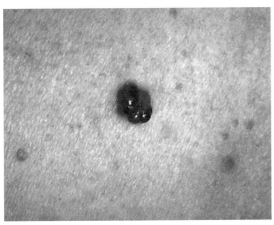

FIGURE 5 - 1 4

Pigmented basal cell carcinoma. (From Callen, J.P., Greer, K.E., Hood, A.F., et al. *Color Atlas of Dermatology*. Philadelphia: W.B. Saunders, 1993, p. 94.)

SQUAMOUS CELL EPITHELIOMA. The squamous cell epithelioma is a skin cancer that occurs most often in middle-aged and older persons, and twice as often in men as in women. It arises from the epidermis and mucosa of sun-exposed, damaged skin, especially from areas such as actinic keratoses, scars, and sites exposed to oils and tars. Its exact appearance depends on the preceding lesion, but the tumor usually begins as a small, hard, red nodule that may appear wartlike. The lesion may also appear ulcerated with a raised, rolled, gray-yellow edge (Fig. 5–15).

This form of cancer is locally invasive and has a high incidence of metastasis. A deep incisional biopsy is necessary for diagnosis, and treatment consists of removal by cautery, curettage, deep cryotherapy, excision, or radiotherapy. The prognosis depends on the duration and the site of the lesion, and

cell epithelioma, also known as basal cell carcinoma and "rodent ulcer," is the most common form of skin cancer in whites. The lesion usually appears on the face, arising from the cells of the epidermis or hair follicles. It starts as a small, smooth, hemispherical, translucent papule covered by thinned epidermis, through which dilated blood vessels and occasional specks of brown or black pigment can be seen (Fig. 5–14). The papule gradually enlarges into a mass of pearly nodules or a papular plaque that may be darkly pigmented, resembling a malignant melanoma (see Fig. 5–16). It can also become an ulcerated lesion surrounded by a nodular rim (rodent ulcer), resembling a keratoacanthoma or squamous cell epithelioma (see Fig. 5–15).

Although metastasis is rare, basal cell epitheliomas can be locally invasive and, without treatment, can cause mutilation or death. Treatment consists of removal of the lesion by curettage and electrosurgery, cryosurgery, excision, Mohs micrographic surgery, and laser surgery. Radiotherapy or excision with or without skin graft may also be performed, depending on the size, location, and type of lesion. The success rate is extremely high, but the client is followed up for 2 years to detect the recurrences that appear in about 5 per cent of the cases. The person most likely to have a basal cell epithelioma is the person who has already had one. Long-term follow-up is essential because of the possibility of recurrence, the development of new lesions, or both (Drake et al., 1992; Young et al., 1993).

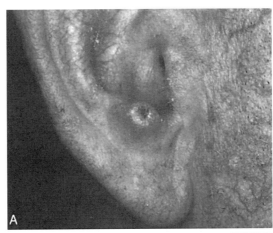

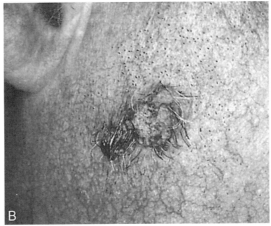

FIGURE 5 - 1 5

A and *B*, Squamous cell carcinoma of the skin. (From Callen, J.P., Greer, K.E., Hood, A.F., et al. *Color Atlas of Dermatology*. Philadelphia: W.B. Saunders, 1993, p. 111.)

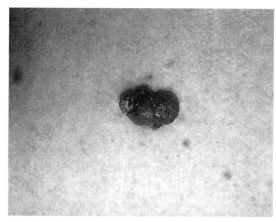

FIGURE 5 – 16

Malignant melanoma. (From Callen, J.P., Greer, K.E., Hood, A.F., et al. *Color Atlas of Dermatology.* Philadelphia: W.B. Saunders, 1993, p. 94.)

higher cure rates are associated with lesions found on unexposed skin (Frankel, 1992; Proper et al., 1990; Young et al., 1993).

Malignant Melanoma

Malignant melanoma is the most common cause of death from diseases arising in the skin. The incidence has increased exponentially during the past 50 years. In 1935, the risk of developing melanoma was 1 : 1500; in the year 2000, the risk is projected to be 1 : 90. In 1992, there were approximately 32,000 new cases and 6700 deaths from melanoma (Drake et al., 1993; National Institutes of Health Consensus Development Panel on Early Melanoma, 1992).

The melanoma lesions are pigmented macules, papules, nodules, patches, or tumors with any of the ABCD warning signs (Fig. 5–16): (1) *a*symmetry, (2) *b*order irregularity, (3) *c*olor variegation, and (4) *d*iameter greater than 6 mm. In some cases, malignant melanomas may be mistaken for rapidly enlarging, deeply pigmented warts, so that biopsy is often necessary for a definitive diagnosis.

The disease is predominantly caused by sunlight or irritation of a mole. Fair-complexioned, redheaded white persons of European descent who sunburn easily or have a history of severe sunburn are most susceptible to the disease. Additionally, people with a family and/or personal history of melanoma and those with many nevi or clinically atypical nevi are at risk. Major subtypes of melanoma are

1. *Lentigo maligna melanoma,* found on ex-

posed skin of fair-complexioned elderly whites

2. *Superficial spreading melanoma,* found on all body surfaces

3. *Nodular melanoma,* found on all body surfaces

4. *Acral lentiginous melanoma,* found on palms, soles, and under the tongue

The disease is highly malignant, producing rapid metastasis through the lymphatic system. Early detection improves prognosis; therefore, older persons should be particularly sensitive to changes in the shape, size, or texture of nevi. Diagnosis is through biopsy, and treatment is through surgical excision. Immunotherapy has become an increasingly popular treatment for high-risk patients with diffuse nodules, particularly the combination of bacillus Calmette-Guérin with chemotherapy. Trials continue in order to demonstrate effectiveness of this therapy (Brozena et al., 1990; Drake et al., 1993; National Institutes of Health Consensus Development Panel on Early Melanoma, 1992; Physicians and Scientists, University College London Medical School, 1992; Young et al., 1993).

Infectious Disorders

Herpes Zoster

Herpes zoster, also known as *shingles,* is an acute viral infection that primarily affects people who are 50 to 75 years of age. According to Knight (1973), if individuals live to 85 years of age, they have a 50 per cent chance of developing herpes zoster. There is evidence that the incidence and severity of the disease is increasing as the population ages (Huff, 1988; Dalziel and Bickers, 1992).

The virus, *herpesvirus varicellae* (varicella zoster virus, VZV), also causes chickenpox in children, and herpes zoster is thought to arise from a reactivation of the varicella virus that has lain dormant in the sensory root ganglia for many years. The disease may occur spontaneously as a result of decreased childhood immunity, or it may result from trauma or disease-related disturbances of immune mechanisms, such as malignancies, radiotherapy, and administration of immunosuppressive drugs (Peto, 1989; Peto and Juel-Jensen, 1988).

The symptoms begin with burning pain, followed by a papular rash lasting 3 to 4 days. The rash becomes edematous, then vesicular and pustular, and finally exhibits erosions and crusting. After the eruption

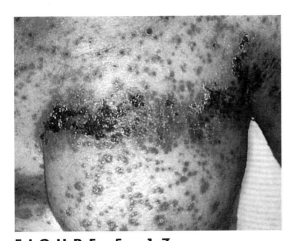

fades, the skin is permanently scarred. There may be chronic pain at the site for many years, a phenomenon known as "postherpetic neuralgia." Herpes zoster is most commonly located in the thoracic area in a unilateral dermatomal or linear distribution, or in the trigeminal, cervical, lumbar, or lumbosacral areas (Fig. 5–17) (Schmader, 1990).

The most effective treatment of acute herpes zoster is the antiviral agent acyclovir (Zovirax). The drug should be used within 48 to 72 hours after the onset of the rash to be effective for relief of pain and promotion of healing. Some studies have found the drug to be helpful in reducing the incidence of postherpetic neuralgia. When postherpetic neuralgia occurs, analgesics, anticonvulsants (carbamazepine), and antidepressants (amitriptyline) as well as mechanical vibration or transcutaneous electrical nerve stimulation may be used for pain relief (Morton and Thomson, 1989; Schmader, 1990; Bowsher, 1992; Robertson and George, 1990; Young et al., 1993).

Psoriasis

Psoriasis affects approximately 1 per cent of the population in the United States and causes the greatest number of repeat visits to the dermatologist per year of any skin disease. The incidence of psoriasis peaks around the age of 30, but it can appear at any age, even over 100 years. There is a second peak in the sixth decade. In an interesting parallel with diabetes mellitus, early onset appears to be more strongly associated with a positive family history. Some surveys have found the disease to occur more commonly in men (Dalziel and Bickers, 1992; Smith et al., 1993; Marks, 1987).

Three major components make up the pathogenesis and etiology of psoriasis: (1) abnormal epidermal proliferation, (2) genetic factors, and (3) inflammation. The cells of the epidermis reproduce more rapidly than normal, both in the lesions and in normal-appearing skin. This characteristic is thought to be inherited because a positive family history is obtained in approximately 40 to 50 per cent of those affected. Human lymphocytic antigen is also associated with the disease. Inflammation is related to the immunological origin that has been surmised for the disorder because abnormalities of both humoral and cellular components of the immune system have been noted (Champion, 1981; Marks, 1987; Young et al., 1993).

The lesion begins as a small, red, scaly, elevated patch on the scalp, elbows, or knees. There may have been a previous history of dandruff or scaling around the ears. Psoriasis is not thought to be a pruritic disorder, but many people complain of mild to moderate itching. Psoriasis may exacerbate after emotional stress, drug ingestion (such as lithium, antimalarials, and some beta-blockers), or sun exposure; however, some people note improvement during the summer months. In some cases, the patches develop within 7 to 14 days after trauma, such as that seen in cuts, burns, or operative sites. Smoking also has been linked with psoriasis (Mills et al., 1992; Dalziel and Bickers, 1992; Young et al., 1993).

Psoriatic plaques vary in size and shape and appear as red, elevated areas of skin covered by a fine scale (Fig. 5–18). They may affect any part of the body, including the scalp, ears, face, trunk, external genitalia, perineal area, limbs, hands and feet, and nails. The appearance of the lesions may vary according to their location. Psoriasis may have a profound effect on the psychological well-being of clients who may limit activities because of their appearance (Farber, 1992a, 1992b; Yasuda et al., 1990; Finlay et al., 1990; McHenry and Doherty, 1992).

Diagnosis of the disease is accomplished through history, observation, and skin biopsy. Because psoriasis is a chronic, lifelong disease, treatment must involve the client's support and cooperation. Clients should be taught that the condition is not contagious and that a healthy lifestyle (good diet, exercise, avoidance of smoking and heavy alcohol intake) is important. Stress management

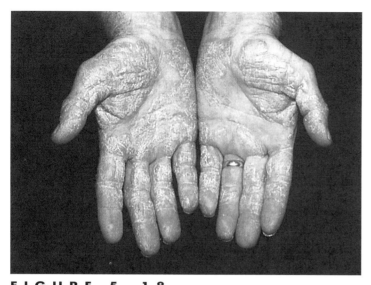

FIGURE 5 – 1 8

Psoriasis of the hands. (From Callen, J.P., Greer, K.E., Hood, A.F., et al. *Color Atlas of Dermatology*. Philadelphia: W.B. Saunders, 1993, p. 120.)

is also helpful. Topical medications are used in an attempt to slow down the rapid growth of epidermal cells; these medications include corticosteroids, tar, and dithranol. Systemic drugs include cytotoxic drugs, such as methotrexate or 6-mercaptopurine. Ultraviolet radiation is also used. Liao and Liao (1992) found acupuncture to be an effective treatment for psoriasis, especially in cases in which traditional management was ineffective. The type of treatment depends on the age, sex, and occupation of the client; the sites affected; the activity and extent of the disease; the presence or absence of complications; and the client's attitude toward the condition (Christensen and Brolund, 1992; Price et al., 1991; Lowe, 1986).

Pressure Sores (Decubitus Ulcers)

Pressure sores, or decubitus ulcers, are localized areas of cellular necrosis resulting from prolonged pressure between any bony prominence and an external object, such as a bed, chair, or cast. The tissues are deprived of blood supply and disintegrate. Areas frequently affected in older persons include the heels, greater trochanter, sacrum, dorsal spine (especially in thin kyphotic persons), scapular spines, and elbows. Long-term pressure increases vulnerability to decubitus ulcer development, as evidenced by the fact that high pressure maintained for a short time is less dangerous than low pressure continued for a long time. Predisposing factors include poor nutrition, aging, immobility, superficial sensory loss, and disturbed

autonomic function (loss of bowel and bladder control). Older people are particularly prone to development of pressure sores because of arteriosclerotic changes in the vessels, loss of subcutaneous tissue and tissue elasticity, senility, and clouding of the sensorium (Perez, 1993; Piloian, 1992; Kelley and Mobily, 1991). Hypotension also has been found to be associated with pressure sore risk in the elderly (Bergstrom and Braden, 1992; Schubert, 1991).

There are two types of pressure sores: *superficial* (benign) and *deep* (malignant). Superficial sores are reddened areas involving only the outer skin layers that are less dangerous than deep sores. They are caused by friction, shearing stresses, trauma, infection, and saturation with urine or other moisturizing agents. The lesions are frequently painful but easily treated and prevented. Treatment consists of keeping the area clean, dry, and free from infection or further pressure; a covering with a nonstick dressing also promotes healing. Good nursing care is the key to prevention, and measures such as frequent turning (every 2 hours), getting the client out of bed into a chair, keeping the vulnerable areas clean and dry, and keeping the weight of the bedcovers off the feet are most effective in warding off superficial pressure sores (Inman et al., 1993).

Deep sores develop quickly as a result of thrombosis of the vessels in deep tissue overlying the bony prominences. The muscle and fat layers are more vulnerable than the dermis, causing deep, large ulcers. The sore begins as a reddening of the skin with unobservable necrosis in the deep underlying tissues. In 1 to 2 days, the lesion bursts through the skin like an abscess, revealing a deep cavity full of black or infected slough, which may go through to the bone. There is a large area of skin loss, resulting in extensive scarring. The appearance of deep pressure sores with an illness can delay recovery and may even be fatal.

Prevention of deep pressure sores is more difficult in the elderly. The risk of developing these lesions is greatest during the 10 days after the onset of illness or admission to the hospital, whichever coincides with the period of greatest immobility. A deep sore that develops early and penetrates deeply is most dangerous to the older person. Nurses should recognize early signs of deterioration, such as apathy, loss of appetite, and incontinence. Some measures that can help to prevent deep pressure sores include the following:

1. Change position every 2 hours.

2. Do not oversedate or undersedate.

3. Avoid or correct malnutrition.

4. Avoid dehydration; maintain blood pressure and cardiac output.

5. Use an alternating-pressure airbed or waterbed.

Treatment consists primarily of reinforcement of preventive measures, including maintenance of fluid and protein stores that are lost through serous and purulent discharge; repair of tissues by giving vitamin supplements; avoidance of general infections, such as pneumonia or cystitis; and remediation of anemia. The lesions should be cleaned and dressed and care should be taken to treat local infection. To promote granulation and healing, the wound should be irrigated with warm saline every day. Irrigation washes out the debris, lowers the growth of anaerobes, promotes the separation of the slough, and decreases the pocketing of infection in deeper tissues. Infection must be eradicated, and the slough must separate before healing can take place (United States Department of Health and Human Services, 1992; Spoelhof and Ide, 1993; Breslow et al., 1993; Ferrell et al., 1993).

More discussion on pressure sores can be found in Chapter 14.

NURSING ASSESSMENT

History

A thorough, accurate nursing history can help to clarify whether a skin condition is a phenomenon of normal aging or a pathological deviation. It can also indicate whether or not an older person is at risk for developing a particular condition and what measures are necessary for prevention. The history should cover all aspects of living and functioning that could affect the condition of the skin. The nurse should investigate the onset, development, and pattern of all skin conditions, accompanying symptoms, past or present systemic diseases, and medications taken. Finally, the general state of health, nutritional status, allergies, level of functioning, and physical and social environments should be determined.

Physical Assessment

Examination of the skin and appendages should be carried out in a warm, well-lighted room (preferably with indirect daylight). The assessment should be systematic and thorough, and care should be taken to

TABLE 5 – 6
Skin Assessment

History
Past and present skin conditions:
  Onset, development, pattern, duration, symptoms
Past and present systemic diseases:
  History and treatment
Drug history:
  Topical, systemic, prescription, nonprescription, allergies
Nutrition:
  Malnourished, obese, diet and eating habits
Functional status:
  Mobility, mental status, activities of daily living capacity
Environment:
  Physical (temperature, climate, use of soaps or other drying agents)
  Social (support systems, work, family interactions)

Physical Assessment
Color:
  Red, jaundiced, brown, gray, cyanotic, pale, blotchy
Temperature:
  Hot, warm, cool
Moisture:
  Dry, oily, or combination of both; moist, clammy
Texture:
  Rough, smooth, scaly, flaky
Edema:
  Location, extent
Thickness:
  Differences among various parts of the body, relationship to itching or redness
Mobility and turgor:
  Supple, pliable, flexible, creases and folds
Lesions:
  Color, size, texture, identifying characteristics, distribution
Hair:
  Amount, distribution, texture, color, dandruff or scaling, odor
Nails:
  Color, length, thickness, splitting, swelling, accumulations

examine the entire skin surface, skin folds, mucous membranes, hair, and nails. It is helpful to examine from the head to the toes, comparing the left and right sides of the body for symmetry. Table 5–6 presents a more detailed history and assessment list.

NURSING DIAGNOSES
Age-Related Changes in the Integument

1. Skin Integrity, Impaired: related to itching, related to physical immobilization, related to alterations in turgor

2. Skin Integrity, Risk for Impaired: related to physical immobilization, related to

pressure, related to skeletal prominence, related to alterations in skin turgor

3. Tissue Integrity, Impaired: related to impaired physical mobility, related to pressure, related to altered circulation

4. Sleep Pattern Disturbance: related to pain or itching

5. Infection, Risk For: related to impaired tissue integrity

NURSING MANAGEMENT

Nursing interventions are aimed at preserving skin integrity and preventing disease or injury. Because the skin is dryer and more fragile in older persons, it should be handled with gentleness and care. Friction, irritation, or mechanical injury should be avoided when bathing, dressing, moving, or turning an older patient. Soap and rubbing alcohol should not be used when bathing or giving a back rub, because these materials tend to dry the skin. Bath water should be lowered in temperature from 110 to 100 to 105°F, and emollients such as Alpha Keri and baby oil may be added for lubrication. It is best to apply lubricants directly to the skin, however, to avoid slipping in the bathtub. Good personal grooming and cleanliness should be stressed, not only to promote healthy skin but also for well-being and comfort. However, baths are not necessary every day for older people, and complete baths two or three times a week supplemented by partial baths are sufficient. Hair and nail care should be included in personal hygiene, and soaking the feet helps to loosen debris under the nails, making cutting of the nails easier.

Older individuals can help promote healthy skin by eating healthy diets high in vitamins and nutrients. Vitamins A and C and protein are necessary for healthy skin cells and supportive tissues. Interventions should include teaching about foods high in these nutrients and helping to ensure that they are included in the diet.

The environment can be modified to promote healthy skin. Staying out of the sun, keeping the air moist with a humidifier, and avoiding exposure to wind and cold help to preserve moist and younger looking skin. Soft, unwrinkled clothing next to the skin minimizes skin irritation and resulting pruritus.

SUMMARY

Normal skin changes, almost more than any other body system, reveal the aging process. Changes generally seen in the skin in older people include thinning of the skin layers, decreased strength and elasticity, decreased vascularity, and delayed healing. The secretions of both the sebaceous and the sweat glands tend to diminish. Hair becomes thinner and grayer, and nails become thicker, more brittle, and hard with diminished growth rates.

Common skin disorders associated with older age include pruritus, neoplastic disorders, herpes zoster, psoriasis, and pressure sores. Skin tags, cherry angiomas, nevi, venous lakes, and lentigos are also common; these cause little discomfort, but the appearance of mottled and spotty skin that they produce may be troublesome to the elderly. Dryness is perhaps the most significant skin problem with aging. It may cause itchiness and scaling and may even lead to other lesions. Treatment with moisturizers and emollients is useful for lubrication.

History and assessment of the skin should focus on past conditions and systemic diseases; drug use; nutrition; the environment; observation of the color, temperature, texture, and thickness of the skin; and any lesions or abnormalities. Nursing care should include the proper use of equipment, encouragement of proper nutrition, avoidance of injury, good hair and nail care, and instruction in self-care and preventive techniques. Prevention is the key to good skin care for older adults.

REFERENCES

Awenat, Y. Leg ulcer clinics: Advanced nursing. *Nurs Stand* 7(suppl):4–7, 1992.

Banov, C.H., Epstein, J.H. and Grayson, L.D. When an itch persists. *Patient Care* 26:75–81, 84–88, 1992.

Bergstrom, N. and Braden, B. A prospective study of pressure sore risk among institutionalized elderly. *J Am Geriatr Soc* 40:747–758, 1992.

Berliner, H. Aging skin. *Am J Nurs* 86:1138–1141, 1986.

Beylot, C. Clinical signs of cutaneous aging. *Revue Fr Gynecol Obstet* 86(6):433–441, 1991.

Bhawan, J., Oh, C.H., Lew, R., et al. Histopathologic differences in the photoaging process in facial versus arm skin. *Am J Dermatopathol* 14:224–230, 1992.

Bornstein, J., Pascal, B. and Abramovici, H. The common problem of vulvar pruritus. *Obstet Gynecol Surv* 48:111–118, 1993.

Bourne, I.H. Treatment of leg ulcers. *J R Soc Med* 85:733–735, 1992.

Bowsher, D. Acute herpes zoster and post herpetic neuralgia: Effects of acyclovir and outcome of treatment with amitriptyline. *Br J Gen Pract* 42:244–246, 1992.

Branchet, M.C., Boisnic, S., Frances, C. and Robert, A.M. Skin thickness changes in normal aging skin. *Gerontology* 36(1):28–35, 1990.

Breslow, R.A., Hallfrisch, J., Guy, D.G., et al. The importance of dietary protein in healing pressure ulcers. *J Am Geriatr Soc* 41:357–362, 1993.

Brozena, S.J., Waterman, D.O. and Fenske, N.A. Malignant melanoma: Management guidelines. *Geriatrics* 45: 55–62, 1990.

Burton, C.S., III. Treatment of leg ulcers. *Dermatol Clin* 11:315–323, 1993.

Cape, R. *Aging: Its Complex Management.* New York: Harper & Row, 1978, pp. 13–15.

Champion, R.J. Psoriasis and its treatment. *BMJ* 282: 343–345, 1981.

Chaum, B.E., Daunter, B. and Evans, R.A. Topical treatment of malignant and premalignant skin lesions by very low concentrations of a standard mixture (BEC) of solasodine glycosides. *Cancer Lett* 59:183–192, 1991.

Christensen, O.B. and Brolund, L. Clinical studies with a novel dithranol formulation (Micanol) in combination with UVB at day-care centres. *Acta Derm Venereol Suppl (Stockh)* 172:17–19, 1992.

Coni, N., Davison, W. and Webster, S. *Lecture Notes on Geriatrics.* Boston: Blackwell Scientific Publications, 1980.

Cuelenaere, C., DeBersaques, J. and Kint, A. Use of topical lithium succinate in the treatment of seborrhoeic dermatitis. *Dermatology* 184:194–197, 1992.

Dalziel, K.L. and Bickers, D.R. Skin aging. *In* Brocklehurst, J.C., Tallis, R.C. and Fillit, H.M. (eds.). *Textbook of Geriatric Medicine and Gerontology.* 4th ed. Edinburgh: Churchill Livingstone, 1992, pp. 898–921.

Downing, D.T., Stewart, M.E. and Strauss, J.S. Changes in sebum secretion and sebaceous glands during aging. *In* Kligman, A.M. and Takese, Y. (eds.). *Cutaneous Aging.* Tokyo: University of Tokyo Press, 1988, pp. 135–148.

Drake, L.A., Ceilley, R.I., Cornelison, R.L., et al. Guidelines for malignant melanoma. *J Am Acad Dermatol* 28: 638–641, 1993.

Drake, L.A., Ceilley, R.I., Cornelison, R.L., et al. Guidelines of care for basal cell carcinoma: The American Academy of Dermatology Committee on Guidelines of Care. *J Am Acad Dermatol* 26:117–120, 1992.

Duncan, W.C. and Fenske, N.A. Cutaneous signs of internal disease in the elderly. *Geriatrics* 45:24–30, 1990.

Efalith Multicenter Trial Group. A double-blind, placebo-controlled, multicenter trial of lithium succinate ointment in the treatment of seborrheic dermatitis. *J Am Acad Dermatol* 26:452–457, 1992.

Elkowitz, E.B. *Geriatric Medicine for the Primary Care Practitioner.* New York: Springer Publishing Company, 1981.

Ensebio, E.B., Graham, J. and Mody, N. Treatment of intractable pruritus ani. *Dis Colon Rectum* 33:770–772, 1990.

Farber, E.M. Ear psoriasis. *Cutis* 50:105–107, 1992a.

Farber, E.M. Facial psoriasis. *Cutis* 50:25–28, 1992b.

Farmer, E.R. and Hood, A.F. Pathology of the Skin. E. Norwalk, CT: Appleton & Lange, 1990.

Fenske, N.A. and Albers, J.E. Cosmetic modalities for aging skin: What to tell patients. *Geriatrics* 45:59–67, 1990.

Fenske, N.A. and Lober, C.S. Skin changes of aging: Pathological implications. *Geriatrics* 45:27–35, 1990.

Ferrell, B.A., Osterweil, D. and Christenson, P. A randomized trial of low-air-loss beds for treatment of pressure ulcers. *JAMA* 269:494–497, 1993.

Finlay, A.Y., Khan, G.K., Luscombe, D.K. and Salek, M.S. Validation of sickness impact profile and psoriasis disability index in psoriasis. *Br J Dermatol* 123:751–756, 1990.

Fitzpatrick, J.E. and Mellette, J.R. Geriatric dermatology. *In* Schrier, R.W. *Geriatric Medicine.* Philadelphia: W.B. Saunders, 1990, pp. 138–148.

Frankel, D.H. Squamous cell carcinoma of the skin. *Hosp Pract* 27:99–102, 105–106, 1992.

Gilchrest, B.A. Pruritus: Pathogenesis, therapy and significance in systemic disease states. *Arch Intern Med* 142:101, 1982.

Gilchrest, B.A. The aging skin. *Dermatol Clin* 4:345–531, 1986.

Gilchrest, B.A. Skin aging and photoaging. *Dermatol Nurs* 2:79–82, 1990.

Grady, D. and Ernster, V. Does cigarette smoking make you ugly and old? *Am J Epidemiol* 135(8):839–842, 1992.

Graham-Brown, R.A.C. and Monk, B.E. Pruritus and xerosis. *In* Monk, B.E., Graham-Brown, R.A.C. and Sarkany, I. (eds.). *Skin Disorders in the Elderly.* London: Blackwell Scientific Publications, 1988, pp. 133–146.

Green, H.A. and Drake, L. Aging, sun damage, and sunscreens. *Clin Plast Surg* 20(1):1–8, 1993.

Griffiths, C.E. The clinical identification and quantification of photodamage. *Br J Dermatol* 127(suppl 41):37–42, 1992.

Guzzo, C.A., Weiss, J.S., Mogavero, H.S., et al. A review of two controlled multicenter trials comparing 0.05% halobetasol propionate ointment to its vehicle in the treatment of chronic eczematous dermatoses. *J Am Acad Dermatol* 25:1179–1183, 1991.

Helfand, A. Foot health for the elderly patient. *In* Reichel, W. (ed.). *Clinical Aspects of Aging.* 2nd ed. Baltimore: Williams & Wilkins, 1983, pp. 303–314.

Holzle, E. Pigmented lesions as a sign of photodamage. *Br J Dermatol* 127(suppl 41):48–50, 1992.

Huff, J.C. Herpes zoster. *Curr Probl Dermatol* 1:1, 1988.

Inman, K.J., Sibbald, W.J., Rutledge, F.S. and Clark, B.J. Clinical utility and cost-effectiveness of an air suspension bed in the prevention of pressure ulcers. *JAMA* 269:1139–1143, 1993.

Itin, P. Intertrigo—A therapeutic problem circle. *Ther Umsch* 46:98–101, 1989.

Jones, P.L. and Millman, A. Wound healing and the aged patient. *Nurs Clin North Am* 25:263–277, 1990.

Kantor, I., Cook, P.R., Cullen, S.I., et al. Double-blind bilateral paired comparison of a 0.05% halobetasol propionate cream and its vehicle in patients with chronic atopic dermatitis and other eczematous dermatoses. *J Am Acad Dermatol* 25:1184–1186, 1991.

Kaplan, R.P. The aging skin. *Compr Ther* 17(8):59–67, 1991.

Karagas, M.R., Stukul, T.A., Greenberg, E.R., et al. Risk of subsequent basal cell carcinoma and squamous cell carcinoma of the skin among patients with prior skin cancer. *JAMA* 267:3305–3310, 1992.

Kelley, L.S. and Mobily, P.R. Iatrogenesis in the elderly. Impaired skin integrity. *J Gerontol Nurs* 17:24–29, 1991.

Kim, J.M. and Su, W.P. Mid dermal elastolysis with wrinkling. *J Am Acad Dermatol* 26(2 Pt 1):169–173, 1992.

Kligman, A.M. Perspectives and problems in cutaneous gerontology. *J Invest Dermatol* 73:39–46, 1979.

Kligman, A.M. and Balin, A.K. Aging of human skin. *In* Balin, A.K. and Kligman, A.M. *Aging and the Skin.* New York: Raven Press, 1989, pp. 1–42.

Knight, V. *Viral and Mycoplasmal Infections.* Philadelphia: Lea & Febiger, 1973, pp. 186–196.

Kulozik, M. and Krieg, T. Changes in collagen connective tissue and fibroblasts in aging. *Z Hautkr* 64(11): 1003–1004, 1007–1009, 1989.

Kurban, R.S. and Bhawan, J. Histologic changes in skin associated with aging. *J Dermatol Surg Oncol* 1:5–12, 1990.

Kurban, R.K. and Kurban, A.K. Common skin disorders of aging: Diagnosis and treatment. *Geriatrics* 48:30–42, 1993.

Lamont, L.J. Venous ulcers: A nursing challenge. *Am Acad Nurse Pract* 3:158–165, 1991.

Lapiere, C.M. The ageing dermis: The main cause for the appearance of "old" skin. *Br J Dermatol* 122(suppl 35):5–11, 1990.

Leyden, J.J. Clinical features of ageing skin. *Br J Dermatol* 122(suppl 35):1–3, 1990.

Liao, S.J. and Liao, T.A. Acupuncture treatment for psoriasis: A retrospective case report. *Acupunct Electrother Res* 17:195–208, 1992.

Lober, C.W. and Fenske, N.A. Photoaging and the skin: Its clinical differentiation and meaning. *Geriatrics* 45: 36–42, 1990.

Lober, C.W. and Fenske, N.A. Cutaneous aging: Effect of intrinsic changes on surgical considerations. *South Med J* 84(12):1444–1446, 1991.

Lombardo, P. Dermatologic disorders in the elderly. *In* Rossman, I. (ed.). *Clinical Geriatrics.* 2nd ed. Philadelphia: J.B. Lippincott, 1979, pp. 338–353.

Lowe, N.J. *Practical Psoriasis Therapy.* Chicago: Year Book Medical Publishers, 1986.

Marghoob, A., Kopf, A.W., Bart, R.S., et al. Risk of another basal cell carcinoma developing after treatment of a basal cell carcinoma. *J Am Acad Dermatol* 28: 22–28, 1993.

Marks, R. *Skin Disease in Old Age.* Philadelphia: J.B. Lippincott, 1987.

Marks, R. Actinic keratosis. A premalignant skin lesion. *Otolaryngol Clin North Am* 26:23–35, 1993.

McHenry, P.M. and Doherty, V.R. Psoriasis: An audit of patients' views on the disease and its treatment. *Br J Dermatol* 127:13–17, 1992.

McMahon, R. The prevalence of skin problems beneath the breasts of in-patients. *Nurs Times* 87:48–51, 1991.

Mills, C.M., Srivastava, E.D., Harvey, I.M., et al. Smoking habits in psoriasis: A case control study. *Br J Dermatol* 127:18–21, 1992.

Moloney, S.J., Edmonds, S.H., Giddens, L.D. and Learn, D.B. The hairless mouse model of photoaging: Evaluation between dermal elastin, collagen, skin thickness and wrinkles. *Photochem Photobiol* 56(4):505–511, 1992.

Monk, B.E. Transcutaneous electronic nerve stimulation in the treatment of generalized pruritus. *Clin Exp Dermatol* 18:67–68, 1993.

Monroe, E.W. Urticaria. *Int Soc Trop Dermatol* 2:32–41, 1981.

Montagna, W. and Carlisle, K. Structural changes in ageing skin. *Br J Dermatol* 122(suppl 35):61–70, 1990.

Morton, P. and Thomson, A.N. Oral acyclovir in the treatment of herpes zoster in general practice. *Aust N Z J Med* 102:93–95, 1989.

National Institutes of Health Consensus Development Panel on Early Melanoma. Diagnosis and treatment of early melanoma. *JAMA* 268:1314–1319, 1992.

Olson, E.A., Abernethy, M.L., Kulp-Shorten, C., et al. A double-blind, vehicle-controlled study evaluating masoprocol cream in the treatment of actinic keratoses on the head and neck. *J Am Acad Dermatol* 24:738–743, 1991.

Oncology 6:87–88, 1992.

Orentreich, N. and Durr, N.P. Nail changes with aging. *In* Balin, A.K. and Kligman, A.M. (eds.). *Aging and the Skin.* New York: Raven Press, 1989, pp. 105–113.

Origoni, M., Garsia, S., Sideri, M., et al. Efficacy of topical oxatomide in women with pruritus vulvae. *Drugs Exp Clin Res* 16:591–596, 1990.

Ortonne, J.P. Pigmentary changes of the ageing skin. *Br J Dermatol* 122(suppl 35):21–28, 1990.

Perez, E.D. Pressure ulcers: Updated guidelines for treatment and prevention. *Geriatrics* 48:39–44, 1993.

Peto, T. Shingles in general practice. *Practitioner* 233: 398–403, 1989.

Peto, T.E.A. and Juel-Jensen, B.E. Varicella zoster virus disease. *In* Monk, B.E., Graham-Brown, R.A.C. and Sarkany, I. (eds.). *Skin Diseases in the Elderly.* London: Blackwell Scientific Publications, 1988, pp. 94–103.

Phillips, T.J. and Dover, J.S. Leg ulcers. *J Am Acad Dermatol* 25:965–987, 1991.

Phillips, W.G. Pruritus: What to do when the itching won't stop. *Postgrad Med* 92:34–36, 43–46, 1992.

Physicians and Scientists, University College London Medical School. Malignant melanoma. *Lancet* 340:948–951, 1992.

Piloian, B.B. Defining characteristics of the nursing diagnosis "high risk for impaired skin integrity." *Decubitus* 5:32–34, 35–38, 42, 1992.

Porth, C. and Kapke, K. Aging and the skin. *Geriatric Nursing* 4:158–163, 1983.

Prawer, S.E. Sun-related skin diseases. *Postgrad Med* 89: 51–54, 59–61, 64–66, 1991.

Price, M.L., Mottahedin, I. and Mayo, P.R. Can psychotherapy help patients with psoriasis? *Clin Exp Dermatol* 16:114–117, 1991.

Proper, S.A., Roes, P.T. and Fenske, N.A. Non-melanomatous skin cancer in the elderly: Diagnosis and management. *Geriatrics* 45:57–62, 65, 1990.

Ries, W.R., Aly, A. and Vrabec, J. Common skin lesions of the elderly. *Otolaryngol Clin North Am* 23:1121–1139, 1990.

Riordan, C.A. The management of venous ulcers of the legs. *Australas J Dermatol* 32:111–116, 1991.

Robertson, D.R. and George, C.F. Treatment of post herpetic neuralgia in the elderly. *Br Med Bull* 46:113–123, 1990.

Robinson, J.K. Skin problems of aging. *Geriatrics* 38:57–65, 1983.

Russell, G. and Bowles, A. Developing a community-based leg ulcer clinic. *Br J Nurs* 1:337–340, 1992.

Sato, K. and Timm, D.E. Effect of aging on pharmacological sweating in man. *In* Kligman, A.M. and Takese, Y. (eds.). *Cutaneous Aging.* Tokyo: University of Tokyo Press, 1988, pp. 127–134.

Schmader, K.E. New weapons against herpes zoster. *Geriatrics* 45:21–23, 1990.

Schubert, V. Hypotension as a risk factor for the development of pressure sores in elderly subjects. *Age Ageing* 20:255–261, 1991.

Segal, R., David, M., Ingber, A., et al. Treatment with bifonazole shampoo for seborrhea and seborrheic dermatitis: A randomized, double-blind study. *Acta Derm Venereol Stockh* 72:454–455, 1992.

Shelley, W. B. and Shelley, E.D. The ten major problems of aging skin. *Geriatrics* 37:107, 1982.

Silverman, S.H., Youngs, D.J., Allan, A., et al. The fecal microflora in pruritus ani. *Dis Colon Rectum* 32:466–468, 1989.

Smith, A.E., Kassab, J.Y., Rowland Payne, C.M. and Beer, W.E. Bimodality in age of onset of psoriasis, in both patients and their relatives. *Dermatology* 186:181–186, 1993.

Spoelhof, G.D. and Ide, K. Pressure ulcers in nursing home patients. *Am Fam Physician* 47:1207–1215, 1993.

Stacey, M.C., Singh, G., Hoskin, S.E. and Thompson, P.J. Aetiology of chronic leg ulcers. *Eur J Vasc Surg* 6: 245–251, 1992.

Taylor, C.R., Stern, R.S., Leyden, J.J. and Gilchrest, B.A.

Photoaging/photodamage and photoprotection. *J Am Acad Dermatol* 22:1–15, 1990.

Tindall, J.P. and Smith, J.G., Jr. Skin lesions of the aged. *JAMA* 186:1039, 1963.

United States Department of Health and Human Services. Clinical practice guideline. *Pressure Ulcers in Adults: Prediction and Prevention.* Rockville, MD: United States Department of Health and Human Services, 1992.

Warren, R., Gartstein, V., Kligman, A.M., et al. Age, sunlight, and facial skin: A histologic and quantitative study. *J Am Acad Dermatol* 25(5 Pt 1):751–760, 1991.

Yasuda, H., Kobayashi, H. and Ohkawara, A. A survey of the social and psychological effects of psoriasis. *Jpn J Dermatol* 100:1167–1171, 1990.

Young, E.M., Jr., Newcomer, V.D. and Kligman, A.M. *Geriatric Dermatology.* Philadelphia: Lea & Febiger, 1993.

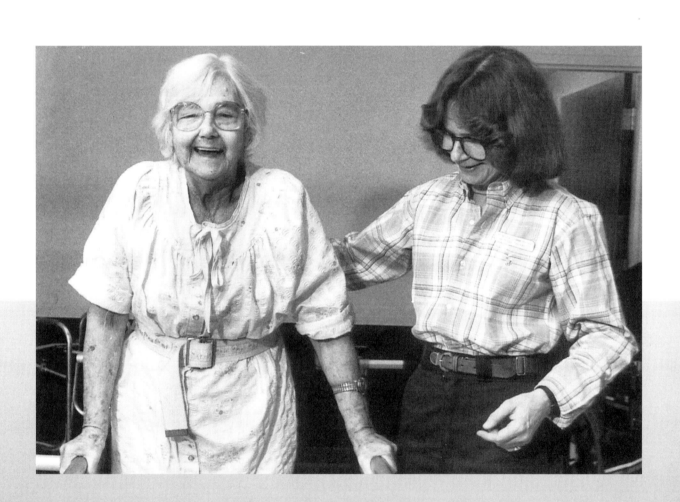

Age-Related Changes in the Musculoskeletal System

MARY ANN MATTESON

OBJECTIVES

Discuss alterations in structure and function associated with normal aging in the bones, joints, and muscles.

Explain the conditions associated with metabolic bone disease, including osteoporosis, osteomalacia, and Paget's disease.

Compare and contrast osteoarthritis, rheumatoid arthritis, and gout.

Describe polymyalgia rheumatica and its cause and treatment.

Formulate a plan for nursing assessment and interventions for older clients with musculoskeletal problems.

Alterations in stature and posture are as characteristic of older age as graying hair and wrinkling skin. An older person is generally depicted as frail, stooped, and bent, with an unsteady gait, maneuvering slowly in the environment. The body appears somewhat wasted, with a rounded belly and thin, fragile extremities. Changes in the musculoskeletal system are responsible for the altered appearance, weakness, and slowed movement that accompany older age.

ALTERATIONS IN STRUCTURE AND FUNCTION

Skeleton

Changes in Stature and Posture

With advancing years, there is a progressive decrease in stature, especially among older women. This decrease is mainly attributed to compression of the spinal column, which results from progressive narrowing of the intervertebral discs and loss of height of individual vertebrae. Disc changes begin during midlife, whereas vertebral changes tend to occur in later life. Height diminishes by approximately 1.2 cm per 20 years, and this tendency toward a smaller stature appears to be universal among all races and sexes. Although aging changes cause shortening of the trunk, the long bones of the extremities remain the same length throughout adult life. Thus, the arms and legs may appear longer in relation to the shortened torso.

Other changes that affect the general appearance are a lengthening and broadening of the nose and ears, probably as a result of the continued growth of cartilage into older age. The shoulders become narrower, and the pelvis becomes wider, producing a "pear-shaped" appearance that is enhanced by an increase in the anteroposterior diameter of the chest (Rossman, 1986).

Distribution of fat and lean body mass changes with advancing age, thereby altering body contours and appearance. The amount of lean body mass decreases, and the amount of subcutaneous fat increases. Subcutaneous fat is also redistributed, so that there is a gradual loss of fat from the face and extremities, and a gain in the amount in the abdomen and hips (Fig. 6–1). Loss of subcutaneous fat in the periphery results in increasingly sharp body contours and deepening hollows, especially around the orbits of the eyes, the axillae, the shoulders, and the ribs. Bony landmarks, such as the tips of the vertebrae, iliac crests, ribs, scapulae, and the bones of the extremities, become more prominent (Evans, 1992; Scileppi, 1985; Rossman, 1986).

Changes in Bone Mass and Metabolism

Skeletal bone provides support, protection, calcium storage, and blood cell production for the body. As with muscle tissue, metabolic processes slow down, and changes in

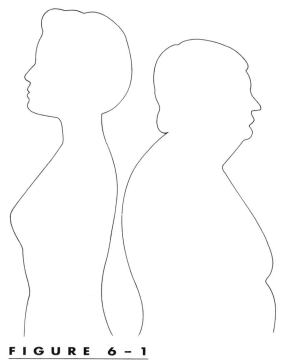

FIGURE 6 – 1

How stature and posture alter with aging. (Illustration by Larue Coats.)

structure occur in bone tissue with older age.

Skeletal bone is made up of three major components, *organic matrix, minerals,* and *cells.* The organic matrix predominantly is composed of collagen fibers. These fibers are responsible for providing the bone's great tensile strength. The mineral component, deposits of calcium and phosphate, further strengthens the organic matrix. Calcium, phosphorus, alkaline phosphatase, and the proper pH must be present for bone mineralization to occur. The cellular component of bone tissue is made up of cells called *osteoblasts, osteocytes,* and *osteoclasts.* Osteoblasts synthesize bone collagen, which makes up the organic matrix, forming new bone tissue. As the osteoblasts synthesize new bone tissue, they become imbedded into the organic matrix and are then known as osteocytes. Osteoclasts promote bone tissue absorption or destruction. All bones have a compact outer shell called the *cortex.* The cortex surrounds the spongy bone-containing sheets of tissue termed *trabeculae.* Cortical bone is chiefly responsible for providing support, whereas trabecular bone provides sites for bone formation and hemopoiesis.

Bone tissue is continuously undergoing change, or *remodeling,* even into older age. Various mechanical and hormonal mechanisms stimulate bone formation and absorption, such as stress, serum levels of vitamin D, parathyroid hormone, and calcium (Francis, 1992). Bone formation and absorption are dynamic processes that occur simultaneously; however, the rate of activity in each process changes with age. From birth to adolescence, bone formation exceeds bone absorption and then equalizes into the mid- to late twenties. Beginning around age 30, bone absorption begins to exceed bone formation, particularly in trabecular bone. The amount of trabecular bone shows a linear decrease beginning in the early thirties and into older age (Fig. 6–2). Men lose 27 per cent of trabecular bone by age 80; women lose 43 per cent by age 90, with a sharp increase occurring immediately after menopause. Cortical bone loss does not begin until age 45 in women and age 50 in men. Not only does cortical bone loss begin earlier in women, but it also occurs at a faster rate than in men (Riggs and Melton, 1986; Francis, 1990; Miller, 1990).

Because loss of trabecular bone begins earlier than cortical bone loss, the ratio of cortical bone to trabecular bone increases with age. At age 15, the average cortical-trabecular bone ratio is 55 to 45; by age 85, it is 70 to 30 (Fig. 6–3). The areas of the skeleton

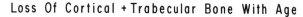

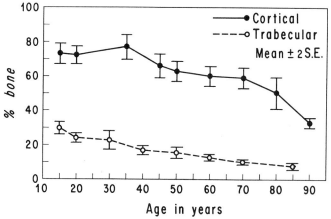

FIGURE 6 – 2

The relative decrease in cortical and trabecular bone with age in apparently normal persons. Note the relatively rapid loss early in life in trabecular bone and comparatively little loss at this age in cortical bone. The situation is reversed after age 35. (From Jowsey, J. *Metabolic Diseases of Bone.* Philadelphia: W.B. Saunders, 1977, p. 43.)

containing the largest amount of trabecular bone are the vertebral bodies, the wrist, and the hip. Because these areas have the highest rate of bone loss with aging, older persons are at risk for sustaining vertebral body compression fractures, Colles' fractures, and femoral neck fractures (Wilmore, 1991; Specht, 1990) (Fig. 6–4).

To understand the changes occurring in bone structure and function with aging, it is helpful to review the interactions among parathyroid hormone, calcium, and vitamin D in relation to bone tissue metabolism. A primary metabolic function of bone tissue is

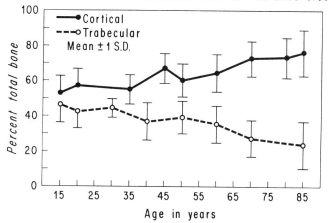

FIGURE 6 – 3

Changes in the proportion of cortical and trabecular bone with age. (From Jowsey, J. *Metabolic Diseases of Bone.* Philadelphia: W.B. Saunders, 1977, p. 44.)

Fracture Rate In Females In Relation To Age

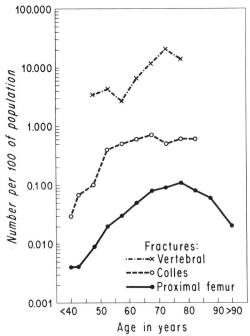

FIGURE 6 – 4

The fracture rate in females in relation to age. Vertebral fractures appear early and are more frequent than either Colles or femoral fractures. (From Jowsey, J. *Metabolic Diseases of Bone.* Philadelphia: W.B. Saunders, 1977, p. 258.)

to maintain calcium homeostasis in the body. Bone tissue provides a storage depot for calcium, and when serum calcium levels fall below normal, a mechanism stimulates release of parathyroid hormone into the bloodstream. Parathyroid hormone in turn stimulates release of calcium from bone tissue into the bloodstream. When serum calcium levels are above normal, calcitonin is released from the thyroid to negate the effect of parathyroid hormone and to promote calcium storage in the bone. Parathyroid hormone, along with vitamin D metabolites, also promotes absorption of dietary calcium intake through the intestinal tract, and it promotes calcium reabsorption from the kidneys. Decreased absorption through the gut has been noted with older age. This phenomenon has been attributed to either a decreased intake of dietary calcium or a decreased proficiency in calcium absorption (Kraenzlin et al., 1990).

Musculature

Changes in Muscle Mass and Structure of Muscle Fibers

A decrease in lean body mass is related to changes in muscle composition and function. Muscle wasting occurs as a result of a de-crease in the number of muscle fibers and general atrophy of organs and tissues. Muscle contours become more prominent as a result of the variable nature of the fiber atrophy. In addition, significant amounts of lipofuscin (age-related waste material) and fat are deposited within the muscle tissue. The density of capillaries per motor unit diminishes; however, oxygen utilization per unit of muscle tissue remains constant.

Regeneration of muscle tissue slows with age, and atrophied tissue is replaced with fibrous tissue. This phenomenon is most noticeable in the muscles of the hands, which become thin and bony, with deep interosseous spaces. The arm and leg muscles also become thin and flabby. Some writers claim that the weakness associated with aging is directly related to muscle atrophy, whereas others state that the degree of wasting is not directly associated with the degree of weakness. However, most studies agree that muscle wasting and diminution of lean body mass are significantly associated with age, race, and sex, chiefly affecting older males of Asian origin (Wilmore, 1991; Hyatt et al., 1990; Grob, 1989a).

Changes in Muscle Function

VOLUNTARY MOVEMENT. Movement slows with older age as a result of changes in both the musculoskeletal and the nervous systems. Slower, more sluggish movement is attributed to a prolongation of the contraction time, latency period, and relaxation period of the motor units in the muscle tissue. Impairment of the extrapyramidal nervous system can also cause slow movements and a decrease in spontaneous and associated movements. The older person also may have an impaired postural system that is slow to stabilize the body before movement is initiated (Woollacott and Manchester, 1993; Merletti et al., 1992; Hicks et al., 1992; Stelmach et al., 1990).

Joints such as the hips, knees, elbows, wrists, neck, and vertebrae become mildly flexed with older age. The increased flexion is caused by changes in the vertebral column, ankylosis (stiffening) of the ligaments and joints, shrinkage and sclerosis (hardening) of the tendons and muscles, and degenerative changes in the extrapyramidal system. Limited movement results from increased muscle rigidity, especially in the neck, shoulders, hips, and knees. The degree of muscle rigidity can be assessed by measuring the amount of resistance to passive movement (Lewis, 1984).

INVOLUNTARY MOVEMENT. Examples of involuntary movements associated with aging are *resting tremors* and *muscular fasciculations.* Resting tremors are manifestations of an impaired extrapyramidal system. Involuntary movements may appear in the extremities or head and neck when an older person is sitting quietly. There may be no obvious cause for these tremors, or they may be associated with drug side effects (especially from psychotropic medications) or neurological disorders. Muscular fasciculations are characterized as flickering movements of muscles in the calves, eyelids, hands, and feet. Fatigue and excessive loss of sodium chloride may exacerbate this phenomenon, but loss of muscle strength and function is the primary cause.

Older persons who are inactive or relatively immobile may experience weakness or paresthesia in the legs as a result of decreased movement. "Restless legs," a phenomenon in which the legs are kept in motion to avoid the discomfort associated with paresthesia, most likely produce unconscious rather than involuntary movements. Restless legs are sometimes related to conditions such as diabetes mellitus, spondylosis, hypoglycemia, hypocalcemia, or alkalosis (hyperventilation) (Grob, 1989a).

STRENGTH AND ENDURANCE. A combination of neural and motor changes alters the strength and endurance of many older people. The decrease in the size and/or number of muscle fibers, particularly type II muscle fibers, results in a reduction in isometric strength, especially in the proximal lower extremities; the back and upper limbs, including hand grip, appear to retain much of their strength, however (Larsson, 1982; Bassey and Harries, 1993; Vandervoort et al., 1993; Reed et al., 1991). Although the decline in strength cannot be stopped as people age, it can be retarded with continued exercise (Roman et al., 1993; Nichols et al., 1993; Greig et al., 1993). Additionally, hormone replacement therapy has been found to increase muscle strength in perimenopausal or postmenopausal women (Phillips et al., 1993).

The decline in muscle mass may parallel the decline in muscle strength, but it does not appear to affect endurance. In fact, endurance may be enhanced in older age (corrected for strength and the capabilities of the cardiopulmonary system) because the type I muscle fibers that affect endurance do not atrophy with age. On the other hand, high-speed performance, which is affected by type II muscle fibers, tends to decline. Therefore, aging athletes with good cardiopulmonary reserve are better able to compete in events that stress endurance rather than bursts of speed (Rogers and Evans,

1993; Sjostrom et al., 1992; Frontera et al., 1991; Laforest et al., 1990).

REFLEXES. Diminished reflexes usually result from the shrinkage and sclerosis of muscles and tendons rather than from changes in the spinal reflex arc. Diminution of tendon jerks, especially in the ankles, may occur, or reflexes may be completely absent. In addition, arm, abdominal, and plantar reflex responses tend to decrease. However, although decreased *flexor* responses are considered a normal phenomenon with aging, an increased *extensor* response (e.g., a positive Babinski response) is still considered abnormal (Grob, 1989a; Carter, 1986).

Joints

Joints, the sites in the body where two or more bones meet, provide motion and flexibility for the human frame. The *freely movable joint* is made up of bones, synovial membrane, cartilage, synovial cavity, tendons, and ligaments (Fig. 6–5). Examples of freely movable joints are elbows, knees, and wrists. Note that the bones are not in direct contact with each other but are protected by articular cartilage, which forms a cushion between the bony surfaces. The synovial membrane, attached at the margins of the articular cartilage, is pouched or folded to allow for joint movement. The membrane surrounds the synovial cavity and secretes synovial fluid (viscous lubricating fluid) into it. The synovial membrane is surrounded by a fibrous joint capsule, which is strength-

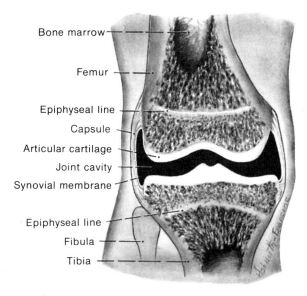

Bone marrow
Femur
Epiphyseal line
Capsule
Articular cartilage
Joint cavity
Synovial membrane
Epiphyseal line
Fibula
Tibia

F I G U R E   6 – 5

Frontal section through the right knee joint. (From Jacob, S.W., and Francone, C.A. *Elements of Anatomy and Physiology.* 2nd ed. Philadelphia: W.B. Saunders, 1989, p. 66.)

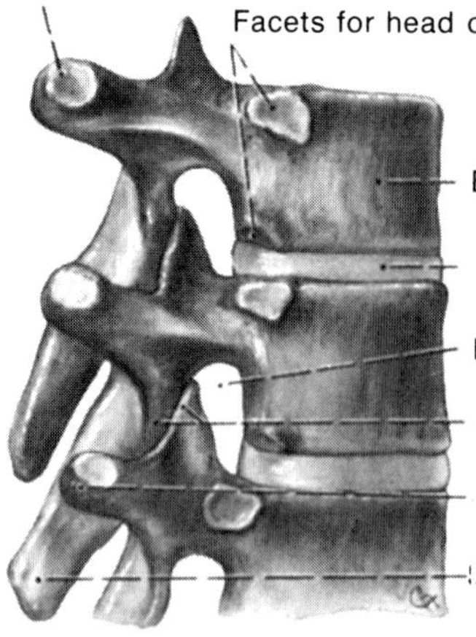

Facet for tubercle of rib

Facets for head of ribs

Body

Intervertebral disc

Intervertebral foramen

Articular processes

Transverse process

Spinous process

FIGURE 6 – 6

Slightly movable joint structure, or a gliding joint, showing articulations between vertebrae. (From Jacob, S.W., Francone, C.A. and Lossow, W.J. *Structure and Function in Man.* 5th ed. Philadelphia: W.B. Saunders, 1982, p. 155.)

ened by ligaments extending from bone to bone. Bursae are disc-shaped, fluid-filled synovial sacs that develop at points of friction around the joints. Their purpose is to decrease friction and to promote ease of motion.

Slightly movable joints are found between the vertebral bodies. They are separated by fibrocartilaginous discs that contain the nucleus pulposa, a fibrogelatinous material that cushions the movements between the vertebrae (Fig. 6–6).

All of these articulating joint surfaces are subject to changes in structure and function with aging. Breakdown of components of the joint capsule results in inflammation, pain, stiffness, and deformity. Arthritis and "rheumatism" are the major causes of structural and functional changes, and almost all older people are affected by these problems in some way (Gardner, 1992). Rainy day predictions are abundant in elderly arthritis sufferers, who frequently dread the discomfort associated with "Mr. Arthur's" visits.

COMMON DISORDERS OF THE AGING MUSCULOSKELETAL SYSTEM

Metabolic Bone Disease

Osteoporosis

Osteoporosis is so ubiquitous in older age that it is generally considered a normal, age-related phenomenon rather than a disease. It is characterized by a decrease in bone mass per unit volume, producing a "porous"-looking skeletal frame that fractures easily when stressed. Senile osteoporosis results from an imbalance in the activity of osteoblasts and osteoclasts, resulting in net loss of bone because more bone is absorbed than is formed (Groessner-Schreiber et al., 1992; Giansiracuso and Kantrowitz, 1982).

Progressive bone loss begins around age 20 but becomes symptomatic only at around age 45 in women and 55 in men. The condition occurs four times more frequently in women than in men, and more often in whites and Northern Europeans. Women also suffer bone loss at a faster rate than men. The difference in incidence among sexes and races is thought to be due to the varying amounts of skeletal bone mass at maturity; men and blacks tend to have a denser bone mass than women and whites. The density of bone mass at maturity seems to be of greater importance in predicting the occurrence of osteoporosis than are genetic, dietary, or environmental influences (Vaananen, 1991; Chesnut, 1990).

TABLE 6 – 1

Risk Factors for Osteoporosis

UNCHANGEABLE	CHANGEABLE
Female	Smoking
Caucasian, Asian	Sedentary life style
Small body structure	Low-calcium diet
Light hair, complexion, eyes	High intake of caffeine, alcohol, protein, phosphorus
Family history of osteoporosis	Estrogen deficiency (surgical oophorectomy, early menopause)
Medical history of:	Excessive exercise (producing secondary amenorrhea)
Rheumatoid arthritis	
Liver disease	
Thyroid problems	
Epilepsy	
Alcoholism	
Anorexia nervosa	
Scoliosis	
Previous bone loss:	
Immobilization	
Hyperparathyroidism	
Malabsorption	
Steroid use: 1 year or more	
Previous osteoporotic fractures (spine, hip, wrist)	
Absence of menstrual cycle for more than 1 year (excluding menopause)	
Menopause before age 40 (without hormonal replacement therapy)	

From Maher, A.B., Salmond, S.W., and Pellino, T.A. *Orthopaedic Nursing.* Philadelphia: W.B. Saunders, 1994, p. 470.

Height

5'6"

5'3"

5'

4'9"

4'6"

4'3"

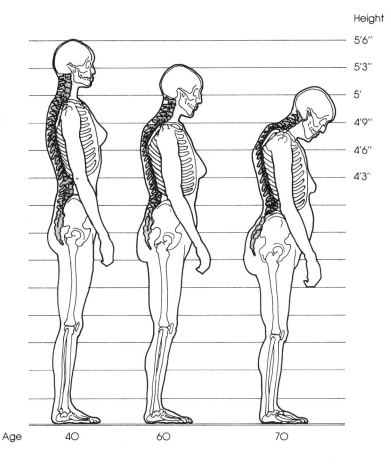

Age   40   60   70

FIGURE 6 – 7

Normal spine at age 40 years and osteoporotic changes at ages 60 and 70. These changes can cause a loss of as much as 6 to 9 inches in height and can result in the so-called dowager's hump *(far right)* in the upper thoracic vertebrae. (Ignatavicius, D.D., Workman, M.L. and Michler, M.A. *Medical-Surgical Nursing: A Nursing Process Approach.* 2nd ed. Philadelphia: W.B. Saunders, 1995, p. 1414.)

The cause of osteoporosis is unknown, but the condition is strongly related to estrogen deficiencies and low serum calcium levels (Table 6–1). Other causes of bone loss are menopause, low body weight, smoking, excessive alcohol consumption, physical inactivity, and nutritional factors (Francis, 1992; Bauer et al., 1993). Riggs et al. (1982) identified two syndromes: type I or *postmenopausal* osteoporosis and type II or *senile* osteoporosis. Postmenopausal osteoporosis affects mainly the trabeculae of the vertebral column in a certain group of women during the early postmenopausal period. This condition seems to be associated with vertebral fractures. Senile osteoporosis affects both trabecular and cortical bone of the vertebrae and articulating bones of the hip in all aging persons. Bone absorption takes place primarily in the trabeculae rather than in the cortex because remodeling occurs at a higher rate in trabecular bone than in cortical bone. Senile osteoporosis seems to be associated with hip fractures, vertebral fractures, or both (Luckerman, 1990).

Major signs and symptoms of osteoporosis are skeletal deformities due to vertebral fractures and pain in the spinal column related to the fractures. Fractures occur when the anterior vertebral bodies become stressed during flexion of the spine and break easily as a result of the loss of the supporting trabecular matrix. Vertebral fractures, called *wedge fractures*, produce acute episodes of sharp pain. They are usually associated with sudden lifting, bending, or falls. The most common sites are the lower thoracic (T12) or upper lumbar (L1) regions, which produce radiating pain around the flank and the abdomen. Collapse of the vertebral body may also be gradual and is accompanied by aching spinal pain or tenderness on percussion and palpation (Lifschitz and Harmon, 1982; Spencer et al., 1986).

Spinal osteoporosis produces changes in height and posture with advancing years (Fig. 6–7). Collapse fractures occurring in the upper thoracic vertebrae may be asymptomatic, but height may diminish by 1 to $1\frac{1}{2}$ inches. Painful collapse of the vertebrae of the lower spine can reduce height by 2 to $2\frac{1}{2}$ inches per episode. *Kyphosis* in the upper dorsal spine produces a "hunchback" or "dowager's hump" and, together with downward angulation of the ribs, produces horizontal folds of skin over the chest and abdomen (Barzel, 1989).

The extremities are also increasingly susceptible to fracture, especially the wrist and the hip. Women older than 45 years of age experience more than one million hip fractures per year. The mean age is 75 years, and 40 per cent of all white women will have experienced hip fractures by 80 to 90 years of age (Alvioli, 1982). As with vertebral fractures, hip fractures occur as a result of decreased resistance to stress and loss of bone mass. Older women tend to fall more frequently as a result of decreased muscle strength, poor coordination, syncopal episodes, and cardiovascular disease. In addition, reduced bone turnover and poor repair of microfractures contribute to the high incidence of fractures. Fracture of one hip appears to signal the likelihood of fractures of the other (Gilmore, 1980; Haberman, 1986).

Aging increases the risk of mortality associated with hip fracture, and the incidence doubles every 5 years after age 50. Estimates of death in the year after hip fracture range from 12 to 30 per cent (Kane et al., 1994; Ochs, 1990). In some cases, the possibility of femoral neck fracture is overlooked in elderly persons who have sustained falls because they are sometimes able to walk after the fracture has occurred. The pain associated with the fracture may also go unnoticed if other injuries are associated with the trauma. Increased pain or "failure to thrive" after the injury may indicate an undiagnosed fractured hip. Thorough follow-up is imperative (Gordon, 1989).

Diagnosis of osteoporosis is made chiefly through the history and the exclusion of other diseases or secondary causes. Secondary causes include hyperparathyroidism, hyperthyroidism, acromegaly, Cushing's disease, diminished physical activity, paralysis, alcoholism, nutritional deficiencies (calcium, vitamin D, phosphate), neoplastic disorders, and renal tubular acidosis. Results of blood tests are normal, including serum calcium, phosphorus, and alkaline phosphatase levels. Another diagnostic measure is made through bone biopsy of the iliac crest; bone turnover is assessed by means of tetracycline labeling. X-ray studies may reveal vertebral compression fractures and a decrease in bone density; however, there must be a 30 to 50 per cent loss of bone mass before bone loss shows up on the radiograph. When a significant loss of bone mass appears on the radiograph, the condition is known as *osteopenia.* This phenomenon may not occur until late in the process of the disease or condition (Nordin, 1983).

Goals for the prevention and treatment of osteoporosis or osteopenia are to inhibit bone resorption and to stimulate bone formation. Clients are encouraged to exercise by either walking or swimming to slow bone loss. Exercise can reduce fracture risk not only by preventing bone loss but also by decreasing the risk of falling and the force of impact by improving strength, flexibility, balance, and reaction time (Smith and Gilligan, 1991). They are also encouraged to avoid strain on the spine, such as occurs with lifting or bending, to prevent compression fractures of the vertebrae. Calcium supplements of 1000 mg per day have had a beneficial effect on bone loss in normal postmenopausal women. Additionally, estrogen replacement can prevent the loss of bone mass after menopause (Ciammella et al., 1993; Palferman, 1993; Balfour and McTavish, 1992; Doren and Schneider, 1992; Reid et al., 1993; Marx et al., 1992).

Osteomalacia

Osteomalacia is defined as a softening of the bones with an excessive accumulation of bone matrix (osteoid) resulting from impaired mineralization of calcium and phosphorus, the major minerals of bone tissue (Francis, 1992). This condition is usually caused by vitamin D deficiencies and is far less common than osteoporosis. Osteomalacia is similar to rickets in children, differing only in the involvement of epiphyseal cartilage (the area where bone growth takes place). In childhood rickets, epiphyseal cartilage is affected, whereas in older adults, only bone matrix is affected because bone growth has ceased.

Vitamin D deficiency in the elderly is most frequently due to malabsorption from the gastrointestinal tract. Dietary deficiencies are rare, but occasionally older persons may have insufficient incomes to provide for an adequate nutritional intake. Housebound elderly may also suffer from vitamin D deficiencies as a result of lack of sunshine. Because vitamin D is stored in the body, deficiencies often do not appear until some time after the stores are depleted.

Vitamin D has two major effects: promotion of calcium absorption through the small bowel and mineralization of bone. A deficiency of vitamin D causes a 20 to 25 per cent decrease in absorption of ingested calcium, which in turn causes a decrease in serum calcium levels. Lowered serum calcium levels trigger release of parathyroid hormone, which not only causes release of calcium from bone tissue but also promotes reabsorption from the renal tubules. Thus,

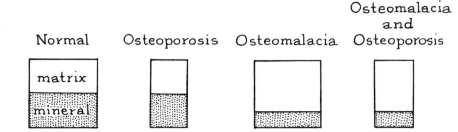

FIGURE 6 - 8

Proportions of unmineralized matrix and mineralized bone in the normal bone and the major groups of metabolic bone disease. (From Rose, C. and Clawson, D.K. *Introduction to the Musculoskeletal System.* New York: Harper & Row, 1970, p. 118.)

there is a decrease in urinary calcium excretion and an increase in serum retention. In addition, parathyroid hormone promotes excretion of phosphorus from the kidneys, resulting in a decreased level of phosphorus in the bloodstream. Eventually, parathyroid hormone is unable to keep up with the fall in serum calcium, so calcium levels also drop. Therefore, in osteomalacia, *serum calcium* and *phosphorus* levels are low as opposed to the normal levels found in osteoporosis. Conversely, the *serum alkaline phosphatase* level is elevated in osteomalacia, for reasons that are not clear; however, this enzyme does originate in the bone and intestinal tract.

Vitamin D is directly responsible for mineralization of bone. When vitamin D is deficient, the onset of mineralization is delayed, leading to an increase in the amount of osteoid (bone matrix). This phenomenon occurs because initiation of mineralization proceeds more slowly than osteoid formation. Therefore, there is an increased amount of *unmineralized matrix* with osteomalacia. Figure 6–8 shows the proportions of unmineralized matrix and mineralized bone in osteoporosis, osteomalacia, and the two conditions together. Note that the level of mineralized bone in osteoporosis is normal, but it is lower in the other two conditions (Rosse and Clawson, 1970; Corless, 1981).

Diagnosis of osteomalacia is made through observation of histological serum, and radiographic changes. Histologically, bone tissues show excessive amounts of osteoid and increased bone resorption. Blood studies reveal decreased amounts of calcium and phosphorus and increased levels of alkaline phosphatase, as previously noted. Radiographs may show decreased bone density as a result of osteoporosis, which frequently accompanies osteomalacia and excessive amounts of unmineralized matrix.

Persons with osteomalacia usually experience vague symptoms of pain, tenderness, and weakness. Pain and tenderness occur in skeletal areas, especially the shoulder bones, thorax, hips, thighs, forearms, and feet. It is aggravated by exercise and active movement. Hip pain may result in an ataxic, waddling gait. Muscle weakness usually occurs proximally and may be mistaken for muscle disorders (Table 6–2).

Treatment generally consists of dietary supplements of calcium and vitamin D. Clients are encouraged to eat foods high in vitamin D content, especially oily fish and margarine, and 800 mg daily of calcium, which is found chiefly in dairy products (Baylink, 1990).

Paget's Disease

Paget's disease, described by Sir James Paget in 1877, is a condition associated with older age in which there is excessive resorption and deposition of bone. It occurs primarily in men older than 40 years, and studies have shown that 1 to 3 per cent of the population older than 50 years are affected (Singer, 1990). The cause of the disease is unknown, but recent thinking favors a virus (Hughes et al., 1992). The disease is characterized by periods of increased bone resorption, which result in replacement of original bone with fibrous material, alternating with periods of increased bone formation, which result in the appearance of "sclerotic" or osteoblastic lesions. The condition is widespread rather than localized to one area and usually involves the sacrum, the lumbar ver-

TABLE 6 - 2

Possible Clinical Signs of Late-Onset Osteomalacia

- Bone pain and tenderness
- Muscle weakness
- Difficulty in walking
- Skeletal deformity

From Alvioli, L.V. and Krane, S.M. *Metabolic Bone Disease and Clinically Related Disorders.* Philadelphia: W.B. Saunders, 1990, pp. 341–342.

tebrae, the skull, the femur, and the pelvis (Singer, 1990).

The most common symptom of Paget's disease is bone pain, although 20 per cent of the victims are asymptomatic. The pain frequently occurs at rest, under pressure, and during the night and is relieved by movement, unlike pain from arthritis, which may occur with movement during the day and is relieved by rest. Disease involving the weight-bearing bones produces the most severe symptoms. When the skull is involved, symptoms may include headaches, intermittent tinnitus and vertigo, and sensorineural hearing loss. In the later stages of the disease, skeletal deformities are common. The most common reason for hospitalization is fracture of the femur, hip, or pelvis (Merkow and Lane, 1990; Singer, 1990).

The diagnosis is usually made through findings on x-ray studies that have been taken for other purposes. Laboratory findings show normal serum calcium and phosphorus levels, but there is an increased serum phosphatase level that is relative to the extent and the activity of the disease (Ouslander and Beck, 1982; Wallach, 1986; Arend et al., 1990). Treatment is symptomatic rather than curative. Calcitonin is the drug of choice for long-term therapy; aspirin and mithramycin may also be given to relieve bone pain and to decrease serum alkaline phosphatase levels (Spencer et al., 1986; Wimalawansa, 1993). Recent studies have found nitrogen-containing bisphosphonates (diphosphonates), such as Tiludronate (chloro-4-phenyl thiomethylene biphosphonate) and dimethyl-aminohydroxypropylidene diphosphonate, to be effective for remission of Paget's disease (Price et al., 1993; Schweitzer et al., 1993; Reginster et al., 1993; Reginster et al., 1992; Ryan et al., 1992).

Muscular Disorders

Polymyalgia Rheumatica and Giant Cell Arteritis

Polymyalgia rheumatica (PMR) and giant cell arteritis (GCA) are two disorders that are closely related and frequently seen together, usually in people over 35 years of age. PMR is a rheumatic disease characterized by diffuse muscular stiffness lasting for 1 month or more. GCA is a condition that involves medium-sized arteries, particularly those branching off the ascending aorta. The disease is characterized by inflammation of the temporal artery, resulting in a

T A B L E   6 – 3
Criteria for Diagnosis of Polymyalgia Rheumatica

1. Age greater than 50 years
2. Shoulder girdle and/or pelvic girdle symptoms of pain and/or stiffness
3. Morning stiffness of > 1 hour's duration
4. Duration of symptoms of at least 4 weeks if untreated
5. No actual muscle weakness found on objective examination
6. No evidence of intrinsic muscle disease, infection, or other collagen-vascular disease
7. Elevated erythrocyte sedimentation rate
8. Relief of symptoms within several days of initiating low-dose corticosteroid therapy

Adapted from Goodwin, J.S. Progress in gerontology: Polymyalgia rheumatica and temporal arteritis. *J Am Geriatr Soc 40*, 1992, p. 516.

unilateral headache, local tenderness, and diminution of the temporal artery pulse. In many cases, people with biopsy-proven GCA present only with symptoms of PMR (Arnold, 1990).

The cause of PMR is unknown, but the onset is frequently initiated by a virus-like illness, consisting of fever and weight loss, usually of less than 2 weeks' duration. Afterward, muscle pain (myalgia) begins in the posterior neck muscles and spreads to the muscles of the shoulders and pelvic girdle. The onset may be either insidious or abrupt. The pain initially may be unilateral but later becomes symmetrical. It may interfere with sleep and is aggravated by exercise. Morning stiffness may last for at least an hour, and the resulting weakness can make getting out of bed or a chair difficult (Table 6–3). Accompanying symptoms are low-grade fever, anorexia, weight loss, depression, malaise, and apathy. Individuals often exhibit tenderness on palpation of the posterior neck, shoulder, and pelvic musculature, and over the flexor surfaces of the elbows, wrists, and knees. Muscle atrophy and joint deformities characteristic of rheumatoid arthritis are absent (Calkins et al., 1986; Giansiracuso and Kantrowitz, 1982).

Initial symptoms of GCA frequently are the same as those of PMR; however, people may also present with a temporal headache that is described as throbbing. The headache is usually unilateral and is accompanied by fever and visual symptoms, such as partial or complete blindness. When an individual presents with symptoms of PMR and symptoms of headache, fever, and visual disturbances, the underlying presence of GCA is suspected. GCA also may cause claudication of the muscles of mastication and a painful burning tongue (Friedlander and Runyon, 1990; Arnold, 1990; Healey, 1990). No specific diagnostic test for PMR or GCA exists; however, an elevated erythrocyte sedimentation rate is present in both diseases (Kyle, 1991a). A biopsy of the temporal arteries should be performed when clinical symptoms of GCA are present (Kaiser, 1993). Administration of prednisone in a single daily dose of 10 to 30 mg or prednisolone, 10 mg for therapeutic purposes, produces such a dramatic clinical improvement that this is thought to be diagnostic of the disease. It is usually necessary to give higher doses (45 to 60 mg per day) of prednisone to patients with GSA (Arnold, 1990; Kyle, 1991b). If a good clinical response is obtained, the drug is used for many months while the dosage is tapered off. Older patients should be monitored for steroid side effects, which include fluid retention, dyspepsia, and spinal osteoporosis leading to vertebral collapse (Bird, 1983; Calkins et al., 1986).

Muscle Cramps

Older people frequently experience muscle cramps after unusual exercise. The cramps occur at night after a day's activity and are characterized by sustained, involuntary, and painful contractions of muscle groups of the calf, foot, thigh, hand, or hip. They result primarily from peripheral vascular insufficiency but may also be related to sodium deprivation or loss, decrease in plasma calcium concentration, toxins, hypoglycemia, or peripheral nerve disease. The pain may be relieved by passive stretch and can often be prevented by soaking in a hot bath at bedtime (Grob, 1989a). Studies on the use of quinine therapy for nocturnal leg cramps have had conflicting results (Fung and Holbrook, 1989; Sidorov, 1993).

Joint Diseases

Osteoarthritis

Osteoarthritis, also known as *hypertrophic arthritis, senescent arthritis, osteoarthrosis,* and *degenerative joint disease,* is a noninflammatory disorder of movable joints. It is characterized by deterioration of articular cartilage and subsequent formation of new bone at the joint surfaces. Degeneration of articular cartilage begins at the age of 20 to 30 and is thought to be a normal response to aging. Although more than 90 per cent of the population are affected by the age of 40, few

people experience symptoms until after the age of 60.

Cartilage is a connective tissue that contains large amounts of collagen fiber and has little or no vascular or nerve supply. Its high water content and the gel-like consistency of its matrix enable it to withstand the forces exerted on the joint during normal function. Cartilage deterioration that occurs with aging generally is a result of accumulated trauma. Initially, cartilage loses its elasticity and becomes dull and opaque; later, it becomes soft and frayed. Loss of water from the cartilage may cause narrowing of the joint spaces. Continuous abrasion results in a progressive loss of cartilaginous surface, leaving the underlying (subchondral) bone exposed. Ulceration of the cartilage and exposure of subchondral bone promote new bone formation and thickening of the cortical bone. *Osteophytes,* or bony spurs, form at the joint margins, and *subchondral cysts* frequently develop (Fig. 6–9). Small pieces of cartilage may break off, resulting in loose bodies in the joint. The synovial membrane may become fibrous, hypertrophic, or inflamed as a result of changes in the cartilage, bony spurs, or loose bodies.

Although osteoarthritis is generally asymptomatic in the young, later stages produce symptoms of pain, stiffness, and joint hypertrophy; however, only a small percentage of persons with joint changes have local symptoms. Symptoms are generally related to the specific joints involved, and the only systemic symptoms associated with osteoarthritis are weakness and muscle wasting from immobility. Pain is usually aggravated by joint motion or weight bearing and may increase before changes in the weather. There is tenderness with palpation. Transient episodes of stiffness occur, especially after periods of inactivity. *Crepitation,* a dry, crackling, grating sound or sensation, is a characteristic associated with degenerative joint movement. There may be some limitation of movement as a result of pain, muscle spasm, muscle contracture, malalignment of joints, or osteophyte formation, and abnormalities of posture and gait can produce muscle pain and soreness.

The course of the disease is slow and progressive, without exacerbations or remissions. Predisposing factors include older age, joint injuries or abnormalities, obesity, and familial tendencies toward the disease. Interestingly, researchers have found that habitual physical activity does not increase the risk of knee osteoarthritis in older men and women (Hannan et al., 1993; Lane et al.,

FIGURE   6 – 9

Progression of joint abnormalities in osteoarthritis. (1) Early degenerative changes in cartilages. (2) More extensive cartilage degeneration and early hypertrophic changes of bone at joint edges. (3) Late state with almost complete destruction of articular cartilages, irregular subchondral bone surfaces, underlying eburnated bone, and extensive hypertrophic spur formation at margins of the joint. (From Sodeman, W.A. and Sodeman, W.A., Jr. *Pathologic Physiology: Mechanisms of Disease.* Philadelphia: W.B. Saunders, 1974, p. 426.)

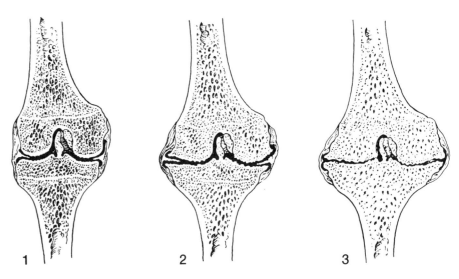

1993; Michel et al., 1992; Panush, 1990; Konradsen et al., 1990; Lane et al., 1990). Major areas affected are the weight-bearing joints (knees, hips, lumbar spine), the cervical spine, and the terminal interphalangeal joints of the hands. Osteoarthritis is rarely found in the wrists, elbows, or feet except after trauma. Joint involvement is unilateral in more than half of all cases, and involvement of one joint does not necessarily precede involvement of the contralateral counterpart (e.g., involvement of the right hip joint does not necessarily indicate future involvement of the left) (Healey, 1990; Hart and Spector, 1993; Slemenda, 1992).

The most frequently affected joint and the major source of disability due to osteoarthritis, particularly in women, is the knee. Cartilage breakdown on the weight-bearing surfaces of the knee joint is usually accompanied by joint enlargement, mild synovitis and effusion, and crepitation on motion. Another disabling site for degenerative joint disease is the hip joint. Risk factors for osteoarthritis of the hip are thought to differ from those of other sites, and osteoarthritis in this area is more likely to be caused by congenital and developmental abnormalities (Felson, 1990b). Degenerative hip disease produces *pain* on motion or weight bearing, which radiates to the groin, buttock, sciatic region, and the middle or inner aspect of the thigh or knee. Limited *motion* of the hip also results, especially abduction, extension, and internal rotation. The leg is often turned outward, accompanied by a flexed and abducted hip. The femoral head may become trapped in the joint capsule. The gait is awkward and shuffling, and sitting or arising from a sitting position is difficult (Grob,

1989b; Cushnagha, and Dieppe, 1991; Healey, 1990; Felson, 1990a).

Degenerative disease of the spine, known as *spondylosis,* is often observed on x-ray studies of middle-aged and older persons. The cervical and lumbar regions of the spine are most frequently involved, producing symptoms such as backache, stiffness, and limitation of motion. The degree of degenerative disease seen on x-ray study is a poor indication of the degree of symptoms manifested in older persons. Some older persons with radiographic evidence of degeneration experience mild symptoms or none at all.

Degeneration of the vertebrae affects primarily the intervertebral discs and the articulating edges of adjacent vertebral bodies. Degeneration of the discs increases the stress on the vertebral bodies, producing osteophyte formation and narrowing of the intervertebral foramina. Osteophyte formation and protrusion of the discs cause compression of the nerve roots or spinal cord in the cervical or lumbar spines in severe cases.

In the cervical spine, the greatest stress is placed on C4 to C6 vertebrae. Because the nerve roots are close to the articulating joints, they are vulnerable to irritation or compression. Persons may experience pain in the shoulders, arms, hands, head, neck, and chest, which is aggravated by active or passive spinal movement, especially rotation and lateral bending. The pain is often accompanied by muscle spasm. Sensory changes, such as burning and numbness, may also occur in relation to the affected nerve root, and may be accompanied by muscle wasting and weakness, decreased tendon reflexes, and occasional fasciculations.

Cervical spondylosis can produce signs of cerebral ischemia, particularly on extension, rotation, or flexion of the neck. This movement causes blockage of the vertebral arteries, which enter at C6 and pass upward through the canal in the transverse processes. The person may exhibit transient episodes of giddiness, syncope, or drop attacks, which are characterized by sudden falling without loss of consciousness. Older persons with this problem should be encouraged to avoid sudden movement of the head and neck to prevent persistent cerebral ischemic lesions.

Vertebral degeneration of the lumbar spine occurs at L5 to S1 in 90 per cent of cases. Prolapse or protrusion of the lumbar intervertebral discs accounts for most low back pain in older persons. The pain is preceded by either an injury from lifting or bending or chronic, intermittent low back pain. Other signs and symptoms include pain in the legs and feet, decreased sensation in the legs and feet, decreased or absent patellar reflex, and weak knee and toe extension. Treatment for vertebral osteoarthritis includes bedrest, analgesics, muscle relaxants, heat, and graded exercises for muscle spasms and for prevention of further injury (Christian, 1982; Grahame, 1992).

Other characteristic signs of osteoarthritis, especially in older women, are *Heberden's nodes*, which are bony protuberances located at the distal interphalangeal joints. Early nodes are soft and cystlike, developing into bony enlargements with angular deformities in which the joints become flexed or displaced laterally (Fig. 6–10). Generally, the nodes are painless, but they may produce local aching, redness, tenderness, clumsiness, and a tight feeling over the area. An inherited trait found chiefly in women, Heberden's nodes are sometimes associated with trauma. Symptoms are limited to the joints in the hand where the nodes occur and are rarely found elsewhere.

Some older persons experience osteoarthritis in the costovertebral joint, located in the area where the intercostal nerve extends from the spine to the rib. The resulting pressure on the intercostal nerves causes pain to be referred to the chest wall or upper abdomen. It is important to keep this phenomenon in mind when assessing an older client for chest pain (Grob, 1989b; Harris, 1993).

Diagnostic tests are generally not definitive in diagnosing osteoarthritis. Results of laboratory studies are usually normal, and radiographs do not always correlate with clinical findings. An older person fre-

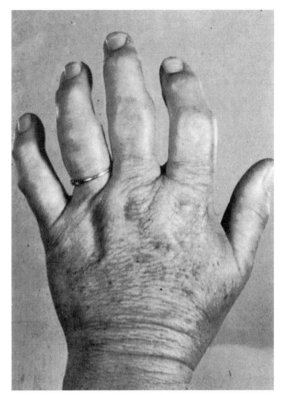

FIGURE 6–10

Hand with Heberden's nodes and deformed joints. (From Schrier, R.W. *Clinical Internal Medicine in the Aged.* Philadelphia: W.B. Saunders, 1982, p. 198.)

quently shows evidence of joint changes on the x-ray study without demonstrating clinical symptoms or may sometimes have clinical symptoms despite a normal x-ray study. However, in a study comparing standard radiography, computed tomography (CT), and magnetic resonance imaging (MRI), MRI was more sensitive in assessing the extent and severity of osteoarthritic changes than either standard radiography or CT (Chan et al., 1991). Changes that can be seen on the x-ray study include joint narrowing, bony sclerosis, osteophytes, and bone cysts (Christian, 1982).

General Treatment Measures

Treatment of osteoarthritis varies according to the anatomical patterns of the disease and the degree of joint deformity. Older persons should be reassured that the disease is not likely to spread or to produce serious disability. Treatment is aimed toward symptomatic relief of pain and prevention of further damage. Therapeutic measures include drugs, rest, weight loss, physical therapy, and surgery (Felson et al., 1992).

DRUG THERAPY. Drugs play a minor

role in the treatment of osteoarthritis and are used principally for pain relief. Drugs of choice are analgesics with anti-inflammatory properties, such as salicylates (aspirin). "Chondroprotective" agents, particularly glutamine sulfate, have recently been used to stop the evolution of the disease as well as for their anti-inflammatory properties. The drugs appear to have few side effects and are suitable for long-term use (Setnikar, 1992; Rovati, 1992). When symptoms become more severe, indomethacin (Indocin), phenylbutazone (Butazolidin), and ibuprofen (Motrin) may be used. It is especially important to observe elderly clients for toxic effects of these drugs, which include nausea and vomiting, epigastric distress, upper gastrointestinal bleeding, rash, edema, anemia, leukopenia, and thrombocytopenia. Because of high-frequency hearing impairment, older persons may be unaware of tinnitus associated with salicylate toxicity; therefore, the nurse should look for other signs or symptoms that indicate overuse, including dizziness, hearing loss without tinnitus, drowsiness or feelings of excitement, and hyperpnea. Many of these drugs produce symptoms associated with senile dementia, such as mental confusion and agitation, in addition to drowsiness, depression, and insomnia (Spencer-Green, 1993). The nurse must be aware of these drug side effects when an acute confusional state or depression occurs in an older person with arthritis.

REST. The use of rest as a therapeutic measure for osteoarthritis is chiefly associated with relief of stress on the affected joints. Work forces and weight bearing should be minimized, and normal joint alignment and motion should be maintained. When there is hip or knee involvement, a sensible modification of strenuous activities is appropriate. People should limit daily activities only as symptoms dictate (Healey, 1990). The use of a cane or crutch can reduce the force of weight bearing by as much as 50 per cent. Obese persons are encouraged to lose weight, especially when the spine and lower extremities are involved. Some periods of rest are recommended, although too much rest can produce stiffness and muscle atrophy. Poor body mechanics associated with faulty work habits can be corrected with proper teaching. Persons with vertebral involvement should avoid hyperflexion and hyperextension, should sleep with a bedboard in a supine position, and should use a cervical collar for immobilization when there is acute pain (Grob, 1989b).

PHYSICAL THERAPY. Although rest is useful for the relief of stress on affected joints, a mild exercise program, particularly isometric exercise or walking, helps to maintain muscle strength and joint motion and to prevent muscle atrophy. Mild exercise, along with dry or moist heat and massage, can provide symptomatic relief of osteoarthritis. Gentle massage over the joints and vigorous massage over the muscles are also effective in preventing atrophy (Allegrante et al., 1993; Peterson et al., 1993; Kovar et al., 1992; Bunning and Materson, 1991; Semble et al., 1990).

SURGERY. When medical treatment and physical therapy fail to relieve symptoms, surgery may be indicated. Severe restriction of joint movement or severe pain in the hip and knees can be relieved by total joint replacement (arthroplasty), often called the "happy operation" because of its high success rate in the relief of pain and immobility. This type of surgery is usually restricted to older adults (older than 65 years) because they are more sedentary and have a shorter life span than younger adults; thus, they are less likely to wear out or damage implants. Total joint replacements are also appropriate for elderly arthritis sufferers because healing time is minimized, providing enough stability to encourage early ambulation with support.

Contraindications for surgery include inadequate medical evaluation and treatment, severe systemic illness (myocardial infarction, bleeding ulcer), infection (in the joint or elsewhere), vascular insufficiency (especially in the lower extremities), poor skin quality, extremely deformed joints, and poor client motivation. Total joint replacement surgery has more than a 95 per cent success rate in older clients. During the immediate postoperative period, it is most important to avoid infections that could spread to the surgical site. Because older persons have a tendency to develop urinary tract infections postoperatively, use of urethral catheters should be avoided if possible. Wound dressings should be changed carefully by use of sterile technique. Clients must also be protected against thromboembolism after arthroplasty and are often given aspirin or warfarin prophylactically. These drugs are contraindicated if there is a history of peptic ulcer.

Older clients are usually hospitalized for 2 to 3 weeks after surgery, or until their general strength has returned, the wound has healed, and they are able to walk with crutches or a walker. Those with hip arthroplasty must avoid full weight bearing for 6 to 12 weeks. Older persons are weaker and more unsteady, and soft tissue healing requires about 6 weeks. Excess activity can

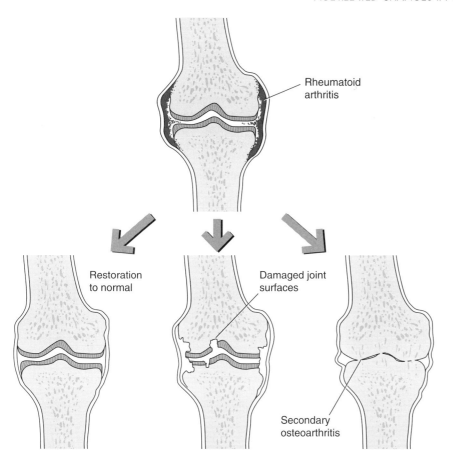

FIGURE 6 – 11
Rheumatoid arthritis, with possible results. (From Adams, J.C. and Hamblen, D.L. *Outline of Orthopaedics*. 11th ed. Edinburgh: Churchill Livingstone, 1990, p. 108.)

cause loosening of the implant, so clients are urged to avoid climbing ladders, lifting, working in the house or yard, and participating in vigorous sports activity. Physical therapy must be carried out not only to teach walking with aids but also to promote muscle strength and joint mobility.

Total joint replacements are used less frequently but with some degree of success for the treatment of arthritis in the shoulders, hands, ankles, and feet. Joint fusions may also be performed when there is extreme pain or deterioration and when a joint is affected unilaterally. Preoperative and postoperative measures and considerations are similar to those associated with total knee and hip replacements (Cracchiolo, 1980; Grahame, 1992; Jerosch and Castro, 1992; Molitor et al., 1991; Cheng et al., 1993).

Rheumatoid Arthritis

Rheumatoid arthritis is a chronic, systemic, progressive disease of unknown origin. The onset of the disease can occur at any age, but it usually begins between the ages of 20 and 60, peaking between 35 and 45. The prevalence of the disease rises with each decade, the largest incidence occurring

after age 60. Women are affected two to three times more frequently than men, and there seems to be a familial tendency toward the disease. Onset is more common in the spring, especially during March. Although the cause is unknown, most scientists be-

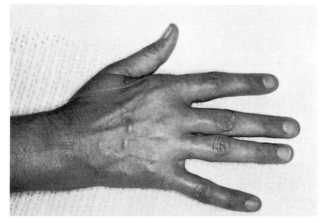

FIGURE 6 – 12
Early rheumatoid arthritic spindling of the fingers. (From Kelley, W.N., Harris, E.D., Jr., Ruddy, S. and Sledge, C.B. *Textbook of Rheumatology*. 2nd ed. Philadelphia: W.B. Saunders, 1985, p. 934.)

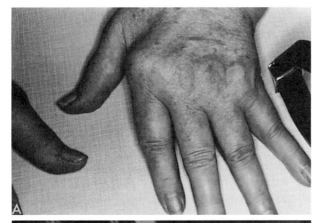

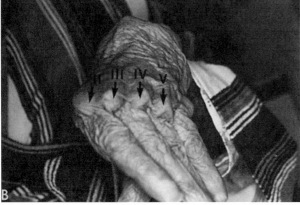

FIGURE   6 – 1 3

A, Early ulnar deviation at the metacarpophalangeal joints without subluxation. *B,* Complete subluxation and marked ulnar deviation in rheumatoid arthritis. (From Kelley, W.N., Harris, E.D., Jr., Ruddy, S. and Sledge, C.B. *Textbook of Rheumatology.* 4th ed. Philadelphia: W.B. Saunders, 1993, p. 889.)

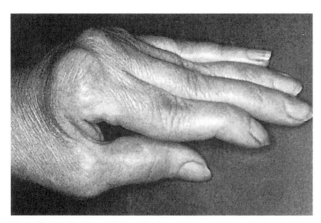

FIGURE   6 – 1 4

Early swan-neck deformity in rheumatoid arthritis. Synovial proliferation and early subluxation of the metacarpophalangeal joints are present as well. (From Kelley, W.N., Harris, E.D., Jr., Ruddy, S. and Sledge, C.B. *Textbook of Rheumatology.* 4th ed. Philadelphia: W.B. Saunders, 1993, p. 890.)

lieve that it is associated with immune (antigen-antibody) factors, called *rheumatoid factors,* in the bloodstream (Healey, 1990; Mannik, 1992). Other speculations on factors that might be involved in triggering the disease are certain types of bacteria, hormonal and reproductive factors in women, low androgen concentrations in men, and genetic factors (Deighton et al., 1993; McCulloch et al., 1993; Bellamy et al., 1992; Spector, 1993).

The disease generally begins with inflammation of the synovial membrane, which later thickens and adheres to the adjacent margins of the articular cartilage. The thickened synovium, or *pannus,* is composed of fibrous tissue containing chronic inflammatory cells. The pannus erodes the cartilage and underlying bone, forming either adhesions between the opposing surfaces of the joint or cysts within the spaces of the bone (Fig. 6–11). Small peripheral joints are usually affected symmetrically, especially the hand, wrist, knee, ankle, elbow, and shoulder. Affected joints in the hands are usually proximal (metacarpophalangeal) rather than distal (distal interphalangeal) as in osteoarthritis (Grob, 1989b).

Systemic involvement in rheumatoid arthritis is characteristic of the disease; the tendon sheaths, bursae, and connective tissues of the heart, lungs, pleura, and arteries are affected. Manifestations of systemic involvement include peripheral neuropathy, leg ulcers, anemia, enlarged spleen, leukopenia, pleuritis, and pericarditis. Rheumatoid nodules, a diagnostic feature of the disease, are subcutaneous masses located over the pressure points of the body, such as the elbows, occiput, sacrum, and heel (Barnes, 1980).

Rheumatoid arthritis is characterized by bony fusion and limited motion of the joints, pain, swelling, and deformity. Initial symptoms include pain and stiffness of involved joints, malaise, and fatigue. Early morning stiffness lasting more than one-half hour is diagnostically significant. Pain or movement may be relieved by rest early in the disease, but later pain may occur spontaneously, even at rest. In the elderly, pain or limitation of movement in the shoulders is more common. Synovitis and synovial effusion produce swelling, warmth, tenderness, edema, and a "boggy" feeling around the joints. A phenomenon called "spindle fingers" results from swelling of the interphalangeal joints (Fig. 6–12). Limited motion is due to synovial effusions, muscle spasms, and contractures. Flexion contractures, which are due to the dominance of flexor muscles, and fibrosis of the joint capsule,

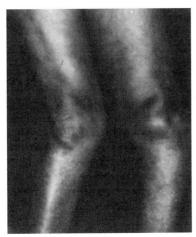

FIGURE 6 – 1 5

Valgus deformity and ligament asymmetry of the knees. (From Kelley, W.N., Harris, E.D., Jr., Ruddy, S. and Sledge, C.B. *Textbook of Rheumatology.* 4th ed. Philadelphia: W.B. Saunders, 1993, p. 1839.)

ligaments, and tendons produce joint deformities of the knees, hips, elbows, and toes. Ulnar deviation of the metacarpophalangeal joints, "swan-neck" deformity, boutonniere (button-hole) deformity, and flexion deformities of the knee are most common (Figs. 6–13 to 6–15) (Gordon et al., 1981; Stevens, 1983).

Laboratory studies show an increase in sedimentation rate and gamma globulin level and the presence of the rheumatoid factor, which occurs in 75 per cent of cases within 2 years after the onset of the disease. Aspirated synovial fluid is inflamed with an increased white blood cell count. X-ray studies show erosion of the articular margins.

The course of the disease is marked by remissions and exacerbations in a downhill, stepwise progression. In younger persons, the disease tends to have a slower, more insidious onset than in older persons. In people older than 60 years, the symptoms are acute, explosive, and widespread; however, the duration is shorter, and there is a greater chance for improvement. In general, the prognosis of the disease is more favorable under the following conditions:

1. Onset in persons older than 40 years
2. Duration of less than 1 year
3. Acute onset
4. Asymmetrical distribution or limited to one joint
5. Absence of rheumatoid nodules or radiographic changes
6. Absent or low titer of rheumatoid factor

Older persons who are males, who have had good joint function, one period of remission, good muscle conditioning, and normal body weight are most likely to have a good prognosis (Giansiracuso and Kantrowitz, 1982). Table 6–4 compares rheumatoid arthritis with osteoarthritis (Hamerman, 1986).

Treatment of older persons with rheuma-

TABLE 6 – 4

Points in Differential Diagnosis of Rheumatoid and Osteoarthritis

	RA	OA
Joints most commonly involved	Proximal interphalangeal Metacarpophalangeal Metatarsophalangeal Knees, hips, wrists, etc. Spine may be involved.	Distal interphalangeal Carpometacarpal of thumb Knee, hip Cervical and lumbar spine
Duration of a.m. stiffness	1 hr to all day	10–30 minutes
Time when pain is most severe	Morning	Evening
Constitutional symptoms	Present	Absent
Tenderness and thickening of synovium	Characteristically present May be severe	May be present May be severe in localized areas (point tenderness)
Synovial fluid	Increased cells Decreased viscosity	Few cells Viscosity normal
X-ray (early changes)	Synovium thickened Erosions at joint margin Subchondral osteoporosis	Cartilage loss Subchondral condensation Osteophytes Cysts

Adapted from Calkins, E., Ford, A.B. and Katz, J.R. *Practice of Geriatrics.* 2nd ed. Philadelphia: W.B. Saunders, 1992, p. 383.

toid arthritis is similar to that of the young: client and family education, psychological support, general rest, local rest (splinting), analgesic and anti-inflammatory medications, physical therapy, occupational therapy, and surgery. Problems with treatment may arise in elderly people who find it difficult to stay ambulatory and remain independent, who have difficulty tolerating supports and braces, or who tolerate drugs poorly (Brewerton, 1979). The aged experience more muscle weakness and atrophy, progressive bone loss, and a greater tendency toward flexion contractures than the young, so judicious use of range-of-motion exercises, isometric exercises for muscle strengthening, and joint splinting is crucial to promote mobility and independence. Although it is important to avoid immobilization in the elderly, rest and splinting are imperative during flare-ups to enhance the action of anti-inflammatory medications and to prevent further damage to the joint. Rest and immobility of inflamed joints actually speed recovery and do not result in permanent loss of joint function as one might assume. Gentle range-of-motion exercises one to two times per day provide enough exercise to maintain function (Sack, 1980a; Sutej and Hadler, 1991; Grob, 1989b).

Drug treatment for all persons with rheumatoid arthritis is aimed toward relief of pain and suppression of inflammation. Because the elderly metabolize drugs differently and because they may have chronic health problems, they are more susceptible to side effects and toxicities of the analgesic and anti-inflammatory agents. The most frequently used drugs for elderly arthritics include the following:

1. Nonsteroidal anti-inflammatory drugs
   Salicylates (aspirin)
   Ibuprofen (Motrin)
   Fenoprofen calcium (Nalfon)
   Naproxen (Naprosyn)
   Sulindac (Clinoril)
   Indomethacin (Indocin)
   Phenylbutazone (Butazolidin)

2. Slow-onset agents
   Anti-malarials (Aralen, Plaquenil)
   D-Penicillamine (Cuprimine)
   Gold sodium thiomalate (Myochrysine)
   Cytotoxic/immunosuppressive agents

3. Corticosteroids

4. Simple analgesics
   Salicylates (aspirin)
   Acetaminophen (Tylenol)
   Codeine

Doses for these drugs are generally lower for older clients, and the goal is to use as few as possible. Major side effects are gastrointestinal disturbances and a potential for gastric ulcer; antacids help to minimize these effects when they are taken concurrently with these drugs (Barnes, 1980; Sack, 1980b).

Several studies have been conducted to evaluate the effectiveness of methotrexate and cyclosporine in the treatment of rheumatoid arthritis. Results have frequently been favorable, but investigators caution about toxic side effects and lack of long-term benefits, especially in older adults (Buchbinder et al., 1993; Walker et al., 1993; Pincus et al., 1992; Alarcon et al., 1992; *Br J Rheumatol*, 1993; Horton et al., 1993; Tishler et al., 1992; Kvien and Husby, 1992).

Gouty Arthritis

Gout is characterized by episodes of acute arthritis, followed by chronic damage to joints and other structures. The disease tends to run in families and is seen primarily in middle-aged men. It is rarely seen before the age of 30, and studies have shown that the highest incidence occurs in the 30s, 40s, and 50s (Villa et al., 1958; Turner et al., 1960; Hall et al., 1967; Grahame and Scott, 1970; Talbott and Yu, 1976).

Hyperuricemia, an excess of uric acid in the blood and tissues, is the major cause of gout. Increased serum uric acid levels are related either to increased formation of uric acid or to decreased excretion of uric acid. Other related factors include sex, age, genetic factors, obesity, higher social class and intelligence, indulgence in alcohol, and high plasma lipid levels. When hyperuricemia is due principally to an inherited metabolic abnormality, the condition is called *primary gout;* when it is due to acquired disease or some environmental factor, it is known as *secondary gout.* Primary gout is seen primarily in men; however, men and women are equally affected by secondary gout (Scott, 1980). Gouty arthritis that begins in older age is associated with a higher incidence in women, a higher likelihood of an underlying blood disorder, and a lower likelihood of inherited and social factors (Grahame, 1992).

An acute attack of gouty arthritis is an inflammatory reaction resulting from the presence of sodium urate crystals within a joint. It most often occurs in the great toe, which is affected in 50 per cent of cases. Acute gout also may appear in other joints, mainly in the periphery, such as the feet and ankles, hands, knees, and elbows. Precipitating factors are loss of body weight, high-fat diet, ingestion of certain drugs (penicillin, thiamine chloride, vitamin B_{12}, insulin, folic acid, sulfa, ergotamine tartrate, and mercurial and thiazide diuretics), joint trauma, emotional turmoil, surgery, or overindulgence in food or alcohol (Scott, 1980; Talbott, 1980).

Each acute episode lasts for a short time and is followed by intervals during which there is freedom from symptoms. Some people have only one or two attacks during their lifetime, whereas others may have repeated occurrences of increasing duration, severity, and frequency, with multiple joint involvement. The affected joint becomes reddened, tender, swollen, and hot (Fig. 6–16). Individuals may have a sensation of discomfort that develops into excruciating pain over a period of hours. Larger joints, such as the knee, may have accumulations of inflammatory effusion. Chalky deposits of urate (tophi) form around joints and areas associated with cartilage, such as the ear (Fig. 6–17); in the elderly, tophi are prone to infection (Scott, 1980; Handy, 1981; Giansiracuso and Kantrowitz, 1982).

Diagnosis is made by means of clinical presentation, serum uric acid levels, identification of uric acid crystals in aspirated synovial fluid, examination of tophi, and radiographs. Serum uric acid levels are elevated

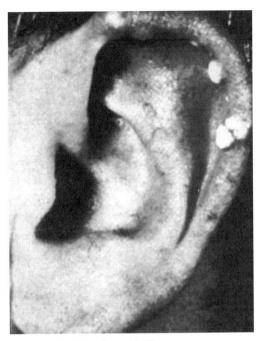

FIGURE 6 – 17

Multiple tophi of the helix. (From Kelley, W.N., Harris, E.D., Jr., Ruddy, S. and Sledge, C.B. *Textbook of Rheumatology.* 2nd ed. Philadelphia: W.B. Saunders, 1985, p. 1362.)

to 8 to 10 mg per 100 ml in gouty arthritis, as opposed to normal levels of 7 mg per 100 ml. Treatment for an initial acute attack is with colchicine, which is 95 per cent effective in providing symptomatic relief. This drug also can provide diagnostic confirmation of the disease. Nonsteroidal anti-inflammatory agents also may be used for the treatment of acute attacks of primary gout, either alone or as an adjunct to colchicine. Allopurinol is the treatment of choice for hyperuricemia in secondary gout; however, it should not be started during an acute flare-up, because allopurinol could make the episode worse (Boyd, 1993; Leong et al., 1992; Vawter and Antonelli, 1992; Levy et al., 1991; Stuart et al., 1991; Edwards, 1991). Prophylactic management usually consists of colchicine, 0.5 mg, and probenemid (Benemid), 0.5 mg every day; weight loss; restriction of foods high in purines (liver, kidney, sweetbreads); and a high fluid intake; however, treatment of asymptomatic hyperuricemia with uric acid–lowering agents is rarely necessary. The drugs must be used judiciously in the elderly because elderly patients tend to experience toxicity and adverse reactions (Scott, 1980; Talbott, 1980;

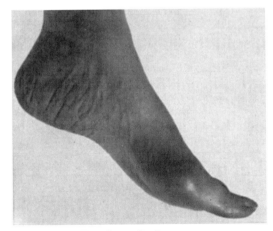

FIGURE 6 – 16

Acute gouty arthritis involving the first metatarsophalangeal joint (great toe) (podagra). (From Wyngaarden, J.B. and Smith, L.H. (eds.). *Cecil Textbook of Medicine.* 17th ed. Philadelphia: W.B. Saunders, 1985, p. 1137.)

Giansiracuso and Kantrowitz, 1982; Levy et al., 1991).

NURSING ASSESSMENT

History

Because musculoskeletal changes often produce profound limitations on mobility and independence in older age, nursing assessment should focus on how these changes influence the functional status of older persons. Information regarding *height and weight at maturity* provides baseline data for measuring changes in stature and posture as well as indications of muscle wasting, obesity, or edema. *Activity and rest patterns,* past and present, should be noted, not only to assess limitations but also to assist in planning for therapeutic interventions. How well a client complies depends on his or her willingness to participate in a therapeutic regimen of rest or activity. An individual who has never exercised or participated in activities may not be willing to begin in later life, especially if the activity is painful or difficult.

Dietary assessment provides information related to musculoskeletal structure and function. A nutritional intake that is low in calcium and vitamin D can adversely affect bone metabolism. Obesity and malnutrition affect mobility, muscle strength, and comfort. The nurse should list all *medications,* including over-the-counter drugs and home remedies. Many arthritis sufferers fall victim to promises of "instant cures" or "miracle drugs," and they may be reluctant to reveal everything they are taking. It is particularly important to note all medications being taken by older clients because these patients are so prone to drug toxicities and side effects.

As noted earlier, an older person's *ability to function in the environment* is crucial to his or her ability to maintain mobility and independence. A checklist of activities of daily living related to independent functioning should include walking, standing, sitting up, lying down, getting out of bed; rising from a sitting position, washing and feeding one's self, and taking care of one's appearance. Several instruments for this assessment are available and are described and/or illustrated in Chapter 2.

Past injuries or illnesses may influence the degree of independent functioning. A hip fracture on the left side may indicate an osteoporotic condition that places an older person at risk for a fracture on the right. A history of *joint pain and stiffness, weakness,* or *fatigue* is frequently associated with the presence of osteoarthritis or rheumatoid arthritis. *Back pain* and *paresthesia* or *numbness* of the lower extremities may be symptoms of vertebral or intervertebral disc degeneration of the lumbar region.

Physical Examination

The first step in examination is to observe the older person's *appearance, stature, and posture.* Observe the client sitting, standing, and walking, and note *body alignment,* gait, and symmetry and flexibility of movement. *Height and weight* provide data that help to determine shortening of the vertebral column, obesity, edema, or severe muscle wasting. Observation of the client's *movement* gives clues to flexibility, agility, and control. Involuntary movements such as tremors, should also be noted and the *range of motion* of all joints should be checked to assess for instability, ankylosis, or contractures. Active range-of-motion movements carried out by the client are assessed for limitations and the ease with which they are performed. Limitations may result from joint deformities or muscle weakness; ease of movement is affected by pain in the muscles or joints. Passive range of motion carried out by the nurse is used to determine resistance to movement, which may indicate joint disorders. *Muscle strength* can be determined during range-of-motion exercises by asking the client to move against the nurse's resistance. Both flexor and extensor muscle groups are assessed for strength in this manner. Progressive muscle weakness is a normal concomitant of older age and should be considered in the assessment for abnormalities.

As stated earlier, *tendon reflexes* diminish or disappear altogether in older age, especially in the distal joint. These should be checked in order to gather baseline data regarding neurological or musculoskeletal deficits. Joints should be inspected and palpated for *swelling, redness, or deformity; crepitation,* or a crackling, grating sensation during movement, should be noted. Swelling, heat, and redness are indicative of rheumatoid arthritis; bony enlargement is indicative of osteoarthritis. Crepitation is produced by grating of the articular cartilages and is indicative of either disorder. Inspection and palpation of the tissues surrounding the joints should be carried out to assess the presence of subcutaneous nodules (Heberden's nodes with osteoarthritis; rheumatoid nodules with rheumatoid arthritis), skin changes (ulceration, discoloration), and mus-

TABLE 6 – 5
Nursing Assessment of the Musculoskeletal System

HISTORY
Height and weight at maturity
Activity and rest patterns
Diet, especially intake of calcium and vitamin D
Medications
Functional status
Environmental aids or barriers
Past history of falls or injuries, especially fractures
Symptoms associated with musculoskeletal problems:
    Pain or stiffness with movement
    Weakness
    Paresthesia
    Numbness
    Muscle cramps, tenderness, or pain
    Joint tenderness
    Fatigue
    Problems with balance
PHYSICAL ASSESSMENT
Height, weight, stature, and posture
Body alignment
Movement (voluntary and involuntary)
Muscle strength and endurance
Reflexes
Joints
    Swelling, redness, deformity, contractures, crepitation
    Condition of surrounding tissues:
        Muscle atrophy
        Subcutaneous nodules
        Skin changes
Use of crutches, walker, cane, prostheses
Evidence of past injuries
    Bruises, burn marks
Activities of daily living
    Walk, stand, sit up, rise from sitting position, lie down, climb, pinch, grasp, lean over
    Comb hair, brush teeth, feed and wash self, cut toenails, turn a page, use a phone and phone book

cle atrophy. The nurse should note whether nodules are firm, soft, movable, or painful. The location of subcutaneous nodules can suggest the type of arthritis present; for example, Heberden's nodes (osteoarthritis) are usually found in the distal interphalangeal joints, and rheumatoid nodules (rheumatoid arthritis) are usually located in pressure point areas (Table 6–5).

NURSING DIAGNOSES
Age-Related Changes in the Musculoskeletal System

1. Activity Intolerance:
   related to weakness, stiffness, and pain secondary to musculoskeletal disorders

2. Pain, Chronic:
   related to musculoskeletal disorders

3. Diversional Activity Deficit:
   related to loss of ability to perform usual or favorite activities secondary to immobility, pain, and weakness

4. Home Maintenance Management, Impaired:
   related to inability to perform household tasks secondary to the effects of musculoskeletal limitations

5. Injury, Risk for:
   related to sensory or motor deficits
   related to lack of awareness of environmental hazards

6. Physical Mobility, Impaired:
   related to musculoskeletal disorders

7. Nutrition Less Than Body Requirements, Altered:
   related to anorexia secondary to chronic pain

8. Self-Care Deficit: Feeding, Bathing/Hygiene, Dressing/Grooming, Toileting:
   related to musculoskeletal disorders

9. Self-Esteem Disturbance:
   related to loss of body function

10. Skin Integrity: Risk for Impaired:
    related to immobility

NURSING INTERVENTIONS AND EVALUATION

Nursing interventions should be aimed toward providing optimal mobility, comfort, and safety. Older clients should be taught the proper use of exercise to promote mobility, muscle strength, and endurance. Exercises can include passive range-of-motion, flexion and stretching movements, walking, swimming, jogging, and aerobics, depending on the level of fitness and functional abilities. Every older person can benefit from some sort of exercise; however, they should avoid fatigue and maintain a proper balance of rest and exercise (see Chapter 14).

Clients must also be aware of proper body mechanics and body alignment to preserve functions and prevent deformity. Assistive and adaptive devices can be provided to promote mobility and independence. Coordination of services also helps older people to live independently in the community by providing support in carrying out activities of daily living. The environment should be modified to enhance safety and independence. Examples are color coding, stair railings, ramps, adequate lighting, and bathroom aids and devices.

Dietary assessment, modification, and teaching may be needed to help older persons lose weight and maintain proper nutrition. The need for calcium and other vitamins and minerals to promote strong bones should be stressed. Discussions about the proper use of medications, their side effects, and their interactions with certain foods are also important nursing interventions.

Effective pain management for those with chronic muscle and joint problems is essential for mobility and well-being. Pain relief is often an individual matter, so many types of interventions or combinations should be tried and evaluated to attain the best results.

Evaluation of outcomes based on nursing diagnoses and goals should also relate to mobility, comfort, and safety. Maintenance of or improvement in movement can be noted through continual reassessment. Adequate pain management may be reflected in a willingness to engage in exercise and activity. Safety in the home can be assessed by means of a home visit and a noticeable decrease in the incidence of falls and injuries.

SUMMARY

Changes and disorders of the musculoskeletal system are associated with altered stature and posture, decreased mobility, injuries, and pain in older age. Normal age-related changes include decreased height, redistribution of lean body mass and subcutaneous fat, increased porosity of bones, muscle atrophy, slowed movement, diminished strength, and stiffening of joints. Common disorders include metabolic diseases, such as osteoporosis, osteomalacia, and Paget's disease; degenerative joint diseases, such as rheumatoid arthritis and osteoarthritis; and muscle disorders, such as polymyalgia rheumatica.

Nursing assessment and interventions are aimed at promoting mobility, comfort, and safety. Clients should be taught to increase their movement and strength through appropriate exercise, relief of pain, and use of necessary aids and adaptive devices. The physical and social environment can be modified to promote safety, mobility, and independence. Evaluation criteria include freedom from injury and improvement or maintenance of function.

REFERENCES

Alarcon, G.S., Lopez-Mendez, A., Walter, J., et al. Radiographic evidence of disease progression in methotrexate treated and nonmethotrexate disease modifying antirheumatic drug treated rheumatoid arthritis patients: A meta-analysis. *J Rheumatol* 19:1868–1873, 1992.

Allegrante, J.P., Kovar, P.A., MacKenzie, C.R., et al. A walking education program for patients with osteoarthritis of the knee: Theory and intervention strategies. *Health Educ Q* 20:63–81, 1993.

Alvioli, L.V. Bone diseases. *In* Wyngaarden, J.B. and Smith, L.H., Jr. (eds.). *Textbook of Medicine.* Philadelphia: W.B. Saunders, 1982, pp. 1318–1353.

Anonymous. An international consensus report: The use of cyclosporin A in rheumatoid arthritis. *Br J Rheumatol* 32(suppl 1):1–3, 1993.

Arend, W.P., Collier, D.H. and Harmon, C.E. Musculoskeletal diseases. *In* Schrier, R.W. (ed.). *Geriatric Medicine.* Philadelphia: W.B. Saunders, 1990, pp. 350–367.

Arnold, W.J. Polymyalgia rheumatica and giant cell arteritis. *In* Hazzard, W.R., Bierman, E.D., Blass, J.P., et al. (eds.). *Principles of Geriatric Medicine and Gerontology.* 2nd ed. New York: McGraw-Hill, 1990, pp. 861–864.

Balfour, J.A. and McTavish, D. Transdermal estradiol: A review of its pharmacological profile, and therapeutic potential in the prevention of postmenopausal osteoporosis. *Drugs Aging* 2:487–507, 1992.

Barnes, C.G. Rheumatoid arthritis. *In* Currey, H.L.F. (ed.). *Mason and Curry's Clinical Rheumatology.* Philadelphia: J.B. Lippincott, 1980, pp. 30–62.

Barzel, U.S. Common metabolic disorders of the skeleton in aging. *In* Reichel, W. (ed.). *Clinical Aspects of Aging.* 3rd ed. Baltimore: Williams & Wilkins, 1989, pp. 330–342.

Bassey, E.J. and Harries, U.J. Normal values for handgrip strength in 920 men and women aged over 65 years, and longitudinal changes over 4 years in 620 survivors. *Clin Sci* 84:331–337, 1993.

Bauer, D.C., Browner, W.S., Cauley, J.A., et al. Factors associated with appendicular bone mass in older women: The Study of Osteoporotic Fractures Research Group. *Ann Intern Med* 118:657–665, 1993.

Baylink, D.J. Osteomalacia. *In* Hazzard, W.R., Bierman, E.D., Blass, J.P., et al. (eds.). *Principles of Geriatric Medicine and Gerontology.* 2nd ed. New York: McGraw-Hill, 1990, pp. 826–836.

Bellamy, N., Duffy, D., Martin, N. and Matthews, J. Rheumatoid arthritis in twins: A study of aetiopathogenesis based on the Australian Twin Registry. *Ann Rheum Dis* 51:588–593, 1992.

Bird, H.A. Polymyalgia rheumatica and temporal arteritis. *In* Wright, V. (ed.). *Bone and Joint Disease in the Elderly.* New York: Churchill Livingstone, 1983, pp. 60–79.

Boyd, R.E. Gout: Modern management of an ancient malady. *J S C Med Assoc* 89:240–243, 1993.

Brewerton, D.A. Rheumatic disorders. *In* Rossman, I. (ed.). *Clinical Geriatrics.* 2nd ed. Philadelphia: J.B. Lippincott, 1979, pp. 451–459.

Buchbinder, R., Hall, S., Sambrook, P.N., et al. Methotrexate therapy in rheumatoid arthritis: A life table review of 587 patients treated in community practice. *J Rheumatol* 20:639–644, 1993.

Bunning, R.D. and Materson, R.S. A rational program of exercise for patients with osteoarthritis. *Semin Arthritis Rheum* 21:33–34, 1991.

Calkins, E. Musculoskeletal diseases in the elderly. *In* Calkins, E., Ford, A.B., and Katz, P.R. (eds.). *The Practice of Geriatrics.* 2nd ed. Philadelphia: W.B. Saunders, 1992, pp. 378–402.

Carter, A.B. The neurological aspects of aging. *In* Rossman, I. (ed.). *Clinical Geriatrics.* 3rd ed. Philadelphia: J.B. Lippincott, 1986, pp. 326–351.

Chan, W.P., Lang, P., Stevens, M.P., et al. Osteoarthritis of the knee: Comparison of radiography, CT and MR imaging to assess extent and severity. *AJR Am J Roentgenol* 157:799–806, 1991.

Cheng, Y.M., Lin, S.Y. and Wu, H.J. Total ankle replacement: Preliminary report of 3 cases. *Kao Hsiung I Hsueh Ko Hsueh Tsa Chih* 9:18–26, 1993.

Chesnut, C.H. Osteoporosis. *In* Hazzard, W.R., Bierman, E.D., Blass, J.P., et al. (eds.). *Principles of Geriatric Medicine and Gerontology.* 2nd ed. New York: McGraw-Hill, 1990, pp. 813–825.

Christian, C.L. Arthritis in the elderly. *Med Clin North Am* 66:1047–1052, 1982.

Ciammella, M., Guareschi, B., Pes, S., et al. Substitution estrogen therapy in the prevention of postmenopausal osteoporosis and cardiovascular diseases: Results of long-term therapy. *Minerva Ginecol* 45:53–55, 1993.

Corless, D. The aging skeleton. *Practitioner* 225:1775–1785, 1981.

Cushnaghan, J. and Dieppe, P. Study of 500 patients with limb joint osteoarthritis: I. Analysis by age, sex, and distribution of symptomatic joint sites. *Ann Rheum Dis* 50:8–13, 1991.

Deighton, C.M., Sykes, H. and Walker, D.J. Rheumatoid arthritis, HLA identity, and age at menarche. *Ann Rheum Dis* 52:322–326, 1993.

Doren, M. and Schneider, H.P. Identification and treatment of postmenopausal women at risk for the development of osteoporosis. *Int J Clinical Pharmacol Ther Toxicol* 30:431–433, 1992.

Edwards, N.L. Drugs to lower uric acid levels: How to avoid misuse in gouty arthritis. *Postgrad Med* 89:111–113, 116, 1991.

Evans, W.J. Exercise, nutrition and aging. *J Nutr* 122:796–801, 1992.

Felson, D.T. The epidemiology of knee osteoarthritis: Results from the Framingham Osteoarthritis Study. *Semin Arthritis Rheum* 20:42–50, 1990a.

Felson, D.T. Osteoarthritis. *Rheum Dis Clin North Am* 16:499–512, 1990b.

Felson, D.T., Zhang, Y., Anthony, J.M., et al. Weight loss reduces the risk for symptomatic knee osteoarthritis in women: The Framingham Study. *Ann Intern Med* 116:535–539, 1992.

Francis, R.M. The pathogenesis of osteoporosis. In Francis, R.M. (ed.). *Osteoporosis: Pathogenesis and Management.* Lancaster, England: Kluwer, 1990, pp. 51–80.

Francis, R.M. Bone aging, osteoporosis, and osteomalacia. *In* Brocklehurst, J.C., Tallis, R.C. and Fillit, H.M. (eds.). *Textbook of Geriatric Medicine and Gerontology.* 4th ed. New York: Churchill Livingstone, 1992, pp. 769–782.

Friedlander, A.H. and Runyon, C. Polymyalgia rheumatica and temporal arteritis. *Oral Surg Oral Med Oral Pathol* 69:317–321, 1990.

Frontera, W.R., Hughes, V.A., Lutz, K.J. and Evans, W.J. A cross-sectional study of muscle strength and mass in 45- to 78-yr-old men and women. *J Appl Physiol* 71:644–650, 1991.

Fung, M.C. and Holbrook, J.H. Placebo-controlled trial of quinine therapy for nocturnal leg cramps. *West J Med* 151:42–44, 1989.

Gardner, D.L. Aging of articular cartilage and joints. *In* Brocklehurst, J.C., Tallis, R.C. and Fillit, H.M. *Textbook of Geriatric Medicine and Gerontology.* 4th ed. New York: Churchill Livingstone, 1992, pp. 792–812.

Giansiracuso, D.F. and Kantrowitz, F.G. *Rheumatic and Metabolic Bone Diseases in the Elderly.* Lexington, MA: The Collamore Press, 1982.

Gilmore, R.L. Recognizing problems of the aging spine. *Geriatrics* 35:83–92, 1980.

Gordon, D.A., Keystone, E.C. and Smythe, H.A. Diagnosis and assessment. *In* Gordon, A.G. (ed.). *Rheumatoid Arthritis.* New York: Medical Examination Publishing Co., 1981, pp. 1–24.

Gordon, J.C. Musculoskeletal injuries in the elderly. *In* Reichel, W. (ed.). *Clinical Aspects of Aging.* 3rd ed. Baltimore: Williams & Wilkins, 1989, pp. 343–361.

Grahame, R. Joint disease in old age. *In* Brocklehurst, J.C., Tallis, R.C. and Fillit, H.M. (eds.). *Textbook of Geriatric Medicine and Gerontology.* 4th ed. New York: Churchill Livingstone, 1992, pp. 813–833.

Grahame, R. and Scott, J.T. Clinical survey of 354 patients with gout. *Ann Rheum Dis* 29:461–468, 1970.

Greig, C.A., Botella, J. and Young, A. The quadriceps strength of healthy elderly people remeasured after eight years. *Muscle Nerve* 16:6–10, 1993.

Grob, D. Common disorders of muscles in the aged. *In* Reichel, W. (ed.). *Clinical Aspects of Aging.* 3rd ed. Baltimore: Williams & Wilkins, 1989a, pp. 296–313.

Grob, D. Prevalent joint diseases in older persons. *In* Reichel, W. (ed.). *Clinical Aspects of Aging.* 3rd ed. Baltimore: Williams & Wilkins, 1989b, pp. 314–329.

Groessner-Schreiber, B., Krukowski, M., Lyons, C. and Osdoby, P. Osteoclast recruitment in response to human bone matrix is age related. *Mech Ageing Dev* 62:143–154, 1992.

Haberman, E.T. Orthopaedic aspects of the lower extremities. *In* Rossman, I. (ed.). *Clinical Geriatrics.* 3rd ed. Philadelphia: J.B. Lippincott, 1986, pp. 538–566.

Hall, A.P., Barry, P.E., Dawber, T.R., et al. Epidemiology of gout and hyperuricemia: A long term population study. *Am J Med* 42:27–37, 1967.

Hamerman, D. Rheumatic disorders. *In* Rossman, I. (ed.). *Clinical Geriatrics.* 3rd ed. Philadelphia: J.B. Lippincott, 1986, pp. 513–522.

Handy, R.C. *Paget's Disease of Bone.* New York: Praeger Publishers, 1981.

Hannan, M.T., Felson, D.T., Anderson, J.J. and Naimark, A. Habitual physical activity is not associated with knee osteoarthritis: The Framingham Study. *J Rheumatol* 20:704–709, 1993.

Hart, D.J. and Spector, T.D. The relationship of obesity, fat distribution and osteoarthritis in women in the general population: The Chingford Study. *J Rheumatol* 20:331–335, 1993.

Healey, L.A. Rheumatology. *In* Cassel, D.K. and Walsh, J.R. (eds.). *Geriatric Medicine.* New York: Springer-Verlag, 1990, pp. 289–298.

Hicks, A.L., Cupido, C.M., Martin, J. and Dent, J. Muscle excitation in elderly adults: The effects of training. *Muscle Nerve* 15:87–93, 1992.

Horton, S., Resman-Targoff, B.H. and Thompson, D.F. Use of cyclosporine in rheumatoid arthritis. *Ann Pharmacother* 27:44–46, 1993.

Hughes, S., Peel-White, A.L. and Peterson, C.K. Paget's disease of bone—Current thinking and management. *J Manipulative Physiol Ther* 15:242–249, 1992.

Hyatt, R.H., Whitelaw, M.N., Bhat, A., et al. Association of muscle strength with functional status of elderly people. *Age Ageing* 19:330–336, 1990.

James, W.H. Rheumatoid arthritis, the contraceptive pill, and androgens. *Ann Rheum Dis* 52:470–474, 1993.

Jerosch, J. and Castro, W.H. Arthroscopy of the elbow joint: Long-term results, complications and indications. *Unfallchirurg* 95:405–411, 1992.

Kaiser, H. Polymyalgia rheumatica. *Z Gerontol* 26:20–23, 1993.

Kane, R.L., Ouslander, J.G. and Abrass, I.B. *Essentials of Clinical Geriatrics.* 3rd ed. New York: McGraw-Hill, 1994.

Konradsen, L., Hansen, E.M. and Sondergaard, L. Long distance running and osteoarthrosis. *Am J Sports Med* 18:379–381, 1990.

Kovar, P.A., Allegrante, J.P., MacKenzie, C.R., et al. Supervised fitness walking in patients with osteoarthritis of the knee: A randomized, controlled trial. *Ann Intern Med* 116:529–534, 1992.

Kraenzlin, M.E., Jennings, J.C. and Baylink, D.J. Calcium and bone homeostasis with aging. *In* Hazzard, W.R., Bierman, E.D., Blass, J.P., et al. (eds.). *Principles of Geriatric Medicine and Gerontology.* 2nd ed. New York: McGraw-Hill, 1990, pp. 799–812.

Kvien, T.K. and Husby, G. Disease modification in rheumatoid arthritis with special reference to cyclosporin A. *Scand J Rheumatol Suppl* 95:19–28, 1992.

Kyle, V. Laboratory investigations including liver in polymyalgia rheumatica/giant cell arteritis. *Baillieres Clin Rheumatol* 5:475–484, 1991a.

Kyle, V. Treatment of polymyalgia rheumatica/giant cell arteritis. *Baillieres Clin Rheumatol* 5:485–491, 1991b.

Laforest, S., St-Pierre, D.M., Cyr, J. and Gayton, D. Effects of age and regular exercise on muscle strength and endurance. *Eur J Appl Physiol* 60:104–111, 1990.

Lane, J.M. and Vigorita, V.J. Osteoporosis—Definition, pathophysiology, diagnosis and treatment. Current concepts review. *J Bone Joint Surg* 65A:274–278, 1983.

Lane, N.E., Michel, B., Bjorkengren, A., et al. The risk of osteoarthritis with running and aging: A 5-year longitudinal study. *J Rheumatol* 20:461–468, 1993.

Larsson, L. Aging in mammalian skeletal muscle. *In* Mortimer, J.A., Pirozzolo, F.J. and Maletta, G.J. (eds.). *Advances in Neurogerontology.* Vol. 3. New York: Praeger Publishers, 1982, pp. 35–43.

Leong, K.H. and Feng, P.H. Gout. *Singapore Med J* 33: 393–394, 1992.

Levy, M., Spino, M. and Read, S.E. Colchicine: A state-of-the-art review. *Pharmacotherapy* 11:196–211, 1991.

Lewis, C.B. Musculoskeletal changes with age. *Clin Management* 4:12–15, 1984.

Lifschitz, M.L. and Harmon, C.E. Musculoskeletal problems in the elderly. *In* Schrier, R.W. (ed.). *Clinical Internal Medicine in the Aged.* Philadelphia: W.B. Saunders, 1982, pp. 182–210.

Mannik, M. Rheumatoid factors in the pathogenesis of rheumatoid arthritis. *J Rheumatol Suppl* 32:46–49, 1992.

Marx, C.W., Dailey, G.E., III, Cheney, C., et al. Do estrogens improve bone mineral density in osteoporotic women over age 65? *J Bone Miner Res* 7:1275–1279, 1992.

McCulloch, J., Lydyard, P.M. and Rook, G.A. Rheumatic arthritis: How well do the theories fit the evidence? *Clin Exp Immunol* 92:1–6, 1993.

Merkow, R.L. and Lane, J.M. Paget's disease. *In* Sculco, T.P. (ed.). *Orthopaedic Care of the Geriatric Patient.* St. Louis: C.V. Mosby, 1985, pp. 253–268.

Merkow, R.L. and Lane, J.M. Paget's disease of bone. *Endocrinol Metab Clin North Am* 19:177–204, 1990.

Merletti, R., Lo Conte, L.R., Cisari, C. and Actis, M.V. Age related changes in surface myoelectric signals. *Scand J Rehabil Med* 24:25–36, 1992.

Michel, B.A., Fries, J.F., Bloch, D.A., et al. Osteophytosis of the knee: Association with changes in weight-bearing exercise. *Clin Rheumatol* 11:235–238, 1992.

Miller, P.D. Osteoporosis and other metabolic bone disease. *In* Schrier, R.W. (ed.). *Geriatric Medicine.* Philadelphia: W.B. Saunders, 1990, pp. 324–340.

Molitor, P.J., Emery, R.J. and Meggitt, B.F. First metacarpal osteotomy for carpo-metacarpal osteoarthritis. *J Hand Surg* 16:424–427, 1991.

Nichols, J.F., Omizo, D.K., Peterson, K.K. and Nelson, K.P. Efficacy of heavy-resistance training for active women over sixty: Muscular strength, body composition, and program adherence. *J Am Geriatr Soc* 41:205–210, 1993.

Nordin, B.E.C. Osteoporosis. *In* Wright, V. (ed.). *Bone and Joint Diseases in the Elderly.* New York: Churchill Livingstone, 1983, pp. 167–180.

Ochs, M. Surgical management of the hip in the elderly patient. *Clin Geriatr Med* 6:571–586, 1990.

Ouslander, J.G. and Beck, J.C. Paget's disease of the bone. *J Am Geriatr Soc* 30:410–414, 1982.

Palferman, T.G. That oestrogen replacement for osteoporosis prevention should no longer be a bone of contention. *Ann Rheum Dis* 52:74–80, 1993.

Panush, R.S. Does exercise cause arthritis? Longterm consequences of exercise on the musculoskeletal system. *Rheum Dis Clin North Am* 16:827–836, 1990.

Phillips, S.K., Rook, K.M., Siddle, N.C., et al. Muscle weakness in women occurs at an earlier age than in men, but strength is preserved by hormone replacement therapy. *Clin Sci* 84:95–98, 1993.

Pincus, T., Marcum, S.B. and Callahan, L.F. Longterm drug therapy for rheumatoid arthritis in seven rheumatology private practices: II. Second line drugs and prednisone. *J Rheumatol* 19:1885–1894, 1992.

Price, R.I., Gutteridge, D.H., Stuckey, B.G., et al. Rapid, divergent changes in spinal and forearm bone density following short-term intravenous treatment of Paget's disease with pamidronate disodium. *J Bone Miner Res* 8:209–217, 1993.

Reed, R.L., Pearlmutter, L., Yochum, K., et al. The relationship between muscle mass and muscle strength in the elderly. *J Am Geriatr Soc* 39:555–561, 1991.

Reginster, J.Y., Colson, F., Morlock, G., et al. Evaluation of the efficacy and safety of oral Tiludronate in Paget's disease of bone: A double-blind, multiple-dosage, placebo-controlled study. *Arthritis Rheum* 35:967–974, 1992.

Reginster, J.Y., Lecart, M.P., Deroisy, R., et al. Paget's disease of bone treated with a five day course of oral Tiludronate. *Ann Rheum Dis* 52:54–57, 1993.

Reid, I.R., Ames, R.W., Evans, M.C., et al. Effect of calcium supplementation on bone loss in postmenopausal women. *New Engl J Med* 328:460–464, 1993.

Riffel, K. Falls: Kinds, causes and prevention. *Geriatr Nurs* 3:165–169, 1982.

Riggs, B.L. et al. Changes in bone mineral density of the proximal femur and spine with aging: Differences between the postmenopausal and senile osteoporosis syndromes. *J Clin Invest* 70:716–723, 1982.

Riggs, B.L. and Melton, L.J., III. Involutional osteoporosis. *New Engl J Med* 314:1676–1686, 1986.

Rogers, M.A. and Evans, W.J. Changes in skeletal muscle with aging: Effects of exercise training. *Exerc Sport Sci Rev* 21:65–102, 1993.

Roman, W.J., Fleckenstein, J., Stray-Gundersen, J., et al. Adaptations in the elbow flexors of elderly males after heavy-resistance training. *J Appl Physiol* 74:750–754, 1993.

Rosse, C. and Clawson, D.K. *Introduction to the Musculoskeletal System.* New York: Harper & Row, 1970.

Rossman, I. The anatomy of aging. *In* Rossman, I. (ed.). *Clinical Geriatrics.* 2nd ed. Philadelphia: J.B. Lippincott, 1986, pp. 3–22.

Rovati, L.C. Clinical research in osteoarthritis: Design and results of short-term and long-term trials with disease-modifying drugs. *Int J Tissue React* 14:243–251, 1992.

Ryan, P.J., Sherry, M., Gibson, T. and Fogelman, I. Treatment of Paget's disease by weekly infusions of 3-aminohydroxypropylidene-1, 1-bisphosphonate (APD). *Br J Rheumatol* 31:97–101, 1992.

Sack, K.E. Arthritis: Specifics on long term management. Part I. *Geriatrics,* 35:32–39, 1980a.

Schweitzer, D.H., Zwinderman, A.H., Vermeij, P., et al. Improved treatment of Paget's disease with dimethylaminohydroxypropylidene bisphosphonate. *J Bone Miner Res* 8:175–182, 1993.

Scileppi, K.P. Aging of the musculoskeletal system. *In*

Sculco, T.P. (ed.). *Orthopaedic Care of the Geriatric Patient.* St. Louis: C.V. Mosby, 1985, pp. 3–11.

Scott, J.T. *Arthritis and Rheumatism.* New York: Oxford University Press, 1980.

Setnikar, I. Antireactive properties of "chondroprotective" drugs. *Int J Tissue React* 14:253–261, 1992.

Sidorov, J. Quinine sulfate for leg cramps: Does it work? *J Am Geriatr Soc* 41:498–500, 1993.

Singer, F.R. Paget's disease of bone. *In* Hazzard, W.R., Bierman, E.D., Blass, J.P., et al. (eds.). *Principles of Geriatric Medicine and Gerontology.* 2nd ed. New York: McGraw-Hill, 1990, pp. 843–848.

Sjostrom, M., Lexell, J. and Downham, D.Y. Differences in fiber number and fiber type proportion within fascicles: A quantitative morphological study of whole vastus lateralis muscle from childhood to old age. *Anat Rec* 234:183–189, 1992.

Slemenda, C.W. The epidemiology of osteoarthritis of the knee. *Curr Opin Rheumatol* 4:546–551, 1992.

Smith, E.L. and Gilligan, C. Physical activity effects on bone metabolism. *Calc Tissue Int* 49(suppl):S50–54, 1991.

Specht, E.E. Orthopedic and foot disorders. *In* Cassel, C.K. and Walsh, J.R. (eds.). *Geriatric Medicine.* New York: Springer-Verlag, 1990, pp. 517–535.

Spector, T.D. Epidemiology of the rheumatic diseases. *Curr Opin Rheumatol* 5:132–137, 1993.

Spencer, H., Sontag, S.J. and Kramer, L. Disorders of the skeletal system. *In* Rossman, I. (ed.). *Clinical Geriatrics.* 3rd ed. Philadelphia: J.B. Lippincott, 1986, pp. 523–537.

Spencer-Green, G. Drug treatment of arthritis: Update on conventional and less conventional methods. *Postgrad Med* 93:129–140, 1993.

Stelmach, G.E., Populin, L. and Muller, F. Postural muscle onset and voluntary movement in the elderly. *Neurosci Lett* 117:188–193, 1990.

Stevens, M.B. Rheumatoid arthritis. *In* Wright, V. (ed.). *Bone and Joint Disease in the Elderly.* New York: Churchill Livingstone, 1983, pp. 39–59.

Stuart, R.A., Gow, P.J., Bellamy, N., et al. A survey of current prescribing practices of antiinflammatory and urate-lowering drugs in gouty arthritis. *N Z Med J* 104:115–117, 1991.

Sutej, P.G. and Hadler, N.M. Current principles of rehabilitation for patients with rheumatoid arthritis. *Clin Orthop* 256:116–124, 1991.

Talbott, J.H. Gouty arthritis. *Geriatrics* 35:69–78, 1980.

Talbott, J.H. and Yu, T.F. *Gout and Uric Acid Metabolism.* New York: Stratton Intercontinental Medical Book Corporation, 1976.

Tishler, M., Caspi, D. and Yaron, M. Methotrexate treatment of rheumatoid arthritis: Is a fortnightly maintenance schedule enough? *Ann Rheum Dis* 51:1330–1331, 1992.

Trentham, D.E. New focus on treatment for rheumatoid arthritis. *Curr Opin Rheumatol* 5:178–183, 1993.

Turner, R.E., Frank, M.J., Van Ausdal, D., et al. Some aspects of the epidemiology of gout. *Arch Intern Med* 106:400–406, 1960.

Vaananen, H.K. Pathogenesis of osteoporosis. *Calcif Tissue Int* 49(suppl):S11–14, 1991.

Vandervoort, A.A., Taylor, A.W. and Brown, W.F. Effects of motor unit losses on strength in older men and women. *J Appl Physiol* 74:868–874, 1993.

Vawter, R.L. and Antonelli, M.A. Rational treatment of gout: Stopping an attack and preventing recurrence. *Postgrad Med* 91:115–118, 127, 1992.

Villa, L., Robecchi, A. and Ballabio, C.B. Physiopathology, clinical manifestations and treatment of gout. *Ann Rheum Dis* 17:9–15, 1958.

Walker, A.M., Funch, D., Dreyer, N.A., et al. Determinants of serious liver disease among patients receiving low-dose methotrexate for rheumatoid arthritis. *Arthritis Rheum* 36:329–335, 1993.

Wallach, S. Paget's disease of bone. *In* Calkins, E., Ford, A.B. and Katz, P.R. (eds.). *The Practice of Geriatrics.* 2nd ed. Philadelphia: W.B. Saunders, 1992, pp. 403–410.

Wilmore, J.H. The aging of bone and muscle. *Clin Sports Med* 10:231–244, 1991.

Wimalawansa, S.J. Long- and short-term side effects and safety of calcitonin in man: A prospective study. *Calcif Tissue Int* 52:90–93, 1993.

Woollacott, M.H. and Manchester, D.L. Anticipatory postural adjustments in older adults: Are changes in response characteristics due to changes in strategy? *J Gerontol* 48:M64–70, 1993.

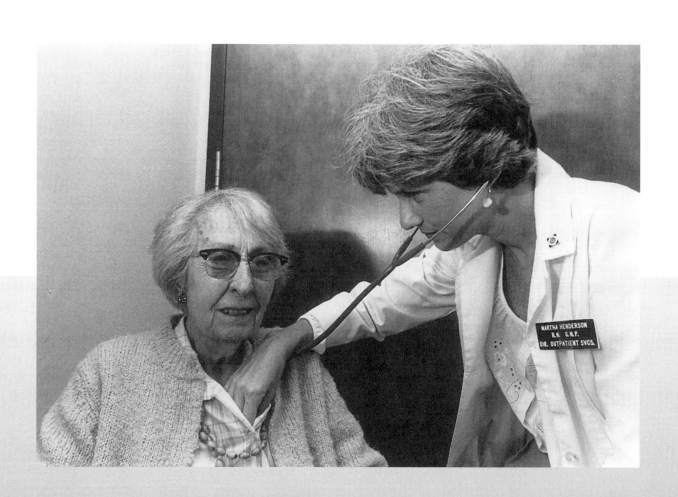

Age-Related Changes in the Cardiovascular System

JOANNE S. HARRELL

OBJECTIVES

List and describe the normal age-related changes in the heart, blood vessels, blood, and pumping ability of the heart.

Discuss the value of exercise in relationship to the aging cardiovascular system.

Review the diseases of the cardiovascular system associated with older age, particularly hypertension, anemia, atherosclerosis, coronary artery disease, angina, acute myocardial infarction, arrhythmias, congestive heart failure, valvular disease, and cerebrovascular and peripheral vascular disease.

Apply the nursing process to the care of older people with cardiovascular changes and diseases.

The high incidence of cardiovascular diseases in the United States makes it somewhat difficult to determine normal age-related changes. Studies indicate that evidence of heart disease can be found in 50 per cent of those aged 65 to 74 and in 60 per cent of those aged 75 and older. In addition, the work the heart is required to perform is less in the aged, who have less lean body mass, so the elderly require less oxygen both at rest and during exercise (Assey, 1993).

NORMAL CHANGES WITH AGING

Heart

Normal anatomical changes in the heart include an increase in a yellow-brown pigment, lipofuscin, in the myocardial fibers, producing a "brown heart." The physiological effects of this pigment have not been clearly described.

Although the overall size of the heart does not increase with age, the thickness of the left ventricular free wall and ventricular septum and the overall weight do increase. Within the myocardium, there are increases in fat, collagen, elastin, and lipofuscin, and progressive loss of myocytes (Kitzman and Edwards, 1990; Wei, 1992). All of these factors contribute to increased stiffness and decreased myocardial contractility in the elderly heart. The stiffness reduces diastolic compliance, thereby limiting the amount of blood that can fill the heart, and the reduced contractility further limits the amount of blood ejected with each heartbeat. Thus, the physiological effect of these normal age-related changes is a reduction of stroke volume in the elderly.

In old age, the coronary arteries become tortuous and dilated and have areas of focal calcification. Coronary collateral vessels may also increase in number, but it is not known if this increase is related to aging alone or is a result of atherosclerosis (Kitzman and Edwards, 1990).

The cardiac valves thicken and stiffen, especially the mitral and aortic valves, which are subject to high pressure for many years. There is some accumulation of lipid, degeneration of collagen, and calcification of the valve fibrosa at the sites of maximum movement of the valve cusps. The increased stiffness at the bases of the aortic valve cusps might be the cause of the common ejection systolic murmur that is often heard in the elderly (Davies, 1992).

The conduction system shows changes with normal aging, which are marked in the sinoatrial (SA) node, located in the right atrium near the vena cava. Pacemaker cells make up about 50 per cent of the mass of the SA node in younger persons but constitute only about 10 per cent of the mass of the SA node in the elderly. Thus, the number of pacemaker cells is decreased, but the amount of fibrous tissue and fat is increased. There are only minor changes in the atrioventricular (AV) node and the right bundle branch of the conduction system with age. However, the left bundle branch passes through connective tissue that is attached to the mitral and aortic valves; the collagen there increases in density and becomes calcified with age, which contributes to a leftward shift of the electrical axis of the electrocardiogram (ECG) with increased age (Davies, 1992).

Electrocardiographic changes can also be demonstrated with age. Some of these changes, such as the loss of the normal sinus rhythm and the decline in the inherent rhythmicity of the SA node, may be explained by the anatomical differences noted earlier. Other changes may be attributed to the increase in size of the left ventricle. These changes include a leftward shift in the frontal plane axis, longer PR and QT intervals, and changes in R and S wave amplitude (Bachman et al., 1981). The QRS complex of adults is wider than that of children (Fisch, 1981), but it may become somewhat narrower with old age (Bachman et al., 1981). The Cardiovascular Heart Study (Kronmal et al., 1992) examined ECGs of 5150 adults older than 65 years for evidence of major ECG abnormalities, which they defined as ventricular conduction defects, isolated major ST-T–wave abnormalities, left ventricular hypertrophy, atrial fibrillation, and first-degree AV block. The prevalence of any major ECG abnormality was 29 per cent overall. However, major ECG abnormalities were found in 37 per cent of those with history of coronary artery disease or hypertension, whereas only 19 per cent of those with no such history had major abnormalities.

Blood Vessels

With advanced age, the aorta also thickens and becomes stiffer and less distensible. The stiffness results from the following degenerative changes: (1) the aortic media thickens, as some elastic tissue is replaced with collagen, and (2) calcification occurs, and cholesterol is taken up into the aortic media and the other large arteries (Assey, 1993). The reduced distensibility is partly compensated for by an increase in the size of the aorta. A further compensatory mechanism is the increase in systolic blood pressure (BP), which sends blood into the larger and stiffer aorta with greater force in the elderly than in young people, who have more flexible arteries. The loss of elasticity of the aorta and large arteries causes an impedance to flow and an increased systemic vascular resistance, so the left ventricle pumps against a greater resistance, contributing to the hypertrophy of that chamber (Assey, 1993).

Other arteries also thicken and become less distensible with age. In the very young, leg arteries have been shown to be much more compliant than the aorta. By the sixth decade, the compliance of the iliac and leg arteries is the same as that of the aorta (Laogun and Gosling, 1984). With advancing age, the smooth muscle of the walls of the arteries becomes less responsive to beta-adrenergic stimulation and to other vasoactive hormones (Assey, 1993). This may explain the blunted cardiovascular response to the stress of exercise.

The baroreceptors, which regulate BP in various positions, are less sensitive in the aged. This probably explains the fairly common finding of orthostatic hypotension in the elderly (Wei, 1992).

Capillary walls also show age-related changes. Capillary endothelial cells lie on a layer of collagen-like material, the basement membrane, which separates these cells from tissue cells. With age, the basement membrane thickens, which may slow the exchange of nutrients and waste products between the blood and tissues (Goldman, 1979).

Blood

The components of the blood also change slightly with age. Blood volume is reduced owing to the drop in plasma volume. There is a 50 per cent reduction in hemopoietic activity in persons over the age of 60, probably because the volume of the bone marrow is less, and some of the hemopoietic tissue is replaced by fat and connective tissue. Erythropoiesis is affected more than leukopoiesis, so there is a slight drop in the number of red blood cells and in hemoglobin and hematocrit values. In addition, the red cells have less flexibility and decreased resistance to osmotic changes. Blood coagulability is increased with age, probably because of increased platelet aggregation and decreased fibrinolytic activity. Table 7–1 indicates the

TABLE 7 – 1

Changes in Blood Components with Age

COMPONENT	CHANGE	IMPLICATIONS OF CHANGE
Erythrocytes	Reduced	} Increased fatigue
Hemoglobin	Reduced	
Hematocrit	Reduced	
Leukocytes	Same	
Neutrophils	Same	
Eosinophils	Same	
Basophils	Same	
Monocytes	Same	
Lymphocytes	Reduced	Decreased resistance to infection

changes in blood components (DeNicola and Casale, 1983).

Pumping Ability of the Heart

Both the isometric contraction phase and the relaxation time of the left ventricle are prolonged with age. The heart spends more time in the contraction phase, which provides a slightly longer systole, to more effectively squeeze out the blood from the stiffer left ventricle. Because the aged left ventricle, which is less distensible, requires a more active filling, the "atrial kick," which is the result of the contraction of the left atrium late in diastole, takes on a special importance. This also possibly explains another normal finding with age, the delay in early diastolic filling. The delay in normal filling time may be due to a slowing down of ventricular relaxation or to the increased stiffness of the left ventricle. The delay allows the heart more time to fill, which gives full opportunity for the active filling caused by the atrial kick and provides an adequate stroke volume in spite of the stiffness of the heart (Wei, 1992).

Formerly, many authors maintained that the left ventricular function of the normal elderly heart was impaired, leading to age-related reductions in cardiac output. However, it is now recognized that those studies were performed on elderly subjects without proper screening for the presence of coronary heart disease (CHD). At present, cardiac physiologists believe that the systolic function of the elderly heart is not impaired (Lewis and Maron, 1992).

The Baltimore Longitudinal Study on Aging, which studied 61 volunteers aged 26 to 79 years who were physically active and free of cardiovascular disease, produced findings that challenge the commonly accepted findings about cardiac output. This study found that with exercise, the heart rate of elderly persons did not increase as much as that of young subjects, but the stroke volume did increase. As a result, the cardiac output of the elderly subjects was not significantly different from that of the young (Rodeheffer and Gerstenblith, 1985). All subjects with cardiovascular disease were excluded through the use of stress ECGs and stress thallium scintigraphy.

In summary, the normal cardiovascular changes with aging include a moderate increase in blood pressure, especially systolic blood pressure; prolonged contraction time; a slow ventricular filling rate; and increased stiffness. There is no evidence for a specific cardiomyopathy of aging. The response of the cardiovascular system to stress, although somewhat blunted in the aged, is still more than adequate in the absence of cardiac pathology (Kitzman and Edwards, 1990; Lewis and Maron, 1992).

CARDIOVASCULAR CHANGES— DUE TO AGE OR DISUSE?

Several new studies indicate that loss of cardiovascular function may be more related to the lack of conditioning than to the effects of age. A Japanese study that controlled for the effects of aging, training, and myocardial ischemia found that all athletes, regardless of age, had the same response as young subjects. This response was a slight early rise in left ventricular end-diastolic volume and a gradual increase in myocardial contractility and heart rate. Healthy aged nonathletes had a similar early response but maintained increased cardiac output only by an increased heart rate. Subjects with heart disease had different patterns of response (Mizutani et al., 1984).

Aging is associated with reduced maximal aerobic power and reduced muscle strength, which are signs of reduced physical fitness. The reductions occur at a rate of 3 to 8 per cent per decade after the second decade of life. Researchers have demonstrated that factors other than age accounted for 84 per cent of the decline in aerobic power seen in older patients (Elward and Larson, 1992). These additional factors may be concurrent disease or merely physical inactivity. Steinhaus et al. (1988) studied 30 healthy young men (aged 20 to 31 years) and 30 healthy older men (aged 50 to 62 years); half of the men in each group reported sedentary lifestyles in the previous 5 years, and half said they often participated in strenuous physical exercise. The researchers found that the active older men had significantly lower resting heart rates, lower resting systolic and diastolic BPs, higher maximal aerobic power, lower maximal exercise diastolic BP, and lower resting heart rates than the inactive young men. Thus, the physiological profiles of the older active men were closer to those of active men who were 30 years younger than to those of older sedentary men. These findings suggest that some of the changes commonly attributed to aging are actually caused by disuse. If this is true, increasing physical exercise could ward off some of the effects of aging.

General and Cardiovascular Benefits of Increased Exercise

Physical training in the elderly can produce profound improvements in the functions necessary for physical fitness (Astrand, 1992a). A large body of research supports the beneficial effects of exercise on strength and aerobic power in older adults. However, there may be additional, less obvious, benefits of an active lifestyle. Although further research is needed, intervention studies have shown that exercise may improve gait, balance, and physical function in the elderly. A training program can normalize glucose intolerance in elderly people and enhance the muscle's sensitivity to insulin. The more physically active a person is, the higher energy intake can be without risking obesity. Because the elderly are at risk for inadequate nutrition, the ability to eat more with less risk of obesity may ensure an adequate intake of essential nutrients. In addition, exercise may promote bone mineral density and thus decrease the risk of fractures in the elderly. It is also possible that regular physical activity can lessen the rate of functional decline in the elderly and possibly improve neurological functioning (Astrand, 1992a; Buchner et al., 1992; Elward and Larson, 1992).

How do older regular exercisers differ from their sedentary counterparts? Elward et al. (1992) studied 561 randomly selected people aged 65 years and older who lived in the community. Compared with the nonexercisers, the exercisers had higher perceptions of current health and a more positive outlook regarding their health; they also had higher incomes and higher educational levels. Further, the exercisers were less likely to report having hypertension, arthritis, or two or more of the following medical conditions: heart disease, hypertension, arthritis, and emphysema. A large study of Dutch men showed that physical activity decreased with age but that total weekly physical activity and specific activators, such as gardening and walking, had favorable associations with cholesterol and systolic BP (Caspersen et al., 1991). Data from the Established Populations for Epidemiologic Studies of the Elderly (EPESE) showed that after 3 years of study, the mortality of those who were moderately or highly active was one half to two thirds the mortality of those who were inactive. The Longitudinal Study of Aging produced similar results: less activity or exercise was associated with a higher risk of mortality (Rakowski and Mor, 1992). The association between walking and reduced mortality was particularly strong in women. The authors strongly recommended that clinicians elicit information on their patient's regular physical activity, and they provided four simple questions to use to assess activity. These questions were suggested:

1. Compared to other persons your age, would you say you are physically more active, less active, or about the same? (Follow up to determine the degree of more or less activity).

2. Do you feel that you get as much exercise as you need, or less than you need?

3. Do you follow a regular routine of physical exercise?

4. How often do you walk a mile or more at a time, without resting? (Probe to determine the number of days per week.)

In 1992, the American Heart Association recognized physical inactivity as a risk factor for coronary artery disease, and summarized the benefits of exercise. Exercise training results in decreased myocardial oxygen

T A B L E   7 – 2
Effects of Habitual Physical Activities

Increase in maximal oxygen uptake and cardiac output
Reduced heart rate at given oxygen uptake
Reduced blood pressure
Reduced heart rate × blood pressure product
Improved efficiency of heart muscle
Improved myocardial vascularization?
Favorable trend in incidences of cardial morbidity and mortality
Increased capillary density in skeletal muscle
Increased mitochondrial density in skeletal muscle
Reduced lactate production at given percentage of maximal oxygen uptake
Reduced perceived exertion at given oxygen uptake
Enhanced ability to utilize free fatty acids as substrate during exercise—is glycogen saving
Improved endurance during exercise
Increases metabolism—advantageous from a nutritional viewpoint
Counteracts obesity
Increases HDL concentrations in blood
Improved structure and function of ligaments, tendons, and joints
Increased muscular strength
Increased production of endorphines
Enhances nerve fiber sprouting to reinnervate muscle fibers
Enhances tolerance to hot environment—increased sweat production
Reduced platelet aggregation?
Counteracts osteoporosis
Can normalize glucose tolerance

Adapted from Astrand, P.-O. "Why exercise?" *Med Sci Sports Exerc* 24(2):153–162, 1992. HDL = high-density lipoprotein.

TABLE 7-3
Contraindications to Physical Activity for the Elderly

Absolute Contraindications

Severe coronary heart disease—unstable angina pectoris and acute myocardial infarction
Decompensated congestive heart failure
Uncontrolled ventricular arrhythmias
Uncontrolled atrial arrhythmias (compromising cardiac function)
Severe valvular heart disease including aortic, pulmonic, and mitral stenosis
Uncontrolled systemic hypertension (e.g., >200/105)
Pulmonary hypertension
Acute myocarditis or infectious illness
Recent pulmonary embolism or deep vein thrombosis

Relative Contraindications

Coronary heart disease
Congestive heart failure
Significant valvular heart disease
Cardiac arrhythmias including ventricular and atrial arrhythmias and complete heart block
Hypertension
Fixed-rate, permanent pacemaker
Cyanotic congenital heart disease
Congenital anomalies of coronary arteries
Cardiomyopathy, including hypertrophic cardiomyopathy and dilated cardiomyopathy
Marfan's syndrome
Peripheral vascular disease
Severe obstructive or restrictive lung disease
Electrolyte abnormalities, especially hypokalemia
Uncontrolled metabolic disease (e.g., diabetes, thyrotoxicosis, myxedema)
Any serious systemic disorder (e.g., mononucleosis, hepatitis)
Neuromuscular or musculoskeletal disorders that would make exercise difficult
Marked obesity
Anemia
Idiopathic long-QT syndrome

(From Van Camp, S.P. and Boyer, J.L. Exercise guidelines for the elderly (part 2 of 2). *Phys Sports Med* 17(5):83–88, 1989. Copyright 1989, McGraw-Hill. Reproduced with permission of McGraw-Hill, Inc.)

demand for the same level of external work; it favorably alters lipid and carbohydrate metabolism, especially if it is accompanied by weight loss; and it enhances the beneficial effects of a low–saturated fat and low-cholesterol diet. "Persons of all ages should include physical activity in a comprehensive program of health promotion and disease prevention, and should increase their habitual physical activity to a level appropriate to their capacities, needs and interest" (Fletcher et al., 1992, p. 341). The physiological advantages produced by exercise are summarized in Table 7–2.

Astrand (1992a) recommended the following prescription for exercise. At least 60 minutes of physical activity daily, not necessarily vigorous, and not necessarily continuous. This regimen can be incorporated into the daily routine of such activities as moving and walking, whether for 1 minute 60 times a day, 12 minutes five times a day, or any combination that totals 60 minutes. Three times a week, more strenuous exercises should be performed for 30 to 45 minutes. Examples of these activities are brisk walking, jogging, cycling, swimming, and aerobic dancing. One of the best exercises for ambulatory elderly persons is walking (Barry et al., 1993). Before beginning an activity program, the patient should be carefully evaluated, with emphasis on a cardiovascular, musculoskeletal, or neurologic condition that would preclude exercise or require treatment before the program is begun (Van Camp and Boyer, 1989). Table 7–3 lists contraindications to physical activity for the elderly.

Nurses should be aware that hospitalized elderly patients also need physical activity. A study of 500 elderly patients in five hospitals showed that no activity order was in effect for 13 per cent of the 3500 patient days reviewed, and when activity was ordered, the patient activity was different from that permitted by the doctor on 41 per cent of the days. Patients who remained in bed or a chair rarely received physical therapy, never had physician orders for exercises, and never performed exercises with the nurses (Lazarus et al., 1991). These results demonstrate the need for nurses to consult with doctors to recommend and initiate activity orders.

DISEASES OF THE CARDIOVASCULAR SYSTEM

Hypertension

The most prevalent cardiovascular disease found in the elderly is hypertension. According to the *Fifth Report of the Joint National Committee on Detection, Evaluation and Treatment of High Blood Pressure* (National Institutes of Health, National Heart Lung and Blood Institute [NIH, NHLBI] 1993), in Americans aged 60 years or older, hypertension is found in 60 per cent of whites, in 61 per cent of Hispanics, and in 71 per cent of non-Hispanic African-Americans. The classification of blood pressure in adults is summarized in Table 7–4. Systolic hypertension is now a well-established independent risk factor for CHD, stroke, and cardiovascular disease.

Because elevated BP is so common in the elderly, this condition used to be considered a normal change with age. However, such elevations are not seen in other, less "ad-

T A B L E   7 – 4

Classification of Blood Pressure for Adults Age 18 and Older*

CATEGORY	SYSTOLIC (mm Hg)	DIASTOLIC (mm Hg)
Normal†	<130	<85
High normal	130–139	85–89
Hypertension‡		
Stage 1 (mild)	140–159	90–99
Stage 2 (moderate)	160–179	100–109
Stage 3 (severe)	180–209	110–119
Stage 4 (very severe)	≥210	≥120

Adapted from National Institutes of Health, National Heart, Lung and Blood Institute. *The Fifth Report of the Joint National Committee on Detection, Evaluation and Treatment of High Blood Pressure.* NIH Pub. No. 932-1088. Bethesda, MD: Public Health Service, 1993.

* Not taking antihypertensive drugs and not acutely ill. When systolic and diastolic pressures fall into different categories, the higher category should be selected to classify the individual's blood pressure status. For instance, 160/92 mm Hg should be classified as stage 2, and 180/120 mm Hg should be classified as stage 4. Isolated systolic hypertension (ISH) is defined as systolic blood pressure (SBP) ≥140 mm Hg and diastolic blood pressure (DBP) <90 mm Hg and staged appropriately (e.g., 170/85 mm Hg is defined as stage 2 ISH).

† Optimal blood pressure with respect to cardiovascular risk is SBP <120 mm Hg and DBP <80 mm Hg.. However, unusually low readings should be evaluated for clinical significance.

‡ Based on the average of two or more readings taken at each of two or more visits following an initial screening.

Note: In addition to classifying stages of hypertension based on average blood pressure levels, the clinician should specify presence or absence of target-organ disease and additional risk factors. For example, a patient with diabetes and a blood pressure of 142/94 mm Hg plus left ventricular hypertrophy should be classified as "stage 1 hypertension with target-organ disease (left ventricular hypertrophy) and with another major risk factor (diabetes)." This specificity is important for risk classification and management.

mm Hg" (United States Department of Health and Human Services, 1980).

Previously the issues of if, when, and how to treat hypertension in the elderly were disputed. However, the value of treating hypertension in the elderly has been well established by large, randomized, controlled studies that are summarized by the *Fifth Report of the Joint National Committee on Detection, Evaluation and Treatment of High Blood Pressure* (NIH, NHLBI, 1993). For example, in the Systolic Hypertension in the Elderly Project (SHEP, 1991) study, there were 35 per cent fewer fatal and nonfatal strokes and 27 per cent fewer myocardial infarctions in the treated group than in the control group. In the elderly, the initial goal of therapy is to reduce the systolic BP to less than 160 mm Hg (if the initial systolic BP is >180 mm Hg) or to reduce systolic BP by 20 mm Hg (if it is between 160 and 179 mm Hg). In patients with isolated systolic hypertension and a systolic BP of 140 to 169 mm Hg, lifestyle modifications may be used as the only therapy or as adjunctive therapy (NIH, NHLBI, 1993).

Lifestyle modifications to reduce BP, include reducing weight if the patient's weight is more than 10 per cent above the ideal weight, moderating daily alcohol intake, reducing dietary sodium, and increasing regular physical activity. In addition, patients with hypertension should be strongly advised to avoid all types of tobacco, not because tobacco has a direct effect on BP, but because it is a strong additional risk factor for cardiovascular disease, and those who smoke may not get maximum protection

vanced" cultures. Data from the Framingham Study indicate that hypertension, regardless of whether it is systolic or diastolic, is a significant risk factor of cardiovascular disease and death in older persons (Kannel, 1992). Systolic-diastolic hypertension (over 160/95 mm Hg) doubles the risk of mortality in men and increases the risk in women by two and one-half times that in normotensives. Borderline systolic-diastolic hypertension (140/90 to 160/95 mm Hg) increases the risk by one and one-half in men and doubles the risk in women. And, contrary to previous beliefs, high systolic pressure may be even more serious than elevated diastolic pressures. "Isolated systolic hypertension greater than 180 increases the risk of stroke and death from coronary disease by two and one-half times in persons aged 65–74 compared to people in the same age group with systolic blood pressures less than 180

T A B L E   7 – 5

Lifestyle Modifications for Hypertension Control and/or Overall Cardiovascular Risk

Lose weight if overweight.

Limit alcohol intake to no more than 1 ounce of ethanol per day (24 ounces of beer, 8 ounces of wine, or 2 ounces of 100 proof whiskey).

Exercise (aerobic) regularly.

Reduce sodium intake to less than 100 mmol per day (<2.3 grams of sodium or <6 grams of sodium chloride).

Maintain adequate dietary potassium, calcium, and magnesium intake.

Stop smoking and reduce dietary saturated fat and cholesterol intake for overall cardiovascular health. Reducing fat intake also helps reduce caloric intake—important for control of weight and type II diabetes.

(From National Institutes of Health, National Heart, Lung and Blood Institute. *The Fifth Report of the Joint National Committee on Detection, Evaluation and Treatment of High Blood Pressure.* NIH Pub. No. 93-1088. Bethesda, MD: Public Health Service, 1993.)

from reducing their BP. Additional dietary modifications that may help reduce BP are to increase the intake of potassium and calcium; however, the evidence is not as strong for those effects. These modifications are shown in Table 7–5. Caffeine may acutely raise BP, but patients develop a tolerance to that effect rapidly, so it is not necessary to limit caffeine unless the patient has other signs of excessive sensitivity to it. Finally, stress management is usually advised for hypertensive patients, although the research literature does not strongly support it (NIH, NHLBI, 1993).

The decision to begin treatment for hypertension is not a nursing decision, but carefully evaluating the patient's response to treatment, teaching the patient about the medications and other forms of therapy, and providing support and reassurance to the patient and family are part of the role of the nurse. The nurse assists elderly patients as they respond to the diagnosis of hypertension.

First-line antihypertensive drug therapy in the elderly is usually diuretics; beta blockers are also used. Both of these types of drugs have been shown in controlled trials to reduce cardiovascular morbidity and mortality. Alternate drugs are calcium antagonists, angiotensin-converting enzyme (ACE) inhibitors, alpha$_1$-receptor blockers, and alpha-beta blockers. Drug therapy should be carried out more cautiously in older patients because they may be more sensitive to volume depletion and sympathetic inhibition than are younger patients (NIH, NHLBI, 1993; Williams and Lowenthal, 1992). Table 7–6 presents more detailed information on antihypertensive medications. Profound or sudden diuresis may lead to urinary retention or incontinence. Long-acting diuretics may cause excessive nocturia and insomnia. With diuretics, the nurse must watch for hypokalemia, increased blood glucose level, and hyperuricemia.

Adverse reactions to antihypertensive drugs are more common in the elderly. Nurses must be aware of the potential problems related to these drugs, such as electrolyte disturbances, glucose intolerance, depression, orthostatic hypotension, and impotence. The Dunedin study showed that elderly subjects receiving antihypertensive medications had an increased incidence of dizziness, fainting, and "blacking-out spells" (Hale et al., 1984). In addition, blood pressure in the elderly is often reduced after

T A B L E 7 – 6
Antihypertensive Medications: Advantages and Precautions

MEDICATION	ADVANTAGES	PRECAUTIONS
Preferred Agents		
Thiazide diuretics	Effective and well tolerated alone and in combination therapy; convenient and inexpensive; may protect against hip fracture.	Monitor for adverse metabolic effects (e.g., hypokalemia) and postural hypotension.
β-Adrenergic blockers	Useful in concomitant therapy for angina or prophylaxis against recurrent myocardial infarction.	Avoid in patients with bronchospasm, bradyarrhythmias, congestive heart failure, diabetes, or peripheral vascular disease.
Calcium antagonists	Very effective and generally well tolerated; useful in concomitant therapy for angina.	Monitor for potential adverse effects on cardiac conduction and adverse interactions with other cardiovascular drugs.
Useful Agents		
Angiotensin-converting enzyme inhibitors	Relatively free of symptomatic and metabolic side effects; useful in concomitant therapy for congestive heart failure.	May be less effective in elderly than in younger patients; cost, impaired taste, and cough may reduce compliance.
Clonidine	Transdermal formulation reduces symptomatic side effects and may enhance compliance with once-weekly administration.	Sedation and dry mouth are common side effects.
Selective α-antagonists	May have favorable effects on serum lipids and symptoms of prostatic hypertrophy.	May precipitate orthostatic hypotension.
Hydralazine	Better tolerated as a step two agent in elderly than in younger patients.	Concomitant diuretic therapy usually required to prevent fluid retention.
Agents to Avoid		
Guanethidine, guanadrel	—	May cause postural hypotension, sedation, and impotence.
Methyldopa	—	May cause postural hypotension, sedation, impotence, hepatic dysfunction, and hemolytic anemia.

Adapted from Burris, J.F. Hypertension management in the elderly. *Heart Dis Stroke* 3:77–83, 1994. Reproduced with permission. Copyright 1994, American Heart Association.

TABLE 7 – 7

Key Points About Hypertension for Clinicians

1. Elderly hypertensive patients benefit from antihypertensive drug therapy.
2. Systolic hypertension is especially prevalent and dangerous in the elderly and should be treated even when diastolic blood pressure is below 90 mm Hg.
3. There is no absolute upper age limit for treatment of hypertension in otherwise relatively healthy elderly persons.
4. Multiple blood pressure determinations are necessary before confirming a diagnosis of hypertension in the elderly, whose blood pressure is often labile.
5. Nonpharmacologic interventions should be instituted in all hypertensive patients and should be the mainstay of therapy in those with borderline and mild hypertension.
6. Drug therapy should be initiated at lower doses and increased in smaller increments and at longer intervals in older compared with younger patients to avoid abrupt and marked falls in blood pressure.
7. Blood pressure should be monitored in the standing as well as seated or supine position in elderly patients, especially when initiating or changing drug therapy, to avoid postural hypotension. Drugs that frequently cause postural hypotension should be avoided.
8. The benefits of antihypertensive therapy have been proven only in relatively healthy, carefully selected elderly patients, and the study results may not be applicable to the frail elderly with multiple medical problems.
9. The principal therapeutic goal in the elderly is maintaining quality of life rather than extending its duration. Therefore, therapy may not be justified if troublesome side effects cannot be avoided.
10. Low doses of diuretics are virtually equally as effective as high doses, produce fewer symptomatic and metabolic side effects, and may be associated with improved outcomes.
11. Diuretics and β-blockers are the principal drugs used in studies of hypertension in the elderly to date. It is not known whether newer drugs such as α-blockers, calcium channel blockers, and angiotensin-converting enzyme inhibitors will produce outcomes that are better, worse, or equal to those achieved so far.
12. Step-down therapy (reduction of the number and dosage of medications) should be attempted after 6 to 12 months of successful treatment. However, complete withdrawal of treatment is rarely possible.

From Burris, J.F. Hypertension management in the elderly. *Heart Dis Stroke* 3:77–83, 1994. Reproduced with permission. Copyright 1994, American Heart Association.

meals. Therefore, to prevent postural hypotension, elderly patients should not take antihypertensives with meals. A summary of the key points about caring for hypertensive elderly patients is given in Table 7–7.

Nurses must also be aware of the potential problems of elderly hypertensive patients. These people are at high risk for target organ damage to the kidneys, brain, and eyes. This means that they have the *potential for complications of hypertension, especially renal failure, transient ischemic attacks (TIAs), cerebrovascular accidents, cerebral hemorrhage, and retinal hemorrhage.* Additional nursing diagnoses are High Risk for Noncompliance related to negative side effects of prescribed therapy versus the belief that no treatment is needed without the presence of symptoms; High Risk for Ineffective Management of Therapeutic Regimen related to lack of knowledge of condition, diet restrictions, medications, risk factors, and follow-up care; and High Risk for Fluid Volume Deficit related to medication (diuretic) (Carpenito, 1993; Jaffe, 1991).

Orthostatic Hypotension

Although orthostatic hypertension is not strictly a disease, this symptom, which is characterized by dizziness and lightheadedness on rising from a chair or bed, is a major cause of morbidity in the elderly. It can cause confusion, falls, and a tendency to avoid activity as a result of insecurity and fear of falling. The baroreceptor reflex is intact in the elderly, but it is often blunted. Even a rather modest cardiovascular abnormality may produce orthostatic hypotension in a person confined to a bed with a subacute or chronic illness.

Many conditions can produce this problem. Disorders of the central or peripheral nervous system, cardiovascular problems,

TABLE 7 – 8

Classification of Orthostatic Hypotension in the Elderly

Autonomic insufficiency based on central nervous system lesions
  Shy-Drager syndrome
  Parkinson's disease
  Cerebrovascular disease
  Wernicke's disease
  Chronic alcoholism
  Medications: phenothiazine, tricyclic antidepressants, methyldopa, clonidine, and other centrally acting psychotropics and antihypertensives
Autonomic insufficiency based on peripheral lesions
Diabetes mellitus
Amyloidosis, vitamin deficiencies, paraneoplastic syndromes
  Medications: ganglionic blocking agents, sympatholytic agents
Cardiovascular abnormalities
  Heart block
  Severe varicose veins
  Intravascular volume depletion secondary to salt and water loss, diuretics
  Blood loss
  Medications: hydralazine, prazosin
Idiopathic orthostatic hypotension

From Rowe, J.W. Altered blood pressure. *In* Rowe, J.W. and Besdine, R.W. (eds.). *Health and Disease in Old Age.* Boston: Little, Brown, 1982, p. 218.

TABLE 7 – 9
Anemia in the Elderly

	NORMAL HEMOGLOBIN	ANEMIC Hb	Hct
Women aged 62–80	13.5 g/100	less than 12 g/100	41%
Men aged 62–80	14.8 g/100	less than 13 g/100	44.8%

From Adler, S.S. Anemia in the aged: Causes and considerations. *Geriatrics* 35:49–59, 1980.

and many medications can cause postural hypotension. Table 7–8 lists some conditions that should alert the nurse to the fact that the person may have a *potential for injury related to postural hypotension.*

Treatment of the person with this problem should begin with a review of all medications being taken and must include a careful measure of BP in various positions. Ideally, the BP should be taken after the person has been lying flat for 1 hour and then after he or she has been standing for 1 or 2 minutes. Isometric exercises and elastic stockings, put on before the person gets out of bed, may help prevent orthostatic hypotension. These patients must be cautioned to get up slowly and to sit on the edge of the bed for a few minutes before standing. It is possible that they may have become volume depleted and may not be getting enough sodium in their diet.

Anemia

Anemia is fairly common in the elderly, but it is not due to aging per se. Rather, it is probably due to the increase in underlying conditions, such as apathy, neglect, and dementia, which can lead to malnutrition and development of chronic infections that predispose to anemia (Mansouri and Lipschitz, 1992). Although anemia may be suspected by a clinical finding of pale conjunctiva, it is easily verified by measuring the hemoglobin and hematocrit. Normal values are shown in Table 7–9.

Even mild anemia may be a clue to an underlying disorder. Diseases that produce anemia include gastrointestinal disturbances (caused by malabsorption of nutrients), chronic inflammatory disorders, autoimmune diseases, cardiac valvular diseases, and drug treatment for chronic diseases.

Atherosclerosis

Atherosclerosis, the principal cause of death in Western civilization, is a progressive systemic disease that generally begins in childhood but does not have clinical manifestations until middle to late adulthood. Our knowledge of the pathogenesis of atherosclerosis has changed greatly in the past 10 years. It is now believed that the development of advanced lesions, that is, atheromatous plaques, is a many-faceted process that requires extensive proliferation of smooth muscle cells within the intima of the artery to cause clinical disease. Three fundamental biological processes are involved:

1. Proliferation of the smooth muscle cells of the intimal lining of the artery, plus accumulation of macrophages and T lymphocytes
2. Formation (by the smooth muscle cells) of large amounts of connective tissue matrix, which includes collagen, elastic fibers, and proteoglycans
3. Accumulation of lipids within the cells and the surrounding connective tissue (the lipids mainly being in the form of cholesterol esters and free cholesterol)

All of this is occurring within the intimal layer of the arterial wall (Ross, 1992). The structure of a normal artery is shown in Figure 7–1.

The earliest signs of changes in the lumen of arteries are fatty streaks, which have been shown to be present by the age of 10 years. Autopsy studies of children who died of other causes have shown that these fatty streaks are located at places in the aorta and the coronary and other arteries where atheromatous plaques develop in adults, that is, at branching areas. Over many years, some of these fatty streaks may progress to foam cells filled with lipid droplets, and then to an atheromatous plaque. An advanced plaque typically contains large amounts of intimal smooth muscle cells, surrounded by collagen and elastic fibers; many, but not all, plaques also contain lipids. These lesions do not cause symptoms or clinical events until the lesion has grown to partially or totally occlude the lumen of the artery or until cracks or fissures develop in the lesions (Ross, 1992).

The three major categories of atherosclerotic disease are coronary, cerebral, and peripheral artery disease. The risk factors for the atherosclerotic diseases have been well established. For adults, the major risk factors are hypertension, smoking, low serum levels

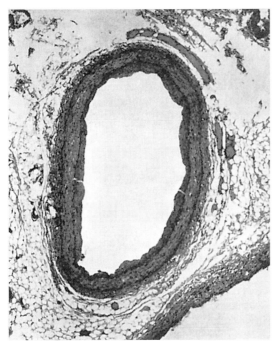

FIGURE 7 – 1

Photomicrograph showing a normal artery seen in cross-section. (By permission of Spain, D.M.; previously published in Scientific American, August 1966; Jacob, S.W. and Francone, G.A. *Elements of Anatomy and Physiology.* 2nd ed. Philadelphia: W.B. Saunders, 1989, p. 199.)

of high-density lipoprotein, high serum levels of low-density lipoprotein, a family history of cardiovascular disease, physical inactivity, glucose intolerance, and high fibrinogen (Kannel, 1992). All of the major risk factors are important in the development of coronary heart disease; however, for stroke, hypertension is particularly important, whereas lipids play a small role. For peripheral arterial disease, cigarette smoking and glucose intolerance are the most important risk factors. In the elderly, some risk factors are not as important as others. For instance, the impact of blood lipid levels, impaired glucose tolerance, and fibrinogen are less in the elderly. However, because the elderly have an increased overall risk of cardiovascular disease, these factors should still be considered. However, even more important risk factors in the elderly are smoking, obesity and weight gain, physical inactivity, and hypertension (Kannel, 1992).

Coronary Artery Disease

In developed countries, cardiovascular disease is the most common cause of death and hospitalization in the elderly, and coronary atherosclerosis is the most common underlying pathology. Autopsy data have shown that 65 to 75 per cent of men aged 50 to 80 years and 60 to 65 per cent of women aged 70 to 80 years have significant coronary stenoses (Rodeheffer and Gerstenblith, 1985), yet less than half this number have clinical evidence of coronary disease. The prevalence and severity of coronary atherosclerosis increase so dramatically with age that more than half of all deaths in people aged 65 years or older are due to coronary disease and about three fourths of all deaths from ischemic heart disease occur in the elderly.

Angina

Angina is chest pain caused by a temporarily insufficient supply of blood to the heart muscle. It commonly occurs with exertion, but a variant of angina occurs at rest. The incidence of angina drops after the age of 80, possibly because of the reduction of physical activity in the very old. The symptoms may be similar to those seen in the young. There may be mild, pressure-like discomfort, with a suffocating, strangling, crushing, or heavy sensation located under the sternum. This sensation often radiates down the inside of the left arm, and it may or may not radiate to the right arm, neck, jaw, or throat. Because of the increased tolerance to pain common in the elderly, the older patient may not experience chest pain at all but may have what has been called "anginal equivalents": breathlessness, faintness, or extreme fatigue. Dyspnea is a common anginal equivalent in the elderly.

Angina may be either stable or unstable. Stable angina usually indicates a pattern of symptoms that recur in a regular fashion, rather predictably. Stable angina may occur for many years, and patients usually have medications prescribed that are effective. Unstable angina, or angina that is characterized by a change in frequency, type, or severity of symptoms, usually requires medical attention.

The treatment for angina pectoris in the older patient is similar to that given to younger patients. It is designed to improve the myocardial oxygen supply-demand ratio. To reduce myocardial oxygen consumption and increase coronary blood flow, sublingual nitroglycerin is given for attacks, and long-acting nitrates are often given to prevent or reduce the frequency of angina. Because of loss of vasomotor and baroreceptor reactivity, the older patient is more likely to have orthostatic hypotension, so a lower dose of nitrates may be indicated (Borst and Lowenthal, 1992). Nitroglycerin should be taken in the sitting position to reduce the chance of postural hypotension. If it is taken when supine, there is an increase in venous side effects and a decrease in the desired cardiac effects.

Long-acting nitroglycerin is frequently prescribed as a topical ointment or in the form of paste patches that are applied to the skin. Nurses must teach patients to remove previous patches when the next one is applied to avoid an accidental overdose. In addition, patients should be instructed to place the patch in an area that will allow for maximum absorption. Some men put the patch on their feet, under their stockings. Although this may be convenient, it could impede absorption in patients who have peripheral vascular disease, which is associated with reduced circulation to the extremities. A better location would be the chest or the inner aspect of the upper arm.

Beta blockers, such as propranolol (Inderal), atenolol (Tenormin), and nadolol (Corgard) are used to decrease myocardial oxygen consumption by reducing the heart rate, BP, and myocardial contractility. These patients must be carefully monitored because resting heart rate is often lower, and the incidence of sinus and AV node dysfunction is greater in the elderly. There is a greater risk of provoking symptomatic bradyarrhythmias, including heart block, with beta blockade. The side effects, such as central nervous system depression, excessive fatigue, and hypoglycemia, may be more common in older than in younger patients.

The relatively new class of drugs, calcium antagonists, act as direct coronary vasodilators. Nifedipine (Procardia) and verapamil (Calan, Isoptin) are examples of drugs that have been used very successfully in elderly patients (Borst and Lowenthal, 1992).

Some lifestyle changes are also recommended for patients with angina. Smoking may exacerbate angina because cigarettes contain nicotine, which stimulates catecholamine release. This phenomenon increases cardiac work and myocardial irritability and causes coronary vasoconstriction and platelet aggregation. Smokers also may have high levels of carbon monoxide in their blood, which reduces the ability of the blood to deliver oxygen to the myocardium.

Patients with angina should also avoid heavy meals, cold weather, and caffeine. They should avoid emotional and physical strain. If sexual activity brings on an anginal attack, prophylactic nitroglycerin used just before maximal exertion may prevent the pain. Patients who also have chronic lung disease should be told that drugs given for an asthma attack may aggravate angina. These agents include some over-the-counter preparations that contain beta-adrenergic drugs. Excessive thyroid replacement may also aggravate angina (Borst and Lowenthal, 1992).

Acute Myocardial Infarction

The clinical presentation of an acute myocardial infarction (AMI) in the elderly may be quite different from that in the young. As in the young, some elderly patients may present with the typical picture of acute, crushing, substernal chest pain that is not relieved by nitroglycerin and rest and is accompanied by hypotension and sweating. However, often the clinical features of AMI in the elderly are quite subtle. Rather than pain, dyspnea and symptoms related to decreased cardiac output, including confusion and mental status changes, may be prominent; (Gerstenblith, 1992). Not only is the clinical presentation different, the clinical course can be much more complicated, and the mortality rate from AMI is higher in the elderly, as is the risk of congestive heart failure, pulmonary edema, and ventricular rupture.

Postural hypotension is a drop in systolic BP, when moving to a standing position, of 20 to 30 mm Hg that is sustained for at least 1 to 2 minutes. Assuming an upright posture produces a pooling of blood in the lower body, which, if unopposed by autonomic responses, results in hypotension. The elderly are particularly prone to postural hypotension because of the age-related loss of elasticity of the carotid sinuses, which combines with hypertension to reduce the sensitivity of the baroreceptors. In addition, there is a reduction in the responsiveness of the sympathetic autonomic system (Borst and Lowenthal, 1992). In persons older than 75 years, the prevalence of postural hypotension is 30 to 45 per cent. Cardiovascular drugs that can cause postural hypotension are alpha and beta blockers, diuretics, vasodilators, and calcium channel blockers.

Medical management of an acute myocardial infarction has changed greatly in the past 10 years. Thrombolytic therapy is now recommended as soon as possible after the infarction, and there is some evidence that elderly patients obtain even greater benefit from this therapy than do younger patients

TABLE 7 – 10
Risk Assessment Measuring Potential Risk for Thrombolytic Therapy

POTENTIAL	RISK FACTORS
Potential for increased mortality	History of angina pectoris, history of previous myocardial infarction, hypertension, congestive heart failure, diabetes mellitus, heart block, bundle branch block
Potential for bleeding complications	Female, low body weight, hypertension, older than 75 years
Potential for heparin complications	Altered bleeding times
Potential for compromise of patient's coagulation system	Altered fibrinogen levels, increased fibrin-degradation products
Potential for allergic reaction	Exposure to streptococci bacteria, exposure to streptokinase
Potential for drug-related hemodynamic compromise	Hypotension, risk of hypotension
Potential for reinfarction	High-grade stenotic lesion, three-vessel disease

From House, M.A. Thrombolytic therapy for acute myocardial infarction: The elderly population. *AACN Clin Issues* 3(2):106–113, 1992.

(Muller and Topol, 1990; O'Connor and Califf, 1992). Unfortunately, studies indicate that many physicians may not consider this relatively aggressive treatment for patients older than 70 years (Hendra and Marshall, 1992). The main cause of mortality and complications with thrombolytic therapy is hemorrhage. Increased age alone should not be a major consideration in the choice of therapy. House (1992) provided guidelines to use to assess the potential risks related to thrombolytic therapy (Table 7–10).

The elderly are also good candidates for percutaneous transluminal coronary angioplasty (PTCA). This noninvasive procedure is particularly useful for those who are at increased risk for a poor outcome from revascularization surgery. PTCA does not require a thoracotomy, general anesthesia, or the prolonged convalescence associated with surgery. Early clinical trials showed that the elderly had more complications and a higher mortality from PTCA than did younger patients, but more recent data indicate that increased age itself is not a contraindication. The elderly have similar long-term benefits from the procedure as younger patients (Gerstenblith, 1992).

In the past 5 years, the use of these new therapies in the elderly has increased, and the use of potentially harmful drugs, such as calcium channel blockers, has declined. This has led to a 10 per cent decrease in mortality due to AMI in the elderly from 1987 to 1990 (Pashos et al., 1993).

The management of elderly AMI patients in the coronary care unit may be difficult. Management may be complicated by confusion, made worse in the elderly by displacement to an unfamiliar environment, disorientation, and the typical presence of disease in other major organ systems. Nursing interventions are similar to those used in younger patients. However, some measures to prevent disorientation are needed, such as more frequent visits by relatives, providing glasses and hearing aids, and keeping a few personal items in the room, even in the coronary care unit.

Cardiac Rehabilitation for the Elderly

Rehabilitation is very important to the elderly cardiac patient. Rehabilitation goals include the preservation and maintenance of physical functional capacity, strength, and coordination, which provide for mobility and self-sufficiency. Mental functional integrity must also be maintained so that the elderly cardiac patient can remain alert and maintain self-respect and self-confidence. A well-planned cardiac rehabilitation program promotes both physical and mental functional capacity, as well as limits or prevents anxiety and depression. It also encourages readjustment to family, community, and society (Carroll and Pollock, 1992).

Teaching about cardiac disease, lifestyle modifications that may be recommended, diet, signs and symptoms of possible complications, and the expected actions and possible side effects of drugs should be part of a rehabilitation program. In addition, such a program should include emotional support of the patient and family as well as information about when to call the health care professional and the importance of continuing physical activity. Group classes are particularly helpful with elderly patients because they provide an opportunity to share experiences and make suggestions.

Physical training begins in the hospital with early ambulation. Nursing research has shown that it requires more energy to use a

TABLE 7 – 1 1

Maximum Heart Rate Predicted by Age and Conditioning*

MAXIMUM HEART RATE, %	AGE, YR														
	20	25	30	35	40	45	50	55	60	65	70	75	80	85	90
Unconditioned															
100%	197	195	193	191	189	187	184	182	180	178	176	174	172	170	168
90%	177	175	173	172	170	168	166	164	162	160	158	157	155	153	152
75%	148	146	144	143	142	140	138	137	135	134	132	131	129	128	127
60%	118	117	115	114	113	112	110	109	108	107	106	104	103	102	101
Conditioned															
100%	190	188	186	184	182	180	177	175	173	171	169	167	165	163	161
90%	171	169	167	166	164	162	159	158	156	154	152	150	149	147	145
75%	143	141	140	138	137	135	133	131	130	128	127	125	124	122	121
60%	114	113	112	110	109	108	106	105	104	103	101	100	99	98	97

From Anderson, J.M. Rehabilitating elderly cardiac patients. *Rehabil Med* 154(5):574–578, 1991.

bedpan than to get on a commode. Patients are usually allowed out of bed soon after an uncomplicated AMI and may walk in the halls within a few days after the infarct. This early ambulation reduces some of the complications of immobility and prevents deconditioning. It also provides the nurse with an opportunity to teach the patient how to monitor the heart rate and to use that information for pacing.

A cardiac rehabilitation program can safely improve cardiac functional capacity, reduce ischemic episodes during ordinary activities, improve psychological outlook, modify cardiovascular risk factors, improve health habits, and decrease morbidity and mortality. A study of the effects of exercise on left ventricular function in 79 patients with coronary artery disease showed that age did not influence left ventricular func-

tion at rest or in response to exercise. Heart function was related to the extent of the disease, not to the age of the subjects (Hakki et al., 1983). Unfortunately, not all patients who have had an MI participate in cardiac rehabilitation. Studies have shown that older women are less likely to be referred for cardiac rehabilitation, although they can have improvements in functional capacity similar to those seen in men (Ades et al., 1992).

Carroll and Pollock (1992) divided the exercise portion of cardiac rehabilitation into three phases. Phase I, the inpatient program, begins as soon after the event as the patient is stable, usually 2 to 4 days for an uncomplicated MI. Activities during this time include progression from self-care activities and range-of-motion exercises to low-level ambulation and stair climbing by the time the patient is discharged from the hospital.

TABLE 7 – 1 2

Comparison of the Exercise Prescription for Cardiac Patients and Healthy Adults

PRESCRIPTION	HEALTHY ADULT	PHASE I	PHASE II	PHASE III
Intensity	50%–85% HRR_{max}	RHR + 20	RHR + 20*; RPE 13	50%–85% HRR_{max}
Frequency	3–5 d/wk	2–3 times/d	1–2 times/d	3–5 times/wk
Duration	20–60 min	MI: 5–20 min	20–60 min	30–60 min
Type of activity	Walk, jog, run, bike, swim, cal, weights, endurance sports	ROM, TDM, bike, 1 flight stairs	ROM, TDM, bike, arm erg, cal, weights	Walk, bike, jog, swim, cal, weights, endurance sports

Adapted from Pollock, M.L. and Wilmore, J.H. Exercise in Health and Disease, 2nd ed. Philadelphia, W.B. Saunders, 1990, p. 741.
* 3–6 wk after surgery or MI, a symptom-limited exercise test is recommended, after which intensity can be based on 60%–70% of maximal heart rate reserve.
MI = myocardial infarction patient; CABG = coronary artery bypass graft surgery patient; HRR_{max} = maximal heart rate reserve; RHR = standing resting heart rate; ROM = range-of-motion exercise; TDM = treadmill; arm erg = arm ergometer; cal = calisthenics; RPE = rating of perceived exertion.

Phase II of rehabilitation begins at discharge and lasts for 8 to 12 weeks. This is a transitional time in which the patient progresses from a restricted, low-level program, to a less restricted, moderate-level training program. The intensity of the training gradually increases so that by the third or fourth week after MI or cardiac surgery, the patient's heart rate during exercise is 20 beats above that during standing rest. After an exercise stress test is performed, the intensity of activity is based on reaching 60 to 70 per cent of the predicted maximal heart rate reserve. Exercises include walking, biking, arm ergometry, mild calisthenics, and in the later stages of phase II, swimming and jogging. Phase III, the long-term program, is often performed in a community-based gymnasium program. The exercises are more varied, and intensity can increase somewhat, up to 80 to 85 per cent of maximal heart rate. Table 7–11 gives sample target heart rates based on the age and the conditioning of the patient.

Although the components of the exercise prescription are the same for the elderly as for the healthy younger adult, there is a difference in the application of the principles of exercise prescription, as is shown in Table 7–12. The elderly need a longer warm-up period because they take longer to reach steady-state levels of heart rate and blood pressure than do younger subjects. They also need a more prolonged cool-down period because of potential problems with orthostatic hypotension and heat dissipation. Low-level aerobic activities and stretching should be included in the cool-down (Carroll and Pollock, 1992).

Surgery for Coronary Artery Disease

Elderly patients with angina that cannot be controlled by medication may be candidates for revascularization surgery. The most common surgery is a coronary artery bypass graft (CABG). In this operation, a blood vessel from another part of the body, usually the saphenous vein, is removed and used as a homograft to carry blood directly from the aorta to the coronary artery distal to the atheromatous plaque that is obstructing the flow of blood, as shown in Figure 7–2. The use of the internal mammary artery for CABG is recommended for elderly patients who do not have diabetes mellitus or severe hyperlipidemia (Azariades et al., 1990). Restenosis is uncommon when the internal mammary artery is used, but it is often seen with saphenous vein grafts.

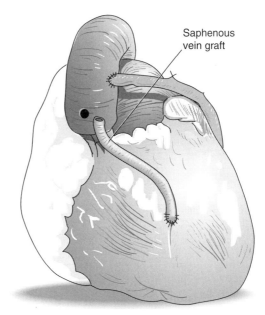

Saphenous vein graft

FIGURE 7 – 2

Nearly completed aortocoronary saphenous vein bypass of the circumflex and anterior descending branches of the left coronary artery.

During the past 10 years, hospital mortality in elderly patients who have undergone CABG has declined to between 2.7 and 7.7 per cent. Typically, mortality is greater in patients older than 75 years, particularly early mortality. Women in this age group are at even higher risk of hospital death than men. Variables that predict perioperative mortality are the same as in younger patients: angina at rest, presence of 70 per cent or more severe stenosis of the left main coronary artery, severe left ventricular dysfunction, and the presence of one or more associated medical disorders. The elderly usually have several associated medical problems. Compared with younger patients, the elderly spend more time in the hospital and are more prone to complications, which include stroke, sternal wound dehiscence, and respiratory failure. However, angina is relieved or diminished in about 80 to 90 per cent of patients older than 65. Thus, advanced age by itself is not a contraindication to surgery (Rutherford and Braunwald, 1992; Smith et al., 1992).

Research has shown that nursing care can significantly improve recovery from cardiac surgery. In a study of 156 patients at two hospitals, patients and spouses assigned to an experimental group received two interventions: (1) supplemental in-hospital education on emotional reactions to surgery and methods of conflict resolution and (2) weekly telephone coaching after discharge to provide support and information. As compared with the control subjects, patients in the experimental group reported significantly greater self-efficacy expectations for walking, and more were walking, lifting, climbing stairs, and returning to work (Gillis et al., 1993).

Arrhythmias

Cardiac arrhythmias in the elderly are important because they are more common, are more often accompanied by cardiac decompensation, and may be harder to treat than in younger patients. Arrhythmias are more serious in the elderly because they compromise the blood supply of organs that may be already seriously impaired by aging and disease and may cause further deterioration of heart function as well as heart failure. Generally, electrophysiology of arrhythmias and the principles of diagnosis and management are the same in the aged as in others (Bexton, 1992).

For any arrhythmia in an elderly patient, the first action is to evaluate the immediate electrical and hemodynamic effects of the arrhythmia on the individual. A rapid identification of the arrhythmia should be made to determine if it is life threatening. If it is identified as ventricular tachycardia, ventricular fibrillation, asystole, or a precursor of these, immediate action is required to terminate the arrhythmia. The next step is to determine how well the patient is tolerating the rhythm. A very rapid heart rate, even if it is sinus tachycardia, may be poorly tolerated in the elderly because the rapid rate reduces the amount of time for cardiac filling, causing a drop in cardiac output. If the person has coronary artery disease or cerebrovascular disease, this drop in output could trigger chest pain, dyspnea, or syncope. Because the person may become hypotensive, the BP should be monitored at intervals during the arrhythmia. An extremely low heart rate could also produce a significant drop in cardiac output, with similar results.

Possible causes of arrhythmias in the elderly are enlargement of the heart chambers and other anatomical changes associated with chronic ischemic heart disease, hypertensive heart disease, cardiomyopathy, or valvular disease. In addition, drug toxicity, heart failure, infection, and electrolyte imbalance, especially low serum potassium level, can all induce arrhythmias (Fenster and Nolan, 1993).

Most of the elderly have normal sinus rhythm (Bexton, 1992; Rials et al., 1992). The incidence of ectopic activity of the heart increases with age, but important arrhythmias and very frequent ectopic beats in the elderly indicate underlying cardiac disease, not normal changes with aging (Harris, 1983). The most common arrhythmias are premature atrial beats, premature ventricular beats, and atrial fibrillation. Precipitating factors for premature ventricular complexes are heavy intake of coffee, smoking, excessive ingestion of alcohol, and ingestion of heavily spiced foods.

Atrial fibrillation occurs in 2 to 5 per cent of asymptomatic ambulatory elderly but more often in hospitalized elderly (Bexton, 1992). It can have particularly severe consequences in the elderly because of the loss of the active contraction of the atrium, the "atrial kick." In the elderly, chronic atrial fibrillation is associated with a significant risk of systemic emboli, which is reduced by long-term anticoagulation with warfarin (Coumadin). The aim of treatment of chronic atrial fibrillation is to control heart rate, which is usually accomplished with beta-adrenergic blockers or verapamil or diltiazem. Although digitalis helps control the ventricular rate in stable patients at rest, it is usually inadequate during exercise or acute illness (Fenster and Nolan, 1993).

Treatment of cardiac arrhythmias is the same in the elderly as in other patients. However, the effect of aging and the presence of concurrent disease may affect the action of antiarrhythmic drugs. Common interactions involving major antiarrhythmic drugs are shown in Table 7–13.

Martin et al. (1984) studied the incidence of arrhythmias in 101 healthy elderly English subjects for 5 years. They found that occasional premature ventricular complexes were very common but were not of concern. However, if premature ventricular complexes occurred at a rate of 10 or more per hour, there was a significant increase in mortality. Atrial fibrillation was also very common, initially occurring in 11 per cent of the subjects but rising with age to 17 per cent by age 84. The third common arrhythmia was bundle branch block, which occurred in over 10 per cent of subjects, the prevalence rising steeply with age. By the end of the study, more than one fourth of the survivors had evidence of disease of the conduction system.

Bradyarrhythmias and conduction disturbances are common in the elderly. The incidence of bundle branch block increases with age. Right bundle branch block, which occurs in about 3.5 per cent of the elderly, is

T A B L E   7 – 1 3
Drug Interactions Involving Major Antiarrhythmic Agents

ANTIARRHYTHMIC DRUG	INTERACTING AGENT	INTERACTION
Digoxin	Quinidine	Increased plasma digoxin concentration
	Amiodarone	Increased plasma digoxin concentration
	Verapamil	Increased plasma digoxin concentration
	Diuretics	Hypokalemia-induced potentiation of digitalis-induced arrhythmias
Verapamil	Beta blockers	Additive effects on depression of sinus node, A-V–conduction system, and left ventricular function
Amiodarone	Warfarin	Potentiation of warfarin anticoagulant effects
	Procainamide	Increased plasma procainamide concentration
	Quinidine	Increased plasma quinidine concentration
Lidocaine	Propranolol	Increased plasma lidocaine concentration
	Cimetidine	Increased plasma lidocaine concentration
	Phenobarbital	Decreased plasma lidocaine concentration
Quinidine	Warfarin	Potentiation of warfarin anticoagulant effects
	Phenobarbital	Decreased plasma quinidine concentration
	Phenytoin	Decreased plasma quinidine concentration
	Diuretics	Exacerbation of orthostatic hypotension; potentiation of hypokalemia-induced arrhythmia, especially torsade de pointes
	Vasodilators	Exacerbation of orthostatic hypotension
	Tricyclic antidepressants	Exacerbation of orthostatic hypotension; additive effects on depression of intraventricular conduction and proarrhythmia
Procainamide	Diuretics	Exacerbation of orthostatic hypotension; potentiation of hypokalemia-induced arrhythmia, especially torsade de pointes
	Vasodilators	Exacerbation of orthostatic hypotension
	Tricyclic antidepressants	Exacerbation of orthostatic hypotension; additive effects on depression of intraventricular conduction and proarrhythmia
Disopyramide	Anticholinergics	Additive anticholinergic side effects
	Diuretics	Potentiation of hypokalemia-induced arrhythmia, especially torsade de pointes
	Tricyclic antidepressants	Additive anticholinergic side effects; additive effects on depression of intraventricular conduction and proarrhythmia
	Verapamil, beta-blockers	Exacerbation of heart failure
Flecainide	Verapamil, beta-blockers	Exacerbation of heart failure
Bretylium	Vasodilators, diuretics	Exacerbation of orthostatic hypotension
Propranolol	Cimetidine	Increased plasma propranolol concentration

From Marinchak, R.A. et al: *Clin Geriatr Med* 4:83–110, 1988.

almost twice as common as left bundle branch block. Uncomplicated right bundle branch block is not associated with increased prevalence of heart disease, but left bundle branch block is nearly always associated with pre-existing organic heart disease. Complete, or third-degree, heart block occurs in about 1 per cent of the elderly and is an indication for insertion of a permanent cardiac pacemaker (Bexton, 1992).

Sick sinus syndrome is an arrhythmia that is more common in the elderly, usually occurring in those in their sixties and seventies. It is characterized either by instances of a very slow heart rate or by the sudden occurrence of a very rapid heart rate alternating with a slow rate. About 60 per cent of elderly with sick sinus syndrome experience a form of tachycardia, which is often accompanied by dizziness or syncope. It may be caused by many drugs, such as digoxin, propranolol, quinidine, lithium, and most sympathetic agents. Sick sinus syndrome is treated by insertion of a permanent pacemaker that provides atrial demand pacing (Rials et al., 1992).

Congestive Heart Failure

Congestive heart failure (CHF) is a clinical syndrome that is defined as a chronic inadequate contraction of the heart muscle, which results in insufficient cardiac output to meet body needs and in circulatory congestion. CHF may be due to systolic or diastolic ventricular dysfunction. The long-term prognosis of CHF depends on the underlying conditions. In the elderly, the most common cause of heart failure is coronary heart disease; other causes are hypertension, valvular heart disease, cardiomyopathy, and aneurism (Centers for Disease Control and Prevention [CDC], 1994; Tighe and Brest, 1992). The prevalence of CHF has increased greatly since 1980, and it is now quite common in the very old. In 1990, the crude death rate for CHF was five times higher for those older than 85 years than for those aged 75 to 84 years and was 18 times higher than for those aged 65 to 74 years (CDC, 1994).

There are several possible explanations for this marked increase in CHF as people age. First, the normal changes of the heart with aging, which slow ventricular filling, may compromise diastolic function and become especially significant during tachycardiac, ischemic, or volume stress. Thus, the left atrial pressure could be increased, and this increased pressure could be transmitted backward to the pulmonary vessels, producing symptoms of shortness of breath and pulmonary edema. Second, there is an increased incidence of diseases in the elderly that predispose them to cardiac failure (Tighe and Brest, 1992; Wei, 1994). Coronary artery disease is the main cause of CHF, but mitral stenosis and insufficiency, calcific aortic stenosis, pulmonary embolism, chronic fibrotic and hemorrhagic pericarditis, subacute bacterial endocarditis, congenital heart disease, thyrotoxicosis, myxedema, bronchitis, and pneumonia can all produce CHF (Rodstein, 1979).

The symptoms of CHF in the elderly include wheezing, cough, dyspnea, and orthopnea, often leading to insomnia and nocturnal wandering. In some patients, the predominating symptoms may be anorexia and nausea. In others, weakness, made worse by chronic malnutrition, may be the major complaint. Weight gain may also be noted as fluid accumulates in the lungs in left-sided heart failure, and in the extremities in right-sided heart failure. Auscultation might reveal moist crackles, or rales, heard best at the end of inspiration. A third heart sound may be heard, caused by the dilatation and noncompliance of the ventricle during rapid filling. Tachycardia is almost invariably present (Tighe and Brest, 1992).

The diagnosis and etiology of CHF may be difficult in the elderly because some of the symptoms, such as dyspnea and ankle edema, may be due to other diseases. Abnormalities of the thoracic cage displace the cardiac apex and complicate palpation. A fourth heart sound is often heard normally in the elderly, and crackles or rales are often heard with chronic lung disease. In addition, there may be no apparent clinical cause for the heart failure. Unfortunately, CHF often presents atypically. Nonspecific signs, such as somnolence, confusion, disorientation, weakness, and fatigue, may be the presenting signs, without dyspnea. In some patients, worsening of pre-existing dementia is an important sign of CHF. Peripheral edema is not a reliable sign of CHF in the elderly, because dependent edema is often seen with immobility (Wei, 1994). A study has shown that CHF is often the precipitating event when elderly persons are admitted with acute confusion (Rockwood, 1989).

In patients with CHF due to systolic dysfunction, treatment consists of rest, digitalis, diuretics, and reduction of afterload and preload. Because prolonged bedrest is dangerous, chair rest is preferred because it enhances diuresis and oxygenation. Preload is reduced with diuretics; afterload may be reduced with vasodilators, particularly nitrates and prazosin. Digitalis is useful in acute CHF, but its role in chronic CHF is controversial. ACE inhibitors, such as captopril and enalapril, have now been shown to be effective in treating CHF; they reduce mortality and may have beneficial synergistic effects with other drugs. In patients with CHD caused solely by diastolic dysfunction, the goal is to enhance ventricular filling. For those patients, calcium antagonists, beta-adrenergic antagonists, and ACE inhibitors may be beneficial (Wei, 1994).

The patient should restrict salt intake to 3 or 4 gm per day or less and eat foods and fruits high in potassium to prevent hypokalemia secondary to the large doses of diuretics that may be required. The elderly person receiving diuretic therapy is also susceptible to calcium and magnesium depletion. Serum levels of potassium, calcium, and magnesium should be monitored regularly (MacLennan et al., 1984a). The impact of CHF on the elderly is severe because it is associated with functional disability due to activity intolerance, long-term drug therapy, and frequent hospitalizations.

Nursing interventions to improve activity tolerance are particularly important because of the diminished cardiac reserve of many elderly, especially those who have led inactive lives. Because prolonged bedrest and inactivity can further reduce that reserve, it is important to encourage some activities but to space them well. During and after activity, the nurse should evaluate the patient's heart rate and watch for shortness of breath, fatigue, or other symptoms.

Valvular Disease

Aortic stenosis is by far the most common and most important valvular lesion in the elderly. It takes one of two forms: (1) calcific aortic stenosis of old age or (2) aortic stenosis, which is either congenital or acquired after rheumatic fever with long-term survival (Channer and Smith, 1992).

To determine the incidence of degenerative calcific valvular disease, Wong et al. (1983) studied 98 subjects aged 65 to 98 years. They diagnosed degenerative calcific valvular disease in 74 per cent of the subjects and heard murmurs in 55 per cent. Only 7 per cent of the subjects had functionally significant disease, and it was not severe in any of those studied. They concluded that degenerative calcific valvular disease is the cause of most systolic murmurs in the elderly, and they are usually hemodynamically unimportant.

Calcific aortic stenosis is caused by degenerative changes in the aortic cusps, sometimes with fusion of the cusps. In patients in whom the degenerative changes are severe, the clinical presentation is one of fatigue, exertional syncope or near-syncope, and angina that may be clinically identical to the angina of coronary artery disease. On auscultation, there is a systolic ejection murmur, which is loudest at the right upper sternal border and is conducted to the neck vessels and above the clavicles. The intensity of the murmur is *not* related to the severity of the disease, because this murmur may be heard in the absence of clinically significant disease. A fourth heart sound is common, whereas the S_2 is soft or absent. Peripheral signs are often misleading in the elderly. Cardiac catheterization is the only sure way to diagnose this condition (Channer and Smith, 1992; Wei, 1994).

Treatment of calcific aortic stenosis is surgery, but only if the lesion is severe enough to produce symptoms. Santiaga et al. (1983) reported on a series of aortic valve replacements in 77 patients older than age 60. The mortality rate for the 55 patients with only aortic valve replacement was 5.5 per cent. The mortality for the entire series, which included patients with multiple valve replacements and concomitant CABG, was 13 per cent. The authors concluded that aortic valve replacement can be carried out safely in the elderly, and the indications should be the same as those used for younger patients.

In the elderly, aortic stenosis that was acquired early in life does not differ much from calcific stenosis of old age, except that it is usually nonprogressive and tends to be milder, so surgery is indicated less often. If it is secondary to rheumatic fever, there is a high likelihood that the mitral valve is also involved (Wei, 1994).

Mitral annulus calcification is a process found almost exclusively in the elderly. It can produce severe hemodynamic abnormalities of the mitral valve. The mobility of the mitral leaflets is limited, causing mitral insufficiency in most patients and occasionally stenosis if the calcific mass is close to the mitral orifice. Medical therapy is recommended because surgical replacement of the mitral valve is difficult owing to the calcium deposits. However, surgery may be needed if medical therapy cannot control the symptoms of CHF. The disease is usually mild to moderate, so mitral valve replacement is seldom required (Channer and Smith, 1992; Wei, 1994).

Mitral insufficiency is very common in the elderly. It may result from mucoid degeneration of the mitral valve, from ruptured chordae tendineae, or from severe papillary muscle dysfunction. In the last two cases, pulmonary hypertension and severe left-sided and right-sided heart failure may occur. This condition is characterized by a loud apical holosystolic murmur that radiates widely to the axilla and even to the neck. Diagnosis and treatment are the same as those in younger patients (Channer and Smith, 1992; Wei, 1994).

Cerebral Vascular Disease

Transient Ischemic Attack

A TIA, called a "little stroke" by some, is characterized by transient focal neurological signs and symptoms that occur suddenly and last a short time, usually less than an hour, and never longer than 24 hours. In about 90 per cent of the aged who have this syndrome, it is caused by a microembolism to the brain from atherosclerotic plaques in the aortocranial arteries. In the remainder, it is caused by mural thrombi; valvular diseases of the heart, especially mitral valve prolapse; vegetations on the heart valves; polycythemia, or some other blood clotting disorder. The presence of a TIA is indicative of an impending stroke in about 25 to 35 per cent of those with this syndrome, but at present, there is no way to clearly identify those who go on to develop a stroke. About a third of those who have a TIA have no residual deficits afterward, and about a third have only one episode (Brust, 1994; Kane-Carlsen, 1990).

The specific signs and symptoms of a TIA vary depending on which vessel is involved, the degree of obstruction of the vessel, and the collateral blood supply. If the anterior (carotid) system is involved, the person may experience ipsilateral blindness, monocular blurring, gradual obscuration of vision, flashes of light, and headaches that may simulate a migraine. If the posterior (vertebrobasilar) system is involved, symptoms may include tinnitus and vertigo, simultaneous bilateral sensory and motor symptoms, and signs of brainstem pathology, including diplopia, facial weakness, ataxia, and "drop attacks" (falling without losing consciousness) (Kane-Carlsen, 1990).

It is important to recognize some symptoms that may be confused with TIAs. The following are *not* part of the syndrome: simple alterations of consciousness, syncope, graying out of vision, lightheadedness, dizziness and giddiness alone, vertigo alone, generalized seizures, and nausea and vomiting alone (Brust, 1994).

Elderly persons who have a TIA may ignore the episode because the symptoms completely resolve. However, they should be seen by a physician so that a major disabling stroke may be prevented. Patients who have a TIA need a complete medical evaluation to determine its cause and to rule out intracranial tumors. The most important diagnostic test is ultrasonographic duplex scanning (Thiele and Strandness, 1994). Studies have shown that carotid endarterectomy is more beneficial than aspirin in patients with TIAs (Brust, 1994). In a recently completed clinical trial of 659 patients with TIAs and incomplete strokes, those randomly assigned to medical treatment (aspirin and anticoagulants) had a 26 per cent occurrence of stroke over 2 years, whereas those who received carotid endarterectomy had only a 9 per cent occurrence of stroke (North American Symptomatic Carotid Endarterectomy Trial) [NASCET], 1991). Patients most likely to benefit from carotid endarterectomy are those with a greater than 80 per cent diameter reduction at the carotid bifurcation. The medical treatment of TIA is presently uncertain (Thiele and Strandness, 1994).

The major role of the nurse in caring for elderly persons with this syndrome is the early identification and referral of people who have these transient symptoms. The nurse may be the first person to whom such vague symptoms are reported. Including auscultation for carotid bruits in the routine assessment of the aged would also lead to early identification of potential problems. The elderly client also needs support and teaching through the diagnostic process, treatment, and possible surgery.

Stroke

Stroke is a syndrome characterized by a sudden or gradual onset of neurological deficits caused by a compromise of the blood supply to a part of the brain. It is the third leading killer in the United States, after heart disease and cancer. About 500,000 Americans suffer a new or recurrent stroke each year. Stroke is the leading cause of serious disability in the United States (American Heart Association, 1993).

The incidence of stroke increases exponentially with age after 55 years of age. In addition to advanced age, the most important risk factor for stroke is hypertension. Other risk factors are a history of TIAs or previous stroke; atherosclerosis, especially in the heart, neck, and legs; and atrial fibrillation. Lifestyle risk factors for stroke are smoking and a high alcohol intake (Mulley, 1992).

Strokes can be classified as thrombotic, embolic, or hemorrhagic. The most common type of stroke in the elderly is the thrombotic stroke, which is associated with atherosclerosis. The most common sites of cerebrovascular atherosclerotic deposits are the bifurcation of the common carotid artery, the origin of the vertebral arteries, and the middle cerebral artery (Thiele and Strandness, 1994; Mulley, 1992).

A survey of stroke patients of all ages found that almost one in three was dead at 3 weeks after the event, with mortality being highest in patients with intracerebral hemorrhage (66 per cent) and subarachnoid hemorrhage (52 per cent) and lower in those with ischemic stroke (15 to 20 per cent). Clinical signs and symptoms on admission that are associated with a poor prognosis are coma, pupillary disturbances, Cheyne-Stokes respirations, dysphagia, and urinary incontinence. Table 7–14 shows how initial impairment of consciousness is related to a patient's chances of surviving stroke. It is important to note that paralysis of limbs is *not* associated with a poor outcome (Mulley, 1992).

In a major stroke, the symptoms are severe and do not disappear. The maximal

TABLE 7 – 14

Effect of Degree of Impairment of Consciousness on Chances of Surviving Stroke

CONSCIOUSNESS LEVEL AT ONSET	% ALIVE AT 1 YEAR
Comatose	15
Semicomatose	30
Somnolent	60
Conscious	90

From Aho, K., Harmsen, M., Hatano, S. et al. Cerebrovascular disease in the community: results of a WHO collaborative study. *Bull WHO* 58:113–130, 1980.

neurological deficits are present at the onset of the stroke. The specific symptoms depend on the location and amount of the brain involved. Symptoms include motor deficits (hemiplegia, dysarthria, dysphagia), sensory deficits (perceptual deficits), language deficits (aphasia), visual deficits, (defects in the visual fields, diplopia, decreased acuity), decreased level of consciousness, intellectual or emotional deficits, and bowel and bladder dysfunction (Leahy, 1991). Other specific symptoms depend on the site of occlusion and which side of the body is involved. Figure 7–3 illustrates the symptoms that may vary with left-sided and right-sided brain damage.

Recovery may take days or months, depending on the amount of brain damage that has occurred. Eventually, a plateau is reached, usually in 3 to 6 months after the event. The focus of nursing care in the first 3 days after the episode includes a complete physical and neurological status examination to provide a baseline measurement and maintenance of life support functions by preventing aspiration and reducing intracranial pressure. Immediate action should be taken to prevent future complications of immobility, such as bedsores and contractures. Later, after the initial "shock" of the stroke is receding, brain edema begins to resolve, and blood flow to the ischemic area begins to improve through collateral circulation. The patient is more attentive to people and the environment and may begin to participate in self-care activities and to learn the extent of his or her deficits. Bedrest should be discontinued when the vital signs have been stable for 48 hours and when the patient is fully awake and alert (Leahy, 1991). Emotional support for the patient and family is especially crucial at this time.

By 2 to 4 weeks after the stroke, cerebral edema should be completely resolved and collateral circulation should be improving. The neurological deficits gradually improve, leaving those that are more or less permanent.

The nursing needs of a stroke patient are complex and varied. Nursing care can be made more precise by recognition of the differences in behavioral responses of patients with left-sided and right-sided brain damage. If the left side of the brain is damaged, right hemiplegia results. Right hemiplegics often have problems with speech and language because the speech center is in the left side of the brain in most people. These patients also tend to be somewhat cautious, anxious, and disorganized when attempting a new task. The American Heart Association

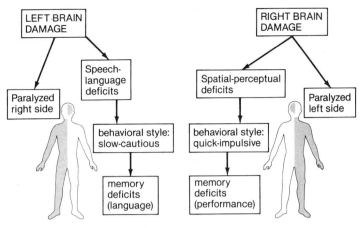

FIGURE 7 – 3

Left-sided and right-sided brain damage in elderly stroke victims. (From Fowler, R.S. and Fordyce, W.E. *Stroke: Why Do They Behave That Way?* Dallas: American Heart Association, 1974, pp. 1–32.)

(Fowler and Fordyce, 1974) makes these suggestions about caring for a right hemiplegic:

1. Do not underestimate the patient's ability to learn and communicate even if he or she cannot use speech.
2. If he or she cannot use speech, try other forms of communication. Pantomime and demonstration are often useful.
3. Do not overestimate the patient's understanding of speech and overload the patient with "static."
4. Do not shout. Keep messages simple and brief.
5. Do not use special voices.
6. Divide tasks into simple steps.
7. Give much feedback and many indications of progress.

If the right side of the brain is damaged, the left side of the body will be paralyzed. Left hemiplegics often have spatial-perception deficits, which can impair their ability to judge distance, size, position, rate of movement, form, and the relation of parts to wholes. These deficits are more subtle than loss of the ability to speak and are often overlooked. In fact, the left hemiplegic can often talk better than he or she can perform. These spatial-perception deficits may have profound effects on the self-care ability of the elderly stroke patient and the family. Patients may not recognize potentially dangerous situations and may overestimate their capacities. They may also have visual field cuts and do not "see" things on the affected (left) side of the body (Fowler and Fordyce, 1974; Mulley, 1992).

American Heart Association suggestions for working with left hemiplegic patients

TABLE 7-15
Possible Complications of Stroke

	INCITING FACTOR(S)	AGGRAVATING FACTOR(S)	PREVENTION	THERAPY
Pressure sores	Prolonged pressure over bony prominences	Poor bed positioning Incontinence	Identify high-risk patient Prescribe regular turning and repositioning	Prescribe intensive nursing care
Peripheral nerve palsy	Traction or pressure injury of peripheral nerve or nerve plexus	Bed and wheelchair positioning Hemiparesis and hemisensory loss	Position properly	Initiate intensive rehabilitation program
Urinary incontinence	Neurogenic bladder	Environmental access Coexisting gynecological or urological disease Medication toxicity	Provide easy access to toilet or commode	Institute bladder schedule Provide incontinence aids Treat coexisting disease
Fecal incontinence	Fecal stasis	Neurogenic bowel Immobility Low fiber diet Dehydration	Encourage early mobilization Increase dietary fiber and fluid intake	Institute bowel program
Adjustment to disability	Brain injury Depression	Inadequate information about deficits and abilities	Ensure early communication regarding prognosis	Provide patient and family education Institute active rehabilitation program
Withdrawal of family support	Stress secondary to impact of illness	Poor premorbid family relationships Inadequate education and involvement of family in therapeutic process	Promote active communication with family Provide programs to involve family in care	Initiate family conferences or family therapy
Depression	Multiple losses Brain injury	Premorbid personality Unrealistic expectations about recovery	Provide early information regarding deficits and prognosis	Set up rehabilitation program to assure sense of progress
Sensory deprivation	Environmental isolation	Dysphasia Hemianopsia Preexisting cognitive and sensory deficits	Provide stimulating environment	Augment sensory input
Medication toxicity	Altered pharmacokinetics and pharmacodynamics	Multiple medications	Review medications Use lowest dosage	Discontinue offending medications
Spasticity	Brain injury	Pain Contractures Anxiety	Position properly	Initiate definitive measures to treat spasticity
Contractures	Immobility	Spasticity Pain	Position properly Prescribe range-of-motion exercises	Institute physical therapy program
Shoulder problems	Hemiparesis	Improper lifting and positioning of flaccid shoulder	Lift and position shoulder properly	Treat specific conditions
Falls	Hemiparesis	Orthostatic hypotension Coexisting musculoskeletal, neurological, or cardiovascular disease Medication toxicity	Institute environmental safety program	Increase environmental safety measures Eliminate possible offending medications
Physical deconditioning	Hemiparesis Immobility	Coexisting chronic diseases	Encourage early rehabilitation	Institute a graded exercise program

From Kelly, J. and Winograd, C.H. A functional approach to stroke management in elderly patients. *J Am Geriatrics Soc* 33:48–60, 1985.

with significant spatial-perceptual deficits include:

1. Do not overestimate their abilities. Spatial-perceptual deficits are easy to miss.
2. Use verbal cues if the patients have difficulty with demonstration.
3. Break tasks into small steps and give much feedback.
4. Watch to see what they can do safely rather than taking their word for it.
5. Minimize clutter around them.
6. Avoid rapid movement around them.
7. Highlight visual reference points.

The elderly stroke patient is subject to many complications. Nursing care should focus on prevention of these complications.

Table 7–15 provides a list of potential problems, factors that might aggravate the problems, and measures to prevent and treat these complications.

The major rehabilitation goals for geriatric stroke victims are to prevent complications from inactivity and to prevent additional strokes and other vascular events. Thus, it is vital to have ways to safely increase activity in these patients. A nursing study of 33 geriatric stroke patients during ambulation validated that they are at risk for activity intolerance but also showed that subjective symptoms, such as dyspnea and weakness, were good predictors of activity intolerance. Other predictors were changes in heart rate and rhythm and in respiratory rate and pattern. The authors concluded that elderly stroke patients can be taught to recognize signs of activity intolerance so they can begin low-risk rehabilitation exercise programs (Mol and Baker, 1991).

Peripheral Vascular Disease—Claudication

A large number of elderly have symptoms of arterial occlusive disease, presenting as weak or absent pedal pulses and cold or even cyanotic feet. In one study of 261 Belgians with an average age of 80, the incidence of arterial occlusive disease was found to be 45 per cent (Petermans, 1984). However, only a minority of people with cold feet and faint pedal pulses suffer from severe symptoms, such as intermittent claudication or rest pain, and even fewer go on to develop frank necrosis and gangrene (Walsh and Nauta, 1989).

The main cause of claudication in the elderly is atherosclerosis. Because this is a systemic problem, the person with claudication is very likely to have other related problems, such as angina, a history of heart attacks, or cerebrovascular disease. The location of the atherosclerotic obstruction determines the location of pain. An obstruction in the femoral artery usually causes calf pain; pain in the gluteal region and thigh or even in the back could be caused by an obstruction higher in the arterial system, perhaps at the bifurcation of the aorta (Walsh and Nauta, 1989).

Some other, less common, causes of ischemia of the legs are diabetes; venous stasis with ulceration; arterial embolization; trauma, especially a fractured femur; and polyarteritis.

Symptoms that may make a nurse suspect that an elderly patient has peripheral vascular disease include complaints of cold feet on warm days, a burning pain in the feet when they are warmed, and intermittent claudication. This latter symptom is very characteristic. The person has leg pain and cramps when walking that are completely relieved with rest. Typically, the pain is induced by walking a specific distance, such as two blocks. This distance is fairly consistent for an individual. If leg pain is present at rest, there is probably advanced obstructive disease complicated by poor collateral flow (Thiele and Strandness, 1994; Walsh and Nauta, 1989).

On physical examination, there are diminished or absent peripheral pulses. In addition, a bruit may be heard over the obstructed artery. The affected leg may have a red or violaceous skin color with mottling. It may show pallor when elevated and redness when dependent and may feel cool to the touch. There is an increased venous filling time. Color is slow to return to the leg after pressure is applied. In addition, trophic changes may be seen in the leg. These include thinning of the skin, loss of hair, thick nails, and decreased muscle mass (Thiele and Strandness, 1994; Walsh and Nauta, 1989).

Most patients with chronic arterial occlusive disease and intermittent claudication are treated conservatively and do not require surgery. In these patients, it is vital to control risk factors, especially cigarette smoking. Patients should be told that if they continue to smoke, their arterial disease will progress, and they may lose a limb. Patients who stop smoking, lose weight (if overweight), and start a regular exercise program can see significant improvement in their symptoms. Diabetes, if present, should be rigidly controlled, because peripheral vascular disease is more common and progresses much faster in those with diabetes. The only medication that has been shown to improve intermittent claudication is pentoxifylline, an agent that lowers blood viscosity by making red blood cells more deformable (Thiele and Strandness, 1994).

If the elderly patient is severely disabled and cannot carry out daily activities because of leg pain, surgical correction may be considered. Surgery can take the form of vascular reconstruction of percutaneous transluminal angioplasty (PTA). The 5-year patency of aortobifemoral grafts is more than 90 per cent, and the surgical mortality is about 1 to 2 per cent. PTA is most effective in cases in which surgery cannot be justified either because of the location of the lesion or because the patient is a poor surgical risk. Although complication rates as high as 50 per cent have been reported with PTA, most are minor, and subsequent surgical intervention was required in fewer than 5 per cent (Walsh and Nauta, 1989). Figure 7–4 shows changes that would be expected in an atherosclerotic plaque with angioplasty.

Some local treatments are important to preserve tissue. The feet must be kept clean, and all trauma should be avoided because healing in the absence of adequate arterial flow would be severely compromised. Thickened nails or skin callosities should be treated by a podiatrist because of the danger of ulceration. Infections should be promptly treated with an appropriate antibiotic. Ulcers may develop as a complication of peripheral vascular disease. If so, skillful nursing care is required, involving regular, gentle cleansing of the ulcer. The ulcer can be firmly bandaged, allowing the blood supply to improve with walking.

Venous Disease

Varicose veins, the simplest of venous disorders, may develop in the elderly as the

TABLE 7–16
Factors That Predispose to Deep Vein Thrombosis

Hypercoagulability
Postoperative state
Fever
Abrupt discontinuation of anticoagulants
Some malignancies, such as cancer of the pancreas
Dehydration
Acute or chronic inflammation (urinary tract infections, cellulitis, bronchopneumonia)

Changes in the Vessel Wall
Trauma, especially hip fractures
Peripheral vascular disease
Degenerative diseases
Pooling
Varicose veins

Venous Stasis
Obesity
Congestive heart failure
Arrhythmias, especially atrial fibrillation
Long-term immobility

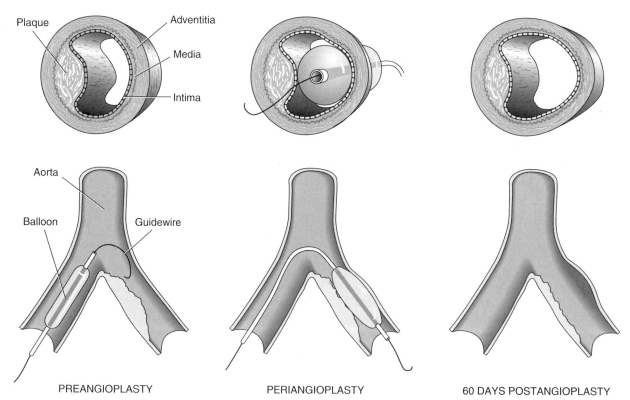

PREANGIOPLASTY   PERIANGIOPLASTY   60 DAYS POSTANGIOPLASTY

FIGURE 7–4

The plaque fracturing and remodeling that occurs with angioplasty in the iliac arteries. (Walsh, D.B., and Nauta, R.J. Peripheral vascular disease in the geriatric patient. In Reichel, W. [ed.]: *Clinical Aspects of Aging.* 3rd ed. Baltimore: Williams & Wilkins, 1989, pp. 106–123. Copyright 1989, Williams & Wilkins.)

veins lose their elasticity and the muscles supporting them weaken. The treatment consists simply of consistent use of elastic stockings to counteract stasis and swelling. Vein ligation and stripping may not be necessary if support hose are worn. Other conservative measures are periodic leg elevation, weight loss if needed, and avoidance of prolonged standing and constrictive clothing. Exercises, as walking, cycling, and swimming, are recommended (Fahey, 1988).

Thrombophlebitis is the inflammation of superficial or deep veins; the incidence increases with advanced age. The symptoms of superficial thrombophlebitis are a red, warm, painful, or tender area under the skin along the course of a vein. It can occur in varicose as well as in normal veins. There is no edema and no danger of emboli, so no anticoagulant therapy is needed. Treatment consists of the application of moist heat, rest, and elevation of the extremity (Fahey, 1988).

Deep vein thrombosis (DVT) is more difficult to diagnose. There may be minimal physical findings, or edema may be present with distended superficial veins, a reddish cyanotic color of the leg, pain, and tenderness. Unfortunately, about half of the patients with clinical signs of DVT have normal veins, whereas others with the problem may have no clinical signs (MacLennan et al., 1984b; O'Neill, 1992).

The danger of DVT is the association with emboli and the possibility of a fatal pulmonary embolus. DVT bosis and pulmonary emboli are the leading causes of morbidity and mortality in hospitalized patients, especially the elderly (Lee et al., 1980).

There are three primary predisposing factors to DVT; venous stasis, hypercoagulability, and injury to the venous wall intima. Effects of these factors are increased by advanced age, surgery, prolonged bedrest, prolonged crossing or strapping of the legs, obesity, and a previous history of DVT (Fahey, 1988; MacLennan et al., 1984b). Table 7–16 lists some factors in the elderly that may predispose to DVT.

Some of these factors, such as dehydration and immobility, can be diagnosed and treated by nurses. Others, such as surgery and the presence of cancer, cannot be treated directly, but their presence can increase our awareness of the potential problem of DVT and pulmonary emboli.

Prevention of DVT begins with treatment of the underlying disorder. In addition, some physicians use prophylactic anticoagulation for patients at risk, but studies have demonstrated real benefit for the elderly only in those with a fractured proximal femur (Fahey, 1988; MacLennan, et al., 1984b). Heparin is usually used because oral anticoagulants are less effective.

Diagnosis of DVT can be difficult. The

TABLE 7–17
Therapy for Peripheral Occlusive Disease

CONDITION	SIGNS AND SYMPTOMS	TREATMENT
Acute arterial occlusions	Drop in temperature below nearest joint distal to occlusion (with acute emboli, there can be a second drop in temperature several inches below the first); pallor, mottling of involved skin	For thrombosis, surgery may be needed for threatened limb; however, improvement without treatment occurs in many cases. For embolism, intravenous heparin (dosage 5,000 units initially, then 300–1,000 units by continuous IV infusion, adjusted inversely with age); embolectomy, preferably under local anesthesia, except when embolus inaccessible (e.g., retinal or cerebral) or unimportant (e.g., splenic); where damage is irreversible, amputation at the lowest possible level is necessary
Chronic arterial occlusions	Claudication after walking; cramping, burning, numbness, rest pains in foot; necrotic signs, e.g., cracks, deep cyanosis, pallor, blackening	Surgical repair (endarterectomy, bypass graft using prosthesis or saphenous vein), when possible; if not possible, amputation at lowest possible level
Venous disorders	Swelling, warmth, cyanosis (severe cases), tenderness in lower third of calf (frequent in deep venous thrombosis)	For deep venous thrombosis (DVT), heparin (initial dose, 3,000–5,000 units IV; maintenance dose, 300–1,000 units per hour by continuous pump infusion for a few days) followed by warfarin sodium (Coumadin, Panwarfin) (initial dose 10 mg per day for 2–3 days until prothrombin time is 1.5–2 times control, then 2.5–10.0 mg per day for 6–8 weeks), unless contraindicated; alternative is dextran 70 (Macrodex) (300–500 ml IV per day) or (where risk of venous embolism great) venous interruption. For postphlebitic syndrome, employ conservative management, e.g., elastic bandages or stockings or, at most, skin grafting of stasis ulcers.

From Couch, N.P. How to establish a diagnosis in peripheral vascular disease. *Geriatric* 36(2):44–52, 1981.

most sensitive test is contrast phlebography, in which the venous system is visualized by the injection of contrast material, or dye, into the superficial veins of the foot or ankle. Other, less invasive, methods are available. These include Doppler ultrasound studies, plethysmography, and fibrinogen scanning (O'Neill, 1992).

Treatment of DVT consists of aggressive anticoagulation, pain control, and bedrest. Heparin is the initial anticoagulant used, followed by an oral anticoagulant. Because aging increases sensitivity to oral anticoagulants, lower doses of warfarin may be given to the elderly. However, recent studies provide conflicting evidence regarding the dose-related effects of oral anticoagulants, so the precise dose to use in the elderly is not clear. Oral anticoagulants should be used for at least 4 weeks (O'Neill, 1992). Nursing care must consist of careful observation for any signs of bleeding as well as alleviation of symptoms of DVT, especially because the elderly are often receiving other drugs that can either interfere with or potentiate the action of the oral anticoagulant.

Table 7–17 summarizes the therapy for arterial and venous peripheral vascular disease.

SPECIAL ISSUES

Smoking Cessation in the Elderly

Smoking cessation is of paramount importance for the elderly. In a study of 1394 men aged 65 to 74 who had been followed for 12 years, the relative risk for CHD was higher in elderly smokers than in nonsmokers. Further, the risk for CDH was 3.6 events per 1000 person-years in elderly smokers, as compared with 1.9 events for middle-aged smokers, prompting the authors to conclude that the dangers of smoking "increase exponentially with age" (Benfante et al., 1991). Another large study showed that in white women, stopping smoking at any age substantially reduced the risk of stroke within 2 to 4 years of quitting. Thus, smoking cessation counseling should be given to smokers at every opportunity and used as a preventive strategy against disease as well as a therapeutic intervention in all elderly patients (Heuser and Hazzard, 1994).

Cardiovascular Disease in Women

Recently, health professionals have become more aware of the importance of cardiovascular disease in women, especially elderly women. Cardiovascular diseases, especially CHD and stroke, are the leading causes of death in women in the United States and cause more deaths than cancer, accidents, and diabetes combined. The age-adjusted death rates from heart diseases in women are four times higher in white women and six times higher in black women than the death rates from breast cancer. By the ages of 75 to 84 years, the death rate from CHD in women is more than 1290 per 100,000 population (Eaker et al., 1993).

Although the risk factors for cardiovascular disease are the same in women as in men, those risk factors may affect women differently. For example, there is some evidence that diabetes, hypertriglyceridemia, low levels of high-density lipoprotein cholesterol, obesity, and sedentary lifestyle seem to be stronger risk factors for women than for men (Eaker et al., 1993). However, more research is needed. Unfortunately, the prevalence of smoking in women has increased, so more elderly women are now likely to be smokers, thus further increasing their risk for cardiovascular disease.

Diagnosis and treatment of cardiovascular disease is more complicated in elderly women than in elderly men. Angina is the predominant initial symptom of CHD in women, but an exercise-based diagnostic test may not be conclusive. Many women, even young women, are unable to exercise to sufficient intensity for a conclusive result, and many older women have concomitant diseases that make such a test impossible. The onset of CHD is about 7 to 10 years later in women than in men. Although the clinical presentation of MI is similar for men and women, treatment tends to be more conservative in women. Mortality from MI is higher in women than in men; mortality is highest in black women. Women have greater operative and postoperative mortality from CABG surgery, and they have lower graft patency (Eaker et al., 1993).

For all of these reasons, prevention of cardiovascular disease is extremely important in women. Prevention should include avoidance of obesity through an active lifestyle, healthful eating (low-fat foods, with plenty of fruits, vegetables, and complex carbohydrates), and no smoking. In addition, postmenopausal use of estrogens has been shown to be associated with a 50 per cent reduction in risk for CHD; the beneficial effect may extend for years after estrogen use is stopped. Estrogens lower levels of low-density lipoproteins and raise levels of beneficial high-density lipoprotein particles (Eaker et al., 1993). Estrogens may also cause dilation of the coronary arteries (Gilligan et al., 1994).

CARDIOVASCULAR NURSING ASSESSMENT OF THE ELDERLY

History

Obtaining a detailed history from an elderly patient may be difficult. The elderly patient may have a poor memory and may have had so many health problems that a history could be very long and complicated. Often, older individuals have diminished pain perception or have learned to ignore or live with symptoms for so long that they may no longer recognize them as important. They may have altered their normal lifestyle to avoid important cardiovascular symptoms, such as dyspnea on exertion, pain, and fatigue (Fields, 1991).

Because of this, it is often helpful to get a picture of the typical daily activities, such as how often the person leaves the house to shop, how often he or she takes walks and how far, and what type of work the individual does around the house (Mezey et al., 1993). It is important to ask if the person's usual activity level has changed in the previous 5 to 10 years to determine whether alterations in exercise tolerance may be the result of cardiovascular problems.

A nutritional history is also important. The person should describe all the food eaten in a day, including condiments, such as boullion cubes, garlic salt, and other sources of sodium. A smoking history is very important for the elderly. The pack-year smoking history can be determined by multiplying the number of packs of cigarettes smoked daily by the total number of years the person has been smoking.

A family history, including brothers, sisters, and children as well as parents, may give some clues to potential cardiovascular problems. It also gives the elderly patient a chance to reminisce and helps establish the rapport that is necessary to help the person relax and promote a climate of trust. The history is more complete if the patient believes the nurse really is interested in him or her as a person. A family history of coronary or cerebral vascular disease, renal vascular hypertension, varicose veins, peripheral vascular disease, or pulmonary emboli should be determined.

Specific questions should be asked to determine the presence or absence of cardiovascular problems. Does the person have a history of high BP? If so, for how long, and what treatment was prescribed (and was the prescription followed? If not, why not?). If the patient is hypertensive, has he or she experienced any headaches or epistaxis?

Dyspnea is a very common sign of cardiac disease in the elderly, so a careful analysis of typical episodes of shortness of breath is warranted. Dyspnea may be an important pain-equivalent symptom of a MI in the elderly (Fields, 1991; Wei, 1994). Does labored breathing occur with exertion or at rest? Does it occur suddenly? Is nocturnal dyspnea or orthopnea present? How many pillows does the person need at night, and has this number changed recently? Is there a history of congestive heart failure? The presence of right-sided heart failure or venous insufficiency may produce edema, so the patient should be asked if shoes, rings, or clothes seem tight at the end of the day. How much swelling is present and where, and does it disappear with rest? (Mezey et al., 1993; Fields, 1991).

Have there been any episodes of chest pain or tightness in the chest? Did the pain radiate to the arms, the shoulders, or the jaw? This type of pain, or pain in the throat and epigastrium, may be due to cardiac ischemia and may be confused with arthritis, hiatal hernia, peptic ulcer, or other common problems of the elderly. Is there any pain in the legs with walking? The location, intensity, duration, and onset of pain should be described, along with any aggravating factors or associated sensory or motor disturbances.

Have there been any dizzy spells, lightheadedness, or vertigo? Do these occur when the patient is standing up, and is any medication being taken for them? Have there been any transient changes in vision or other signs of cerebral insufficiency? Does the person cough or wheeze? If so, when, and if a cough is present, what is the amount, color, and consistency of the sputum?

Has the person had any episodes of thumping or racing heart or markedly irregular heart beats? When do these occur, what seems to bring them on, and how long do the episodes last? Most importantly, are there any associated symptoms, such as weakness, dyspnea, and faintness?

Finally, it is important to find out all the medications the person is currently taking for any reason, both prescribed and over-the-counter drugs. The nurse should try to find out which of the drugs the person is actually taking, and how often. Many elderly take drugs only when they feel sick and try to "do without" as long as possible.

Physical Examination

Inspection and palpation of the neck is particularly important in the elderly. A prominent arterial pulsation above the right clavicle, caused by kinking of the right common carotid artery, is often found. If the neck veins are distended when they are inspected with the patient sitting at a 45-degree angle, heart disease and congestive heart failure may be present. The carotid arteries should be auscultated for bruits, which may indicate arterial stenosis and increased risk of stroke. As in all patients, it is important to palpate only one carotid artery at a time and gently, to avoid stimulating the vagal receptors in the neck or dislodging any atherosclerotic plaques that may be present.

Examination of the heart and chest of elderly clients is more difficult because of the greater incidence of pulmonary emphysema, kyphoscoliosis, and other rib cage deformities. The precordial pulsations should be examined, but these are often difficult to see or palpate. In addition, the heart borders are harder to palpate or percuss, and the heart sounds may be distant or diminished. Because of the difficulty in localizing heart murmurs in the elderly, it is essential to palpate the chest for a thrill, the palpable component of a murmur (Mezey et al., 1993; Tighe and Brest, 1992).

On auscultation, extra sounds may be heard in the normal older person. Alterations in the heart sounds have the same significance in the elderly as in younger patients. An easily heard S_4 gallop, especially when it is accompanied by a palpable presystolic lift, is an abnormal finding in an elderly patient. It suggests that the left ventricle is noncompliant, and it may be caused by hypertension, aortic stenosis, cardiomyopathy, or left ventricular ischemia. An S_3 gallop is always abnormal. It can occur with volume overload of the left ventricle and thus is a sign of congestive heart failure (Fields, 1991).

When a murmur is heard, it is important to carefully describe the site where it was heard; whether the sound radiated; and the timing (in systole or diastole), pitch, duration, character, and intensity. The intensity of a murmur is indicated by grade, mea-

sured on a scale of I to VI. Grade I/VI is the softest audible sound, V/VI is the loudest heard with a stethoscope on the chest, and VI/VI is so loud it is heard with the stethoscope off the chest. The character of the murmur describes whether it is harsh, blowing, rumbling, crescendo, or decrescendo.

A soft systolic ejection murmur, occurring late in systole and heard best at the base of the heart, is often found. As many as 60 to 80 per cent of very old patients may have systolic murmurs. These murmurs generally originate from the aortic area and may be due to the dilation of the aortic annulus and ascending aorta or to the thickening or calcification of the aortic cusps. This type of murmur is short in duration, peaks early in systole, and is soft, usually grade I to grade II/VI. If such a murmur is heard, it is important to ask about associated symptoms. Other, more serious, causes of systolic murmurs are aortic stenosis, mitral regurgitation, and idiopathic hypertrophic subaortic stenosis (Fields, 1991).

A diastolic murmur is always abnormal in the elderly. A diastolic decrescendo blowing murmur heard best along the left sternal border almost always indicates aortic regurgitation, which may not be clinically significant. A diastolic rumble, heard best at the apex of the heart, indicates mitral stenosis, a condition that may be first diagnosed when the patient is elderly. This rumble may be accompanied by atrial fibrillation (Fields, 1991).

Peripheral pulses, including brachial, radial, femoral, popliteal, posterior tibial, and dorsalis pedis, should be carefully examined. The arteries may be quite firm as a result of arteriosclerotic changes in the vessel walls, or peripheral pulses may be very faint, or even absent. Pulses are commonly graded as follows: 0 = absent, 1 + = greatly diminished, 2 + = slightly diminished, 3 + = *normal*, and 4 + = bounding. The skin temperature should be noted, and any trophic changes, such as thin, shiny, taut skin; decreased hair distribution; and nail changes should be recorded. If these are found, the affected leg should be elevated for about a minute, then lowered to the floor. If the foot turns pale or gray when elevated, and dark red, dusky, and mottled when dependent, the person may have significant peripheral vascular disease.

The legs must be carefully inspected for stasis dermatitis, varicosities, and leg ulcers. Dependent edema may be determined by applying pressure *over a bone* in the foot or lower leg.

TABLE 7 – 18
Cardiovascular Nursing Assessment of the Elderly

History

History of cardiovascular problems (hypertension, heart attacks, congestive heart failure)
Family history of cardiovascular problems
Typical daily activities and changes in exercise tolerance
Symptoms: dyspnea, edema, chest pain, tightness in chest, pain in legs with walking, dizziness, lightheadedness, transient changes in vision, thumping or racing heart, irregular heart rate or palpitations, confusion, blackouts, syncope, fatigue, shortness of breath, dyspnea, orthopnea
Medications
Diet
Life stressors

Physical Assessment

Inspection and palpation
　Neck vein distention
　Carotid artery bruits
　Trophic changes in legs
Palpation of arterial pulses
　Radial, brachial, femoral, popliteal, dorsalis pedis, posterior tibialis
Auscultation of blood pressure
　Both arms
　Lying, sitting, standing
Auscultation of the heart
　Systole and diastole (extra sounds and murmurs)
　Rhythm
　Extra sounds and murmurs
Percussion
　Heart size

Finally, a BP measurement should be taken in both arms while the patient is lying, sitting, and standing. The normal range is 100/60 to 140/90 mm Hg, with less than 10 mm Hg difference between arms (Berger and Fields, 1980). Because of the common presence of peripheral vascular abnormalities, the BP is often different in the arms. This difference should be noted, and the arm with the highest pressure should be noted on the chart and consistently used for routine BP checks (Table 7–18).

NURSING DIAGNOSES

1. Alterations in Comfort: pain related to cardiac ischemia, impaired circulation in the extremities, and cardiac surgery

2. Activity Intolerance related to decreased cardiac output, fear of recurrent angina, impaired ability of peripheral vessels to supply tissue with oxygen, arterial spasms, pain, hemiplegia, physical deconditioning, and fatigue

3. Grieving: Denial, Anger, and Depression related to actual or perceived losses secondary to cardiac condition

4. Potential Sexual Dysfunction related to decreased libido or erectile dysfunction secondary to medication side effects

5. Knowledge Deficit related to lack of understanding about disease, prognosis, course, treatment, risk factors (obesity, smoking, alcohol), postoperative and follow-up care, and cognitive deficits

6. Altered Tissue Perfusion: Peripheral related to thrombus, compromised circulation, venous congestion

7. Altered Tissue Perfusion: Cerebral related to interruption of cerebral blood flow, fall in blood pressure, orthostatic hypotension, and cerebral edema

8. Decreased Cardiac Output related to increased preload and/or impaired myocardial contractility, and/or excessively increased afterload

9. Potential Alteration in Respiratory Function related to immobility

10. Impaired Gas Exchange related to ventilation/perfusion imbalance, and/or fluid in alveoli

11. Risk for Impaired Skin Integrity related to compromised peripheral circulation

12. Potential for Injury related to decreased sensation in superficial tissues

13. Nutrition: Less than Body Requirements, Altered related to nausea and anorexia secondary to venous congestion of gastrointestinal tract and fatigue

14. Potential Home Maintenance Management related to inability to perform activities of daily living secondary to breathlessness and fatigue

15. Potential Fluid Volume Excess: Edema related to compensatory kidney mechanisms and excessive sodium intake in diet

16. Potential Fluid Volume Deficit: Dehydration related to excessive diuresis

17. Alteration in Thought Processes related to impaired cerebral circulation and damage to brain structures

18. Self-care Deficits related to neuromuscular impairment, indifference, decreased attention span, and fatigue

19. Potential Alterations in Bowel Elimination: Constipation related to immobility and interruption of normal lifestyle and schedule

20. Impaired Physical Mobility related to neuromuscular impairment, activity intolerance, and fatigue
21. Impaired Communication related to damage to left hemisphere brain structures and impairment of left hemisphere cerebral circulation
22. Ineffective Management of Therapeutic regimen (Individual) related to insufficient knowledge of low-salt diet, drug therapy, activity program, and signs and symptoms of complications
23. Powerlessness related to progressive nature of condition

NURSING INTERVENTIONS AND EVALUATION

Nursing interventions should begin with strategies to prevent the development of cardiovascular disease and to promote a healthy lifestyle. Exercise, especially walking, is beneficial to people of all ages and can be tailored to the abilities of each older individual. Improvements in diet, such as minimizing saturated fats and salt intake, can also help to fight cardiovascular disease. Older people should be encouraged to stop smoking, if possible, and to drink alcohol in moderation. The adage that "you can't teach an old dog new tricks" is not always true for older people, and many are able to change habits if they believe it is to their benefit.

For older clients with cardiovascular disease, the goal is to maximize functional abilities, thereby increasing mobility and independence in carrying out activities of daily living. Older clients and their families should be taught strategies for management of medication, management of diet and stress, and maintenance of a proper balance of rest and activity. Concerns, both spoken and unspoken, about the effects of the illness on sexuality should be explored. Health professionals cannot assume that because people are older they do not have an active sex life. Informal and formal support systems in many cases make the difference between living relatively independently in the community and living relatively dependently in a nursing home. Referrals to social service agencies can facilitate the process of obtaining formal supports, such as Meals on Wheels, homemakers services, home health services, and telephone services. The American Heart Association provides information and support for older clients with cardiovascular diseases and their families.

Evaluation of nursing care is based on whether the goals of functional independence, or at least prevention of deterioration, are met. The nurse should determine whether medications are managed correctly, the diet is appropriate, and a proper balance of exercise and rest is achieved. Stress and anxiety should be minimized, and adequate support systems should be maintained for older clients.

SUMMARY

Normal age-related changes occur in the heart, the blood vessels, and the blood, and in the pumping ability of the heart. Generally, there is a stiffening and decreased elasticity of the tissues and a decrease in cardiac output and blood volume. Several studies have shown that regular physical exercise can retard the changes in the cardiovascular system that occur with age.

Commonly occurring cardiovascular diseases in older age include hypertension, anemia, atherosclerosis, myocardial infarction and angina, cardiac arrhythmias, congestive heart failure, valvular disease, cerebrovascular disease, and peripheral vascular disease. In some cases, the classic symptoms of the diseases are altered or absent in the elderly, so that accurate assessment and diagnosis are imperative. Older people should not be ruled out of active rehabilitation programs solely because of age, because they often respond well to treatment. Nursing interventions should focus on prevention of further disease by helping older people to minimize risk factors by stopping smoking, eating a balanced diet low in salt and cholesterol, maintaining an active lifestyle, exercising regularly, and managing stress.

REFERENCES

Ades, P.A., Waldman, M.L., Polk, D.M. and Coflesky, J.T. Referral patterns and exercise response in the rehabilitation of female coronary patients aged > 62 years. *Am J Cardiol* 69:1422–1425, 1992.

Alder, S.S. Anemia in the aged: Causes and considerations. *Geriatrics* 35(4):49–59, 1980.

American Heart Association. *Heart and Stroke Facts: 1994 Statistical Supplement.* AHA, 1993.

Anderson, J.M. Rehabilitating elderly cardiac patients. *Rehabil Med* 154(5):574–578, 1991.

Assey, M.E. Heart disease in the elderly. *Heart Dis Stroke* 2:330–334, 1993.

Astrand, P.-O. Physical activity and fitness. *Am J Clin Nutr* 55:1231S–1236S, 1992a.

Astrand, P.-O. "Why exercise?" *Med Sci Sports Exerc* 24(2):153–162, 1992b.

Azariades, M.F., Fessler, B.S., Floten, H.S. and Starr, A. Five-year results of coronary bypass grafting for patients older than 70 years: Role of internal mammary artery. *Ann Thorac Surg* 50:940–945, 1990.

Bachman, S., Sparrow, D. and Smith, L.K. Effect of aging on the electrocardiogram. *Am J Cardiol* 48(3):513–516, 1981.

Barry, H.C., Rich, B.S.E. and Carlson, R.T. How exercise can benefit older patients: A practical approach. *Physician Sports Med* 21(2):124–140, 1993.

Benfante, R., Reed, D. and Frank, J. Does cigarette smoking have an independent effect on coronary heart disease incidence in the elderly? *Am J Public Health* 81(7):897–899, 1991.

Berger, J.J. and Fields, W.L. Heart and cardiovascular system. *In* Pocket Guide to Health Assessment. New York: Reston, 1980, pp. 68–76.

Bexton, R.S. Cardiac arrhythmias. *In* Brocklehurst, J.C., Tallis, R.C. and Fillet, H.M. (eds.). *Textbook of Geriatric Medicine and Gerontology.* 4th ed. Edinburgh: Churchill Livingstone, 1992, pp. 231–239.

Borst, S.E. and Lowenthal, D.T. Cardiovascular drugs in the elderly. *Cardiovasc Clin* 22:161–173, 1992.

Brott, T. Prevention and management of medical complications of the hospitalized elderly stroke patient. *Clin Geriatr Med* 7(3):475–482, 1991.

Brust, J.C.M. Stroke. *In* Hazzard, W.R., Bierman, E.L., Blass, J.P., et al. (eds.). *Principles of Geriatric Medicine and Gerontology.* 3rd ed. New York: McGraw-Hill, 1994, pp. 1027–1333.

Buchner, D.M., Beresford, S.A., Larson, E.B., et al. Effects of physical activity on health status in older adults: II. Intervention studies. *Annu Rev Public Health* 13:469–488, 1992.

Carpenito, L.J. *Handbook of Nursing Diagnoses.* 5th ed. Philadelphia: J.B. Lippincott, 1993.

Carroll, J.F. and Pollock, M.L. Rehabilitation and lifestyle modification in the elderly. *Cardiovas Clin* 22:209–227, 1992.

Caspersen, C.J. et al. The prevalence of selected physical activities and their relation with coronary heart disease risk factors in elderly men: The Zutphen study, 1985. *Am J Epidemiol* 133:1078–1092, 1991.

Centers for Disease Control and Prevention. Mortality from congestive heart failure—United States, 1980–1990. *MMWR Morb Mortal Wkly Rep* 43(5):77–81, 1994.

Chakka, S. and Kessler, K.M. Changes with aging as reflected in noninvasive cardiac studies. *Cardiovas Clin* 22:1992, 35–47.

Channer, K.S. and Smith, G.H. Valvular heart disease in old age. *In* Brocklehurst, J.C., Tallis, R.C. and Fillit, H.M. *Textbook of Geriatric Medicine and Gerontology.* 4th ed. Edinburgh: Churchill Livingstone, 1992, pp. 220–230.

Davies, M.J. Pathology of the aging heart. *In* Brocklehurst, J.C., Tallis, R.C. and Fillit, H.M. *Textbook of Geriatric Medicine and Gerontology.* 4th ed. Edinburgh: Churchill Livingstone, 1992, pp. 181–187.

DeNicola, P. and Casale, G. Blood in the aged. *In* Platt, D. (ed.). *Geriatrics 2.* New York: Springer-Verlag, 1983, pp. 252–292.

Eaker, E.D., Chesebro, J.H., Sacks, F.M. et al. Cardiovascular disease in women. *Circulation* 88:1999–2009, 1993.

Elward, K. and Larson, E.B. Benefits of exercise for older adults: A review of existing evidence and current recommendations for the general population. *Clin Geriatr Med* 8(1):35–50, 1992.

Elward, K., Larson, E. and Wagner, E. Factors associated with regular aerobic exercise in an elderly population. *J Am Board Fam Pract* 5:467–474, 1992.

Fahey, V.A. *Vascular Nursing.* Philadelphia: W.B. Saunders, 1988.

Fenster, P.E. and Nolan, P.E. Antiarrhythmic drugs. *In* Bressler, R. and Katz, M.D. (eds.). *Geriatric Pharmacology.* New York: McGraw-Hill, 1993, pp. 105–149.

Fields, S.D. Special considerations in the physical exam of older patients. *Geriatrics* 46(8):39–44, 1991.

Fisch, C. The electrocardiogram in the aged. *Cardiovasc Clin* 12(1):65–74, 1981.

Fletcher, G.F. et al. Benefits and recommendations for physical activity programs for all Americans. *Circulation* 86(1):340–344, 1992.

Fowler, R.S. and Fordyce, W.E. *Stroke: Why Do They Behave That Way?* Dallas: American Heart Association, 1974, pp. 1–31.

Gerstenblith, G. Diagnosis and management of ischemic heart disease in the elderly. *In* Brocklehurst, J.C., Tallis, R.C. and Fillit, H.M. *Textbook of Geriatric Medicine and Gerontology.* 4th ed. Edinburgh: Churchill Livingstone, 1992, pp. 206–213.

Gilligan, D.M., Quyyumi, A.A. and Cannon, R.O. Effects of physiological levels of estrogen on coronary vasomotor function in postmenopausal women. *Circulation* 89:2545–2551, 1994.

Gillis, C.L., Gortner, S.R., Hauck, W.W. et al. A randomized clinical trial of nursing care for recovery from cardiac surgery. *Heart Lung* 22:125–133, 1993.

Goldman, R. Decline in organ function with aging. *In* Rossman, I. (ed.). *Clinical Geriatrics.* 2nd ed. Philadelphia: J.B. Lippincott, 1979, pp. 23–59.

Green, J.S. and Crouse, S.F. Aging, cardiovascular function, and endurance exercise: A review of the literature. *Med Exerc Nutr Health* 2:299–309, 1993.

Hakki, A.H., DePace, N.L. and Iskandrian, A.S. Effect of age on left ventricular function during exercise in patients with coronary artery disease. *Jap Heart J* 24(1):3–20, 1983.

Hale, W.E., Stewart, R.B. and Marke, R.G. Central nervous system symptoms of elderly subjects using antihypertensive drugs. *J Am Geriatr Soc* 32:5–10, 1984.

Harris, R. Cardiovascular diseases in the elderly. *Med Clin North Am* 67(2):379–393, 1983.

Hendra, T.J. and Marshall, A.J. Increased prescription of thrombolytic treatment to elderly patients with suspected acute myocardial infarction associated with audit. *BMJ* 304:423–425, 1992.

Heuser, M.D. and Hazzard, W.R. Geriatric medicine. *JAMA* 271(21):1675–1677, 1994.

House, M.A. Thrombolytic therapy for acute myocardial infarction: The elderly population. *AACN Clin Issues* 3(2):106–113, 1992.

Jaffe, M. *Geriatric Nursing Care Plans.* El Paso, TX: Skidmore-Roth Publishing, 1991.

Kane-Carlsen, P.A. Transient ischemic attacks: Clinical features, pathophysiology and management. *Nurse Pract* 15(7):9–14, 1990.

Kannel, W.B. Hypertension, blood lipids, and cigarette smoking as co-risk factors for coronary heart disease. *Ann NY Acad Sci* 304:128–139, 1987.

Kannel, W.B. Epidemiology of cardiovascular disease in the elderly: An assessment of risk factors. *In* Lowenthal, D.T. (ed.). *Geriatric Cardiology.* Philadelphia: F.A. Davis, 1992, pp. 9–22.

Kitzman, D.W. and Edwards, W.D. Age-related changes in the anatomy of the normal human heart. *J Gerontol Med Sci* 45(2):M33–39, 1990.

Kronmal, R.A., Furberg, C.D., Manolio, T.A. et al. Major

electrocardiographic abnormalities in persons aged 65 years and older (The Cardiovascular Health Study). *Am J Cardiol* 69:1329–1335, 1992.

Laogun, A.A. and Gosling, R.G. In vivo arterial compliance in man. *Clin Phys Physiol Measur* 3(3):201–212, 1984.

Lazarus, B.A., Murphy, J.B., Coletta, E.M. et al. The provision of physical activity to hospitalized elderly patients. *Arch Intern Med* 151:2452–2456, 1991.

Leahy, N.M. Complication in the acute stages of stroke. *Nursing Clin North Am* 26(4):971–983, 1991.

Lee, B.Y. et al. Non-invasive detection and prevention of deep-vein thrombosis in the geriatric patient. *J Am Geriatr Soc* 28:171–175, 1980.

Lewis, J.F. and Maron, B.J. Cardiovascular consequences of the aging process. *Cardiovasc Clin* 22:25–34, 1992.

MacLennan, W.J., Shepherd, A.N. and Stevenson, I.H. Disorders of the heart. *In The Elderly.* New York: Springer-Verlag, 1984a, pp. 28–41.

MacLennan, W.J., Shepherd, A.N. and Stevenson, I.H. Disorders of the vascular system. *In The Elderly.* New York: Springer-Verlag, 1984b, pp. 42–58.

Mansouri, A. and Lipschitz, D.A. Anemia in the elderly patient. *Med Clin North Am* 76(3):619–630, 1992.

Martin, A. et al. Five year follow-up of 101 elderly subjects by means of long-term ambulatory cardiac monitoring. *Eur Heart J* 5(7):592–596, 1984.

Meischke, H., Eisenberg, M.S. and Larsen, M.P. Prehospital delay interval for patients who use emergency medical services: The effects of heart-related medical conditions and demographic variables. *Ann Emerg Med* 22(10):1597–1601, 1993.

Mezey, M.D., Rauckhorst, L.H. and Stokes, S.A. *Health Assessment of the Older Individual.* 2nd ed. New York: Springer Publishing Company, 1993, pp. 81–96.

Mizutani, Y., Nakano, S., Ote, N. et al. Evaluation of effects of aging, training and myocardial ischemia on cardiac reserve by exercise echocardiography. *Jpn Circ J* 48(9):969–979, 1984.

Mol, V.J. and Baker, C.A. Activity intolerance in the geriatric stroke patient. *Rehabil Nursing* 16(6):337–343, 1991.

Muller, D.W.M. and Topol E.J. Selection of patients with acute myocardial infarction for thrombolytic therapy. *Ann Intern Med* 113:949–960, 1990.

Mulley, G.P. Stroke. *In* Brocklehurst, J.C., Tallis, R.C. and Fillet, H.M. (eds.). *Textbook of Geriatric Medicine and Gerontology.* 4th ed. Edinburgh: Churchill Livingstone, 1992, pp. 365–388.

National Institutes of Health, National Heart, Lung and Blood Institute. *Fifth Report of the Joint National Committee on Detection, Evaluation and Treatment of High Blood Pressure.* NIH Publ. No. 93-1088, Bethesda: MD, Public Health Service 1993, pp. 1–49.

North American Symptomatic Carotid Endarterectomy Trial Collaborators. Beneficial effect of carotid endarterectomy in symptomatic patients with high-grade stenosis. *N Engl J Med* 325:445–449, 1991.

O'Connor, C.M. and Califf, R.M. Aggressive therapy of acute MI in the elderly. *Hosp Pract (Off Ed)* Feb 15:59–70, 1992.

O'Connor, G.T., Morton, J.R., Dielh, M.J. et al. Differences between men and women in hospital mortality with coronary artery bypass surgery. *Circulation* 88(5):2104–2110, 1993.

O'Neill, P.A. Venous thrombotic disease. *In* Brocklehurst, J.C., Tallis, R.C. and Fillit, H.M. (eds.). *Textbook of Geriatric Medicine and Gerontology.* 4th ed. Edinburgh: Churchill Livingstone, 1992, pp. 249–257.

Pashos, C.L., Newhouse, J.P. and McNeil, B.J. Temporal

changes in the care and outcomes of elderly patients with acute myocardial infarction, 1987 through 1990. *JAMA* 270(15):1832–1836, 1993.

Pepine, C.J. and Pepine, A. Intervention therapy for coronary artery disease in the elderly. *Cardiovasc Clin* 22:175–187, 1992.

Petermans, J. Prevalence of disease of the large arteries in an elderly Belgian population: Relationship with some metabolic factors. *Acta Cardiol* 34(5):365–372, 1984.

Rakowski, W. and Mor, V. The association of physical activity with mortality among older adults in the longitudinal study of aging (1984–1988). *J Gerontol Med Sci* 47(4):M122–M129, 1992.

Rials, S.J., Marinchak, R.A. and Kowey, P.R. Arrhythmias in the elderly. *Cardiovas Clin* 139–157, 1992.

Rockwood, K. Acute confusion in elderly medical patients. *J Am Geriatr Soc* 37:150–154, 1989.

Rodeheffer, R.J. and Gerstenblith, G. Effect of age on cardiovascular function. *In* Johnson, H.A. (ed.). *Relations Between Normal Aging and Disease.* New York: Raven Press, 1985, pp. 85–100.

Rodstein, M. Heart disease in the aged. *In* Rossman, I. (ed.). *Clinical Geriatrics.* 2nd ed. Philadelphia: J.B. Lippincott, 1979, pp. 181–203.

Ross, R. The pathogenesis of atherosclerosis. *In* Braunwald, E. (ed.). *Heart Disease: A Textbook of Cardiovascular Medicine.* 4th ed. Philadelphia: W.B. Saunders, 1992, pp. 1106–1124.

Rutherford, J.D. and Braunwald, E. Chronic ischemic heart disease. *In* Braunwald, E. (ed.). *Heart Disease: A Textbook of Cardiovascular Medicine.* 4th ed. Philadelphia: W.B. Saunders, 1992, pp. 1292–1364.

Salive, M.E., Coroni-Huntley, J., LaCorix, A.Z. et al. Predictors of smoking cessation and relapse in older adults. *Am J Public Health* 82(9):1268–1271, 1992.

Santiaga, J.T. et al. Aortic valve replacement in the elderly. *JAMA* 31:211–212, 1983.

SHEP Cooperative Research Group. Prevention of stroke by antihypertensive drug treatment in older persons with isolated systolic hypertension. *JAMA* 265:3255–3264, 1991.

Smith, J.M., Rath, R., Feldman, D.J. and Schreiber, J.T. Coronary artery bypass grafting in the elderly: Changing trends and results. *J Cardiovasc Surg* 33:468–471, 1992.

Steinhaus, L.A., Dustman, R.E., Ruhlings, R.O. et al. Cardio-respiratory fitness of young and older active and sedentary men. *Br J Sports Med* 22(4):163–166, 1988.

Thiele, B.L. and Strandness, D.E., Jr. Peripheral vascular disease. *In* Hazzard, W.R., Bierman, E.L., Blass, J.P., et al. (eds.). *Principles of Geriatric Medicine and Gerontology.* 3rd ed. New York: McGraw-Hill, 1994, pp. 533–540.

Tighe, D. and Brest, A.N. Congestive heart failure in the elderly. *Cardiovasc Clin* 22:127–138, 1992.

United States Department of Health and Human Services. *Statement on Hypertension in the Elderly.* Bethesda, MD: National Institutes of Health, April 1980, pp. 1–7.

Van Camp, S.P. and Boyer, J.L. Exercise guidelines for the elderly (part 2 of 2). *Physician Sports Med* 17(5):83–88, 1989.

Walsh, D.B. and Nauta, R.J. Peripheral vascular disease in the geriatric patient. *In* Reichel, W. (ed.). *Clinical Aspects of Aging.* 3rd ed. Baltimore: Williams & Wilkins, 1989, pp. 106–123.

Wei, J.Y. Age and the cardiovascular system. *Mech Dis* 327(24):1735–1739, 1992.

Wei, J.Y. Disorders of the heart. *In* Hazzard, W.R., Bierman, E.L., Blass, J.P., et al. (eds.). *Principles of Geriatric Medicine and Gerontology.* 3rd ed. New York: McGraw-Hill, 1994, pp. 517–532.

Williams, L. and Lowenthal, D.T. Hypertension in the elderly. *Cardiovas Clin* 49–61, 1992.

Wong, M., Chuna, T. and Pravin, M.S. Degenerative calcific valvular disease and systolic murmurs in the elderly. *J Am Geriatr Soc* 31:156–163, 1983.

Young, R.F. and Kahana, E. Gender, recovery from late heart attack, and medical care. *Women Health* 20(1):11–31, 1993.

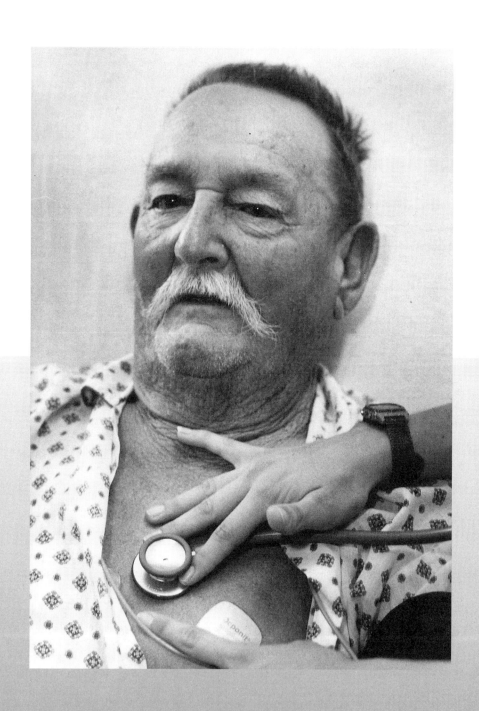

Age-Related Changes in the Respiratory System

JOANNE S. HARRELL

OBJECTIVES

List and describe normal anatomical and functional changes in the aging lung.

❖

Discuss factors that may further decrease lung function in the elderly—specifically smoking, obesity, immobility, and surgery.

❖

Compare and contrast the effect of respiratory diseases on older persons, particularly chronic obstructive pulmonary disease, asthma, pneumonia, tuberculosis, lung cancer, and sleep apnea.

❖

Conduct a pulmonary assessment on an older person.

The lungs comprise the organ of the body that, in addition to the skin, is most exposed to the environment. Smoke, bacteria, and multiple irritants are inhaled daily for many years. In addition, the lung has a subtle way of healing, so that even a large injury can leave an extremely small residual scar (Liebow, 1964; Thurlbeck, 1991). Also, the elderly frequently have other diseases that may affect lung function. Changes in the neuromuscular and cardiovascular systems can profoundly affect respiratory function. For these reasons, it is difficult to differentiate the effects of environment and disease from the effects of age. In addition, many of the studies of the effects of aging have been cross-sectional rather than longitudinal, and many early studies included smokers, so the true effects of aging may not have been clearly identified. Further, the aging process closely mimics changes in lung tissues associated with a disease process, such as emphysema (Johnson and Dempsey, 1991). In spite of these limitations, the effects of age on the lungs have been widely discussed. Thurlbeck (1991) suggests that it is perhaps better to consider these findings descriptions of aged lungs rather than the effects of aging on the lungs.

Although the function of the pulmonary system decreases with age, the loss involves the reserve necessary during stress. The losses are not great enough to interfere with ordinary activity. Even this decrease in reserve can be kept to a minimum if elderly people actively maintain fitness (Hodgkin et al., 1993; Knudson, 1991).

NORMAL CHANGES WITH AGING

Anatomical Changes

Extrapulmonary Changes

Aging produces changes in the respiratory system itself and in related systems that collectively result in a moderate decline in lung function. Skeletal deformities, such as kyphoscoliosis, may develop with age. The thorax becomes shorter and the anterior-posterior diameter increases with age. In addition, osteoporosis of the ribs and vertebrae and calcification of the costal cartilages contribute to chest wall stiffness. This stiffness produces a decline in chest wall compliance. Authors have reported that the muscles of respiration, particularly the diaphragm and intercostal muscles, weaken with age (King and Schwarz, 1982). However, more recent studies have found conflicting results that indicate that age-related changes in the respiratory muscles are minimal, and loss in their strength may be related more to atrophy associated with a sedentary lifestyle (Johnson and Dempsey, 1991; Crapo, 1993). This combination of increased stiffness of the chest wall and potential or possible diminished muscle strength reduces the efficiency of breathing, so that the aged have reduced maximal inspiratory and expiratory force. More muscle work is needed to move air in and out of the lung (Kenney, 1989).

Intrapulmonary Changes

Within the lung itself, an opposite process is occurring in the lung parenchyma and conducting airways. There is a progressive loss of lung elastic recoil with age. This elastic recoil normally opposes the elastic forces in the chest wall. Both of these forces are reduced in the aged, so that the effects of each are balanced. The loss of elastic recoil is not due to a change in the amount of elastin but is probably related to the decrease in the cross-linking of the collagen of the elastic fibers in the lung (Kenney, 1989; Johnson and Dempsey, 1991). The lungs become more compliant because of the loss of elastic forces (Weiss, 1982), which partially compensates for the decreased chest wall compliance, making it somewhat easier for the weakened respiratory muscles to move the stiffer chest wall.

There are significant changes within the

lung parenchyma. The lung parenchyma is composed of terminal bronchioles, alveolar ducts, and many alveoli arranged in grape-like clusters. Surrounding these alveoli are capillaries (Fig. 8–1). It is here that the vital transfer of oxygen and carbon dioxide occurs. The number of alveoli remains constant in the healthy aging person, but alveolar changes occur. The alveoli enlarge; the alveolar walls become thinner, resulting in a loss of alveolar septal tissue; and there are fewer capillaries present. This loss of alveolar structure gives aged lungs some of the microscopic characteristics of emphysematous lungs and is sometimes called "senile lung." Thus, the effective alveolar surface area that is vital to gas exchange is reduced from 70 to 75 square meters (m^2) at the age of 20 years to about 60 m^2 at the age of 70 years (Crapo, 1993; Murray, 1986).

As a result of these changes, the mechanics of breathing are modified in the aged. As the chest wall becomes less mobile, chest wall compliance is reduced, and dynamic lung compliance becomes more frequency-dependent. That is, the elderly are less able to provide adequate force to *move air rapidly*. There is a decrease in the maximal force available for both inspiration and expiration. Because the work of breathing is increased, the elderly tend to make greater use of all respiratory muscles, especially the diaphragm. This increased reliance on the diaphragm makes the elderly more sensitive to changes in intra-abdominal pressure, such as that caused by a large meal or body position (Kenney, 1989).

Finally, the pulmonary vessels stiffen with age, causing a small reduction in pulmonary arterial pressure. This pulmonary stiffness could also account for an increased perfusion to the apex of the lungs of elders, which contributes to a perfusion-diffusion imbalance (Johnson and Dempsey, 1991).

Functional Changes

The anatomical changes have significant effects on lung function. There are changes in the volume of air moved, in the rate of air flow, and in actual gas exchange.

Lung Volumes

Lung volumes are measured with pulmonary function tests (PFTs). The commonly measured volumes are defined in Table 8–1. Normal adult values and comparable values for the elderly are shown.

One of the most significant lung volumes for nursing care is tidal volume (V_T), which

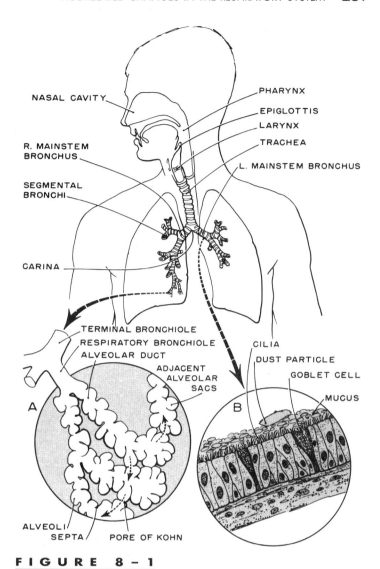

FIGURE 8–1

Anatomy of lung parenchyma. (From Price, S.A. and Wilson, L.M.) *Pathophysiology: Clinical Concepts of Disease Process.* New York: McGraw-Hill, 1982.)

is simply the amount of air moved with a normal, or typical, breath. A large part of V_T, the portion of air that moves from the mouth through the terminal bronchioles, is not in contact with alveoli and therefore does not participate in gas exchange. This is a major part of the "dead space" in the lung. This dead space volume is related to body size and can be conveniently estimated from body weight. The amount of dead space in the lung is approximately equal to an individual's weight in pounds. Thus, if a person weighs 200 pounds, about 200 cc of the V_T is dead space ventilation. V_T, which can be simply measured with a spirometer, should be relatively unchanged in the aged.

Another simple and useful measure is minute ventilation, the amount of air that is

TABLE 8-1

Lung Capacities and Volumes

| MEASUREMENT | SYMBOL | AVERAGE VALUES | | DESCRIPTION |
		Adult Man	Elderly Man	
Tidal volume	V_T	500 ml	500 ml	Amount of air inhaled or exhaled with each breath (value listed is for resting conditions)
Inspiratory reserve volume	IRV	3100 ml	2800 ml	Amount of air that can be forcefully inhaled after taking a normal tidal volume inhalation
Expiratory reserve volume	ERV	1200 ml	1000 ml	Amount of air that can be forcefully exhaled after taking a normal tidal volume exhalation
Residual volume	RV	1200 ml	1800 ml	Amount of air left in the lungs after a forced exhalation
Total lung capacity	TLC	6000 ml	6000 ml	Maximal amount of air that can be contained in the lungs after a maximal inspiratory effort: $TLC = V_T + IRV + ERV + RV$
Vital capacity	VC	4800 ml	4300 ml	Maximal amount of air that can be expired after a maximal inspiration: $VC = V_T + IRV + ERV$ (should be 80% of TLC)
Inspiratory capacity	IC	3600 ml	3100 ml	Maximal amount of air that can be inspired after a normal expiration: $IC = V_T + IRV$
Functional residual capacity	FRC	2400 ml	2800 ml	Volume of air remaining in the lungs after a normal tidal volume expiration: $FRC = ERV + RV$

Adapted and reproduced with permission from Forster, R.E., II, Dubois, A.B., Briscoe, W.A. and Fisher, A.B. *The Lung: Physiologic Basis of Pulmonary Function Tests,* 3rd ed. © 1986 by Year Book Medical Publishers, Inc., Chicago.

moved in 1 minute. It is determined by multiplying the V_T by the number of respirations in 1 minute. There are conflicting reports on changes in respiratory rate with age in adults, but it appears that there is little if any significant age effect in normal subjects at rest (Crapo, 1993).

Changes in lung volume occur with age. Although total lung volume remains fairly constant, age influences the subdivisions of this volume (Fig. 8–2). Residual volume (RV, the volume of air that remains in the lung after a maximal expiration) increases with age, probably because of the loss of elastic forces in the lung. This increased RV encroaches on and reduces the vital capacity (VC). Studies have shown that VC decreases

about 25 per cent in the aged, with a loss of 26 ml per year in men and 21 ml per year in women (Crapo, 1993). At the same time, functional residual capacity (FRC) also rises (Knudson, 1991; Stark and Lipscomb, 1983; Murray, 1986). The reduction in VC is thought to be largely related to the loss of chest wall mobility, which increases the RV in the lungs. VC is related to height and is smaller in women, but the rate of reduction with age is more rapid in men. The drop in

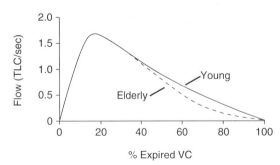

FIGURE 8-2

Age-related changes in lung volume. (Redrawn from Allen, S.C. Aging and the respiratory system. *In* Brocklehurst, J.C., Tallis, R.C. and Fillit, H.M. [eds.]. *Textbook of Geriatric Medicine and Gerontology.* 4th ed. Edinburgh: Churchill Livingstone, 1992, p. 740.)

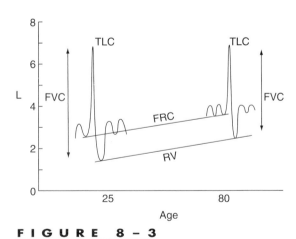

FIGURE 8-3

Comparison of maximal expiratory flow-volume curves of young (aged 25 to 35 years) and elderly (aged 65 to 75 years) subjects. To compensate for size, flow is expressed as TLC (total lung capacity) per second and volume is expressed as percentage expired VC (vital capacity). (From Knudson, R.J. Physiology of the aging lung. *In* Crystal, R.G. and West, J.B. [eds.]. *The Lung: Scientific Foundations.* New York: Raven Press, 1991, p. 1752.)

forced vital capacity (FVC) is illustrated in Figure 8–3. This reduction becomes more rapid in both sexes after 45 years of age. The ability to take maximally deep breaths (inspiratory capacity) also decreases with age (Mauderly, 1981). Studies show that the maximal expiratory flow diminishes with age only at low volumes (Knudson, 1991).

Air Flow Rates

Not only are lung volumes changed with age, the rate at which air is moved is also reduced. Air flow is dependent on airway size and resistance, muscle strength, and elastic recoil. All the indices of air flow (FVC, forced expiratory volume in 1 second [FEV_1], and forced expiratory flow [FEF]) decrease with age (Crapo, 1993). Both forced expiratory volume (FEV) and maximal voluntary ventilation (MVV) are decreased. The FEV is defined as the amount of air expelled from the lungs after a maximal inspiration. The MVV is the amount of air a person can breathe in and out, as rapidly as possible, in a given time. Both of these show a 50 per cent decline from the third to the ninth decades. Both tests depend on the ability to move air, which in turn depends on airway resistance, compliance of the thoracic cage, and muscle strength (Feuer, 1981).

The proportion of the FEV a person can expel in 1 second is a good measure of bronchial obstruction and airway resistance. A drop of 25 to 30 ml per year in FEV_1 has been reported (Brandstetter and Kazemi, 1983; Starke and Lipscomb, 1983; Murray, 1986; Knudson, 1991). This drop is shown in Figure 8–3. In the "six cities studies," Ware et al. (1990) found an accelerated decline of FEV_1 and FVC with age, which was more evident in longitudinal analyses. At age 75 years, the annual rate of loss of function in the longitudinal analysis was double that of the cross-sectional analysis. The rate of loss of FVC and FEV_1 was greater in men, in taller people, and in those with higher baseline values.

In summary, FEV_1 and VC fall with age, and RV, FRC, and the RV/TLC (total lung capacity) ratio increase. The tendency for lung volume to increase because of loss of elastic recoil is offset by stiffness in the chest wall and reduced muscle power, so the overall TLC remains relatively unchanged (Knudson, 1991).

Airway Closure and Distribution of Ventilation

The loss of elastic recoil (increased compliance) leads to a dynamic collapse of the air-ways on expiration, with trapping of gas in the lungs and a decrease in flow rates due to increased resistance. Small airways (diameter of less than 1 mm) without cartilaginous support are kept open by the guy-rope effect of the elastic tissue surrounding them and by subatmospheric intrapleural pressure. Airway stability is promoted by airway surfactant. The decrease in elastic recoil with age reduces the stability of the small airways, which leads to a tendency for those airways to close, especially at low tidal volumes (Kenney, 1989).

Early airway closure at low lung volumes is also due to an age-related increase in the closing lung volume, or closing capacity. Closing capacity is the lung volume at which small airways begin to close during a forced expiration. This closing volume may be greater than the total volume of gas remaining in the lungs at the end of a normal breath, the FRC. This leads to early closure of the airways and less efficient matching of ventilation with perfusion (Kenney, 1989; Knudson, 1991).

This early airway closure, which has been shown to increase with age and with shallow breathing, may also be increased in the supine position (Mauderly, 1981). A practical application in nursing care of this knowledge of airway closure is a reinforcement of the need to encourage deep breathing in the elderly and to keep them out of bed as much as possible, because airways tend to collapse in the elderly when they breathe at low volumes and are in the supine position.

Gas Exchange

Gas exchange is determined by the distribution of ventilation and blood flow. When ventilation and perfusion match well, gas exchange is maximal, and the arterial blood is saturated with oxygen. In adults, it is more common to report arterial oxygen tension (PaO_2) than oxygen saturation. Oxygen tension has been shown to fall with age at a rate of 4 mm Hg per decade. Knudson (1991) provides the following equation to estimate PaO_2 changes with age in subjects older than 20 years:

$$PaO_2 = 100.1 - (0.323 \times age)$$

Thus, at age 25, the PaO_2 would be 92 mm Hg, whereas it would be expected to be 86 mm Hg at the age of 45, 79 mm Hg at the age of 65, and 73 mm Hg by the age of 85 (Murray, 1986) (Fig. 8–4).

This drop in arterial oxygen is probably related to the increased closing volume of the elderly during quiet tidal breathing.

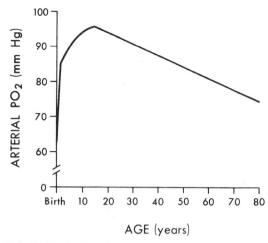

FIGURE 8 – 4

Arterial PO_2 as a function of age from birth to 80 years. (From Murray, J.F. *The Normal Lung*. Philadelphia: W.B. Saunders, 1986.)

Blood flow continues to the areas that have lost ventilation from the small airways leading to them, resulting in ventilation and perfusion that are not matched. This imbalance is especially marked in the recumbent position (Murray, 1986). In addition, there is reduced alveolar surface for gas exchange. Another factor is the age-related reduction of hemoglobin, which is necessary to carry oxygen (Wahba, 1983). Arterial pH and PCO_2 do not change with age (Crapo, 1993; Knudson, 1991).

Control of Ventilation

Ventilation is normally regulated by a central controller in the brain that coordinates information fed to its various centers and modulates the activity of the respiratory muscles. There are two major sensors: the central chemoreceptor and the peripheral chemoreceptors. The *central chemoreceptor*, located in the medulla, increases ventilation in response to respiratory acidosis (high PCO_2), causing a lowering of arterial PCO_2. It is responsible for three fourths of the ventilatory response to carbon dioxide. The *peripheral chemoreceptors*, which respond more rapidly, are located in the carotid bodies at the bifurcation of the common carotid arteries and in the aortic bodies. The carotid bodies, which are most important, respond to decrease in arterial PO_2 and pH by increasing ventilation. The peripheral receptors are solely responsible for the increase in ventilation that follows hypoxemia (King and Schwarz, 1982). Thus, either hypoxia or hypercapnia will normally increase the rate and depth of breathing (minute ventilation).

The responses of the normal elderly to either hypoxia or hypercapnia appear to be blunted in the aged (Crapo, 1993). In a study of healthy older people (mean age, 70), the ventilatory response to either stimulus was half that of younger persons (mean age, 25) (Peterson et al., 1981). Another study showed less increase in both heart rate and ventilatory response to hypoxia and hypercapnia in healthy elderly persons (King and Schwarz, 1982). One small study of the effect of aging on respiratory responses to carbon dioxide found that ventilation responses to increasing carbon dioxide in the aged were lower, but there was no statistically significant difference (Rubin et al., 1982). In a review of studies of gas transport and aging, Horvath and Borgia (1984) found conflicting results and stressed the need for longitudinal rather than cross-sectional studies before an adequate assessment of age-related changes in function, lung capacity, or adaptive potential can truly be predicted. However, most current studies support the finding of a decreased homeostatic response to lowered oxygen content and increased carbon dioxide (Crapo, 1993).

This diminished response to hypoxia and hypercarbia has great clinical significance for nurses. The usual clinical signs of increased need for oxygen include increases in respiratory rate and volume and increased heart rate and blood pressure. These responses are all blunted in the aged (Crapo, 1993). Therefore, additional cues, such as changes in mentation and affect, must be used. An elderly patient who normally has a low arterial oxygen level could have clinically significant arterial hypoxemia (PO_2 less than 60 mm Hg) with a relatively minor pulmonary insult. In addition, these patients may respond more slowly to treatment. Ivanov (1983) compared the effects of oxygen deprivation on young (19 to 32 years of age) and old (60 to 89 years of age) men. He found not only that the respiratory system in old people functions under greater initial strain when it is first exposed to hypoxic conditions but also that return to normal arterial blood levels after the exposure was delayed.

Lung Host Defense

In addition to the respiratory functions already discussed, the lung has important nonrespiratory functions, which include purifying the air and maintaining an infection-

T A B L E   8 – 2
Effects of Aging on the Respiratory System

RESPIRATORY ABNORMALITY	PHYSIOLOGICAL BASIS	CLINICAL DISORDERS
Decline in bellows function	Increased chest wall stiffness Loss of elastic recoil Decreased respiratory muscle strength Increased airway collapsibility	"Senile" emphysema
Abnormal gas exchange	Ventilation-perfusion mismatch Reduced diffusing capacity for carbon monoxide Increasing alveolar-arterial oxygen gradient	Arterial hypoxemia Decreased exercise tolerance
Abnormal breathing pattern	Diminished responsiveness to hypoxemia and hypercapnia Changing set point for ventilation due to fluctuating level of wakefulness	Cheyne-Stokes breathing Periodic breathing
Upper airway obstruction	Decreased airway muscle tone due to loss of wakefulness stimulus, decreased metabolic respiratory drive	Snoring, sleep apnea, hypopnea, oxygen desaturation
Altered lung host defense	Decreased ciliary action Impaired cough mechanism Decreased IgA production ? Decreased phagocytic function of alveolar macrophages	Increased susceptibility to infection (pneumonia and chronic bronchitis)

From King, T.E. and Schwarz, M.I. Pulmonary function and disease in the elderly. *In* Schrier, R.S. (ed.). *Clinical Internal Medicine in the Aged.* Philadelphia: W.B. Saunders, 1982.

free lung tissue. An early study found that there were no qualitative changes in the healing process with aging (Kleinerman, 1964). King and Schwarz (1982) state that no systematic evaluation of lung host defenses of elderly persons has been reported. However, there is an increased occurrence of respiratory infections in the elderly, and several authors discuss the possible factors.

Cell-mediated immunity and humoral antibody formation decline with age in some individuals; this may be related more to diseases than to age, however (King and Schwarz, 1982). In addition, several defense mechanisms are altered with age. First, the *cough mechanism* is impaired in the elderly, in volume, force, and flow rate. This impairment may be related to the weakened respiratory muscles. Second, because older patients have fewer cilia and *ciliary action* is less effective, the "mucociliary escalator," which cleanses the lungs by moving inhaled particles up and out of the respiratory tract at a rate of about 2 cm an hour, is less effective. As a result, inhaled particles are not cleared readily from the tracheobronchial tree. A third factor is the *decrease in immunoglobulin A (IgA).* This is the secretory immunoglobulin of nasal and respiratory mucosal surfaces, which has neutralizing action against viruses. The fourth factor is the defective activity of *alveolar macrophages,* phagocytic cells that ingest foreign material that reaches the alveoli; this factor affects smokers especially (King and Schwarz, 1982; Wahba, 1983; Kenney, 1989).

One study of the influence of age on bronchiomucociliary transport found that in 19 nonsmoking subjects, the mucociliary clearance was significantly lower in older subjects. However, the researchers suggest that because the results varied considerably within each age group, factors other than age may have an effect on mucociliary clearance (Puchelle et al., 1979). In summary, it is possible that the elderly may have reduced host defenses against pulmonary insults.

Thus, it is evident that multiple changes in the elderly affect pulmonary function. These are summarized in Table 8–2.

Effects of Exercise

The capacity to exercise is determined by many factors in addition to pulmonary function. A decrease in cardiac output and skeletal muscle function, the presence of joint and circulatory and respiratory system diseases, and an overall drop in fitness all contribute to the decrease in exercise tolerance that is commonly seen in the elderly. Muscle power decreases with age, and poor muscle coordination increases the energy expenditure for a given load. Also, physiological dead space increases, so total ventilation increases, increasing the likelihood for breathlessness with exercise (Stark and Lipscomb, 1983; Johnson and Dempsey, 1991).

A longitudinal study has shown that the ventilatory cost of submaximal work increases significantly between age 64 and age 70, with an even higher rate of change

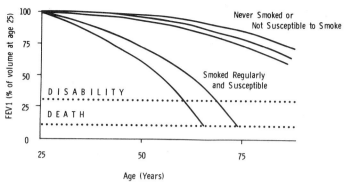

FIGURE 8 – 5

Gradual decline in 1-second forced expiratory volume (FEV₁) in nonsmokers or individuals not susceptible to smoke. Note the more rapid decline in FEV₁ in smokers susceptible to the effects of smoke. (From Stark, J.E. and Lipscomb, D.J. Physiological and pathological aspects of the respiratory system. In Platt, D. [ed.]. *Geriatrics 2.* New York: Springer-Verlag: modified from Fletcher, C. and Peto, R. The natural history of chronic airflow obstruction. *Br Med J* 1:1645–1648, 1977.)

than has been shown in cross-sectional studies. Both heart rate and respiratory rate were greatly increased with exercise (Patrick et al., 1983). Brischetto et al. (1984) also showed that the ventilatory response to exercise was much higher in the elderly than in a matched younger sample.

Older studies have shown that with age, there is a decrease in maximal oxygen consumption (Mauderly, 1981). This was found even in subjects who remained physically active and has been shown to be present in both longitudinal and cross-sectional studies. However, Yerg and associates (1985) compared 14 master athletes (age 63) with 14 healthy male control subjects of the same age. They showed that maximal oxygen consumption was significantly greater in the aged athletes, whereas there was less hyperventilation with exercise. In a related experiment, they studied 11 healthy men and women, also aged 63, before and after 12 months of endurance training. They found that the increased ventilatory response and decreased maximal oxygen uptake seen with age can be reduced by endurance training. A series of studies by Johnson and Dempsey (1991) showed that fit elderly subjects can maintain blood gas homeostasis even during intense exercise. Knudson (1991) states that "the ventilatory or gas-exchanging capabilities of the aging respiratory system are not limiting factors to maximal oxygen consumption" (p. 1757). He attributes the decline in aerobic work capacity to a decrease in mitochondrial activity at the level of the exercising muscle, as well as to sedentary

lifestyles leading to a loss of fitness and muscle mass.

So, although we cannot modify age, we can modify fitness by training. In the elderly, the pulmonary and cardiac reserves are limited by age. Thus, it becomes increasingly important not to limit them also by inactivity. "Training in the elderly, perhaps more than in young people, will help provide the cardiopulmonary reserve necessary to withstand future insults to the cardiopulmonary system" (Keltz, 1984).

Factors That May Further Decrease Lung Function

Smoking, obesity, and immobility are often seen in the elderly. These all decrease lung function. In addition, surgery places the aged at particular risk for pulmonary complications.

Smoking

It is well known that smoking damages the lungs. The annual decrease in FEV₁ that is seen in the elderly may be increased ninefold in some heavy smokers, although not in all. Normal people have a drop of 20 to 30 ml per year in FEV₁. Individuals who are susceptible to the effects of smoking have an annual loss of 50 to 160 ml. A 20 pack-year history of smoking leads to a marked decrease in VC, FEV/VC per cent, and maximal breathing capacity (King and Schwarz, 1982; Wahba, 1983). Figure 8–5 shows the effects of smoking on FEV₁ for those who are susceptible.

Ciliary action is inhibited by tobacco smoke, which also causes an increased production of mucus. Inhaled cigarette smoke also causes bronchoconstriction. Airway resistance may double after the smoking of one cigarette, and this may last for as long as 30 minutes (Cherniack and Cherniack, 1983). In addition, closing volume increases (Murray, 1986). This means that more lower lung area will not be ventilated because the small airways close earlier.

Even nonsmokers may be significantly harmed by long exposure to cigarette smoke. Nonsmokers who are exposed to side-stream smoke and who have pre-existing heart or lung diseases are at increased risk for complications of those diseases. In addition, the lungs of nonsmoking spouses of heavy cigarette smokers have been shown to have many of the same characteristics as those of smokers: pulmonary function tests show evidence of chronic obstructive pulmonary disease. Elders who have been exposed to passive smoking for long periods may also have an increased risk for lung cancer (Taylor et al., 1985).

Fortunately, it has been shown that stopping smoking can reverse many of these harmful effects (Bosse et al., 1981). Even long-time smokers may show a significant improvement in lung function after they stop smoking.

Most studies have examined the health consequences of smoking on young and middle-aged adults. There is evidence that a long history of smoking can have a cumulative impact on physical decline, affecting the cardiovascular and pulmonary systems and also reducing some cognitive abilities (Hill and Fisher, 1993). A study of more than 14,000 adults 65 years of age or older showed that current smokers reported higher frequencies of chronic disease than did former or never smokers. Further, although a number of the current smokers in the study had survived beyond age 85, their health care needs and functional disability were extremely high (Colsher et al., 1990). "Smoking cessation in later life may not only prolong life but may play a more important role in relieving current symptoms of chronic disease, extending functional capacity, and reducing health care costs—with the subsequent potential for life satisfaction" (Hill and Fisher, 1993, pp. 196–197).

Obesity

Lung and chest wall compliance and some lung volumes (FRC, ERV, VC) are markedly reduced by obesity, further increasing the work of breathing, which is already compromised by age. The obese also have decreased ventilation of the lower parts of their lungs, possibly due to early airway closure and lower arterial oxygen tension (PaO_2) (Wahba, 1983; Jenkins and Moxham, 1991).

Immobility

The inactivity that accompanies certain diseases, such as stroke and arthritis, can further jeopardize lung function in the aged. Bedrest is particularly harmful because the supine position increases the closing volume in adults, which predisposes to early airway closure and atelectasis in the dependent parts of the lung (Mauderly, 1981).

Surgery

Elderly patients are at high risk for pulmonary complications. In a retrospective review of postoperative pulmonary problems, it was found that among patients who died within 6 weeks of surgery, pulmonary complications occurred in 33 per cent of those aged 20 to 59 and in 46 per cent of those aged 60 or older. In another study, pulmonary complications were shown to occur three times more often in patients older than 60 years (Campbell, 1977).

The effects of anesthesia and surgery on the lung tend to mimic the effects of age. Postoperative lung functions are impaired in all patients. There is an early phase of respiratory depression because of the lingering effects of premedication and anesthetic agents. During this time, tidal volume and respiratory rate fall, resulting in mild to moderate hypoventilation, which may produce hypoxemia and moderate increases in PCO_2. Subsequently, although the respiratory rate increases and the PCO_2 decreases, tidal volume may remain low, which increases dead space ventilation. Hypoxemia is produced not only by this hypoventilation but also because of retained secretions and atelectasis that result from intraoperative depressed respiration, absent sigh and cough reflexes, and a high fraction of inspired oxygen (Campbell, 1977).

The changes in pulmonary function with surgery, which may last for 10 to 14 days, include decreases in VC, V_T, and inspiratory and expiratory reserve volume; there is a generalized loss in alveolar volume and alveolar collapse, which is atelectasis (Campbell, 1977; Wahba, 1983).

Nursing care is clearly required to prevent pulmonary complications in the elderly. A stir-up regimen, including turning, coughing, deep breathing, and incentive spirometry, is essential. Because gas exchange is improved in the seated position (Wahba, 1983), the patient should be up in a chair as soon as possible, and early ambulation is vital. The nurse should check the preoperative PETs and be aware of the patient's normal VC and V_T. These can be used as guides in incentive spirometry. The target volume for incentive spirometry can initially be set at about a quarter to a third of the preoperative VC and gradually raised.

A study of 177 surgical patients aged 65 and older found that those who performed poorly on a preoperative test of exercise capacity had significantly more pulmonary and cardiovascular complications than did those who were more physically fit (Gerson et al., 1990). Thus, the nurse should evaluate the exercise capacity of elderly patients before surgery to target those with the greatest potential for complications for intensified preoperative and postoperative nursing care.

Finally, the nutritional status of the patient must be evaluated. Wahba (1983) says there is clear evidence that undernourished patients breathe shallowly, do not sigh, and have poor ventilatory responses to carbon dioxide. However, these factors can be reversed with appropriate dietary intake.

RESPIRATORY DISEASES COMMON TO THE AGED

The most common and important pulmonary problems in the elderly include chronic obstructive pulmonary disease (COPD), adult-onset asthma, pneumonia, tuberculosis, lung cancer, and pulmonary embolism (Reichel, 1983). Pulmonary embolism is covered in Chapter 7 (cardiovascular disease). In addition, sleep apnea has been shown to be fairly common in the aged.

Chronic Obstructive Pulmonary Disease

COPD is common in the elderly, especially in men, with a peak incidence in the sixth and seventh decades. In men, age-adjusted prevalence rates for COPD have been stable since 1980; however, in women, the prevalence of COPD has increased by 35 per cent between 1979 and 1985 (Hodgkin et al., 1993). Some of the changes characteristic of aging are similar to those seen in COPD, but there are important differences. First, COPD is a progressive disease, whereas the changes with aging seem to be normal physiological changes. Second, patients with COPD are usually symptomatic and have the physical signs of chronic lung diseases, such as labored breathing, wheezing, use of accessory muscles of respiration, and chronic cough (Block, 1979). COPD is characterized by airway obstruction, small airways disease, or the clinical presence of a chronic productive cough that has no other cause. COPD is predominantly a disease of cigarette smokers; the majority of COPD patients smoke. However, because only about 15 per cent of smokers have symptomatic air flow obstruction, it has been suggested that some people may have a genetic predisposition to airway injury (Canadian Thoracic Society Workshop Group, 1992; Mahler, 1993). Other causes of COPD are environmental pollution, recurrent infections, and bronchial irritation (Reichel, 1983). In the elderly, COPD can also result from chronic asthma (Bloom and Barreuther, 1993; Traver et al., 1993).

COPD is classically divided into two types: type A, emphysema, and type B, chronic bronchitis, although one individual often has both types (mixed COPD), and it may be difficult to separate them clinically. Both are characterized by a *limitation of expiratory air flow*. They are second only to heart disease as a cause of disability (Hodgkin et al., 1993).

Emphysema

Emphysema can be truly diagnosed only in a postmortem examination because it is defined morphologically as abnormal and permanent dilation of the terminal air spaces of the lungs, combined with destruction of the alveolar wall. A presumptive diagnosis can be made on the basis of the clinical picture and PFTs. Clinically, the patient has chronic dyspnea on exertion, with or without cough, and progressive disability due to unrelenting dyspnea. Early in the disease, there are no characteristic physical findings. Later, the patient is often anxious, thin, and sometimes emaciated; the chest is large and hyperinflated, and the patient struggles to breathe. Pursed-lip breathing may be used in an unconscious effort to get rid of the excess trapped air. If there is a cough, it is usually nonproductive. The patient has a prolonged expiratory phase of breathing, often with wheezes, and is *not* cyanotic (Block, 1979; King and Schwarz, 1982; Petty, 1983).

PFT show large lung volumes because of overdistention. RV is increased because of trapping of air on expiration due to the large, floppy alveoli, which have lost much of their elastic recoil. The ability to expel air quickly is severely limited, so FEV_1 is markedly reduced.

Interestingly, the loss of alveoli is accompanied by a loss of pulmonary capillaries, so the distribution of ventilation and perfusion is relatively well maintained. The patient with pure emphysema is not cyanotic and does not have hypoxemia (PO_2 below 60 mm Hg) or carbon dioxide retention until the disease is terminal. In spite of this, the dyspnea experienced is profound (Petty, 1983).

Chronic Bronchitis

Chronic bronchitis is diagnosed when an individual has a chronic productive cough on most days for at least 3 consecutive months in a year for 2 successive years, in the absence of any other known condition that could produce these symptoms (Cherniack and Cherniack, 1983; Weiss, 1982; Reichel, 1983; Stark and Lipscomb, 1983). A person with chronic bronchitis is usually somewhat obese, has a chronic cough, and complains of frequent "chest colds." Cyanosis, cardiomegaly, and cor pulmonale are often present in these patients but not in those with only emphysema. These patients often have severe hypoxemia and elevated carbon dioxide (Block, 1979; Stark and Lipscomb, 1983).

Chronic bronchitis is more common in men than in women, probably because in the past more men than women smoked. It outranks all other respiratory diseases as a crippler and a killer. In a well-established case, there is hypertrophy of the bronchial mucous glands and the globlet cells, and effective cilia are reduced. The major etiologic factor is cigarette smoking, although environmental pollution and occupation may also play a role in the development of the disease. The prevalence of the disease is highest in industrial areas, especially in men who work in dusty occupations, such as coal mining (Cherniack and Cherniack, 1983).

The onset of this disease is usually insidious, appearing as a chronic cough that the person may attribute to smoking. Breathing problems may not become apparent to the individual until after 30 years of smoking. It is important to understand that a "cigarette cough" is not normal but is an early sign of bronchitis. It may disappear if the smoking is stopped early enough. The course of the disease may be slow, with death due to bronchopneumonia, respiratory insufficiency, and right-sided heart failure occurring 20 to 35 years after the onset of symptoms (Cherniack and Cherniack, 1983).

Complications of COPD

Cor pulmonale is hypertrophy of the right ventricle resulting from lung diseases. It is characterized by high pulmonary artery pressures. Apparently, high pulmonary artery pressures develop in patients with COPD as a result of long-standing hypoxemia, polycythemia, and respiratory acidosis. The patient with cor pulmonale may have severe cyanosis, unexplained drowsiness, engorged neck veins, heptomegaly, and fluid retention with dependent edema (King and Schwarz, 1982).

Other complications of COPD include su-

praventricular and ventricular *arrhythmias,* secondary *polycythemia, pulmonary embolism,* and rarely *spontaneous pneumothorax. Sleep apnea* occurs in perhaps 80 per cent of patients with COPD, leading to periods of serious nocturnal hypoxia. *Peptic ulcer disease* also occurs more frequently in these patients (10 to 35 per cent) than in the average population (3 per cent) (King and Schwarz, 1982).

A common and serious complication is *acute respiratory failure,* sometimes occurring in combination with or as a result of some of the other complications. It is defined as arterial hypoxemia (PO less than 50 mm Hg) and hypercapnia (PCO_2 greater than 50 mm Hg). Precipitating causes include (1) respiratory infection; (2) carbon dioxide narcosis caused by respiratory depression after the administration of oxygen; (3) oversedation; (4) congestive heart failure; and (5) pulmonary embolism (King and Schwarz, 1982). Patients with these problems are usually in a critical care unit, and a discussion of their care is beyond the scope of this book.

Nursing Care for COPD Patients

Medical therapy for COPD is primarily aimed at controlling symptoms and complications (King and Schwarz, 1982). Nursing care supports these goals and includes finding ways to help patients adapt to this chronic illness and live their lives as fully as possible in spite of the disability. In a study of 123 elderly COPD patients, the link between severity of disease and their quality of life was weak. Symptoms of dyspnea and wheezing were related to quality of life, but scores on PFTs were unrelated (Schrier et al., 1990). This suggests that helping patients and families find ways to lessen symptoms and cope with the disease can have a major impact on their lives. Some coping techniques that have been suggested for COPD patients are relaxation techniques, activity modification and energy conservation, social support, increased knowledge and education, monitoring of the intensity of dyspnea, contracting for goals, and changing one's attitude toward disease (Mahler, 1993).

Primary nursing interventions should be directed toward helping the patient stop smoking. Cigarette smoke has a profound inhibitory effect on mucociliary clearance, but at the same time it stimulates production of excess mucus. In addition, it acts as a bronchoconstrictor; airway resistance may double after smoking one cigarette, and this effect may last as long as 30 minutes (Cherniack and Cherniack, 1983). Mahler (1993) says "cessation of cigarette smoking is certainly the single most important intervention for elderly patients with COPD" (p. 171).

Another major focus for nursing care is controlling the exacerbation of symptoms. Adequate hydration is important for those with chronic bronchitis because mucus tends to be thick and difficult to expectorate. If modified postural drainage is required, a family member may be taught to help the patient with simple exercises over pillows in bed. Some patients with chronic bronchitis require oxygen at home. In this case, the patient and family need instruction in the safe use of oxygen and must be told to keep the flow rate of oxygen low, about 2 liters per minute, certainly never more than 4 liters per minute, because of the danger of suppressing the breathing reflex. In patients with a chronically high carbon level, breathing is stimulated by the relatively low oxygen tension in the blood; if this is raised to a level that would be normal in others, the breathing reflex could be blunted or even lost, and the patient may stop breathing.

The nurse should focus on helping the patient develop a lifestyle that minimizes energy expenditure while allowing as much activity as possible. The patient can be taught to be aware of breathing and not to hold the breath at intervals when shaving or putting on make-up as most people do. Patients with COPD may be embarrassed by their obvious dyspnea and may avoid going out in public. When they do go out, it is important for them to plan ahead, allowing plenty of time to get ready. Rushing only increases the patient's dyspnea. Participating in a discussion with a group of people with the same problem may help these patients feel less unusual and give them an opportunity to share ideas about how to save energy and breath.

Early and aggressive treatment of a respiratory infection is vital for patients with COPD. Thus, patients should be taught to report an increase in the amount of sputum and especially any change in its color. These signs, with or without fever, may indicate that the patient may need an antibiotic such as tetracycline or ampicillin (Reichel, 1983). Cough suppressants and analgesics should be avoided in these patients because they may cause sputum retention and depress respirations. Sedatives and tranquilizers must also be avoided because they may depress respiration. Expectorants and antispasmotics appear to have little value in COPD patients (Freeman, 1978). Intermittent positive-pressure breathing has been shown to have no benefit for COPD patients and may even be harmful (King and Schwarz, 1982).

Patients should be taught proper breathing techniques, with emphasis on the need to breathe slowly, using the abdominal muscles to facilitate lung emptying during expiration. Nurses often recommend purse-lip breathing, but studies have failed to demonstrate that this improves breathing efficiency. Many patients adopt this breathing pattern spontaneously, and there is no need to interfere. General physical conditioning exercises that improve muscle tone may be necessary because the patient may suffer from extreme breathlessness and disability (Reichel, 1983). It is important to maintain activity at the highest possible level for the patient's psychological and physical benefit.

An excellent patient teaching booklet, *Shortness of Breath: A Guide to Better Living and Breathing,* is available (Moser et al., 1991). Although not specific to the elderly, it is accurate, up to date, and very readable, full of helpful and entertaining illustrations.

Asthma

Acute and chronic asthma may occur in the elderly. Asthma is characterized by hyperactive airways and produces an increased resistance to expiratory flow and hyperinflation of the lungs. Asthma has been considered a disease of the young, and COPD a disease of the elderly. However, asthma is now recognized as relatively common in the elderly. Two large epidemiological studies indicate that asthma prevalence is between 8 and 10 per cent in childhood, declines to about 5 per cent in early adulthood, and increases to 7 to 9 per cent in the elderly (Bardana, 1993). Common estimates of the incidence of new-onset asthma after age 65 vary from 1 to 3 per cent. However, one study of elderly asthmatics in a pulmonary referral clinic showed that asthma developed in 48 per cent of them at age 65 or older (Braman et al., 1991).

Commonly, elderly who have asthma late in life have been considered to have "intrinsic" asthma, which does not have allergic or environmental triggers; as opposed to "extrinsic" asthma, which is more common in children. Some dispute this, saying that all asthma has some allergic basis (Smyrnios and Irwin, 1993). In childhood, the severity of asthma correlates strongly with IgE levels and the presence of a skin-sensitizing antibody. However, neither of these tests is as useful in the elderly, probably because of decrease in allergic response with aging (Bardana, 1993; Traver et al., 1993).

Respiratory infections are a common precipitating factor, but exposure to dust, cigarette smoke, polluted air, or even a change in temperature can precipitate an attack. These patients may have fairly continuous symptoms. Symptoms of asthma in the elderly include paroxysms of dyspnea, often occurring at night, as well as wheeze and cough. These symptoms can be markedly improved with bronchodilator or corticosteroid therapy (Smyrnios and Irwin, 1993).

In an acute exacerbation of the disease, there is bronchoconstriction, tracheobronchial mucosal edema, and increased secretion of thick, tenacious mucus. Ventilation-perfusion mismatch can result from local obstruction of airways, and there may even be complete obstruction of airways by large mucous plugs.

The symptoms of asthma, which may develop gradually or suddenly, include a sensation of chest tightness and expiratory wheezing. There are varying degrees of dyspnea, which is more common at night in the elderly asthmatic (Traver et al., 1993). As the symptoms become more severe, wheezing is present on both inspiration and expiration. A productive cough, often worse after exertion or at night, may be the major complaint. Initially, the sputum is clear and mucoid, but it may become green, gray, or yellow with infection or stasis. The patient may use accessory muscles in the struggle to breathe and almost always has tachypnea. Tachycardia is also commonly seen in an acute attack. On auscultation, coarse breathe sounds with a prolonged expiratory phase and of course wheezes are heard. In a severe and prolonged case, these may be hypoxia and hypercapnia (Sherter et al., 1984).

Treatment of asthma is the same in the elderly as in the young. It includes initial and periodic monitoring of lung function through spirometry, cessation of smoking, removal of animals if the person is allergic to them, and good bronchial hygiene to improve airway clearance because many patients with advanced disease may have problems mobilizing airway secretions. Such hygiene measures include adequate oral hydration and humidification of inspired air. Inhaled bronchodilators and corticosteroids are the drugs of choice for asthmatics; they are effective in the larger doses now available and have relatively few side effects (Traver et al., 1993). However, the elderly may have problems using the devices properly because of poor coordination, weakness, or impaired cognitive function (Woodhouse and Wynne, 1992). Thus, it is important to teach the proper use of the equipment and have the patient regularly demonstrate the use of all prescribed inhalers.

The elderly asthmatic has some special problems because of the common presence of other chronic diseases. The hypoxemia characteristic of moderate to severe asthma may exacerbate cardiac ischemia. Also, beta blockers such as propranolol (Inderal), commonly used for angina, make asthma worse and should be avoided if possible. Some individuals have an allergic response to aspirin. Because many elderly use aspirin regularly for arthritis, this could be a problem. Finally, the elder's mental status may be adversely affected, especially if the asthma is poorly controlled and partially disabling. It is vital to relieve fear and anxiety by providing control over the asthma attacks. Adherence to the therapeutic regimen is particularly important in elderly asthmatics. Treatment is usually successful, and the decline in lung function after treatment is similar to that found in "healthy" elderly (Traver et al., 1993).

Because asthma responds well to treatment, it is important for the nurse to recognize that it can coexist with COPD. In the Lung Health Study, bronchial reactivity (hyperactive airways) was present in two thirds of patients with early COPD (Mahler, 1993). Unfortunately, treatable disorders of the airway are often undiagnosed in the elderly, perhaps because of the high prevalence of other forms of respiratory disease and cardiac failure that may have similar clinical presentations (Dow and Holgate, 1990). Dow (1992) reports that about 15 per cent of patients older than 65 will not be able to perform spirometric diagnostic tests reliably and suggests that additional tests, such as symptom scores and distance walked without dyspnea or wheezing, be used to diagnose patients with chronic air flow limitation. Nurses can carefully observe elders for these symptoms, and question them further, because the elderly tend to underreport symptoms of dyspnea.

Drug Therapy

Drugs for COPD and asthma can be divided into two groups, bronchodilators and anti-inflammatory agents. Bronchodilators, used in most COPD and in virtually all asthma patients, include beta-adrenergic agonists, theophylline, and anticholinergic agents. Bronchodilators act mainly to relax the smooth muscle of the airways. In addition, theophylline may have minor anti-inflammatory effects on the airways. The beta-adrenergic agonists also stabilize mast

TABLE 8 – 3

Beta$_2$-Adrenergic Bronchodilators Available in the United States

DRUG	DOSAGE FORM	STRENGTHS
Metaproterenol (Alupent)	Tablets	10 mg and 20 mg
	Oral solution	10 mg/5 ml
	MDI	650 μg/spray
	Nebulizer solution	5%
Terbutaline (Bricanyl, Brethaire)	Tablets	2.5 mg and 5 mg
	MDI	200 μg/spray
	Injection	1 mg/ml
Albuterol (Proventil, Ventolin)	Tablets	2 mg and 4 mg
		4-mg extended release
	Oral solution	2 mg/5 ml
	MDI	90 μg/spray
	Dry powder rotohaler	200 μg/capsule
	Nebulizer solution	0.5% (5 mg/ml)
Bitolterol (Tornalate)	MDI	370 μg/spray
Pirbuterol (Maxair)	MDI	200 μg/spray

MDI = metered dose inhaler.

From Bloom, J.W. and Barreuther, A.D. Drug therapy of airways obstructive diseases. *In* Bressler, R. and Katz, M.D. (eds.). *Geriatric Pharmacology.* New York: McGraw-Hill, 1993. Copyright 1993, McGraw-Hill.

cells, inhibiting the release of chemical mediators of bronchospasm and improving mucociliary clearance of the airways (Bloom and Barreuther, 1993).

Beta-adrenergic stimulants are the cornerstone of therapy for asthmatic patients (Table 8–3). The most common side effects are tremor and palpitations, and these effects are greater when the drug is given orally or intravenously than when it is inhaled. In the past, oral doses were commonly used, particularly in the elderly. However, the current recommended mode of administration is through inhalation. Oral administration is much less effective in asthmatics, and it is associated with a greater frequency of side effects than metered dose inhalers (MDIs) are (Bloom and Barreuther, 1993; Traver et al., 1993). Even in acute asthma, studies show there is no difference in the effectiveness between inhaled and intravenous terbutaline (Bloom and Barreuther, 1993).

The major problem with the use of MDIs is improper inhalation technique. Allen and Prior (1986) studied the use of MDIs in elderly patients and found that only 60 per cent used appropriate technique, and in only 10 per cent was the technique ideal. Patients must be taught carefully and observed at frequent intervals. According to Bloom and Barreuther (1993), the appropriate technique is as follows:

1. Shake the MDI.
2. Tilt head slightly back.
3. Breathe out slowly, but not forcibly, to a volume just below normal resting volume.
4. Put mouthpiece in the mouth between the teeth, and pointed above the tongue.
5. Begin to inhale slowly through the mouth and *then* activate the inhaler.
6. Continue to inhale to total lung capacity.
7. Hold breath for at least 10 seconds.

Theophylline has been the most commonly used bronchodilator for many years, but at present, there is much controversy as to its role; there is a trend to use it as a second- or third-line choice for therapy. Theophylline is well absorbed from the gastrointestinal tract, and its bioavailability is not affected by age; it is cleared from the body through the liver. The major problem with the drug is the high frequency of toxic effects, which is even higher in the elderly. Common side effects are nausea, tremor, headache, agitation, and insomnia, which are especially common when therapy is instituted. More severe side effects are seizures and life-threatening cardiac arrhythmias. Accepted therapeutic levels are 10 to 20 μg per ml, but it may be better to keep the range to 10 μg per ml in the elderly (Bloom and Barreuther, 1993; Traver et al., 1993). Bloom and Barreuther (1993) conclude that there is little or no additional benefit to be gained from adding theophylline to a regimen that uses adequate doses of inhaled beta-adrenergic agonists. Furthermore, they note that theophylline may be even less effective in the elderly than in younger asthmatics.

Anticholinergics, particularly ipratropium bromide (Atrovent), are less effective as bronchodilators in asthmatics, but they may be more effective in patients with COPD. No drug interactions have been reported with its use, and the only important side effect is cough (Bloom and Barreuther, 1993).

Corticosteroids, major anti-inflammatory agents, are commonly used in treating asthma. Because inhaled corticosteroids have few of the major side effects associated with oral use, Bloom and Barreuther (1993) recommend that elderly asthmatics be switched from oral to inhaled preparations such as beclomethasone dipropionate (Vanceril, Beclovent), but their use in COPD is not clear.

Pneumonia

Lower respiratory tract infections are a major cause of morbidity in the elderly. Pneumonia and influenza are the fifth leading cause of death in people older than 65. Death rates from pneumococcal pneumonia are estimated to be three to five times higher in those older than 65. More than two thirds of those admitted to hospitals with pneumonia are older than 65 (Fox, 1993). Most elderly patients with pneumonia will require hospitalization and will have a longer hospital stay because of coexisting illness. Elderly patients with pneumonia are also more likely to have bacteremia, empyema, and meningitis (Fein et al., 1991). Some of the reasons for this are the deterioration of the body's immune defenses, a weakened cough reflex, the presence of other chronic diseases, a general debilitated condition, and late diagnosis (Niederman, 1993; Sims, 1990).

Initial symptoms in the elderly may differ from those in younger patients. High spiking fevers, productive cough, and an elevated white blood cell count may not be seen. Instead, the initial cues may be an altered mental status, tachypnea, and evidence of dehydration. Most patients will have increasing cough and sputum, some fever, hyperventilation, and chest pain. The lack of typical symptoms in an elderly patient with pneumonia has been associated with a higher mortality rate (Niederman, 1993). One of the most important early signs of pneumonia is tachypnea. A study of nursing home patients found that respiratory rate for stable patients who did not have an infection was 16 to 25 per minute. However, when pneumonia or other respiratory tract infections developed, the respiratory rate increased above that range. Importantly, tachypnea was present 24 to 48 hours before any other signs of infection (Niederman, 1993). This finding reinforces the importance of monitoring respiratory rate carefully and frequently.

Pneumonia is often categorized according to the source, that is, community-acquired or nosocomial. The most common causative agent for community-acquired pneumonia is *Streptococcus pneumoniae;* these patients are more likely to present a typical clinical picture. Patients with COPD in the community often have *Haemophilus influenzae* pneumonia. *Staphylococcus aureus* is often seen in pneumonias that develop after the flu. Pneumonias acquired in the hospital are often caused by gram-negative organisms; those acquired in nursing homes are frequently due to *Klebsiella pneumoniae* and *S. aureus* (Fox, 1993). In the elderly, these bacteria often colonize from the mouth or may be aspirated. In addition, the impaired mucociliary clearance and weakened immune system of-

ten seen in elders make them highly susceptible (Niederman, 1993; Sims, 1990).

In a study of 166 patients hospitalized for pneumonia, it was found that age had no effect on the symptoms of a well-established case of pneumonia. However, the outcome did vary with age. Hospital stay was 5.7 days in patients younger than 60 years but was 9.8 days in those 60 to 79 and 11.3 days in those older than 79. In addition, mortality rose with age, from 6 per cent in those in their 60s, up to 11 per cent in those 70 and older (Fedullo and Swinburne, 1985).

Elderly patients with pneumonia are likely to be hospitalized "if they are expected to have a complicated course, if a coexisting disease (such as diabetes or CHF) is likely to decompensate as a result of the infection, or if specific supportive measures are needed that can only be provided in a hospital. In the latter category are intravenous medications, oxygen, chest physiotherapy, and close monitoring of vital signs" (Niederman, 1993, p. 308). Other important forms of therapy are hydration to replace reduction in fluid intake that may be due to confusion. Mucolytics and mucokinetics may also be used. The patient's fluid balance should be carefully watched; many antibiotics promote fluid retention, which may not be well tolerated in patients with decreased cardiac function. In addition, the nurse should be alert for indications that the antibiotic is causing a reaction with other medications the patient is taking (Niederman, 1993). Mortality in pneumonia in the elderly is often due to secondary or underlying causes, such as congestive heart failure (Fox, 1993).

Because this problem is so prevalent in the elderly, one of the major concerns of a geriatric nurse should be to prevent pneumonia. Keeping elders up, active, and well nourished is of primary importance. People who are in bed most of the time and those fed by hand or by feeding tube are at increased risk for aspiration pneumonia and must be carefully and frequently observed for early changes in lung function, such as cough, and especially for increase in respiratory rate and changes in respiratory pattern.

Nurses should take special precautions to prevent aspiration by patients hospitalized for pneumonia. Thus, use of hypnotics and sedatives should be kept to a minimum. Also, if a nasogastric tube is needed, a small-bore tube and small amounts of fluid should be used; if dilution of feedings is needed, sterile water and not tap water should be used (Fox, 1993).

Colds and flu may lead to pneumonia, so they should be treated early. The incidence of upper respiratory infections, such as the common cold, pharyngitis, and acute laryngitis, is less in older than in younger persons, but these diseases are important because they can predispose to pneumonia. Influenza may be a serious threat to life in the elderly, primarily because of the complications of bronchitis and pneumonia. The symptoms of uncomplicated flu are the same in the elderly as in the young; sudden onset, chills, fever headache, cough, sore throat, myalgia, and malaise.

The primary way to prevent pneumonia for community-dwelling elderly is through flu vaccinations, which have been shown to be effective in reducing the occurrence of pneumonia (Foster et al., 1992). The U.S. Public Health Service's Advisory Committee on Immunization Practices recommends annual revaccination of those older than 65 as well as of younger individuals with chronic diseases. It takes 2 to 3 weeks for the influenza vaccine to achieve effectiveness, and the overall success rate is 45 to 65 per cent (Foster et al., 1992).

Tuberculosis

Although tuberculosis (TB) is not the major health hazard it was in the first half of the 20th century, it still occurs, and 60 per cent of cases occur in patients older than 45 years. Because many elderly were exposed to TB as children, reactivation may occur in later years. More than 90 per cent of newly reported cases of active TB in the United States involve a reactivation of dormant disease. Susceptibility is increased by alcoholism, malnutrition, diabetes, use of immunosuppressive drugs, and cardiovascular disease. An additional risk factor is living in close quarters with other susceptible individuals. In elderly residents of nursing homes, shelters, or prisons, new TB infections are often a common problem, producing serious disease and even death (Umeki, 1991).

The clinical picture of TB is familiar: fever, night sweats, weight loss, anorexia, and hemoptysis. However, this typical picture may not be seen in the elderly, and TB is often missed in this population. The elderly patient with TB may show the classic TB symptoms of cough, fever, and general fatigue, but these may also be associated with other chronic diseases common in the elderly. Dyspnea and night sweats are not commonly associated with TB in the elderly. Because of the large disease burden carried by many elders, and a low index of suspicion for TB by their health care providers,

the diagnosis of TB may be made only at autopsy (Allen, 1992; Umeki, 1991).

Diagnosis is based on chest x-rays or on demonstration of acid-fast bacilli in the sputum. X-rays show shadows in the upper lobes, as in younger patients, but those aged 60 are also likely to have involvement of the middle and lower lobes (Umeki, 1991; Allen, 1992). Skin tests are not helpful because results are often negative in the aged with TB, possibly because of their reduced immune system activity (Mostow, 1983; Stark and Lipscomb, 1983).

Treatment with modern chemotherapy is effective, and a cure rate of almost 100 per cent can be achieved *if the disease is diagnosed* and chemotherapy is correctly prescribed, and *if the prescribed drugs are taken faithfully* for the recommended 6 to 18 months. Drug therapy consists of three major drugs: rifampin, isoniazid (INH), and ethambutol (Allen, 1992; Fox, 1993; Umeki, 1991).

All of these drugs may have significant toxic effects. INH causes hepatitis in the elderly, so liver function must be carefully monitored. Early signs of this problem are anorexia, nausea, vomiting, fatigue, malaise, and weakness. Another adverse reaction to INH is peripheral neuropathy, especially in malnourished, bedridden elderly and in those predisposed to neuritis, such as diabetics and alcoholics. Rifampin, when used in combination with INH, can also cause liver damage. The major adverse reactions to rifampin are gastrointestinal and include anorexia, nausea, epigastric distress, and vomiting. The most severe and dangerous toxic effect of ethambutol is a potential for retinal damage. Patients should be evaluated by an ophthalmologist before being prescribed this drug (Umeki, 1991).

Formerly, all patients with TB were hospitalized for long periods. This is no longer necessary unless it is likely that the patient will not take the prescribed drugs or there are complications. Patients may be in the hospital for 1 to 2 weeks while therapy is instituted. The patient is usually placed in isolation for the first 2 weeks of therapy. In addition, when an active case of TB is detected, household and other close contacts must be tested for infection. For nursing home residents, this often means that other residents and most of the staff should be tested (Allen, 1992).

Nursing care for the elderly patient with TB includes teaching the patient and family about the disease and drugs and providing psychological support. The patient may view this diagnosis as a stigma and feel like an outcast, because TB patients were formerly placed in sanatoriums, far removed from family and friends. They often need nutritional support and may require consultation from a dietitian and a social worker. In addition, the nurse must be alert for early signs of drug toxicity, as described before.

One important aspect of the nursing care of the elder with TB is assessment of compliance with the drug regimen. Nurses are often in a position to find out whether the patient is actually taking all the drugs prescribed and in the way they were recommended. Close adherence to the drug regimen for a long time is difficult but essential if the disease is to be cured.

Cancer of the Lung

Lung cancer, a major disease of the elderly, was responsible for more than 150,000 deaths in the United States in 1990. From 1950 to 1993, the overall age-adjusted death rate for lung cancer increased from 13.0 to 50.3 per 100,000 people, with a fourfold increase for men and a sevenfold increase for women. Although the overall death rate for lung cancer is higher in men than in women, the rate of increase for men started to slow in the 1980s, whereas it increased sharply in women during that time. As shown in Figure 8–6, the death rate from lung cancer in women has been higher than their death rate from breast cancer for several years (Boring et al., 1993). The cohort of women born from 1931 to 1940, in whom the prevalence of smoking peaked at about 44 per cent, is likely to have the highest prevalence of lung cancer. Thus, the death rate from lung cancer in elderly women will no doubt continue to rise. As with other malignant neoplasms, lung cancer is more common with advancing age; the peak mortality from lung cancer is seen in those 75 to 84 (Allen, 1992).

There are five types of bronchogenic carcinoma. These include (1) epidermoid (squamous), (2) adenocarcinoma, (3) alveolar cell, (4) small cell (oat cell), and (5) large cell (undifferentiated). Overall 5-year survival for the major histological types of cancer is shown in Table 8–4. In a survey of elderly men, the most common histological type was squamous cell carcinoma (30 per cent), closely followed by small cell carcinoma (24 per cent), adenocarcinoma (22 per cent), and large cell carcinoma (22 per cent). Mixed carcinoma was seen in 2 per cent, and alveolar carcinoma was rare (Allen, 1992).

Although the rate of tumor growth is somewhat slower in the elderly than in younger lung cancer patients, it is still a lethal disease, with an average survival in the elderly of only about 25 weeks for small cell cancer and about 48 weeks for non–small cell cancer (Findlay et al., 1991; Ishida et al., 1990). Survival for small cell cancer is especially low, with a life expectancy often given in weeks or months instead of years. Unfortunately, this virulent type of cancer accounts for about 20 per cent of all bronchogenic carcinomas (Hoffman et al., 1984). Lung cancer, especially small cell, is likely to metastasize. Common sites of metastasis are the central nervous system, liver, and bones (Allen, 1992).

Common signs and symptoms of lung cancer are shown in Table 8–5. These may be related to the primary lung tumor or to the spread of the tumor. Common symptoms are cough, streaky hemoptysis, and

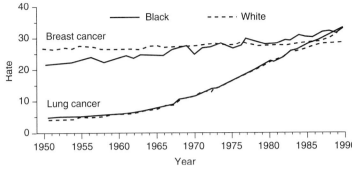

FIGURE 8 – 6

Age-adjusted lung and breast cancer death rates for women, by race—United States, 1950 to 1990.

T A B L E   8 – 4

Overall 5-Year Survival Percentage for the Major Histological Types of Lung Cancer

HISTOLOGICAL TYPE	5-YEAR SURVIVAL PERCENTAGE		PERCENTAGE RESECTABLE
	All Cases (N = 2155)	Resected (N = 835)	
Epidermoid carcinoma	25	37	60
Adenocarcinoma	12	27	38*
Large cell carcinoma	13	27	38*
Small cell carcinoma	1	0	11

* Combined in the report of the American Joint Committee for Cancer Staging and End Results Reporting.

From Matthews, M.J. and Gordon, P.R. Morphology of pulmonary and pleural malignancies. In Straus, M.J. (ed.). *Lung Cancer: Clinical Diagnosis and Treatment.* New York: Grune & Stratton, 1977; Mountain, C.F., Carr, D.T., Martini, N., et al. *Staging of Lung Cancer 1979.* American Joint Committee for Cancer Staging and End Results Reporting. Chicago: Task Force on Lung Cancer, 1980.

TABLE 8 – 5
Common Signs and Symptoms of Lung Cancer

Symptoms Due to Central or Endobronchial Growth of the Primary Tumor
Cough
Hemoptysis
Wheeze and stridor
Dyspnea from obstruction
Pneumonitis from obstruction (fever, productive cough)

Symptoms Due to Peripheral Growth of the Primary Tumor
Pain from pleural or chest wall involvement
Cough
Dyspnea on a restrictive basis
Lung abscess syndrome from tumor cavitation

Symptoms Related to Regional Spread of the Tumor in the Thorax by Contiguity or by Metastasis to Regional Lymph Nodes
Tracheal obstruction
Esophageal compression with dysphagia
Recurrent laryngeal nerve paralysis with hoarseness
Phrenic nerve paralysis with hemidiaphragm elevation and dyspnea
Sympathetic nerve paralysis with Horner's syndrome
Eighth cervical and first thoracic nerves with ulnar pain and Pancoast's syndrome
Superior vena cava syndrome from vascular obstruction
Pericardial and cardiac extension with resultant tamponade, arrhythmia, or cardiac failure
Lymphatic obstruction with pleural effusion
Lymphangitic spread through lungs with hypoxemia and dyspnea

From Cohen, M.H. Signs and symptoms of bronchogenic carcinoma. In Straus, M.J. (ed.). *Lung Cancer: Clinical Diagnosis and Treatment.* New York: Grune & Stratton, 1977, pp. 85–94.

chest pain. With the exception of hemoptysis, these symptoms are often ignored by the elderly. Often fairly common symptoms are a new onset of localized wheezing, worsening dyspnea, and obstructive pneumonia. Unfortunately, these are usually seen late in the disease after it is well established. In addition, endocrine and metabolic abnormalities such as hypercalcemia, inappropriate antidiuretic hormone secretion, and Cushing's syndrome may be caused by hormones manufactured by the lung tumor (Allen, 1992).

Chest x-ray usually shows the tumor, and occasionally the tumor is found early by x-ray before any symptoms have been noted. For this reason, annual chest x-rays may be indicated for those at increased risk. Cell type and stage of the disease are determined by cytological study of sputum and fiberoptic bronchoscopy; this information helps guide decisions about prognosis and treatment. Computed tomography of the thorax or nuclear magnetic resonance scanning may be used to visualize deep structures (Allen, 1992).

Smoking accounts for 87 per cent of all lung cancer deaths (Boring et al., 1993). Lung cancer is also associated with long-term exposure to a number of other carcinogenic pollutants such as asbestos, uranium, nickel, chlormethyl ether, and chromium. Asbestos and uranium exposure apparently act synergistically with cigarette smoke.

Treatment of lung cancer consists primarily of resection of the lesion. Allen (1992) recommends that surgical resection of the tumor be done in the elderly whenever possible; in some studies, the results of resection in those older than 70 have been as good as in younger patients. Although only have 15 per cent have a truly resectable tumor at the time of diagnosis, surgery can reduce the tumor mass and increases the efficacy of later radiotherapy or chemotherapy. Further, surgery offers the only possibility of a true cure. Radiotherapy may be used with surgery and is also an important alternative for those who are unable or unwilling to have surgery. Radiotherapy is particularly helpful in those with squamous cell cancer and is as well tolerated by the elderly as by younger patients.

Currently, there is much controversy over the role of chemotherapy in the treatment of the most virulent form of lung cancer, small cell carcinoma. Some authors conclude that chemotherapy should be used in the elderly because there is little difference in survival rates for young and old subjects (Johnson, 1993). However, others say aggressive chemotherapy is not justified because of the high occurrence of toxic effects in elders and the short mean survival of 25 weeks (36 weeks for intensive treatment, 16 weeks for those with less intensive treatment) (Findlay, et al., 1991).

Nursing care of the elder with lung cancer is no different from that given young patients. The older person is perhaps more likely to have thought about the possibility of death. The idea of dying of cancer may be particularly frightening because of the fear of pain and the possibility that there may be no family and few friends to provide support. The patient needs to be reassured that excessive pain is not common in most cancers, and that the pain that is present can be controlled without significantly changing the ability to function and think. Hospice care is particularly helpful for the elderly patient with lung cancer.

Sleep Apnea

Apnea, defined as the cessation of breathing for 10 seconds or longer, commonly occurs during sleep. It may be accompanied by underventilation and oxygen desaturation. The most commonly accepted criterion for diagnosis of sleep apnea is 5 periods of documented apnea per hour of sleep, that is, an apnea index of 5. By use of this criterion, large-scale studies have shown that 24 per cent of community-dwelling elders and 43 per cent of nursing home patients have sleep apnea (Ancoli-Israel et al., 1991a, 1991b; Fleury, 1992; Schwartz and Smith, 1989). Obesity and increasing age, especially in men and postmenopausal women, are strongly associated with nocturnal desaturation.

The sleep apnea syndromes are a group of disorders associated with an abnormality in the central regulation of breathing (central apnea) or with an obstruction to air flow in the upper airways (occlusive apnea). In the elderly, central regulation may be impaired by microinfarcts, poor perfusion, or hormonal changes. Occlusive apnea is caused by collapse of the upper airway at sleep onset and is related to obesity and neurogenic depression of pharyngeal muscle tone (Ancoli-Israel et al., 1991a, b).

It is possible that sleep-related breathing disorders contribute to the high frequency of cardiac, hemodynamic, and nervous system dysfunctions and to functional deficits in the elderly. On the other hand, these disorders may also be secondary to many pulmonary cardiac, endocrine, and neurological diseases that occur in the elderly. Ancoli-Israel (1991a) has shown a strong relationship between dementia and sleep apnea, especially when both are severe. Currently, it is not clear whether sleep apnea increases mortality and morbidity in those older than 65. These may be associated with only the more severe forms of the disease. It is possible that the definition used (apnea index of 5) may not be applicable to the elderly. Clearly, longitudinal studies are needed (Ancoli-Israel et al., 1991b; Fleury, 1992).

Sleep apnea is characterized by snoring and nocturnal arousals. These individuals are usually unaware of the sleep abnormality except for the spouse's complaints about the snoring. Some may complain of either excessive daytime sleepiness or insomnia, but many are asymptomatic.

The high frequency of sleep-related breathing disorders has significance for nursing. These disorders are frequently ac-companied by insomnia; as a result, the elder may use hypnotics or alcohol to help induce sleep. Alcohol has been found to increase the occurrence, duration, and severity of oxygen desaturation of both symptomatic and asymptomatic sleep apnea patients and so should be avoided in these patients. Sedative and hypnotic drugs have also been implicated in these disorders. Benzodiazepines have less of an impact on respiration than barbiturates or other hypnotics, but they can cause or worsen sleep apnea. Wooten (1992) recommends that long-acting sedatives such as flurazepam (Dalmane) be avoided in the elderly. Table 8–6 lists common doses of benzodiazepine hypnotics.

The nurse should be aware of the high frequency of sleep apnea and should carefully monitor the respiratory pattern of the elderly at night. Patients may need to be referred to a sleep laboratory for diagnosis and specific treatment to prevent or reduce the occurrence of this debilitating condition. Obese elders with sleep apnea should be strongly encouraged to lose weight, because even modest reductions in weight have been shown to cause pronounced reductions in the frequency of apnea and hypopnea (Schwartz and Smith, 1989).

PULMONARY ASSESSMENT

History

For an adequate assessment of the pulmonary status of the elderly, the nurse must determine these important points: presence and extent of symptoms that indicate pulmonary disease or impairment; presence of environmental factors that interfere with res-

T A B L E   8 – 6

Benzodiazepine Hypnotics Commonly Used for Insomnia in Older Patients

Long-acting Agents	Approximate Dose Equivalents
Quazepam (Doral)	15 mg
Flurazepam (Dalmane)	15 mg
Diazepam (Valium, Valrelease)	4 mg
Short-acting Agents	
Estazolam (ProSom)	1 mg
Temazepam (Restoril)	15 mg
Alprazolam (Xanax)	0.5 mg
Oxazepam (Serax)	15 mg
Triazolam (Halcion)	0.25 mg

From Bachman, D.L. Sleep disorders with aging. Evaluation and treatments. *Geriatrics* 47(9):53–61, 1992.

T A B L E   8 – 7
Nursing Assessment of the Respiratory System

History
History of respiratory diseases (chronic obstructive pulmo-
   nary disease, asthma, tuberculosis)
Smoking history
Symptoms: cough, breathlessness or dyspnea, wheezing,
   hemoptysis, chest pain, orthopnea

Physical Assessment
Inspection
   Posture
   Shape of chest; symmetry of chest expansion
   Respirations (rate, rhythm, depth, length)
   Capillary refill of nail beds
   Skin color
   Sputum (color, odor, amount, consistency)
Palpation
   Ribs (tenderness)
   Skin temperature, turgor, moisture
Percussion
   Areas of dullness or flatness, hyperresonance
   Bilateral comparisons
Auscultation
   Breath sounds (rales, rhonchi, wheezes)

piratory function, especially smoking; and extent to which the person's usual lifestyle and activities of daily living have changed or are limited. In addition, it is important to determine the respiratory diseases the patient has had in the past as well as all other chronic diseases (Table 8–7).

Symptoms to Look For

The major symptoms of respiratory disorders are cough, often associated with sputum production, and shortness of breath. Other, less common symptoms are hemoptysis, chest pain, cyanosis, and an abnormal breathing pattern (Stiesmeyer, 1993). The history can obtain important information about all of these except the abnormal breathing patterns, which must be directly observed.

Cough must be carefully assessed. It is important to know whether the cough occurs daily or is intermittent and whether it has lasted for months or years. How long do the periods of coughing last? When do they occur? What brings them on? Are they debilitating? Most important, do they produce *sputum?* The patient should also be asked whether phlegm is brought up from the chest, because many patients who deny cough will admit to producing phlegm, and it has the same clinical significance. The amount, color, and consistency of the sputum should be very carefully determined, because this is one of the most important aspects of the examination in a pulmonary

patient. Remember that the diagnosis of chronic bronchitis is made primarily on the basis of the history of cough and sputum.

Breathlessness, or *dyspnea,* is one of the most frequent complaints in the elderly. A study of people aged 70 showed that 45 per cent of them had exertional dyspnea, and of those with dyspnea, 64 per cent of the men and 48 per cent of the women had an identifiable illness of the cardiopulmonary system. It is important to determine under what circumstances the person has dyspnea. Caird and Judge (1979) suggest a simple grading system, shown in Table 8–8. The distance the person can walk on a flat surface, at a reasonable pace without stopping, is a good indication of breathlessness.

The occurrence of nocturnal dyspnea and orthopnea usually, but not always, indicates a cardiac element in the breathlessness. A denial of dyspnea or replacement of dyspnea by fatigue as a major symptom is more common in elderly patients with heart disease than in those whose dyspnea is due to respiratory disease. It may also be a sign of a new acute process. "In the elderly patient with respiratory disease the recent onset of extreme fatigue usually signifies not the worsening of respiratory function, but the onset of an acute infection" (Caird and Judge, 1979).

An *elevated respiratory rate* has been shown to be a sensitive indicator of respiratory dysfunction and is an important sign of impending respiratory failure. Thus, it is important to count the respiratory rate. If the rate is more than 28 per minute, there will usually be other signs of labored breathing, such as use of accessory muscles and supraclavicular retractions (Alex and Tobin, 1993).

Cyanosis is a poor indicator of respiratory distress. A relatively late sign, it correlates roughly with arterial oxygen saturation (SaO_2) of less than 78 per cent. However, cyanosis may also be due to peripheral causes, such as low cardiac output and pe-

T A B L E   8 – 8
Grades of Dyspnea

1. Short of breath hurrying on level or walking up hills or
   stairs
2. Short of breath walking on level with people of same
   age
3. Short of breath walking on level at own pace
4. Short of breath on washing or dressing
5. Short of breath while sitting quietly

From Caird, F.I. and Judge, T.G. *Assessment of the Elderly Patient.* Philadelphia: J.B. Lippincott, 1979, p. 34.

ripheral vasoconstriction, or to the presence of abnormal pigments like methemoglobin; in those cases, it is not associated with arterial hypoxemia. Another poor indicator or respiratory distress is a bedside estimate of V_T, which is not useful because it is difficult to measure and thus can be variable (Alex and Tobin, 1993).

Chest pain in the elderly is not always due to myocardial ischemia. It may be pleuritic and may be seen in pneumonia, pulmonary infarction, rib fractures, costochondritis, and pulmonary hypertension, or it may be simply muscle pain after severe coughing. Complaints of pleuritic pain are not common in the elderly, even with severe pneumonia. The reason for this blunted pain sensation in the elderly is not clear. The pain of rib fracture, however, can be intense (Stiesmeyer, 1993). Again, it is important to ask specific questions if there is a complaint of pain. What brings it on? What relieves it? Is it dull, sharp, stabbing, constant, intermittent? Is it related to breathing cycles? How long has it been a problem?

Another symptom that may be of help is the occurrence of *wheezing.* Many people with chronic bronchitis complain of wheezing, which may vary from week to week with infectious processes but does not vary much from day to day or hour to hour. It is often worse in winter. The wheezing of asthma, however, is more episodic and tends to vary from day to day; when present, it frequently disturbs sleep.

Risk Factors and History of Diseases

The smoking history must be clearly identified in pack-years. That is, the age at which smoking was started and the average number of cigarettes smoked should be determined. If the person has been smoking for 50 years and has averaged 1½ packs a day, the person has a 75 pack-year history of smoking. Such a long history is not uncommon in elderly men. If they do not smoke but live with someone who does, the inhalation of secondhand smoke is an environmental hazard.

Other environmental conditions that could have an impact on respiratory function are living in a highly industrial area with air pollution for a long time, a history of working with asbestos in any form, and working as a miner. Any previous occupation that involved prolonged exposure to dust, smoke, or fumes should be noted. Even farming is associated with the development of a variety of respiratory diseases. The elderly often have pets, and these can also exacerbate respiratory diseases (Cherniack and Cherniack, 1983).

Elders should be asked whether they have any chronic diseases, such as hypertension, cardiac disease, or arthritis, as well as any respiratory diseases. It is important to find out whether the person has a recent history of pneumonia, flu, frequent colds, bronchitis, or contact with TB.

Physical Examination

The pulmonary examination is typically presented in four phases: inspection, palpation, percussion, and auscultation.

Inspection (Observation)

Inspection of the elderly usually reveals some musculoskeletal changes. Kyphosis is commonly seen, especially in elderly women. This accentuation of the thoracic curve, caused by osteoporotic collapse of the spinal vertebrae, gives the person the impression of leaning forward. There may also be a widening of the anterior-posterior distance of the chest, giving a barrel-chest appearance. This may be a normal finding with age and should be differentiated from the barrel chest seen in COPD by looking for abnormal pulmonary findings on percussion and auscultation (Mezey et al., 1980).

The quality, rate, and rhythm of quiet respirations should be observed. They are normally the same for all adults regardless of age; rate varies from 8 to 16 per minute, and V_T from 400 to 800 ml. In addition, respirations should be *evaluated during sleep* for abnormal patterns. *Obstructed breathing* is seen in patients with COPD and is characterized by a slow rate and increased volume, perhaps with wheezing also present. *Gasping respiration* consists of irregular, quick inspirations associated with an extension of the neck, followed by a long expiratory pause. This is characteristic of severe cerebral hypoxia and is common in patients with severe cardiac failure. *Cheyne-Stokes* respiration is a cyclic pattern of alternating apnea and hyperpnea. It is sometimes seen in healthy elderly persons but is usually found during sleep in patients with COPD, cardiac failure, or cerebrovascular insufficiency (King and Schwarz, 1982). Sleep apnea may also occur. As discussed earlier, this disorder is fairly common in the elderly and may cause oxygen desaturation as well as sleep disturbance.

It is also important to observe the patient while coughing to determine the strength of the cough reflex. A weak cough may signal a greater potential for serious trouble from a respiratory infection. Sputum should also be examined and the color and consistency carefully noted. If the sputum is clear or mucoid, there is no severe current infection (Caird and Judge, 1979).

Palpation

The trachea is often deviated in the elderly, but this may be due to scoliosis and so does not have the same significance as when it is found in the young. Also, because chest expansion is limited in the elderly, using a tape measure to try to determine it is a waste of time. Because rib fractures are common in the elderly, it is important to palpate for areas of point tenderness. Even a slight blow or fall could cause an undetected fracture (Mezey et al., 1980).

Percussion

Percussion is similar in the young and the old, except that the lungs of the elder may sound more resonant. Impairment of percussion—that is, dull or flat sounds—indicates consolidation or effusion.

Auscultation

The lungs of the elderly may be difficult to auscultate because the patient may not be able to take the deep and frequent breaths that are needed. The sounds heard over the normal lung are no different in younger and older adults. If structural deformities such as kyphosis or barrel chest are present, the breath sounds may be distant in those areas. Crackles, also called rales and rhonchi, and wheezes are heard only if disease is present (Caird and Judge, 1979; Mezey et al., 1980).

NURSING DIAGNOSES

1. Activity Intolerance related to compromised respiratory function, dyspnea, and fatigue
2. Airway Clearance, Ineffective related to pain, tracheobronchial secretions, exudate, bronchospasm, and increased pulmonary secretions
3. Anxiety related to breathlessness, fear of suffocation, and fear of recurrence
4. Breathing Pattern, Ineffective related to increased pulmonary secretions, stiff chest wall, reduced physiological responses to decreased PO_2 and increased

PCO_2, and shortness of breath with exercise (and obesity, if present)
5. Pain, Acute or Chronic related to hyperthermia, malaise, cough, and pulmonary disease
6. Communication, Impaired Verbal related to dyspnea
7. Fluid Volume Deficit, High Risk for related to increased insensible fluid loss secondary to fever and hyperventilation
8. Gas Exchange, Impaired related to carbon dioxide retention and excess mucus production
9. Infection, High Risk for: Respiratory related to decreased cough mechanism, impaired mucociliary escalator, decreased IgA, and less efficient alveolar macrophages
10. Knowledge Deficit related to lack of understanding about disease, prognosis, course, treatment, risk factors (smoking, environmental hazards), and complications
11. Nutrition, Altered: Less Than Body Requirements related to anorexia, dyspnea, and abdominal distention secondary to air swallowing
12. Oral Mucous Membrane, Altered related to mouth breathing and frequent expectoration
13. Powerlessness related to loss of control and the restrictions that the condition may place on lifestyle
14. Skin Integrity, Impaired: High Risk for related to prescribed bedrest
15. Sleep Pattern Disturbance related to cough, inability to assume recumbent position, and sleep apnea

NURSING INTERVENTIONS AND EVALUATION

Nursing interventions for pulmonary problems are focused on teaching and counseling related to risk factors, medication management, and keeping the airway as clear as possible (interventions related to specific nursing diagnoses are described in Chapter 14). The major risk factors for respiratory diseases are smoking and environmental toxins. Older clients should be helped in their attempt to stop smoking, either by behavior modification methods or smoking cessation programs. It can be done! The elderly should not be eliminated from these programs simply because of age. The environment should be modified, if necessary, to prevent exacerbations of existing lung diseases. Examples are the use of air conditioners and filters to remove pollutants, humidifiers or dehumidifiers (whichever is appropriate), and temperature control.

Older people who are at risk for the development of pneumonia should be urged to have flu vaccinations, and colds and upper respiratory infections should be treated with caution. Those who are isolated should be checked to see whether their homes are properly heated and whether there is enough food. Medications for various lung diseases may cause side effects, so the clients and families must be taught about their administration, actions, and side effects. This is a particular problem for older clients with pneumonia who are at high risk for confusion.

Breathing exercises help to increase the depth and strength of respirations. The nurse should be sure that older clients are administering oxygen and respirators correctly, especially in the home, where their use is increasing every day. It is also important to have patients demonstrate their use of inhalers to allow the nurse to evaluate their technique as well as the efficacy of the drug. Psychosocial support is also needed to help relieve the anxiety associated with breathlessness.

Evaluation is based on goals related to elimination of risk factors, medication management, and unimpaired respirations. The number of cigarettes smoked per day can be measured, and decreases as well as cessation should be applauded. The environment should be conducive to adequate exchange in the lungs and prevention of lung disease. Older clients and their families should be able to demonstrate proper medication management and to explain the uses and side effects of the drugs.

SUMMARY

Because the lungs are constantly exposed to the environment and lung diseases are common in older age, it is difficult to distinguish the effects of the environment and disease from normal aging changes. Changes that occur with normal aging include reduction of alveolar surface area, loss of elastic recoil, decrease in vital capacity and oxygen saturation, decline in lung host defense, and reduction in exercise tolerance. Risk factors that further decrease lung function are smoking, obesity, immobility, and surgery. Respiratory diseases common in the aged are COPD, asthma, pneumonia, tuberculosis,

cancer of the lung, and sleep apnea. Nursing interventions should focus on minimizing risk factors, managing medications, and keeping the airway as clear as possible.

REFERENCES

Alex, C.G. and Tobin M.J. Noninvasive monitoring of respirations. *In* Mahler, D.A. (ed). *Pulmonary Disease in the Elderly Patient*. New York: Marcel Dekker, 1993, pp. 27–60.

Allen, S.C. Aging and the respiratory system. *In* Brocklehurst, J.C., Tallis, R.C. and Fillit, H.M. (eds). *Textbook of Geriatric Medicine and Gerontology*. 4th ed. Edinburgh: Churchill Livingstone, 1992, pp. 739–768.

Allen, S.C. and Prior, A. What determines whether an elderly patient can use a metered dose inhaler correctly? *Br J Dis Chest* 80:45–49, 1986.

Ancoli-Israel, S., Klauber, M.R., Butters, N., et al. Dementia in institutionalized elderly: Relation to sleep apnea. *J Am Geriatr Soc* 39:258–261, 1991a.

Ancoli-Israel, S., et al. Sleep-disordered breathing in community-dwelling elderly. *Sleep* 14(6):486–495, 1991b.

Bachman, D.L. Sleep disorders with aging: Evaluation and treatment. *Geriatrics* 47(9):53–61, 1992.

Bardana, E.J. Editorial: Is asthma really different in the elderly patient? *J Asthma* 30(2):77–79, 1993.

Block, E.R. Pitfalls in diagnosing and managing pulmonary diseases. *Geriatrics* 34(2):70–79, 1979.

Bloom, J.W. and Barreuther A.D. Drug therapy of airways obstructive diseases. *In* Bressler, R. and Katz, M.D. (eds.): *Geriatric Pharmacology*. New York: McGraw-Hill, 1993.

Boring, C.C., Squires, T.S., Tong, T. and Heath, C.W. Mortality trends for selected smoking-related cancers and breast cancer—United States, 1950–1990. *MMWR* 42(44):857–863, 1993.

Bosse, R., Sparrow, D., Rose, C.L. et al. Longitudinal effect of age and smoking cessation on pulmonary function. *Am Rev Respir Dis* 123:378–381, 1981.

Braman, S.S., Kaemmerlen, J.T. and Davis S.M. Asthma in the elderly: A comparison between patients with recently acquired and long-standing disease. *Ann Rev Respir Dis* 143:336–340, 1991.

Brandstetter, R.D. and Kazemi, H. Aging and the respiratory system. *Med Clin North Am* 67(2):419–431, 1983.

Brischetto, M.J., Millman, R.P., Peterson, D.D., et al. Effect of aging on ventilatory response to exercise and CO_2. *J App Physiol* 56(5):1143–1150, 1984.

Caird, F.I. and Judge, T.G. Respiratory system. *Assessment of the Elderly Patient*. 2nd ed. Philadelphia: J.B. Lippincott, 1979, pp. 33–37.

Campbell, J.C. Detecting and correcting pulmonary risk factors before operation. *Geriatrics* 32(5):54–57, 1977.

Canadian Thoracic Society Workshop Group. Guidelines for the assessment and management of chronic obstructive pulmonary disease. *Can Med Assoc J* 147(4):420–428, 1992.

Cherniack, R.M. and Cherniack, L. *Respiration in Health and Disease*. 2nd ed. Philadelphia, W.B. Saunders, 1983.

Colsher, P.L., Wallace, R.B., Pomrehn, P.R., et al. Demographic and health characteristics of elderly smokers: Results from established populations for epidemiologic studies of the elderly. *Am J Prev Med* 6:61–70, 1990.

Crapo, R.O. The aging lung. *In* Mahler, D.A. (ed.). *Pulmonary Disease in the Elderly Patient*. New York: Marcel Dekker, 1993, pp. 1–25.

Dow, L. The epidemiology and therapy of airflow limitation in the elderly. *Drugs & Aging* 2(6):546–559, 1992.

Dow, L. and Holgate, S.T. Assessment and treatment of obstructive airways disease in the elderly. *Br Med Bull* 46(1):230–245, 1990.

Fedullo, A.J. and Swinburne, A.J. Relationship of patient age to clinical features and outcome for in-hospital treatment of pneumonia. *J Gerontol* 47(1):29–33, 1985.

Fein, A.M., Feinsilver, S.H. and Niederman, M.S. A typical manifestation of pneumonia in the elderly. *Clin Chest Med* 12(2):319–336, 1991.

Feuer, M.M. Pulmonary disease: Aging and pharmacology. *In* Jarvic, L.F., Greenblatt, D.J. and Herman, D. (eds.). *Aging.* Vol. 16: *Clinical Pharmacology and the Aged Patient.* New York: Raven Press, 1981, pp. 157–186.

Findlay, M.P.N., Griffin, A.M., Raghavan, D., et al. Retrospective review of chemotherapy for small cell lung cancer in the elderly: Does the end justify the means? *Eur J Cancer* 27(12):1597–1601, 1991.

Fleury, B. Sleep apnea syndrome in the elderly. *Sleep* 15(6 Suppl):539–541, 1992.

Foster, D.A., Talsma, A., Furumoto-Dawson, A., et al. Influenza vaccine effectiveness in preventing hospitalization for pneumonia in the elderly. *Am J Epidemiol* 126(3):296–306, 1992.

Fox, R.A. Treatment recommendations for respiratory tract infections associated with aging. *Drugs & Aging* 3(1):40–48, 1993.

Freeman, E. The respiratory system. *In* Brocklehurst, J.C. (ed.). *Textbook of Geriatric Medicine and Gerontology.* 2nd ed. New York: Churchill Livingstone, 1978, pp. 433–451.

Gerson, M.C., Hurst, J.M., Hertzberg, V.S., et al. Prediction of cardiac and pulmonary complications related to elective abdominal and noncardiac thoracic surgery in geriatric patients. *Am J Med* 88:101–107, 1990.

Hill, R.D. and Fisher, E.B. Smoking cessation in the older chronic smoker: A review. *In* Mahler, D.A. (ed.). *Pulmonary Disease in the Elderly Patient.* New York: Marcel Dekker, 1993, pp. 189–218.

Hodgkin, J.E., Connors, G.L. and Bell, C.W. (eds.). *Pulmonary Rehabilitation: Guidelines to Success.* 2nd ed. Philadelphia: J.B. Lippincott, 1993.

Hoffman, P.C., Albain, K.S., Bitran, J.D., et al. Current concepts in small cell carcinoma of the lung. *CA* 34(5):269–281, 1984.

Horvath, S.M. and Borgia, J.F. Cardiopulmonary gas transport and aging. *Am Rev Respir Dis* 129(2):568–571, 1984.

Ishida, T., Yokoyama, H., Kaneko, S., et al. Long-term results of operation for non–small cell lung cancer in the elderly. *Ann Thorac Surg* 50:919–922, 1990.

Ivanov, L.A. Effect of hypoxia on external respiratory function in old age. *Hum Physiol* 9(2):126–133, 1983.

Jenkins, S.C. and Moxham, J. The effects of mild obesity on lung function. *Respir Med* 85:309–311, 1991.

Johnson, B.D. and Dempsey, J.A. Demand vs capacity in the aging pulmonary system. *Exerc Sport Sci Rev* 19:171–210, 1991.

Johnson, D.H. Treatment of the elderly patient with small-cell lung cancer. *Chest* 103:72S–74S, 1993.

Keltz, H. Pulmonary function and disease in the aged. *In* Williams, T.F. (ed.). *Rehabilitation in the Aging.* New York: Raven Press, 1984, pp. 13–22.

Kenney, R.A. The respiratory and cardiovascular systems. *In Physiology of Aging: A Synopsis.* Chicago: Year Book Medical Publishers, 1989, pp. 49–66.

King, T.E. and Schwarz M.I. Pulmonary function and disease in the elderly. *In* Schrier, R.S. (ed.). *Clinical Internal Medicine in the Aged.* Philadelphia: W.B. Saunders, 1982, pp. 124–148.

Kleinerman, J. Reparative process of the lung. *In* Cander, L. and Moyer, J.H. (eds.). *Aging of the Lung.* New York: Grune & Stratton, 1964, pp. 77–88.

Knudson, R.J. Physiology of the aging lung. *In* Crystal, R.G. et al. (eds.). *The Lung: Scientific Foundations.* New York: Raven Press, 1991, pp. 1749–1759.

Liebow, A.A. biochemical and structural changes in the aging lung: Summary. *In* Cander, L. and Moyer, J.H. (eds.). *Aging of the Lung.* New York: Grune & Stratton, 1964, pp. 97–104.

Mahler, D.A. Chronic obstructive pulmonary disease. *In* Mahler, D.A. (ed.). *Pulmonary Disease in the Elderly Patient.* New York: Marcel Dekker, 1993, pp. 159–188.

Mauderly, J.L. Lung-thorax system. *In* Masaro, E.J., Adelman, R.C. and Roth, G.S. (eds.). *CRC Handbook of Physiology in Aging.* Boca Raton, FL: CRC Press, 1981, pp. 197–214.

Mezey, M.D., Rauckhorst, L.H. and Stokes, S.A. Assessment of the cardiac, vascular, respiratory, and hematopoietic systems. *Health Assessment of the Older Individual.* New York: Springer-Verlag, 1980, pp. 71–85.

Moser, K.M., Rees, A.L., Sassi-Dambrom, D.E., et al. *Shortness of Breath: A Guide to Better Living and Breathing.* 4th ed. St. Louis: C.V. Mosby, 1991.

Mostow, S.R. Infectious complications in the elderly COPD patient. *Geriatrics* 38(10):42–48, 1983.

Murray, J.F. Aging. *The Normal Lung.* 2nd ed. Philadelphia: W.B. Saunders, 1986, pp. 339–359.

Niederman, M.S. Pneumonia in the elderly. *In* Mahler, D.A. (ed.). *Pulmonary Disease in the Elderly Patient.* New York: Marcel Dekker, 1993.

Patrick, J.M., Bassey, E.J. and Fentem, P.H. The rising ventilatory cost of bicycle exercise in the seventh decade: A longitudinal study. *Clin Sci* 65(5):521–526, 1983.

Peterson, D.D., Pack, A.I., Silage, D.A., et al. Effects of aging on ventilatory and occlusion pressure responses to hypoxia and hypercapnea. *Am Rev Respir Dis* 124(4):387–391, 1981.

Petty, T.L. Respiratory diseases. *In* Steinberg, F.U. (ed.). *Care of the Geriatric Patient.* 6th ed. St. Louis: C.V. Mosby, 1983, pp. 105–117.

Puchelle, E., Sahm, J.H. and Bertrand, A. Influence of age on bronchial mucociliary transport. *Scand J Respir Dis* 60(6):307–313, 1979.

Reichel, J. Pulmonary problems in the elderly. *In* Reichel, W. (ed.). *Clinical Aspects of Aging.* Baltimore: Williams & Wilkins, 1983.

Rubin, S., Tack, M. and Cherniack, N.S. Effect of aging on respiratory responses to CO_2 and inspiratory resistive loads. *J Gerontol* 37(3):306–312, 1982.

Schrier, A.C., Dekker, F.W., Kaptein, A.A. and Dijkman, J.H. Quality of life in elderly patients with chronic nonspecific lung disease seen in family practice. *Chest* 98:894–899, 1990.

Schwartz, A.R. and Smith P.L. Sleep apnea in the elderly. *Clin Geriatr Med* 5(2):315–329, 1989.

Sherter, C.B., Depew, C.C. and Mattay, R.A. Pulmonary diseases and disorders of respiration. *In* Covington, T.R. and Walker, J.I. (eds.). *Current Geriatric Therapy.* Philadelphia: W.B. Saunders, 1984, pp. 104–139.

Sims, R.V. Bacterial pneumonia in the elderly. *Emerg Med Clin North Am* 8(2):207–220, 1990.

Smyrnios, N.A. and Irwin, R.S. Wheeze and cough in the elderly. *In* Mahler, D.A. (ed.). *Pulmonary Disease in the Elderly Patient.* New York: Marcel Dekker, 1993, pp. 113–158.

Stark, J.E. and Lipscomb, D.J. Physiological and pathological aspects of the respiratory system. *In* Platt, D. (ed.). *Geriatrics 2.* New York: Springer-Verlag, 1983, pp. 294–314.

Stiesmeyer, J.K. A four-step approach to pulmonary assessment. *AJN* 93(8):22–28, 1993.

Taylor, L.D., Greenberg, S.D. and Buffler, P.A. Health effects of indoor passive smoking. *Texas Med* 81(5), 1985.

Thurlbeck, W.M. Morphology of the aging lung. *In*

Crystal, R.G. and West, J.B. (eds.). *The Lung: Scientific Foundations*. New York: Raven Press, 1991, pp. 1743–1748.

Traver, G.A., Cline, M.G. and Burrows, B. Asthma in the elderly. *J Asthma* 30(2):81–91.

Umeki, S. Age-related changes in the manifestations of tuberculosis: Implications for drug therapy. *Drugs & Aging* 1(6):440–457, 1991.

Wahba, W.M. Influence of aging on lung function—clinical significance of changes from age twenty. *Anesth Analg* 62:764–776, 1983.

Ware, J.H., Dockery, D.W., Louis, T.A., et al. Longitudinal and cross-sectional estimates of pulmonary function decline in never-smoking adults. *Am J Epidemiol* 132(4):685–700, 1990.

Weiss, S.T. Pulmonary system. *In* Rowe, J.W. and Besdine, R.W. (eds.). *Health and Disease in Old Age*. Boston: Little, Brown, 1982, pp. 369–379.

Woodhouse, K.W. and Wynne, H.A. The pharmacology of aging. *In* Brocklehurst, J.C., Tallis, R.C. and Fillit, H.M. (eds.). *Textbook of Geriatric Medicine and Gerontology*. 4th ed. Edinburgh: Churchill Livingstone, 1992, pp. 130–135.

Wooten, V. Sleep disorders in geriatric patients. *Clin Geriatr Med* 8(2):427–439, 1992.

Yerg, J.E., Seals, D.R., Hagberg, J.M., et al. Effect of endurance exercise training on ventilatory function in older individuals. *J Appl Physiol* 58(3):791–794, 1985.

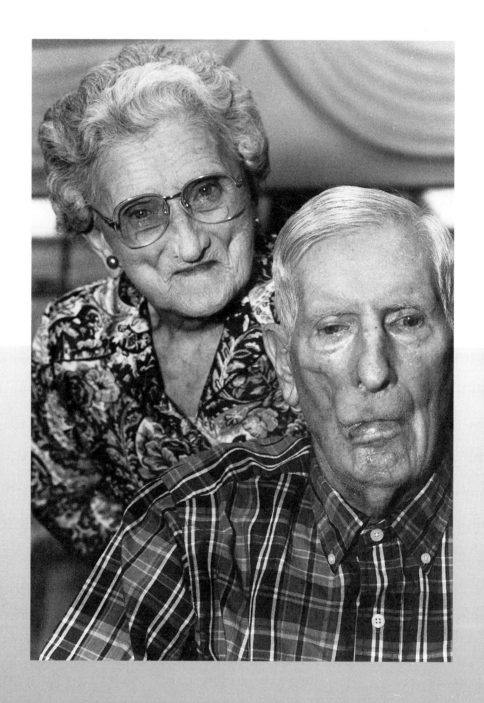

Age-Related Changes in the Neurological System

ADRIANNE DILL LINTON
MARY ANN MATTESON

 OBJECTIVES

Describe the normal age-related changes in the structure of the neurological system, particularly neuronal losses, synaptic changes, and changes in the composition of the brain and nerve cells.

❖

Discuss the normal age-related changes in the functional abilities of the neurological system, including reaction time, proprioception, thermoregulation, and EEG and sleep patterns.

❖

Define and distinguish between delirium and dementia.

❖

Distinguish among the types of dementia, including dementia of the Alzheimer's type, vascular dementia, dementia due to HIV disease, dementia due to head trauma, dementia due to Parkinson's disease, dementia due to Huntington's disease, dementia due to Pick's disease, dementia due to Creutzfeldt-Jakob disease, dementia due to other general medical conditions, substance-induced persisting dementia, dementia due to multiple etiologies, and dementia not otherwise specified.

❖

Examine the structural abnormalities in the neurological system associated with older age, especially normal pressure hydrocephalus, subdural hematoma, and brain tumors.

❖

Apply the concepts of nursing assessment and intervention to the care of older persons with neurological changes and disorders.

No body system is as misunderstood as the neurological system in relation to normal aging. Lay people and professionals alike believe that senility is inevitable with aging, rarely viewing the phenomenon of impaired mental capacities as a pathological process. Disparaging remarks are often made about confused elderly who may be actually suffering from acute illnesses or chronic disabilities. Although changes do occur in the neurological system, it cannot be assumed that senility is a normal concomitant of aging.

ORGANIZATION OF THE NEUROLOGICAL SYSTEM

The major function of the nervous system is integrative, referring to the process of selecting incoming sensory information and channeling it to cause appropriate motor responses (Guyton, 1991). The nervous system is divided into two parts: the central nervous system (CNS), consisting of the brain and the spinal cord, and the peripheral nervous system, consisting of the cranial, spinal, and peripheral nerves. The peripheral nervous system provides input to the CNS through sensory receptors and output through motor endings to effectors (muscles and glands). Communicating networks within the central nervous system and various brain centers process incoming sensory information in order to direct appropriate conscious and unconscious responses.

Peripheral efferent nerve fibers distributed to smooth muscle, cardiac muscle, and glands are known as the autonomic nervous system (ANS). The ANS consists of the sympathetic and parasympathetic systems and is involved in regulation of behavioral and neuroendocrinological mechanisms of the body with responsibilities for maintaining a constant internal environment (temperature, fluid balance, and ionic composition of the blood). The parasympathetic system is concerned with body functions such as digestion, excretion, and intermediary metabolism. The sympathetic system is involved in the regulation of stress reactions.

The nervous system is composed of two major types of cells: neurons and neuroglia. The neurons are the basic units of the nervous system and are responsible for conducting nerve impulses from one part of the body to another. The neuroglia provide the supporting structure for nervous tissue and consist of blood vessels, connective tissue, and supporting cells.

Nerve impulses are carried from one cell to another at the synaptic junctions. The transmission is usually carried from the axon of one cell to the dendrites of another. Large nerve fibers, which are long neuron processes such as axons, are insulated by a myelin sheath. Myelin is 80 per cent lipid, and it increases the rate at which impulses are conducted along nerve fibers. Transmission of electrical impulses at the synapse requires the intervention of chemical mediators, or neurotransmitters. Over 40 chemicals are known or thought to be neurotransmitters, including acetylcholine, dopamine, serotonin, and norepinephrine (Fig. 9–1) (Guyton, 1991).

NORMAL CHANGES IN STRUCTURE AND FUNCTION

Structure

With aging, there is thought to be a steady loss of neurons in the brain and spinal cord. Although neurons are postmitotic cells that are not reproduced when lost, they are replaced by neuroglial cells. Neuroglial cells, which do proliferate, make up the supporting structure of nervous tissue. Estimates of neuronal loss are conflicting, but there is evidence of losses ranging from 10 to 60 per cent in the neocortex, cerebellum, and hippocampus. Subcortical structures, except for the locus ceruleus, seem to have less dramatic neuronal cell loss. In the cortical structures, the greatest losses are in the inferior temporal gyrus and the tip of the temporal lobe. Increased dendritic growth in some neurons of the cerebral cortex and hippocampus may represent compensation for neuronal loss in specific areas (Poirier and Finch, 1994). Plaques and tangles are found in the aging brain.

Deposits of lipofuscin, a yellow-brown pigment, have been found in the neuronal cytoplasm with aging, particularly in the lower brain structures, such as the thalamus and brainstem. The effect on cell functioning is not known, but lipofuscin accumulations may be an indication of cell damage with age, possibly caused by free radical reactions (Lewis, 1992). It is interesting to note, however, that the areas of the brain showing the largest accumulations of lipofuscin have the smallest amounts of neuronal loss.

Neuronal losses do not necessarily affect brain function, but they may have an influence on brain weight. Brain atrophy has been reported, based on cross-sectional studies. Poirier and Finch (1994) reported that longitudinal computed tomography (CT) scans have revealed atrophy primarily in selected areas and do not support the notion of extensive generalized atrophy with normal aging. Lauter's study, cited in Oxman and Baynes' (1992) review of studies on brain weights, reported only a 7 to 8 per cent decrease.

The appearance and configuration of the brain change with age. There is a decrease in the cortical area due to narrowing and flattening of the gyri (brain folds) and widening and deepening of the sulci (valleys between the brain folds). The loss of hemispheric volume occurs at a faster rate in men than in women. The general shrinkage of brain size results in greater separation from the skull and enlargement of the ventricles (Lewis, 1992). Water and protein content increase as lipid content decreases, owing to losses of lipid-rich myelin (Poirier and Finch, 1994).

In addition to neuronal cell loss, changes take place among neurons and supporting cells. Intracellular accumulations of lipofuscin pigment occur not only in the cytoplasm of the neurons but in the glial cells as well. There is a loss of ribonucleic acid (RNA), mitochondria, and enzymes in the cytoplasm and a decrease in the size of the nuclei. The axons degenerate, with a loss of myelin and swellings of the axis cylinders—a process called "dying back."

The changes in synaptic transmissions are not only affected by dendritic atrophy but

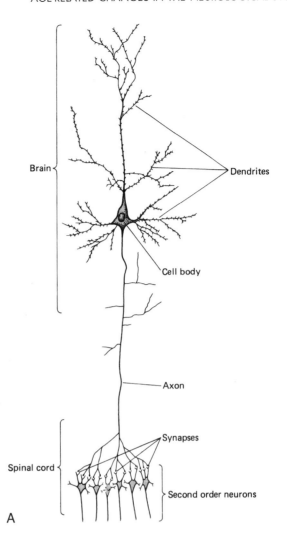

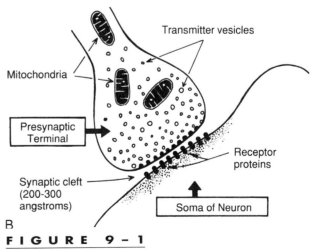

FIGURE 9 – 1

A, Structure of a large neuron of the brain, showing its important functional parts. *B,* Physiological anatomy of the synapse. (From Guyton, A.C. *Basic Neuroscience: Anatomy and Physiology.* 2nd ed. Philadelphia: W.B. Saunders, 1991.)

are also influenced by changes in the chemical neurotransmitters. The major neurotransmitters are classified as inhibitory, excitatory, or modulatory. They influence excitation or inhibition of firing rates and information coding at the synapse, or they modulate other neurotransmitters (Poirier and Finch, 1994). With aging, the synthesis and metabolism of the major neurotransmitters are diminished, causing a slowing of many neural processes, especially in the central processes where conduction over multisynaptic pathways may be delayed (Bannon et al., 1992). In addition, there is a decrease in receptors in specific areas of the brain.

It must be noted that changes in the brain composition, cells, and synapses associated with aging do not necessarily have an effect on thinking and cognition. Little correlation has been noted between cerebral atrophy and cognitive loss, and frequently persons maintain a "sharp mind" in later life in spite of physiological evidence that might indicate otherwise.

Changes in the nerve cells of the spinal column are similar to those in the brain, especially those related to neuronal loss and atrophy. There is a 30 to 50 per cent loss of anterior horn cells in the lumbosacral area, and a 30 per cent loss of myelinated nerve fibers in the posterior roots and peripheral nerves by age 90 years. Larger nerve fibers are progressively lost in the sympathetic chain, possibly accounting for the increased incidence of postural hypotension in older age. The efferent system also loses its largest fibers, resulting in diminished conduction velocity and prolonged muscle action potentials.

Loss of neurons, slowed conduction of nerve impulses, and loss of peripheral nerve functions all have an effect on the efficiency with which the autonomic nervous system performs in older age. Maintenance of body homeostasis becomes more difficult, so that recovery from stress is prolonged and incomplete. Stressors such as heat, cold, and extreme exercise can be particularly harmful, even life-threatening.

Changes in Functional Abilities of the Neurological System

Reaction Time

The general slowing and wasting of the nervous system seems to produce a decrement in the ability to react quickly to stimuli. Reaction time, or the lag between the stimulation and the initiation of a response, increases with aging (Madden, 1992; Mucig-

nat et al., 1991; Reuben, 1992; Shaw, 1992). It appears that the simpler the movement or the action required, the less the change in reaction is noted. According to Welford (1980), there are three types of movement related to reaction time: (1) repetitive movements of tapping between two targets; (2) simple unaimed movement; and (3) more elaborate movements, such as writing or tracing. Repetitive movements show fewer decrements with aging because they are simple movements that require little in the way of decision making. On the other hand, more elaborate movements require increasingly greater reaction times because more choices are required between two or more responses to various signals. In addition, the time between signals and responses increases when complex intermediate steps are necessary in order to relate signals to their corresponding responses. Spatial transpositions, which occur when the spatial layout of signal sources is different from the corresponding responses (e.g., mirror image or left to right), also increase reaction time. Thus, the nature of the signals and the complexity and types of responses required significantly influence the degree of change in reaction times of elderly people.

It might be assumed that slowed responses to stimuli would impair the performance of older adults in such activities as operating machines, automobiles, or other complex instruments. However, it has been found that elderly people are willing to give up speed in favor of accuracy (Geary and Wiley, 1991; Carr et al., 1992), and they tend to respond more slowly but more precisely. Without the pressure of time, older persons are capable of performing as well as younger persons. If the quality of performance does decrease, other causes should be considered, such as motivation, health, or environmental influences.

Proprioception

How well older persons retain their ability to maintain an upright position without falling depends on how well they continue to integrate three functions: balance, posture, and moving equipoise. Balance is the ability to stand steadily, posture is the alignment of body segments in proper relation to one another, and moving equipoise is the control of equilibrium in movements. In addition, muscle-joint sense, which results from muscle spindle and tendon proprioception, provides information about the length, tension, and speed of muscle activity. Muscle-joint sense is monitored in various levels of the brain, e.g., reflex antigravity support in the brain stem, righting reflexes controlling posture and balance in the midbrain, and integration of patterned movements in the cerebral cortex. Older people typically demonstrate diminished joint position sense (Barrett et al., 1991; Ferrell et al., 1992).

BALANCE. With age, postural control decreases because of loss of sensory cues of pressoreceptors, declining function of stretch reflexes that initiate from muscle spindles, and slowed processing of information (Ring et al., 1989; Pyykko et al., 1990; Teasdale et al., 1991; Hu and Woollacott, 1994). Elderly people come to depend on visual control to maintain postural stability. Manchester and colleagues (1989) found that older adults were less stable when peripheral vision was occluded. Postural sway increases, affecting women more dramatically than men (Ring et al., 1989; Stelmach et al., 1989a; Burl et al., 1992; Maki et al., 1994). In addition, stabilizing processes are slower (Manchester et al., 1989; Stelmach et al., 1989b; Stelmach et al., 1990).

Age-related changes place the older person at risk for falls. Specific problems that may contribute to impaired balance include dizziness, lightheadedness, and vertigo. Falls may result from syncope or drop attacks associated with postural hypotension or changes in arterial blood flow, normal pressure hydrocephalus, cervical spondylitis, and lumbar stenosis (Tinetti, 1989; Patla et al., 1992). Fallers have been found to have less control of lateral stability (Maki et al., 1994).

DIZZINESS. The central nervous system is constantly integrating sensory messages in order to provide information required for maintaining balance and movement and for interacting with objects in the environment. Sensory messages are received through vision, vestibular sensation, joint position sense, touch-pressure sensation, and hearing. Persons who receive incorrect or insufficient information or who fail to integrate the information correctly may experience dizziness. Jonsson and Lipsitz (1994, p. 1165) define dizziness as "an unpleasant sensation of insecure balance." It may result from visual, proprioceptive, labyrinthine, or psychophysiological disturbances. Older persons who are prone to decreased sensory input are especially likely to develop dizziness. Dizziness can be categorized into four types: (1) vertigo, (2) near syncope, (3) disequilibrium, and (4) nonspecific dizziness.

Vertigo produces a rotational sensation in which persons feel that either they or the environment are spinning. This is less common in the elderly than other forms of diz-ziness and is related to disorders of the vestibular system. The onset of vertigo is often instantaneous, and it may be accompanied by nausea, vomiting, and a staggering gait.

Near syncope produces a sensation of impending faint or loss of consciousness. Complaints of impending faint are usually due to an inadequate supply of blood or nutrients to the entire brain, which may occur in older persons with postural hypotension. This sensation may be accompanied by pallor, roaring in the ears, dimness of vision, and diaphoresis.

Disequilibrium is the loss of balance without an abnormal sensation in the head. It occurs when persons are walking and disappears when they sit down. The phenomenon of disequilibrium is due to a disorder of motor system control.

Nonspecific dizziness is described as a vague lightheadedness other than vertigo, near syncope, or disequilibrium.

Age-related changes that may contribute to dizziness include decreased visual perception, increased threshold for vestibular and proprioceptive sensory organ response, and loss of proprioceptive receptors. Aging alone may not explain dizziness, but it may be more easily triggered when the individual has visual loss. To compensate for the sensation of lightheadedness, the older person may use a broad-based, tentative gait with shortened steps. Dizziness may be so severe that the person is unable to walk without assistance (Jonsson and Lipsitz, 1994).

SYNCOPE. Syncope is brief loss of consciousness with loss of postural tone, which resolves spontaneously. Syncopal attacks result from a failure of baroreceptor mechanisms in the neck or inadequate cerebral blood flow. In elderly people, syncope is frequently associated with coughing, micturition, or position changes. Cough syncope occurs more frequently in middle age than old age, especially in male smokers who suffer from emphysema and bronchitis. This problem generally occurs in large, barrel-chested individuals whose severe cough generates a Valsalva maneuver causing wooziness, collapse, and loss of consciousness. Some elderly persons who are hypotensive may also suffer from cough syncope (Gandy, 1994; Jonsson and Lipsitz, 1994). Micturition syncope can occur after voiding a large amount of urine.

Orthostatic hypotension implies a fall of 20 mm Hg or more in the systolic blood pressure when a person moves to an upright position. This condition is also called postural hypotension and postural syncope. Age-related changes that contribute to orthostatic hypotension are decreased cerebral blood flow, impaired baroreflex sensitivity, decreased cardiac output, and decreased efficiency of fluid regulation with a tendency toward hypovolemia (Jonsson and Lipsitz, 1994). Many drugs taken by elderly people, such as vasodilators, antihypertensives, diuretics, neuroleptics, dopaminergics, and antidepressants, decrease cardiac output, thereby increasing the risk of orthostatic hypotension.

The occurrence of these phenomena, which increases with age, is due to an impairment of homeostatic mechanisms responsible for systemic arteriolar constriction and possibly venous reservoirs. Deficient baroreceptors, the pooling of blood in the periphery, and an uncompensated decrease in cardiac output result in decreased cerebral blood flow and syncope.

Depending on the cause of the syncope, many simple interventions can be prescribed. Older persons should be taught to rise slowly from the toilet to prevent a fainting episode related to micturition syncope. They should also rise slowly from bed or chair to prevent syncope related to orthostatic hypotension. Dorsiflexing the ankles several times before standing may also minimize postural hypotension. Fluid intake should be sufficient to maintain adequate hydration, and the use of drugs that cause orthostatic hypotension should be re-evaluated and possibly discontinued. If there is evidence of carotid sinus hypersensitivity, the individual should avoid extreme neck rotation and tight collars (Gandy, 1994; Jonsson and Lipsitz, 1994).

MOTOR ACTIVITY. As discussed in Chapter 6, motor activity tends to change with aging, especially posture, movement, and reflexes. Reflexes decrease, chiefly in proximal areas of the lower extremities, where ankle jerks may be completely absent. Motor activity slows, and there may be some difficulty with fine movement. Joints become more rigid in a flexed position, and muscle power declines. The gait is often characterized by a shortened stride, shuffling, and decreased arm swing (Williams and Bird, 1992). Pathy (1992) reported that one third of people over age 75 years have gait impairment.

Benign essential tremor affecting the hands and head is common among older persons (Sweeney, 1993). Age-related tremors are intermittent, are exaggerated by movement and emotion, and rarely appear at rest. These tremors usually do not significantly interfere with activities of daily living. When there is a strong family history of essential tremor, the onset may be at any age. Essential tremor may be confused with idiopathic parkinsonism or drug-induced parkinsonism (Pathy, 1992; McDowell, 1994).

Thermoregulation

Elderly people are at great risk for developing episodes of hypothermia and hyperthermia. Stories of the deaths of older persons during extreme hot or cold spells are abundant in the news. Particularly susceptible are elderly people living in isolation.

HYPOTHERMIA. General hypothermia is described as a state of low body temperature in which the rectal temperature is 35°C (95°F) or below. It is so prevalent among elderly people that it is one of the most important causes of death in Great Britain in the winter. Elderly people who live in mild climates, however, are also susceptible to hypothermia during the cooler months (Thomas, 1988; Kramer et al., 1989; Kane et al., 1994). Multiple factors are involved in the etiology of hypothermia. Social influences play important roles in cold exposure, including inadequate income, social isolation, inadequate housing, and physical inability to maintain heating appliances. Other factors are a decline in heat production with age, loss of fat and subcutaneous tissue, impaired thermoregulation mechanisms (decreased shivering and vasoconstriction), and an inability to feel cold as intensely as the young, resulting in little motivation to seek warmth.

Pathological causes of hypothermia include alcoholism, diabetes, cardiovascular and cerebrovascular diseases, sepsis, and bronchopneumonia. Other causes include falls, fractures, confusion, and ingestion of drugs (Table 9–1). Drugs that predispose to hypothermia are alcohol, barbiturates, tranquilizers, reserpine, tricyclic antidepressants, salicylates, acetaminophen, and general anesthetics (Woodhouse et al., 1989; Hirsch, 1992; Abrass, 1994; Kane et al., 1994).

Older persons who are suffering from hypothermia have a gray appearance due to a combination of pallor and cyanosis. The skin is cold to the touch in both exposed and unexposed areas; the face appears puffy, the voice is husky, and there is slowed thinking. When the body temperature falls below 32°C, there is clouding of consciousness and drowsiness. As the body temperature decreases, older persons are more likely to become comatose.

All body systems function in an increasingly sluggish manner—heart and respiratory rates decrease, reflexes are slower, and muscles become hypotonic. Shivering ceases, but there may be an involuntary flapping

TABLE 9-1

Factors Predisposing to Hypothermia

- Decreased heat production
  Hypothyroidism
  Hypoglycemia
  Starvation and malnutrition
  Immobility and decreased activity (e.g., stroke, arthritis, parkinsonism)
- Increased heat loss
  Decreased subcutaneous fat
  Exposure to cold (immersion)
- Thermoregulatory impairment
  Hypothalamic and CNS dysfunction
    Heat trauma
    Hypoxia
    Tumor
    Cerebrovascular disease
  Drug-induced impairment
    Alcohol
    Barbiturates
    Major and minor tranquilizers
    Glutethimide
    Reserpine
    Tricyclic antidepressants
    Salicylates, acetaminophen
    General anesthetics
  Old age
- Miscellaneous
  Sepsis
  Cardiovascular disease
  Bronchopneumonia

Data from Kane, R.L., Ouslander, J.G. and Abrass, I.B. *Essentials of Clinical Geriatrics.* 3rd ed. New York: McGraw-Hill, 1994. Copyright, 1994. Reproduced with permission of McGraw-Hill, Inc.

tremor in the arms and legs. Tissue anoxia results from poor arterial circulation and slow, shallow respirations.

Mild-to-moderate hypothermia (body temperature of 32°C to 35°C) is treated with gradual warming of the body at a rate of about 0.5° per hour (Dexter, 1990). A warm environment and wrapping the person in blankets are usually adequate. Rapid rewarming can be dangerous, as cold blood is shunted to the core, possibly triggering cardiac dysrhythmias. Severe hypothermia (body temperature lower than 32°C) is treated more vigorously as a medical emergency. The patient should be handled gently because of myocardial irritability. Antidysrhythmics are usually ineffective and may cause complications when the temperature rises. Core rewarming with peritoneal dialysis and inhalation rewarming are commonly employed (Kane et al., 1994). Efforts are made to correct dehydration and acidosis. Broad-spectrum antibiotics may be ordered to treat potential sepsis. The prognosis depends more on the severity of the underlying clinical condition than on temperature at the time of diagnosis or the rate of rewarming (Hirsch, 1992). Since elderly people often have chronic medical conditions, their mortality rate from hypothermia is higher (Abrass, 1994).

HYPERTHERMIA. Of the several heat-related disorders, heat stroke is the most serious among elderly people. In the United States, 5000 people die from heat stroke each year—two thirds of them over age 60 years. Deaths are greatest during prolonged heat waves (Abrass, 1994). Heat stroke is due to an impairment of the thermoregulatory function, resulting in excessive storage of heat in the body from an inability to dissipate the heat by radiation, convection, and sweat evaporation. Transfer of body heat from the core to the periphery decreases owing to an inability to make circulatory adjustments. It has long been thought that older people sweat less than younger people. Recent studies suggest that less sweating is not a consequence of normal aging but is due to other factors that affect thermoregulation (Sagawa et al., 1988; Tankersley et al., 1991). Older people are also at increased risk for hyperthermia when taking phenothiazines, anticholinergics, and tranquilizers, which further decrease sweat gland activity (Abrass, 1994; Bressler and Katz, 1994).

Heat exhaustion, which generally precedes heat stroke, is manifested by dizziness, weakness, nausea and vomiting, diarrhea, feelings of warmth, headache, and dyspnea. As the temperature rises above 40.6°C, the classic signs and symptoms of heat stroke appear: psychosis, delirium, loss of consciousness, and hot, dry skin (Kane et al., 1994). There is a widening pulse pressure, decreased cardiac output, and low peripheral resistance, progressing to circulatory failure and eventual death. In older persons, some of the signs may not be present owing to compromised cardiac function associated with aging. Older persons are also at high risk for dehydration due to impaired renal and cardiovascular mechanisms and depressed sensorium.

Heat exhaustion is treated by moving the person to a cooler environment, removing excess clothing, and using fans. Severe hyperthermia is treated with cold water sponging and baths with vigorous massage to avoid peripheral vasoconstriction induced from the external cooling. The aged are at high risk for circulatory shock as a result of the traumatic nature of the treatment. Intravenous fluids are given to counteract water or sodium depletion; however, older persons in this condition should be observed continuously for signs of pulmonary edema when given intravenous fluids. Estimates of mortality range from 17 to 80 per cent, depending on the duration and severity of the hyperthermia. The risk is greatest for those who present in shock or coma (Hirsch, 1992; Abrass, 1994; Kane et al., 1994).

Changes in the Electroencephalogram

The continuous electrical activity of the brain is recorded on the electroencephalogram (EEG), which shows patterns or undulations called brain waves. Intensity and frequency of brain waves vary, and their character is highly dependent on the degree of activity in the cerebral cortex. For example, changes can be noted between sleep and wakefulness by observing the wave patterns on the EEG. Although brain waves are usually irregular, distinct patterns often appear. The distinct patterns are known as alpha, beta, theta, and delta waves (Guyton, 1991); the changes associated with normal aging are usually related to the alpha waves.

Alpha waves are found predominantly over the occipital and parietal regions of the brain. These rhythmic waves occur at a frequency of 8 to 13 cycles per second (cps) and are found during wakefulness, disappearing entirely during sleep. In older people, the mean alpha rhythm slows. Beta activity is unchanged with age, but theta and delta rhythms (rarely seen in young people) are commonly reported over the temporal region in elderly people (Fozard et al., 1992; Mayeux and Schofield, 1994).

It must be noted that there is little relationship between measures of intellectual functioning and changes in the EEG with healthy aging people. However, severely demented elderly persons may show bursts of EEG activity that are different in frequency or amplitude from the norm. Diffuse slowing of activity may also indicate pathology associated with intellectual deterioration. In people with Alzheimer's disease, the EEG may reveal decreased posterior dominant alpha rhythm (Folstein and Folstein, 1994; Mayeux and Schofield, 1994).

Sleep Changes

According to Guyton (1991), sleep is "a state of unconsciousness from which a person can be aroused by sensory or other stimuli." Two kinds of sleep are slow-wave sleep and REM sleep. Slow-wave sleep is characteristic of the deep, restful, dreamless sleep experienced most of the night. REM sleep takes place at intervals during the night and is associated with dreaming as well as rapid eye movements. REM sleep is

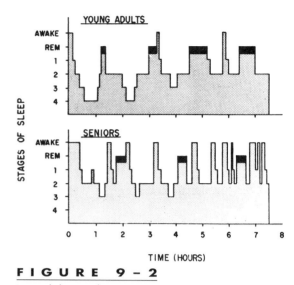

F I G U R E   9 – 2

Normal sleep cycles. As we get older, it takes us longer to fall asleep and we have less deep sleep, more awakenings, and less REM sleep. (From Ancoli-Israel, S. and Kripke, D.F. Sleep and aging. *In* Calkins, E., Ford, A.B. and Katz, P.R. (eds.). *Practice of Geriatrics.* 2nd ed. Philadelphia: W.B. Saunders, 1992.)

characterized by irregular, high-frequency beta waves, which reflect lack of synchrony in the firing of neurons. For this reason, REM sleep may be called desynchronized sleep.

There are four stages of slow-wave sleep. During stage 1, low-voltage, high-frequency beta waves with short spindle-shaped bursts of alpha waves appear on the EEG. From stages 2 to 4, wave frequency progressively slows until there are only 2 to 3 waves per minute. These slow waves are called delta waves. With older age, there is a decrease in the amount of deep slow-wave sleep, which is most commonly found in the early part of sleep. Other changes are a slowing of EEG spindle activity, which is consistent with the general slowing of alpha waves, and a decrease in the absolute and relative amount of REM sleep, so that older persons have more difficulty recalling dreams upon arousal (Fig. 9–2). They generally prefer to sleep on the right side and change positions less frequently than younger people (Haponik, 1994).

In general, older persons take longer to fall asleep and may awaken more frequently at night. Frequent awakenings are associated with the decrease in the amount of deep slow-wave sleep in addition to other factors such as nocturia, anxiety, or physical disorders. They often nap during the day. Total sleep time may decrease somewhat in the aged, but because they wake frequently and spend a longer time awake, they may spend a longer amount of time in bed. Older persons are generally considered "light sleepers" because the transition between sleep and wakefulness is usually abrupt. Although elderly people complain that they have difficulty going to sleep, have insufficient and restless sleep, and have frequent wakings, their total sleep time decreases only slightly when compared with that of younger people (Morgan, 1992; Haponik, 1994; Kane et al., 1994).

Sleep disorders in elderly people include disturbances in initiating and maintaining sleep, excessive somnolence, sleep-wake cycle disturbances, abnormal sleep behaviors, and obstructive sleep apnea. Insomnia may be associated with depression, drugs, and alcohol intake (Haponik, 1994; Kane et al., 1994). Assessment of older individuals' sleep patterns and habits can provide a basis for intervention. A thorough sleep history should include questions regarding a typical night's sleep, daytime functioning, and details of drug and alcohol use. It is helpful to find out what time older persons go to bed, how long it takes them to fall asleep, how often they awaken during the night, and what time they wake in the morning. A sleep diary kept for several weeks can help identify sleep patterns. Questions related to daytime functioning include how the individuals feel when they get up in the morning, how often they nap during the day, and whether they fall asleep during daytime activities such as watching television or reading. Since drugs (corticosteroids, theophylline, beta blockers), alcohol, and food (especially caffeine) can affect sleep, the time and frequency of administration should be noted. Sedatives-hypnotics, antihistamines, tranquilizers, methyldopa, and tricyclic antidepressants may cause excessive drowsiness (Haponik, 1994). In addition, symptoms of cardiovascular, musculoskeletal, and urologic disorders may disrupt sleep.

Several measures can be used to promote sleep in the elderly. Efforts should be made to retain usual sleep patterns or rituals, which are often disrupted in hospital and nursing home settings. Progressive relaxation and imagery training may be helpful (Ancoli-Israel and Kripke, 1992; Haponik, 1994). Distressing symptoms such as dyspnea and joint pain should be treated.

The elderly should be encouraged to exercise in the afternoon or early evening and to avoid naps, if possible. Stimulants should be avoided 3 to 4 hours before bedtime, but a light bedtime snack—preferably warm milk—may be quite beneficial. Warm milk contains tryptophan, a natural sedative. Alcohol at bedtime may hasten falling asleep, but later sleep becomes more fragmented.

Measures to treat sleep apnea include weight loss, sleeping upright or on the side, and use of continuous positive airway pressure (CPAP) during sleep.

Drugs should be avoided or used with utmost caution. Major categories of sleep medications include benzodiazepines (flurazepam, diazepam), hypnotics (chloral hydrate), antihistamines (Benadryl), and other agents (tryptophan). Benzodiazepines have lower addiction rates and weak interactions with other drugs; however some, such as flurazepam, have very long half-lives in older people and tend to accumulate over several days or weeks. Long-acting benzodiazepines tend to cause daytime sedation and ataxia that may lead to falls. For elderly people, one third to one half the usual adult dose is recommended. Sedatives-hypnotics should be used only temporarily. The best hypnotics are short-acting, with minimum effect on sleep stages. Chloral hydrate is widely used, but doses in excess of 1.0 gm may cause CNS depression and confusion in the older person. Estazolam is an appropriate sleep medication because the duration of action is 6 to 8 hours, and daytime sedation is minimized (Frankhauser, 1993). Over-the-counter sleep medications frequently contain scopolamine, which can cause confusional episodes or toxic delirium. Excessive use of aspirin for inducing sleep can produce salicylate side effects. Benadryl is often an effective sleep medication that has few side effects. Tryptophan can also be effective (Ancoli-Israel and Kripke, 1992).

The milieu of the bedroom and/or sleeping area can sometimes be manipulated to promote sleep. The room should be cool (not below 60°F), and the bedsheets and pillowcases should be clean and comfortable. The bed should be made every morning, and it is best to use it only during nighttime sleeping hours, keeping the time in bed to a minimum. If older persons cannot fall asleep after 10 to 15 minutes, they should turn on the light and read or watch television for diversion. It is useful to arise at the same time every morning to strengthen circadian cycling and to promote regular times for sleep onset (Ancoli-Israel and Kripke, 1992; Haponik, 1994).

COMMON AGE-RELATED DISORDERS IN THE NEUROLOGICAL SYSTEM

Disorders that had been classified as organic mental disorders are now classified into three categories: (1) delirium, dementia, and amnestic and other cognitive disorders;

(2) mental disorders due to a general medical condition; and (3) substance-related disorders. The *Diagnostic and Statistical Manual,* 4th edition *(DSM-IV),* defines the characteristics of the first category as follows:

- Delirium: "A disturbance of consciousness and a change in cognition that develop over a short period of time."
- Dementia: "Multiple cognitive deficits that include impairment in memory."
- Amnestic disorder: "Memory impairment in the absence of other significant cognitive impairments."

Delirium

Delirium is characterized by a rapid impairment of intellectual function resulting from a widespread disturbance of brain metabolism. The essential features of delirium, as defined in the *DSM-IV* (American Psychiatric Association, 1994), are disturbances in consciousness and cognition that are not explained by a known or evolving dementia. Delirium is also characterized by a rapid onset and evidence that it is a direct physiological consequence of a general medical condition, substance intoxication or withdrawal, drug effects, exposure to a toxin, or a combination of these factors. During hospitalization for general medical conditions, approximately 10 per cent of people over age 65 years exhibit delirium on admission, and another 10 to 15 per cent develop delirium during hospitalization (Lipowski, 1994).

Disturbance in consciousness is reflected in the inability to focus, sustain, or shift attention in a normal manner. The level of consciousness may fluctuate from drowsiness to stupor or coma, or the individual may be restless or hyperactive. Perceptual disturbances may precipitate misinterpretation of environmental cues, causing illusions or hallucinations (usually visual). Cognitive changes may also appear as memory impairment, disorientation, or language disturbance. Wandering attention is closely linked with an inability to maintain goal-directed thinking and behavior, leading to disorganized thinking, incoherent speech, and perseveration of speech and behavior. Other symptoms of delirium include anxiety, depression, irritability, anger, apathy, euphoria, sudden mood changes, sleep disturbances, and fear.

Delirium due to general medical conditions may be caused by hypoxia; fluid, electrolyte, and acid-base imbalances; hepatic or renal disease; systemic infection; thiamine deficiency; postoperative states; hypertensive encephalopathy; postictal states; and head

TABLE 9–2

Drugs That Can Cause or Contribute to Delirium and Dementia

ANALGESICS	**CARDIOVASCULAR**
Narcotic	Atropine
Codeine	Digitalis
Meperidine	Diuretics
Morphine	Lidocaine
Pentazocine	
Propoxyphene	**HYPNOTICS**
Nonnarcotic	Barbiturates
Indomethacin	Benzodiazepines
	Chloral hydrate
ANTIHISTAMINES	
Diphenhydramine	**HYPOGLYCEMICS**
Hydroxyzine	Insulin
	Sulfonylureas
ANTIHYPERTENSIVES	
Clonidine	**PSYCHOTROPIC**
Hydralazine	**DRUGS**
Methyldopa	Antianxiety drugs
Propranolol	Benzodiazepines
Reserpine	Antidepressant drugs
	Lithium
ANTIMICROBIALS	Tricyclics
Gentamicin	Antipsychotics
Isoniazid	Chlorpromazine
	Haloperidol
ANTIPARKINSONISM DRUGS	Thiothixene
Amantadine	Thioridazine
Bromocriptine	
Carbidopa	**OTHERS**
L-Dopa	Cimetidine
Trihexyphenidyl and other	Steroids
anticholinergics	

From Kane, R.L., Ouslander, J.G. and Abrass, I.B. *Essentials of Clinical Geriatrics.* 3rd ed. New York, McGraw-Hill, 1994. Copyright, 1994. Reproduced with permission of McGraw-Hill, Inc.

injury (American Psychiatric Association, 1994). Substance-induced delirium may be caused by substance intoxication or withdrawal from a substance (Table 9–2). In many cases, a number of variables contribute to delirium, in which case the patient is said to have delirium due to multiple etiologies. Delirium caused by other factors such as sensory deprivation, sensory overload, or others not yet identified is classified delirium not otherwise specified.

Differential diagnosis is important so that proper treatment can be initiated. Treatment of underlying conditions may reverse the confusional state, but it may be several weeks before normal mental functioning is restored. Meanwhile, the patient must be protected from harm. A calming environment with one constant caregiver may be reassuring. Restraints are discouraged, and drugs should be used sparingly. Soft lighting, music, and familiar objects may be soothing (Foley, 1992).

Dementia

Defined broadly, dementia is an observable, irreversible decline in mental abilities

T A B L E   9 – 3
Potentially Reversible Causes of Dementia

D —Drugs
E —Emotional disorders
M—Metabolic or endocrine disorders
E —Eye and ear dysfunction
N —Nutritional deficiencies
T —Tumor and trauma
I —Infections
A —Arteriosclerotic complications (i.e., myocardial infarction, heart failure) and alcohol

From Lamy, P.P. *Prescribing for the Elderly.* Littleton, MA: PSG Publishing Company, 1980.

(Emery and Oxman, 1994); however, some potentially reversible causes are listed in Table 9–3. It is usually progressive and results in functional impairment (Oxman and Baynes, 1994). One system for classifying dementias differentiates between cortical and subcortical dementias. Alzheimer's disease is a cortical dementia. Examples of subcortical dementias are those associated with Huntington's disease, Parkinson's disease, progressive supranuclear palsy, multiple sclerosis, acquired immunodeficiency syndrome, lacunar state, sarcoidosis, and hydrocephalus (Ross and Cummings, 1994) (Table 9–4).

T A B L E   9 – 5
DSM-IV Diagnostic Criteria for Dementia

A. The development of multiple cognitive deficits manifested by both
  (1) memory impairment (impaired ability to learn new information or to recall previously learned information)
  (2) one (or more) of the following cognitive disturbances:
    (a) aphasia (language disturbance)
    (b) apraxia (impaired ability to carry out motor activities despite intact motor function)
    (c) agnosia (failure to recognize or identify objects despite intact sensory function)
    (d) disturbance in executive functioning (i.e., planning, organizing, sequencing, abstracting)
B. The cognitive deficits in Criteria A1 and A2 each cause significant impairment in social or occupational functioning and represent a significant decline from a previous level of functioning.
C. The deficits do not occur exclusively during the course of a delirium.

From American Psychiatric Association. *Diagnostic and Statistical Manual of Mental Disorders.* 4th ed. Washington, D.C., 1994.

Specific criteria for a diagnosis of dementia as defined by the *DSM-IV* are in Table 9–5.

Some patients have both dementia and delirium, but dementia is not diagnosed if

T A B L E   9 – 4
Cortical and Subcortical Dementias: A Comparison of Neuropsychologic and Neuropsychiatric Features

FEATURE	CORTICAL DEMENTIA	SUBCORTICAL DEMENTIA
Memory	More severe than subcortical Impaired recognition and retrieval	Less severe than cortical Relatively intact recognition; impaired retrieval
	Poor response to verbal cues Impaired automatic memory Impaired effort demanding memory Remote memory impaired but in early stages, recalls information learned earlier in life Intact procedural memory	Good response to verbal cues Intact automatic memory Impaired effort demanding memory Impaired remote memory over patient's entire life Impaired procedural memory
Language and speech	Language impaired Speech normal	Language generally intact Impaired speech and writing mechanics Preserved semantics and syntax
Visuospatial function	Impaired extrapersonal spatial manipulation	Impaired egocentric spatial manipulation
Attention and concentration		Poorer performance on tests of attention and concentration
Executive function	All aspects impaired	Most aspects impaired
Bradyphrenia (slowness of thought)	Less severe than subcortical	More severe than cortical
Mood changes	Depression not common	Depression very common Manic episodes less common
Personality changes	Unaware	May include apathy, self-neglect, irritability
Psychosis	Delusions common	Delusions common

From Ross, G.W. and Cummings, J.L. Cortical and subcortical dementias. *In* Emery, V.O.B. and Oxman, T.E. (eds.). *Dementia Presentations, Differential Diagnosis, and Nosology.* Baltimore: The Johns Hopkins University Press, 1994.

T A B L E   9 – 6

Key Features Differentiating Delirium from Dementia

FEATURE	DELIRIUM	DEMENTIA
Onset	Acute, often at night	Insidious
Course	Fluctuating, with lucid intervals during day; worse at night	Generally stable over course of day
Duration	Hours to weeks	Months or years
Awareness	Reduced	Clear
Alertness	Abnormally low or high	Usually normal
Attention	Hypoalert or hyperalert, distractible; fluctuates over course of day	Usually normal
Orientation	Usually impaired for time, tendency to mistake unfamiliar for familiar place and persons	Often impaired
Memory	Immediate and recent impaired	Recent and remote impaired
Thinking	Disorganized	Impoverished
Perception	Illusions and hallucinations (usually visual) relatively common	Usually normal
Speech	Incoherent, hesitant, slow, or rapid	Difficulty in finding words
Sleep-wake cycle	Always disrupted	Often fragmented sleep
Physical illness or drug toxicity	Either or both present	Often absent, especially in Alzheimer's disease

Modified by Kane, R.L., Ouslander, J.G. and Abrass, I.B. *Essentials of Clinical Geriatrics.* 3rd ed. New York: McGraw-Hill, 1994; from Lipkowski, 1987. Copyright, 1994. Reproduced with permission of McGraw-Hill, Inc.

cognitive symptoms are present only during delirium. Key features differentiating delirium and dementia are compared in Table 9–6.

Dementias are classified by the *DSM-IV* as dementia of the Alzheimer's type, vascular dementia, dementia due to human immunodeficiency virus (HIV) disease, dementia due to head trauma, dementia due to Parkinson's disease, dementia due to Huntington's disease, dementia due to Pick's disease, dementia due to Creutzfeldt-Jakob disease, dementia due to other general medical conditions, substance-induced persisting dementia, dementia due to multiple etiologies, and dementia not otherwise specified (Table 9–7).

Dementia of the Alzheimer's Type

Alzheimer's disease (AD) is a chronic, progressive, degenerative illness associated with neuropathological changes for which no cure or treatment has yet been found. It is the most common cause of dementia in elderly people. The average duration of the disease is usually about 5 years, but it sometimes lasts much longer. It is thought to be the fourth or fifth leading cause of death in the United States, although death is usually attributed to accompanying disorders and diseases, such as pneumonia, accidental trauma, infections, vascular disease, and cancer, rather than to AD itself (Reichman and Cummings, 1992; Blennow et al., 1994).

The onset of the disease is insidious and usually occurs after age 55 years, with few cases appearing before age 49 years. The incidence is estimated at 2 to 4 per cent of people aged 65 to 75 years and may be as high as 47 per cent in people over age 85 years (American Psychiatric Association, 1994; Evans et al., 1989, cited in Wisniewski et al., 1994). AD is represented in about 50 per cent of all older persons with dementia. When the onset is before age 65 years, AD is generally considered early onset, or "presenile." Immediate relatives of people with presenile AD are at greater risk for developing dementia, but the disease is thought to be rarely inherited. The inherited form of the disease is carried as a dominant trait; it is caused by an abnormal gene in chromosome 21 (Reichman and Cummings, 1992; American Psychiatric Association, 1994; Blennow et al., 1994; Wisniewski et al., 1994).

A definitive diagnosis of AD can be made only at autopsy, at which the distinctive neurological changes in the brain can be noted. The hallmark characteristics include neurofibrillary tangles, argyrophilic plaques, and granulovacuolar bodies. Argyrophilic plaques are lesions occupying the neutrophils that have the same approximate distribution as neurofibrillary tangles. Tangles and plaques are lesions in the cytoplasm of pyramidal nerve cells in the cortex. They are masses of coarse fibers made up of clustered pairs of helical filaments that run through the perikaryon and displace other organelles. Plaques and tangles are identical to those found in normal aging, but they increase significantly in the cerebral cortex with AD. Concentrations of these plaques in the neocortex are directly correlated with the presence and type of dementia; high concentrations of argyrophilic plaques are also correlated with low levels of choline acetyltransferase. Thus, much research is presently directed at investigating the relationship of these enzyme levels to the presence of dementia. Granulovacuolar degeneration of pyramidal neurons in the hippocampus may affect more than 60 per cent of these cells. Granulovacuolar bodies are lesions in the neuronal cytoplasm that are uncommon in normal aging, so their appearance is especially helpful in diagnosing senile dementia (Lewis, 1992; Erkinjuntti et al., 1994).

Clinical diagnosis of Alzheimer's disease is based chiefly on a thorough history to determine the onset and course of the disease. Efforts may be made to rule out any underlying physical or emotional factors that produce symptoms that mimic the disease, such as depression, vascular disorders, endocrinological disorders, or metabolic disorders (Fig. 9–3). Studies such as computed axial tomography (CT) scans, magnetic resonance imaging (MRI), positron emission tomography (PET scans), single photon emission computed tomography (SPECT scans), EEGs, and lumbar puncture and other invasive procedures are occasionally used to rule out vascular or tissue lesions or infections, but they do not provide definitive proof of the presence of Alzheimer's disease. In the middle stages of AD, the EEG may show theta-range slowing, and imaging studies may reveal mild cerebral atrophy. Later findings include delta-range slowing on EEG, whereas imaging studies detect cortical atrophy, sulcal enlargement, and ventricular dilatation. Unfortunately, these findings are not specific to AD (Reichman and Cummings, 1992). PET scans reveal areas in the brain with metabolic changes that allow prediction of the functional problems that are most likely to emerge as the disease progresses. The SPECT scan permits location of brain areas with abnormal acetylcholine receptors. The location of receptor changes appears to be specific to AD and Pick's disease and may therefore aid in differential diagnosis (National Institutes on Aging, 1991).

SYMPTOMS AND CLINICAL MANIFESTATIONS. The course of AD is insidious, smooth, and progressive. Major symptoms include impaired memory (especially recent memory), disorientation, impaired abstract thinking, impaired judgment and impulse control, and changes in personality and affect. Specific stages of the disease have been noted, and the symptoms become progressively worse with each stage.

Stage 1: Normal. Reisberg et al. (1992, 1988) describe the progression of AD through seven major stages (Table 9–8). In stage 1, the individual exhibits no subjective or objective evidence of cognitive impairment in an interview. Occupational and social abilities remain intact.

Stage 2: Forgetfulness. The patient reports functional decline in memory, but there is no objective evidence of impairment. Common complaints include forgetting names and appointments and misplacing things. Occupational and social abilities remain intact, and others are unaware of any loss of function.

TABLE 9 – 7
Features of Specific Dementias

DEMENTIA OF THE ALZHEIMER'S TYPE	VASCULAR DEMENTIA
The course is characterized by gradual onset and continuing cognitive decline. The cognitive deficits in Criteria A1 and A2 are not due to any of the following: (1) other central nervous system conditions that cause progressive deficits in memory and cognition (e.g., cerebrovascular disease, Parkinson's disease, Huntington's disease, subdural hematoma, normal pressure hydrocephalus, brain tumor) (2) systemic conditions that are known to cause dementia (e.g., hypothyroidism, vitamin B_{12} or folic acid deficiency, niacin deficiency, hypercalcemia, neurosyphilis, HIV infection) (3) substance-induced conditions	Focal neurological signs and symptoms (e.g., exaggeration of deep tendon reflexes, extensor plantar response, pseudobulbar palsy, gait abnormalities, weakness of an extremity) or laboratory evidence indicative of cerebrovascular disease (e.g., multiple infarctions involving cortex and underlying white matter) that is judged to be etiologically related to the disturbance.
DEMENTIA DUE TO OTHER GENERAL MEDICAL CONDITIONS	SUBSTANCE-INDUCED PERSISTING DEMENTIA
There is evidence from the history, physical examination, or laboratory findings that the disturbance is the direct physiological consequence of one of the following medical conditions: dementia due to HIV disease, dementia due to head trauma, dementia due to Huntington's disease, dementia due to Pick's disease, dementia due to Creutzfeldt-Jakob disease, dementia due to normal pressure hydrocephalus, etc.	There is evidence from the history, physical examination, or laboratory findings that the deficits are etiologically related to the persisting effects of substance use (e.g., a drug of abuse, a medication).

From *Diagnostic and Statistical Manual of Mental Disorders.* 4th ed. American Psychiatric Association: Washington, D.C., 1994.

Stage 3: Early Confusional. In the early confusional stage, the patient is able to perform routine tasks in familiar settings but has functional decrements in the ability to perform complex psychomotor tasks. People who have long been productive may find that they are unable to complete tasks or maintain schedules.

Stage 4: Late Confusional. The late confusional stage is marked by deficient performance in the complex tasks of daily life. Tasks such as cooking and managing money become increasingly difficult. The patient can still bathe, dress, and travel to familiar locations but is likely to need some assistance to live independently in the community. Pau-

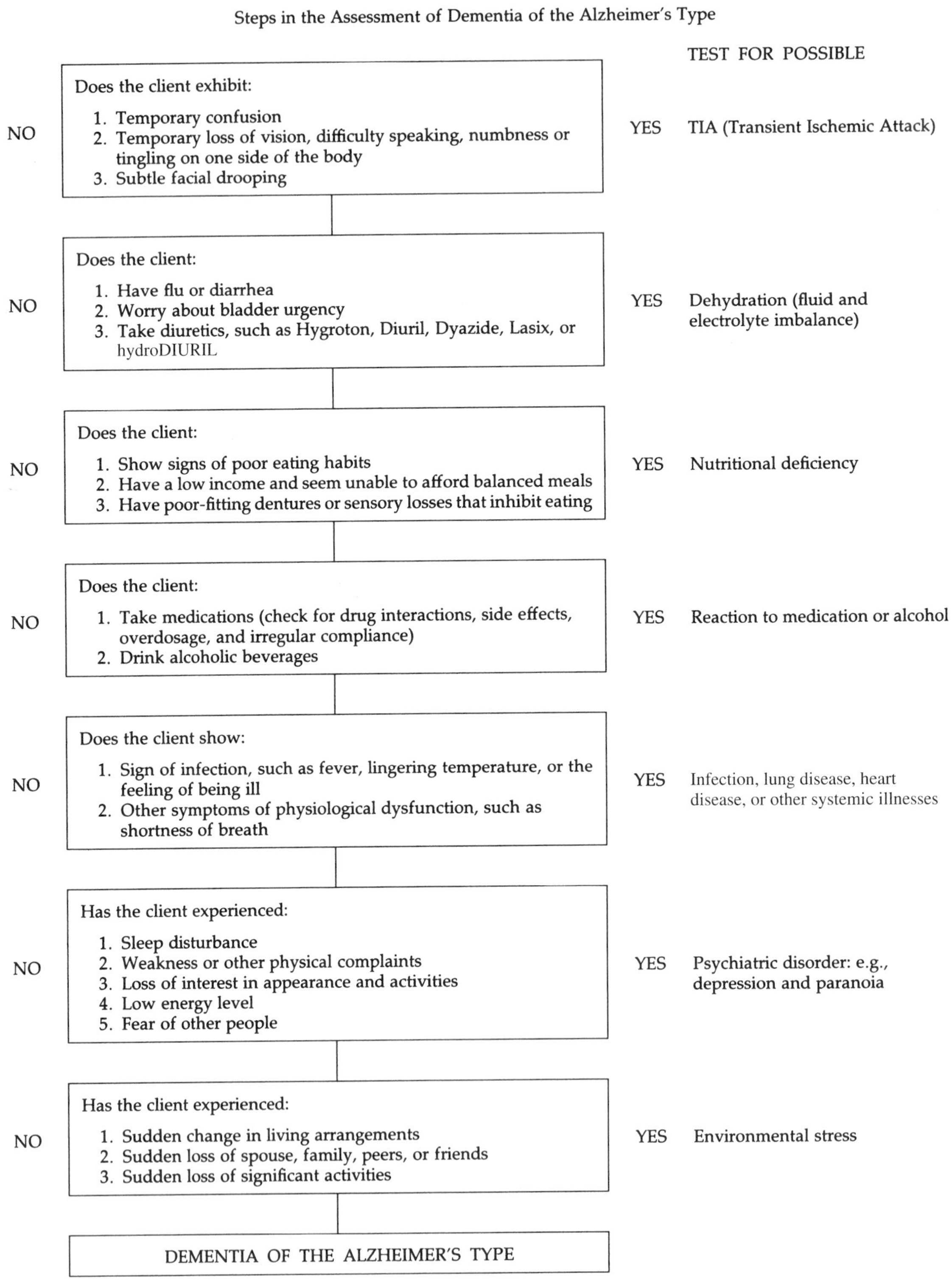

Steps in the Assessment of Dementia of the Alzheimer's Type

TEST FOR POSSIBLE

NO | Does the client exhibit:
1. Temporary confusion
2. Temporary loss of vision, difficulty speaking, numbness or tingling on one side of the body
3. Subtle facial drooping

YES | TIA (Transient Ischemic Attack)

NO | Does the client:
1. Have flu or diarrhea
2. Worry about bladder urgency
3. Take diuretics, such as Hygroton, Diuril, Dyazide, Lasix, or hydroDIURIL

YES | Dehydration (fluid and electrolyte imbalance)

NO | Does the client:
1. Show signs of poor eating habits
2. Have a low income and seem unable to afford balanced meals
3. Have poor-fitting dentures or sensory losses that inhibit eating

YES | Nutritional deficiency

NO | Does the client:
1. Take medications (check for drug interactions, side effects, overdosage, and irregular compliance)
2. Drink alcoholic beverages

YES | Reaction to medication or alcohol

NO | Does the client show:
1. Sign of infection, such as fever, lingering temperature, or the feeling of being ill
2. Other symptoms of physiological dysfunction, such as shortness of breath

YES | Infection, lung disease, heart disease, or other systemic illnesses

NO | Has the client experienced:
1. Sleep disturbance
2. Weakness or other physical complaints
3. Loss of interest in appearance and activities
4. Low energy level
5. Fear of other people

YES | Psychiatric disorder: e.g., depression and paranoia

NO | Has the client experienced:
1. Sudden change in living arrangements
2. Sudden loss of spouse, family, peers, or friends
3. Sudden loss of significant activities

YES | Environmental stress

DEMENTIA OF THE ALZHEIMER'S TYPE

FIGURE 9 – 3

Assessment of dementia of the Alzheimer's type. (From Denco, S., Owen, M.L. and Toseland, R.W. Alzheimer's disease and related disorders: Assessment and intervention. *Health Soc Work*, Summer, 1984, pp. 212–226.

TABLE 9-8
Common Findings at Each Stage of Alzheimer's Disease

Stage 1. NORMAL
   No subjective or objective evidence of cognitive impairment
Stage 2. FORGETFULNESS
   No objective evidence of impairment but subjective concern about memory loss
Stage 3. EARLY CONFUSIONAL
   Can do routine tasks in familiar settings
   Decreased ability to perform in demanding employment and social interactions
   Deficit in memory and ability to concentrate
   Difficulty with serial 7's
Stage 4. LATE CONFUSIONAL
   Increasing difficulty performing complex tasks of daily life including money management
   Can bathe, dress, and travel in familiar settings
   Paucity of speech may begin
Stage 5. EARLY DEMENTIA
   Unable to recall phone number
   Can recall own name and names of spouse and children
   No assistance required with eating or toileting
   Difficulty choosing proper clothing
   May require coaxing to bathe
   Difficulty subtracting 3's from 20
Stage 6. MID-DEMENTIA
   More deliberate gait; smaller steps
   Progressive deficits in independent dressing, bathing, and toileting
   Eventual urinary and fecal incontinence
Stage 7. LATE DEMENTIA
   Progressive loss of speech, locomotion, and consciousness

city of speech may be seen in this stage or in stage 5.

Stage 5: Early Dementia. In early dementia, basic activities of daily living can no longer be accomplished independently. The selection of mismatched clothing is characteristic of this stage. Once clothing is provided, the patient is able to dress independently. The patient must be encouraged or assisted to bathe and requires help to manage more complex tasks. Driving skills decline, so the patient may elect or be forced to give up driving.

Stage 6: Mid-Dementia. Mid-dementia is characterized by progressive deficits in independent dressing, bathing, and toileting. In addition, the ability to speak in complete sentences declines. The patient's gait may change to more deliberate and smaller steps. There are five substages: 6A, 6B, 6C, 6D, and 6E. The substages may or may not be sequential, and behaviors of more than one substage may be present simultaneously.

SUBSTAGE 6A. There is decreased ability to put on clothing properly. Examples of behaviors in this substage are putting on layers of clothing rather than changing them, inability to tie shoelaces, and putting shoes on the wrong feet.

SUBSTAGE 6B. The ability to bathe independently decreases. The patient may exhibit fear of bathing and be unable to adjust the water, get in and out of the tub, or shower, wash, or dry.

SUBSTAGE 6C. The ability to toilet independently declines. Patients at this stage can usually control elimination but have difficulty with the mechanics of toileting. They may forget to flush the toilet, have difficulty removing clothing or redressing, and fail to clean properly after toileting.

SUBSTAGE 6D. The major event marking substage 6D is the appearance of urinary incontinence. Within a few months after toileting difficulties begin, patients experience urinary incontinence without urinary tract infection or other pathology. The patient is apparently unable to respond to urinary urgency.

SUBSTAGE 6E. Fecal incontinence, typical of substage 6E, may occur simultaneously with substages 6B and 6C or may follow them.

Stage 7: Late Dementia. The final stage of AD is marked by loss of speech, locomotion, and consciousness. Stage 7 has seven substages.

SUBSTAGE 7A. The patient's vocabulary is limited to fewer than a half-dozen words.

SUBSTAGE 7B. Intelligent vocabulary is limited to a single word, sometimes "yes" or "no." Once speech is lost, the patient may resort to grunting or screaming.

SUBSTAGE 7C. This substage is marked by loss of the ability to walk. An abnormal gait (small, deliberate steps) may have appeared in stage 6. By this time, the patient may lean forward, backward, or toward one side when standing. Impaired ambulation usually precedes loss of other voluntary motor abilities.

SUBSTAGE 7D. The patient is no longer able to sit unassisted.

SUBSTAGE 7E. The ability to smile is lost. The patient has deliberate eye movements in response to stimuli but does not recognize familiar people or objects. Many patients can still chew and swallow. The grasp reflex is intact.

SUBSTAGE 7F. The patient loses the ability to hold up the head.

Behavioral Symptoms. These are common with AD and are often a major source of stress for caregivers. Frequently reported symptoms are delusions, visual hallucinations, wandering, purposeless activity, hiding or storing things in inappropriate places, verbal outbursts, physical threats or violence, frequently awakening during the night, tearfulness, anxiety about upcoming events, and fear of being alone. Not all patients exhibit all these symptoms, though multiple symptoms are common. Various symptoms may appear and disappear throughout the course of the illness. Delusions and sleep disturbances are most common in stage 5. Activity disturbances (wandering, purposeless activity, overeating, and inappropriate activity) and aggressiveness tend to be seen in stages 5 and 6. Behavioral symptoms resolve by stage 7.

Personality and Affect Changes. Personality changes may be manifested as an accentuation or caricature of a previous personality. Subtle behavior changes may be seen in the early stages, such as lack of spontaneity and initiative, loss of a previously sharp sense of humor, lack of energy and enthusiasm, or decreased interest in work, family, or recreation.

Affective problems include tearfulness, anxiety, and depression. Depression may occur early in the disease when the individual is aware of the progressive deficits.

TREATMENT. Medical treatment of AD has focused on management of the symptoms, because at this time no known cure exists. Treatments include behavioral interventions, environmental adaptations, education, and drug therapy. In general, other strategies should be tried before pharmacological intervention. In the early stages, patients can be helped to simplify their lives (Dawson et al., 1993). Notes and lists can provide the needed clues to manage everyday activities. Patients and their families need education to understand AD and to plan for the eventual decline. Patients may have unfinished business that they need to resolve. Plans must be made for management of the patient's finances. Psychotherapeutic interventions (discussed in Chapter 22) are sometimes helpful in the early stages. They should focus on determining the patient's concerns and offering practical coping measures (Table 9–9).

Management of behavior problems begins with thorough assessment to identify possible causes. For example, agitation might be related to fear, pain, constipation, or a urinary tract infection. Correction of the underlying problem can eliminate the symptom. General guidelines for dealing with problem behaviors include simplifying tasks and maintaining a consistent routine. The care-

TABLE 9–9
Key Principles in the Management of Dementia

- Optimize the patient's function
  Treat underlying medical conditions (e.g., hypertension, Parkinson's disease)
  Avoid use of drugs with CNS side effects (unless required for management of psychological or behavioral disturbances)
  Assess the environment and suggest alterations, if necessary
  Encourage physical and mental activity
  Avoid situations stressing intellectual capabilities; use memory aids whenever possible
  Prepare the patient for changes in location
  Emphasize good nutrition
- Identify and manage complications
  Wandering and other hazards
  Behavioral disorders
  Depression
  Agitation or aggressiveness
  Psychosis (delusions, hallucinations)
  Incontinence
- Provide ongoing care
  Reassessment of cognitive and physical function
  Treatment of medical conditions
- Provide medical information to patient and family
  Nature of the disease
  Extent of impairment
  Prognosis
- Provide social service information to patient and family
  Community health care resources (day centers, homemakers, home health aides)
  Legal and financial counseling
- Provide family counseling for
  Identification and resolution of family conflicts
  Handling anger and guilt
  Decisions on respite or institutional care
  Legal concerns
  Ethical concerns

From Kane, R.L., Ouslander, J.G. and Abrass, I.B. *Essentials of Clinical Geriatrics.* 3rd ed. New York: McGraw-Hill, 1994. Copyright, 1994. Reproduced with permission of McGraw-Hill, Inc.

giver needs to remain calm and approach the patient in a nonthreatening way. Arguing is usually ineffective, but distraction can be used to redirect the patient's attention. The patient may be able to complete a task if it is begun for him. Directions should be short and include only one step at a time. Agitation and frustration can develop into a catastrophic reaction when the patient's inability to cope with a situation is overwhelming.

Caregivers must be sensitive to the patient's abilities and not impose unrealistic expectations. Reality orientation has been traditionally recommended; however, this intervention has become questionable and controversial as a worthwhile or therapeutic endeavor. Experiences of family members and nursing personnel have shown that in many cases reality orientation is ineffective and leads to frustration in both patients and caregivers. We studied the management of problem behaviors by matching interventions with the patient's cognitive level using Piaget's classification system. Results demonstrated that interventions derived in this way can be effectively employed while psychotropic drugs are being withdrawn.

Wandering may be aimless or purposeful but is worrisome to caregivers who imagine the patient becoming lost. Complicated or concealed locks may be needed to prevent unsafe wandering. Sometimes an official-looking sign that says "STOP" or "DO NOT ENTER" will deter the patient from pursuing a particular path. Patients who tend to wander should wear medical alert tags engraved "memory impaired." If a patient leaves the safe environment, a caregiver should follow the person, fall into step, and strike up a friendly conversation. Once the patient is distracted, he or she can usually be redirected casually back to the home or nursing facility. Drugs are not effective with wandering. They only sedate the patient, increasing the risk of falls and injury (Jarvik et al., 1992).

Controversy exists over the role of medications in alleviating the symptoms of AD. Pharmacological treatment has been directed primarily toward the management of behavioral symptoms. The medication should be given for the patient's benefit, not the caregiver's. Drugs should be used cautiously with lower initial doses, longer titration intervals, and lower final dosages. The side effects of certain drugs can produce discomfort and may aggravate the dementia, so the benefits and risks must be weighed. Clients should be observed for drug interactions, keeping in mind that their physical condition affects drug action. Finally, drugs should never be used as the only method of treatment but should be used in conjunction with psychological, social, and environmental therapies (Jarvik et al., 1992; McAllister and Powers, 1994).

Types of drugs that may be employed for treatment of symptoms include neuroleptics, antipsychotics, sedatives-hypnotics, and antidepressants. Neuroleptics such as haloperidol, thiothixene, and thioridazine may be employed in the treatment of psychotic symptoms. These drugs are not without risk, however, since older people with dementia are especially susceptible to adverse effects of neuroleptics, particularly confusion and extrapyramidal reactions (Reichman and Cummings, 1992; Mayeux and Schofield, 1994; McAllister and Powers, 1994). Other adverse effects of neuroleptics are sedation, orthostatic hypotension, psychomotor slow-

ing, blurred vision, and dry mouth. Agitation and activity disturbances may respond to neuroleptics, benzodiazepines, and non-benzodiazepine sedatives-hypnotics. One to two mg of haloperidol is usually adequate; over 4 mg is rarely indicated (Jarvik et al., 1992). Benzodiazepines and sedatives-hypnotics may be used for sleep disturbances, but they should be reserved for situations when other approaches fail. Short-acting drugs (oxazepam, lorazepam) are preferred over long-acting drugs (flurazepam, diazepam) because long-acting drugs are more likely to cause daytime sedation (Reichman and Cummings, 1992).

Researchers are seeking drugs that might slow or stop the cognitive decline of AD by restoring deficient neurotransmitters, reversing neuronal dysfunction, or slowing neuronal damage. Potential cognitive enhancers include cholinergic agents, nootropics, and a variety of other drugs. The most promising of the cholinergic agents is tacrine (Cognex), a cholinesterase inhibitor. While taking tacrine, some early AD patients have shown moderate, though not overwhelming, improvement in cognition as measured by the Clinical Global Impression of Change and the cognitive subscale of the Alzheimer's Disease Assessment Scale. Adverse effects include elevated transaminase levels, nausea and vomiting, diarrhea, dyspepsia, myalgia, anorexia, and ataxia. In addition, some patients on tacrine experience confusion, insomnia, agitation, and depression. During clinical trials, 8 per cent of subjects had to be withdrawn from the drug due to elevated transaminase levels—a sign of hepatotoxicity. Nootropics, including piracetam and tenilsetam, are being studied for possible improvement in the acquisition, storage, and retrieval of information. Ergoloid mesylate (Hydergine) has been widely used, but its value is not well supported. Calcium channel blockers, noradrenaline, vitamins, and clonidine are among the other agents being studied in the treatment of Alzheimer's disease (McAllister and Powers, 1994).

Electroconvulsive therapy has been tried with some success in the treatment of depression in dementia patients (McAllister and Powers, 1994).

Nursing care and home management are the major foci of treatment, with emphasis on environmental manipulation. Caregivers are advised to provide a structured environment with a routine that is dependable and contains relatively little change. Social support should be provided, and often the use of touch can be very reassuring. Table 9–10 summarizes nursing care of clients with Al-

T A B L E   9 – 1 0
Nursing Care Plan for the Patient with Alzheimer's Disease

FUNCTIONAL DISABILITY	NURSING GOAL	NURSING INTERVENTIONS
Altered cognitive and perceptual abilities	Establish effective verbal and nonverbal communication with the patient	Adapt approach and expectations to patient's abilities.
		Gently approach the patient with an open, friendly, relaxed manner and expression. Alzheimer's patients mirror the affect of those around them.
		Always identify yourself and look directly at the patient to be sure you have his or her attention.
		Speak in a clear, low-pitched voice. High-pitched tones convey anxiety and tension.
		Use short and simple words, sentences, and questions and ask only one question at a time.
		Use yes/no questions and avoid those that require choices.
		Break down tasks into individual steps and ask the patient to do them one at a time.
		If the patient reacts catastrophically to a situation, remain calm and try to remove the patient from the upset.
		Carefully assess the patient's nonverbal behavior, since the patient may not be able to verbalize pain or discomfort. Closely observe body cues such as posture, grimacing, sudden changes in behavior, and increased restlessness.
	Provide a safe, structured environment	Provide consistent caregivers.
		Provide a room that allows careful observation.
		Never leave anything that might harm the patient at the bedside.
		Keep siderails up and the bed in a low position. Check the patient frequently at night.
		Assess the degree of ataxia; help with walking if necessary.
		Establish a schedule of care.
		Label items, using visual cues.
Alteration in exercise activity patterns	Maintain mobility and exercise as much as possible appropriate to the patient's level of fitness	Encourage walking if patient is able.
		Bedridden patients require active and passive range-of-motion exercises.
		Avoid restraints, if possible.
	Provide cognitive stimulation in the environment	Avoid isolating the patient.
		Soft music from a radio or tape recorder may be very soothing.
		Patient may enjoy television.
Altered bowel and bladder patterns	Maintain bowel and bladder continence for as long as possible	Determine the usual pattern and offer the bedpan or urinal or walk to the bathroom as the pattern indicates.
		Limit the fluids the patient consumes at bedtime to prevent nighttime incontinence.
		Avoid using laxatives but encourage high-fiber diets to help maintain bowel regularity. Observe subtle signs of constipation since patient may not be able to tell.
Altered nutritional/ metabolic patterns	Maintain optimal nutritional status	Encourage well-balanced meals appropriate to eating abilities—"finger foods" if necessary.
		Plan a high-caloric diet if the patient is hyperactive. Encourage fluids during the day to prevent dehydration.
		Limit the number of foods you place in front of the patient at one time, as too many foods can be overwhelming.
		Observe for swallowing difficulties that may put the patient at risk for aspiration.
		Enteral or parenteral feeding may be required in later stages of the disease.
Altered sleep/rest patterns	Maintain normal day/night patterns	Encourage the patient to stay awake during the day.
		If the patient is on psychotropics to control agitation, periodically assess their effectiveness and look for side effects.
		Schedule tests and treatments for the morning and afternoon, so the patient can wind down in the late afternoon and evening. This helps avoid overstimulation before bedtime.
		If the patient wakes during the night and becomes confused and agitated, reorient in a soft, soothing manner to avoid precipitating extreme agitation and loss of control.

From Pajk, M. Alzheimer's disease in patient care. *Am J Nurs* 84:218–219, 1984.

zheimer's disease based on specific functional impairments.

Vascular Dementia

Vascular dementias are associated with ischemic cerebral injury. There are several types of vascular dementias, the most common being multi-infarct dementia (MID) (Jarvik et al., 1992). MID is a vascular disorder in which there is occlusion of multiple large and small cerebral blood vessels. Between 10 per cent and 20 per cent of all dementia cases are vascular in origin, and the incidence is closely associated with the presence of hypertension. Other factors contributing to the disease are arrhythmias, myocardial infarction, transient ischemic attacks, atrial fibrillation, snoring, carotid bruits, alcoholism, peripheral vascular disease, diabetes mellitus, obesity, and smoking. The usual age of onset is between 55 and 70 years, with an average age of 65 years. The disease occurs more frequently in men than in women.

The disease is different from Alzheimer's disease in its presentation and tissue pathology. It typically occurs earlier than AD, and the onset is usually abrupt. Destruction of brain tissue resulting from small emboli or strokes may be localized or diffuse, so scattered areas of the brain may be involved; however, focal neurological signs are frequently present. There are diffuse, irregular, asymmetrical regions of cerebral softening and hemorrhage with evidence of atherosclerotic disease (Jarvik et al., 1992; Reichman and Cummings, 1992; American Psychiatric Association, 1994; Kane et al., 1994; Kobayashi, 1994).

CLINICAL PRESENTATION AND SYMPTOMS. Persons with vascular dementia demonstrate a stepwise and paroxysmal deterioration of intellectual function that is associated with a clear-cut succession of strokes and infarcts to the brain. In general, a single stroke does not cause dementia, but an initial episode of delirium may be associated with the onset of a stroke, with clouding of consciousness and disorientation. Although there is improvement within a few weeks, residual disability remains. Fluctuation of mental status, characterized by episodes of acute confusional states and general intellectual deterioration, results in memory loss, problems with concentration and comprehension, and disturbances in abstract thinking, judgment, impulse control, and personality. Specific changes depend on the areas of the brain affected. Focal

TABLE 9 – 11
Modified Hachinski Ischemia Score

CHARACTERISTIC	POINT SCORE
Abrupt onset	2
Stepwise deterioration	1
Somatic complaints	1
Emotional incontinence	1
History or presence of hypertension	1
History of strokes	2
Focal neurological symptoms	2
Focal neurological signs	2

Note: This tool has been validated on a small number of demented patients by autopsy findings. A score of 4 or more is consistent with multi-infarct dementia (now called vascular dementia).

From Rosen, W.G., Terry, R.D., Fuld, P.A., et al. Pathological verification of ischemic score in differentiation of dementia. *Ann Neurol* 7:486–488, 1980. Reprinted with permission.

neurological signs may include limb weakness, asymmetrical reflexes, extensor plantar responses, dysarthria, and small-stepped gait.

Preservation of insight and personality may lead to depression as the afflicted individuals recognize their disabilities. Emotional lability that is so characteristic of stroke patients is also present. About one half have disordered breathing during sleep (Erkinjuntti et al., cited in Haponik, 1994). The underlying vascular pathology, such as hypertension, may produce symptoms of palpitations, anxiety, fatigue, difficulty in sleeping, hypochondriasis, irritability, headache, chest pains, and giddiness. It is interesting to note that these symptoms are also physiological symptoms of depression (Cohen and Eisdorfer, 1992; Jarvik et al., 1992; Reichman and Cummings, 1992; American Psychiatric Association, 1994; Kane et al., 1994).

DIAGNOSIS AND TREATMENT. An accurate history of the onset and course of the illness is as important in diagnosing vascular dementia as it is in Alzheimer's disease. Predisposing factors such as vascular disease and hypertension should also be considered. The examiner should look for focal signs and symptoms, emotional lability, and intellectual deterioration as diagnostic cues.

The Hachinski ischemia score is a useful tool to identify vascular dementias (Table 9–11). A score of 7 or more is compatible with vascular dementia (Reichman and

Cummings, 1992). Brain imaging also provides diagnostic information. The CT scan may reveal areas of lucency compatible with infarcts. Increased signal intensity on the MRI also reveals ischemic areas (Reichman and Cummings, 1992). The diagnostic value of PET scans and studies of regional metabolism continues to be explored (Rossor, 1992).

Treatment is generally aimed at the underlying vascular pathology. Antihypertensive medications are given to alleviate elevated blood pressure. Occasionally a thromboendarterectomy is done when bilateral carotid disease is present, which promotes intellectual improvement and decreased incidents of transient ischemic attacks and strokes. However, this procedure does not affect the rate of survival. Antiplatelet therapy, often low-dose aspirin, may be prescribed to decrease the risk of further infarction. Major tranquilizers may be administered for acute confusional states. Drug therapy for arrhythmias may be ordered (Jarvik et al., 1992; American Psychiatric Association, 1994; Kobayashi, 1994).

Dementia Due to Pick's Disease

The onset, course, and clinical presentation of Pick's disease are so similar to those of Alzheimer's disease that the two are often categorically linked and treated in the same manner. Pick's disease has some subtle differences from Alzheimer's, and it is important to have some knowledge of a condition that is almost exclusively associated with aging. Investigators disagree as to whether Pick's and Alzheimer's disease can be differentiated by brain imaging studies or neuropsychological tests (Kirshner, 1994). This condition is more frequently found in women than in men, predominantly between ages 50 and 60 years. The onset is slow and insidious and progresses to death; the average duration of the illness is 4 years. There is evidence of autosomal dominant inheritance (Jarvik et al., 1992).

A major difference between Alzheimer's disease and Pick's disease lies in the pathological process. The former is characterized by diffuse involvement of higher brain structures, whereas the latter is characterized by extreme atrophy of localized cortical areas. Anterior parts of the frontal, temporal, and parietal lobes shrink. The posterior parts of some gyri remain normal, creating what is referred to as a "knife-edge" appearance. The cell pattern in affected areas is disorganized, and the loss of neurons is extensive. As a result, focal cortical impairments such as motor or sensory aphasia may appear. Senile plaques, neurofibrillary tangles, and granulovacuolar degeneration, which are so characteristic of Alzheimer's disease, may be found with Pick's disease but are much less common (Lewis, 1992). Silver-staining inclusion bodies, called Pick bodies, are found in neurons with Pick's disease (Kirshner, 1994).

Characteristics that differentiate Pick's dementia from other dementias are swelling and pallor of affected neurons with loss of Nissl bodies and the formation of argyrophilic inclusions in affected neurons (Lewis, 1992). The specific diagnosis is usually confirmed on autopsy (American Psychiatric Association, 1994).

SYMPTOMS AND CLINICAL PRESENTATION. The symptoms of the disease are similar to those of Alzheimer's disease, with progressive impairment of cognition, memory, and orientation. Early symptoms are personality changes, inappropriate social behavior, loss of insight, and anomia. Language disorders are common, eventually leading to mutism. Depression and apathy may also accompany the disease. See Table 9–12 for differential diagnoses of various types of dementias.

TREATMENT. Because there is no known cure for Pick's disease, treatment is aimed toward management of the symptoms. Modification of the home environment and work with family caregivers are important in the early stages. Institutionalization may be necessary in the later stages (Jarvik et al., 1992).

Dementia Due to Huntington's Disease

Huntington's disease is a progressive degenerative disorder that affects cognition, emotion, and movement (American Psychiatric Association, 1994). It is mentioned here because it is a dementia that usually begins in young adulthood and middle age, but there are juvenile and late-onset forms. The onset occurs between the ages of 35 and 42 years, and the disease has an average duration of 15 years. The outcome is fatal. The disease is inherited through an autosomal dominant gene; men and women are equally affected. A person whose parent had Huntington's disease has a 50 per cent chance of developing the disease. A genetic test can determine an individual's risk (American Psychiatric Association, 1994).

The extrapyramidal and subcortical areas of the brain and nervous system are af-

TABLE 9-12
Differential Diagnosis of Various Types of Dementia

	DEPRESSIVE DISORDERS	VASCULAR DEMENTIA	ALZHEIMER'S DISEASE, SENILE ONSET	ALZHEIMER'S DISEASE, PRESENILE ONSET	PICK'S DISEASE
FACTORS					
Usual age of onset	Any age	55–70 years average: 65 years	70+ years average: 75 years	50–60 years average: 56 years	50–60 years average: 50 years
Sex distribution	Early life: more women Late life: more men	Men:women = 3:1	Men:women = 2:3	Men:women = 2:3	Men:women = 2:3
Duration	Varies from weeks to years	Varies from days to many years; average: 4 years	Varies from months to years; average: 5 years	Average: 4 years	Average: 4 years
Mode of onset	Gradual or sudden: precipitating stress often apparent	Gradual or acute	Insidious	More sudden and less gradual	Slow and insidious
Course	Self-limited, but tendency to recur	Intermittent, fluctuating	Slowly or rapidly progressive	Rapidly progressive	Progressive and fatal
Prognosis	Responsive to drugs or ECT	Varies depending on multiple factors	Poor (in moderate or severe cases)	Very poor	Very poor
Outcome	Usually recovery: sometimes suicide or regression to paranoid level	Death from CVA, heart disease, or infection	Death from general organ failure; infection		
Hereditary and precipitating factors	Involution; previous history of depression	Some familial tendency	Multiple genetically determined factors	Multifactorial inheritance, genetic factors causing premature aging	Degenerative process
Signs of brain damage	None	Diffuse or focal	Diffuse, generalized	Diffuse, generalized, more severe than in senile onset	Circumscribed atrophy; frontal, temporal, or parietal lobes
Impairment of higher cortical functions	No structural impairment	Some isolated impairments: e.g., aphasia, apraxia, agnosia	Progressive dementia	Involvement of cerebral associative areas; transcortical aphasia, apraxia, agnosia, etc.	Focal cortical impairments; e.g., motor or sensory aphasia
Neuromuscular	Psychomotor retardation or agitation	Paralyses; minor extrapyramidal signs	Tremors, uncertain gait, variable muscular rigidity, incontinence	Transient or progressive paresis; unsteady gait; increased muscle tone; occasional tremors, incontinence	Primitive reflexes; extrapyramidal signs; attacks of muscular hypotonia, incontinence
Seizures	None	Epileptiform attacks	Rare	Occasional	Rare
Medical	Physiological concomitants of depression (sleep, appetite, weight, energy)	Common history of CVA; headaches, dizziness, and syncope (in 50%); transient ischemic attacks; arteriosclerosis in heart, kidney, legs, etc.	Infections, contractures, fractures, decubitus ulcers		
NEUROPATHOLOGY					
Macroscopic	None characteristic	Large or small areas of softening and hemorrhage	Diffuse generalized shrinkage of brain, especially gray matter; dilated ventricles; internal hydrocephalus	General cerebral atrophy; dilated ventricles; internal hydrocephalus	Circumscribed lobar atrophy, mostly orbitofrontal or temporal

Table continued on following page

TABLE 9–12

Differential Diagnosis of Various Types of Dementia *Continued*

	DEPRESSIVE DISORDERS	VASCULAR DEMENTIA	ALZHEIMER'S DISEASE, SENILE ONSET	ALZHEIMER'S DISEASE, PRESENILE ONSET	PICK'S DISEASE
Microscopic	None characteristic	Granular atrophy of cortex diffusely with hypertensive cardiovascular disease; destruction of neurons, nerve fibers, and glia; focal neuronal and selective cortical degeneration Secondary gliosis Senile plaques not typical	Neuronal degeneration and shrinking; most damage in upper layers of cortex; deposition of lipofuscin and intracellular fibrils Moderate gliosis, especially in outer layer of cortex Senile plaques	Diffuse loss of neurons, especially in cortex layers 3 and 5; disturbed cortical layers Neuron degeneration: pyknosis; granulovacuolar bodies; Alzheimer's neurofibrillary change Gliosis more severe than in senile onset Senile plaques throughout cortex	Progressive atrophy of neurons; no predilection for cortical layers; neuron degeneration; increased pigment pyknosis; swollen cells; argyrophilic cytoplasmic inclusions Gliosis prominent Senile plaques rare
Vascular	None characteristic	*Large arteries:* atherosclerosis *Small vessels:* endothelial proliferation, medial hypertrophy, and intima hyalinization	Endothelial degeneration; media fibrosis; adventitial proliferation; vascular loops	Degenerative changes of endothelial and adventitial cells	Endothelial proliferation; hyaline degeneration
PSYCHIATRIC SYMPTOMATOLOGY					
Orientation	Intact, except in depressive stupor	Episodes of acute confusion; lucid intervals	Progressive disorientation in all spheres Loss of time perspective		
Perception	Occasional auditory hallucinations	Auditory and visual during acute exacerbations	Various types of hallucinations in advanced stages	Occasional hallucinations	
Intellect and thought	No mental impairment Delusions consistent with affect Insight varies	Lacunar types of intellectual deficit; Delusions: rare Insight present in early stages	Progressive, generalized dementia Delusions depend on degree of regression and premorbid personality No insight	Progressive dementia and loss of abstraction Aphasia, alexia, agnosia, asymbolia, agraphia, apraxia No insight	*Frontal lobe* syndrome: progressive loss of abstraction *Aphasic* syndrome: aphasia, alexia, etc. *Alogic* syndrome: agnosia, apraxia, etc. No insight
Memory	Transient memory problems due to CNS slowing	Varying deficits of recent and remote memory, of retention and recall Confabulations: rare	Progressive impairment of all memory functions Confabulations of presbyophrenic type	Progressive impairment of all memory functions Confabulations: rare	Progressive impairment of all memory functions Confabulations: common
Affect	Depression; guilt; low self-esteem	Emotional lability; anxiety and depression Later: blunting of affect	Depends on subtype: Simple: apathy Depressed: agitated Delirious: Anxious Paranoid: hostile Presbyophrenic: shallow euphoria	Variable at first; later, apathy	Apathy and indifference
Psychomotor	Retardation, sometimes agitation	Hypoactive or hyperactive or restless agitation		Hyperactive; repetitive, primitive motor behavior; extrapyramidal signs	Hypo- or hyperkinetic; primitive reflexes; stereotyped activity; preservation; echolalia; logoclony
Personality changes	Transient regressive changes	Regressive changes are intermittent or slowly progressive	Progressive deterioration of social behavior and personal habits		

From Verwoerdt, A. *Clinical Geropsychiatry.* 2nd ed. Baltimore: Williams & Wilkins, 1981, pp. 72–76. Copyright, Williams & Wilkins.

fected, producing characteristic symptoms of choreiform, or brief, dancing, jerky movements, gait disturbances, and bradykinesia, accompanied by memory loss, irritability, paranoia, and impaired impulse control. Patients have impaired language fluency but do not make many perseverative errors (Fozzard, 1992). Psychotic behavior, severe dementia, urinary incontinence, and an inability to communicate or swallow characterize the final stages of the disease. Death usually results from heart failure or pulmonary complications caused by asphyxiation or aspiration of food. Table 9–13 describes the stages of Huntington's disease and the accompanying decline in function.

The only available medical treatment is administration of drugs to manage the psychotic and depressive symptoms and decrease choreiform movements. Drugs most frequently used are haloperidol, fluphenazine, and reserpine to minimize choreiform movements, mild tranquilizers such as diazepam to lower anxiety, and antidepressants for depression. Genetic counseling is also provided for families of the afflicted individuals to prevent further incidence of the disease (Fozzard et al., 1992; Jarvik et al., 1992; Martin and Turker, 1994).

Nursing care; physical, occupational, and speech therapy; and social services can help with the problems of dysphagia, malnutrition, impaired communication, functional disabilities, and behavioral abnormalities. Table 9–14 provides strategies for coping with these problems. The Huntington's Disease Foundation of America provides information and support for caregivers to help them cope with this difficult situation. In addition, the Foundation supports research studies to understand the disease more fully.

Dementia Due to Creutzfeldt-Jakob Disease

Creutzfeldt-Jakob disease is a neurodegenerative disorder that results in dementia and severe neurological impairment. The onset usually occurs between ages 40 and 60 years, and a small percentage of patients have a familial component. This rare disease occurs in only 1 in 1 million people. Creutzfeldt-Jakob disease is caused by prions which are also called "slow viruses." There have been some documented reports of iatrogenic transmission by way of corneal transplants and human growth hormone therapy, but most cases are of unknown etiology (Martin and Turker, 1994). The classic manifestations are dementia, involuntary movements, and periodic EEG activity, but individual presentations vary. Prodromal symptoms (fatigue, anxiety, disturbances in sleep and concentration) precede motor dysfunction and rapidly progressive dementia. The duration of the disease has been variously reported as 2 to 9 months. The histopathology of the brain disorder is similar to that seen in Alzheimer's disease. Tissue studies are needed for a definitive diagnosis (American Psychiatric Association, 1994). There is no known treatment (Jarvik et al., 1992).

Dementia Due to Parkinson's Disease

Parkinsonism, characterized by tremor at rest, slowness and weakness of voluntary movement, and rigidity, is second only to stroke as the most common neurological disorder in elderly persons. The term "parkinsonian syndrome" is often used to describe extrapyramidal movement disorders whether or not Parkinson's disease is actually present. Parkinson's disease is in fact the major cause of parkinsonism; however, the administration of major tranquilizers, such as haloperidol and phenothiazines, may produce similar symptoms. Parkinson's disease is found worldwide and is estimated to affect one half to 1 million Americans. The onset is usually between ages 55 and 60 years, but it sometimes occurs as early as 30 years of age (Mutch, 1992).

The disease is degenerative, involving the basal ganglia and the extrapyramidal nervous system. The basal ganglia contain short anatomical pathways that connect the basal ganglionic structures to the cerebral cortex. This interconnecting system has an important role in modifying posture for cortically induced movements. The major pathology in Parkinson's disease is related to the loss of cells in the substantia nigra, a structure in the basal ganglia; these cells are rich in dopamine. The 90 per cent or more loss of dopamine produces the symptoms of parkinsonism. Symptoms do not usually appear until there is a loss of 70 per cent of the neurons. Some patients have diffuse cortical atrophy, but most do not. Plaques and tangles are commonly found at autopsy.

SYMPTOMS AND CLINICAL PRESENTATION. Parkinson's disease is characterized by tremor; a slow, progressive rigidity of the limbs and trunk; and decreased voluntary movements. The tremor is typically rapid, rhythmic, and increased by stress. It usually begins in one arm and progresses to other parts of the body (Poirier and Finch,

T A B L E   9 – 1 3
Progressive Stages of Huntington's Disease

	ENGAGEMENT IN OCCUPATION	CAPACITY TO HANDLE FINANCIAL AFFAIRS	CAPACITY TO MANAGE DOMESTIC RESPONSIBILITIES	CAPACITY TO PERFORM ACTIVITIES OF DAILY LIVING	CARE CAN BE PROVIDED AT
Stage 1	Usual level	Full	Full	Full	Home
Stage 2	Lower level	Requires slight assistance	Full	Full	Home
Stage 3	Marginal	Requires major assistance	Impaired	Mildly impaired	Home
Stage 4	Unable	Unable	Unable	Moderately impaired	Home or extended care facility
Stage 5	Unable	Unable	Unable	Severely impaired	Total care facility only

From *Huntington's Disease: The Challenge of Care and Coping*. New York: Huntington's Disease Foundation of America, 1983.

1994). There is a flexion posture of the neck, trunk, and limbs, with cogwheeling on passive movement.

Bradykinesia (slowness of voluntary movement) occurs and may become so severe that the person is unable to initiate movements. Individuals have an expressionless face; whispered, muffled, and monotonous speech; excessive salivation; and limited ocular mobility. Handwriting becomes progressively smaller until it may be illegible. Older persons have particular difficulty with balance and may experience frequent falls. Depression is common, and it is thought to be related to decreased serotonin rather than simply a response to a debilitating illness (Bunting and Fitzsimmons, 1991; Habermann-Little, 1991). Because the disease involves the lower brain primarily, mental capacities are not necessarily impaired. Estimates of dementia with Parkinson's range from 20 to 60 per cent. Dementia due to Parkinson's disease is characterized by slowed motor and cognitive function, executive dysfunction, and memory impairment (American Psychiatric Association, 1994).

Drugs used to treat Parkinson's disease frequently produce side effects similar to those characteristic of dementia: confusion, disorientation, depression, excitement, and hallucinations (Jarvik et al., 1992; Hodgson et al., 1993).

Diagnosis of the disease may be difficult in elderly people because many of the usual signs and symptoms may be altered or masked. For example, the characteristic tremor may be completely absent, especially when the arms are resting in the person's lap. The flexed posture of the head, shoulders, and thorax; joint rigidity; and bradykinesia may be mistaken for changes associated with aging. In addition, the immobile appearance of the face may be considered a result of depression or deafness rather than Parkinson's disease.

TREATMENT. Drug therapies include dopaminergics (levodopa, amantadine), MAO-B inhibitors (selegiline), and anticholinergics (Table 9–15). Once the loss of natural dopamine exceeds 90 per cent, levodopa is no longer effective. Anticholinergics are most therapeutic for tremors in the early stages of the disease; however, they have little effect on rigidity, akinesia (absence of movements), and loss of postural reflexes. Drugs with anticholinergic effects that have been used include trihexyphenidyl (Artane), antihistamines (Benadryl), antidepressants (Tofranil), procyclidine (Kemadrin), orphenadrine (Disipal), and benztropine (Cogentin). In some cases, the anticholinergic drugs, especially procyclidine and orphenadrine, are useful for treating drug-induced parkinsonism. Side effects that cause anticholinergics to be problematic for elderly people include drowsiness, mental confusion and hallucinations, constipation, blurred vision, urinary retention, and aggravation of glaucoma (Montgomery and Lipsy, 1993; Shlafer, 1993).

Like levodopa, amantadine is used in the earlier stages of the disease and has been found to improve akinesia, rigidity, and tremor. It is thought to act by releasing dopamine from the intact dopaminergic terminals that remain in the basal ganglia. Unfortunately, it has a fading effect, which is a major drawback in treatment. Side effects of the drug are slurred speech, tremor, ataxia, confusion, insomnia, depression, and restlessness. In addition, amantadine may exacerbate congestive heart failure (Montgomery and Lipsy, 1993).

Levodopa increases the level of dopamine in the brain and is very effective in relieving the symptoms of Parkinson's disease. Levodopa is commonly combined with carbidopa, which prevents the peripheral breakdown of levodopa (Hodgson et al., 1993). Although this drug does not provide a cure, there is rapid improvement in gait, posture, balance, dressing, and handwriting, and life expectancy is prolonged somewhat (Fig. 9–4). Initial doses are generally smaller in older people than in the young and are then increased slowly. Side effects of L-dopa include nausea and vomiting, cardiac arrhythmias, postural hypotension, dyskinesias (orofacial movements or choreiform movements involving the head, trunk, or limbs), hallucinations, increased libido, and unresponsiveness. Older people who take levodopa for a long period of time may show marked decreases in intellectual capacity and, in many cases, may develop dementia. Long-term treatment may also produce a diminished effectiveness of the drug in addition to an "on-off" syndrome in which the effects intensify or disappear. It must be noted that L-dopa is not effective for the treatment of drug-induced parkinsonism, because the causative drugs block its effect on dopamine receptors in the nigrostriatal system (McDowell, 1992; Hodgson et al., 1993; Montgomery and Lipsy, 1993; Shlafer, 1993; McDowell, 1994).

A recent addition to the drugs available for Parkinson's disease is selegiline hydrochloride (Eldepryl), which may slow the progression of symptoms. It may also be used to boost the effectiveness of levodopa compounds. Side effects frequently include nausea and dizziness. Confusion, hallucinations, and vivid dreams may occur, and the patient may demonstrate signs of CNS depression or overstimulation. Selegiline should never be given with meperidine, because the interaction may cause a fatal reaction (Hodgson et al., 1993; Montgomery and Lipsy, 1993).

The transplantation of adrenal medullary tissue was once thought to be a promising way to provide dopamine replacement. This procedure has not fulfilled the early expectations, and researchers have turned to studying the value of transplanting fetal substantia nigra or genetically altering cells to make them capable of producing dopamine (McDowell, 1994).

A low-protein diet has been proposed in the treatment of Parkinson's disease. The value of this dietary restriction is under study (Yen, 1990).

In addition to drug treatment, physical and occupational therapy and social work services may be useful adjuncts for relieving symptoms and promoting functional status and independence. Exercise is generally encouraged, but there is limited evidence of long-term benefits of physical therapy in relation to the progression of Parkinson's

TABLE 9–14
Care of the Patient with Huntington's Disease

PROBLEM	CAUSE	MANAGEMENT
Dysphagia (difficulty swallowing solids and liquids leading to gagging and choking)	Lack of tongue and breathing control	Dysphagia therapy. While eating, patient should (1) Use sitting position, leaning slightly forward (2) Hold breath before swallowing and cough after each mouthful swallowed (3) Avoid liquids that are too thick (milkshakes) or too thin (watery drinks); use liquids with texture (pineapple juice) (4) Avoid hard or crumbly foods that are difficult to manipulate
Poor nutrition	Swallowing difficulties	(1) Take daily vitamin and mineral tablet; high-calorie protein supplements (2) Eat slowly (3) 5–6 small meals are better than 3 large meals (4) Avoid empty calories (5) Use powdered milk supplements for cooking and thickening (6) Use breakfast drinks and bars for snacks/supplements
Communication	Poor control of oral and respiratory muscles	(1) Spend time with patient and develop discernible signals (2) Talking boards or yes/no cards (3) Create relaxed environment; don't rush communications; keep conversations simple
Functional disabilities	Choreiform movements	(1) Pad wheelchairs and beds; use shin guards to prevent bruising (2) Use wrist weights to aid hand and arm coordination (3) Explore use of aids and assistive devices (4) Explore use of alternative sitting and sleeping devices (beanbag chairs, hammocks) (5) Keep clothing light and simple
Behavioral problems	Neurological changes	(1) May have to isolate or sedate abusive patient (2) Never use restraints (3) Encourage activity for passive patients (4) Use patience and understanding

From *Huntington's Disease: The Challenge of Care and Coping.* New York: The Huntington's Disease Foundation of America, 1983.

disease (McDowell, 1994). Some small studies have reported improved gait pattern with specific physiotherapies. Speech therapy has also been recommended for some, but evidence of benefits is lacking (Weiner and Singer, 1989; Bagley et al., 1991). Training in activities of daily living with the help of grab bars and handles, eating aids, and dressing aids promotes independence. The environment can be modified for safety and convenience; for example, chairs and beds should be firm and of sufficient height to

TABLE 9–15
Drugs Used to Treat Parkinson's Disease

DRUG (BRAND NAME)	USUAL DOSAGES	MECHANISM OF ACTION	POTENTIAL SIDE EFFECTS
levodopa (Dopar, Larodopa)	2000–5000 mg/day in divided doses	Increases availability of dopamine by providing metabolic precursor	Nausea, vomiting, anorexia Dyskinesias Orthostatic hypotension Behavioral disturbances Vivid dreams and hallucinations
carbidopa; levodopa (Sinemet)	40/400 to 200/2000* mg/day in divided doses	Increases dopamine availability by providing metabolic precursor and decreasing peripheral dopamine metabolism	As above
amantadine (Symmetrel)	100–300 mg/day†	Increases dopamine release	Delirium and hallucinations
bromocriptine (Parlodel)	1–1.5 mg tid or qid (initial); gradually increase to maximum of 100–200 mg in divided doses	Directly activates dopaminergic receptors	Behavioral changes Hypotension Nausea
anticholinergic agents‡ trihexyphenidyl (Artane, Apo-Trihex)	2–20 mg/day in divided doses	Decreases effects of acetylcholine and helps restore balance between cholinergic and dopaminergic systems	Dry mouth Constipation Urinary retention Blurred vision Exacerbation of glaucoma Tachycardia Confusion Behavioral changes
benztropine mesylate (Cogentin)	0.5–8 mg/day in divided doses	Inhibits type B monoamine oxidase	As above Nausea
seligiline (Eldepryl)	10 mg/day in one dose	Delays onset of disability, especially during first 12 months	Confusion Agitation Insomnia Involuntary movements

* Left number represents carbidopa; right number, levodopa.
† Eliminated by kidney; dosages should be adjusted when renal function is diminished.
‡ Several other anticholinergic agents are available.
From Kane, R.L., Ouslander, J.G. and Abrass, I.B. *Essentials of Clinical Geriatrics*. 3rd ed. New York: McGraw-Hill, 1994. Copyright, 1994. Reproduced with permission of McGraw-Hill, Inc.

enable the person to rise to a standing position. Social workers can help obtain services for older persons with Parkinson's disease, such as home help, and Meals-on-Wheels to promote independence as well (Weiner and Singer, 1989; Marr, 1991; McDowell, 1992; McPherson, 1992; Taira, 1992; McDowell, 1994).

Substance-Induced Persisting Dementia

Dementia associated with the persisting effects of drug use can be related to substance intoxication or substance withdrawal (see Table 9–2). It occurs in people who have had substance dependence or exposure involving alcohol, inhalants, sedatives, hypnotics, anxiolytics, anticonvulsants, intrathecal methotrexate, lead, mercury, carbon monoxide, organophosphate insecticides, industrial solvents, or other unknown substances. The onset of symptoms is usually insidious and slowly progressive. Even if substance abuse stops, the dementia is usu-

ally permanent and may continue to worsen (American Psychiatric Association, 1994).

Dementia Due to HIV Disease

The neuropathological change associated with human immunodeficiency virus (HIV) disease is diffuse, multifocal destruction of white matter and subcortical structures that results in dementia. Typical manifestations are forgetfulness, slowness, poor concentration, and difficulties with problem solving. The patient may become apathetic and withdrawn and may have delusions and hallucinations. Motor effects include tremor, impaired rapid repetitive movements, ataxia, hypertonia, and impaired pursuit and saccadic eye movements (American Psychiatric Association, 1994).

Dementia Due to Head Trauma

When dementia follows head trauma, it is usually nonprogressive and may be marked by various cognitive impairments, behavioral disturbances, and motor or sensory deficits, depending on the area of the brain injured (American Psychiatric Association, 1994).

Dementia Due to Other General Medical Conditions

A number of specific conditions discussed earlier are known to cause dementia. Other conditions that may cause dementia include structural brain lesions, endocrine conditions, nutritional deficiencies, infectious conditions, renal and hepatic dysfunction, other neurologic disorders, and less common central nervous system injuries such as electrical shock and intracranial radiation (American Psychiatric Association, 1994).

Dementia Due to Multiple Etiologies

It is not uncommon for dementia to have more than one etiology.

Dementia Not Otherwise Specified

A dementia that does not meet the criteria for any of the specific types is classified as dementia not otherwise specified. This diagnosis may be used when a specific etiology cannot be established because of inadequate evidence.

Structural Abnormalities

Normal Pressure Hydrocephalus

Persons in their late fifties occasionally are diagnosed as having normal pressure hydrocephalus (NPH), communicating hydrocephalus, or idiopathic hydrocephalus. Five to six per cent of all persons with dementia are thought to have normal pressure hydrocephalus. The disorder may occur as a result of previous head trauma, subarachnoid hemorrhage, meningitis, or changes in the skull related to Paget's disease. The flow of cerebrospinal fluid (CSF) is obstructed at the level of the arachnoid granulations that normally absorb the fluid. The ventricles enlarge, compressing cerebral tissue, but the cerebrospinal fluid pressure is normal. The disorder may also be manifested by an insidious onset and progressive course with no apparent cause (Reichman and Cummings, 1992; Wallach, 1992).

Major symptoms appear in a distinctive triad, which is diagnostic of the disorder. First, gait disturbances occur in many forms. Spastic ataxia is characterized by an increase in deep tendon reflexes of the lower extremities and unsteadiness in walking; apraxia is characterized by difficulty in walking in which the feet appear glued to the floor.

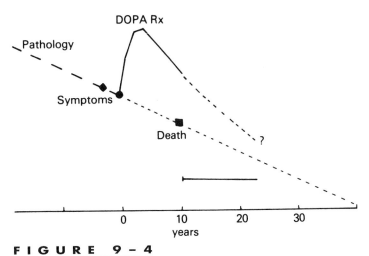

FIGURE 9–4

The impact of levodopa therapy on Parkinson's disease: a hypothetical concept of the effects of chronic levodopa treatment. The underlying pathology (of unknown cause) is believed to progress over many years irrespective of therapy. After an initial period, it becomes severe enough to cause symptoms. Before levodopa, pathological changes and disability progressed to cause death on average 10 years after onset. Levodopa therapy results in considerable initial symptomatic improvement but no change in pathology. Despite some loss of benefit after a few years of treatment, life expectancy is prolonged, but this means that new aspects and consequences of the progression of the disease are likely to emerge. (From Denham, M.J. Management of Parkinson's disease in the elderly. In The Treatment of Medical Problems in the Elderly. Baltimore: University Park Press, 1980.)

Second, the patient demonstrates relatively rapidly progressing dementia, in which there is impaired memory, apathy, inattention, and decreased spontaneity. Third, urinary incontinence appears late in the disorder, and patients are generally unaware of their incontinence.

Diagnosis is made through a careful, accurate history and radiography. CT and MRI scans typically reveal enlargement of the ventricle that is out of proportion to the degree of atrophy. Radionuclide cisternography and CSF pressure monitoring may be used to study the pattern of CSF flow (Kane et al., 1994).

Treatment is provided through a surgical shunt, which produces a dramatic alleviation of symptoms in about 50 per cent of patients. The best surgical candidates are those with typical gait disturbances, dementia, and urinary incontinence (Jarvik et al., 1992).

Subdural Hematoma

Older persons who present with symptoms similar to those of Alzheimer's disease may in some cases be misdiagnosed because a fall or injury resulting in a subdural hematoma has been overlooked. Decreased responsiveness and dullness with increased drowsiness are major symptoms; confusion and cognitive impairment may also be present. A subdural hematoma may also cause a worsening mental status in older people with Alzheimer's disease or other dementias. Neurological signs of increased intracranial pressure may not be evident because of a widening of the subarachnoid space.

A history of a recent fall may alert the nurse to a possible head injury and hematoma. Diagnosis is made through a CT scan. Surgery may be attempted in an effort to remove the hematoma; however, the mortality rate is around 70 per cent.

Slowly progressing symptoms 3 or more weeks after a head injury are typical of chronic subdural hematoma. Like acute subdural hematoma, the symptoms are insidious. Chronic hematoma, which often can be evacuated with craniostomy drainage, carries a much better prognosis, with a mortality rate of only 15 per cent (Vollmer and Eichler, 1994).

Brain Tumors

The incidence of both primary and metastatic brain tumors decreases with older age, although tumors are more likely to be malignant than benign. It is thought that the decreased incidence is due to less precise neurological diagnoses in elderly people, the tendency to attribute the signs and symptoms to cerebrovascular disease, and the reluctance to investigate suspected brain tumors in the elderly on the assumption that surgical intervention is either not indicated or too dangerous. Primary brain tumors are usually hemispheric and aggressive in the aged, and signs and symptoms depend on the location and growth of the lesion. Various symptoms include sudden motor paralysis, adult-onset seizures, disturbance of mood and memory, weakness, and sensory disturbances. Motor weakness, mental changes, memory disturbances, and personality changes are primary symptoms in older persons. Headache and papilledema are less common in older people than in younger people. Diagnosis is made through CT, MRI, or magnetic resonance spectroscopy (MRS) scans. Treatment consists of surgical removal of benign and malignant tumors; in addition, corticosteroids, chemotherapy, and radiation may be used for malignant tumors.

Prognosis for surgical removal is good for benign tumors diagnosed early, but it is poorer for older persons with malignant tumors. Surgical outcomes depend more on tumor type and the person's overall health than on age (Litchman and Posner, 1994; Roberts, 1992).

Metastatic brain tumors arise predominantly from the primary sites of the lung, breast, skin, colon, and kidney. Diagnosis is done through CT scan, and treatment is surgical for persons with solitary metastatic tumors if the general condition and location of the lesion are appropriate. Prognosis depends on the type of primary carcinoma, the extent of the surgery, and the sex and age of the patient. Women have a better prognosis than men.

NURSING ASSESSMENT

Assessment of functions related to the nervous system may be time-consuming but is essential to providing appropriate nursing care for elderly people. At the conclusion of the baseline neurological assessment, the nurse should be able to:

- Describe changes in neural function in the client as the result of the aging process and chronic diseases and the patient's response to these changes.

- Formulate tentative nursing diagnostic statements in relation to the functional patterns of health perception–health maintenance, cognition and perception, and activity and rest.

- Refer the patient to other health professionals for further assessment of selected neurological problems, such as gait disturbance, tremor, or impaired mental status.

Assessment of neurological status is indicated in the following situations:

1. Admission to a long-term care facility
2. New patient encounter in an outpatient facility or wellness center
3. Geriatric consultation
4. Diagnosis of a neurological impairment
5. New onset of a "behavioral problem" or behavior change
6. Recent accident that may affect neurological function
7. New medical or health problem that may subsequently affect neurological function

Although it is important to gather baseline data to monitor the client's adaptation to illness and response to treatment, it may not be possible or desirable to complete the assessment during the first encounter. Older persons may become fatigued more easily or may need more time to build a trusting relationship than younger persons. Time constraints may limit data gathering due to slowed responses or limited time allowed during the first encounter. In some cases it is desirable to assess over a period of time and in various locations to validate assessment results or to note the effect of the environment on the assessment situation. Priorities frequently must be set when carrying out a neurological assessment. Factors influencing the setting of priorities are the prevalence of the problem, the effect of the problem on functional ability, the effect of the problem on client goals, the ease with which data can be gathered, and the potential for solving the problem.

The nervous system has unique characteristics that influence assessment. First, since it is not possible to observe directly neuronal structure or activity, indirect measures of neurological function must be used. Because neurological functions interrelate with other body system functions, the integrity of the other systems must be considered. Thus, one test that might indicate a cognitive impairment, for example, should be validated with another.

Second, all neuronal functions are associated with a refractory period, so fatigue must be considered in the assessment. For example, repetitive testing of a simple reflex over a short period of time, such as pupillary response or deep tendon reflex, may result in an inaccurate conclusion that the reflex is sluggish when in reality an inadequate refractory period has elapsed.

Third, the nervous system is characterized by considerable redundancy. Because of this phenomenon, the body often is able to compensate for neuronal loss. Thus, a loss of structural integrity does not necessarily lead to a concomitant loss of function. In addition, many different methods may be used to assess a particular domain of function. For example, the simple act of undressing can reveal loss of fine motor function, confusion, visual defects, loss of balance and equilibrium, and stiffness and rigidity.

Finally, data gathered must be compared with age-adjusted standards to account for the changes of normal aging.

History

In the history, data should be gathered in the areas of speech and communication, movement, cognition, personality and emotional state, and functional status. The past medical history documents disorders, illnesses, or injuries, as well as medications that may be related to neurological symptoms. A family history of particular diseases is important for the neurological history because they are frequently genetically determined. Families can provide data about the onset, duration, and type of symptoms, especially in the dementing disorders. The functional assessment explores the effects of the patient's condition on everyday life and the extent of impairment imposed.

Physical Assessment

A thorough physical assessment of the neurological system includes examination of level of consciousness, mental status, cranial nerves, ability to communicate, movement and coordination, reflexes, the peripheral nervous system, functional status, and potential for rehabilitation. Tables 9–16 and 9–17 illustrate the components of the history and physical assessment in the neurological examination. Assessment of the level of consciousness is discussed in more detail in

TABLE 9 – 16
Nursing Assessment of Neurological Changes and Disorders

HISTORY
Family history of neurological diseases (Alzheimer's disease, vascular dementia, Huntington's disease, Parkinson's disease)
Symptoms:
  Changes in speech and communication
  Changes in sleep patterns
  Alterations in mental status (orientation, reasoning, judgment, cognition, hallucinations)
  Alterations in emotional status (depression, anxiety, hostility)
  Personality changes
  Loss of balance, dizziness, falls
PHYSICAL ASSESSMENT
Level of consciousness
Mental status
Speech and language (dysarthria, dysphagia)
Cranial nerves (see Table 9–17)
Gait, balance, coordination, tremor
Reflexes:
  Corneal reflex, Babinski reflex
  Grades of reflexes
    0 absent
    1 decreased
    2 normal
    3 increased
    4 spasticity
Sensory system
Functional assessment

TABLE 9-17
Cranial Nerves

NUMBER	NERVE	FUNCTION	TESTING
I	Olfactory	Sense of smell	Smell tobacco, coffee (don't use pungent substance)
II	Optic	Vision	Visual acuity—Snellen's chart
			Visual fields—confrontation
			Funduscopic—ophthalmoscope
III	Oculomotor	Pupillary constriction	Pupil size, shape, reaction to light, and accommodation
		Elevation of upper lid	Relationship of lid to pupil
		Most of extraocular movements	Pursuit movements
IV	Trochlear	Downward, inward movement of eye	Pursuit
V	Trigeminal	Motor—temporal and masseter muscles (chewing)	Attempt to open closed jaw
		Lateral movement of jaw	
		Sensory-facial (includes corneal)	Light touch with pin
			Corneal reflex
VI	Abducens	Lateral movement of eye	Pursuit

III Inferior oblique   III Superior rectus

III Medial rectus   VI Lateral rectus

IV Superior oblique   III Inferior rectus

The numbers correspond to the cranial nerve number. The names are the muscles resulting in the shown deviation.

NUMBER	NERVE	FUNCTION	TESTING
VII	Facial	Motor—muscles of facial expression	Keep eyes closed
			Show teeth
VIII	Acoustic	Hearing (cochlear division)	Listen to watch tick, or finger rub.
		Balance (vestibular division)	Gait. Romberg. Heel-to-toe.
IX	Glossopharyngeal	Sensory—pharynx and posterior tongue	Gag reflex.
		Motor—pharynx	Bilateral palate rise with "ah."
			Swallowing
X	Vagus	Sensory—pharynx and larynx	Gag reflex.
		Motor—pharynx	Bilateral palate rise with "ah."
			Swallowing.
XI	Spinal accessory	Motor—sternocleidomastoid and upper portion of trapezius	Shoulder shrug
XII	Hypoglossal	Motor—tongue	Protrude tongue and move it side to side

From Meyd, C.H. Assessment of the nervous system. *In* Eliopoulis, C. (ed.). *Health Assessment of the Older Adult*. Menlo Park, CA: Addison-Wesley, 1984, p. 155.

Chapter 14, and the mental status examination is described in Chapters 2 and 14.

NURSING DIAGNOSES

1. *Communication, Impaired Verbal:* related to aphasia and impaired ability to speak words

2. *Family Coping: Compromised, Ineffective:* related to caregiver burden of demented relatives

3. *Family Coping: Disabling, Ineffective*

4. *Health Maintenance, Altered:* related to functional dependency, confusion, and immobility

5. *Home Maintenance Management, Impaired:* related to chronic debilitating disease, impaired mental status, unavailable support system, sensory deficits, and immobility

6. *Physical Mobility, Impaired:* related to neuromuscular impairment, musculoskeletal impairment, decreased motor agility, and muscle weakness

7. *Nutrition, Altered: Less than Body Requirements:*
   related to chewing or swallowing difficulties, confusion

8. *Self-Care Deficit: Feeding, Bathing/Hygiene, Dressing/Grooming, Toileting:*
   related to mental or motor impairment

9. *Sensory-Perceptual Alterations: Kinesthetic, Perception:*
   related to neuropathies, immobility

10. *Sleep Pattern Disturbance:*
    related to medications (tranquilizers, sedatives, hypnotics) and confusion

11. *Thought Processes, Altered:*
    related to delirium or dementia

12. *Violence, Risk for Self Directed or Directed at Others:*
    related to inability to control behavior secondary to dementia

---

NURSING INTERVENTIONS AND EVALUATION

Nursing interventions for neurological disorders are aimed at maintaining functional independence in older clients for as long as possible, providing support for family members, and helping caregivers with the management of the symptoms of the dementing diseases. An ongoing evaluation of the mental and emotional status of the client helps determine whether the condition is acute or reversible and aids in measuring the losses in mental function in the chronic dementias. Caregivers can be referred to a number of national organizations such as the Alzheimer's Disease and Related Disorders Association or the Huntington's Disease Society of America for information on the disease, research findings, and specific strategies for care.

Evaluation is based on the success with which the older clients are able to maintain function and the attainment of social supports for both clients and families.

SUMMARY

Age-related changes in the nervous system are frequently attributed to disease states, and therefore many people believe that these changes are an inevitable consequence of older age. In fact, the normal changes that take place have little effect on thinking and cognition. Structural changes that occur with normal aging include loss of neurons and brain weight, accumulations of lipofuscin in the neuronal cytoplasm, slowed synaptic transmissions, and loss of peripheral nerve function. Functional changes include slowed reaction time, a decline in proprioceptive capacities, impaired thermoregulation, and changes in electroencephalographic and sleep patterns.

Disorders of the nervous system are mainly responsible for the conditions of delirium and dementia. These conditions cause impairments in cognition, reasoning, judgment, and orientation, which in turn cause declines in functional status. Because the burden of care often falls on families of impaired older persons, the nurse should provide support and encouragement to them.

REFERENCES

Abrass, I.B. Disorders of temperature regulation. *In* Hazzard, W.R., Bierman, E.L., Blass, J.P., et al. (eds.). *Principles of Geriatric Medicine and Gerontology.* 3rd ed. New York: McGraw-Hill, 1994, pp. 1191–1196.

Albert, M.S. Cognition and aging. *In* Hazzard, W.R., Bierman, E.L., Blass, J.P., et al. *Principles of Geriatric Medicine and Gerontology.* 3rd ed. New York: McGraw-Hill, 1994, pp. 1013–1020.

American Psychiatric Association. *Diagnostic and Statistical Manual of Mental Disorders.* 4th ed. Washington, D.C., 1994.

Ancoli-Israel, S. and Kripke, D.F. Sleep and aging. *In* Calkins, E., Ford, A.B. and Katz, P.R. (eds.). *Practice of Geriatrics.* 2nd ed. Philadelphia: W.B. Saunders, 1992, pp. 331–338.

Bagley, S., Kelly, B., Tunnicliffe, N., et al. The effect of visual cues on the gait of independently mobile Parkinson's disease patients. *Physiotherapy* 77(6): 415–420, 1991.

Bannon, M.J., Poosch, M.S., Xia, J., et al. Dopamine transporter MRNA content in human substantia nigra decreases precipitously with age. *Proc Natl Acad Sci USA* 89(15): 7095–7099, 1992.

Barrett, D.S., Cobb, A.G. and Bentley, G. Joint proprioception in normal, osteoarthritic and replaced knees. *J Bone Joint Surg Br* 73(1): 53–56, 1991.

Blennow, K., Wallin, A. and Gottfries, C. Clinical subgroups of Alzheimer disease. *In* Emery, V.O.B. and Oxman, T.E. (eds.). *Dementia Presentations, Differential Diagnosis, and Nosology.* Baltimore: The Johns Hopkins University Press, 1994, pp. 95–107.

Boss, B.J. Normal aging in the nervous system: Implications for SCI nurses. *Sci Nurs* 8(2): 42–47, 1991.

Bressler, R. and Katz, M.D. *Geriatric Pharmacology.* New York: McGraw-Hill, 1993.

Buchner, D.M., Beresford, S.A., Larson, E.B., et al. Effects of physical activity on health status in older adults. *Annu Rev Public Health* 13:469–488, 1992.

Bunting, L.K. and Fitzsimmons, B. Depression in Parkinson's disease. *J Neurosci Nurs* 23(3): 158–164, 1991.

Burl, M.M., Williams, J.G. and Nayak, U.S. Effects of cervical collars on standing balance. *Arch Phys Med Rehabil* 73(12): 1181–1185, 1992.

Carr, D., Jackson, T.W., Madden, D.J. and Cohen, H.J. The effect of age on driving skills. *J Am Geriat Soc* 40(6): 567–573, 1992.

Cohen, D. and Eisdorfer, C. Depression. *In* Calkins, E., Ford, A.B. and Katz, P.R. (eds.). *Practice of Geriatrics.* 2nd ed. Philadelphia: W.B. Saunders, 1992, pp. 285–294.

Dawson, P., Wells, D.L. and Kline, K. *Enhancing the Abilities of Persons with Alzheimer's and Related Dementias.* New York: Springer Publishing Company, 1993.

Dexter, W.W. Hypothermia. Safe and efficient methods of rewarming the patient. *Postgrad Med* 88(8):55–58, 61–64, 1990.

Erkinjuntti, T., Hachinski, V.C. and Sulkava, R. Alzheimer disease and vascular dementia: Differential diagnosis. *In* Emery, V.O.B. and Oxman, T.E. (eds.). *Dementia Presentations, Differential Diagnosis, and Nosology.* Baltimore: The Johns Hopkins University Press, 1994, pp. 208–231.

Ferrell, W.R., Crighton, A. and Sturrock, R.D. Age-dependent changes in position sense in human proximal interphalangeal joints. *Neuroreport* 3(3): 259–261, 1992.

Foley, J.M. Delirium. *In* Calkins, E., Ford, A.B. and Katz, P.R. (eds.). *Practice of Geriatrics.* 2nd ed. Philadelphia: W.B. Saunders, 1992, pp. 305–308.

Folstein, M.F. and Folstein, S.E. Neuropsychiatric assessment of syndromes of altered mental state. *In* Hazzard, W.R., Bierman, E.L., Blass, J.P., et al. *Principles of Geriatric Medicine and Gerontology.* 3rd ed. New York: McGraw-Hill, 1994, pp. 221–228.

Fozzard, J.L., Mulin, P.A., Giambra, L.M., et al. Normal and pathological age differences in memory. *In* Brocklehurst J.C., Tallis, R.C. and Fillit, H.M. (eds.). *Textbook of Geriatric Medicine and Gerontology.* 4th ed. Edinburgh: Churchill-Livingstone, 1992, pp. 94–109.

Frankhauser, M.P. Anxiolytic drugs and sedative-hypnotic agents. *In* Bressler, R. and Katz, M.D. (eds.) *Geriatric Pharmacology.* New York: McGraw-Hill, 1993, pp. 165–206.

Gandy, S.E. Other degenerative disorders of the nervous system. *In* Hazzard, W.R., Bierman, E.L., Blass, J.P., et al. (eds.). *Principles of Geriatric Medicine and Gerontology.* 3rd ed. New York: McGraw-Hill, 1994, pp. 1063–1069.

Geary, D.C. and Wiley, J.G. Cognitive addition: Strategy choice and speed of processing differences in young and elderly adults. *Psychol Aging* 6(3): 474–483, 1991.

Guyton, A.C. *Textbook of Medical Physiology.* 8th ed. Philadelphia: W.B. Saunders, 1991.

Haberman-Little, B. An analysis of the prevalence and etiology of depression in Parkinson's disease. *J Neurosci Nurs* 23(3): 165–169, 1991.

Haponik, E.F. Sleep problems. *In* Hazzard, W.R., Bierman, E.L., Blass, J.P., et al. (eds.). *Principles of Geriatric Medicine and Gerontology.* 3rd ed. New York: McGraw-Hill, 1994, pp. 1213–1228.

Hirsch, C.H. Hypo- and hyperthermia. *In* Calkins, E., Ford, A.B. and Katz, P.R. (eds.). *Practice of Geriatrics.* 2nd ed. Philadelphia: W.B. Saunders, 1992, pp. 266–275.

Hodgson, B.B., Kizior, R.J. and Kingdon, R.T. *Nurse's Drug Handbook.* Philadelphia: W.B. Saunders, 1993.

Hu, M. and Woollacott, M.H. Multisensory training of standing balance in older adults: Kinematic and electromyographic postural responses. *J Gerontol* 49(2): M62–M71, 1994.

Hyams, D.E. Cerebral blood flow and autoregulation in the elderly. *In* Brocklehurst, J.C., Tallis, R.C. and Fillit, H.M. (eds.). *Textbook of Geriatric Medicine and Gerontology.* 4th ed. Edinburgh: Churchill-Livingstone, 1992, pp. 280–289.

Jacob, S.W. and Francone, C.A. *Elements of Anatomy and Physiology.* 2nd ed. Philadelphia: W.B. Saunders, 1989.

Jarvik, L.F., Lavertsky, E.P. and Neshkes, R.E. Dementia and delirium in old age. *In* Brocklehurst, J.C., Tallis, R.C. and Fillit, H.M. (eds.). *Textbook of Geriatric Medicine and Gerontology.* 4th ed. Edinburgh: Churchill-Livingstone, 1992, pp. 326–348.

Jonsson, P.V. and Lipsitz, L.A. Dizziness and syncope. *In* Hazzard, W.R., Bierman, E.L., Blass, J.P., et al. (eds.). *Principles of Geriatric Medicine and Gerontology.* 3rd ed. New York: McGraw-Hill, 1994, pp. 1165–1182.

Kane, R.L., Ouslander, J.G. and Abrass, I.B. *Essentials of Clinical Geriatrics.* 3rd ed. New York: McGraw-Hill, 1994.

Kertesz, A. Language deterioration in dementia. *In* Emery, V.O.B. and Oxman, T.E. (eds.). *Dementia Presentations, Differential Diagnosis, and Nosology.* Baltimore: The Johns Hopkins University Press, 1994, pp. 123–138.

Kirshner, H.S. Progressive aphasia and other focal presentations of Alzheimer disease, Pick disease, and other degenerative diseases. *In* Emery, V.O.B. and Oxman, T.E. (eds.). *Dementia Presentations, Differential Diagnosis, and Nosology.* Baltimore: The Johns Hopkins University Press, 1994, pp. 108–122.

Kobayashi, S. The relation of hypertension to vascular dementia. *In* Emery, V.O.B. and Oxman, T.E. (eds.). *Dementia Presentations, Differential Diagnosis, and Nosology.* Baltimore: The Johns Hopkins University Press, 1994, pp. 195–207.

Kramer, M.R., Vandijk, J. and Rosin, A.J. Mortality in elderly patients with thermoregulatory failure. *Arch Intern Med* 149(7): 1521–1523, 1989.

Lewis, P.D. The neuropathology of old age. *In* Brocklehurst, J.C., Tallis, R.C. and Fillit, H.M. (eds.). *Textbook of Geriatric Medicine and Gerontology.* 4th ed. Edinburgh: Churchill-Livingstone, 1992, pp. 258–279.

Lipowski, Z.J. Delirium (acute confusional states). *In* Hazzard, W.R., Bierman, E.L., Blass, J.P. et al. (eds.). *Principles of Geriatric Medicine and Gerontology.* 3rd ed. New York: McGraw-Hill, 1994, pp. 1021–1026.

Litchman, C.D. and Posner, J.B. Brain tumors in the elderly. *In* Hazzard, W.R., Bierman, E.L., Blass, J.P., et al. (eds.). *Principles of Geriatric Medicine and Gerontology.* 3rd ed. New York: McGraw-Hill, 1994, pp. 1095–1102.

Madden, D.J. Four to ten milliseconds per year: Age-related slowing of visual word identification. *J Gerontol* 47(2): P59–P68, 1992.

Maki, B.E., Holliday, P.J. and Topper, A.K. Deterioration in postural balance may lead to falls: A prospective study of postural balance and risk of falling in an ambulatory and independent elderly population. *J Gerontol* 49(2): M72–M84, 1994.

Manchester, D., Woollacott, M., Zederbauer-Hylton, N. and Marin, O. Visual, vestibular and somatosensory contributions to balance control in the older adult. *J Gerontol* 44(4): M118–M127, 1989.

Marr, J. The experience of living with Parkinson's disease. *J Neurosci Nurs* 23(5):325–329, 1991.

Martin, G.M. and Turker, M.S. Genetics of human disease, longevity, and aging. *In* Hazzard, W.R., Bierman, E.L., Blass, J.P., et al. (eds.). *Principles of Geriatric Medicine and Gerontology.* 3rd ed. New York: McGraw-Hill, 1994, pp. 19–36.

Matteson, M.A., Linton, A.D., Cleary, B.L., et al. Management of problem behaviors associated with dementia. *The Gerontologist.* Submitted for publication.

Mayeux, R. and Schofield, P.W. Alzheimer's disease. *In* Hazzard, W.R., Bierman, E.L., Blass, J.P., et al. (eds.). *Principles of Geriatric Medicine and Gerontology.* 3rd ed. New York: McGraw-Hill, 1994, pp. 1035–1050.

McAllister, T.W. and Powers, R. Approaches to the treatment of dementing illness. *In* Emery, V.O.B. and Oxman, T.E. (eds.). *Dementia Presentations, Differential Diagnosis, and Nosology.* Baltimore: The Johns Hopkins University Press, 1994, pp. 355–383.

McDowell, F.H. Neurologic diseases: Part II—Parkinson's disease and other disorders. *In* Calkins, E., Ford, A.B. and Katz, P.R. (eds.). *Practice of Geriatrics.* 2nd ed. Philadelphia: W.B. Saunders, 1992, pp. 319–330.

McDowell, F.H. Parkinson's disease and related disorders. *In* Hazzard, W.R., Bierman, E.L., Blass, J.P., et al.

(eds.). *Principles of Geriatric Medicine and Gerontology.* 3rd ed. New York: McGraw-Hill, 1994, pp. 1051–1062.

McPherson, M.L. Management of Parkinson's disease. *J Home Health Care Prac* 4(4): 31–35, 1992.

Montgomery, E.B. and Lipsy, R.J. Treatment of Parkinson's disease. *In* Bressler, R.B. and Katz, M.D. (eds.). *Geriatric Pharmacology.* New York: McGraw-Hill, 1993, pp. 309–328.

Morgan, K. Sleep in normal and pathological aging. *In* Brocklehurst, J.C., Tallis, R.C. and Fillit, H.M. (eds.). *Textbook of Geriatric Medicine and Gerontology.* 4th ed. Edinburgh: Churchill-Livingstone, 1992, pp. 122–129.

Mucignat, C. Effect of age on the orientation of attention: Effect of changing the interval between signal and stimulus. *Bull Soc Ital Biol Sper* 67(5): 521–527, 1991.

Mucignat, C., Castiello, U., Umilta, C. and Tradardi, V. Effect of age on the orientation of attention: Effect of changing the interval between signal and stimulus (abstract). *Boll Soc Itali Biol Sper* 67(5): 521–527, 1991.

Mutch, W.J. Parkinsonism and other movement disorders. *In* Brocklehurst, J.C., Tallis, R.C. and Fillit, H.M. (eds.). *Textbook of Geriatric Medicine and Gerontology.* 4th ed. Edinburgh: Churchill-Livingstone, 1992, pp. 411–429.

National Institutes on Aging. *Special Report on Alzheimer's Disease.* Washington, D.C.: NIA, 1991.

Oxman, T.E. and Baynes, K. Boundaries between normal aging and dementia. *In* Emery, V.O.B. and Oxman, T.E. (eds.). *Dementia Presentations, Differential Diagnosis, and Nosology.* Baltimore: The Johns Hopkins University Press, 1994, pp. 3–18.

Pathy, M.S.J. Neurological signs in old age. *In* Brocklehurst, J.C., Tallis, R.C. and Fillit, H.M. (eds.). *Textbook of Geriatric Medicine and Gerontology.* 4th ed. Edinburgh: Churchill-Livingstone, 1992, pp. 302–306.

Patla, A.E., Frank, J.S. and Winter, D.A. Balance control in the elderly: Implications for clinical assessment and rehabilitation. *Can J Public Health* July–Aug, Suppl 2, S29–S33, 1992.

Poirier, J. and Finch, C.E. Neurochemistry of the aging human brain. *In* Hazzard, W.R., Bierman, E.L., Blass, J.P., et al. (eds.). *Principles of Geriatric Medicine and Gerontology.* 3rd ed. New York: McGraw-Hill, 1994, pp. 1005–1012.

Pyykko, I., Jantti, P. and Aalto, H. Postural control in elderly subjects. *Age Ageing* 19(3):215–221, 1990.

Reichel, W. and Rabins, B. Evaluation and management of the confused, disoriented, or demented elderly patient. *In* Reichel W. (ed.). *Clinical Aspects of Aging,* 3rd ed. Baltimore: Williams & Wilkins, 1989, pp. 137–150.

Reichman, W.E. and Cummings, J.L. Dementia. *In* Calkins, E., Ford, A.B. and Katz, P.R. (eds.). *Practice of Geriatrics.* 2nd ed. Philadelphia: W.B. Saunders, 1992, pp. 295–304.

Reisberg, B. Functional assessment staging (FAST). *Psychopharmacology Bulletin* 24(4): 653–659, 1988.

Reisberg, B. Functional assessment staging in Alzheimer's disease: Reliability, validity, and ordinality. *In International Psychogeriatrics,* Vol. 4, Supp. 1. Springer, 1992, pp. 55–69.

Reuben, D. The physician and the aging driver. *In* Calkins, E., Ford, A.B. and Katz, P.R. (eds.). *Practice of Geriatrics.* 2nd ed. Philadelphia: W.B. Saunders, 1992, pp. 197–203.

Ring, C., Nayak, U.S. and Isaacs, B. The effect of visual deprivation and proprioceptive change on postural sway in healthy adults. *J Am Geriat Soc* 37(8): 745–749, 1989.

Robbins, A.S. Hypothermia and heat stroke: Protecting the elderly patient. *Geriatrics* 44(1): 73–77, 1989.

Roberts, M.A. Intracranial tumours. *In* Brocklehurst, J.C., Tallis, R.C. and Fillit, H.M. (eds.). *Textbook of Geriatric Medicine and Gerontology.* 4th ed. Edinburgh: Churchill-Livingstone, 1992, pp. 450–454.

Ross, G.W. and Cummings, J.L. Cortical and subcortical dementias. *In* Emery, V.O.B. and Oxman, T.E. (eds.). *Dementia Presentations, Differential Diagnosis, and Nosology.* Baltimore: The Johns Hopkins University Press, 1994, pp. 141–161.

Rossor, M.N. Neurochemistry of the aging brain and dementia. *In* Brocklehurst, J.C., Tallis, R.C. and Fillit, H.M. (eds.). *Textbook of Geriatric Medicine and Gerontology.* 4th ed. Edinburgh: Churchill-Livingstone, 1992, pp. 290–301.

Sagawa, S., Shiraki, K., Yousef, M.K. and Miki, K. Sweating and cardiovascular responses of aged men to heat exposure. *J Gerontol* 43(1): M1–M8, 1988.

Shaw, N.A. Age-dependent changes in central somatosensory conduction time. *Clin Electroencephalogr* 23(2): 105–110, 1992.

Shlafer, M. *The Nurse Pharmacology and Drug Therapy.* Redwood City, CA: Addison-Wesley, 1993.

Stelmach, G.E., Phillips, J., DiFabio, R.P. and Teasdale, N. Age, functional postural reflexes, and voluntary sway. *J Gerontol* 44(4):B100–B106, 1989a.

Stelmach, G.E., Teasdale, N., DiFabio, R.P. and Phillips, J. Age-related decline in postural control mechanisms. *Int J Aging Hum Dev* 29(3):205–223, 1989b.

Stelmach, G.E., Zelaznik, H.N. and Lowe, D. The influence of aging and attentional demands on recovery from postural instability. *Aging* 2(2): 155–161, 1990.

Sweeney, P.J. Understanding tremors. *Emerg Med* 25(1): 88–89, 1993.

Taira, F. Facilitating self-care in clients with Parkinson's disease. *Home Health Care Nurse* 10(4):23–27, 1992.

Tankersley, C.G., Smolander, J., Kenney, W.L. and Fortney, S.M. Sweating and skin blood flow during exercise: Effects of age and maximal oxygen uptake. *J Appl Psychol* 71(1):236–242, 1991.

Teasdale, N., Stelmach, G.E. and Breunig, A. Postural sway characteristics of the elderly under normal and altered visual and support surface conditions. *J Gerontol* 46(6): B238–B244, 1991.

Thomas, D.R. Accidental hypothermia in the Sunbelt. *J Gen Intern Med* 3(6): 552–554, 1988.

Tinetti, M.E. Instability and falling in elderly patients. *Semin Neurol* 9(1): 39–45, 1989.

Toledo, L.W. The postanesthesia patient with Parkinson's disease. *J Post Anesth Nurs* 7(1): 32–37, 1992.

Vollmer, D.G. and Eichler, M.E. Head injury. *In* Hazzard, W.R., Bierman, E.L., Blass, J.P., et al. (eds.). *Principles of Geriatric Medicine and Gerontology.* 3rd ed. New York: McGraw-Hill, 1994, pp. 1079–1088.

Wallach, S. Paget's disease of the bone. *In* Calkins, E., Ford, A.B. and Katz, P.R. (eds.). *Practice of Geriatrics.* 2nd ed. Philadelphia: W.B. Saunders, 1992, pp. 403–410.

Weiner, W.J. and Singer C. Parkinson's disease and nonpharmacologic treatment programs. *J Am Geriatr Soc* 37(4): 359–363, 1989.

Welford, A.T. Sensory, perceptual, and motor processes in older adults. *In* Birren, J.E. and Sloane, R.B. (eds.). *Handbook of Mental Health and Aging.* Englewood Cliffs, N.J.: Prentice-Hall, 1980.

Williams, K. and Bird, M. The aging mover: A preliminary report on constraints to action. *Int J Aging Hum Dev* 34(3):241–255, 1992.

Wisniewski, H.M., Wegiel, J., Morys, J. and Bobinski, M. Alzheimer dementia neuropathology. *In* Emery, V.O.B. and Oxman, T.E. (eds.). *Dementia Presentations, Differential Diagnosis, and Nosology.* Baltimore: The Johns Hopkins University Press, 1994, pp. 79–94.

Woodhouse, P., Keatings, W.R. and Coleshaw, S.R. Factors associated with hypothermia in patients admitted to a group of inner city hospitals. *Lancet* 2: 1201–1205, 1989.

Yen, P.K. Does a low protein diet help with Parkinson's? *Geriatr Nurs* 11(1): 48, 1990.

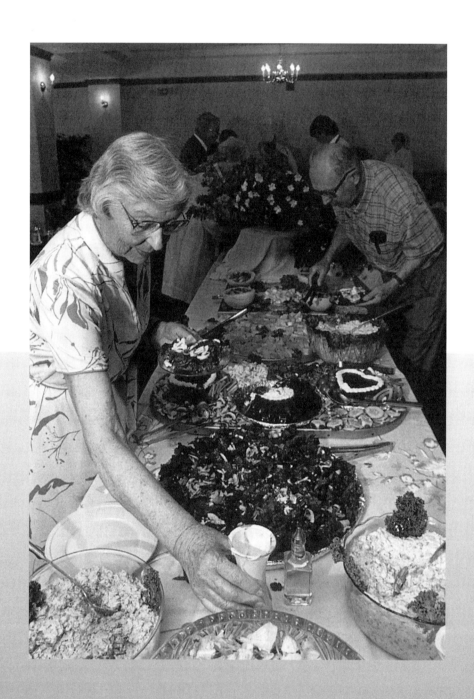

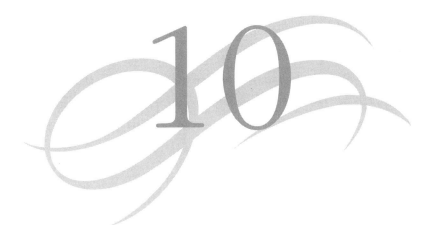

Age-Related Changes in the Gastrointestinal System

ADRIANNE DILL LINTON

OBJECTIVES

Identify normal changes in structure and function of the gastrointestinal system.

❖

Describe common disorders of the gastrointestinal system and discuss their causes and treatment.

❖

Demonstrate nursing assessment of the structure and function of the gastrointestinal tract.

❖

Formulate nursing diagnoses related to nursing assessment of the gastrointestinal tract.

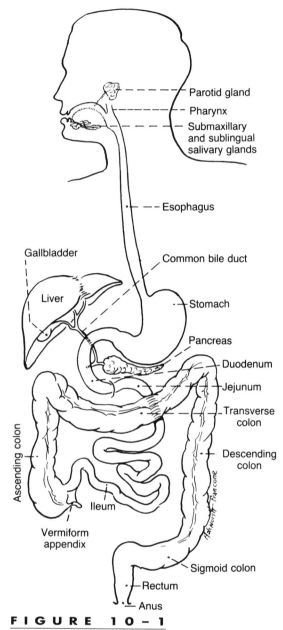

FIGURE 10 – 1

Organs of the gastrointestinal system. (From Jacob, S.W. and Francone, C.A. *Elements of Anatomy and Physiology.* 2nd ed. Philadelphia, W.B. Saunders, 1989.)

Older people are notorious for having complaints related to the functioning of their digestive systems. Television, magazine, and newspaper advertisements are filled with remedies for anything from gastric upset to constipation, usually aimed toward elderly consumers. The major question is, do older people really have changes in the gastrointestinal system that cause major problems with digestion and elimination?

NORMAL STRUCTURE AND FUNCTION

The gastrointestinal or digestive system consists of a long, muscular tube that begins at the lips and ends at the anus and includes the mouth, pharynx, esophagus, stomach, and small and large intestines. Glands located outside the intestinal tract, which empty their secretions into the tube, are the salivary glands, liver, gallbladder, and pancreas (Fig. 10–1). The major functions of the digestive system are the digestion and absorption of ingested food and the elimination of solid wastes.

NORMAL CHANGES IN STRUCTURE AND FUNCTION

Oral Cavity

Stereotypes surrounding geriatric dentition have propagated the unattractive picture of the edentulous, drooling old person who is undernourished because of an inability to chew or taste nutritional foods. Fortunately, studies do not substantiate this myth and have shown that most problems associated with the oral cavity are due to pathological processes and not to normal aging. Older persons today retain more of their natural dentition. From 1957 to 1987, the percentage of Americans age 65 years and older who were edentulous declined from around 55 per cent to about 40 per cent. This decline is attributed to changing attitudes about loss of teeth with age, increased fluoridation, and increased availability and use of dental services by elderly people (Gordon, 1990; Nelson and Castell, 1990).

If normal aging changes do occur in the oral cavity, oral function is affected only minimally. There may be increased growth of dentine, fibrosis of the root pulp, increased thickness of cementum, gingival retraction, and loss of bone density in the alveolar ridge (Mjor, 1986; Walls, 1992; Carranza, 1990). Changes in the oral mucosa are chiefly due to a loss of mucosal elasticity, which is consistent with losses of elastic tissue throughout the body, and thinning of the mucosa. The enamel of the crowns of the teeth often shows attrition. Thinning and staining of the enamel cause the teeth to appear darker or yellow. The tongue may appear smooth and lobular, and varicosities may appear on the ventral surface (Tyron, 1986; Ferguson and Devlin, 1992).

In spite of the minimal changes that occur on the tongue, data regarding decrements in gustation are equivocal. Recent studies have shown that the sensation of taste does not noticeably decrease with age, and the changes that do occur are modest (Kalu and Masoro, 1986; Ferguson and Devlin, 1992; Reinus and Brandt, 1992). It is thought that there may be some increase in taste thresholds for individual amino acids, salt, and sugars, causing bitter tastes to predominate (Deems et al., 1991).

Xerostomia (dry mouth) has frequently been associated with normal aging, but research does not support the concept of age-related salivary gland dysfunction. The total salivary flow remains adequate in the healthy older person despite some decrease in saliva production by the submandibular salivary glands (Baum and Ship, 1990; Walls, 1992; Gordon, 1990; Ferguson and Devlin, 1992; Tenovuo, 1992). Decreased salivation may be found in some older persons, but this should not be considered an inevitable consequence of older age. It is more likely due to a disease process, abnormal physiological state, or drug therapy (Rogers and Duvall, 1989; Baum and Ship, 1990). Changes in swallowing are rare and are usually associated with a disease process (Baum and Bodner, 1983).

Esophagus

Esophageal function is essentially preserved with aging. Soergel and associates (1964) coined the term "presbyesophagus" to describe the presence of an abnormal frequency of nonperistaltic contractions and inadequate relaxation of the lower esophageal sphincter, resulting in decreased esophageal motility. This phenomenon was thought to be related to a decrease in esophageal muscle mass, similar to deterioration of the muscle mass in other body organs. However, it is now thought that abnormal esophageal motility is more likely to be due to the consequences of the high prevalence of neurological diseases in elderly people rather than to the process of normal aging (Gibbons and Levy, 1989). Ekberg and Feinberg (1991) found radiographic evidence of swallowing abnormalities in elderly subjects who had no dysphagia. Ren and colleagues (1993) studied coordination of the glottis and upper esophageal sphincter during swallowing in aged subjects and found these functions to be preserved in elderly people. This and other studies led Curless and James (1992) to conclude that there are not adequate data to show that swallowing is significantly impaired in normal older people.

Stomach

The major changes in the stomach with older age are related to the gastric mucosa and the secretion of hydrochloric acid. By age 70 years, atrophy of the gastric mucosa becomes increasingly common. This is thought to be related to a change in the ratio of the cells secreting gastrin to cells secreting somatostatin. (Gastrin is a hormone that stimulates the secretion of gastric juices, whereas somatostatin is a hormone that inhibits the secretion of gastrin.) The final result is a diminished capacity of the stomach to secrete hydrochloric acid, a condition known as hypochlorhydria. It is generally accepted that decreased acid secretion is an age-related change, but it is not found universally (Gibbons and Levy, 1989).

Small Intestine

The small intestine, with its enormous surface area, has as its major function the absorption of nutrients. Many gerontologists claim that there is a diminished rate of absorption with aging due to the decrease in height and increase in breadth of the intestinal villa, resulting in a significant decrease in mucosal surface area.

Although villous atrophy may have an impact on absorption, the functional consequences of age-related changes are debatable at this time. Absorption in the small intestine is affected by factors other than structure, including the material ingested, intestinal motility and blood flow, and gastric emptying. Absorption of vitamin A is actually improved in the elderly, whereas vitamin D and calcium absorption may be impaired. Older people do not usually demonstrate evidence of malabsorption (Nelson and Castell, 1990).

Large Intestine

Although studies are inadequate, some age-related changes have been noted in the large intestine. First, there is an increased tortuosity (twisting) of blood vessels that may compromise the blood flow to the colon. In addition, there may be diminished motility in the colon; however, bowel habits do not change predictably with age as has been generally thought.

The notion that constipation is more common in elderly than in young people is not supported by good data. When older people do have constipation, it may be caused by drug therapy, dehydration, inadequate dietary fiber, and a number of disorders (Singleton, 1990). Read (1992) suggests that fecal impaction in the older person may be due to inability to detect the fecal mass in the rectum until it is too large to expel. This would be consistent with Vierling's (1982) finding that a greater volume of rectal distention was needed to produce discomfort in the older person. On the other hand, Nelson and Castell (1990) found no differences in perceptions of rectal distention in healthy older subjects.

Pancreas

Several changes in the pancreas have been noted in older age, especially on autopsy. The weight of the pancreas decreases or remains unchanged, and acinar atrophy is noted (Nelson and Castell, 1990; Braganza, 1992). Fibrotic changes are observed in blood vessels. The incidence of dilation and distention of the pancreatic ducts increases 8 per cent per decade after 60 years of age. There is frequent prolapse of the entire gland and calcification of the pancreatic ves-

sels. Deposits of lactoferrin and lipofuscin have been found in the pancreas as in other organs of the body. Despite these changes, the production of bicarbonate, amylase, and trypsin remains adequate because the pancreas has a large reserve capacity. Some studies have found normal response to pancreatic stimulation (Gullo, 1992). Other studies revealed decreased volume of pancreatic secretions and decreased production of amylase, trypsin, bicarbonate, and/or phospholipase (Fikry, 1968; Bartos and Groh, 1969; Laugier and Sarles, 1985). (Older studies must always be examined to determine the characteristics of the sample studied. Many older studies collected data only from ill elderly people.) A decrease in the production of lipase may result in subclinical abnormalities of fat absorption. There is also a diminished output of exocrine secretions, which causes an impairment in the pancreatic reserve.

Liver and Biliary Tract

The liver begins to lose weight and mass after a person attains age 50 years. The shape of the liver changes gradually to conform to the shape of surrounding structures. There is some decline in blood flow, with estimates ranging from 0.3 to 1.5 per cent per year (Nelson and Castell, 1990; James, 1992). The decrease in size is due to a decrease in hepatic cells, which tend to change in size and character. The nuclear volume, as well as the size of individual hepatocytes, increases. In addition, there is an increase in fibrous tissue in the liver. Hepatic protein synthesis is compromised, and there are changes in the enzymes involved in a variety of metabolic pathways in the liver. For example, synthesis of cholesterol and total bile acid diminish with age. Standard liver function tests do not change significantly, but there is evidence of decreased storage capacity and slower clearance of numerous substances, including the benzodiazepines (Nelson and Castell, 1990). James (1992) reports that the metabolism of drugs probably declines as much as 30 per cent from adulthood to old age.

COMMON DISORDERS

Gerodontic Disorders

Major problems in the oral cavity that are more common in older age include xerostomia (dry mouth), burning and painful tongue, temporomandibular joint pains, periodontal diseases, and oral lesions. Root caries, found almost exclusively in older people, occurs where the tooth root is exposed by receding gingiva (Ferguson and Devlin, 1992). Disorders of the oral cavity are frequently due to systemic, local, and physiological changes, such as nutritional deficiencies, dehydration, atrophy, decreased elasticity and reparative capacity of tissue, hypertension, decreased circulation, shortness of breath, and decreased glandular secretions (Katz and Meskin, 1986). Tooth loss increases with age so that approximately 40 per cent of persons over age 65 years are edentulous; the percentage increases dramatically among people over age 75 years. Periodontal diseases are the primary cause of tooth loss.

Xerostomia

Xerostomia, or dry mouth due to decreased salivary secretions, occurs in approximately 20 per cent of the population over 65 years of age. Saliva is important for providing the primary protection for all oral tissues. It contains lubricatory factors to keep oral tissues hydrated, pliable, and insulated; buffering acids; and proteins that regulate oral bacterial colonization patterns, thereby modulating dental disease and preventing systemic infections originating from the mouth. It provides for mechanical cleansing of the mouth. Other salivary proteins keep the secretions supersaturated with calcium and phosphate, allowing for remineralization of caries (cavities). Saliva also provides a medium by which the sense of taste is stimulated.

Salivary flow of major salivary glands does not decrease as a normal consequence of aging (Ship and Baum, 1990; Ferguson and Devlin, 1992; Wu et al., 1993). Functions of minor salivary glands often decline, but it is unclear whether this would contribute to dry mouth symptoms. Major causes of dry mouth are obstructive nasal diseases that promote mouth breathing, drugs, vitamin B complex deficiency, diabetes, dehydration, radiotherapy, anxiety, and fear. Drugs that are often the culprits include anticholinergics, diuretics, some opiates, antidepressants, antipsychotics, tranquilizers, antihistamines, decongestants, antihypertensives, antineoplastics, and antispasmodics (Gordon, 1990; Ferguson and Devlin, 1992). The problem is extremely disturbing to those who experience it; it can result in altered taste sensation, increased vulnerability of the oral mucosa, oral pain, dysphagia, and impaired clearance of the bacteria prominent in causing caries. The oral mucosa appears dry, atrophic, inflamed or pale, and translucent. In addition, sore spots may develop under dentures due to lack of lubrication, interfering with denture retention. The incidence of dental plaque formation and dental caries can increase, especially if sucking on hard candies is used to relieve dry mouth (Elkowitz, 1981; Minaker and Rowe, 1982).

Treatment of xerostomia is minimally effective. It is helpful to stop drugs that may be causing dry mouth and substitute other drugs or treatments. Drinking more water or use of mouthwash may provide some relief. Saliva stimulants, such as citric fruit drops or lemon swabs, are rarely successful. Artificial saliva agents are most effective. These include 10 per cent glycerine in distilled water and artificial saliva or Xerolube— both over-the-counter products (Ferguson and Devlin, 1992; Holm-Pedersen and Lee, 1986).

Disorders of the Tongue

Disorders of the tongue may include structural changes, pain (glossodynia), and a burning sensation (glossopyrosis). The tongue is a good indicator of a variety of systemic problems. For example, a red, beefy tongue might indicate the presence of monilial infections or iron deficiency anemia; a flat tongue surface may point to pernicious anemia. Nutritional anemias related to deficiencies of folic acid, iron, and/or vitamin B_{12} account for many of the problems associated with a burning or painful tongue. Other conditions that may be associated with oral burning sensations are psychiatric illness, menopause, diabetes mellitus, and various oral and dental conditions (Mott et al., 1993). The term "burning mouth syndrome" is used to describe symptoms that cannot be explained. The sensation typically is present on waking and gradually increases during the day (Ferguson and Devlin, 1992; Walls, 1992). Symptoms include glossitis, fissures at the corners of the mouth, and atrophy of the tongue's papillae. In many cases, the tongue may become enlarged when there are absent or missing teeth. The increased masticatory function transferred from the teeth to the tongue causes hypertrophy as the tongue compensates for the decreased ability to chew (Elkowitz, 1981; Minaker and Rowe, 1983).

Burning tongue is treated according to the

cause of the problem. Therefore, if infections exist, they are treated appropriately; if malnourishment is the cause, vitamins and diet therapy are the treatment. If dry mouth is the cause, treatments include mouthwashes and changes in drug regimens, as noted earlier. The client is advised to avoid smoking and the use of alcohol. When there is no identifiable cause, burning mouth sensation sometimes improves with the use of low-dose tricyclic antidepressants. Some clients have spontaneous remissions (Mott et al., 1992). Sometimes the cause of the problem is elusive, making treatment difficult.

Temporomandibular Joint Syndrome

The temporomandibular joint (TMJ) provides the hinge on which the movement of the mandible is guided. Over a period of years the joint may sustain damage from continuous grinding of the teeth, malocclusion, chewing hard foods, sustaining local head and neck disorders, trauma, and wide yawning. Changes in the temporomandibular joint may also result from partial or complete tooth loss. Osteoarthritis and other degenerative joint diseases can affect the TMJ, usually unilaterally, resulting in ability to open the mouth excessively wide, jaw clicking, ear discomfort, muscle spasms, crepitation, and hearing difficulties. Some clients have vertigo or tinnitus (Yoder, 1989; Baum and Ship, 1990; Lund and Westesson, 1991).

When degenerative joint disease is the cause of TMJ problems, treatment usually consists of analgesic and anti-inflammatory agents. Drugs of choice are aspirin, ibuprofen, and naproxen. Other drugs, such as indomethacin and phenylbutazone, are effective but have uncomfortable side effects and should be used with caution. Physical therapy, including biofeedback, topical heat, dental splints, bite blocks, and range of motion exercises are sometimes helpful. A soft diet is recommended. Psychotherapy may be prescribed for some patients (Yoder, 1989). Surgery is generally not indicated for older adults (Kamen, 1983).

Oral Lesions

The incidence of malignant lesions of the oral cavity peaks in the seventh decade, and 90 per cent of the malignancies are squamous cell carcinoma. Malignant lesions are associated with use of tobacco and alcohol and with iron deficiency. The incidence of oral cancers has been reported to increase in people with syphilis, oral candidiasis, and the herpes simplex virus type II (Walls, 1989). They usually occur on the lower lip, the lateral and inferior surfaces of the tongue, the gingiva, and the floor of the mouth. The most important oral cancer detection procedure is careful inspection of the oral mucosa. Early malignant lesions may appear as leukoplakia, an exophytic growth, a red patch, or an ulcer. Painless lesions that persist for more than one month are suspicious for malignancy (Walls, 1989; Ferguson and Devlin, 1992).

The first sign of cancer may be a lump in the neck. Lesions found in the posterior tongue or pharyngeal region may produce an earache, followed by dysphagia, dysphasia, or difficulty in chewing. Treatment depends on the location, size, and type of lesion, and usually consists of either surgery or radiation or a combination of the two. Chemotherapy is less often used (Walls, 1989).

Periodontal Disease

Periodontal diseases, such as periodontitis (pyorrhea) and gingivitis, are the primary cause of tooth loss in elderly people. Their inflammatory nature produces destruction of the bone that supports the teeth, resulting in a progressive loosening and ultimate shedding of teeth. The major causes of periodontitis are local irritation (including ill-fitting dental work), mouth breathing, food impurities, oral sepsis, malocclusions, malnutrition, endocrine imbalance, diabetes, leukemia, diphenylhydantoin (Dilantin), hypovitaminosis, scurvy, and pellagra. Advanced periodontitis can lead to impaired mastication owing to discomfort and increased tooth mobility, and to gastrointestinal disorders. There is a risk of associated bacteremia, with endocarditis and vertebral osteomyelitis (Adams and Nystrom, 1986).

The most effective treatment for periodontal disease is preventive removal of plaque and calculus, good oral hygiene, and good nutrition. Other types of treatment may be geared toward the specific cause of the problem. Surgery is sometimes indicated in severe cases (Otomo-Corgel, 1990).

Oral Candidiasis

Acute and chronic oral candidiasis occur in older people. Acute candidiasis ("thrush") is manifested by white or cream-colored plaques on the oral mucosa that can be stripped from the surface. It is often associated with antibiotic or immunosuppressive therapy and is treated with oral antifungal agents (Walls, 1989; Reinus and Brandt, 1992).

Chronic candidiasis is associated with acrylic-based dentures and with iron and folate deficiencies. The space between the upper denture and the mucosa apparently creates an environment that fosters candidal growth on the palatal mucosa. Chronic candidiasis may be accompanied by angular cheilitis: painful fissures at the corners of the mouth. Treatment requires oral antifungal therapy, thorough cleansing and overnight soaking of dentures, and correction of dental flaws that shelter organisms (Walls, 1989).

Disorders of the Esophagus

Three disorders associated with the esophagus that are related to aging are dysphagia, hiatus hernia, and carcinoma. Esophageal dysfunction is usually secondary to diseases of the nervous system that cause neuromuscular incoordination, such as Parkinson's disease, amyotrophic lateral sclerosis, pseudobulbar palsy, peripheral neuropathy, diabetes mellitus, and stroke. Because symptoms are often absent, there may be pulmonary aspiration, painless dysphagia, and progressive protein-calorie malnutrition (Minaker and Rowe, 1982).

Dysphagia

Dysphagia, once thought to be a normal concomitant of aging and part of the phenomenon of "presbyesophagus," is now considered to have pathological origins. Among elderly people in long-term care, about one third have some dysphagia (Curless and James, 1992; Shaker et al., 1993). Causes of dysphagia may be extraesophageal or intraesophageal, but they are usually vascular, structural, or neurogenic in nature. Vascular dysphagia may be due to dilation or aneurysm of the aorta. Neurogenic dysphagia may be caused by stroke, Parkinson's disease, myasthenia gravis, and a number of other conditions (Curless and James, 1992). Structural or neurogenic abnormalities may involve any portion of the esophagus, affecting the initiation of the swallowing mechanism or the ability to propel food into the stomach. The esophagus may be either dilated or constricted, and there is increasing

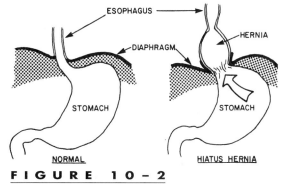

FIGURE 1 0 – 2

Diaphragmatic hernia.

irritation to the mucous membranes due to food stasis.

It is important to note the types of substances that cause difficulty. The client who has dysphagia only for solids is more likely to have a mechanical swallowing problem, whereas difficulty with both solids and liquids suggests a motility disorder. Some clients swallow solids and semisolids more easily than liquids. Evaluation by a speech therapist may help determine appropriate treatment (Curless and James, 1992). Severe pain may occur with swallowing, which can waken an individual from sleep and mimic the symptoms of angina.

Treatment may consist of correction of the underlying disorder, swallowing therapy, dilatation, or cricopharyngeal sphincterotomy. Impaired esophageal motility may be treated with nitrates, anticholinergics, calcium channel blockers, or sedatives (Reinus and Brandt, 1992). Prolonged enteral feedings are sometimes necessary. For stroke patients with severe dysphagia, percutaneous endoscopic gastrostomy is preferred by many physicians (Curless and James, 1992).

Hiatus Hernia

Age, obesity, and the female sex are highly associated with the occurrence of hiatus hernia. There are three types: sliding, rolling, and combination. With a sliding hernia, the upper part of the stomach and cardioesophageal junction rise up through the diaphragm by direct herniation through the hiatus. A rolling hernia, which is less common, is characterized by the herniation of the upper stomach through the hiatus alongside the esophagus while the cardioesophageal junction maintains a normal relationship to the diaphragm (Fig. 10–2). If both the gastroesophageal junction and the gastric fundus are displaced, the hernia is called a combination hiatus hernia (Curless and James, 1992).

Most hiatus hernias are asymptomatic; however, if symptoms do occur, they are usually related to reflux esophagitis, a condition resulting from gastric juices regurgitating into the lower esophagus and irritating the esophageal lining. Symptoms in the older person may include regurgitation, flatulence, and acid vomiting, but many older people are asymptomatic. Heartburn is more commonly reported by younger than older clients (Curless and James, 1992). Bending over or lying down may aggravate the symptoms. If reflux esophagitis becomes severe enough, peptic ulceration or stricture may occur, and occult bleeding may lead to iron deficiency anemia.

Treatment is generally conservative, since there is a high morbidity and mortality with surgery. Strictures may be relieved by endoscopic esophageal dilation. Antireflux surgery is done in a small percentage of cases. Older persons with hiatus hernias are advised to decrease intra-abdominal pressure from tight clothing, avoid lifting or straining, and elevate the heads of their beds 4 to 6 inches. In addition, they should lose weight if obese; eat small, frequent meals; and avoid eating before going to bed. Smoking and alcohol consumption are discouraged because they promote reflux and impair healing. Antacids are recommended, along with H_2 receptor antagonists or omeprazole, a proton pump inhibitor. Anticholinergics, nitrates, calcium antagonists, and theophylline should be avoided because they decrease lower esophageal sphincter pressure (Curless and James, 1992).

Esophageal Carcinoma

The incidence of esophageal carcinoma increases with age, with two times as many men affected as women. It is the most common cause of esophageal obstruction and progressive dysphagia in elderly people. The lesions may occur at the junction of the pharynx and the esophagus, the crossing at the left main bronchus, or the lower end of the esophagus. For symptoms to occur, 60 per cent of the lumen must be stenotic. The most common symptoms are dysphagia, substernal distress, and weight loss. By the time the client has dysphagia, the disease is usually quite advanced. Regurgitation and aspiration may occur, producing respiratory symptoms. Hoarseness and lymphadenopathy may develop. Use of alcohol and tobacco contribute to the development of esophageal cancer in the United States. Other risk factors are achalasia, long-standing esophageal injury, gastric surgery, and hiatus hernia. In some parts of the world, dietary deficiencies are believed to be causative (Klumpp and Macdonald, 1992).

Surgical removal of the tumor is determined by its location and extent and the overall condition of the individual. Only about 20 per cent of the patients are candidates for potentially curative resection. Operative mortality rates have improved, but long-term survival is still 12 to 22 per cent. Surgical risk is greatest for those aged 75 years or over. Preoperative and postoperative radiotherapy have been employed, and various approaches continue to be evaluated. Surgery with postoperative adjuvant radiotherapy apparently has effected some cures. The role of chemotherapy in treating esophageal cancer is still being explored. Some researchers recommend intense chemotherapy with radiotherapy with or without surgery (Ahlgren, 1992; Gomes, 1992; Harter, 1992), whereas others report that chemotherapy may improve symptoms but does not significantly affect life expectancy (Reinus and Brandt, 1992). Sometimes palliative procedures using radiotherapy are done to relieve dysphagia. Palliative measures include radiotherapy, laser therapy to burn away obstructive lesions, insertion of a prosthetic tube, and gastrostomy to promote nutrition (Vierling, 1982; Curless and James, 1992).

Disorders of the Stomach

The most common age-related disorders of the stomach are gastritis, peptic ulcer disease, and carcinoma. Although symptoms of epigastric distress and sensations of gassiness are thought to be frequent phenomena in elderly people, it must not be assumed that these are normal concomitants of older age. An underlying pathological cause must be ruled out.

Gastritis

Gastritis may be acute or chronic, and in at least 50 per cent of cases there are related organic disorders. Acute erosive gastritis may be caused by overwhelming stress or the ingestion of irritants, including NSAIDs (nonsteroidal anti-inflammatory drugs) and alcohol. The widespread use of NSAIDs for arthritic aches and pains places the older person at risk for erosive gastritis and subsequent hemorrhage (Reinus and Brandt, 1992; Shetty and Woodhouse, 1992). Treatment of acute erosive gastritis may include H_2 receptor antagonists, omeprazole, sucralfate, or misoprostol. Some sources recommend antiulcer therapy for elderly clients who take NSAIDs regularly (James, 1992).

There are three types of chronic gastritis:

1. Superficial, in which there is inflammation, edema, and increased mucus production.
2. Atrophic, with thinning of the mucosa and prominence of blood vessels, and highly associated with hypochlorhydria or achlorhydria, pernicious anemia, and gastric carcinoma.
3. Hypertrophic, accompanied by a swollen, spongy mucosa with ulcerations and erosions.

Atrophic gastritis is most common in the elderly. It usually results in a decrease in hydrochloric acid secretion, which leads to decreased absorption of iron and vitamin B_{12} and proliferation of alimentary tract bacterial flora. The final result is bacterial overgrowth. If symptoms occur, there are likely to be mild or severe epigastric pains, which can be relieved by alkali or food. The patient may also have dyspepsia, distention, nausea, and vomiting (Reinus and Brandt, 1992). Frequent feedings of a bland diet free of spices but containing vitamins and iron are recommended. Dilute hydrochloride for achlorhydria and magnesium hydroxide also provide some relief. Sodium bicarbonate should be avoided because it may cause rebound acidity.

Chronic atrophic gastritis is associated with drug abuse, circulatory disturbances, nutritional deficiency, and local or distant infection. The two types of this condition, A and B, distinguish its etiology and associated disorders. Type A gastritis denotes the presence of antibodies against the parietal cells of the stomach; it is associated with pernicious anemia and other autoimmune phenomena. In type B disease, antibodies are not present, and there is no association with pernicious anemia. *Helicobacter pylori* is believed to play a role in the development of type B gastritis (James, 1992). However, there is an increased incidence of dyspepsia and gastric and duodenal ulcers with type B. Both types may predispose to gastric cancer. Symptomatic gastritis is treated like peptic ulcer disease (Reinus and Brandt, 1992).

Peptic Ulcer Disease

The prevalence, complications, and mortality of peptic ulcer disease are high among elderly people (James, 1992). The most striking characteristic of peptic ulcer disease in older people is the atypical presentation of symptoms. Pain is less typical and poorly localized, or it may present as left-sided or lower chest discomfort. There may be other nonspecific manifestations, such as anorexia, weight loss, general debility, anemia, nausea, and painless vomiting. In some cases the disease is not discovered until major complications occur (e.g., acute upper gastrointestinal hemorrhage, perforation, or pyloric stenosis) (Achkar, 1992; James, 1992).

Gastric ulcers are more common in elderly people than duodenal ulcers, and they occur even though there is a high prevalence of decreased hydrochloric acid secretions in the stomach. Men are as vulnerable to peptic ulcer disease as women among the aged, which differs from the situation in young people, in whom the ratio of women to men is approximately 5:1 to 10:1. The initial presentation can occur beyond age 60 years. The cause may be related to the chronic use of aspirin, steroids, or NSAIDs, such as ibuprofen (Motrin), indomethacin (Indocin), or phenylbutazone (Butazolidin). Decreasing gastric mucosal blood flow may contribute to ulceration in elderly people (James, 1992; Shetty and Woodhouse, 1992).

Gastric ulcers are prone to be cancerous, whereas duodenal ulcers generally are not. Diagnosis is made through endoscopy and double contrast radiography. A biopsy is performed to rule out malignancy. Treatment is conservative in elderly people and includes bedrest, H_2 receptor antagonists, omeprazole, anti-*H. pylori* agents, and cytoprotectives. Antacids are not used as widely as they once were because of the potential adverse effects of the mineral salts of which they are made (James, 1992; Reinus and Brandt, 1992). Cimetidine, a histamine H_2 receptor antagonist, is a drug frequently used for treatment of peptic ulcer disease, but it may cause confusion in elderly people owing to its prolonged half-life (Reinus and Brandt, 1992). Conservative treatment is effective in about 50 per cent of the cases. Surgery may be performed if complications such as bleeding or obstructions occur. Despite the risks of surgery in the older person, it can be life-saving and should not be withheld simply because of the patient's age (James, 1992; Reinus and Brandt, 1992).

Carcinoma

Stomach cancer is a common malignancy of older age, especially in the sixth and seventh decades. Older men are twice as likely to have the disease as older women. The mortality rate is high, largely due to the fact that early detection is difficult. There may be nonspecific early symptoms, such as weight loss, anorexia, malaise, anemia, or change in bowel habits, especially diarrhea; or a more characteristic picture may emerge, with symptoms of dysphagia, dyspepsia, nausea and vomiting, and hematemesis. Diagnosis is made through endoscopy, with biopsies and brushings for cytology (James, 1992). Surgical intervention may be performed but in most cases is palliative. Massive resections are not recommended for elderly persons. Chemotherapy may be given preoperatively (neoadjuvant therapy) or postoperatively (adjuvant therapy). Early combinations of chemotherapeutic agents have not affected survival significantly, but researchers are hopeful that newer combinations will be more effective. Radiotherapy has been used alone or with surgery, but results have been variable (Caudry, 1992; James, 1992; Reinus and Brandt, 1992; Schein, 1992a, b; Vezeridis and Wanebo, 1992).

Disorders of the Small Intestine

In general, age alone is not thought to cause significant changes in small intestine structure or function (Lipski and James, 1992; Fox 1992b). Two disorders of the small intestine encountered in the older patient are malabsorption and vascular disease.

Malabsorptive Disorders

Malabsorptive disorders may result from atrophy of the small intestinal mucosa, bacterial overgrowth, vascular ischemia, inflammatory bowel disease, radiation-induced enteritis, motility disorders, pancreatic disease, drugs, celiac disease, and some systemic diseases such as scleroderma and rheumatoid arthritis (Lipski and James, 1992; Fox 1992b). There may be decreased absorption of vitamins A and B_{12} and B-complex, folic acid, and glucose, producing symptoms of weight loss, diarrhea, or anemia. Younger persons may complain of changes in bowel habits, but elderly people may show only secondary consequences, such as symptoms due to anemia. Steatorrhea, a symptom of malab-sorption, is not common in elderly persons (Lipski and James, 1992). Effective treatment of malabsorption depends on accurate diagnosis and may employ drug and diet therapy and nutritional supplementation. If bacterial overgrowth is the precipitating factor in malabsorptive disorders, treatment is accomplished with antibiotics.

Vascular Ischemia

Vascular disease of the small intestine increases with older age. It may be caused by occlusion of the mesenteric vessels, thrombosis, or states associated with low cardiac output (shock, recurrent myocardial infarction, or sepsis), and it results in ischemia. Acute embolism of the mesenteric vessels produces the classic symptoms of abdominal pain, abdominal distention, and fever, although the symptoms may be less dramatic in the elderly patient (Fox, 1992b). Symptoms related to thrombosis of the mesenteric vessels, especially the veins, are not as dramatic, and older persons may have nonspecific complaints of abdominal pain. Treatment consists of replacement of intravascular volume, correction of metabolic acidosis, and surgery. The mortality rate with massive resection is high, especially among elderly persons. If a large part of the small intestine is resected, long-term total parenteral nutrition may be needed (Fox, 1992b; Lipski and James, 1992).

Disorders of the Large Intestine

The major age-related disorders of the large intestine are diverticular disease, carcinoma, and changes in bowel habits (constipation and diarrhea).

Diverticular Disease

Diverticular disease, including diverticulitis and diverticulosis, is extremely common among the elderly, and by age 80 years at least 40 per cent of persons are afflicted. A colonic diverticulum is a herniation of the colonic mucosa through the otherwise normal colonic wall, with weakness or abnormalities of intracolonic pressure or both. There is also a pronounced thickening of the longitudinal and circular muscle layers (Fig. 10–3). Diverticular disease has three phases:

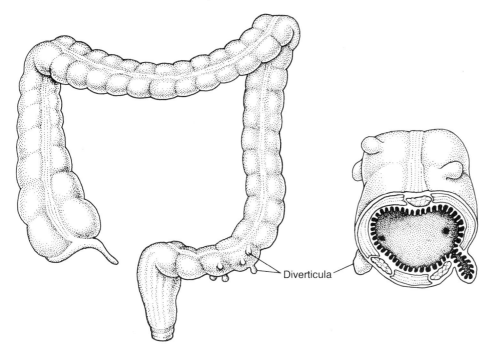

Diverticula

FIGURE 10 – 3

Diverticula (*sing.*, diverticulum), abnormal outpouchings or herniations in the intestinal wall. (From Ignatavicius, D.D. and Bayne, M.V. *Medical-Surgical Nursing: A Nursing Process Approach.* 2nd ed. Philadelphia, W.B. Saunders, 1995, p. 1651.)

1. Prediverticular state, characterized by muscular thickening and luminal narrowing of the colon.
2. Diverticulosis, consisting of diverticula without complications.
3. Diverticulitis, producing inflammation in the area of the diverticulum.

The major cause of diverticular disease is thought to be the absence of dietary fiber. The most significant symptom is a dysfunction of bowel habits, particularly diarrhea, constipation, or alternating diarrhea and constipation. Other symptoms include abdominal pain, rectal bleeding, and nausea and vomiting. In many cases of diverticulosis, older persons are asymptomatic and require no treatment. A high-fiber diet with added bran or bulking agents relieves symptoms in 85 per cent of the clients who have no inflammation. Antibiotics (metronidazole and gentamicin) may be given if inflammation is present, and antispasmodics may be given for colicky pain. Surgery is performed for diverticulitis that does not respond to conservative treatment, which consists of rest, nasogastric suction, and antibiotics. Surgery may also be performed for abscess, perforation, fistula, or obstruction (Shearman et al., 1989; Brocklehurst, 1992; Farmer, 1992).

Cancer

Cancer of the colon and rectum is one of the most common malignancies in both men and women over age 70 years, and it is the most common cancer causing death. It is thought to be related to lack of dietary fiber and, more importantly, to eating red meat. Increased risk factors for colon cancer include age over 40 years, family history of colon cancer, history of previous polyps or colon cancer, history of breast or uterine cancer, history of inflammatory bowel disease, and familial polyposis. Dietary intake of fat, protein, and fiber is also thought to influence the development of colorectal cancer (Alabaster, 1992). Symptoms include changes in bowel habits, anemia, weakness, mucous discharge, rectal bleeding, and intestinal obstruction. Pain is less common in older people than in younger people (Brocklehurst, 1992).

The disease can be successfully treated with surgery if detected early; however, it is frequently diagnosed too late because symptoms may go unnoticed. Preoperative radiotherapy may be useful in decreasing lymph node metastases. Surgical treatment should not be withheld on the basis of age alone, but the risks are higher in very old people (Brocklehurst, 1992). Health care professionals recommend that people age 50 years and over have annual stool tests for occult blood and flexible sigmoidoscopy every 2 to 3 years. More aggressive screening should be done in high-risk populations (Schein, 1992a, b). At least 80 per cent of colonic cancers have positive occult blood tests at the time of diagnosis. The Hemoccult Slide Test is a simple, inexpensive, accurate test that can be used at home and sent to the physician (Siegel, 1992).

Changes in Bowel Habits

Changes in bowel habits are actually symptoms rather than disease states, but they are listed as separate entities because they are so bothersome to elderly people. An in-depth discussion is found under Alterations in Elimination in Chapter 14.

Diarrhea

Diarrhea is defined as an increased fluidity, volume, or frequency of bowel movements (Shearman et al., 1989). The most common causes in elderly people are fecal impactions, bacterial and viral infections, dietary indiscretions (too much fruit, especially bananas), and medications. Chronic diarrhea can result from diverticulitis, thyrotoxicosis, diabetes with autonomic neuropathy, steatorrhea, gastric and hepatic disease, and, occasionally, ulcerative colitis. Diagnosis is based on the duration of the condition, the presence of blood in the stool, a recent history of constipation, a medical and drug history, and recent changes in dietary habits. Clients should be checked for signs and symptoms of volume depletion, such as tachycardia, postural hypotension, poor skin turgor, absence of axillary sweat, and an increase in the hematocrit or BUN level, as well as changes in serum potassium. Treatment is aimed at providing support, relieving symptoms, and treating the underlying condition. The client is supported by replacing fluid and electrolyte losses, and symptomatic relief is provided by giving antidiarrheals to decrease the number of bowel movements or to improve the consistency of the stool. The underlying condition may be treated medically or surgically. Depending on the condition, drug therapy may include antimicrobials, corticosteroids, and enzyme preparations (Rankin, 1992).

Constipation

Constipation is a phenomenon in which there is a decrease in the frequency of bowel movements, accompanied by a prolonged and difficult passage of stool, followed by a sensation of incomplete evacuation. It is not a normal concomitant of older age (Fig. 10-4), and one should look for specific causes of the condition, such as decreased motility, malignancy, obstruction, poor nutrition, decreased fluid intake, hypothyroidism, hypercalcemia, depression, or medications (Table 10-1). Nevertheless, 30 per cent of people over age 60 years take a cathartic at least once a week (Woodhouse and Wynne, 1992). A major complication of constipation is fecal impaction and megacolon. Treatment of constipation consists of increased physical activity, a high-fiber diet, increased fluids, laxatives, and enemas (Table 10-2). Preferred laxatives for the elderly are senna, bisacodyl, lactulose, natural gums, and dioctyl sodium sulfosuccinate. Immobile clients who are prone to fecal impactions may require enemas or suppositories twice weekly (Brocklehurst, 1992).

Disorders of the Pancreas

The pancreatic diseases most likely to affect elderly persons are acute and chronic pancreatitis and pancreatic carcinoma.

Pancreatitis

Pancreatitis is usually secondary to other disorders of the gastrointestinal tract, such as gallbladder disease, penetrating peptic ulcer, pancreatic infections and infestations, or alcohol ingestion. Abdominal surgery or trauma, invasive procedures, and drugs, including steroids, diuretics, hypotensives, NSAIDs, antibiotics, estrogens, and possibly anesthetic agents, have all been implicated (Shearman et al., 1989; Brocklehurst, 1992). The classic symptom of acute pancreatitis is sudden, excruciating abdominal pain, radiating to the back and chest and relieved by sitting up; at times the pain can be severe enough to produce shock. Elderly people often have an atypical clinical presentation, so that the pain may be more prominent in the lower abdomen than in the epigastric area, or pain may be absent. Also, some older people exhibit acute confusion progressing to coma (Brocklehurst, 1992). Loss of consciousness can also occur. If the disease is asymptomatic and goes unrecognized, death may result. Blood tests reveal an increase in white blood cells, amylase, and lipase; these tests produce the most definitive diagnosis.

The prognosis is poor, but treatment con-

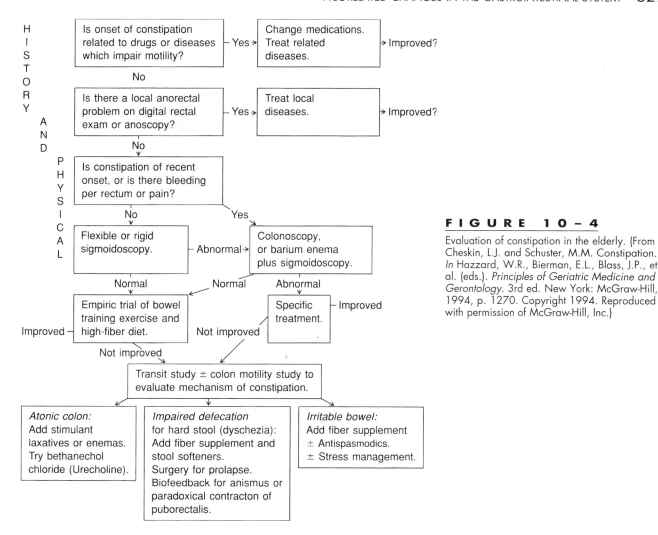

FIGURE 10-4

Evaluation of constipation in the elderly. (From Cheskin, L.J. and Schuster, M.M. Constipation. In Hazzard, W.R., Bierman, E.L., Blass, J.P., et al. (eds.). *Principles of Geriatric Medicine and Gerontology*. 3rd ed. New York: McGraw-Hill, 1994, p. 1270. Copyright 1994. Reproduced with permission of McGraw-Hill, Inc.)

sists of nasogastric suction, intravenous fluid and electrolyte replacement, and analgesics. Antibiotics may be given but are questionably effective in preventing sepsis. Blood or plasma may be required. If transient diabetes mellitus develops, it is usually treated with insulin (Shearman et al., 1989; Brocklehurst, 1992).

Chronic pancreatitis results from repeated acute episodes. Abdominal pain is the major symptom, in addition to malnutrition, deficiency of the fat-soluble vitamins, osteomalacia, and tetany. Treatment consists of a high-carbohydrate, high-fat, alcohol-free diet and supplements of vitamin B complex, vitamins A, D, E, and K, and pancreatic extracts.

Pancreatic Cancer

Pancreatic cancer, most often adenocarcinoma, usually appears in persons aged 60 to 80 years and peaks in the ninth decade. Risk factors are cigarette smoking, high-fat diet, alcoholism, and exposure to volatile hydrocarbons. The initial symptoms are vague and nonspecific, so that diagnosis is frequently made during the advanced stages of the disease. Weight loss, anorexia, upper abdominal distress (especially epigastric pain radiating to the back), steatorrhea, and progressive jaundice may occur, but the most significant symptom is depression or anxiety. Up to 76 per cent of older persons with pancreatic cancer experience depressive symptoms; therefore, this diagnosis is considered if there are unexplained psychiatric complaints. Because the disease is generally inoperable when it is diagnosed, the survival rate is less than 2 per cent for 5 years (Shearman et al., 1989; Braganza, 1992).

If the tumor is located in the head of the pancreas, resection may be attempted. Otherwise, surgery may be performed only

TABLE 10-1

Causes of Constipation

Bowel disorders	Bowel obstruction Neoplasm Stricture Irritable bowel syndrome Anal lesions Hemorrhoids Fissures Colorectal dysmotility
Neurologic disorders	Spinal cord injury Parkinson's disease Dementia
Endocrine and metabolic disorders	Diabetic autonomic neuropathy Hypothyroidism Hypercalcemia Hypokalemia
Habits	Inadequate intake of fluids or fiber Poor toilet habits Laxative abuse
Activity	Immobility
Psychological factors	Depression
Drugs	Antacids: aluminum hydroxide gel, calcium carbonate Anticholinergics Antidepressants: tricyclics, lithium Antihypertensives: calcium channel blockers Narcotic analgesics Nonsteroidal anti-inflammatory drugs Sympathomimetics: pseudoephedrine

to bypass the obstructed common duct to promote drainage and relieve jaundice and pruritus. This bypass may be done during endoscopic retrograde cholangiopancreatography or by percutaneous transhepatic cholangiography, thereby sparing the patient major abdominal surgery (Braganza, 1992). Chemotherapy has not demonstrated effectiveness. Clinical trials are under way to evaluate the use of chemotherapy with radiotherapy as surgical adjuvants. Other new therapies being investigated in the treatment of pancreatic cancer are immunotherapy and monoclonal antibodies (Schein, 1992a, b). If analgesic medications are not effective in relieving pain, a splanchnic nerve block may be performed (Brandt, 1986; Sklar, 1986).

Disorders of the Liver

Although cirrhosis is the hepatic disease most highly associated with older age, hepatitis is also mentioned here because of its atypical presentation in elderly people (Woodhouse and James, 1993).

Hepatitis

There are four types of viral hepatitis: A, B, C, and D. Hepatitis A is acute, self-limited, and usually subclinical, but fever and gastrointestinal symptoms may occur. Fatalities are rare but are more common in elderly persons. Hepatitis B occurs more frequently in the elderly, with a sudden intense onset, followed by a more prolonged course that may become chronic. There is increased morbidity and mortality with the B virus; however, recovery is usually complete. Hepatitis C probably accounts for most posttransfusion hepatitis. The hepatitis D virus can replicate only in the presence of the hepatitis B virus, and it increases the severity of the hepatitis B infection (James, 1992).

Older people may have acute, chronic, or nonspecific reactive hepatitis, which is associated with chronic illness (atherosclerotic or hypertensive cardiovascular disease). Acute viral hepatitis is more severe with prolonged jaundice, and a high mortality rate is associated with the disease, especially among elderly people (Shearman et al., 1989). In this instance, high mortality is usually related to malnutrition and delay in hospital admission. Chronic hepatitis can result from viral hepatitis, usually Type B, or hepatotoxic injury from drugs or chemicals. Older persons may have atypical symptoms and are especially likely to experience an acute confusional state (Vierling, 1982).

The aims of treatment for hepatitis are adequate nutrition, relief of symptoms, and avoidance of further liver injury by inappropriate drugs. A low-fat, high-carbohydrate diet is recommended. Any hepatotoxic drugs are discontinued. Corticosteroids and immunosuppressants may be prescribed for chronic active hepatitis but not for chronic persistent hepatitis (Shearman et al., 1989). Corticosteroids must be used cautiously in elderly people to avoid side effects such as osteopenia, bone fractures, hypertension, and diabetes (Brandt, 1986).

Cirrhosis

The incidence of cirrhosis increases after age 45 years because of long-standing liver disease (Vierling, 1982). The course of the disease is chronic and progressive, ultimately resulting in severe liver failure and death. Cirrhosis is almost always related to chronic alcoholism but may be associated with viral hepatitis B, drugs and toxins, biliary obstruction, metabolic disorders, and hepatic inflammation (Shearman et al., 1989).

The liver is large and tender in the early stages and becomes small and fibrotic in the later stages of the disease. Symptoms include jaundice, clay-colored stools, and feminization in men. Eventually portal hypertension develops, with enlarged esophageal varices, enlarged abdominal wall veins, and a palpable spleen. Later, ascites may develop.

Treatment is aimed at maintaining nutrition, controlling encephalopathy, and avoiding further insults to the liver. Clients are put on modified bedrest and fed a high-carbohydrate, low-fat diet. Dietary protein allowance depends on the presence of complications, especially encephalopathy. Vitamin B complex and vitamin K may be prescribed, although some researchers believe there is no evidence that supplements and special diets are necessary except when ascites is present (Shearman et al., 1989; Winkelman, 1992). Hepatotoxic drugs and alcohol should be avoided. If ascites develops, treatment consists of sodium restriction, diuretics, management of fluid and electrolyte balance, and paracentesis. Hemorrhage from esophageal varices may be treated with balloon tamponade, nasogastric suction, surgery, or endoscopic sclerotherapy. Vasopressin may be given to decrease portal pressure. Mortality and morbidity rates for cirrhotic clients who undergo abdominal surgery are high (Shearman et al., 1989; Winkelman, 1992).

Disorders of the Gallbladder

Cholelithiasis (gallstones) is common in the elderly; however, the condition is usually asymptomatic and rarely requires treatment (Fox, 1992a). If symptoms do occur, they may be similar to those experienced in the young: dyspepsia with fatty intolerance, attacks of cholecystitis, and episodes of obstructive jaundice when the stones enter the common bile duct. Some older people have less acute symptoms and delay seeking treatment. Acute cholecystitis can produce mild-to-severe discomfort, right upper quadrant pain, and belching.

Treatment is conservative and includes a low-fat diet, bland foods in small amounts, and avoidance of fried, greasy, and spicy foods. Drug therapy may include antispasmodics, analgesics, antibiotics, sedatives, and bile salts to increase bile flow. Other treatment options are dissolution therapy, lithotripsy, endoscopic cholecystectomy, and cholecystectomy. Unless the gallbladder is removed, there is a risk of recurrence. Surgery is safer for elderly clients now than in the past, especially if the procedure is done on an elective rather than an emergency basis. Nevertheless, very old or frail people are usually treated conservatively (Shearman et al., 1989; Zuccaro, 1992).

TABLE 10 – 2
Drugs Used to Treat Constipation

TYPE	EXAMPLES	MECHANISM OF ACTION
Stool softeners or lubricants	Dioctyl sodium succinate Mineral oil	Soften and lubricate fecal mass
Bulk-forming agents	Bran Psyllium mucilloid	Increase fecal bulk and retain fluid in bowel lumen
Osmotic cathartics	Milk of magnesia Magnesium sulfate or citrate	Poorly absorbed salts retain fluid in bowel lumen; increase net secretions of fluid in small intestine
Stimulants or irritants	Cascara Senna Bisacodyl Phenolphthalein	Alter intestinal mucosal permeability; stimulate muscle activity and fluid secretions
Enemas	Tap water Saline Sodium phosphate Oil	Induce reflex evacuations
Suppositories	Glycerin Bisacodyl	Cause mucosal irritation

From Ouslander, J.G: Incontinence. *In* Hazzard, W.R., Andres, R. and Richter, J.E. (eds.). *Principles of Geriatric Medicine and Gerontology.* 2nd ed. New York: McGraw-Hill, 1994, p. 1247. Copyright 1994. Reproduced with permission of McGraw-Hill, Inc.

ASSESSMENT

A thorough assessment of the gastrointestinal system includes an accurate history of oral hygiene and dietary and elimination habits. Physical assessment includes inspection and palpation of the oral cavity, and inspection, auscultation, percussion, and palpation of the upper and lower abdomen. (Note the deviation from the usual order of inspection, palpation, percussion, and auscultation.) Table 10–3 gives a more detailed description of the history and assessment process.

NURSING DIAGNOSES

1. Chronic or Acute Pain
related to oral lesions, gastrointestinal disorders, malignancy

T A B L E   1 0 – 3
Assessment of the Gastrointestinal System

HISTORY
Oral Cavity, Mouth, Pharynx, and Larynx
Complaints of disturbances in the sense of taste
Pain or bleeding of the tongue, lips, or gums
Abnormalities of salivation
Dental problems
Dentures
  Ability to chew
Last dental examination
Difficult or painful swallowing of liquids and/or solids
Sore throat
Hoarseness
Lump in throat

Upper and Lower Gastrointestinal Tract
Diet, especially liquids
Appetite; anorexia; weight loss; appetite changes
Intolerance to certain foods
Nausea (circumstances, time of day, relation to meals)
Vomiting (type, color, quantity, relation to meals)
Heartburn, epigastric pain
Pain (type, location, intensity, duration)
Jaundice
Bowel habits; use of laxatives
Flatulence; tarry stools; bloody stools

PHYSICAL ASSESSMENT
Oral Cavity, Mouth, Larynx, and Pharynx
Face (anterior and side view)
  Observe for asymmetry, pigmentations, masses, ulcers, inflammatory lesions, lacerations
  Describe location, size, and depth of deviations
Lymph nodes
  Palpate cervical chain of lymph nodes, starting with the posterior cervical region through the submandibular, sublingual, and anterior cervical areas
Lips
  Observe for normal and abnormal changes
  Compress lips gently to palpate for masses
Teeth
  Observe caries, missing teeth, dentures
Buccal mucosa
  Observe color, masses, or inflammatory lesions
  Examine alveolar ridges in edentulous patients, palpating for any unusual lumps or bumps
Tongue
  Examine ventral and dorsal aspects of tongue
  Grasp tongue with a 2 by 2 gauze pad and examine the lateral borders and base of the tongue and the floor of the mouth
Palate
  Observe for lesions or masses
  Observe uvula for deviation
Throat
  Note condition, color, vascularity, and evidence of postnasal drip

Upper and Lower Gastrointestinal Tract
Inspection
  Observe for scars, striae, dilated veins, lesions, masses, color changes, increased pigment, tautness
  Note contour, especially symmetry, herniations along midline, swelling
  Check movement and rigidity; look for arterial pulsations, peristalsis
Auscultation
  Listen for bowel sounds, vascular bruits, and rubs
Percussion
  Check for tympany (normal abdominal sounds) and dullness (solid viscera)
Palpation
  Assess for rebound tenderness or pain, organomegaly

2. Constipation or Colonic Constipation
   related to neuromuscular impairment, intestinal obstruction, megacolon, painful defecation, drug side effects, immobility, inadequate intake of fluids and fiber, metabolic problems

3. Perceived Constipation
   related to inappropriate use of aids to elimination based on custom or lack of information

4. Diarrhea
   related to gastrointestinal disorders, infectious processes, adverse effects of laxatives or other drugs

5. Bowel Incontinence
   related to neuromuscular impairment, diarrhea, fecal impaction, cognitive impairment

6. Fluid Volume Deficit (Active Loss)
   related to abdominal cancer, hemorrhage, diarrhea

7. Risk for Fluid Volume Deficit
   related to decreased fluid intake, drug effects, inability to obtain fluids due to immobility, abnormal loss of fluid through diarrhea or vomiting

8. Knowledge Deficit
   of oral hygiene and dental care, diet, nutrition, self-medication

9. Nutrition, Altered: Less Than Body Requirements
   related to chewing difficulties, anorexia, difficulty in procuring or inability to procure food

10. Nutrition, Altered: More Than Body Requirements
    related to imbalance of intake vs. activity expenditures secondary to lack of basic nutritional knowledge, decreased activity patterns, and decreased metabolic needs

NURSING INTERVENTIONS

Nursing interventions based on nursing diagnoses include providing good mouth care and referral to a dentist, if necessary, modifying the diet, implementing regimens for regular bowel elimination, and relieving pain and discomfort. All interventions must have a central focus of patient and family teaching to promote self-care and health maintenance whenever possible. Chapter 14 presents an in-depth discussion of the preceding nursing diagnoses, interventions, and evaluation of care.

SUMMARY

Studies have shown that normal age-related changes in the gastrointestinal system are difficult to identify. Diminished functional capacity may be associated with normal aging; however, decreased functioning is more often linked to pathological problems. Some age-related changes that probably occur in the gastrointestinal system include decreases in the blood flow to the organs, the size of the organs, and motility.

Pathological problems most commonly found in the gastrointestinal system in older age include periodontal disease of the mouth, malignant lesions, dysphagia, hiatus hernia, gastritis, peptic ulcer disease, malabsorption syndromes, diverticular disease, pancreatitis, hepatitis, cirrhosis, cholelithiasis, and cholecystitis. These disease states produce problems with nutrition and elimination, resulting in pain, discomfort, anorexia, constipation, and diarrhea. The nurse should provide measures to relieve these problems through direct interventions and patient teaching to promote the highest level of functioning.

REFERENCES

Achkar, E. Peptic ulcer disease. In Achkar, E., Farmer, R.G. and Fleshler, B. (eds.). Clinical Gastroenterology. 2nd ed. Philadelphia: Lea & Febiger, 1992, pp. 234–249.

Adams, R.A. and Nystrom, G.P. Periodontal disease. In Tyron, A.F. (ed.). Oral Health and Aging. Littleton, MA: PSG Publications, 1986, pp. 271–286.

Ahlgren, J.D. Esophageal cancer: Chemotherapy and combined modalities. In Ahlgren, J. and Macdonald, J. (eds.). Gastrointestinal Oncology. Philadelphia: J.B. Lippincott, 1992, pp. 135–146.

Alabaster, O. Colorectal cancer: Epidemiology, risks, and prevention. In Ahlgren, J. and Macdonald, J. (eds.). Gastrointestinal Oncology. Philadelphia: J.B. Lippincott, 1992, pp. 243–259.

Bartos, V. and Groh, J. The effect of repeated stimulation of the pancreas on the pancreatic secretion in young and aged men. Gerontol Clin 11:56, 1969.

Baum, B.J. Age changes in salivary glands and salivary secretion. In Holm-Pedersen, P. and Harald Loe, H.: Geriatric Dentistry. Copenhagen: Munksgaard, 1986, pp. 114–120.

Baum, B.J. Dental and oral disorders. In Abrams, W.B. and Berkow, R. (eds.). The Merck Manual of Gerontology. Rahway, NJ: Merck Sharp & Dohme Research Laboratories, 1990, pp. 466–475.

Baum, B.J. and Bodner, L. Aging and oral motor function: Evidence for altered performance among older persons. J Dent Res 62:2–6, 1983.

Baum, B.J. and Ship, J.A. The oral cavity. In Hazzard, W.R., Andres, R. and Richter, J.E. (eds.). Principles of Geriatric Medicine and Gerontology. 2nd ed. New York: McGraw-Hill, 1990, pp. 413–421.

Braganza, J.M. The pancreas. In Brocklehurst, J.C., Tallis, R.C. and Fillit, H.M. (eds.). Textbook of Geriatric Medicine and Gerontology. 4th ed. Edinburgh: Churchill Livingstone, 1992, pp. 527–535.

Brandt, L.J. Pancreas, liver and gall bladder. In Rossman, I. (ed.). Clinical Geriatrics. 3rd ed. Philadelphia: J.B. Lippincott, 1986, pp. 302–325.

Brocklehurst, J.C. The large bowel. In Brocklehurst, J.C., Tallis, R.C., and Fillit, H.M. (eds.). Textbook of Geriatric Medicine and Gerontology. 4th ed. Edinburgh: Churchill Livingstone, 1992, pp. 569–591.

Carranza, F.A. (1990). Aging and the periodontium. In Glickman's Clinical Periodontology. 7th ed. Philadelphia: W.B. Saunders, 1990.

Caudry, M. Gastric cancer: Radiotherapy and approaches to locally unresectable or recurrent disease. In Ahlgren, J. and Macdonald, J. (eds.). Gastrointestinal Oncology. Philadelphia: J.B. Lippincott, 1992, pp. 181–187.

Curless, R. and James, O.F.W. The oesophagus. In Evans, J.G. and Williams, T.F. (eds.). Oxford Textbook of Geriatric Medicine. Oxford: Oxford University Press, 1992, pp. 196–211.

Deems, D.A., Doty, R.L., Settle, R.G. et al. Smell and taste disorders: A study of 750 patients from the University of Pennsylvania Taste and Smell Center. Arch Otolaryngol 117:(5):519–528, 1991.

Douglas, C.W., Jetta, A.M., Fox, C.H. et al. Oral health status of the elderly in New England. J Gerontol 48(2): M39–M46, 1993.

Ekberg, O. and Feinberg, M.J. Altered swallowing function in elderly patients without dysphagia: Radiologic findings in 56 cases. Am J Roentgenol 156(6):1181–1184, 1991.

Elkowitz, E.B. Geriatric Medicine for the Primary Care Practitioner. New York: Springer, 1981.

Farmer, R.G. Diverticular disease of the colon. In Achkar, E.A., Farmer, R.G. and Fleshler, B. (eds.). Clinical Gastroenterology. 2nd ed. Philadelphia: Lea & Febiger, 1992, pp. 362–366.

Ferguson, M.W.F. and Devlin, H. Aging and the orofacial tissues. In Brocklehurst, J.C., Tallis, R.C. and Fillit, H.M. (eds.). Textbook of Geriatric Medicine and Gerontology. 4th ed. Edinburgh: Churchill Livingstone, 1992, pp. 558–561.

Fikry, M.E. Exocrine pancreatic function in the aged. J Am Geriatr Soc 16:463, 1968.

Fox, R.A. Diseases of the gallbladder. In Brocklehurst, J.C., Tallis, R.C. and Fillit, H.M. (eds.). Textbook of Geriatric Medicine and Gerontology. 4th ed. Edinburgh: Churchill Livingstone, 1992a, pp. 558–561.

Fox, R.A. Diseases of the small bowel. In Brocklehurst, J.C., Tallis, R.C. and Fillit, H.M. (eds.). Textbook of Geriatric Medicine and Gerontology. 4th ed. Edinburgh: Churchill Livingstone, 1992b, pp. 562–568.

Gibbons, J.C. and Levy, S.M. Gastrointestinal diseases in the elderly. In Reichel, W. (ed.). Clinical Aspects of Aging. 3rd ed. Baltimore: Williams & Wilkins, 1989, pp. 188–198.

Gomes, M.N. Esophageal cancer: Surgical approach. In Ahlgren, J. and Macdonald, J. (eds.). Gastrointestinal Oncology. Philadelphia: J.B. Lippincott, 1992, pp. 89–121.

Gordon, S.R. Oral and dental problems. In Schrier, R.W. (ed.). Geriatric Medicine. Philadelphia: W.B. Saunders, 1990, pp. 129–137.

Gullo, L. Diseases of the exocrine pancreas. In Evans, J.G. and Williams, T.F. (eds.). Oxford Textbook of Geriatric Medicine. Oxford: Oxford University Press, 1992, pp. 241–256.

Harter, K.W. Esophageal cancer: Management with radiation. In Ahlgren, J. and Macdonald, J. (eds.). Gastrointestinal Oncology. Philadelphia: J.B. Lippincott, 1992, pp. 123–143.

Holm-Pedersen, P. and Loe, H. *Geriatric Dentistry*. Copenhagen: Munkegaard, 1986.

Jacob, S.W., Francone, C.A. and Lossow, W.J. *Structure and Function in Man*. 5th ed. Philadelphia: W.B. Saunders, 1982.

James, O.F.W. The stomach. *In* Evans, J.G. and Williams, T.F. (eds.). *Oxford Textbook of Geriatric Medicine*. Oxford: Oxford University Press, 1992, pp. 215–225.

Kalu, D.N. and Masoro, E.J. Metabolic and nutritional aspects of aging. *Gerodontics* 2(4):121–126, 1986.

Kamen, S. Oral care of the geriatric patient. *In* Steinberg, R.U. (ed.). *Care of the Geriatric Patient*. St. Louis: C.V. Mosby, 1983.

Katz, R.V. and Meskin, L.H. The epidemiology of oral diseases in older adults. *In* Holm-Pedersen, P. and Loe, H. (eds.). *Geriatric Dentistry*. Copenhagen: Munksgaard, 1986.

Klumpp, T.R. and Macdonald, J.S. Esophageal cancer: Epidemiology and pathology. *In* Ahlgren, J. and Macdonald, J. (eds.). *Gastrointestinal Oncology*. Philadelphia: J.B. Lippincott, 1992, pp. 71–80.

Laugier, R. and Sarles, H. The pancreas. *Clin Gerontol* 14(7), 1985.

Lipski, P.S. and James, O.F.W. Small intestine. *In* Evans, J.G. and Williams, T.F. (eds.). *Oxford Textbook of Geriatric Medicine*. Oxford: Oxford University Press, 1992, pp. 226–235.

Lund, H. and Westesson, P.L. Clinical signs of temporomandibular joint internal derangement in adults. An epidemiological study. *Oral Surg Oral Med Oral Pathol* 72(6):637–641, 1991.

Mackenzie, I.C., Holm-Pedersen, P. and Karring, T. Age changes in the oral mucous membranes and periodontium. *In* Holm-Pedersen, P. and Loe, H. (eds.). *Geriatric Dentistry*. Copenhagen: Munksgaard, 1986, pp. 102–109.

Mercado, M.D. and Falkner, K.D. The prevalence of craniomandibular disorders in completely edentulous denture-wearing subjects. *J Oral Rehabil* 18(3):231–242, 1991.

Minaker, K.L. and Rowe, J.W. Gastrointestinal system. *In* Rowe, J.W. and Besdine, R.W. (eds.). *Health and Disease in Old Age*. St. Louis: Little, Brown, 1982.

Mjor, I.A. Age changes in the teeth. *In* Holm-Pedersen, P. and Loe, H. (eds.). *Geriatric Dentistry*. Copenhagen: Munksgaard, 1986, pp. 94–100.

Mott, A.E., Grushka, M. and Sessle, B.J. Diagnosis and management of taste disorders and burning mouth syndrome. *Dent Clin North Am* 37(1):33–71, 1993.

Nelson, J.B. and Castell, D.O. Aging of the gastrointestinal system. *In* Hazzard, W.R., Andres, R. and Richter, J.E. (eds.). *Principles of Geriatric Medicine and Gerontology*. 2nd ed. New York: McGraw-Hill, 1990, pp. 593–608.

Otomo-Corgel, J. Periodontal management of geriatric patients. *In* Carranza, F.A., Jr. (ed.). *Glickman's Clinical Periodontology*. 7th ed. Philadelphia: W.B. Saunders, 1990.

Rankin, G.B. Diarrhea. *In* Achkar, E.A., Farmer, R.G. and Fleshler, B. (eds.). *Clinical Gastroenterology*. 2nd ed. Philadelphia: Lea & Febiger, 1992, pp. 82–88.

Read, N.W. Colonic disease in elderly people. *In* Evans, J.G. and Williams, T.F. (eds.). *Oxford Textbook of Geriatric Medicine*. Oxford: Oxford University Press, 1992, pp. 236–242.

Reinus, J.F. and Brandt, L.F. The upper gastrointestinal tract. *In* Brocklehurst, J.C., Tallis, R.C. and Fillit, H.M. (eds.). *Textbook of Geriatric Medicine and Gerontology*. 4th ed. Edinburgh: Churchill Livingstone, 1992, pp. 507–526.

Ren, J., Shaker, R., Zamir, Z. et al. Effect of age and bolus variables on the coordination of the glottis and upper esophageal sphincter during swallowing. *Am J Gastroenterol* 88(5):665–669, 1993.

Robbins, J., Hamilton, J.W., Lof, G.L. and Kempster, G.B. Oropharyngeal swallowing in normal adults of different ages. *Gastroenterology* 103(3):823–829, 1992.

Rogers, V.C. and Duvall, D.J. Geriatric dentistry. *In* Reichel, W. (ed.) *Clinical Aspects of Aging*. 3rd ed. Baltimore: Williams and Wilkins, 1989, pp. 464–473.

Schein, P. Gastric cancer: Radiotherapy and approaches to locally unresectable or recurrent disease. *In* Ahlgren, J.D. and Macdonald, J.S. (eds.). *Gastrointestinal Oncology*. Philadelphia: J.B. Lippincott, 1992a, pp. 189–193.

Schein, P. Gastrointestinal cancer: A global perspective. *In* Ahlgren, J.D. and Macdonald, J.S. (eds.). *Gastrointestinal Oncology*. Philadelphia: J.B. Lippincott, 1992b, pp. 3–11.

Serfaty, V., Nemcovsky, C.E., Friedlander, D. and Gazit, E. Functional disturbances of the masticatory system in an elderly population group. *Cranio* 7(1):46–51, 1989.

Shaker, R., Ren, J., Podvrsan, B. et al. Effect of aging and bolus variables on pharyngeal and upper esophageal sphincter motor function. *American Journal of Physiology* 264(3 Pt 1):G427–432, 1993.

Shearman, D.J.C., Finlayson, N.D.C. and Carter, D.C. *Diseases of the Gastrointestinal Tract and Liver*. 2nd ed. Edinburgh: Churchill Livingstone, 1989.

Shetty, H.G.M. and Woodhouse, K.W. Non-steroidal anti-inflammatory drugs and the gastrointestinal tract. *In* Evans, J.G. and Williams, T.F. (eds.). *Oxford Textbook of Geriatric Medicine*. Oxford: Oxford University Press, 1992, pp. 179–195.

Ship, J.A. and Baum, B.J. Is reduced salivary flow normal in old age? *Lancet* 336:1507, 1990.

Siegel, R.S. Screening for colorectal cancer. *In* Ahlgren, J.D. and Macdonald, J.S. (eds.). *Gastrointestinal Oncology*. Philadelphia: J.B. Lippincott, 1992, pp. 293–297.

Singleton, J.W. Management of constipation and diarrhea. *In* Schrier, R.W. (ed.). *Geriatric Medicine*. Philadelphia: W.B. Saunders, 1990, pp. 434–439.

Sklar, M. Gastrointestinal diseases. *In* Calkins, E., Davis, P.J. and Ford, A.B. (eds.). *The Practice of Geriatrics*. Philadelphia: W.B. Saunders, 1986, pp. 555–575.

Soergel, K.H., Zboralske, F.E. and Amberg, J.R. Presbyesophagus: Esophageal motility in nonagenarians. *J Clin Invest* 43:1472, 1964.

Tenovuo, J. Oral defense factors in the elderly. *Endodont Dent Traumatol* 8(3):93–98, 1992.

Tyron, A.F. *Oral Health and Aging*. Littleton, MA: PSG Publishing Company, 1986.

Vezeridis, M.P. and Wanebo, H.J. Gastric cancer: Surgical approach. *In* Ahlgren, J.D. and Macdonald, J.S. (eds.). *Gastrointestinal Oncology*. Philadelphia: J.B. Lippincott, 1992, pp. 159–170.

Vierling, J.M. Physiology and diseases of the digestive system in the aged. *In* Schrier, R.W. (ed.). *Clinical Internal Medicine in the Aged*. Philadelphia: W.B. Saunders, 1982.

Walls, A.W.G. Prevention in the aging dentition. *In* Murray, J.J. (ed.). *The Prevention of Dental Disease*. 2nd ed. Oxford: Oxford Medical Publications, 1989, pp. 303–326.

Walls, A.W.G. The aging mouth. *In* Evans, J.G. and Williams, T.F. (eds.). *Oxford Textbook of Geriatric Medicine*. Oxford: Oxford University Press, 1992, pp. 179–195.

Winkelman, E.I. Cirrhosis. *In* Achkar, E.A., Farmer, R.G. and Fleshler, B. (eds.). *Clinical Gastroenterology*. 2nd ed. Philadelphia: Lea & Febiger, 1992, pp. 581–603.

Woodhouse, K.W. and James, O.F.W. Hepatobiliary disease. *In* Evans, J.G. and Williams, T.F. (eds.). *Oxford Textbook of Geriatric Medicine*. Oxford: Oxford University Press, 1993, pp. 256–267.

Woodhouse, K.W. and Wynne, H.A. The pharmacology of aging. *In* Brocklehurst, J.C., Tallis, R.C. and Fillit, H.M. (eds.). *Textbook of Geriatric Medicine and Gerontol-*

ogy. 4th ed. Edinburgh: Churchill Livingstone, 1992, pp. 129–142.

Wu, A.J., Atkinson, J.C., Fox, P.C. et al. Cross-sectional and longitudinal analyses of stimulated parotid salivary constituents in healthy, different-aged subjects. *J Gerontol* 48(5):M219–M224, 1993.

Yoder, M.G. Geriatric ear, nose, and throat problems. *In*

Reichel, W. (ed.). *Clinical Aspects of Aging.* 3rd ed. Baltimore: Williams and Wilkins, 1989, pp. 454–463.

Zuccaro, G. Gallstones and benign biliary tract disorders. *In* Achkar, E.A., Farmer, R.G. and Fleshler, B. (eds.). *Clinical Gastroenterology.* 2nd ed. Philadelphia: Lea & Febiger, 1992, pp. 509–517.

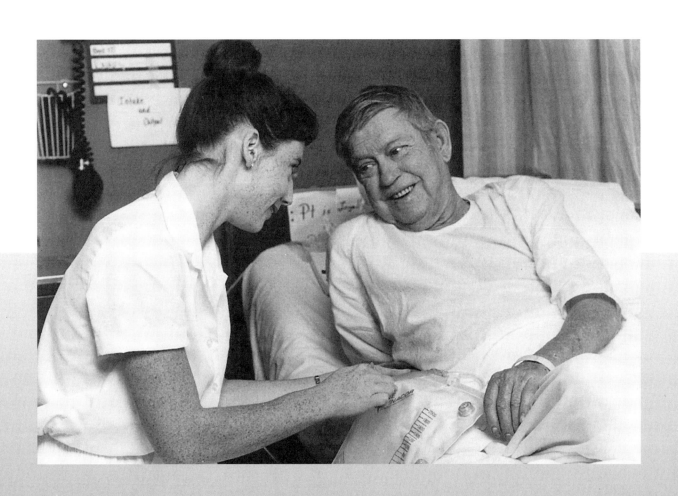

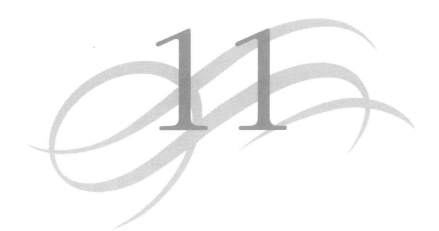

Age-Related Changes in the Genitourinary System

DOROTHY J. BRUNDAGE
ADRIANNE DILL LINTON

OBJECTIVES

List and describe the normal age-related changes in the kidney, ureters, bladder, urethra, prostate, vagina, and external genitalia.

Discuss the effect of these changes on urological functioning in older age.

Differentiate the common disorders of the genitourinary system associated with aging—specifically, acute and chronic renal failure, benign prostatic hypertrophy, prostate and bladder cancer, urinary tract infections, urinary retention and incontinence, and vaginitis.

Conduct an assessment of an older person with urological problems.

NORMAL STRUCTURE AND FUNCTION
NORMAL CHANGES IN STRUCTURE AND FUNCTION
Kidney
Ureters
Bladder
Urethra
Prostate
Vagina
External Genitalia
COMMON DISORDERS
Acute Renal Failure
Chronic Renal Failure
Benign Prostatic Hypertrophy
Prostate Cancer
Bladder Cancer
Urinary Tract Infections
Urinary Retention
Urinary Incontinence
Vaginitis
NURSING ASSESSMENT
History
Physical Assessment
NURSING DIAGNOSES
NURSING INTERVENTIONS AND EVALUATION

The changes in the genitourinary system, particularly changes related to urinary elimination, present problems to older people and challenges to nurses. Elderly people may have difficulty in maintaining bladder control, which may create great embarrassment. They try to avoid their embarrassment by avoiding public places or long trips, or limiting their liquid intake. The problem can lead to other conditions that can produce greater and greater limitations and ultimately a completely dysfunctional state of mind and body. Nurses are challenged to help older people maintain optimal functioning of the genitourinary system, particularly as related to elimination, in order to prevent unnecessary deterioration.

NORMAL STRUCTURE AND FUNCTION

The genitourinary system functions to eliminate bodily wastes formed in the kidneys and, in men, to provide a pathway for sperm in the reproductive process. The system components are the kidneys, ureters, urinary bladder, and urethra (Fig. 11–1). The normal functioning of this system depends on the interrelated activities of the circulatory, endocrine, and nervous systems.

The kidneys, which are paired organs located in the back abdominal wall on either side of the vertebral column, are each composed of approximately 1 million units called nephrons. The nephron is made up of two components: (1) a vascular component, or glomerulus, and (2) a tubular component.

FIGURE 11–1

Organs of the urinary system. (From Ignatavicius, D.D. and Bayne, M.V. *Medical-Surgical Nursing: A Nursing Process Approach.* 2nd ed. Philadelphia: W.B. Saunders, 1995, p. 2012.)

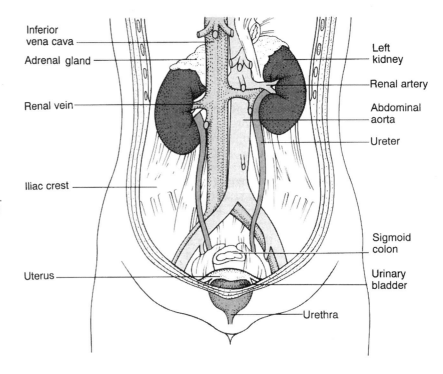

The glomerulus protrudes into the side of Bowman's capsule, a blind sac lined with epithelial cells. On the other side, the tubule originates from Bowman's capsule and consists of the proximal convoluted tubule, Henle's loop, the distal convoluted tubule, and the collecting duct (Fig. 11–2).

The kidneys excrete end-products of metabolism, excess amounts of normal bodily substances, and foreign substances such as drugs. Fluid and electrolyte balances are regulated by the kidneys. The kidney produces renin, various prostaglandins, erythropoietin, and active forms of vitamin D. The process of urine formation, which takes place in the nephrons, includes glomerular filtration, solute reabsorption and secretion, urine concentration and dilution, and urinary acidification and alkalinization. The urine collects in the renal pelvis and then flows through the ureter into the bladder, from which it is eliminated via the urethra (Fig. 11–3).

NORMAL CHANGES IN STRUCTURE AND FUNCTION

Kidney

Nephron

Anatomical and physiological changes occur in the kidney with aging. The kidney's adaptive capacity is decreased, but the built-in extra capacity permits the aging kidney to maintain homeostasis. This lessened reserve makes the aging person more vulnerable when changes due to trauma or disease are superimposed on the changes due to aging. Both cardiovascular and intrinsic renal changes are involved and are important considerations in clinical diagnosis and treatment.

According to Fillit and Rowe (1992), the anatomical changes in the nephron include loss of whole nephrons; progressive loss of renal mass, primarily in the cortex; increase in interstitial tissue; decrease in the number of identifiable glomeruli, primarily in the cortex (by degeneration and sclerosis); and thickening of the glomerular and tubular basement membranes. Both the proximal and distal convoluted tubules decrease in length and volume. Diverticula occur in the distal tubules. These may be the origin of simple retention cysts commonly found in elderly people. The large renal blood vessels show sclerotic changes that are more prominent in hypertensive individuals. Changes in small blood vessels are minimal in normotensive people (Levi and Schrier, 1990). Arteriolar-glomerular alterations revealed in

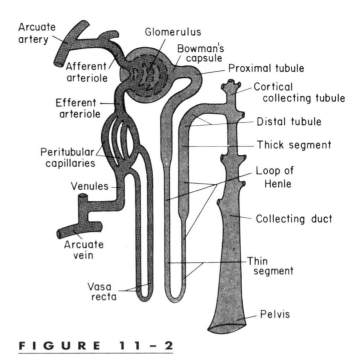

FIGURE 1 1 – 2

Basic structure of a nephron. (From Guyton, A.C. *Textbook of Medical Physiology.* 8th ed. Philadelphia: W.B. Saunders, 1991.)

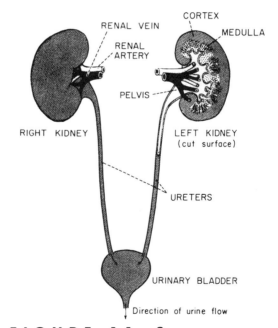

FIGURE 1 1 – 3

General organizational plan of the urinary system. The urine, formed by the kidney, collects in the renal pelvis and then flows through the ureter into the bladder, from which it is eliminated via the urethra. (Half the left kidney has been sliced away.) Note that the structure shows regional differences. The outer portion, which has a granular appearance, contains all the glomeruli. The collecting ducts form a large portion of the inner kidney, giving it a striped, pyramidal appearance, and they drain into the renal pelvis. (From Guyton, A.C. *Textbook of Medical Physiology.* 8th ed. Philadelphia: W.B. Saunders, 1991.)

TABLE 11–1
Differences in Renal Blood Flow and Glomerular Filtration Rate with Aging

	VALUES IN ADULTS	VALUES IN ELDERLY
Renal blood flow	600 ml/min/1.73 m²	300 ml/min/1.73 m²
Glomerular filtration rate	120 ml/min/1.73 m²	65.3 ml/min/1.73 m²

From Rowe, J.W. Renal system. *In* Rowe, J.W. and Besdine, R.W. (eds.). *Health and Disease.* Boston: Little, Brown, 1982, pp. 165–183.

microangiographical and histological studies include hyalinization and collapse of the glomerular tuft and obliteration of the lumen of the preglomerular arteriole, resulting in diminished blood flow. Another change is the development of connections between the afferent and efferent arterioles, which allows the blood to bypass the sclerosed glomeruli. Blood flow to the medullary area is maintained via the vasa recta (Levi and Schrier, 1990).

Age-related physiological changes include a decreased filtering surface area, with no change in permeability of the glomerular basement membrane (Rowe, 1986b). Progressive decreases in renal blood flow (RBF) and glomerular filtration rate (GFR) are associated with the age-related decrease in cardiac output, renal mass, and filtering surface (Table 11–1). The creatinine clearance also decreases with age (Levi and Schrier, 1990; Fillit and Rowe, 1992) (Table 11–2). When the dosage of a drug is critical, the creatinine clearance value, not the serum creatinine level, should be used as the criterion for renal function. The serum creatinine level does not increase with the decrease in GFR because the muscle mass from which creatinine arises falls with age. Serum creatinine levels overestimate renal function in older persons.

The kidney's endocrine functions change with age. Plasma renin and plasma aldosterone levels decrease in the normotensive person. The conversion of 1-OH-cholecalciferol to 1-25-(OH)₂-cholecalciferol is decreased.

This may be the cause of the decrease in intestinal absorption of calcium seen in normal subjects and subjects with osteoporosis. A decrease in erythropoietin may contribute to anemia.

The vasoconstrictor response is not affected by age, but there may be changes in the vasodilating system. There is less compensatory renal hypertrophy in the aging kidney, and therefore the kidney is less able to compensate for function lost after a unilateral nephrectomy.

Tubules

Changes in the tubules decrease the tubular transport mechanisms. The ability to concentrate and dilute the urine in response to water or salt excess or deprivation is diminished. As a related problem, excretion of drugs is altered (Beers, 1992). The transport maximum declines at a rate parallel to the decline in GFR. This change results in a higher renal threshold for glucose. An older person may have an elevated blood glucose level but no evidence of glycosuria. The change in tubular transport is also reflected in the specific gravity and maximum osmolarity of the urine, the ability to dilute the urine, and the ability to handle acid-base loads.

The adaptive mechanisms for maintaining the constant blood volume and the composition of the extracellular fluid are impaired. Decreased ability to concentrate the urine is related to the decreased number of nephrons, the increased osmotic load each remaining nephron must handle, the mild osmotic diuresis that accompanies this change, and the decreased renin and aldosterone levels. The loop of Henle develops a defect in the thick ascending limb that decreases the medullary hypertonicity. This change may also contribute to the kidney's impaired ability to concentrate the urine.

The diurnal rhythm of urine production is lost; the rate of urine production is the same over 24 hours. Nocturia may be an expected outcome.

The water balance is affected by the inability of the loop of Henle, the distal convoluted tubule, and the collecting ducts to concentrate the urine and an age-related decrease in response to antidiuretic hormone (ADH). These factors are important when water intake is limited (overnight dehydration before tests) and when water losses are increased (fever, vomiting, diarrhea). The use of contrast agents with their high osmolarity in the presence of dehydration may lead to acute renal failure in elderly people. The decreased GFR augments the potential

TABLE 11–2
Differences in Creatinine Clearance with Aging

		VALUES IN ADULTS	VALUES IN ELDERLY
Creatinine clearance	Men: 85–125 ml/min/1.73 m² Women: 75–115 ml/min/1.73 m²		96.9 ± 2.9 ml/min/1.73 m²

From Rowe, J.W. Renal system. *In* Rowe, J.W. and Besdine, R.W. (eds.). *Health and Disease.* Boston: Little, Brown, 1982, pp. 165–183.

for injury from such agents or hypotension caused by hypovolemia.

An aged person's response to a decrease in salt intake is slow. A salt-losing tendency in illness is compounded by inadequate salt intake and may result in impaired cardiac, renal, and mental function. Careful administration of salt-containing fluids is required in elderly persons who are volume depleted.

Dehydration can cause an acute confusional state. Although reduced thirst sensation has been documented in the elderly, dehydration problems arise more from a physical difficulty in obtaining and drinking fluids. Altered mental status can contribute to decreased water intake. People who are incontinent also tend to restrict their intake in an attempt to avoid the problem. Fluid losses also occur with vomiting and diarrhea.

A decrease in the ability to taste salt may result in an increased salt intake without an appropriate increase in water. Dehydration with hyperosmolarity results. If an excess of sodium is ingested, resulting in volume overload, the kidney is less able to handle the problem owing to the decrease in GFR. Problems occur when the older person increases salt in the diet or receives it in intravenous fluids, medications, or sodium-containing contrast agents.

Water intoxication may result in hyponatremia. This may occur because of the decreased ability to excrete water related to decreased RBF and excess secretion of ADH. Medications that increase ADH secretion (vasopressin, chlorpropamide, carbamazepine, aspirin, and acetaminophen) should be used with caution.

An excess of potassium may occur because of decreased renin and aldosterone levels and decreased GFR. Normal excretion of potassium and retention of sodium is altered. Other factors that may contribute to hyperkalemia are gastrointestinal bleeding, intravenous administration of potassium-containing salts, acidosis, and potassium-sparing diuretics such as spironolactone.

Problems in acid excretion by the kidney are probably associated with the tubular and collecting ducts defects in excreting ammonium. They do not appear to be related to the decrease in GFR.

Changes in the kidney's function with aging alter the renal excretion of drugs. Drugs excreted in an unchanged form are likely to be excreted more slowly. Renal disease may cause an accumulation of drugs and their toxic metabolites. A low-protein intake may result in low serum albumin levels with less binding of the drug, thereby making more free drug available.

Drug dosages of digitalis, aminoglycosides, and other antibiotics should be calculated using the creatinine clearance. A decrease in clearance means an increase in the drug's half-life for drugs that are excreted primarily by the kidney. The creatinine clearance is not very practical for routine use. Equations and nomograms have been developed that estimate a person's creatinine clearance from sex, weight, age, and serum creatinine level. The equation suggested by Levi and Schrier (1990) is:

$$\text{Estimated creatinine clearance} = \frac{(140 - \text{age}) \times \text{weight in kilograms}}{72 \times \text{serum creatinine level}}$$

For women, multiply the figure obtained by .85 (Lindeman, 1992).

In general, the dosage is reduced and the dosing interval remains constant, or the dosage remains constant and the dosing interval is increased.

Ureters

The major defects in the ureters are related to the vesicoureteral junction and the possible reflux of urine into the ureter and subsequently into the renal pelvis. Bilateral obstruction of the ureters can occur when the uterus is prolapsed, causing pressure on the ureters.

Bladder

Age-related changes in the bladder include replacement of smooth muscle and elastic tissue with fibrous connective tissue, and the formation of trabeculae, diverticula, and pseudodiverticulitis. The bladder muscles weaken, and incomplete emptying may occur. There is a decrease in the force of the urine stream. Bladder capacity decreases, and frequency of urination increases. The ability to postpone voiding declines (Brandeis et al., 1992). Bladder outlet changes may cause obstruction in the male (benign prostatic hypertrophy) or incontinence in the female (relaxation of pelvic musculature). Overstretching of the bladder wall may occur with urinary retention. Tumors of the bladder may occur.

Phases of the urination process include (1) bladder fills until the person senses the desire to void, (2) person voluntarily controls and postpones urination, (3) person empties bladder at the appropriate time and place. Incontinence may occur with neurogenic disease, overflow in the absence of a lesion, or selected drug therapy. Stress incontinence may occur with a sudden increase in intra-abdominal pressure. Interference in the urination process may arise from alterations in the sphincter muscle, neural controls, outlet size, muscle strength, or sensation of need to void. Defects in peripheral innervation may occur with prostatic surgery, alcoholism, and diabetes mellitus. Uninhibited bladder contractions may occur for reasons not well understood (Augspurger, 1990; Brocklehurst et al., 1992).

Urethra

There may be difficulty in opening or closing the bladder outlet. Decreased closing pressure may be caused by loss of striated muscle that makes up the external sphincter (Brocklehurst et al., 1992). Both men and women may experience difficulty in starting the urinary stream. In men the problem is usually benign prostatic hypertrophy. In women the problem is related to childbirth or surgery that weakens the pelvic musculature. Urethral stenosis or stricture may occur in aging women. Diminished estrogen secretion affects all tissues of the perineal area including the urethra.

Prostate

The major change in the prostate that occurs with aging is hypertrophy. Any enlargement can decrease or obstruct the urinary flow. Such a change predisposes the person to urinary tract infections, especially after the use of instruments to examine the urinary tract. In response to the narrowed outlet the bladder wall muscle hypertrophies in order to increase the pressure to empty it. The outcome of such hypertrophy may be bladder diverticuli, residual urine after voiding, overflow incontinence, vesicoureteral reflux, and eventually renal damage.

Vagina

The tissues of the vagina atrophy because of estrogen deficiency. Secretions diminish; vaginal pH rises; the normal flora are altered; the lining is thinner, drier, less elastic, and more easily traumatized. The length and width of the vagina diminish. The outcome frequently is painful intercourse, vaginal infections, and pruritus.

External Genitalia

The labia atrophy, shrinking in size owing to loss of estrogen and progesterone stimulation. They are subject to irritation (pruritus

vulvae) and infection. Vaginal stenosis may occur. Alterations in sexual response associated with aging include a delay in lubrication of the vagina as well as production of a smaller amount. Painful uterine cramps may occur with orgasm. With the vaginal changes already described, intercourse may be painful. Impaired sexual function in men may be attributed to altered blood flow to the penis, physical discomforts of chronic illnesses, depression, and the effects of drugs, including alcohol (Butler et al., 1992). In the older man, erections develop more slowly, there is greater difficulty maintaining an erection, and the unresponsive refractory period is prolonged (Brown and Cooper, 1992). (See Chapter 12.)

COMMON DISORDERS

This section discusses some of the most common genitourinary problems of the elderly. Each part includes a brief description with prevalence, pathophysiology, clinical presentation, methods of diagnosis and treatment, and prognosis.

Acute Renal Failure

Acute renal failure (ARF) is a sudden decrease in GFR caused by disease of the blood vessels, glomeruli, tubules, or interstitial tissue. ARF may be caused by intrinsic, prerenal, or postrenal problems. The resulting decrease in function may or may not be reversible.

The elderly are particularly at risk for ARF because the more common inciting events occur more frequently in the elderly, who may have multiple impairments. Such events are dehydration, diabetes mellitus, multiple myeloma, congestive heart failure, major surgery, sepsis, and atherosclerosis (Fillit and Rowe, 1992).

Intrinsic problems causing ARF include arterial or venous thromboembolic events, cortical necrosis, acute tubular necrosis (ATN) from nephrotoxic agents (contrast media, nonsteroidal anti-inflammatory drugs, and antibiotics, including aminoglycosides, penicillins, and cephalosporins), and acute glomerulonephritis (Levi and Schrier, 1990). Prerenal causes include hypotension, sepsis, volume depletion, congestive heart failure, and increased vascular resistance. Postrenal causes include urinary tract obstruction from tumors, prostatism, calculi, papillary necrosis, or blood clots.

The presenting signs and symptoms seen

most frequently are azotemia, oliguria, hypotension or hypertension, hyperkalemia, acidosis, and altered mental status. Nonoliguric failure may occur and is manifested by elevated serum BUN and creatinine without oliguria for several days after a brief hypotensive episode or exposure to nephrotoxic agents. Renal function normally improves gradually (Fillit and Rowe, 1992).

Diagnostic studies include renal function tests. A high degree of suspicion helps. A history of exposure to contrast media or renal insufficiency is important. It is especially important to detect contributing factors such as urinary obstruction or strictures of renal blood vessels (Fillit and Rowe, 1992; Lindeman, 1992).

Treatment is similar to that for a younger person. Electrolyte and hemoglobin values are monitored. Reversible causes such as obstruction are addressed promptly; catheterization, placement of a nephrostomy tube, or placement of a stent to facilitate urine flow may be employed (Lindeman, 1992). Antibiotics are ordered if infection is present. Either hemodialysis or peritoneal dialysis is instituted early to treat hyperkalemia, volume overload, and azotemia. Sodium bicarbonate is given to correct acidosis. Diet prescriptions include protein and potassium restrictions and sufficient calories to prevent catabolism. Sodium is not usually markedly restricted. Dosage adjustments are made for essential drugs while the patient is oliguric. Fillit and Rowe (1992) recommend using blood studies to monitor progress rather than inserting a catheter to measure output because of the increased risk of infection associated with indwelling catheters.

The aged kidney can recover from episodes of transient and reversible acute renal failure (ARF). However, the mortality rate is about 50 per cent. Survival is less in older people than in younger people.

Chronic Renal Failure

Chronic renal failure (CRF) is a permanent loss of renal function. The causes in the older patient include age-dependent diseases such as chronic glomerulonephritis, diabetic nephropathy, hypertensive nephropathy, polycystic kidney disease, obstructive uropathy, and multiple myeloma. Other causes are nephrotoxic agents and volume depletion (Fillit and Rowe, 1992). Mild or moderate renal failure can progress to end-stage renal disease.

The picture of CRF may include azotemia, oliguria, hypertension, nausea and vomiting, edema, itching and dry skin, fatigue, malaise, weakness, cognitive and personality changes, and infection. However, many elderly people with CRF present with decompensation of pre-existing medical conditions rather than symptoms of uremia (Levi and Schrier, 1990). A flat plate x-ray of the abdomen will reveal if the kidneys are small or contracted (chronic renal failure) or normal or enlarged (polycystic kidney disease, diabetes mellitus, or obstructive uropathy). Other useful studies are excretory urograms, ultrasonography, and renal scans. Percutaneous renal biopsy may be done, although it carries some risks of complications that must be considered (Fillit and Rowe, 1992). Typical blood chemistries are as follows:

Blood urea nitrogen	>70–80 mg/dl
Serum creatinine	<6–8 mg/dl
Creatinine clearance	<20 ml/min
Serum potassium	3.5–6 mEq/liter
Serum phosphate	>5 mg/dl
Serum calcium	8.0–10.5 mg/dl

The serum creatinine level does not rise in proportion to the loss of renal function. It is important to identify any reversible components: Obstruction should be relieved and infection treated.

Treatment of CRF is two-pronged, focusing on managing the effects of the condition and on correcting any reversible contributing factors. Management includes controlling hypertension, anemia, and acidosis and adjusting serum levels of potassium, calcium, and phosphate. Drug dosages are adjusted because of the altered elimination that can lead to toxicity. Anemia is treated with oral or parenteral iron supplements and is monitored via serum iron and ferritin. Transfusions of packed red blood cells and administration of erythropoietin may be ordered (Fillit and Rowe, 1992; Lindeman, 1992). Dietary modifications are generally less strict than in younger people, but they may include moderate restrictions of protein and sodium. Potassium is more restricted.

Dialysis is the treatment of choice, either at home or in a dialysis center, and the number of older people on dialysis is increasing (Kutner et al., 1992). Excessive delay of initiating dialysis increases the risks of disabling effects of uremia (Levi and Schrier, 1990). Since the arteriovenous fistula often matures more slowly in elderly people, it should be created as soon as possible after making a decision that hemodialysis will be used. Creation of the fistula is sometimes difficult in the older person because of peripheral vascular changes. If hemodialysis is used, special attention must be paid to cardiovascular and pulmonary status, control of diabetes, ocular changes, nutrition, and anticoagulation. Often psychological adjustment is very good.

Cardiac disease may make hemodialysis too dangerous for some people. Also, some patients are not good candidates for anticoagulation therapy, as required with hemodialysis. In these and other situations, peritoneal dialysis may be recommended. Results of continuous ambulatory peritoneal dialysis in elderly people compare favorably with those seen in younger patients. Severe depression or dementia may preclude such treatment. For patients who are unwilling or unable to try continuous ambulatory peritoneal dialysis, in-center dialysis may be an alternative.

Renal transplantation has been successful in patients over age 60 years (Lindeman, 1992). Cadaveric donors are used more frequently. As experience with older patients increases, the major problem resulting seems to be the lack of available organs. Complications are more common in elderly people, and death usually results from infection, cardiovascular disease, or stroke (Fillit and Rowe, 1992; Lindeman, 1992). Fatal rupture of colonic diverticula is more common in the elderly transplant patient. Steroid diabetes increases the risk of infection.

The outcome depends on the presence or absence of other organ or bodily system disease. Psychological factors and the support of family are also important.

Benign Prostatic Hypertrophy

An enlargement of the prostate of unknown etiology is called benign prostatic hypertrophy (BPH). Aging is a factor in this entity, which undoubtedly has a hormonal basis (Brendler et al., 1994; Diokno and Hollander, 1992). Researchers are exploring the roles of the testis, intracellular dihydrotestosterone, and androgen/estrogen synergism in the development of BPH (Donohue et al., 1990). There is no apparent relationship between BPH and cancer of the prostate, although some factors such as age are shared (Mebust et al., 1992). BPH occurs in more than 80 per cent of men over age 60 years. Half of them have urinary difficulties, and 10 per cent of those need surgery.

Most often BPH is asymptomatic. Enlargement of the intracapsular tissue may obstruct the bladder outlet. The location of the enlargement is more important than the amount. Patients present with urinary tract infections, incontinence, difficulty in starting urine flow, retention of urine, dysuria, posturination dribbling, decreased force and size of urine stream, frequency, nocturia, and ur-

gency. These last three may not be related to the severity of the disease. Over time, obstruction can lead to bladder decompensation, overflow incontinence, hydronephrosis, and renal failure (Diokno and Hollander, 1992).

Diagnostic procedures may include urinalysis, urine culture and sensitivity smears, suprapubic percussion for bladder distention, digital rectal examination to assess prostate size and texture, retrograde pyelogram to study urinary structures and detect diverticula and reflux, transrectal ultrasonography, cystourethrography to visualize urine flow through the urethra, cystoscopy to evaluate outlet obstruction, and uroflowmetry (more than 15 ml per minute is normal; less than 10 ml per minute reflects obstruction) (Blacklock and Higgins, 1992; Diokno and Hollander, 1992; Donohue et al., 1990). In addition, an ultrasound-guided transrectal biopsy may be done. A chart of voiding frequency and volumes may be helpful in assessing the condition.

Treatment options in common use include balloon dilatation of the bladder neck and prostatic urethra, placement of a stent in the prostatic urethra, pharmacological therapy, and surgery. Additional studies are needed to assess the long-term benefits of balloon dilatation because study results have varied (Donatucci et al., 1993; Hernandez-Graulau, 1993; Petrovich et al., 1993; Vale et al., 1993). Moseley (1992) asserts that anterior commissurotomy through the fibromuscular stoma is the key to successful balloon dilatation. Hald and Nordling (1992) reviewed 17 studies of patients who were treated with stents; while noting that most of the studies were small, they concluded that the stent provided a useful alternative to catheterization when surgery was not advisable. Drug therapy may employ alpha-adrenergic blockers or antiandrogenic agents. Alpha-adrenergic blockers decrease the sympathetic stimulation of the bladder neck and prostate gland. The use of antiandrogens improves urinary flow rates, presumably by decreasing prostate size, and shows promise in clinical trials (Diokno and Hollander, 1992; Jonler et al., 1994).

Indications for surgery include complete urinary retention, renal insufficiency caused by obstruction, recurrent urinary tract infections, bladder stones, and recurrent gross hematuria (Denis et al., 1992). Four types of prostatectomy are used: transurethral resection (TUR), suprapubic prostatectomy, retropubic prostatectomy, and perineal prostatectomy. Which procedure is used depends on the size of the prostate, the location of the

TABLE 11-3

Results of Various Treatments for Benign Prostatic Hypertrophy in Men with Moderate Symptoms of Prostatism

	TURP	TUIP	OPEN PROSTATECTOMY	WATCHFUL WAITING	BALLOON DILATATION	ALPHA-ADRENERGIC BLOCKERS
Chance for improvement of symptoms	80% Range: 78–83%	88% Range: 75–96%	98% Range: 94–99.8%	42% Range: 31–55%	57% Range: 37–76%	74% Range: 59–86%
Degree of symptom improvement	73%	85%	79%	<32%	51%	51%
Mean peak flow rates (ml/sec) pretreatment post-treatment	8 15	8 18	8 23	9 8	7 13	8 13
Chance of further treatment within 5 yr	8.1% Range: 6.8–9.6%	3.4% Range: 1.1–9.6%	0.4% Range: 0.04–4.2%	26.4% Range: 7.2–55.5%	20.1% Range: 9.2–35.2%	50% probability >10% but <26%

TURP, transurethral prostatectomy; TUIP, transurethral incision of the prostate.
Figures represent a summary of published studies (1960–1990) reviewed by the Agency for Health Care Policy and Research.
Modified with permission from Brendler, C., et al. Surgical treatment for benign prostatic hyperplasia. *Cancer Suppl* 70(1):372, 1992.

enlargement, whether surgery of the bladder is needed, and the age and physical condition of the patient. Newer procedures that are being studied include transurethral laser prostatectomy, transrectal microwave hyperthermia, transurethral microwave hyperthermia, transurethral thermal therapy, and transurethral incision of the prostate (TUIP)

(Kletscher and Oesterling, 1992). These alternative treatments are most likely to be used at this time for patients who are poor surgical risks. Denis et al. (1992) observed that various surgical alternatives are probably appropriate for some types of patients but not others, and that the best choice must be sought for the individual. Table 11–3 com-

TABLE 11-4

Complications of Surgical Treatment for Benign Prostatic Hypertrophy

COMPLICATION	TUIP	TURP	OPEN PROSTATECTOMY
Overall complications	14.0% (2.9–35.5%)*	16.1% (5.8–32.1%)	21.7% (7.3–43.6%)
Total incontinence	0.1% (0.02–1.9%)	0.8% (0.6–1.2%)	0.4% (0.2–0.6%)
Impotence†	12.6% (3.9–24.5%)	15.7% (3.3–34.8%)	19.0% (0.8–12.1%)
Retrograde ejaculation	39%	68%	72%
Pain Days of injectable medications Days of oral medications	0–2 2–3	0–2 2–4	2–4 7–10
Blood transfusion	<1%	5%	NA
Need for operative treatment of surgical complications	2.9% (2.1–4.2%)	3.3% (0.8–11.7%)	4.2% (0.8–12.1%)
Chance of death in 30–90 days‡	1% (0.2–1.9%)	1.5% (1.3–1.7%)	2% (0.9–5.3%)

TUIP: transurethral incision of the prostate; TURP: transurethral resection of the prostate; NA, not available.
* 95% confidence interval.
† Because sexual function usually has been evaluated subjectively, further prospective objective data are needed to determine the actual risk of impotence after surgical prostatectomy.
‡ For reference, the chance of death for a 67-year-old man during a period of 90 days is approximately 0.8%.
Modified with permission from Brendler, C. et al. Surgical treatment for benign prostatic hyperplasia. *Cancer Suppl* 70(1):372, 1992.

pares results of various treatments for BPH. If there is weakness of the detrusor muscle and a hypotonic bladder, surgery will not improve the urine flow rate.

This condition has a good prognosis, but postoperative complications of TUR include hemorrhage, urinary retention, urethral stricture, bladder neck contracture, and total urinary incontinence (Doll et al., 1992) (Table 11–4). Impotence rates after surgery for BPH have been reported at between 5 per cent and 34 per cent. Lindner et al. (1991) reported an impotence rate of 11.8 per cent in 210 prostatectomy patients. Impotence is most likely to occur after perineal prostatectomy for cancer. Retrograde ejaculation may occur.

Prostate Cancer

Cancer of the prostate is the third most frequent cause of cancer deaths in men over 55 years of age (Brendler, 1994; Diokno and Hollander, 1992). Unsuspected carcinoma is found in approximately 10 per cent of prostate glands operated on for prostate enlargement (Lee et al., 1992). Most often it is adenocarcinoma. The incidence of prostatic cancer increases with age, but tumors appearing in younger men are more lethal. The etiology is not clear. It is a slow-growing tumor and, on occasion, inactive. The active form may be confined to the prostate, invade the capsule, or metastasize to nearby tissues: nodes, liver, lung, and bone. Metastases spread by local growth or by hematogenous or lymphatic routes.

There are no early symptoms. When symptoms occur they include a firm mass or nodule found on rectal examination; increased levels of serum acid phosphatase, prostatic specific antigen (PSA), and prostatic acid phosphatase (PAP); and a positive bone scan or node when the tumor has moved beyond the capsule. Patients may have obstructive symptoms, or hematuria may occur.

Diagnosis is made by digital rectal examination. Tissue samples may be obtained for study by transrectal fine-needle aspiration or by transperitoneal or transurethral biopsy. Flam et al. (1992) recommended transrectal ultrasound as the best approach to study the prostate when cancer is suspected. Staging is done to guide the selection of appropriate therapy. A variety of staging systems are used. Recent recommendations from the American Urological Association propose staging based on tumor volumes (Graham et al., 1992). Procedures used to stage the cancer may include chest radiographs, bone scans, excretory urography, computed to-

mography, magnetic resonance imaging, and transurethral ultrasonography. Pelvic lymph nodes should be examined. Helpful biological markers used in staging include PSA and PAP. They are also important in detecting residual or recurrent disease (Diokno and Hollander, 1992; Lee et al., 1992).

Treatment depends on the stage and may include surgery (radical prostatectomy) (Link and Freiha, 1991; Mettlin et al., 1994), radiation therapy, hormone treatment, chemotherapy, and watchful waiting. If cancer is found in those over age 80 years, careful observation may be the treatment of choice. External beam radiation or implanted interstitial radioactive seeds may be used if surgery is not feasible. Hormone suppression by orchiectomy, estrogens, or antiandrogen drugs (flutamide, cyproterone, luteinizing hormone–releasing hormone, leuprolide acetate, diethylstilbestrol) may inhibit growth of the tumor (Goldspiel and Kohler, 1990; Goldenberg and Bruchovsky, 1991). Chemotherapy is least effective and is used as a last resort (Hirsch and Schwartz, 1992).

The prognosis is good if the tumor is found early. Localized disease is curable. Inactive disease should be watched closely. The virulence of the tumor seems to be less in older men. However, disease stabilization has occurred with some chemotherapeutic agents used alone or in combination with hormonal agents (Donohue et al., 1990; Schellhammer et al., 1992). Impotence is a potential complication of radical prostate surgery, external beam radiation therapy, and hormonal therapy. Before nerve-sparing techniques were available, the incidence of impotence with radical prostatectomy was very high. New surgical techniques have greatly decreased this complication. In addition, a number of treatment options are available for older patients who do experience post-treatment impotence. They include drug therapy, vacuum suction and penile constriction devices, intracavernosal injection therapy, venous ligation, and placement of penile prostheses (Telang and Farah, 1992). Cure is unlikely if the tumor has spread beyond the capsule, but it may be treated as a chronic condition that can often be managed for a long time (Donohue et al., 1990).

Bladder Cancer

Bladder cancer is the second most common form of all genitourinary tumors. Most tumors occur in people over the age of 50 years; they are five times more common in men (Carroll, 1992; Skinner and Skinner, 1994). The incidence increases with age. Environmental factors associated with the occurrence of these tumors include industrial exposure (dye, rubber, leather), paint, organic chemicals, electrical cable manufacture, and aluminum production. Cigarette smoking is believed to account for at least 50 per cent of all bladder cancer. The total amount smoked is more significant than the patient's current smoking status. Painless gross hematuria is the most common presenting symptom, but the patient may have signs of bladder irritation or asymptomatic pyuria (Skinner and Skinner, 1994). Bleeding with clot formation may cause urinary retention. Early diagnosis is very important. Diagnosis is made with an excretory urogram, cystourethroscopy, and transurethral resection (TUR) or biopsy.

Treatment depends on staging, which is categorized as superficial, invasive (no metastases), or metastatic. Metastases occur in the lymph nodes, liver, lungs, and bone. Some physicians treat the symptoms with antibiotics on a trial basis, a practice criticized by Skinner and Skinner (1994), who caution that this only delays diagnosis. TUR with fulguration of the tumor is used for superficial tumors with or without intravesical chemotherapy (thiotepa, doxorubicin, BCG, mitomycin C). Treatment options for invasive, nonmetastatic disease include radical cystectomy with urinary diversion or definitive radiation therapy. Adjuvant chemotherapy may be advised for patients with more advanced disease. Systemic chemotherapy using various combinations of agents (cisplatin, methotrexate, vinblastine, and doxorubicin) is used for metastatic disease (Carroll, 1992; Skinner and Skinner, 1994). The prognosis in superficial disease is 60 to 80 per cent survival at 5 years. Survival is less in the other two stages.

Urinary Tract Infections

Infections of the urinary tract (UTI) are common health problems in elderly people. They include urethritis, cystitis, and pyelonephritis. The prevalence increases with age. Risk factors include urinary stasis (decrease in fluid intake, less frequent washout of bladder and urethra), increase in urine pH, institutionalization, concomitant disease, sexual activity (postmenopausal changes increase the susceptibility of women), and catheterization or other instrumentation.

Bacteria enter through the urethra and ascend the urinary tract. They may cause bacteremia. On the other hand, septicemia may cause pyelonephritis. Anatomical abnormalities in the urinary tract predispose a person to UTI. Organisms involved frequently are *Escherichia coli, Proteus, Enterobacter, Klebsiella,* *Pseudomonas, Staphylococcus aureus, Candida,* and anaerobes.

Most patients are asymptomatic, but some have fever, vomiting, or signs of other illness, or the classic signs may be present: frequency, dysuria, and urgency. Hematuria may be present. Foul urine odor may be present with infection, but this is sometimes noted in the absence of bacteriuria. If pyelonephritis is the problem, the picture may not be the same as that seen in a younger person (fever, chills, flank pain). This is a medical emergency because septicemia may develop.

Diagnosis is made difficult in the absence of fever and reduced recognition of pain. Urine from a clean-catch specimen is examined for bacteriuria and pyuria and by Gram stain and culture. The significance of bacteriuria in elderly people is in question. The prevalence of bacteriuria among community-dwelling women age 80 years and over is about 25 per cent; for men, the rate is estimated at 5 to 10 per cent. Fifty per cent of severely impaired institutionalized elderly people have bacteriuria, and the rate rises to nearly 100 per cent with long-term indwelling catheterization. The presence of pyuria has traditionally been used to differentiate infection from colonization, but this is not helpful in elderly people since virtually all who have bacteriuria also have pyuria (Nicolle, 1994). If this infection is a relapse or reinfection, a urological abnormality should be suspected, and an excretory urogram should be obtained after the infection has cleared to look for obstruction or reflux.

For symptomatic urinary infections, an appropriate drug can be started once the infecting organism has been identified. Most antimicrobial drugs are effective for the short-term therapy needed; high blood levels of effective drugs are needed to treat pyelonephritis. Asymptomatic bacteriuria in elderly persons is generally not treated unless there is evidence of renal disease, urinary tract abnormalities, or clinical signs of sepsis (Fillit and Rowe, 1992; Levi and Schrier, 1990; Nicolle, 1994). The indiscriminate use of broad-spectrum antimicrobials to treat asymptomatic bacteriuria invites the emergence of resistant organisms, especially among elderly institutionalized patients who tend to harbor gram-negative organisms in the oropharynx (Nicolle, 1994). On occasion, infection-suppressive agents such as methenamine mandelate (Mandelamine) or acidifying agents such as vitamin C are used.

The prognosis for simple UTI is good, although recurrence is very common. However, in a chronically ill, debilitated patient the prognosis may be limited. Rousseau

TABLE 11-5

Prospective Studies Reporting the Association Between Asymptomatic Bacteriuria and Survival in Elderly People

STUDY	POPULATION	NO. OF SUBJECTS	PROPORTION BACTERIURIC		OBSERVATIONS
Sourander and Kasanen	Random sample >65 yr, Turka, Finland	405	Women: Men:	33% 11%	Increased mortality in bacteriuric women; at 5 yr, 51% versus 29% survival
Dontas et al.	Residents of Athens home for aged	342	Women: Men:	28% 14%	Significantly increased survival at 10 yr for nonbacteriuric men and women
Nordenstam et al.	Representative sample, Goteborg, Sweden, age 70 yr	1966	Women: Men:	18% 2.5%	No significant difference in mortality between bacteriuric and nonbacteriuric at 5 or 10 yr when stratified for underlying disease
Heinamaki et al.	>85 yr population, Tampere, Finland	561	27%		No difference in mortality between bacteriuric and nonbacteriuric
Nicolle et al.	Male nursing home population	91	Persistent: Intermittent:	25% 34%	No difference in mortality between bacteriuric and nonbacteriuric

From Nicolle, L.E. Urinary tract infection. *In* O'Donnell, P.D. (ed.). *Geriatric Urology.* Boston: Little, Brown, 1994, p. 406.

(1990) reported studies that demonstrated increased mortality among elderly people with asymptomatic bacteriuria, but others (Fillit and Rowe, 1992; Nicolle, 1994) argue that there is no consistent support for this claim (Table 11–5). It is noted that less than 1 per cent of nursing home deaths are attributed to urinary tract infections. Morbidity has not been widely studied, but these infections account for only a small number of hospital admissions (Nicolle, 1994).

Urinary Retention

Urinary retention may be an acute problem, developing rapidly, or a more chronic one that develops over time. Inability to urinate is not an uncommon problem in elderly people. Causes include phimosis, paraphimosis, meatal stenosis, urethral trauma or stricture, BPH, cancer of the prostate, bladder tumor, bleeding with clot formation, intrapelvic tumors in women, prolapse of the uterus, neurological impairment (diabetes mellitus, nerve damage related to neoplasms), and fecal impaction. Drugs may also cause urinary retention (see Table 11–6).

The patient with retention is unable to void and has a palpable suprapubic mass with discomfort. There may be some dribbling urination. Diagnostic procedures include catheterization, cystoscopy, and excretory urography. The onset, duration, and precipitating factors should be identified. If retention has been prolonged and azotemia has developed, postobstructive diuresis may occur. The fluid lost should be monitored and replaced. The retained urea, salt, and water are excreted. Treatment may include urethral dilatation, local application of estrogens, pharmacotherapy (Table 11–7), or surgery to correct the urinary tract abnormality; if it is not correctable, then intermittent catheterization is used. For the patient at home, a clean technique of catheterization is used. Prognosis depends on the cause of the retention.

Urinary Incontinence

Incontinence is a condition in which involuntary losses of urine occur, causing a social or hygienic problem. It is difficult to estimate the prevalence of urinary incontinence because many people fail to report it. The prevalence among nursing home residents is estimated at 50 per cent. McDowell and colleagues (1994) studied frail elders who lived at home. Forty-one per cent of those interviewed reported urinary incontinence, compared with 59 per cent of those seen in a geriatric assessment unit and 16 per cent of those who saw private physicians. Harrison and Memel (1994) found a reported rate of 53 per cent among community-dwelling women aged 20 and older. These findings suggest that urinary incontinence may be much more common than the often-quoted estimates of 15 to 30 per cent (Broderick and Wein, 1994; Furner et al., 1994). Unquestioning acceptance of incontinence in the aged is inappropriate. It is not an expected, permanent outcome of aging, but age-related factors increase the risk of variables that can lead to incontinence. These factors are weakened pelvic floor, benign prostatic hypertrophy and increased incidence of urinary tract infections, fecal incontinence, and impaired

TABLE 11–6
Drugs That May Cause Various Degrees of Urinary
Retention or Obstructive Symptoms

Brain level: antiepileptics
  Carbamazepine
  Clonazepam
  Opioids and other narcotics
  Phenytoin
Spinal cord level: polysynaptic inhibitors (effect on blad-
  der is compensated for by reduced outlet resistance)
  Baclofen
Bladder level
  Anticholinergic agents
  Antihistamines
  Antiparkinsonism drugs
    Benztropine
    Biperiden
    Cycrimine
    Levodopa
    Procyclidine
    Trihexyphenidyl
  Beta-adrenergic agonists (not common)
  Calcium antagonists
    Flunarizine
    Nifedipine
    Terodiline
  Diuretics
  Ganglionic blocking agents
  Musculotropic relaxants
    Diazepam
    Dicyclomine
    Flavoxate
    Oxybutynin
  Prostaglandin inhibitors (not common)
  Psychiatric drugs
    Phenothiazines
    Tricyclic antidepressants
  Others
    Bromocriptine
    Hydralazine
    Isoniazid
    Theophylline
Bladder outlet level
  Alpha-adrenergic agonists
  Beta-adrenergic blocking agents (by potentiating alpha-
    adrenergic receptors)
  Estrogen combinations
  Others
    Amphetamines
    Levodopa
    Tricyclic antidepressants, particularly imipramine

From Bissada, N.K. and Finkbeiner, A.E. Urologic manifestations of drug therapy. *Urol Clin North Am* 15:725, 1988.

TABLE 11–7
Drugs Used to Treat Urinary Retention

ACTION	CLASSIFICATION	EXAMPLES
Increase bladder contractility	Cholinergics	bethanecol (Urecholine)
	Prostaglandins (bladder instillation)	prostaglandin E$_2$
	Alpha-adrenergic antagonists	phenoxybenzamine (Dibenzyline) prazosin (Minipres) terazosin (Hytrin)
Decrease bladder outlet resistance	Alpha-adrenergic antagonists	phenoxybenzamine (Dibenzyline) prazosin (Minipres) terazosin (Hytrin)

but some people have multiple contributing factors, some of which may lead to established incontinence. Established incontinence is basically due to one of two problems: fail-

TABLE 11–8
Drugs That May Cause Urinary Incontinence or Reduce Bladder Storage
Function

Bladder level
  Alpha-adrenergic agonists (minimal effect)
  Anticholinesterases
    Distigmine
    Neostigmine
  Beta-adrenergic blocking agents
  Direct smooth muscle stimulants
    Angiotensin
    Bradykinin
    Ergotamine
    Histamine
    5-Hydroxytryptamine
    Oxytocin
    Prostaglandins
    Vasopressin
  Ganglionic stimulants
    Lobeline
    Nicotine
    Tetramethylammonium
  Opioid antagonists (methadone)
  Parasympathomimetics
    Arecholine
    Bethanechol
    Carbachol
    Dehydromuscarone
    Furtrethonium
    Methacholine
    Muscarine
    Mecarone
  Prostaglandins
  Others
    Digitalis
    Furosemide
    Metoclopramide
    Metronidazole
Testosterone
Thioridazine (nocturnal enuresis)
Valproic acid
Bladder outlet level
  Alpha-adrenergic blocking agents
    Alpha-methyldopa
    Clonidine
    Guanethidine
    Phenoxybenzamine
    Phentolamine
    Prazosin
    Reserpine
  Beta-adrenergic agonists
    Isoproterenol
    Terbutaline
  Smooth-muscle relaxants
    Chlordiazepoxide
    Diazepam
    Methocarbamol
    Orphenadrine
  Striated-muscle relaxants
    Baclofen (Lioresal)
    Dantrolene
    Hydramitrazine (Lisidonil)
  Others
    Bromocriptine
    Bupivacaine
    Demecarium
    Isoflurophate
    Ketanserin
    Levodopa
    Lithium
    Phenothiazines
    Phenytoin
    Progesterone

From Bissada, N.K. and Finkbeiner, A.E. Urologic manifestations of drug therapy.
Urol Clin North Am 15:725, 1988.

mobility. Many drugs that are often prescribed for elderly people affect voiding.

Whether transient or established, urinary incontinence should be considered remediable until proved otherwise. Causes of transient incontinence include infection, atrophic vaginitis and urethritis, fecal impaction, immobility, drug therapy (Table 11–8), hyperglycemia, delirium, and depression (Broderick and Wein, 1994; Augspurger, 1990). Identification and treatment of the underlying problem should relieve the incontinence,

TABLE 11-9
Nursing Assessment of the Genitourinary System

HISTORY
Personal or family history of disease of the urogenital
  system
Recent surgery or illnesses (hypertension, diabetes melli-
  tus, cardiac disease)
Symptoms:
  Urine (frequency, amount, timing, sensation, control,
    color, appearance)
  Bladder (feeling of fullness, distention)
  Pain (flank, back, costovertebral angle, abdomen, pel-
    vis, scrotum)
  Medications
  Sexual activity

PHYSICAL ASSESSMENT
Inspect for hydration (edema, skin turgor)
Inspect suprapubic area for distention
Measure and observe urine (cloudiness, sediment, concen-
  tration, odor, pH, blood, glucose, protein, specific grav-
  ity)
Check for vaginal or urethral discharge
Palpate and percuss abdomen for size of bladder

---

ure to empty the bladder or failure to store urine. The bladder may not empty owing to decreased bladder contractility (as with diabetic neuropathy) and/or increased bladder outlet resistance (as in prostate hypertrophy). Failure to empty leads to urinary retention and overflow. Failure to store urine, as in stress incontinence and detrusor instability, can be attributed to increased bladder pressure, decreased bladder outlet resistance, or both. The most common cause of urinary incontinence is detrusor instability manifested by abnormal bladder contractions of uncertain etiology. The term "functional incontinence" is used to describe the situation in which the bladder functions normally but the patient voids inappropriately. Treatments for established incontinence may include drug therapy, surgery, and behavioral therapy (O'Donnell, 1994). These are discussed in greater detail in Chapter 14. Nursing care includes assessment of the patient, which often includes maintenance of voiding records, implementation of prescribed therapy, and evaluation of outcomes. The nurse is the key person in planning and implementing strategies to deal with functional incontinence. The first step may be convincing the patient and family that improvement is probably possible.

Vaginitis

Inflammation of the vaginal tissues is associated with the age-related changes known as atrophic or senile vaginitis. Such changes increase the susceptibility to trauma and infection. The vaginal walls are thin and easily traumatized, thus permitting the introduction of microorganisms. Pruritus may lead to areas of excoriation. Coitus or douching may cause injury. All elderly women are at risk unless they are receiving estrogen replacement therapy.

Patients complain of vaginal bleeding, pruritus, and dyspareunia. A vaginal examination will help rule out other problems. Estrogen cream applied nightly for 3 to 4 months is the usual treatment. If there is a concurrent infection, an antibacterial or antifungal cream is used also.

NURSING ASSESSMENT

History

Questions specific to the genitourinary tract are included in a nursing assessment (Table 11-9). Determine whether the patient has a personal or family history of diseases of the urogenital system. Recent illness or surgery is particularly important. Ask about hypertension, diabetes mellitus, and cardiac disease. Have there been neurological, gynecological, or urological problems? Ask about symptoms directly related to the urinary pattern: any changes in frequency, amount, timing, sensation, control, and appearance of the urine. Ask what medications the person is taking. Assess activity level and personal hygiene. Ask about fluid intake. What causes problems? Ask specifically about pain in the flank, back, costovertebral angle, abdomen, pelvis, or scrotum. Tactfully inquire about sexual activities and interests. Is impotence or dyspareunia a problem? Review results of pertinent renal function studies. Such studies include serum creatinine and blood urea nitrogen levels, creatinine clearance rate, excretory urogram, renal scans, computed tomography, magnetic resonance imaging, and ultrasound studies.

Physical Assessment

Assess the person's hydration status. Is there edema or evidence of dehydration? Is the suprapubic area distended? Are there changes in the external genitalia? Are there visible changes in the urine: hematuria, cloudiness, high concentration or dilution? Measure urine pH, blood (if present), glucose, and protein, and measure the specific gravity. Is there any sediment? Additional studies on the urine may include culture and sensitivity determinations, and cytology examination. Any vaginal or urethral discharge should be examined.

The abdomen should be percussed over

the bladder area. Dullness may be present if the bladder is very full.

Palpate the abdomen for the bladder. The prostate is palpated on rectal examination. The uterus, fallopian tubes, and ovaries are palpated during a bimanual vaginal examination. Palpate the scrotum, flanks, and abdomen for masses. Note any tenderness. Normally the kidneys are not palpable.

Abnormalities in blood flow to the kidneys may cause bruits. Listen with a stethoscope in the epigastric area.

NURSING DIAGNOSES

1. Comfort, Alteration in
   related to pruritus, vaginitis

2. Fluid Volume Deficit, Potential
   related to excessive fluid losses, decreased fluid intake

3. Self-Care Deficit: Toileting
   related to incontinence

4. Sexual Dysfunction
   related to aging changes, malignancies, and other problems of the bladder, prostate, uterus, and vagina

5. Tissue Perfusion, Renal Altered
   related to acute renal failure, chronic renal failure

6. Urinary Elimination, Altered
   related to incontinence, malignancies, effects of drugs or surgery

7. Urinary Retention (Chronic)
   related to benign prostatic hypertrophy, effects of drugs, surgery, or instrumentation

NURSING INTERVENTIONS AND EVALUATION

Nursing interventions for older clients with changes or disorders in the genitourinary system are related to the problems of urinary incontinence, chronic renal failure, and sexual dysfunction (Cormack, 1985; Hoffart, 1986; Newman et al., 1986; Belcher, 1992; Brundage, 1992; Gray, 1992). Urinary incontinence has many causes—physiological, psychological, and environmental, and nursing interventions must be geared toward the cause. If problems with toileting occur, the nurse must determine the factors that interfere with self-care and remove any barriers that exist. These may include clearing pathways, providing assistance in ambu-

lating, providing adequate lighting, allowing privacy, and providing sufficient space in toilet areas. Commodes and urine-containment devices at the bedside are also useful. Interventions for urinary incontinence resulting from physiological and psychological causes are discussed in Chapter 14.

Nurses should help older persons with renal failure to manage their medication intake, making sure that nephrotoxic drugs are avoided. The serum levels of K^+ and Ca^{++} should be monitored, and abnormal levels should be reported. Dietary intake and fluids should be allowed within restrictions. Emotional support and teaching is aimed toward helping older clients and their families adapt to the short- and long-term management of acute and chronic renal failure. These include dialysis, any nutritional and fluid restrictions, medication regimens, renal transplantation (if an option), self-monitoring skills, and sexual dysfunction related to renal disease.

Sexual dysfunction can result from age-related or pathological changes in the genitalia, prostate disorders, or renal failure. The nurse should help older clients and their partners to understand the normal changes of aging and should discuss expected alterations in sexual functioning, if necessary. Some older clients may be referred to a professional counselor.

Evaluation should be based on measures of achievement of self-care, understanding of the condition, and maintenance of the highest level of functioning.

SUMMARY

The changes in the genitourinary system that occur with aging, particularly the difficulty in maintaining urinary continence, present challenging problems to nurses, older clients, and their families. These problems can be embarrassing, isolating, and debilitating. Normal anatomical and physiological changes include loss of nephrons and renal mass, sclerotic changes in the renal blood vessels and diminished renal blood flow, decreased creatinine clearance, and a decline in the endocrine functions of the kidney. Bladder changes include replacement of the smooth muscle and elastic tissue with fibrous connective tissue, reduction in bladder capacity, and loss of bladder control. In women, the external genitalia and vagina may atrophy and become less elastic; in men, there may be alterations in blood flow to the penis with resultant diminished erectile capacity.

Common disorders associated with the

genitourinary system in older age are acute and chronic renal failure, benign prostatic hypertrophy, cancer of the prostate and bladder, urinary tract infections, urinary retention and incontinence, and vaginitis. Treatment and nursing care are geared toward maintaining continence, functional independence, and self-care.

REFERENCES

Augspurger, R.R. Urinary incontinence and catheters in the elderly male and female. *In* Schrier, R.W. (ed.). *Geriatric Medicine*. Philadelphia: W.B. Saunders, 1990, pp. 156–167.

Beck, L.H. Aging changes in renal function. *In* Hazzard, W.R., Bierman, E.L., Blass, J.P. et al. (eds.). *Principles of Geriatric Medicine and Gerontology*. 3rd ed. New York: McGraw-Hill, 1994, pp. 615–624.

Beers, M.H. Medication use in the elderly. *In* Calkins, E., Ford, A.B. and Katz, P.R. (eds.). *Practice of Geriatrics*. 2nd ed. Philadelphia: W.B. Saunders, 1992, pp. 33–49.

Belcher, A.E. *Cancer Nursing*. St. Louis: Mosby–Year Book, 1992.

Blacklock, N.J. and Higgins, J.R.A. The prostate. *In* Brocklehurst, J.C., Tallis, R.C., & Fillit, A.M. (eds.). *Textbook of Geriatric Medicine and Gerontology*. 4th ed. Edinburgh: Churchill-Livingstone, 1992, pp 647–655.

Brandeis, G.H., Yalla, S.V., and Resnick, N.M. Urinary incontinence. *In* Calkins, E., Ford, A.B., & Katz, P.R. (eds.). *Practice of Geriatrics*. 2nd ed. Philadelphia: W.B. Saunders, 1992, pp. 220–228.

Brendler, C. Disorders of the prostate. *In* Hazzard, W.R., Bierman, E.L., Blass, J.P. et al. (eds.). *Principles of Geriatric Medicine and Gerontology*. 3rd ed. New York: McGraw-Hill, 1994, pp. 657–664.

Brendler, C., Schlegel, P., Dowd, J. et al. Surgical treatment for benign prostatic hyperplasia. *Cancer* (Suppl.) 70(1):371–373, 1992.

Brocklehurst, J.C., Tallis, R.C. and Fillit, H.M. (eds.). *Textbook of Geriatric Medicine and Gerontology*. 4th ed. Edinburgh, Churchill Livingstone, 1992.

Broderick, G.A. and Wein, A.J. Pharmacologic therapy for incontinence. *In* O'Donnell, P.D. (ed.). *Geriatric Urology*. Boston: Little, Brown, 1994, pp. 285–299.

Brown, A.D.G. and Cooper, T.K. Gynecological disorders in the elderly—sexuality and aging. *In* Brocklehurst, J.C., Tallis, R.C., & Fillit, H.M. (eds.). *Textbook of Geriatric Medicine and Gerontology*. 4th ed. Edinburgh: Churchill-Livingstone, 1992). pp 656–665.

Brundage, D.J. *Renal Disorders*. St. Louis: Mosby–Year Book, 1992.

Burkart, J.M. and Canzanello, V.J. Renal disease. *In* Hazzard, W.R., Bierman, E.L., Blass, J.P. et al. (eds.). *Principles of Geriatric Medicine and Gerontology*. 3rd ed. New York: McGraw-Hill, 1994, pp. 637–655.

Burns, P.A., Pranikoff, K., Nochajski, T.H. et al. A comparison of effectiveness of biofeedback and pelvic muscle exercise treatment of stress incontinence in older, community-dwelling women. *J Gerontol* 48(4): M167–M174, 1993.

Butler R.N., Lewis, M.I. and Sunderland, T. Psychology of aging. *In* Brocklehurst, J.C., Tallis R.C. & Fillit, H.M. *Textbook of Geriatric Medicine and Gerontology*. 4th ed. Edinburgh: Churchill Livingstone, 1992, pp 91–93.

Calkins, E., Ford, A.M. and Katz, P.R. (eds.). *Practice of Geriatrics*. 2nd ed. Philadelphia: W.B. Saunders, 1992.

Carroll, P.R. Urothelial carcinoma: Cancers of the bladder, ureter and renal pelvis. *In* Tanagho, E.A. and McAninch, J.W. (eds.). *Smith's General Urology*. 13th ed. Norwalk, CT: Appleton & Lange, 1992, pp. 341–358.

Cormack, D. (ed.). *Geriatric Nursing: A Conceptual Approach*. Oxford: Blackwell Scientific Publications, 1985.

Couillard, D.R., Deckard-Janatpour, K.A. and Stone, A.R. The vaginal wall sling: A compressive suspension procedure for recurrent incontinence in elderly patients. *Urology* 43(2):203–208, 1994.

Denis, L., Lepor, H., Dowd, J. et al. Alternatives to surgery for benign prostatic hyperplasia. *Cancer* (Suppl.) 70(1):374–378, 1992.

Diokno, A.C. and Hollander, J.B. Prostate gland disease. *In* Calkins, E., Ford, A.M. and Katz, P.R. (eds.). *Practice of Geriatrics*. 2nd ed. Philadelphia: W.B. Saunders, 1992, pp. 462–473.

Dixon, C.M. and Lepor, H. Laser ablation of the prostate. *Semin Urol* 10(4):273–277, 1992.

Doll, H.A., Black, N.A., McPherson, K. et al. Mortality, morbidity, and complications following transurethral resection of the prostate for benign prostatic hypertrophy. *J Urol* 147(6):1566–1573, 1992.

Donohue, R.E., Davis, M.A. and Crawford, E.D. Diseases of the prostate. *In* Schrier, R.W. (ed.). *Geriatric Medicine*. Philadelphia: W.B. Saunders, 1990, pp. 168–178.

Dreicer, R. and Williams, R.D. Management of prostate care. *In* O'Donnell, P.D. (ed.). *Geriatric Urology*. Boston: Little, Brown, 1994, pp. 125–145.

Ekengren, J. and Hahn, R.G. Continuous versus intermittent flow irrigation in transurethral resection of the prostate. *Urology* 43(3):328–332, 1994.

Fillit, H.M. and Rowe, J.W. The aging kidney. *In* Brocklehurst, J.C., Tallis, R.C. and Fillit, H.M. (eds.). *Textbook of Geriatric Medicine and Gerontology*. 4th ed. Edinburgh: Churchill Livingstone, 1992, pp. 612–628.

Finkbeiner, A.E. and Bissada, N.K. Urologic effects of concurrent medical therapy. *In* O'Donnell, P.D. (ed.). *Geriatric Urology*. Boston: Little, Brown, 1994, pp. 413–420.

Flam, T.A., Brawer, M.K., Cooper, E.H. and Javadpour, N. Diagnosis and markers in prostatic cancer. *Cancer* (Suppl.) 70(1):357–358, 1992.

Furner, S.E., Grant, M.D. and Brody, J.A. The aging population. *In* O'Donnell, P.D. (ed.). *Geriatric Urology*. Boston: Little, Brown, 1994, pp. 3–12.

Goldenberg, S.L. and Bruchovsky, N. Use of cyproterone acetate in prostate cancer. *Urol Clin North Am* 18(1):111–122, 1991.

Goldspiel, B.R. and Kohler, D.R. Flutamide: An antiandrogen for advanced prostate cancer. *Drug Intelligence and Clinical Pharmacy* 24(6):616–623, 1990.

Gormley, G.J., Stoner, E., Bruskewitz, R.C. et al. The effect of finasteride in men with benign prostatic hyperplasia. *N Engl J Med* 327(17):1185–1191, 1992.

Graham, S.D., Bostwick, D.G., Hoisaeter, A. et al. Report of the committee on staging and pathology. *Cancer* (Suppl.) 70(1):359–361, 1992.

Gray, M. *Genitourinary Disorders*. St. Louis: Mosby–Year Book, 1992.

Hald, T. and Nordling, J. Nonsurgical, nonpharmacologic treatment of benign prostatic hypertrophy. *Cancer* (Suppl.) 70(1):346–350, 1992.

Harrison, G.L. and Memel, D.S. Urinary incontinence in women: Its prevalence and its management in a health promotion clinic. *Br J Gen Pract* 44(381):149–152, 1994.

Hernandez-Graulau, J.M. Transurethral balloon divulsion of prostate. *Urology* (Suppl.) 41(1):43–48, 1993.

Hirsch, J.D. and Schwartz, R.W. Prostate cancer. *In* Herfindal, E.T., Gourley, D.R. and Hart, L.L. (eds.). *Clinical Pharmacy and Therapeutics*. Baltimore: Williams and Wilkins, 1992.

Hoffart, N. Chronic renal failure. *In* Carnevali, D.L. and Patrick, M. (eds.). *Nursing Management for the Elderly*.

2nd ed. Philadelphia: J.B. Lippincott, 1986, pp. 519–531.

Jonler, M., Riehman, M. and Bruskewitz, R.C. Benign prostatic hyperplasia: Current pharmacologic treatment. *Drugs* 47(1):66–81, 1994.

Kletscher, B.A. and Oesterling, J.E. Transurethral incision of the prostate: A viable alternative to transurethral resection. *Semin Urol* 10(4):265–272, 1992.

Kutner, N.G., Cardenas, D.D. and Bower, J.D. Rehabilitation, aging and chronic renal disease. *Am J Phys Med Rehabil* 71(2):97–101, 1992.

Lee, F., Torp-Pedersen, S., Cooner, W., Drago, J. Detection and screening for prostate cancer. *Cancer* (Suppl.) 70(1):359–361, 1992.

Levi, M. and Schrier, R.W. Renal disease. *In* Schrier, R.W. (ed.). *Geriatric Medicine*. Philadelphia: W.B. Saunders, 1990, pp. 189–206.

Lindeman, R.D. Renal and electrolyte abnormalities. *In* Calkins, E., Ford, A.B. & Katz, P.R. *Practice of Geriatrics*. 2nd ed. Philadelphia, W.B. Saunders, 1992, pp. 436–453.

Lindner, A., Golomb, J., Korzcak, D. et al. Effects of prostatectomy on sexual function. *Urology* 38(1):26–28, 1991.

Link, P. and Freiha, F.S. Radical prostatectomy after definitive radiation therapy for prostate cancer. *Urology* 37(3):189–192, 1991.

McDowell, B.J., Silverman, M., Martin, D. et al. Identification and intervention for urinary incontinence by community physicians and geriatric assessment teams. *J Am Geriatr Soc* 42(5):501–505, 1994.

Mebust, W., Bostwick, D., Grayhack, J. et al. Scope of the problem. *Cancer* (Suppl.) 70(1):369–370, 1992.

Mettlin, C., Murphy, G.P. and Menck, H. Trends in treatment of localized prostate cancer by radical prostatectomy: Observations from the Commission on Cancer, National Cancer Database, 1985–1990. *Urology* 43(4):488–492, 1994.

Moseley, W.G. Balloon dilatation of prostate: Keys to sustained favorable results. *Urology* 39(4):314–318, 1992.

Newling, D.W.W., McLeod, D., Soloway, M. et al. Distant disease. *Cancer* (Suppl.) 70(1):365–367, 1992.

Newman, E., Price, M. and Magney, J. *Care of the Disabled Urinary Tract: Prevention of Renal Deterioration*. Springfield, IL: Charles C Thomas, 1986.

Nicolle, L.E. Urinary tract infection. *In* O'Donnell, P.D. (ed.). *Geriatric Urology*. Boston: Little, Brown, 1994, pp. 399–412.

Nissenson, A.R., Gentile, D.E., Soderblom, R. et al. Continuous ambulatory peritoneal dialysis in the elderly—regional experience. *In* Maher, J.F. and Winchester, J.F. (eds.). *Frontiers in Peritoneal Dialysis*. New York: Field, Rich, and Associates, 1986, pp. 312–317.

O'Donnell, P.D. Behavioral therapy for incontinence. *In* O'Donnell, P.D. (ed.). *Geriatric Urology*. Boston: Little, Brown, 1994, pp. 301–308.

Perez-Marrero, R. and Emerson, L.E. Balloon-expanded titanium prostatic urethral stent. *Urology* (Suppl.) 41(1):38–42, 1993.

Peters, D.H. and Sorkin, E.M. Finasteride. A review of its potential in the treatment of benign prostatic hypertrophy. *Drugs* 46(1):177–208, 1993.

Petrovich, Z., Ameye, F., Baert, L. et al. New trends in the treatment of benign prostatic hyperplasia and carcinoma of the prostate. *Am J Clin Oncol* 16(3):187–200, 1993.

Plawecki, H.M. and Brewer, S. The elderly hemodialysis patient. *ANNA J* 13(3):146–149, 1986.

Psihramis, K.E. and Dretler, S.P. Urinary retention. *In* Hoffer, E.P. (ed.). *Emergency Problems in the Elderly*. Oradell, NJ: Medical Economics Books, 1985, pp. 97–115.

Quinlan, D.M., Epstein, J.I., Carter, B.S. and Walsh, P.C. Sexual function following radical prostatectomy: Influence of preservation of neurovascular bundles. *J Urol* 145(5):998–1002, 1991.

Resnick, M.I. and Palmer, R.M. Surgical decisions. *In* O'Donnell, P.D. (ed.). *Geriatric Urology*. Boston: Little, Brown, 1994, pp. 13–24.

Rousseau, P. Chronic urethral catheterization in nursing homes. *Geriatr Consult* Sept/Oct, 12–14, 1990.

Rowe, J.W. Renal and lower urinary tract disease in the elderly. *In* Calkins, E., Davis, P.J. and Ford, A.B. (eds.). *The Practice of Geriatrics*. Philadelphia: J.B. Lippincott, 1986a, pp. 339–349.

Rowe, J.W. Renal system. *In* Rowe, J.W. and Besdine, R.W. (eds.). *Health and Disease*. Boston: Little, Brown, 1986b, pp. 165–183.

Schellhammer, P., Debruyne, F., Altwein, J. et al. Locoregional disease. *Cancer* (Suppl.) 70(1):362–364, 1992.

Schnelle, J.F., Newman, D., White, M. et al. Maintaining continence in nursing home residents through the application of industrial quality control. *Gerontologist* 33(1):114–121, 1993.

Schrier, R.W. *Geriatric Medicine*. Philadelphia: W.B. Saunders, 1990.

Schroder, F.H. Endocrine therapy: Where do we stand and where are we going? *Cancer Surv* 11:77–94, 1991.

Skinner, E.C. and Skinner, D.G. Management of bladder cancer. *In* O'Donnell, P.D. (ed.). *Geriatric Urology*. Boston: Little, Brown, 1994, pp. 157–165.

Spear, K.A., Bollard, G.A. and Summers, J.L. Early discharge of transurethral prostatectomy patients with an indwelling Foley catheter. *Urology* 43(3):333–336, 1994.

Tanagho, E.A. and McAninch, J.W. (eds.). *Smith's General Urology*. 13th ed. Norwalk, CT: Appleton and Lange, 1992.

Telang, D.J. and Farah, R.N. Management of impotence after treatment of carcinoma of the prostate. *Henry Ford Hosp Med J* 40:111–113, 1992.

Tunkel, A.R. and Kaye, D. Urinary tract infections. *In* Hazzard, W.R., Bierman, E.L., Blass, J.P. et al. (eds.). *Principles of Geriatric Medicine and Gerontology*. 3rd ed. New York: McGraw-Hill, 1994, pp. 625–635.

Vale, J.A., Miller, P.D. and Kirby, R.S. Balloon dilatation of the prostate—should it have a place in the urologist's armamentarium? *J Res Soc Med* 86(2):83–86, 1993.

Wasserman, N.F., Reddy, P.K., Zhang, G. et al. Transurethral balloon dilatation of the prostatic urethra: Effectiveness in highly selected patients with prostatism. *Am J Roentgenol* 157(3):509–512, 1991.

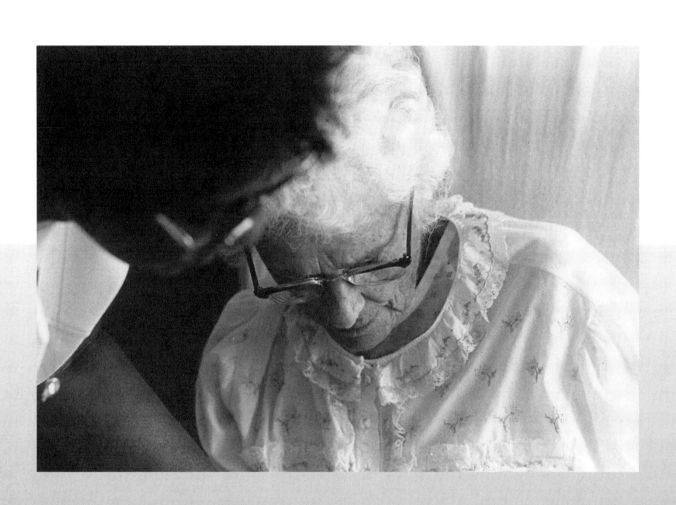

12

Age-Related Changes in the Endocrine System

ADRIANNE DILL LINTON
PAULINE LEE
MARY ANN MATTESON

OBJECTIVES

Discuss the normal age-related changes that occur in hormone production; the pituitary, parathyroid, and thyroid glands; the adrenal cortex; the gonads; and the pancreas.

❖

Describe the diagnosis, symptoms, and treatment of type II diabetes mellitus.

❖

Compare and contrast the symptoms and treatments of the various thyroid disorders.

❖

Demonstrate a breast self-examination for older women.

❖

Apply the nursing process in the care of older clients with endocrine disorders.

The endocrine system is made up of various tissues and glands whose function is to produce and secrete hormones into the bloodstream. The major hormone-secreting glands are the hypophysis (pituitary), thyroid, parathyroids (four), pancreatic islets, pineal gland, ovaries (two), testes (two), and suprarenal or adrenal glands (two) (Fig. 12–1). Hormones are released in low concentrations and are transported to other parts of the body, where they exert regulatory effects on cellular processes. Their purpose is to coordinate body activities, control growth and development, and maintain homeostasis. The endocrine system also acts with the nervous system to bring about various responses to changes in the external and internal environment. The endocrine glands and their secretions are listed in Table 12–1.

NORMAL CHANGES IN STRUCTURE AND FUNCTION

Hormone Production

Alterations with aging occur in both the reception and the production of hormones. Not only is there a change in the target tissue and sensitivity to hormonal stimulation, but there is also a decrease in the hormonal secretory rate and metabolic degradation rate with aging. Changes in plasma levels of hormones vary. For example, levels of estrogen, aldosterone, calcitonin, prolactin (in women), growth hormone, and plasma renin activity decrease, whereas levels of follicle-stimulating hormone (FSH), luteinizing hormone (LH), and norepinephrine increase. Plasma levels of thyroxine (T4), thyrotropin (TSH), cortisol, insulin, testosterone, and epinephrine remain unchanged. Hormone levels that are variably reported as normal or decreased are parathyroid hormone and 25-hydroxyvitamin D. Hormonal responses to stimuli may also vary with age. For example, T4 and T3 levels respond normally to stimulation of TSH, whereas testosterone has a decreased response to gonadotropin (Davis and Davis, 1992).

Pituitary Gland

The pituitary gland, or hypophysis, which consists of an anterior and a posterior segment, is about 1 cm in diameter and weighs 0.5 to 1 gm. The posterior pituitary gland does not actually produce any hormones, but it stores two hormones, oxytocin and antidiuretic hormone (ADH), whose release is governed by nerve impulses from the hypothalamus. The major function of ADH is to reduce the volume and increase the concentration of urine in the kidneys. The primary action of oxytocin (pitocin) is to influence the lactating breast to release milk from the glandular cells into the ducts.

The anterior pituitary gland produces thyroid-stimulating hormone (TSH), (FSH), (LH), human growth hormone (hGH, somatotropin), prolactin, and adrenocorticotropin (ACTH). These hormones, with the exception of growth hormone, control the activities of their target glands—the thyroid, adrenal cortex, ovaries, testes, and mammary glands. Human growth hormone exerts effects on almost all body tissues. Hypothalamic releasing and inhibitory hormones or factors secreted within the hypothalamus control the release of anterior pituitary hormones. Known releasing and inhibiting hormones include TSH-releasing hormone, corticotropin-releasing hormone, growth hormone–releasing hormone, growth hormone inhibitory hormone, gonadotropin-releasing hormone, and prolactin inhibitory factor. There are probably other releasing and inhibitory hormones that have not yet been recognized (Fig. 12–2) (Guyton, 1991).

The pituitary gland reaches maximum size during middle age and then gradually diminishes. There is a decrease in cell mass and weight because of atrophy, fibrosis, and

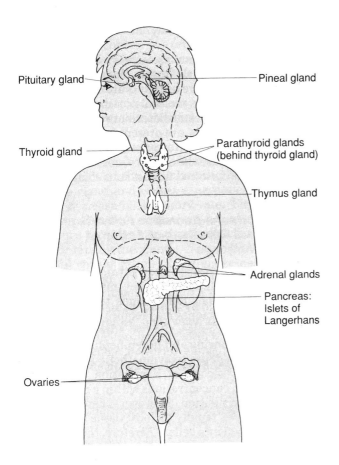

Pituitary gland

Pineal gland

Thyroid gland

Parathyroid glands
(behind thyroid gland)

Thymus gland

Adrenal glands

Pancreas:
Islets of
Langerhans

Ovaries

FIGURE 12–1

The anatomical loci of the principal endocrine glands of the body. (From Guyton, A.C. Philadelphia: W.B. Saunders, *Textbook of Medical Physiology*. 8th ed. 1991, p. 811.)

decreased vascularity. Some incidental small adenomas or areas of hyperplasia may appear after age 40.

Thyroid Gland

The thyroid gland is composed of two lobes lying on either side of the trachea that are connected at the midline by a thin isthmus extending over the anterior surface of the trachea. Two hormones responsible for the major functions of the thyroid are triiodothyronine (T3) and T4. TSH, secreted by the anterior pituitary, stimulates iodine uptake by the thyroid gland as well as the synthesis and ultimate release of T3 and T4. The actions of T3 and T4 are to raise the basal metabolic rate, develop the central nervous system, stimulate all aspects of glucose and fat metabolism, increase the demand for vitamins, increase the rates of secretion of other endocrine glands, and enhance normal sexual functioning. Among the many effects of thyroid activity are enhanced glycolysis and gluconeogenesis; increased insulin secretion; increased fatty acids in the plasma; decreased cholesterol, phospholipid, and triglyceride levels in the plasma; increased blood flow and cardiac output; increased

rate and strength of heartbeat; increased systolic blood pressure; increased secretion of digestive juices; and increased intestinal motility.

TABLE 12–1

Important Endocrine Glands and Their Hormones

Anterior pituitary	Islets of Langerhans
Growth hormone	Insulin
Adrenocorticotropin	Glucagon
Thyroid-stimulating	Ovaries
hormone	Estrogens
Follicle-stimulating	Progesterone
hormone	Testes
Luteinizing hormone	Testosterone
Prolactin	Parathyroid glands
Posterior pituitary	Parathormone
Antidiuretic hormone	Placenta
Oxytocin	Human chorionic gona-
Adrenal cortex	dotropin
Cortisol	Estrogens
Aldosterone	Progesterone
Thyroid gland	Human somatomammotro-
Thyroxine	pin
Triiodothyronine	
Calcitonin	

From Guyton, A.C. *Textbook of Medical Physiology*. 8th ed. Philadelphia: W.B. Saunders, 1991, pp. 810–811.

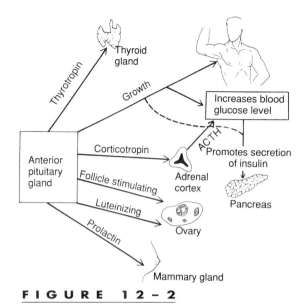

FIGURE 12 – 2

Metabolic functions of the anterior pituitary hormones. (From Guyton, A.C. Philadelphia: W.B. Saunders, *Textbook of Medical Physiology*. 8th ed. 1991, p. 820.)

Age-related changes in the thyroid include diminished glandular substance, infiltration of lymphocytes, and fibrosis. There is an increased incidence of nodules and small, firm goiters. Because renal iodide clearance decreases, there is an increase in plasma inorganic iodide concentrations. Thyroid iodide clearance rates decrease, although radioactive iodine uptake by the thyroid remains constant. T4 levels tend to remain the same in the old and the young, but T3 levels tend to decline with older age. The inverse relationship between the T4 and the TSH levels is maintained (Barzel, 1989). The basal metabolic rate begins a gradual and significant decline at about 20 to 30 years; however, this decline parallels the loss in metabolizing tissues and lean body mass, so that the metabolic rate per unit of lean body mass appears to undergo no important change with age (Barzel, 1989).

Adrenal Cortex

The adrenal cortex is the outer layer of the two adrenal glands, which rest on top of the kidneys. The major types of hormones secreted by the adrenal cortex are the corticosteroids: mineralocorticoids, glucocorticoids, and androgens. Aldosterone, the principal mineralocorticoid, regulates the fluid and electrolyte balance by increasing the reabsorption of sodium and decreasing the reabsorption of potassium by the kidneys. Cortisol, the principal glucocorticoid, influences the metabolism of glucose, protein, and fat, is required for a normal response to stress, and exerts anti-inflammatory and antiallergic actions. The androgenic hormones have the same effects as testosterone.

The stress response occurs in the hypothalamic-pituitary-adrenal axis. When the body is stressed, there is an increase in the neural and hormonal input into the hypothalamus. Corticotropin-releasing factor is then secreted into the hypothalamic-hypophyseal portal tract and is then transmitted to the anterior pituitary gland. ACTH release is stimulated, causing a two- to sevenfold increase in plasma cortisol, which in turn regulates the metabolic response of the stressed person.

Changes in the adrenal cortex are of major importance in the hypothalamic-pituitary-adrenal axis and the stress response because alterations in the regulation of cortisol responsiveness may have immediate clinical consequences. However, it has been found that older people normally have little change in the hypothalamic-pituitary-adrenal axis. They maintain normal rhythmic patterns of cortisol secretion and normal levels of plasma cortisol (Barton et al., 1993; Barzel, 1989; Greenspan et al., 1993).

Aldosterone secretion has been variously reported as decreased and as well preserved in healthy older persons (Barton et al., 1993; Barzel, 1989; Greenspan et al., 1993; Beck, 1994; Belchetz, 1992). Some sources report decreased circulating plasma renin activity and blunted response of the renin-angiotensin-aldosterone axis in older people (Beck, 1994; Abernathy and Andrawis, 1992). Beck (1994) cited evidence that the total renin concentration remains stable, but *active* renin concentration declines. A study by Weidman et al. (cited in Beck, 1994) measured renin concentration in old and young subjects, receiving low-sodium and high-sodium diets, in supine and upright positions. The greatest declines in plasma renin level were in older subjects receiving low-sodium diets when in the upright position. This positional decline in renin is probably a factor in the increased time needed by many older people to adapt to position changes.

Gonads

The gonads serve two basic functions: they secrete sex steroids (predominantly testosterone from the testes and estradiol and progesterone from the ovaries) and they produce gametes (sperm and ova). In general, production of the sex steroids from the

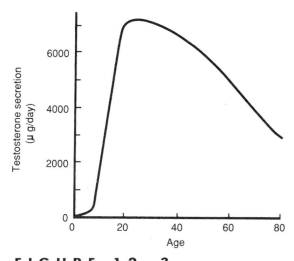

FIGURE 12 – 3

Approximate rates of testosterone secretion at different ages. (From Guyton, A.C. Philadelphia: W.B. Saunders, *Textbook of Medical Physiology.* 8th ed. 1991, p. 892.)

gonads is stimulated by the secretion of LH from the pituitary, and production of gametes is stimulated by FSH, also secreted from the pituitary. Sex steroids are responsible for the establishment and maintenance of secondary sex characteristics, whereas gametes are responsible for reproduction (Guyton, 1991).

Changes in the Older Male

In the aging male, the primary changes occur in the testes rather than in the hypothalamic-pituitary axis. Testicular volume decreases, there is some sclerosis of the tubules, and the numbers of Leydig's and Sertoli's cells decline. Spermatogenesis is somewhat impaired, so there is a decrease in the number of spermatozoa, but reproduction can take place even into very old age. Degenerative and atrophic changes occur in the epididymis, seminal vesicles, and prostate gland, with loss of epithelial cells. Testosterone secretion declines beginning around age 40 as depicted in Figure 12–3. There is an increase in estrogen values, which increases the ratio of estrogen to testosterone. There are increases in both LH and FSH, which suggests that the decline in testicular function is related to changes in the testicle rather than in regulatory structures (Barzel, 1989; Davis and Davis, 1992; Terry and Halter, 1994).

Erectile dysfunction may occur with older age, but it is more likely to be a result of factors other than decreased testosterone. For example, psychosocial factors, dis-

eases, and chronic illnesses (Table 12–2) and drugs (Table 12–3) frequently inhibit sexual responses in older males. Sex is more likely if there is a willing partner available and if there has been no interruption in sexual activity during the middle years.

Sexual responses normally become slower and less intense with aging. For example, erection may take longer to achieve and may be less full than in younger men. Erection can be maintained for extended periods without ejaculation; however, if erection is lost without ejaculation, a secondary refractory period may result. The ejaculatory force is decreased, along with the volume of the semen. The refractory period lasts for an extended amount of time, and there is rapid loss of the erection (Table 12–4) (Brown and Cooper, 1992; Butler and Lewis, 1992; Gill and Ducharme, 1992; Levy, 1994).

Changes in the Older Female

Menopause, the cessation of menses, is the most striking change in aging women. It begins at approximately age 40 with gradually decreasing follicular sensitivity to gonadotropins and reduced estrogen production (Birkenfeld and Kase, 1993). Although the mean age for the occurrence of menopause is 51, it may occur prematurely before the age of 40 in about 8 per cent of women. During the perimenopausal period, the men-

TABLE 12 – 2

Diseases Associated with Sexual Dysfunction

Endocrine	Vascular
Hypothyroidism	Hypertension
Hyperthyroidism	Sickle cell anemia
Addison's disease	Leriche's syndrome
Pituitary adenoma	Aortoiliac disease
Hypogonadism	Coronary heart disease
Metabolic	Genital
Diabetes mellitus	Peyronie's disease
Hemochromatosis	Phimosis
Renal failure	Hepatic
Alcoholism	Cirrhosis
Neurologic	Other
Dementia	Obstructive pulmonary
Stroke	disease
Multiple sclerosis	Chronic infections
Postconcussion	
Spinal cord injury	
Pelvic nerve lesions	
Limbic system lesions	

Adapted from Korenman, S.G. Erectile dysfunction (impotence). *In* Guyton, A.C. *Textbook of Medical Physiology.* 8th ed. Philadelphia: W.B. Saunders, 1994, pp. 1251–1258; Barzel, U.S., Gambert S.R. and Tsitouras, P.D. (eds.). *Contemporary Geriatric Medicine.* Vol. 1. New York: Plenum Medical Book Co., 1983.

TABLE 12-3
Medical and Surgical Treatments Associated with Sexual Dysfunction*

Surgical
Abdominal-perineal resection
Rectal anastomosis
Radical prostatectomy
Castration
Lumbar sympathectomy

Medical
Antihypertensive agents
  Diuretics: amiloride, chlorthalidone, spironolactone, thiazides
  Beta-adrenergic blocking agents: atenolol, labetalol, metoprolol, pindolol, propranolol, timolol
  Direct vasodilators: hydralazine, minoxidil
  Centrally acting antiadrenergics: clonidine, guanabenz, guanfacine, methyldopa
  Peripherally acting antiadrenergics: doxazosin, guanadrel, guanethidine, prazosin, reserpine, terazosin
  Calcium channel blockers: verapamil
Drugs affecting the central nervous system (CNS)
  Antianxiety agents/hypnotics: alprazolam, diazepam
  Antipsychotics: chlorpromazine, chlorprothixene, fluphenazine, haloperidol, mesoridazine, perphenazine, pimozide, thioridazine, thiothixene, trifluoperazine
  CNS stimulants: amphetamines/anorexiants
  Antidepressants: amitriptyline, amoxapine, desipramine, doxepin, imipramine, isocarboxazid, maprotiline, nortriptyline, pargyline, phenelzine, protriptyline, tranylcypromine, trazodone
  Narcotic analgesics
Antiarrhythmics: amiodarone, digoxin, disopyramide, mexiletine
Gastrointestinal agents
  H_2 antagonists: cimetidine, nizatidine, ranitidine
  Others: anticholinergics, metoclopramide, propantheline
Anticonvulsants: barbiturates, carbamazepine, ethosuximide, phenytoin, primidone
Anti-infective agents: ethionamide, ketoconazole
Miscellaneous agents: acetazolamide, baclofen, clofibrate, danazol, disulfiram, estrogens, interferon, levodopa, lithium, naproxen, progesterone

* Includes erectile dysfunction (impotence), loss of libido, and failure of ejaculation.
Data from Bressler, R. and Katz, M.D. *Geriatric Pharmacology.* New York: McGraw-Hill, 1993, p. 272. Reproduced with permission of McGraw-Hill, Inc.

strual cycle increases in length and variability. Menstruation may be either fertile or infertile, depending on the hormone levels. Menopause is said to follow a 1-year period of amenorrhea (Buxton et al., 1992; Walsh and Schiff, 1990).

Menopause is just one facet of the larger climacteric, which is the long transition phase extending many years before and after the last menstrual event. The climacteric encompasses endocrine, somatic, and psychological changes and involves an intricate relationship between the ovarian and hypothalamic-pituitary factors. The aging ovary decreases production of estrogen to about 20 per cent of the premenopausal period, resulting in increased levels of the gonadotropins FSH and LH. There are two mechanisms by which this occurs:

1. Because the ovary is less responsive to stimulation by FSH and LH, there is an increase in the production of these hormones to compensate for the diminished ovarian response.

2. LH and FSH are regulated by negative feedback from estrogen, which inhibits their production. When estrogen levels are diminished, there is no negative feedback, resulting in increased LH and FSH levels.

The production of the ovarian hormones estradiol and progesterone decreases after menopause. The ovary continues to produce androstenedione (from which estrone is in turn produced; estrone is in turn converted to estradiol), but the adrenal cortex produces by far the bulk of androstenedione. Ovarian testosterone production does not change during the perimenopausal period or after menopause (Birkenfeld and Kase, 1993). Androstenedione is peripherally converted to estrogen in skin and fat, and it is the primary source of postmenopausal estrogen.

The estrogen deficiency that accompanies menopause produces changes in the vulva, vagina, cervix, uterus, fallopian tubes, ovaries, and pelvic and supportive ligaments and tissue. Atrophy of subcutaneous fat, epithelium, and associated glands and loss of elasticity occur in the entire pelvic region. Atrophy of the vaginal epithelium causes the vaginal walls to thin, and vaginal secretions become more alkaline. These changes make the vaginal tissues more vulnerable to infections. The ovaries, uterus, cervix, and fallopian tubes decrease in size, and there is a shortening of the vaginal vault. Breast tissue becomes involuted, and this is accompanied by a decrease in the number of mammary ducts and a disappearance of the alveoli. Atrophy of the urogenital tract can lead to excessive dryness, bleeding, inflammations and infections, and atrophic and hypertrophic lesions. These may be treated with estrogen, antimicrobials, corticosteroids, and antipruritics (Barzel, 1989; Buxton et al., 1992; Homesley, 1994).

Only 20 to 30 per cent of all older women seek medical attention for symptoms associated with menopause. This may be explained by variations in levels of endogenous estrogens or by the perceptions of many women that menopausal symptoms are expected and do not require medical intervention. Because so many women do not seek medical attention for menopausal symptoms, the percentage of women who

T A B L E   1 2 – 4

Phase-Specific Changes in the Sexual Response Cycle of Aging Men

TARGET TISSUE	PHASE OF SEXUAL RESPONSE			
	Excitement	Plateau	Orgasm	Resolution
Breast	Nipple erection less discernible	—	—	Nipple erection lost more slowly
Skin	Sex flush does not occur as frequently	Sex flush does not occur as frequently	—	—
Muscle	Degree of myotonia decreased	Degree of myotonia decreased	—	—
Rectum	—	—	Rectal sphincter contractions decreased in frequency	—
Penis	Erection may be less full; erection requires two to three times as much time as necessary for younger males; erection can be maintained for extended periods without ejaculation; if erection is lost without ejaculation, there may be a secondary refractory period (rare in men under 50 years)	Color change at coronal ridge not observed in men over 60 years of age	Ejaculatory force is decreased (expulsion of semen 6 to 12 inches versus 12 to 14 inches in younger men); volume of semen decreases; fewer contractions with orgasm	Refractory period lasts for extended period; rapid loss of erection
Scrotum	Decreased evidence of vasocongestion; less tensing of scrotal sac evident	—	—	Slow involution of vasocongestion
Testes	Testes do not elevate fully to perineum; less contractile tone of cremasteric musculature observed; rare vasocongestive increase in size	—	—	Testicular descent extremely rapid

Summary of findings from *The aging male. In* Masters, W. and Johnson, V. *Human Sexual Response.* Boston: Little, Brown, 1966, pp. 248–270. From Woods, N.F. Human sexuality and the healthy elderly. *In* Brown, M. (ed.). *Readings in Gerontology.* 2nd ed. St. Louis: C.V. Mosby, 1978, pp. 69–87.

experience "hot flashes" is uncertain. Estimates range from 50 to 75 per cent. In 85 per cent of women, they persist for 1 year, and in 25 to 50 per cent they persist for more than 5 years. Hot flashes are accompanied by increased perspiration, increased skin blood flow or vasodilation, decreased core temperature, and a 10 to 15 per cent increase in pulse rate. The symptoms are caused by acute estrogen withdrawal. Even with natural menopause, estrogen levels typically rise and fall rather than decline steadily. Hypothesized causes of hot flashes include instability of the thermoregulatory center in the hypothalamus, surges in LH, and decreased noradrenergic neuronal function in the hypothalamus (Buxton et al., 1992; Walsh and Schiff, 1990). The latter theory is supported by the effectiveness of clonidine in the treatment of hot flashes (Marshburn and Carr, 1994). Treatment for hot flashes may also include administration of estrogen alone or with progesterone (Walsh and Schiff, 1990).

Hormone replacement is used not only for treatment of hot flashes but also for prevention and treatment of atrophic vaginitis. In addition to the symptomatic relief provided by estrogen replacement therapy (ERT), benefits include increased high-density lipoprotein and decreased low-density lipoprotein levels. The benefits, risks, and side effects of estrogen therapy continue to be controversial. Among the many adverse effects of ERT are headache, nausea, mastalgia, slight impairment of glucose tolerance, hypertension, increased risk of thromboembolism, increased risk of gallbladder disease, edema, weight gain, and dermatitis. Estrogen also causes endometrial hyperplasia and contributes to the development of endometrial adenocarcinoma. Estrogen can be effectively administered by the oral, topical (vaginal), and transdermal routes. Although vaginal administration provides some relief from vaginitis, systemic absorption via this route is questionable. Because of its inhibitory effect on the development of estrogen-induced endometrial hyperplasia, progestin should be added to the regimen for the woman who retains her uterus and who is receiving long-term ERT (Birkenfeld and Kase, 1993).

HRT (hormone replacement therapy) describes use of both estrogen and progesterone.

There are relative and absolute contraindications to ERT. Relative contraindications are chronic liver disease, uterine leiomyomata, poorly controlled hypertension, a history of thromboembolic disease, and acute intermittent porphyria. Absolute contraindications are known or suspected endometrial or breast cancer (unless the therapy is specifically employed for the treatment of metastatic cancer), undiagnosed genital bleeding, active thromboembolic disease, and a history of estrogen-induced thromboembolic disease (Walsh and Schiff, 1990). Caution should be used in administering estrogens to patients who have cerebrovascular or coronary artery disease (Shlafer, 1993).

The menopause does not necessarily signal an end to sexuality. According to Masters and Johnson (1966), a postmenopausal woman "is capable of full sexual performance and pleasure, provided she is regularly exposed to effective stimulation." Although some women do report changes in libido, menopause is most likely not the cause. Other variables, such as frequency of coitus, increased age, nonavailability of sexual partners, presence or absence of dyspareunia (difficult or painful coitus), and psychosocial variables are more likely to blame. Physical conditions that may affect sexual function include cardiac disease, stroke, diabetes mellitus, arthritis, recurrent cystitis and urethritis, Parkinson's disease, and pulmonary disease. In addition, women who have had traumatic injuries or surgical procedures, such as hysterectomies, mastectomies, and ostomies, may have changes in body image that affect sexual interest and enjoyment.

Many women have heightened sexual interest because of the lessened fear of pregnancy, more leisure time, and fewer distractions—such as children—at home. Although the testosterone level does not rise, its effect is probably less mitigated by estrogen than in the premenopausal period.

Masters and Johnson (1966) assembled baseline data in their now-classic work. They found that sexual responses in older women, as in older men, are characterized by a gradual decrease in the duration and intensity of the response. A major change affecting sexual intercourse is the diminished rate and amount of vaginal lubrication (see summary of changes in Table 12–5). However, continuation of sexual activity throughout the climacteric may delay and prevent some of the atrophic vaginal changes associated with aging, including decreased lubrication and accompanying discomfort.

Parathyroid Glands

The parathyroid glands, which are located behind the thyroid gland, are responsible for secretion of parathyroid hormone (PTH). PTH promotes calcium and phosphate mobilization from bone, calcium reabsorption and phosphate excretion by the kidneys, and, indirectly calcium and phosphate absorption from the gastrointestinal tract. Parathyroid secretion is primarily regulated by the serum calcium concentration through negative feedback. Because half of the circulating calcium is bound to serum proteins such as albumin, the total serum calcium concentration varies directly with the serum albumin concentration (Barzel, 1989; Guyton, 1991).

Parathyroid glands appear to have increased interstitial fatty tissue with older age; however, whether changes in parathyroid function accompany this increase is unclear. Studies of serum calcium level in the elderly have yielded inconsistent results. There does seem to be a small decrease at menopause, but the level still remains within the normal range. The PTH level rises, which is normally associated with a low serum calcium level, but in the elderly this phenomenon may be related to reduced renal PTH excretion, regardless of calcium level (Barzel, 1989). The rise in PTH may, however, pose a risk for bone demineralization. Serum levels of vitamin D may fall, but many studies in this area have been flawed by the inclusion of subjects who were rarely exposed to sunlight (Davis and Davis, 1992). In older people, there is a decline in the absorption efficiency of calcium from the small intestine. This alone would not generally be clinically significant, but it can be important if the individual has diminished gastric acid, which is needed for calcium absorption, or consumes less than the recommended intake of calcium sources. The kidneys appear to remain capable of conserving calcium through reabsorption in the proximal tubule. Serum calcitonin concentration decreases with aging, but this is probably not a major factor in calcium metabolism (Baylink and Jennings, 1994).

Pancreas

The two major types of tissue that make up the pancreas are the acini and the islets of Langerhans. Acini secrete digestive juices

TABLE 12 – 5
Phase-Specific Changes in the Sexual Response Cycle of Aging Women

TARGET TISSUE	PHASE OF SEXUAL RESPONSE			
	Excitement	Plateau	Orgasm	Resolution
Breast	Vasocongestive increase in size less pronounced, especially in more pendulous breasts	Engorgement of areola less intense	—	Loss of nipple erection slowed
Skin	Sex flush does not occur as frequently	Sex flush does not occur as frequently	—	—
Muscle	Degree of myotonia decreases with age	Degree of myotonia decreases with age	—	—
Urethra and urinary bladder	—	—	Minimal distention of meatus*	—
Rectum	—	—	Contraction of rectal sphincter only with severe tension levels	—
Clitoris	—	—	—	Retracts rapidly; tumescence lost rapidly
Labia majora	No women past age 51 demonstrated flattening, separation, and elevation of labia majora	—	—	—
Labia minora	Vasocongestion reduced	Labial color change (sex skin) usually pathognomonic of orgasm decreased in frequency among women 61 years of age and older	—	—
Bartholin's glands	—	Reduction in amount of secretions and activity, especially among postmenopausal women	—	—
Vagina	Rate and amount of vaginal lubrication decreased; lubrication occurs 1 to 3 minutes after stimulation; vaginal expansion in breadth and width decreases	Inner two thirds of vagina may still be expanding during this phase; vasocongestion of orgasmic platform reduced in intensity	Postmenopausal orgasmic platform contracts 3 to 5 times versus 5 to 10 times in younger women	Rapid involution and loss of vasocongestion
Cervix	—	—	—	Dilation of cervix not noted
Uterus	Uterine elevation and tenting of transcervical vagina develop more slowly and are less marked	Uterine elevation and tenting of transcervical vagina develop more slowly and are less marked	Some women report painful contractions with orgasm	—

* Mechanical irritation of urethra and bladder may occur as a result of thinning of vagina, which minimizes protection of these structures during thrusting.
Summary of findings from The aging female. In Masters, W. and Johnson, V. *Human Sexual Response.* Boston: Little, Brown, 1966, pp. 233–247. Adapted from Woods, N.F. Human sexuality and the healthy elderly. In Brown, M. (ed.). *Readings in Gerontology.* 2nd ed. St. Louis: C.V. Mosby, 1978, pp. 69–87.

into the duodenum. About 2 per cent of the glandular tissue of the pancreas is made up of the islets of Langerhans, which are scattered throughout. The islets secrete two polypeptide hormones—insulin and glucagon. Alpha, beta, delta, and PP cells are found in the islets. The alpha cells form glucagon, and the beta cells form insulin. The delta cells produce somatostatin, which is thought to inhibit the secretion of glucagon and insulin. PP cells secrete pancreatic polypeptide—a hormone of uncertain function (Guyton, 1991).

It is generally thought that there is a decrease in glucose tolerance with advancing age (Andres, 1992; Goldberg and Coon, 1994; Davis and Davis, 1992). Glucose metabolism involves both islet cell (beta cell) responsivity (insulin secretion) and insulin action at the target organs (insulin resistance). Age-related decreases in glucose tolerance are likely to occur at both sites. Figure 12–4 shows the decline in oral glucose tolerance with older age—specifically, the elevated blood glucose concentration that occurs after an oral glucose challenge and the corresponding decline in insulin secretion with advancing age.

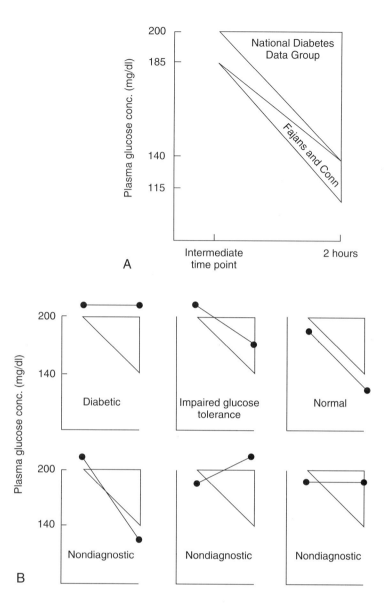

FIGURE 12–4

A, The NDDG standards for interpreting the oral glucose tolerance test (OGTT) are depicted in comparison with the old Fajans and Conn criteria. The shift upward toward higher glucose levels in the new versus the old criteria is apparent at both the intermediate and the 2-hour time points. *B*, The diagnostic categories for results of the OGTT according to the NDDG criteria. These have been related to the actual cutoff points defining the diagnostic triangle in *A*. (Redrawn from Goldberg, A.P. and Coon, P.J. Diabetes mellitus and glucose metabolism in the elderly. *In* Hazzard, W.R., Bierman, E.L., Blass, J.P. et al. (eds.). *Principles of Geriatric Medicine and Gerontology.* 3rd ed. New York: McGraw-Hill, 1994, pp. 831. Reproduced with permission of McGraw-Hill, Inc.)

PATHOLOGICAL CHANGES AND COMMON DISORDERS

Non–Insulin-Dependent Diabetes Mellitus (Type II)

Diabetes mellitus is a chronic condition characterized by abnormal glucose, fat, and protein metabolism and vascular and nervous system disease (Goldberg and Coon, 1994). The National Diabetes Data Group (NDDG) (1979) classified diabetes mellitus into type I (insulin-dependent diabetes, or IDDM) and type II (non–insulin-dependent diabetes, or NIDDM) based on the presence or absence of adequate amounts of insulin. Type I diabetes mellitus is characterized by insulin deficiency and dependence on insulin therapy to prevent ketoacidosis and death. Formerly known as "juvenile diabe-

tes," IDDM has its onset usually before age 20, but it sometimes develops in elderly people. Type II diabetes represents defects in insulin secretion as well as tissue resistance to insulin (Davis and Davis, 1992; Fernando and Coulton, 1992). It often begins in middle age, usually in obese individuals. The vast majority of people over age 65 who have diabetes have type II diabetes. A third category, impaired glucose tolerance, is used by some for individuals whose blood glucose level is above normal but is not high enough to be considered diabetes mellitus (Davis and Davis, 1992; Fernando and Coulton, 1992).

The prevalence of diabetes increases with age. Estimates of prevalence among the elderly range from 10 to 25 per cent (Campbell and Mooradian, 1993; Davis and Davis,

1992; Goldberg and Coon, 1994). Diabetes mellitus has sometimes been called a model for accelerated aging because physical changes typical of diabetes resemble age-related changes. Scientists have postulated that people with diabetes experience more rapid senescence than those who are free from the disease, and a diabetic is generally accepted as being 10 years or more older than his chronological age (Table 12–6). Pathological changes that occur prematurely include aging of the islet cells in the pancreas, development of cataracts, decrease in bone mass, and atherosclerosis. It has been argued that many variables common in aging, rather than the aging process itself, decrease glucose tolerance. These factors include obesity, decreased physical activity, increased prevalence of diseases, increased drug use, and less than optimal carbohydrate intake (Andres, 1992; Fernando and Coulton, 1992).

Diagnosis and Symptoms

Diagnosis of type II diabetes mellitus becomes difficult in the elderly because of the decrease in glucose tolerance that usually accompanies older age. The fasting plasma glucose concentration normally increases 1 mg/dl per decade, and the 2-hour postglucose load increases 5.3 mg/dl per decade. Using the old Fajans and Conn criteria, an estimated 40 to 70 per cent of the elderly would be diagnosed as having diabetes mellitus. There has been debate about whether to adjust the criteria for the elderly. The NDDG added the classification "impaired glucose tolerance" for people whose fasting and 2-hour glucose levels fall within certain parameters that had previously been called borderline diabetes or had been accepted as a normal variation of aging. A diagnosis of

diabetes mellitus is made only if fasting hyperglycemia is present (i.e., a blood glucose level >140 mg/dl) or if the 2-hour postprandial plasma glucose level is greater than 200 mg/dl. A diagnosis of impaired glucose tolerance is made on the basis of a fasting glucose level of less than 140 mg/dl and a 2-hour glucose level of 140 to 200 mg/dl. With this classification system, no age-specific adjustments are made. The work of Stern et al. (1993) provides support for using the NDDG criteria rather than relying on a single oral glucose tolerance test result. In their study, reliance on a single glucose tolerance test result resulted in overestimation of the prevalence of type II diabetes (Fig. 12–4).

Andres (1992) cautioned that steps must be taken to ensure an accurate glucose tolerance test result. The test should not be performed when the patient is very ill. He or she should consume at least 150 gm per day of carbohydrates for 3 days before the test. Also, medications that affect the results of the glucose tolerance test must be discontinued.

It has long been thought that early detection and good management of hyperglycemia could delay or prevent some of the complications of diabetes. Therefore, general health screenings usually include some measure of blood glucose level. There has been discussion of the most appropriate methods to be used to screen for diabetes. Hanson et al. (1993) compared methods used to screen 2092 subjects. They concluded that the fasting blood glucose level has the best screening properties, but that HbA1C, HbA1, and quantitative urine glucose levels were useful as well. Another study found that the sensitivity of the fasting blood glucose level decreased with increasing age but continued to be a useful tool in screening the elderly (Blunt et al., 1991).

The clinical presentation of diabetes mellitus in the older person is often atypical. The patient may present with weight loss, fatigue, pruritis vulvae, urinary tract infection, incontinence, recurrent infections, poor wound healing, and seizures. Some patients are diagnosed with diabetes mellitus when they are treated for diabetes complications, such as cataract, nephropathy, neuropathy, foot ulcers, peripheral vascular disease, or even hypoglycemic nonketotic coma. Other asymptomatic people are diagnosed during routine screening. The classic symptoms of polydipsia, polyuria, and polyphagia may be completely absent in older persons (Fernando and Coulton, 1992; Goldberg and Coon, 1992; Mersey, 1989) (Table 12–7).

TABLE 12–6
Diabetes Mellitus as a State of Accelerated Aging

Fibroblast cell culture	Decreased replication and culture viability
Collagen	Abnormal formation; apparent increase in polymerization and aging
Capillary basement	Increased rate of age-related thickening
Arterial smooth muscle endothelial cells	Increased age effects on lipid metabolism

From Lipson, L.G. *Diabetes Mellitus in the Elderly: Special Problems, Special Approaches.* New York: Pfizer Pharmaceuticals, 1985, p. 6.

TABLE 12-7
Clinical Symptoms and Signs of Diabetes Mellitus in the Elderly Patient

Common
1. Unexplained weight loss, fatigue, slow wound healing, mental status
2. Cataracts, microaneurysms, and retinal detachment
3. Recurrent bacterial or fungal infections of skin (pruritus vulvae in women), intertriginous areas, and urinary tract
4. Neurologic dysfunction, including paresthesias, dysesthesias, and hypoesthesias, muscle weakness, and pain (amyopathy), and cranial nerve palsies (mononeuropathy), and autonomic dysfunction of the gastrointestinal tract (diarrhea), cardiovascular system (postural hypotension), reproductive system (impotence), and bladder (atony, overflow incontinence)
5. Arterial disease (macroangiopathy) involving the cardiovascular system (silent ischemia, angina, and myocardial infarction), cerebral vasculature (transient ischemia and stroke), or peripheral vaculature (diabetic foot, gangrene)
6. Small-vessel disease (microangiopathy) involving the eyes (macular disease, hemorrhages, exudates), kidneys (proteinuria, glomerulopathy, uremia), and nervous system (mononeuropathy)
7. Comorbid endocrine-metabolic abnormalities, including obesity, hyperlipidemia, and osteoporosis
8. A family history of NIDDM or IDDM and a history of gestational diabetes or large babies

Rare
1. Classical polyuria, polydipsia, and polyphagia as in young persons with IDDM
2. Lesions of the skin, such as diabetic dermopathy, Dupuytren's contractures, and facial rubeosis

From Goldberg, A.P. and Coon, P.J. Diabetes mellitus and glucose metabolism in the elderly. *In* Hazzard, W.R., Bierman, E.L., Blass, J.P. et al. (eds.). *Principles of Geriatric Medicine and Gerontology.* 3rd ed. New York: McGraw-Hill, 1994, pp. 825–845. IDDM = insulin-dependent diabetes mellitus; NIDDM = non–insulin-dependent diabetes mellitus.

Treatment

The goals of treatment for diabetes mellitus are to relieve symptoms, control hyperglycemia, and prevent acute and chronic complications with minimal interference with the quality of life (Fernando and Coulton, 1992; Goldberg and Coon, 1992) (Fig. 12–5).

The treatment is essentially the same as that given in other age groups—that is, diet, exercise, medication, and prevention and/or treatment of complications. It was once thought that good glucose control was unnecessary because the older patient would not live long enough to develop long-term complications. With the increasing life expectancy, this assumption is no longer valid. Older persons should be afforded the same treatment options as younger persons. As in any clinical situation, the risks of poor control must be weighed against the potential benefits of good control (Fernando and Coulton, 1992).

DIET. Maintaining normal weight is the mainstay of treatment of people with type II diabetes (Goldberg and Coon, 1992). Obesity is highly associated with the onset of the disease, and weight reduction has an extremely positive effect on reducing symptoms, eliminating or reducing the need for medications, and maintaining control of diabetes. Evidence is growing that high dietary fat intake significantly predicts conversion from impaired glucose tolerance to NIDDM (Marshall et al., 1994). A longitudinal intervention study of severely obese subjects demonstrated that weight loss prevented the progression from impaired glucose tolerance to NIDDM. Only one of 109 subjects on a weight-loss program developed NIDDM, as compared with six of 27 in the control group (Long et al., 1994). A proper diet should begin with a careful history of what the person is eating. This promotes modification of eating habits without making drastic changes, which may make adherence difficult.

There are varying views about the appropriate diet for the older person with NIDDM. More liberal plans caution against prescribing dramatic changes but advise low-fat, high-fiber meals without simple sugars and with moderate amounts of salt. Stacpoole (1992) reported that there is a short-term rise in triglyceride levels after a low-fat, high-carbohydrate diet is initiated, but that the triglyceride and total cholesterol levels fall over time, and the high-density lipoprotein level remains at desirable levels. Others recommend a more traditional diet with complex carbohydrates and fiber contributing 55 to 60 per cent of the daily caloric intake, and less than 30 per cent of the calories being derived from fat (<10 per cent from saturated fats) (Campbell and Mooradian, 1993; Davis and Davis, 1992; Fernando and Coulton, 1992; Goldberg and Coon, 1994).

Unfortunately, sustained changes in dietary practices are difficult to achieve. Close et al. (1992) compared the 7-day food records of people with diabetes and people without diabetes. They found only three patients with diabetes who met the prescribed carbohydrate and fat intake criteria. Most subjects with diabetes consumed approximately the same nutrients as those without diabetes, except that they had higher intakes of protein and lower intakes of sugar and alcohol. Campbell et al. (1990) compared the outcomes of an intensive educational approach to dietary change with a more con-

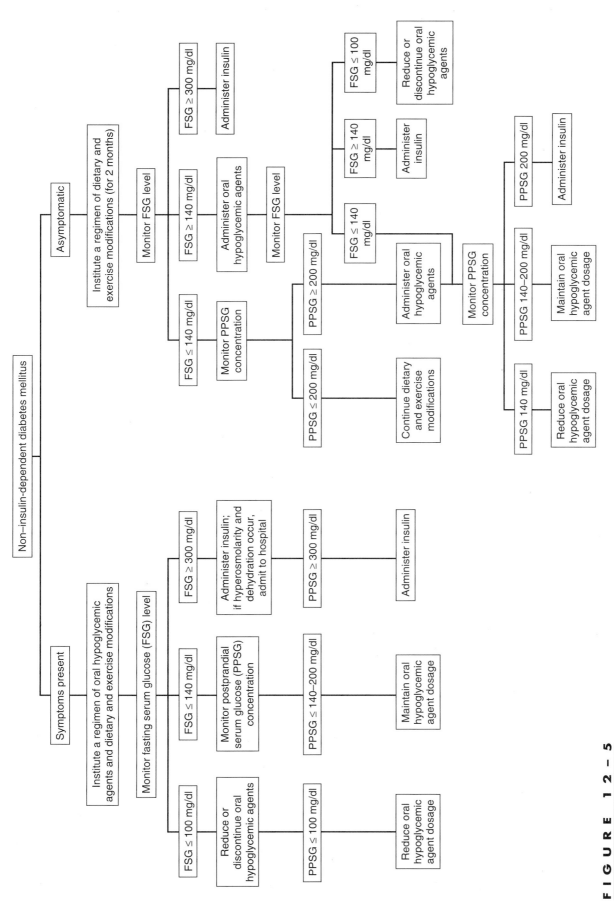

F I G U R E 1 2 – 5

A suggested approach to blood glucose control of elderly patients with non-insulin-dependent diabetes mellitus.

ventional approach. Dietary compliance improved significantly in the group with intensive education; however, improved glycemic control was transient in both groups.

Milne et al. (1994) compared the effects of three different diets (weight management, high carbohydrates and fiber, and modified lipid) on metabolic control of NIDDM. They found few differences in the outcomes, but glycosylated hemoglobin level fell significantly during the recruitment phase of the study and remained lower throughout the study.

Despite the complexities of a diabetes diet, Arnold et al. (1993) found that patients with NIDDM were significantly less likely than those with IDDM to have seen a dietitian for counseling and instruction. More than half of those who had not seen a dietitian reported that no physician had referred them for dietary instruction.

EXERCISE. Regular exercise helps to control weight and promotes vigorous health. Muscular exercise can lower the daily blood glucose level, reduce the urinary glucose concentration, and lower the daily insulin requirement. It is not clear whether this effect is due to an increased affinity of insulin for its receptor, to an increased number of insulin receptors, or primarily to metabolic factors. Depending on their level of mobility, older people may engage in regular activities, such as walking, jogging, stationary bicycling, or swimming. Exercises that require straining or breathholding should be avoided. The focus on strength training should emphasize high-repetition, low-tension activity. The exercise program must be based on the patient's physical status, as determined by an exercise treadmill test and the physical examination. Physical activity must be initiated in a slow, progressive manner. Sometimes, the health care provider must first help the patient overcome the fear of exercise (Goldberg and Coon, 1994).

MEDICATION. If diet and exercise do not control hyperglycemia, drug therapy is indicated. Drugs do not replace diet and exercise but are used in conjunction with them. The sulfonylureas are the most commonly used oral drugs for diabetes. The oral sulfonylureas may act by stimulating insulin production and by decreasing tissue resistance to insulin, but they are ineffective in the absence of functioning beta cells. First-generation sulfonylureas are tolbutamide (Orinase), acetohexamide (Dymelor), tolazamide (Tolinase), and chlorpropamide (Diabenase). Second-generation sulfonylureas are glipizide (Glucotrol) and glyburide (DiaBeta, Micronase). In general, second-generation drugs are preferred for the elderly because

the risk of adverse effects is somewhat lower. A comparative study of glyburide versus glipizide in elderly people with NIDDM concluded that both were suitable for properly selected elderly patients, and both were associated with a low incidence of hypoglycemia (Rosenstock et al., 1993). These findings were corroborated by Birkeland et al. (1994) in a long-term randomized placebo-controlled, double-blind study. A study by Noyes et al. (1992) also confirmed the efficacy of glyburide and glipizide but found that glyburide was slightly less expensive, a factor that is worth considering in the treatment of elderly people (Table 12–8).

Drugs that are excreted in the urine (acetohexamide, chlorpropamide, and glyburide) pose a threat to the elderly, who may have impaired renal function that permits accumulation of the drug or its metabolites. In addition, chlorpropamide and tolbutamide can cause the syndrome of inappropriate antidiuretic hormone with hyponatremia, especially, in females, in people over age 60, and in patients taking thiazide diuretics (Campbell and Mooradian, 1993; Goldberg and Coon, 1994; Shlafer, 1993). Although any sulfonylurea can cause hypoglycemia, the risk seems to be lower with second-generation drugs. Also, second-generation drugs have not been associated with hyponatremia (Goldberg and Coon, 1994). Early studies indicated that oral sulfonylureas were associated with increased risk of cardiovascular mortality, but those findings are controversial (Campbell and Mooradian, 1993; Shlafer, 1993). Oral sulfonylureas can also cause hypoglycemia in addition to the following side and adverse effects: gastrointestinal upset, nausea, vomiting, diarrhea, abdominal pain, confusion, ataxia, and hepatic dysfunction. Allergic reactions manifested by urticaria, fever, and sometimes blood dyscrasias may occur. The patient's drug profile must be considered because many drugs, including aspirin, alcohol, beta blockers, clofibrate, thiazide diuretics, and monamine oxidase inhibitors, interact with the sulfonylureas.

Oral drugs are usually started at the lowest possible dose, then increased at 1- to 2-week intervals until the desired clinical response is attained. They are usually taken 30 minutes before meals. The goal of therapy is to maintain the serum glucose level at between 100 and 140 mg/dl and postprandial levels of below 200 mg/dl (Davis and Davis, 1992; Goldberg and Coon, 1993). The Diabetes Control and Complications Trial supported the value of good glucose control in people with type I diabetes, and many believe that the same outcomes can be ex-

TABLE 12-8

Commonly Used Drugs Affecting Glucose Tolerance in Older Persons

WORSEN HYPERGLYCEMIA	POTENTIATE HYPOGLYCEMIA
1. Intrinsic hyperglycemic action 　　Diuretic (thiazide, chlorthalidone, furosemide) 　　Glucocorticoids 　　Estrogens 　　Nicotinic acid 　　Phenothiazines 　　Phenytoin 　　Sympathomimetic agents 　　Lithium 　　Growth hormone 　　Sugar-containing medications (cough syrup) 　　Isoniazid 2. Increased sulfonylurea metabolism 　　Alcohol 　　Rifampin	1. Intrinsic hypoglycemic action 　　Insulin 　　Alcohol 　　Salicylates 　　Monoamine oxidase inhibitors 2. Altered sulfonylurea pharmacology 　　Interfere with metabolism: bishydroxycoumarin, pyrazolone derivatives, (e.g., phenylbutazone), chloramphenicol, monoamine oxidase inhibitors 　　Decrease renal excretion: salicylates, cimetidine, probenecid, allopurinol, phenylbutazone, sulfonamides 　　Displace from albumin-binding site: salicylates, clofibrate, pyrazolone derivatives, sulfonamides 3. Impeded glucoregulation 　　Beta blockers 　　Alcohol 　　Guanethidine

Adapted from Goldberg, A.P. and Coon, P.J. Diabetes mellitus and glucose metabolism in the elderly. In Hazzard, W.R., Bierman, E.L., Blass, J.P. et al. (eds.) Principles of Geriatric Medicine and Gerontology. 3rd ed. New York: McGraw-Hill, 1994, pp. 825–845.

pected with good control of type II diabetes. Therefore, different standards of control are not generally recommended for people with type II diabetes.

Failure of oral drug therapy may be associated with disease progression, acute illness, lack of adherence to dietary and exercise prescriptions, or weight gain. Efforts should be made to improve glycemic control through diet and exercise before insulin therapy is initiated because of the increased risk of hypoglycemia with insulin therapy, especially during the night. However, when oral sulfonylureas and conservative management no longer maintain satisfactory control, insulin therapy is necessary. Insulin therapy has been demonstrated to improve glycemic control and lower very low-density lipoprotein on a long-term basis after secondary failure to oral agents (Lindstrom et al., 1994). A variety of regimens are being studied that include insulin therapy alone and combinations of oral sulfonylureas and insulin. Combination therapy may pose special disadvantages for the elderly, who often already have problems with polypharmacy. A meta-analysis of studies of combination therapy led Pugh et al. (1992) to conclude that combinations produce modest improvement over insulin therapy alone in glycemic control, achieve control with lower insulin doses, and provide better control than do single agents for obese patients with higher fasting C peptide levels. Montgomery (1992) criticized many combination trials for lack of proper controls, inadequate duration of treatment, and failure to compare combination treatments with intensive insulin treat-

ment with multiple daily injections. Researchers continue to test the efficacy of new drugs in the management of NIDDM that act by inhibiting the release or action of counter-regulatory hormones, inhibiting postprandial glucose increase, increasing tissue sensitivity to insulin, and inhibiting gluconeogenesis (Bressler and Johnson, 1992).

Some researchers recommend using insulin alone when oral drug therapy fails (Davidson, 1992; Genuth, 1992; Riddle, 1992). Davis and Davis (1992) reported that 25 per cent of their patients with type II diabetes were able to maintain normal fasting blood glucose and glycosylated hemoglobin levels with one or two daily injections of intermediate and regular insulin. A common insulin regimen would start with one or two daily doses of an intermediate-acting insulin, with a dose of 10 to 20 units in the morning. Bedtime insulin may be inappropriate because many elderly people do not have the "dawn" phenomenon.

The major concern with insulin therapy is the risk of hypoglycemia, which leads in some people to cardiac dysrhythmias (Lindstrom et al., 1992). Other problems associated with insulin therapy in the elderly are delayed excretion, hyperinsulinemia, weight gain, and possibly sodium and fluid retention (Campbell and Mooradian, 1993; Koivisto, 1993). Other factors that must be considered with insulin therapy are the ability of the older person to prepare and self-administer insulin and the willingness of the patient to accept parenteral therapy. When patients are taking insulin, they need to be able to monitor blood glucose

TABLE 12-9

Insulin Injection Aids

Syringe magnifiers	Needle and vial holders
Insul-eze	Dos-Aid
Magni-Guide	Holdease
Syringe magnifier	Inject-Aid
Dose gauges	Insul-eze
Andros IDM	Load-Matic
Click-Count Syringe	Insulin Needle Guide
Count-a-dose	Magni-Guide
Dos-Aid	Vial Center Aid
Insulgauge	Insulin pens
	Autopen
	Novo Pen
	Novolin Pen

From Bressler, R. and Katz, M.D. *Geriatric Pharmacology.* New York: McGraw-Hill, 1993, p. 420.

levels. Periodic measurements of glycosylated hemoglobin or serum fructosamine levels can be obtained to evaluate blood glucose control over time. Whereas urine testing is generally considered unreliable for evaluating glycemic control, glycosuria usually indicates hyperglycemia and thus may provide some useful data.

In addition to hyperglycemia, the person who has diabetes is at risk for microvascular and macrovascular disease, neuropathy, nephropathy, and peripheral neuropathy. Ketoacidosis is not common in the elderly, but it may occur and is more often fatal than in younger people. Ketoacidosis may be precipitated by infection, myocardial infarction, and poorly managed diabetes. Hyperglycemic nonketotic coma is sometimes the first manifestation of diabetes mellitus in the older person. This condition is treated with intravenous fluids, small doses of regular insulin, and potassium replacement.

Because of the wide variation in absorption from injection sites, the patient is advised to rotate sites in the same anatomical region. Absorption is best from the abdomen. Unless the patient is thin, the medication can be injected at a 90-degree angle. Various devices are available to facilitate self-injection for people with visual or motor impairments (Table 12-9).

PREVENTION AND TREATMENT OF COMPLICATIONS. The major complications associated with diabetes in older people include atherosclerosis of large blood vessels, microvascular disease of the kidneys and retina, and neuropathy. Effects of these complications include vascular insufficiency and gangrene, hypertension, myocardial infarction, stroke, renal disease, and blindness

(Goldberg and Coon, 1994). The increased prevalence of stroke in the known diabetic population, the undiagnosed diabetic population, and those with impaired glucose tolerance is well documented (Bell, 1994). Self-monitoring of blood glucose levels should be carried out by elderly diabetics to control the disease and to prevent complications. Blood glucose testing is more accurate than urine testing, especially in the elderly because they have higher thresholds before blood glucose concentrations are reflected in the urine. Most people can learn blood glucose testing, although motor and visual impairments must be considered. Some devices are easier to use than others, and some people who cannot distinguish colors can see digital readouts. Clients feel more in control, and they receive good feedback and incentives to adhere to diet and exercise regimens. Benefits of controlled diabetes mellitus include an improved sense of well-being, decreased lethargy, less blurring of vision, fewer symptoms of hyperglycemia (especially polyuria), lower levels of lipids and glycemia, fluid and electrolyte balance, better metabolic balance, avoidance of volume depletion, and possibly a decrease in long-term complications.

General health practices may also help prevent or delay complications. For example, there is some evidence that smoking promotes the progression of diabetic nephropathy in people with type I diabetes (Sawicki et al., 1994). Because smoking is known to cause vasoconstriction, it may aggravate the circulatory changes typical of diabetes. People who have diabetes are therefore particularly encouraged to stop smoking. Data obtained from the 1989 National Health Interview Survey revealed that the prevalence of smoking in people with diabetes mellitus was slightly higher (although not statistically significant) than that in people who did not report having diabetes. The highest prevalence was among black and Hispanic males with diabetes (Ford et al., 1994).

FOOT CARE. Foot care is particularly important for older persons who have diabetes. Vascular changes and neuropathy lead to muscle wasting, loss of sensation, and inadequate tissue perfusion. Therefore, the feet are susceptible to injury or progressive ischemia that could result in gangrene and amputation. Diabetes is the most common disease that causes foot disorders (Gudas, 1992), and diabetic foot problems often require hospitalization. All older persons with diabetes mellitus and their families should be instructed in daily cleansing, protection from injury, and avoidance of extremes of heat and cold. It would also be beneficial for older people with diabetes to visit a podiatrist at regular intervals, especially when there is any problem with nails, calluses, or injury from improper footwear.

SPECIAL PROBLEMS IN MANAGING THE TREATMENT OF OLDER DIABETICS. In planning the care and treatment of older diabetics, it is important to consider the normal and pathological changes associated with aging (Table 12–10). Dietary planning must account for changes in the perceptions of taste and smell, as well as difficulties in preparing food and eating. Social and economic factors may also influence the nutrition of older diabetics, especially those who are poor and living alone.

Drugs cleared through the kidney, including oral sulfonylureas and insulin, remain in the body longer, so that serum concentrations of these drugs may accumulate, producing increased pharmacological effects. In addition, insulin degradation, which occurs largely in the liver, diminishes with age, reflecting a decrease in hepatic function. Alterations in renal function influence urine testing by increasing the plasma glucose

TABLE 12–10
Factors That May Interfere with or Alter Control of the Diabetic State

1. Alterations in the senses
   a. Diminished vision
   b. Diminished smell
   c. Altered taste perception
2. Difficulties in preparing food and eating
   a. Tremor
   b. Arthritis
   c. Poor dentition
   d. Alterations in gastrointestinal function
3. Altered renal and hepatic function
4. Diminished exercise and mobility
5. Effects of other diseases
   a. Other chronic diseases
   b. Neoplasms
   c. Infection
6. Neuropsychiatric problems
   a. Depression
   b. Cognitive impairment
7. Social factors
   a. Lack of education
   b. Poor dietary habits
   c. Living alone
   d. Poverty
8. Drugs
   a. Other medications
   b. Alcoholism

From Lipson, L.G. *Diabetes Mellitus in the Elderly: Special Problems, Special Approaches.* New York: Pfizer Pharmaceuticals, 1985, p. 9.

threshold before it spills into the urine, as noted earlier.

Exercise is important because it increases insulin sensitivity, improves glucose tolerance, promotes weight loss, and lowers plasma lipid levels and blood pressure in some people (Goldberg and Coon, 1994). Diminished mobility associated with older age can produce a decrease in exercise. Less physical activity can in turn increase the need for oral hypoglycemic agents or insulin. It is important to encourage as much physical activity as possible in older diabetics (Goldberg and Coon, 1994).

Other diseases, including chronic diseases, neoplasms, and infections, may have an impact on the control of diabetes in older adults. The incidence of chronic disease increases with age, especially hypertension, atherosclerosis, and arthritis. A high proportion of the older population with diabetes mellitus also has hypertension, which can aggravate the microvascular and macrovascular complications.

Many drugs commonly used by older people interact with hyperglycemic agents. Beta blockers that are used as antihypertensives and antidysrhythmics are particularly problematic. They inhibit insulin secretion, but they also lower serum glucose levels, prolong recovery from hypoglycemia, and inhibit the tachycardia that is normally a sign of hypoglycemia. Therefore, people with diabetes who take beta blockers may experience hypoglycemia without the usual symptoms and may delay seeking appropriate treatment. These effects occur even with ophthalmic beta blockers. If systemic beta blockers are indicated, selective $beta_1$ blockers like atenolol are recommended because they have less impact on serum glucose. Other drugs that enhance the hypoglycemic effects of drugs used to treat diabetes include nonsteroidal anti-inflammatory drugs, sulfonamides, ethanol, ranitidine, cimetidine, and chloramphenicol (Lehne, 1994; Shlafer, 1993). A number of other drugs counteract the hypoglycemic effects of drugs used to treat diabetes. They include calcium channel blockers, combination oral contraceptives, glucocorticoids, phenothiazines, and thiazide diuretics (Lehne, 1994; Shlafer, 1993). The fact that so many drugs affect serum glucose levels poses a challenge to the physician in managing osteoarthritis, hypertension, infections, and cancer. Special care must be taken to teach older clients about drug interactions and side effects. One additional interaction that must be mentioned is the disulfiram-like action resulting from combining first-generation sulfonylureas (especially tolbutamide) with alcohol. The result may simply be flushing and palpitations but may include hypotension and vomiting (Lehne, 1994).

Cognitive factors, such as dementia or depression, can interfere with eating habits and proper management of diabetes. Confused older people may eat sporadically, paying little attention to proper diet. They may not be able to manage their medications nor be able to prevent complications such as infection. Infections and abnormal serum glucose level may produce more confusion, further exacerbating the problem. Older persons who are depressed also may eat sporadically, skip meals, and pay little attention to food intake. If their medications are not adjusted, hypoglycemia may result.

Social factors, such as lack of education, poor dietary habits, isolation, and poverty may influence the older person's ability to cope with diabetes. Care must be taken with teaching and management of the symptoms of the disease, so that interventions are tailored to the special needs of the individual. A patient's motivation to modify lifestyle and adhere to the diabetic regimen is of the utmost importance and must be assessed and encouraged.

Thyroid Disease

Hyperthyroidism

Estimates of the incidence of hyperthyroidism among the elderly range from 0.7 (Davis and Davis, 1992) to 2.0 per cent (Miller, 1992). The prevalence is believed to be seven times higher in people over age 60 than in younger people (Gregerman and Katz, 1994). The condition typically affects women in greater proportions than men. About half of the cases of hyperthyroidism in the elderly are due to toxic nodular goiter. Other causes are toxic adenoma and iodine ingestion (Miller, 1992).

The symptoms of hyperthyroidism are frequently minimal or atypical in the elderly and may lack the typical restlessness, hyperactivity, and nervous appearance. Approximately 1/3 of patients have no palpable nodularity, and exophthalmia is uncommon (Kane et al., 1994). Among the signs and symptoms reported in the elderly are weight loss, tremor, palpitations, and heat intolerance. The skin is typically warm and moist and has a fine texture. Anorexia is the only symptom in some people. Some pathological conditions, such as congestive heart failure, profound myopathy, or a psychiatric disorder of recent onset, may represent masked hyperthyroidism (Barzel, 1989; Gregerman

and Katz, 1994; Kane et al., 1994). It is important that older patients who present with these diagnoses be evaluated for possible underlying thyroid disease (Table 12–11).

Diagnosis of hyperthyroidism is difficult in the elderly, not only because symptoms are often absent or atypical but also because symptoms of other diseases are frequently present and may confuse the picture. In general, an older person with hyperthyroidism shows elevations of serum T4 concentration, resin T3 uptake, and serum free T4 and a decreased TSH level. A small percentage of elderly patients with hyperthyroidism have normal or only slightly elevated serum T4 levels (Davis and Davis, 1992). Radioactive iodine uptake tests are not routinely performed for diagnostic purposes but may be used to help determine the appropriate dose for radiation therapy (Barzel, 1989).

Treatment is accomplished chiefly through the administration of radioactive iodine,

TABLE 12–11

Clinical Features of Hyperthyroidism in the Elderly

SYMPTOM	FREQUENCY (%)
Hyperhidrosis	38
Heat intolerance	63
Weight loss	69
Palpitation	63
Angina pectoris	20
Respiratory symptoms consistent with congestive heart failure	66
Polyphagia	11
Anorexia	36
Increased stool frequency	12
Constipation	26
Tremor/nervousness	55
SIGN	
Hyperkinesis	25
Apathy	16
Cachexia/chronically ill appearance	39
Classical skin changes (warm, fine, moist)	81
Proptosis	8
Lid lag	35
Extraocular muscle palsy	22
Impalpable or normal-sized thyroid gland	37
Multinodular thyroid gland	20
Solitary thyroid nodule	21
Diffuse thyroid enlargement	22
Atrial fibrillation (AF)	39
Supraventricular tachycardia (rate > 120 beats/min)	11
Brisk deep tendon reflexes, shortened relaxation phase	26

From Davis, P.J. and Davis, F.B. Endocrine diseases. In Calkins, E., Ford, A.B. and Katz, P.R. (eds.). Practice of Geriatrics. 2nd ed. Philadelphia: W.B. Saunders, 1992, p. 485.

which is easy to administer and avoids the risk of surgery. Traditionally, antithyroid drugs have been administered to restore a euthyroid state, and beta-adrenergic blockers have been used to control the cardiac manifestations of hyperthyroidism. Radioactive iodine is then prescribed to destroy the overactive gland. Many physicians are reluctant to expose the patient to radiotherapy until the euthyroid state is achieved out of concern for possible thyroid storm caused by the release of thyroid hormones from the radiation-damaged thyroid gland (Davis and Davis, 1992). Gregerman and Katz (1994), however, asserted that the dangers of radiation are "largely anecdotal" and that there is no reason to delay that treatment. Thyroidectomy is rarely recommended for hyperthyroidism in the elderly unless the gland enlarges enough to compromise the airway (Table 12–12).

Hypothyroidism

Hypothyroidism is difficult to recognize in the elderly because the symptoms so closely resemble the process of aging. The prevalence rate of hypothyroidism among the elderly has been estimated to be from 2.3 to 14.4 per cent (Barzel, 1989; Davis and Davis, 1992).

Hypothyroidism in older people is caused by failure of the diseased or damaged thyroid gland to secrete an adequate amount of thyroid hormone. This failure is most often due to autoimmune thyroiditis, in which the body develops an immunological reaction to the thyroid. It may also be a consequence of radiation or drug treatment for hyperthyroidism.

Signs and symptoms of hypothyroidism in the elderly are anorexia, constipation, weight gain, muscular weakness and pain, joint stiffness and aching, mild anemia, depression, hoarse voice, cold intolerance, facial puffiness, scaly yellowish skin, coarse hair, bradycardia, slow relaxation of reflexes, delirium, and slow speech, thought, and movement (Gregerman and Katz, 1994). A majority of older persons do not have any symptoms except debilitation and apathy, so that diagnosis is difficult. In addition, many of the clinical signs and symptoms associated with hypothyroidism may be attributed to other age-related problems (Table 12–13) (Gregerman and Katz, 1994). Diagnosis is usually based on the presence of symptoms and on laboratory findings of elevated serum TSH concentrations and decreased free T4 levels (Gregerman and Katz, 1994). Low total T4 levels (including total T4 and thyroid-binding proteins) alone are not diagnostic in depressed or seriously ill people (Kane et al., 1994).

Treatment is based on replacement of thyroid hormone through oral administration of L-thyroxine. The maintenance dose is lower in the elderly than in younger patients, and therapy should be instituted slowly and cautiously. Most younger people require 0.15 to 0.2 mg of L-thyroxine daily, whereas some older persons need as little as 0.05 mg. The variability is great, however, so that dosages should be individually determined. According to Cunningham and Barzel (1984), lean body mass is a better predictor of thyroid

TABLE 12–12

Therapeutic Alternatives for Hyperthyroidism in the Elderly

MODALITY	DOSAGE	THERAPEUTIC GOAL	ONSET OF CLINICAL EFFECT
Propylthiouracil*	300–450 mg po daily	Inhibition of thyroid hormonogenesis†	2–8 weeks
Iodide	1–3 drops SSKI po 1–3 times daily‡	Inhibition of thyroid hormone release Inhibition of thyroid hormonogenesis	Hours
Propranolol§	10–40 mg po‖ qid	Damping of peripheral manifestations of hyperthyroidism	Hours to days, depending upon dose

* Methimazole may be substituted (30–45 mg po daily). Either thioamide drug may be administered as a single daily dose or in divided dosage.

† Propylthiouracil also acts to inhibit conversion in extrathyroidal tissues of thyroxine (T_4) to triiodothyronine (T_3); whether this is a clinically significant action is unclear. Methimazole does not affect conversion of T_4 to T_3.

‡ In situations where oral administration is impractical, iodide may be administered IV as NaI, 250- to 500-mg bolus daily.

§ Caution is advised in treating thyrotoxicosis in the setting of heart failure with beta-blocking agents. Experience with other beta blockers in managing hyperthyroidism is limited. Dosage is titrated against heart rate.

‖ In situations where oral administration is impractical, propranolol may be administered IV, 0.5- to 1.0-mg bolus, titrating against heart rate (e.g., maintenance of rate at ≤ 120/min).

Adapted from Davis, P.J. and Davis, F.B. Endocrine disorders. In Calkins, E., Ford, A.B. and Katz, P.R. (eds.). *Practice of Geriatrics.* 2nd ed. Philadelphia: W.B. Saunders, 1992, p. 487.

SSKI = saturated solution of potassium iodide; po = orally; IV = intravenously.

TABLE 12-13
Clinical Features of Hypothyroidism in Elderly Individuals*

Psychiatric manifestations and dementia	Musculoskeletal disorders
Depression	Osteoarthritis
Paranoia	Painful extremities
Delirium	Myopathy: muscle weakness, difficulty with repetitive movements
Central nervous system	
Hypothermia	Gastrointestinal disorders
Hearing loss and tinnitus	Constipation
Vertigo	Cardiovascular conditions
Myxedema coma	Hypercholesterolemia and hyperlipidemia
Cerebellar function	
Ataxia	Atherosclerosis
Neuromuscular function	Cardiomegaly
Impaired chest wall mechanics	Pericardial effusion
Upper airway disturbances	Hypertension
Peripheral nervous system	Renal and electrolyte abnormalities
Paresthesias	Hyponatremia (uncommon)
Carpal tunnel syndrome	SIADH
Skin	Hematologic changes
Thickening, scaling, dryness ("parchment like")	Macrocytic anemia
	Responses to drugs
Fluid-filled sacs beneath lower eyelids	Increased drug sensitivity
	Prolonged recovery from anesthesia
Diffuse loss of scalp hair	

* About ⅔ of the elderly with hypothyroidism are asymptomatic or present only with debilitation and apathy.
SIADH = syndrome of inappropriate antidiuretic hormone.
Adapted from Gregerman R.I. and Katz, M.S. Thyroid diseases. In Hazzard, W.R., Bierman, E.L., Blass, J.P. et al. (eds.). *Principles of Geriatric Medicine and Gerontology.* 3rd ed. New York: McGraw-Hill, 1994, pp. 807–824.

hormone dose requirement than age or weight. Caution should be used when prescribing thyroxine for older persons with heart disease, who may experience cardiac dysrhythmias or myocardial infarction (Gregerman and Katz, 1994). The initial dose is usually 0.025 mg, which is increased by 0.025 mg at 2- to 4-week intervals until the patient's TSH and T4 levels are normal (Barzel, 1989; Davis and Davis, 1992; Gregerman and Katz, 1994). The average daily maintenance dose for an older person is 0.115 mg. Any medication therapy requires special monitoring in the hypothyroid patient because the rate of metabolism may be slowed, and the drug may accumulate and become toxic. Hypnotic drugs may induce myxedema coma in a hypothyroid person (Kane et al., 1994).

Thyroid Carcinoma

Thyroid cancer, a relatively rare phenomenon, occurs twice as often in the elderly as in the young. The major types of carcinoma of the thyroid are papillary carcinoma, follicular carcinoma, C cell carcinoma, and anaplastic carcinoma. The incidence of anaplastic carcinoma increases with age, so that by

age 80 nearly half of the cases are the anaplastic type (Gregerman and Katz, 1994; Miller, 1992).

Symptoms of thyroid carcinoma include a new, rapidly enlarging, solitary mass or nodule; pain; hoarseness; dysphasia; and hemoptysis. Most lesions are benign. However, if there is a history of therapeutic irradiation of the head, neck, or upper chest, there is an increased risk of both benign and malignant thyroid nodules. Diagnosis is made through needle biopsy. Thyroid scans, ultrasound study, and soft tissue radiography may also be employed in evaluating thyroid nodules.

Surgery is often the treatment of choice for thyroid cancer, depending on the client's general health state and the type of tumor. Papillary or follicular thyroid carcinomas are relatively slow growing, and in very old people with relatively short life expectancies, treatment may be carried out with TSH suppression therapy (Gregerman and Katz, 1994). The prognosis is more favorable for people under 40 than for those over 40. The survival rates for follicular, papillary, and medullary thyroid cancers are quite high, whereas anaplastic tumors are almost universally fatal (Gregerman and Katz, 1994; Kane et al., 1994; Miller, 1992).

Cancer of the Female Reproductive System

The incidence of malignant female reproductive system tumors increases with age. Breast cancer is the most frequently diagnosed malignancy of the reproductive system (Giuliano, 1994); endometrial cancer is the most frequently diagnosed malignancy of the reproductive tract (Hacker, 1994). Additional sites of postmenopausal primary cancers are the vulva, vagina, uterine cervix, and ovaries.

Breast Cancer

Cancer of the breast ranks second to lung cancer in mortality statistics related to female deaths caused by malignant tumors (American Cancer Society, 1994; Giuliano, 1994). The incidence of diagnosed breast cancer is 60/100,000 women aged 65 and under; after age 65, the incidence rises to 320/100,000 women (Muss, 1994). The most significant predisposing factor identified thus far is a family history that includes premenopausal breast cancer in a woman's mother, sister, or daughter (Giuliano, 1994). Additional significant risk factors include a long reproductive phase (early menarche and/or late menopause), nulliparity or late parity, and a prior history of breast, reproductive tract, or colon cancer. A multitude of other risk factors have been identified (e.g., obesity, use of oral contraceptives or postmenopausal estrogen, and alcohol consumption) but have not been validated by extensive research.

The initial suspicion of breast cancer may be raised by palpation of a mass during breast self-examination or during physical examination by a primary health care provider, or a mass may be detected via screening mammography and subsequent sonography. However, biopsy of the suspicious tissue provides the only mechanism for definitive diagnosis (Giuliano, 1994).

The American Cancer Society recommends a three-pronged approach to early detection of cancer for women over 50: monthly breast self-examination, yearly examination and palpation by a professional health care provider, and yearly mammogram (American Cancer Society, 1994). All women should be taught to perform breast self-examination by either the circular, vertical strip, or wedge method (Fig. 12–6). It is easier to palpate the breasts of postmenopausal women than those of premenopausal women because of the older woman's progressive atrophy of breast tissue and the lack of confusing findings related to pregnancy and to the menstrual cycle. However, research indicates that women over 60 report less tendency to perform breast self-examination and demonstrate significantly less sensitivity to lumps in breast models than do younger women (Rutledge, 1992), which suggests the importance of assessing the older woman's ability to accurately palpate her breasts. These findings, coupled with the highest incidence of breast cancer in the older age population, also reinforce the importance in the older woman of both mammography and regular examination by a professional health care provider.

After the diagnosis of breast cancer is confirmed by biopsy, staging of the tumor by the tumor-nodes-metastases system (Table 12–14) indicates the treatment options. Initial treatment is primarily surgical, with the extent of surgery and additional treatment dependent on many factors: stage and type of the cancer, age and physical status of the patient, and judgment of the physician.

Postmastectomy and chemotherapy/radiation treatment for breast cancer traditionally rules out use of ERT to mitigate menopausal sequelae. Thus, affected women are deprived of the protective effects of estrogen on cardiovascular health and bone density. Prohibition of ERT for women with histories of breast cancer is based predominantly on the theory that estrogen may stimulate dormant cancer cells and activate new tumor formation. Cobleigh et al. (1994) challenged the theory as unsubstantiated by numerous studies and recommended additional clinical trials of ERT, particularly in combination with tamoxifen, for patients who had breast cancer.

Cancer of the Cervix, Uterus, and Ovary

Routine use of the Papanicolaou test has resulted in early detection of, and treatment for, most cases of precancerous uterine cervical cancer in situ. Therefore, the incidence of invasive cervical cancer has decreased markedly to a predicted 15,000 cases for 1994 (American Cancer Society, 1994). In contrast, 31,000 new cases of uterine endometrial cancer were anticipated during the same period. Although endometrial cancer may be detected by the Papanicolaou test, about 50 per cent of the tests fail to do so (American Cancer Society Cancer Response System, 1994c; Hacker, 1994). Ovarian cancer is the second most prevalent of female reproductive tract malignancies; 24,000 new cases were predicted for 1994. Vulvar cancer is relatively rare and is included in the 5300 new cases predicted for the "other" category of female genital cancers (American Cancer Society, 1994).

The characteristics most commonly associated with endometrial cancer are postmenopausal status, obesity, hypertension, and high-fat diet. Additional risk factors are long menstrual history (early menarche and/or late menopause), history of abnormal uterine bleeding or infertility or nulliparity, diabetes mellitus, and prolonged estrogen stimulation of the endometrium. Because of the latter, progesterone is currently added to ERT for its protective effect on the endometrium (American Cancer Society Cancer Response System, 1994c; Hacker, 1994). Because no reliable screening mechanisms have been identified, biopsy of uterine tissue samples obtained via fractional dilation and curettage is recommended at the time of menopause and at subsequent but unspecified intervals for all women identified as being at high risk. Additional tests may be indicated for advanced carcinoma to determine the extent of involvement before surgery. Magnetic resonance imaging has not been found to be accurate enough to warrant its expense in the evaluation process for endometrial cancer.

The clinical staging system (Table 12–15) used for endometrial cancer was developed

Here's what you should do to check for changes in your breasts.

Do breast self-examination (BSE) once a month. Become familiar with how your breasts usually look and feel. Do BSE to look for any change from what looks and feels normal for you. Pick a certain day—such as the first day of each month—to remind you to do BSE.

Remember, BSE is not a substitute for routine mammograms or regular breast examinations by a health practitioner.

1 Stand in front of a mirror that is large enough for you to see your breasts clearly. Check each breast for anything unusual. Check the skin for puckering, dimpling, or scaliness. Look for a discharge from the nipples.

Do steps 2 and 3 to check for any change in the shape or contour of your breasts. As you do these steps, you should feel your chest muscles tighten.

2 Watching closely in the mirror, clasp your hands behind your head and press your hands forward.

3 Next, press your hands firmly on your hips and bend slightly toward the mirror as you pull your shoulders and elbows forward.

4 Gently squeeze each nipple and look for a discharge.

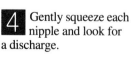

5 Raise one arm. Use the pads of the fingers of your other hand to check the breast and the surrounding area–firmly, carefully, and thoroughly. Some women like to use lotion or powder to help their fingers glide easily over the skin. Feel for any unusual lump or mass under the skin.

Feel the tissue by pressing your fingers in small, overlapping areas about the size of a dime. To be sure you cover your whole breast, take your time and follow a definite pattern: lines, circles, or wedges.

Some research suggests that many women do BSE more thoroughly when they use a pattern of up-and-down lines or strips. Other women feel more comfortable with another pattern. The important thing is to cover the whole breast and to pay special attention to the area between the breast and the underarm, including the underarm itself. Check the area above the breast, up to the collarbone and all the way over to your shoulder.

LINES: Start in the underarm area and move your fingers downward little by little until they are below the breast. Then move your fingers slightly toward the middle and slowly move back up. Go up and down until you cover the whole area.

CIRCLES: Beginning at the outer edge of your breast, move your fingers slowly around the whole breast in a circle. Move around the breast in smaller and smaller circles, gradually working toward the nipple. Don't forget to check the underarm and upper chest areas, too.

WEDGES: Starting at the outer edge of the breast, move your fingers toward the nipple and back to the edge. Check your whole breast, covering one small wedge-shaped section at a time. Be sure to check the underarm area and the upper chest.

6 It's important to repeat step 5 while you are lying down. Lie flat on your back, with one arm over your head and a pillow or folded towel under the shoulder. This position flattens the breast and makes it easier to check. Check each breast and the area around it very carefully using one of the patterns described above.

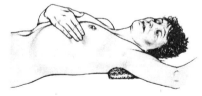

7 Some women repeat step 5 in the shower. Your fingers will glide easily over soapy skin, so you can concentrate on feeling for changes underneath.

> If you notice a lump, a discharge, or any other change during the month–whether or not it is during BSE–contact your doctor.

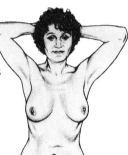

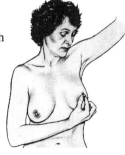

FIGURE 12-6

Technique for breast self-examination.

T A B L E   1 2 – 1 4

Breast Cancer: Staging and Treatment

STAGE	TUMOR	AXILLARY LYMPH NODES	METASTASES	TREATMENT
I	<2 cm, no fixation	Negative	None	*I and II* Mastectomy with axillary lymph node dissection
IIA	>2 cm, <5 cm, no fixation	Negative or positive	None	OR Conservative surgery (lumpectomy, partial or segmental mastectomy, quadrantectomy) with axillary lymph node dissection, radiation therapy
IIB	OR >2 cm, <5 cm, fixation to underlying fascia/muscle	Positive, fixed to one another	None	OR Conservative surgery with axillary lymph node dissection, without radiation therapy OR Mastectomy or conservative surgery with axillary lymph node dissection, chemotherapy, and/or hormonal therapy
IIIA	>5 cm, no fixation	Positive, multiple; may be attached to other structures	None	*IIIA and IIIB* Modified radical mastectomy with axillary lymph node dissection
	OR >5 cm, no fixation	Positive	Supraclavicular, infraclavicular lymph nodes	AND Chemotherapy: Cyclophosphamide, methotrexate, fluorouracil (CMF) CMF plus prednisone (CMFP) Methotrexate, fluorouracil, citrovorum factor AND/OR
IIIB	>5 cm, fixation to underlying fascia/muscle	Positive, may include substernal nodes	As IIIA, may include chest wall	Hormonal therapy: Estrogen receptor positive only—tamoxifen if tumor is estrogen receptor positive
IV	Any size, fixation to chest wall or skin, edema, skin ulceration	Positive	Distant structures (e.g., bones, lungs, liver, brain)	*IV* Modified radical or radical mastectomy, lymph node dissection plus surgery to remove a single metastasis; possibly removal of adrenal, pituitary glands AND Chemotherapy as for stage III, plus paclitaxel, bone marrow transplantation AND/OR Hormonal therapy: Tamoxifen, estrogens, androgens

by the International Federation of Gynecologists and Obstetricians (FIGO) (Hacker, 1994). Although a more extensive FIGO surgical staging system has been developed, Hacker indicated that its widespread use is currently unlikely. Treatment includes either hysterectomy or a combination of hysterectomy and radiation therapy and may include chemotherapy or hormonal therapy. Although the overall 5-year survival rate for endometrial cancer is 83 per cent (American Cancer Society, 1994), the prognosis for women over 60 years of age is significantly less favorable than for women under 60 (Hacker, 1994). Hacker postulates that the difference is attributable to the tendency toward better-differentiated, less invasive tumors in the younger group of women.

Ovarian cancer is most likely to occur after menopause, in women between 65 and 84 years of age. Risk factors include family history of ovarian cancer and personal history of obesity or of previous cancer of breast, reproductive tract, or colorectal tract. Because of difficulty in detection at an early stage, the death rate from ovarian cancer is the highest of all female reproductive system cancers: 13,600 deaths were predicted for 1994 (American Cancer Society, 1994). Because of the complexity of ovarian tissue, many types of tumors are possible. Adenocarcinoma is the most common. Although research indicates that a combination of tumor marker elevated serum CA125 level and transvaginal sonography may be effective in detecting ovarian cancer in its early stage,

T A B L E   1 2 – 1 5
Endometrial Cancer: FIGO Clinical Staging

STAGE	EXTENT OF TUMOR GROWTH	INVOLVEMENT OF OTHER STRUCTURES
0	Carcinoma in situ	None
I	Carcinoma confined to corpus (body) of uterus	None—does not include uterine cervix
II	Carcinoma confined to uterine corpus and cervix	Does not extend beyond the uterus
III	Carcinoma extends beyond the uterus	Does not extend beyond the true pelvis
IV	Carcinoma extends beyond the true pelvis	May involve mucosa of rectum and/or bladder
IVA	Carcinoma extends beyond the true pelvis	Metastasis to adjacent organs
IVB	Carcinoma extends beyond the true pelvis	Metastasis to distant organs

FIGO = International Federation of Gynecologists and Obstetricians

results have not yet reached the accuracy level necessary for their use as routine screening techniques (Berek, 1994). Because ovaries normally atrophy and become non-palpable after menopause, the first indication of ovarian cancer may be ovarian palpability after menopause. Subjective symptoms are rare until a tumor becomes large enough to affect other pelvic structures. Diagnosis requires laparoscopic surgery to examine the ovary and to remove tissue for biopsy; the ovary itself is often removed. Additional and extensive testing is performed to determine local and distant metastases. Depending on the stage of the tumor, treatment ranges from simple ovarectomy if tumor growth is confined to the ovary to removal of the entire reproductive tract and pelvic viscera if the tumor growth extends throughout the pelvic cavity. Distant tumor growth may be included in surgical treatment. Aggressive chemotherapy follows surgery for metastatic cancer; single-agent therapy is commonly employed for older patients who are unable to tolerate more toxic combination chemotherapy (Berek, 1994).

NURSING ASSESSMENT

Nursing assessment of the endocrine system is centered mainly on the diseases that commonly occur—diabetes mellitus, thyroid disorders, and breast cancer. Information regarding sexuality, menstruation and child-

bearing, and menopause is also elicited (Table 12–16).

History

Diabetes Mellitus

A recent history of fatigue, generalized weakness, excessive appetite and thirst, and rapid weight loss may indicate type I or type II diabetes mellitus. Obesity may be associated with type II diabetes mellitus.

T A B L E   1 2 – 1 6
Nursing Assessment of the Endocrine System

History
Family history of diabetes mellitus, thyroid disease, or cancer
Symptoms
  Diabetes mellitus
    Fatigue, generalized weakness, excessive appetite, thirst, rapid weight loss, obesity
  Hypothyroidism
    Decreased tolerance to cold, lethargy, constipation, muscle weakness, pain, stiffness, loss of sense of smell or nasal stuffiness, answers questions slowly and inappropriately
  Hyperthyroidism
    Angina, confusion, emotional lability, weakness, fatigue, weight loss, increased cold tolerance, decreased heat tolerance
  Breast cancer
    Changes in appearance of breast, tenderness, mass, discharge
Sexual history and functioning
  Availability of a partner, interest, ease of intercourse
Menstruation, childbearing, and menopause
  Gynecological care
  Menstruation history
  Number of pregnancies
  Menopause
    Age of onset
    Symptoms: "hot flashes," chills, sweating, palpitations, headaches, irritability, depression

Physical Assessment
Diabetes mellitus:
  Thinning of skin and subcutaneous tissue in lower extremities
  Skin infections, foot ulcers
  Decreased temperature sensation
  Cataracts: diabetic retinopathy
  Diminished patellar and Achilles reflexes
Hypothyroidism:
  Lifeless, dry hair
  Coarse, dry, and thickened skin
  Prominent lips and nostrils
  Sparse eyebrows with loss of outer one-third margin
  Enlarged heart; congestive heart failure
  Husky and weak voice
Hyperthyroidism:
  Skin warm, damp, fine, smooth
  Exophthalmia or staring eyes
  Tremors of tongue or hands
  Tachycardia or atrial fibrillation
Breast examination:
  Symmetry, contour, swelling, dimpling, changes in nipples
  Lumps, thickening, hard knots

Thyroid Disorders

HYPOTHYROIDISM. Older clients should be questioned about symptoms such as decreased tolerance to cold, lethargy, and constipation. They may also complain about muscle weakness, pain, stiffness, and loss of sense of smell or nasal stuffiness. Their answers to questions may be slowed and inappropriate.

HYPERTHYROIDISM. There may be a history of cardiovascular symptoms, such as angina pectoris and atrial fibrillation. Other symptoms include confusion, depression, emotional lability, weakness, fatigue, weight loss, increased cold tolerance, and decreased heat tolerance.

Breast Cancer

Clients should be asked whether they have noticed changes in appearance of breast or the presence of a mass, tenderness, or discharge. Family history is noted.

Sexuality

Information regarding sexual activity should include the availability of a partner, interest, and ease of intercourse. Men should be questioned about erectile dysfunction.

Menstruation, Childbearing, and Menopause

A menstrual and pregnancy history should be obtained in women. Inquiries about gynecological care should also be made. Information about menopause includes age of onset and symptoms such as hot flashes, chills, sweating, and palpitations. Other complaints to be investigated include headaches, irritability, and depression.

Physical Assessment

Diabetes Mellitus

Older clients with diabetes mellitus may appear chronically ill and fatigued. There may be thinning of the skin and subcutaneous tissue in the lower extremities with plantar redness of the feet. Skin infections and foot ulcers may be present. An examination of the eye may reveal cataracts or retinopathy. Neuropathy can result in diminished patellar and Achilles tendon reflexes as well as decreased temperature sensation.

Thyroid Disorders

HYPOTHYROIDISM. The nurse should observe for lifeless, dry hair and coarse, dry, and thickened skin. The lips and nostrils may appear prominent, and the eyebrows are sparse with loss of the outer third of the margin. The voice is often husky and weak. There may be evidence of an enlarged heart or congestive heart failure.

HYPERTHYROIDISM. The skin appears warm, damp, fine, and smooth with excessive perspiration. The eyes may have the bulging appearance of exophthalmia or may appear to be staring. Tremors may occur in the tongue when it is extended from the mouth, or in the hands when the arms and fingers are extended. Tachycardia or atrial fibrillation also occurs with hyperthyroidism.

Examination of the Breasts

Older women may have large, pendulous breasts that make examination difficult. The nurse should observe for symmetry, changes in contour, swelling, dimpling of the skin, and changes in the nipple. The nurse should also palpate for lumps, thickening, and hard knots in the clockwise direction. Self-breast examination should be taught to all older women (see Fig. 12–6).

NURSING DIAGNOSES

1. Anxiety related to erectile dysfunction diagnosis of breast cancer, symptoms of menopause

2. Bowel Elimination, Alterations in: Constipation related to hypothyroidism

3. Fear related to diagnosis of breast cancer

4. Knowledge Deficit related to lack of skill in carrying out breast examination or diabetes care; lack of understanding of sexuality in the aged

5. Noncompliance related to negative side effects of prescribed treatment of diabetes

6. Nutrition, Alterations in: Less Than Body Requirements related to symptoms of diabetes

7. Self-Concept, Disturbance in: Body Image related to mastectomy

8. Self-Concept, Disturbance in: Self-Esteem, Role Performance related to impotence

9. Sexual Dysfunction related to impotence, lack of knowledge, or change or loss of body part secondary to mastectomy

10. Thought Processes, Alteration in related to confusion secondary to thyroid disease

---

NURSING INTERVENTIONS AND EVALUATION

Nursing interventions are mainly associated with teaching and counseling related to care of older persons with diabetes mellitus and thyroid disease, symptoms of menopause, and problems with sexuality. Drug management, especially the preparation and administration of insulin, is often difficult for older persons with sensory and motor deficits. In many cases, family members or community nurses must be involved in the preparation of medications to be sure that proper doses and schedules are maintained.

Counseling may be necessary to help older clients to adjust to changes in lifestyle, such as diet modification and exercise. Older people are willing to modify their diets and to engage in exercise programs if they are able and see the need to do so. Dietary changes and exercise regimens should be developed based on individual preferences and abilities, cultural background, and previously held attitudes and beliefs.

Older people may have difficulty in discussing intimate matters related to sexuality. Careful discussion may reveal attitudes and beliefs that may be untrue and that interfere with satisfactory sexual functioning. Nurses must also examine their own attitudes toward sexuality in the elderly and must be aware that sexuality is a normal part of life at any age.

Evaluation is based on the amount of compliance and ability to carry out drug, dietary, and exercise regimens. In addition, older clients should be able to express satisfaction with their sexual outlets.

SUMMARY

The endocrine system is made up of tissues and glands whose function is to produce and secrete hormones into the bloodstream. Age-related changes occur in both the reception and the production of hormones and affect the functioning of the pituitary and thyroid glands, adrenal cortex, gonads, parathyroid glands, and pancreas. Major changes occurring in the older male include decreases in testicular volume and spermatogenesis; however, serum testosterone levels remain constant. Females experi-

ence menopause, decreased serum estrogen levels, and atrophy of the subcutaneous tissues of the breast and external genitalia. Sexual responses tend to become slower and are less intense in both men and women in older age.

Pathological changes in the endocrine system that commonly occur with older age include type II diabetes mellitus, thyroid disorders, and cancer of the breast and reproductive organs. Treatment is aimed toward proper management of medications, diet and exercise, and sexual counseling.

REFERENCES

Abernathy, D.R. and Andrawis, N. Hypertension in the elderly. In Calkins, E., Ford, A.B. and Katz, P.R. (eds.). *Practice of Geriatrics.* 2nd ed. Philadelphia: W.B. Saunders, 1992, pp. 454–461.

Akinmokun, A., Harris, P., Home, P.D. and Alberti, K.G. Is diabetes always diabetes? *Diabetes Res Clin Prac* 18(2):131–136, 1992.

Alberti, K.G. Problems related to definitions and epidemiology of type 2 (non-insulin-dependent) diabetes mellitus: Studies throughout the world [review]. *Diabetologia* 36(10):978–984, 1993.

American Cancer Society. *Cancer Facts and Figures—1994.* Atlanta, GA: American Cancer Society, 1994.

American Cancer Society Cancer Response System. *Breast Cancer: Advanced.* Publ. No. 407077. Atlanta, GA: American Cancer Society, 1994a.

American Cancer Society Cancer Response System. *Breast Cancer: Staging.* No. 407075. Atlanta, GA: American Cancer Society, 1994b.

American Cancer Society Cancer Response System. *Endometrial Cancer: Organ/Site Description.* No. 417257. Atlanta, GA: American Cancer Society, 1994c.

American Cancer Society Cancer Response System. *Endometrial Cancer: Staging.* No. 417272. Atlanta, GA: American Cancer Society, 1994d.

American Cancer Society Cancer Response System. *Endometrial Cancer: Treatment.* No. 417275. Atlanta, GA: American Cancer Society, 1994e.

American Cancer Society Cancer Response System. *Ovarian Cancer: Treatment.* No. 458076. Atlanta, GA: American Cancer Society, 1994f.

American Cancer Society Cancer Response System. *Vulvar Cancer: Staging.* No. 480076. Atlanta, GA: American Cancer Society, 1994g.

Andres, R. Diabetes and aging. In Brocklehurst, J.C., Tallis, R.C. and Fillit, H.M. (eds.). *Textbook of Geriatric Medicine and Gerontology.* 4th ed. Edinburgh: Churchill-Livingstone, 1992, pp. 724–728.

Arnold, M.S., Stepien, C.J., Hess, G.E. and Hiss, R.G. Guidelines vs practice in the delivery of diabetes nutrition care. *J Am Diet Assoc* 93(1):34–39, 1993.

Barton, R.N., Horan, M.A., Weijers, J.W.M. et al. Cortisol production rate and the urinary excretion of 17-hydroxycorticosteroids, free cortisol, and 6 beta-hydroxycortisol in healthy elderly men and women. *J Gerontol* 48(5):M213–M218, 1993.

Barzel, U.S. Endocrinology and aging. In Reichel, W. (ed.). *Clinical Aspects of Aging.* 3rd ed. Baltimore: Williams & Wilkins, 1989, pp. 373–381.

Baylink, D.J. and Jennings, J.C. Calcium and bone homeostasis and changes in aging. In Hazzard, W.R., Bierman, E.L., Blass, J.P. et al. (eds.). *Principles of Geri-*

atric *Medicine and Gerontology.* 3rd ed. New York: McGraw-Hill, 1994, pp. 879–896.

Beck, L.H. Aging changes in renal function. *In* Hazzard, W.R., Bierman, E.L., Blass, J.P. et al. (eds.). *Principles of Geriatric Medicine and Gerontology.* 3rd ed. New York: McGraw-Hill, 1994, pp. 615–624.

Belchetz, P.E. Pituitary and adrenal disorders in old age. *In* Brocklehurst, J.C., Tallis, R.C. and Fillit, H.M. (eds.). *Textbook of Geriatric Medicine and Gerontology.* 4th ed. Edinburgh: Churchill Livingstone, 1992, pp. 694–700.

Bell, D.S.H. Stroke in the diabetic patient. *Diabetes Care* 17(3):213–219, 1994.

Berek, J.S. Epithelial ovarian cancer. *In* Berek, J.S. and Hacker, N.F. (eds.). *Practical Gynecologic Oncology.* 2nd ed. Baltimore: Williams & Wilkins, 1994, pp. 327–375.

Blesch, K.S. and Prohaska, T.R. Cervical cancer screening in older women: Issues and interventions. *Cancer Nurs* 14(3):141–147, 1991.

Birkeland, K.I., Furuseth, K., Nelander, A. et al: Long-term randomized placebo-controlled double-blind therapeutic comparison of glipizide and glyburide. Glycemic control and insulin secretion during 15 months. *Diabetes Care* 17(1):45–49, 1994.

Birkenfeld, A. and Kase, N.G. The management of the postmenopausal woman. *In* Glass, R.H. (ed.). *Office Gynecology.* 4th ed. Baltimore: Williams & Wilkins, 1993, pp. 285–300.

Blunt, B.A., Barrett-Connor, E. and Wingard, D.L. Evaluation of fasting plasma glucose as screening test for NIDDM in older adults. Rancho Bernardo Study. *Diabetes Care* 14(11):989–993, 1991.

Braganza, J.M. The pancreas. *In* Brocklehurst, J.C., Tallis, R.C. and Fillit, H.M. (eds.). *Textbook of Geriatric Medicine and Gerontology.* 4th ed. Edinburgh: Churchill Livingstone, 1992, pp. 527–535.

Bressler, R. and Johnson, D. New pharmacological approaches to therapy of NIDDM [review]. *Diabetes Care* 15(6):792–805, 1992.

Bressler, R. and Katz, M.D. *Geriatric Pharmacology.* New York: McGraw-Hill, 1993.

Brown, A.D.G. and Cooper, T.K. Gynaecological disorders in the elderly—Sexuality and aging. *In* Brocklehurst, J.C., Tallis, R.C. and Fillit, H.M. (eds.). *Textbook of Geriatric Medicine and Gerontology.* 4th ed. Edinburgh: Churchill Livingstone, 1992, pp. 656–665.

Butler, R.N. and Lewis, M. Sexuality. *In* Abrams, W.B. and Fletcher, A.J. (eds.). *The Merck Manual of Geriatrics.* Rahway, NJ: Merck Sharp & Dohme Research Laboratories, 1992, pp. 631–642.

Buxton, B.H., Schinfeld, J.S. and Ryan, G.M. Gynecologic problem. *In* Calkins, E., Ford, A.B. and Katz, P.R. (eds.). *Practice of Geriatrics.* 2nd ed. Philadelphia: W.B. Saunders, 1992, pp. 474–482.

Campbell, L.V., Barth, R., Gosper, J.K. et al. Impact of intensive educational approach to dietary change in NIDDM. *Diabetes Care* 13(8):841–847, 1990.

Campbell, S. and Mooradian, A.D. Diabetes mellitus. *In* Bressler, R. and Katz, M.D. (eds.). *Geriatric Pharmacology.* New York: McGraw-Hill, 1993.

Chalmers, T.C. Oral hypoglycemic agents? Negative. *Hosp Pract (Off Ed)* 27(Suppl[1]):32–34, 1992.

Close, E.J., Wiles, P.G., Lockton, J.A. et al. Diabetic diets and nutritional recommendations: What happens in real life? *Diabet Med* 9(2):181–189, 1992.

Cobleigh, M.A., Berris, R.F., Bush, T. et al. Estrogen replacement therapy in breast cancer survivors. *JAMA* 272(7):540–545, 1994.

Coleman, E.A., Feuer, E.J. and The NCI Breast Cancer Screening Corsortium. Breast cancer screening among women from 65 to 74 years of age in 1987–1988 and 1991. *Ann Intern Med* 117(11):961–966, 1992.

Coulston, A.M., Mandelbaum, D. and Reaven, G.M. Dietary management of nursing home residents with non-insulin-dependent diabetes mellitus. *Am Clin Nutr* 51(1):67–71, 1990.

Cunningham, J.J. and Barzel, U.S. Lean body mass is a predictor of the daily requirement for thyroid hormone in older men and women. *J Am Geriatr Soc* 32:204–209, 1984.

Davidson, M.B. Rational use of sulfonylureas. *Postgrad Med* 92(2):69–70, 1992.

Davies, I. Aging and the endocrine system. *In* Brocklehurst, J.C., Tallis, R.C. and Fillit, H.M. (eds.). *Textbook of Geriatric Medicine and Gerontology.* 4th ed. Edinburgh: Churchill Livingstone, pp. 666–674.

Davis, P.J. and Davis, F.B. Endocrine diseases. *In* Calkins, E., Ford, A.B. and Katz, P.R. (eds.). *Practice of Geriatrics.* 2nd ed. Philadelphia: W.B. Saunders, 1992, pp. 483–501.

Fernando, D.F.S. and Coulton, A.F.M. Diabetes—Management in old age. *In* Brocklehurst, J.C., Tallis, R.C. and Fillit, H.M. (eds.). *Textbook of Geriatric Medicine and Gerontology.* 4th ed. Edinburgh: Churchill Livingstone, 1992, pp. 729–738.

Ford, E.S., Malarcher, A.M., Herman, W.H. and Aubert, R.E. Diabetes mellitus and cigarette smoking. *Diabetes Care* 17(7):688–692, 1994.

Freedman, T.G. Social and cultural dimensions of hair loss in women treated for breast cancer. *Cancer Nurs* 17(4):334–341, 1994.

Funnell, M.M. and Merritt, J.H. The challenges of diabetes and older adults [review]. *Nurs Clin North Am* 28(1):45–60, 1993.

Genuth, S. Management of the adult onset diabetic with sulfonylurea drug failure. *Endocrinol Metab Clin North Am* 21(2):351–370, 1992.

Gill, K.M. and Ducharme, S. Sexual concerns of the elderly. *In* Calkins, E., Ford, A.B. and Katz, P.R. (eds.). *Practice of Geriatrics.* 2nd ed. Philadelphia, W.B. Saunders, 1992, pp. 276–282.

Giovannucci E., Ascheria, A., Rimm, E.B. et al. A prospective cohort study of vasectomy and prostate cancer in U.S. men. *JAMA* 269(7):873–877, 1993.

Giuliano, A.E. Breast disease. *In* Berek, J.S. and Hacker, N.F. (eds.). *Practical Gynecologic Oncology.* 2nd ed. Baltimore: Williams & Wilkins, 1994, pp. 481–515.

Glass, R.H. (ed.). *Office Gynecology.* 4th ed. Baltimore: Williams & Wilkins, 1993.

Goldberg, A.P. and Coon, P.J. Diabetes mellitus and glucose metabolism in the elderly. *In* Hazzard, W.R., Bierman, E.L., Blass, J.P. et al. (eds.). *Principles of Geriatric Medicine and Gerontology.* 3rd ed. New York: McGraw-Hill, 1994, pp. 825–845.

Granda, C. Nursing management of patients with lymphedema associated with breast cancer therapy. *Cancer Nurs* 17(3):229–235, 1994.

Greenspan, S.L., Rowe, J.W., Maitland, L.A. et al. The pituitary-adrenal glucocorticoid response is altered by gender and disease. *J Gerontol* 48(3):M72–M77, 1993.

Gregerman, R.I. and Katz, M.S. Thyroid diseases. *In* Hazzard, W.R., Bierman, E.L., Blass, J.P. et al. *Principles of Geriatric Medicine and Gerontology.* 3rd ed. New York: McGraw-Hill, 1994, pp. 825–845.

Groop, L.C. Sulfonylureas in NIDDM. *Diabetes Care* 15(6):737–754, 1992.

Grunberger, G. Maintenance of sulfonylurea responsiveness in NIDDM. *Diabetes Care* 15(5):696–699, 1992.

Gudas, C.J. Common foot problems in the elderly. *In* Calkins, E., Ford, A.B. and Katz, P.R. (eds.). *Practice of Geriatrics.* 2nd ed. Philadelphia: W.B. Saunders, 1992, pp. 420–428.

Guyton, A.C. *Textbook of Medical Physiology.* 8th ed. Philadelphia: W.B. Saunders, 1991.

Hacker, F.F. Uterine cancer. *In* Berek, J.S. and Jacker, N.F. (eds.). *Practical Gynecologic Oncology.* 2nd ed. Baltimore: Williams & Wilkins, 1994, pp. 285–326.

Hanson, R.L., Nelson, R.G., McCance, D.R. et al. Comparison of screening tests for non-insulin-dependent diabetes mellitus. *Arch Intern Med* 153(18):2133–2140, 1993.

Hardy, K.J., Burge, M.R., Boyle, P.J. and Scarpello, J.H.B. A treatable cause of recurrent severe hypoglycemia. *Diabetes Care* 17(7):722–724, 1994.

Harris, M.I., Klein, R., Welborn, T.A. and Knuiman, M.W. Onset of NIDDM occurs at least 4–7 years before clinical diagnosis. *Diabetes Care* 15(7):815–819, 1992.

Horsley, J.S. Breast diseases. *In* Shingleton, H.M. and Hurst, W.G. (eds.). *Postreproductive Gynecology.* New York: Churchill Livingstone, 1990, pp. 355–395.

Hodgson, B.B., Kizior, R.J. and Kingdon, R.T. *Nurse's Drug Handbook.* Philadelphia: W.B. Saunders, 1993.

Homesley, H.D. Geriatric gynecology. *In* Hazzard, W.R., Bierman, E.L., Blass, J.P. et al. (eds.). *Principles of Geriatric Medicine and Gerontology.* 3rd ed. New York: McGraw-Hill, 1994, p. 474.

Hosker, J.P., Kumar, S., Gordon, C. et al. Diet treatment of newly presenting type 2 diabetes improves insulin secretory capacity, but has no effect on insulin sensitivity. *Diabet Med* 10(6):509–513, 1993.

Jacobson, A.M., de Groot, M. and Samson, J.A. The evaluation of two measures of quality of life in patients with type I and type II diabetes. *Diabetes Care* 17(4):267–274, 1994.

Johnson, J.L. and Felicetta, J.V. Hypothyroidism: A comprehensive review. *J Am Acad Nurse Pract* 4(4):131–138, 1992.

Kane, R.L., Ouslander, J.G. and Abrass, I.B. *Essentials of Clinical Geriatrics.* 3rd ed. New York: McGraw-Hill, 1994.

Klein, R., Klein, B.E., Moss, S.E. and Linton, K.L. The Beaver Dam Eye Study. Retinopathy in adults with newly discovered and previously diagnosed diabetes mellitus. *Ophthalmology* 99(1):58–62, 1992.

Kinney, J.C. and Keenan, P.W. A survey of breast cancer detection methods in long-term facilities. *J Gerontol* 17(4):20–22, 1991.

Koivisto, V.A. Insulin therapy in type II diabetes [review]. *Diabetes Care* 16(Suppl[3]):29–39, 1993.

Lebovitz, H.E. Are oral hypoglycemic agents likely to benefit NIDDM patients? Affirmative. *Hosp Pract (Off Ed)* 27(suppl[1]):26–31, 1992.

Lehne, R.A. *Pharmacology for Nursing Care.* Philadelphia: W.B. Saunders, 1994.

Levy, J.A. Sexuality and aging. *In* Hazzard, W.R., Bierman, E.L., Blass, J.P. et al. (eds.). *Principles of Geriatric Medicine and Gerontology.* 3rd ed. New York: McGraw-Hill, 1994, pp. 115–124.

Lindstrom, T., Eriksson, P., Olsson, A.G. and Arnquist, H.J. Long-term improvement of glycemic control by insulin treatment in NIDDM patients with secondary failure. *Diabetes Care* 17(7):719–721, 1994.

Lindstrom, T., Jorfeldt, L., Tegler, L. and Arnquist, H.J. Hypoglycemic and cardiac arrhythmias in patients with type 2 diabetes mellitus. *Diabet Med* 9(6):536–541, 1992.

Long, S.D., O'Brien, K., MacDonald, K.G. et al. Weight loss in severely obese subjects prevents the progression of impaired glucose tolerance to type II diabetes. *Diabetes Care* 17(5):372–375, 1994.

Marshall, J.A., Hoag, S., Shetterly, S. and Hamman, R.F. Dietary fat predicts conversion from impaired glucose tolerance to NIDDM. *Diabetes Care* 17(1):50–55, 1994.

Marshburn, P.B. and Carr, B.R. The menopause and hormone replacement therapy. *In* Hazzard, W.R., Bierman, E.L., Blass, J.P. et al. (eds.). *Principles of Geriatric Medicine and Gerontology.* 3rd ed. New York: McGraw-Hill, 1994, pp. 867–878.

Masters, W.H. and Johnson, V.E. *Human Sexual Response.* Boston: Little, Brown, 1966.

McGuire, E.J., DeLancey, J.O.L. and Elkins, T. Female genitourinary disorders. *In* Abrams, W.B. and Fletcher, A.J. (eds.). *The Merck Manual of Geriatrics.* Rahway, N.J.: Merck Sharp & Dohme Research Laboratories, 1990, pp. 831–840.

Meneilly, G.S., Dawson, K. and Tessier, D. Alterations in glucose metabolism in the elderly patient with diabetes. *Diabetes Care* 16(9):1241–1248, 1993.

Mersey, J.H. Diabetes mellitus in the elderly patient. *In* Reichel, W. (ed.). *Clinical Aspects of Aging.* Baltimore: Williams & Wilkins, 1989, pp. 382–389.

Miller, A.M. and Champion, V.L. Mammography in women >50 years of age: Predisposing and enabling characteristics. *Cancer Nurs* 16(4):260–269, 1993.

Miller, M. Diseases of the thyroid. *In* Brocklehurst, J.C., Tallis, R.C. and Fillit, H.M. (eds.). *Textbook of Geriatric Medicine and Gerontology.* 4th ed. Edinburgh: Churchill Livingstone, 1992, pp. 701–716.

Milne, R.M., Mann, J.I., Chisholm, A.W. and Williams, S.M. Long-term comparison of three dietary prescriptions in the treatment of NIDDM. *Diabetes Care* 17(1): 74–80, 1994.

Montgomery, P.A. Combination use of sulfonylureas and insulin in the treatment of noninsulin dependent diabetes mellitus. *Pharmacotherapy* 12(4):292–299, 1992.

Muss, H.B. Breast cancer. *In* Hazzard, W.R., Bierman, E.L., Blass, J.P. et al. (eds.). *Principles of Geriatric Medicine and Gerontology.* 3rd ed. New York: McGraw-Hill, 1994, pp. 481–494.

Noyes, M.A., Carter, B.L., Helling, D.K. et al. Evaluation of glipizide and glyburide in a health maintenance organization. *Ann Pharmacol* 26(10):1215–1220, 1992.

Pastors, J.G., Blaisdell, P.W., Balm, T.K. et al. Psyllium fiber reduces rise in postprandial glucose and insulin concentrations in patients with non-insulin-dependent diabetes. *Am J Clin Nutr* 53(6):1431–1435, 1991.

Patterson, W.B., Yancik, R. and Carbone, P.P. *In* Calkins, E., Ford, A.B. and Katz, P.R. (eds.). *Practice of Geriatrics.* 2nd ed. Philadelphia: W.B. Saunders, 1992, pp. 523–540.

Pugh, J.A., Wagner, M.L., Sawyer, J. et al. Is combination sulfonylurea and insulin therapy useful in NIDDM patients? A metaanalysis. *Diabetes Care* 15(8): 953–959, 1992.

Riddle, M.C. Combining insulin and sulfonylureas. A therapeutic option for type II diabetes. *Postgrad Med* 92(2):89–90, 1992.

Riddle, M., Hart, J., Bingham, P. et al. Combined therapy for obese type II diabetes: Suppertime mixed insulin with daytime sulfonylureas. *Am J Med Sci* 303(3): 151–156, 1992.

Rosenstock, J., Corrao, P.J., Goldberg, R.B. and Kilo, C. Diabetes control in the elderly: A randomized, comparative study of glyburide versus glipizide in non-insulin-dependent diabetes mellitus. *Clin Ther* 15(6): 1031–1040, 1993.

Roysarkar, T.K., Gupta, A., Dash, R.J. and Dogra, M.R. Effect of insulin therapy on progression of retinopathy in noninsulin-dependent diabetes mellitus. *Am J Ophthalmol* 115(5):569–574, 1993.

Rutledge, D.N. Effects of age on lump detection accuracy. *Nurs Res* 41(5):306–308, 1992.

Sanders, L.R. Pituitary, thyroid, and adrenal disturbances in the elderly. *In* Schrier, R.W. (ed.). *Clinical Internal Medicine in the Aged.* Philadelphia: W.B. Saunders, 1989, pp. 475–487.

Sane, T., Helve, E., Yki-Jarvinen, H. and Taskinen, M.R. One-year response to evening insulin therapy in non-insulin-dependent diabetes. *J Intern Med* 231(3):253–260, 1992.

Sawicki, P.T., Didjurgett, U., Muhlhauser, I. et al. Smoking is associated with progression of diabetic nephropathy. *Diabetes Care* 17(2):126–131, 1994.

Schrier, R.W. *Clinical Internal Medicine in the Aged.* Philadelphia: W.B. Saunders, 1989.

Shingleton, H.M. and Hurt, W.G. (eds.). *Reproductive Gynecology.* New York: Churchill Livingstone, 1990.

Shlafer, M. *The Nurse, Pharmacology, and Drug Therapy.* 3rd ed. Redwood City, CA: Addison Wesley Publishing Co., 1993.

Smith, D.E. and Wing, R.R. Diminished weight loss and behavioral compliance during repeated diets in obese patients with type II diabetes. *Health Psychol* 10(6):378–383, 1991.

Stacpoole, P.W. Should NIDDM patients be on high-carbohydrate, low-fat diets? Affirmative. *Hosp Pract (Off Ed).* 27(suppl 1):6:6–10, 1992.

Stenchever, M.A. (ed.). *Office Gynecology.* St. Louis: C.V. Mosby, 1992.

Stern, M.P., Valdez, R.A., Haffner, S.M. et al. Stability over time of modern diagnostic criteria for type II diabetes. *Diabetes Care* 16(7):978–983, 1993.

Terry, L.C. and Halter, J.B. *In* Hazzard, W.R., Bierman, E.L., Blass, J.P. et al. (eds.). *Principles of Geriatric Medicine and Gerontology.* 3rd ed. New York: McGraw-Hill, 1994, p. 791.

Trilling, J.S. Screening for non-insulin-dependent diabetes mellitus in the elderly [review]. *Clin Geriatr Med* 6(4):839–848, 1990.

Walsh, B.W. and Schiff, I. Menopause and ovarian hormone therapy. *In* Abrams, W.B. and Fletcher, A.J. (eds.). *The Merck Manual of Geriatrics.* Rahway, N.J.: Merck Sharp & Dohme Research Laboratories, 1990, pp. 831–840.

Wolffenbuttel, B.H., Drossaert, C.H. and Visser, A.P. Determinants of injecting insulin in elderly patients with type II diabetes mellitus. *Patient Educ Counsel* 22(3):117–125, 1993.

Wyatt, G., Kurtz, M.E. and Liken, M. Breast cancer survivors: An exploration of quality of life issues. *Cancer Nurs* 16(6):440–448, 1993.

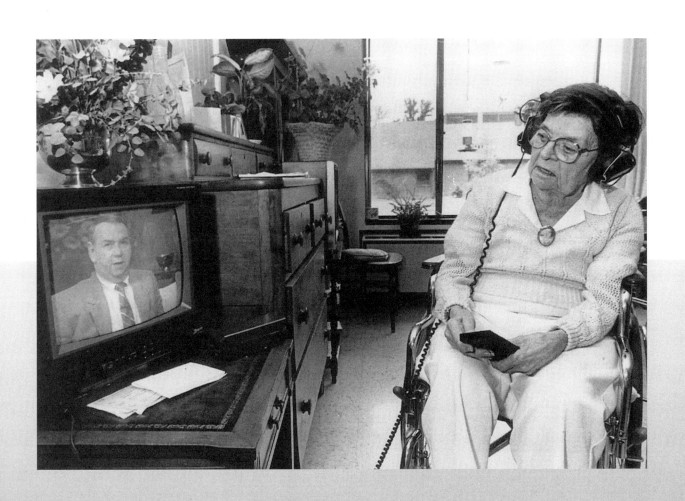

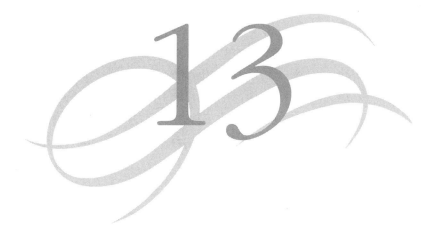

Age-Related Changes in the Special Senses

BRENDA LEWIS CLEARY

OBJECTIVES

Describe the normal age-related changes in vision, hearing, taste, smell, and touch.

❖

Discuss the impact of sensory changes on an older adult.

❖

Recognize common age-related disorders of the eye, including cataracts, glaucoma, senile macular degeneration, diabetic retinopathy, and senile entropion and ectropion.

❖

Compare and contrast the changes in hearing with age.

❖

Identify changes in touch, vibration, and pain sensitivity with age.

❖

Assess an older client for sensory changes and develop appropriate nursing interventions.

Sensory changes can have a great impact on the lifestyle of older persons, substantially altering the quality of life and independence they once took for granted. Visual and hearing impairments may interfere with written and verbal communication, enjoyment of previously meaningful activities, and important social interactions. Older persons may become socially isolated because they are unable to endure the strain of attempting to hear a muted or indistinguishable conversation or because they cannot see well enough to provide their own transportation to social activities. It is important to understand the sensory changes associated with aging to help the elderly adjust and function at their highest possible level.

People of all ages require a minimum of stimulation of sense organs to evoke any sensory experience. The minimum physical energy needed to activate a particular sensory system is known as the *absolute threshold*. It is determined by finding a range of intensities over which the physical energy moves from having no effect to having a complete effect. The absolute threshold is generally considered to be the value at which the stimulus is perceived 50 per cent of the time. The threshold varies among individuals and also within an individual from time to time, depending on physical condition, motivational state, and the conditions under which the observations are made (Rich, 1990). With advanced aging, it is generally thought that greater sensory inputs are required to evoke responses. Thus,

the absolute threshold is higher for the elderly than it is for the young.

Sensory decrements, like absolute threshold levels, vary among and within individuals. The senses of vision, hearing, taste, smell, and touch may all be affected by the changes of aging, but vision and hearing changes are the most dramatic and have the greatest impact.

VISION

Every sense organ responds to a particular type of physical energy. The eye is sensitive to light, a portion of electromagnetic energy that travels in waves through space. The colors that are perceived by the eye travel at varying wavelengths (the distance from the crest of one wave to the crest of the next) that are related to the colors of the rainbow. The red end of the rainbow is produced by longer wavelengths and the violet end by short wavelengths. Light enters the eye through the transparent *cornea* and is focused on the *retina* by the *lens*. The *pupil* regulates the amount of light entering the visual system and is controlled by the autonomic nervous system. The retina is composed of three layers: (1) the rods and cones, which convert light energy into nerve impulses; (2) the bipolar cells, which make synaptic connections with the rods and cones; and (3) the ganglion cells, which contain the fibers forming the optic nerve. The *fovea*, located on the retina, is the most sensitive portion of the eye and plays a major role in visual perception (Rich, 1990) (Fig. 13–1).

Changes in Structure and Function

Structural Changes

The external structures of the eye consist of the *orbital cavity*, the *extrinsic ocular muscles*, the *eyelids*, the *conjunctiva*, and the *lacrimal apparatus*. Changes occurring in the orbital areas are similar to those that occur with aging in other parts of the body. There is a graying of the eyebrows and eyelashes and a wrinkling and loosening of the skin around the eyelids, which is due to loss of tonus and decreased elasticity of the eyelid muscle. Loss of orbital fat causes the eyes to sink deeper into the orbit and limits upward gaze. Tear secretions may diminish, producing a condition known as "dry eyes." This phenomenon may cause discomfort and irritation for older people and can be relieved by the use of eyedrops or "artificial tears."

The internal structures of the eye are the

sclera (fibrous protective coat), *cornea* (transparent tissue serving as refractive surface), *choroid* (vascular pigmented middle layer), *ciliary body, iris, pupil, lens,* and *retina* (inner layer containing visual receptor cells). The eyeball is divided into two cavities: (1) the anterior cavity, which consists of anterior and posterior chambers, located in front of the lens, and (2) the posterior cavity, located behind the lens. The anterior cavity contains a fluid called the *aqueous humor,* and the posterior cavity contains a soft, jelly-like material called the *vitreous humor.*

Age-related changes in the cornea produce a decrease in the number of endothelial cells. Corneal sensitivity is often diminished, so that the elderly may be less aware of injury or infection. The corneal reflex also may be diminished or absent in relatively healthy older individuals, as evidenced by a study conducted by Rai and Elias-Jones (1979). They found that although two thirds of elderly subjects with either unilateral or bilateral absence of corneal reflexes were diagnosed as having cerebrovascular disease, one third of the subjects had no evidence of neurological disease. It was concluded that too much significance should not be given to the absence of a corneal reflex in older persons. Another phenomenon characteristic of aging is the *arcus senilis* (Fig. 13–2), which is found on the periphery of the cornea. It is a grayish-yellow ring surrounding the iris and is thought to be caused by an accumulation of lipids.

The ciliary body is an anterior continuation of the choroid lining of the sclera. It contains the ciliary muscle, which governs the convexity of the lens, and the ciliary processes, which produce the aqueous humor. With aging, the ciliary body secretes less aqueous humor; however, because there is generally less outflow of fluid from the anterior and posterior chambers, intraocular pressure remains relatively stable. The length of the ciliary muscle tends to decrease owing to atrophy, and the lost muscle tissue is replaced with connective tissue. Because ciliary muscle action is responsible for the changing curvature of the lens, the focusing ability of the lens is compromised when deterioration of the muscle takes place. The process of focusing the image on the retina is known as *accommodation,* and the inability to focus properly is called *presbyopia.*

Accommodation is also difficult because the lens becomes less elastic, larger, and more dense as a result of continued production of new cells and accumulation of old and dead cells within the lens capsule. Increased density of the lens, together with the

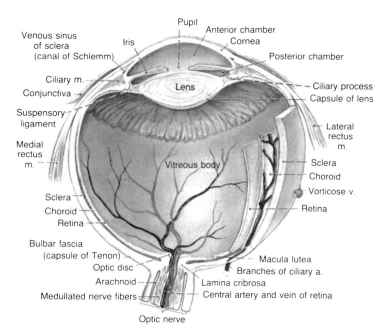

FIGURE 13–1

Midsagittal section through the eyeball, showing layers of retina and blood supply. (From Jacob, S.W., Francone, C.A. and Lossow, W.J. *Structure and Function in Man.* Philadelphia: W.B. Saunders, 1986.)

accumulation of loosened, degenerated cells on the iris, cornea, and lens capsule, causes increased scattering of light and sensitivity to glare. The lens also becomes progressively yellowed and opaque, probably owing to absorption of ultraviolet light over the years. Although there is poorer discrimination at all ages for blues and greens than for reds and yellows, the aged have particular diffi-

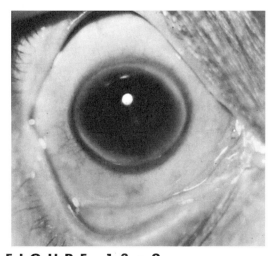

FIGURE 13–2

Corneal arcus. (From Scheie, H.G. and Albert, D.M. *Textbook of Ophthalmology.* 9th ed. Philadelphia: W.B. Saunders, 1977, p. 459.)

culty in this respect. This phenomenon is thought to be related to the fact that the effect of age is greatest on short wavelengths of light (violet, blue, green), which are filtered by the yellowed lenses (Corso, 1971). The generous use of warm (yellow, orange, red) contrasting colors can greatly increase the ease with which elderly persons manipulate their environments and carry out activities of daily living. It must be noted, however, that although the elderly do have difficulty with blue-green discrimination, general color vision defects either are of genetic origin or are indicative of a pathological process (Kline et al., 1982; Mashiah, 1978).

The iris, which is a diaphragm containing the pupil, loses its pigment with age, so that most older people appear to have grayish or light blue eyes. The pupil becomes progressively smaller with advancing age; by age 60, it is one third of the size it was at age 20. Decreased pupil size results in a smaller amount of light reaching the retina, and the light must pass through the densest, most opaque area of the lens (Corso, 1981; Marmour, 1981).

In the posterior cavity, the vitreous gel begins to liquefy and collapse. Bits of condensation and debris may become visible as "floaters," a common occurrence with aging. Although the condition is not pathologically significant nor does it impair vision, it may be a source of annoyance to older people. The retina also begins to degenerate owing to local ischemia and loss of neurons.

Functional Changes

Major visual changes with aging include decreased visual acuity, decreased tolerance of glare, decreased ability to adapt to dark and light, and decreased peripheral vision. All of these changes in visual function are related to changes in eye structure that affect the quality and intensity of the light reaching the retina (Rich, 1990).

A large-scale study of 5335 subjects revealed that functional blindness increased with age to 17 per cent in those 90 years of age and older, whereas visual impairment rose to 39 per cent. Residence in a nursing home, diabetes, history of glaucoma or cataracts, and socioeconomic factors were significantly associated with functional blindness and visual impairment (Salive et al., 1992).

There is a general decline in visual acuity with older age, and almost everyone over age 55 must wear eyeglasses for either reading or distance vision. However, failure of visual function is not inevitable with older age, and a large percentage of elderly people retain excellent visual acuity. Only about 16 per cent have 20/50 vision or worse, impairing the ability to drive, although glare is a contributing factor; only 5 per cent are unable to read. Milne (1979) observed visual acuity over a 5-year period in almost 500 subjects ranging in age from 63 to 90 years. Visual acuity worsened in 26 per cent and actually improved in 25 per cent of the subjects studied. They noted that the incidence of progressive vision impairment was highest in the oldest subjects.

Glare is a particular problem to older people and is one of the major reasons, along with poor adjustment to dark and light, that the elderly frequently give up night driving. Oncoming lights produce light scattering in the cornea and lens, rendering the elderly virtually blind at times. Sunlit rooms in which window light reflects on shiny floors are equally difficult to negotiate (Fig. 13–3). Rooms should be well lighted with soft, incandescent rather than fluorescent lighting to minimize glare. Sheer curtains and rugs can be used to reduce window glare.

Because dark and light adaptation take longer with advancing age, the elderly are at greater risk for falls and injuries. Entering and leaving a theater, going to the bathroom at night, and moving from a well-lighted room to a dark room can therefore be most dangerous for elderly people. Interestingly, the dark-adapted eye makes use of the rods rather than the cones and is much more sensitive to blue-green wavelengths than to the longer red wavelengths. Because red light stimulates the cones but not the rods, older persons may see well enough by red light to function in the dark. In addition, the time required for dark adaptation in red light is greatly reduced. This phenomenon is noteworthy because older people can be encouraged to keep a red light on in darkened rooms at all times to improve the rate of dark adaptation and to increase visibility at night.

Loss of peripheral vision is a common occurrence with aging and greatly limits social interactions and physical activities. Older persons may not communicate with others sitting next to them because they are out of their range of vision. At the table, they may spill food and drinks located on their visual periphery, or they may not be able to find objects placed out of visual range. Driving also can be hazardous because of their inability to see oncoming motorists. In a study of 397 volunteers from the Baltimore Longitudinal Study of Aging, Kline et al. (1992) found that visual problems of driving increased with age along five dimensions: (1) unexpected vehicles, (2) vehicle speed, (3)

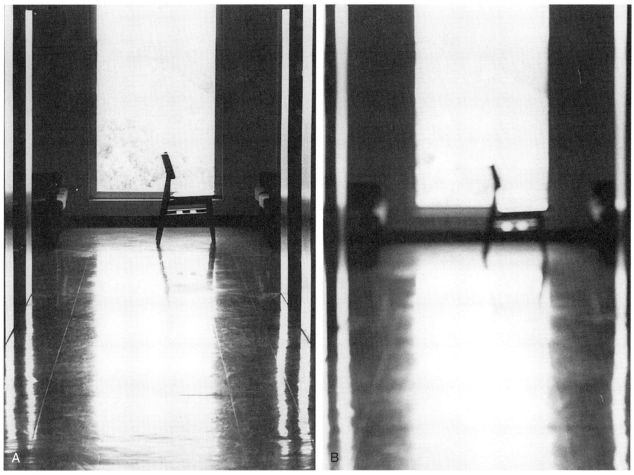

FIGURE 13–3

Age-related changes in visual acuity are demonstrated in *B*, which is a photographic simulation of the scene in *A* as a 70- to 80-year-old person might see it. Elderly people have an increased susceptibility to glare. (Photographs by Steve Matteson.)

dimly lit displays, (4) windshield problems, and (5) sign reading. Marx et al. (1992) surveyed 103 nursing home residents and reported that the half of the sample with low vision were more dependent on caregivers for performing activities of daily living. It is important that elderly people be made aware of these limitations so that they can compensate for them.

Common Disorders and Diseases

The most prevalent disorders of the visual system with older age are *cataracts, glaucoma, senile macular degeneration,* and *diabetic retinopathy.* These diseases can result in varying degrees of blindness, but half of all cases of blindness can be treated if they are found early. Overall, more than 500,000 United States citizens are legally blind, owing to glaucoma (12.5 per cent), macular degeneration (11.7 per cent), cataracts (8.3 per cent), optic atrophy (7 per cent), and diabetic reti-

nopathy (6.6 per cent), and most of these conditions are preventable or treatable (Grimes et al., 1992). The Framingham Eye Study (Liebowitz et al., 1980) found that the visual disorder with the highest incidence in persons over 65 was cataracts, followed by senile macular degeneration, diabetic retinopathy, and glaucoma (Table 13–1). In addition, the study showed that the incidence

TABLE 13–1

Prevalence of Blinding Disease

Age (years)	65–74	75+
Cataracts (%)	28	40
Diabetic retinopathy (%)	2	6
Glaucoma (%)	3	4–5 (10% > 85)
Macular degeneration (%)	8–11	20

Data from Pizzarello, L.D. The dimensions of the problem of eye disease among the elderly. *Ophthalmology* 94:1191–1195, 1987.

of cataracts had the greatest increase with advancing age, followed by macular degeneration. The results of this cross-sectional survey differed somewhat from those of the Duke Longitudinal Studies of Aging (Anderson and Palmore, 1974), which did not show an increase in the incidence of cataracts longitudinally in a relatively healthy group of older adults. Rather, the increase in the incidence of glaucoma was more significant in older age. It is interesting to note, however, that in a later longitudinal study by Milne (1979), the incidence of cataracts increased significantly with age (from 15 per cent at the original examination to 36 to 46 per cent after 5 years) and had an important association with decreased visual acuity.

Cataracts

Senile cataracts are the most common cause of adult blindness. Most cataracts develop bilaterally in persons older than 50 years and are to some degree present in all individuals older than 70 years; the incidence increases with diabetes and tends to be familial. The disorder is characterized by a clouding or opacity of the normally clear, crystalline lens. Structural changes in the proteins of the lens cause liquefication and swelling within the lens capsule. There is a gradual loss of vision in one or both eyes, with symptoms of excessive glare, general darkening of vision, and loss of acuity from dimness and distortion. Ophthalmoscopic examination reveals a haziness of the lens, an inability to see the fundus in detail, and a reduced red reflex (Lichtenstein, 1992).

Surgical removal of the cataract is the treatment of choice, depending on the needs of the individual. The location of the cataract, the degree of visual impairment, and the effect on the individual's ability to carry out activities of daily living all influence the decision to operate. Surgery is almost always performed before a cataract becomes "ripe"—that is, when water is drawn into the lens with resultant swelling. Changes in visual acuity postoperatively are typically dramatic; however, a major limiting factor is the coexistence of retinal disease (Lichtenstein, 1992).

Two types of surgical procedures are used to remove cataracts: (1) intracapsular extraction, and (2) extracapsular extraction. Intracapsular extraction involves removal of the lens intact in its capsule through a wide incision in the cornea. In an extracapsular extraction, the contents of the lens are aspirated through a large-bore needle inserted through a small incision in the cornea, leaving the posterior portion of the lens capsule

behind (Grimes et al., 1992). The condition in which the lens is absent from the eye is known as *aphakia*.

Because removal of the lens contents or capsule deprives the eye of focusing power, some type of replacement is necessary. There are three ways to provide focusing power for the visual system. The first is an intraocular lens, a surgically implanted lens positioned in place of the natural lens. The intraocular lens implant is highly desirable because it is most like a natural lens; however, it does represent a foreign body in the eye and may cause problems over time. Therefore, this type of procedure is best indicated in people older than 70 years, who may also have difficulty with eyeglasses or contact lenses. Contact lenses are the second type of lens replacement and are the next best treatment for aphakia. They are particularly appropriate and safe for younger persons. Hard or soft lenses may be used; the long-wearing type are best because they require care only once a month. Eyeglasses are the third and least effective means of treating aphakia, although they are the simplest, safest, and most proven method. Persons using aphakic eyeglasses may have difficulty with depth perception and peripheral vision; they may also complain of double vision if they have had surgery in only one eye.

Glaucoma

Glaucoma is an insidious, chronic condition that has been characterized as a "thief in the night" because it robs its victims of vision without any noticeable symptoms. Three to four per cent of all people older than 40 have glaucoma, but at least half of them are unaware of it. Rich (1990) noted that for persons of all ages, glaucoma is the leading cause of blindness in the United States, affecting 12 to 30 per cent of all cases. The disease is more common, severe, and difficult to treat in blacks.

Characteristic signs of glaucoma are high intraocular pressure, degeneration and cupping of the optic disc, atrophy of the optic nerve head, and loss of visual field. All conditions must be present to make the diagnosis of glaucoma; increased intraocular pressure without concomitant damage to the optic disc and optic nerve head is defined as *ocular hypertension*. Increased intraocular pressure is caused by a defect in the outflow of aqueous humor from the anterior and posterior chambers into the venous system; damage to the optic disc and nerve head is due to the high intraocular pressure. Normal intraocular pressure is 10 to 21 mm Hg; any measurement over 21 mm Hg is viewed suspiciously, although it is not necessarily diagnostic of glaucoma (Rich, 1990; Langston, 1990).

Glaucoma is classified according to the cause of the obstruction of the aqueous outflow. These causes are classified as follows:

1. Primary or secondary (primary is genetic in origin; secondary is caused by other ocular disorders—tumor, inflammation, trauma—that obstruct aqueous outflow)

2. Open-angle or closed-angle (*angle* is the point in the anterior chamber where the iris inserts into the corneoscleral junction)

3. Congenital or developmental (disease develops during gestation or the first year of life, but signs and symptoms may not appear until adulthood)

Primary open-angle glaucoma, also known as *simple, ordinary,* or *chronic glaucoma,* is the major cause of visual impairment. It is a slow, progressive, painless, bilateral disease that is genetic in origin. An obstruction in the aqueous outflow system causes an increase in intraocular pressure and destruction of bundles of optic nerve fibers at the nerve head. Loss of peripheral vision, or "tunnel vision," is a significant symptom that usually occurs late in the disease. Central visual acuity remains intact and is a poor index of damage. Diagnosis is made through measurement of the intraocular pressure combined with the characteristic visual field defects and damage to the optic disc. Treatment includes eye drops, such as pilocarpine, timolol, or epinephrine, or oral acetazolamide (Diamox). The drugs act to decrease the secretion of aqueous fluid and to enhance aqueous outflow (Rich, 1990). A recent study, by Netland et al. (1993), of 54 subjects suggested that calcium channel blockers may also be a useful treatment, particularly for enhancing optic nerve blood flow. Response to medical treatment is good, but it is important to diagnose the disease early to prevent further deterioration.

Angle-closure or *narrow-angle glaucoma* is fairly rare, occurring in only 5 per cent of all cases of primary glaucoma. It is an inherited condition that causes anatomical shallowing of the anterior chamber and narrowing of the angle. The disease is characterized by an acute onset brought on by some type of stress or other condition that thickens the iris and obstructs the angle, resulting in a sudden blockage of outflow channels. Symptoms include extreme pain, localized in and around the eye, blurred or foggy vision, and colored halos around lights. Treatment is directed toward decreasing the intraocular pressure. Topical, oral, and intravenous medications are given immediately, followed by surgical iridectomy 4 to 6 hours later. Analgesics are also given for pain. Immediate treatment is the key to prevention of permanent blindness (Rich, 1990).

Senile Macular Degeneration

The macula, located on the retina, is functionally the most important part of the eye. It is the area that contains the *fovea,* the central focusing point for the optic system of the eye. With aging, the function of the macula is compromised by a decreased blood supply, an accumulation of waste products, and tissue atrophy; systemic disease, genetic inheritance, and nutritional factors can also contribute to macular impairment (Eifrig and Simons, 1983). Degenerative changes of the macula are usually bilateral and increase significantly with age. Rich (1990) identified macular degeneration as the second leading cause of blindness; Langston (1990) and Woods (1992) further identified it as the leading cause of new cases of legal blindness in the United States and the industrialized world. The prevalence of macular degeneration was 9 per cent in the Framingham study.

Visual loss related to the neovascular type of senile macular degeneration results from the growth of abnormal blood vessels under the retina, which cause irreversible damage to the macula. Because the loss is central, reading and recognition of objects are impaired, whereas side vision and mobility remain intact. Eyeglasses are not effective in improving vision; however, results from a clinical trial of photocoagulation treatment with an argon laser showed a dramatic decrease in visual loss in this form of senile macular degeneration. The laser seals off the damaged vessels and prevents bleeding, fluid leakage, scar tissue formation, and nerve tissue destruction. The investigators concluded that 90 per cent of cases of legal blindness related to neovascular senile macular degeneration can be prevented or significantly delayed by appropriately timed laser treatment. They noted that treatment must be carried out early in the disease to be effective (National Eye Institute, 1983). Unfortunately, most cases of macular degeneration in general remain untreatable (Langston, 1990).

Diabetic Retinopathy

Diabetic retinopathy is the most common ocular complication of diabetes mellitus and is responsible for 10 to 15 per cent of all

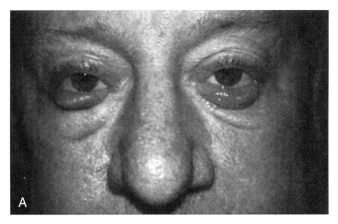

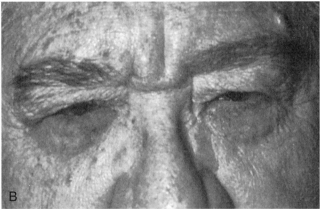

FIGURE 13-4

A, Ectropion. The lid margin turns outward, exposing the palpebral conjunctiva. The eye does not drain satisfactorily, and tearing occurs. *B*, Entropion. The lid margin turns inward, and lower lashes may irritate the conjunctiva and lower cornea. Entropion can be demonstrated by asking the patient to shut the eyes tightly and then open them. Both ectropion and entropion are more common in elderly people. (From Iliff, C.E., Iliff, W.J. and Iliff, N.T. *Oculoplastic Surgery*. Philadelphia: W.B. Saunders, 1979, pp. 128, 136.)

blindness is rare. Visual deterioration is more rapid in older patients with diabetes, as evidenced by the fact that 3 per cent of patients younger than 60 and 20 per cent of those older than 60 with diabetic retinopathy are legally blind. The goal of treatment is to delay or retard visual impairment. Medical and surgical treatment methods include control of blood glucose levels, laser photocoagulation (the treatment of choice according to Rich [1990] for proliferative retinopathy), and vitrectomy to remove the blood-stained vitreous.

Senile Entropion and Ectropion

Two other disorders that are not necessarily threatening to visual integrity but are most troublesome and uncomfortable for older people are *senile entropion* and *senile ectropion* (Fig. 13-4). Entropion, a complete inversion of the lower lid, is caused by a general weakening and wasting of the muscles, fat, and skin surrounding the orbit of the eye, resulting in decreased support of the lower lid against the globe. The eye may become irritable, watery, and prone to conjunctivitis, or it may develop keratitis or corneal ulceration from the constant rubbing of the eyelashes against the eyeball (Rich, 1990). Temporary relief can be obtained by strapping the lid outward with a short strip of adhesive. For permanent correction, surgery or cautery is the treatment of choice.

Senile ectropion, also called involutional, atonic, relaxation, or senescent ectropion, is an outward turning of the eyelid margin from its position of contact with the globe. It may occur as a result of facial nerve paralysis; however, with increasing age, it may simply be the result of atrophy of eyelid tissues. Ectropion is due to relaxation and loss of muscle tone, which results in laxity of the lid. The lid is in a good position but no longer has any snap and can easily be pulled away from the globe. The lid becomes elongated, leading to conjunctival hypertrophy and keratonization. Ectropion may also result from mechanical weighting of the lids from growths or lesions. Surgical treatment is aimed toward shortening the lid to produce better tone (Rich, 1990).

cases of acquired blindness in the United States. Because the incidence of diabetic retinopathy is related to the duration of the diabetes, the longer an individual has diabetes, the greater his or her chances of developing retinopathy. The disease has the same characteristics of diabetes elsewhere in the body. There is early damage to the retinal capillaries, progressive growth of abnormal small vessels, and leaking and hemorrhage of the retinal vasculature into the vitreous body. The results are scarring, contracture, and finally, retinal detachment. The course of the disease is slow and chronic, and it appears in two stages: (1) nonproliferative (background retinopathy) and (2) proliferative. Only 17 per cent of patients who are treated progress to the proliferative stage, which is a poor prognostic sign (Lichtenstein, 1992).

The major symptom of diabetic retinopathy is central visual impairment; complete

HEARING

The ear has two functions: hearing and maintenance of balance. Hearing is achieved through the vibration of sounds transmitted through the tympanic membrane, or eardrum. The vibrations are then conveyed to the inner ear and are transformed into tiny nerve impulses to the brain. Equilibrium is controlled through the hairs located in the inner ear that innervate fibers of the vestibular branch of the eighth cranial, or acoustic, nerve.

The three parts of the ear are (1) the external ear, (2) the middle ear, and (3) the inner ear (Fig. 13–5). The external ear, consisting of the *auricle* and the *external auditory canal,* conducts sound to the *tympanic membrane* (eardrum) and protects the deeper parts of the ear. The middle ear consists mainly of an air space in the temporal bone, which is bounded laterally by the tympanic membrane. This space contains three bones—the *malleus,* the *incus,* and the *stapes,* which are responsible for transmitting sound vibrations from the tympanic membrane to the middle ear and for reducing the amplitude of large vibrations. The inner ear is made up of the *osseous (bony) labyrinth,* which contains the *semicircular canals,* the *vestibule,* and the *cochlea,* and the *membranous labyrinth,* which contains the *semicircular ducts,* the *utricle,* the *saccule,* and the *cochlear duct.* The *organ of Corti* with its sensitive hair cells lies at the base of the cochlear duct. The cochlea is the essential organ of the auditory system.

The ear is sensitive to mechanical energy or pressure changes among the molecules in the atmosphere. The vibration of molecules produces sound waves, which are the stimuli for hearing. Sound waves have two main characteristics—*frequency* and *amplitude.* Frequency is measured by the number of vibra-

tions or cycles per second; amplitude is the amount of compression and expansion of the sound waves. Frequency is related to the pitch of a sound, so that the higher the vibration frequency, the higher the perceived pitch. *Hertz* (Hz) is used to denote cycles per second. Amplitude is related to the loudness of a sound, so that the greater the intensity with which the sound pressure strikes the eardrum, the louder the tone. Intensity of sound is measured in decibels (dB). Table 13–2 shows the relative intensities of some common sounds. Sound waves differ from light waves in that light waves

TABLE 13 – 2
Decibel Levels for Normal Sounds

DECIBEL LEVEL AT 1000 Hz	
160	Bursting of eardrum
140	Severe pain
120	Pain threshold; thunder
100	Damage to hearing after prolonged exposure; average factory, loudest passages of orchestra for close listener
80	Class lecture, loud radio
60	Conversational speech
40	Very soft music, typical living room
20	Very quiet room
0	Threshold of hearing

Adapted from Nave, C.R. and Nave, B.C. *Physics for the Health Sciences.* 3rd ed. Philadelphia: W.B. Saunders, 1985; Goodhill, V. *Evaluation of the aging ear. Emerg Med* 24(15): 165–166, 1992.

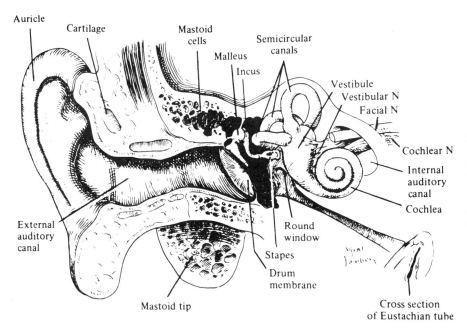

Auricle
Cartilage
Mastoid cells
Malleus
Incus
Semicircular canals
Vestibule
Vestibular N
Facial N
Cochlear N
Internal auditory canal
Cochlea
External auditory canal
Round window
Stapes
Drum membrane
Mastoid tip
Cross section of Eustachian tube

FIGURE 13 – 5
The peripheral auditory apparatus. The cochlea is turned slightly to show its coils. The eustachian tube runs forward as well as downward and inward. (From Davis, H. and Silverman, S.R. *Hearing and Deafness.* New York: Holt, Reinhart and Winston, 1970.)

are specified in terms of length of the wave, whereas sound waves are specified on the basis of the number of waves per unit of time. When dimensions of light and color are compared with sound and tone, hue can be likened to pitch and brightness can be equated with loudness.

Changes in Structure and Function

Structural Changes

The external ear exhibits changes with aging similar to those seen in other parts of the body. The skin of the auricle often becomes dry and lax with increased wrinkling. There is also increased itching and dryness in the external auditory canal. The tragi (hairs on the lateral external auditory canal) of adult males become longer, coarser, and more noticeable beginning with the third and fourth decades. The ceruminal glands, which are modified apocrine sweat glands, decrease in number and activity, producing drier cerumen (ear wax). The dried cerumen may result in impactions within the external auditory canal, especially in older men, whose large tragi become imbedded in the accumulated wax and prevent the natural dislodging of the cerumen.

In the middle ear, some degeneration of the bony joints may take place, but there is no apparent effect on sound transmission. The eardrum thickens, and there may be scarring accumulated over the years from infections, injuries, or other disorders. The most severe changes caused by aging take place in the inner ear, and affect sensitivity to sound, understanding of speech, and maintenance of equilibrium. Degeneration of the vestibular structures, including loss of hair cells and myelinated nerve fibers, and atrophy of the cochlea, including the simultaneous loss of cochlear neurons, atrophy of the organ of Corti, and atrophy of the stria vascularis, are the major age-related changes that produce deficits in equilibrium and hearing (Mhoon, 1990; Goodhill, 1992).

Functional Changes

In the United States, 13 to 14 million people have hearing loss sufficient to affect their everyday living. Some degree of hearing loss is an almost inevitable consequence of advancing age, although elderly persons should be screened for correctible disorders. In 1975, the Department of Health, Education, and Welfare estimated that 23 per cent of all persons aged 65 to 74 years have a hearing impairment, and 40 per cent of those older than 75 have a hearing loss (Powers and Powers, 1978; Goodhill, 1992).

Furthermore, institutionalized elderly have greater impairments than active, ambulatory older people in the community. It is estimated that 30 per cent of all community-residing and 90 per cent of all institutionalized elderly persons over age 65 have a hearing impairment (Rappaport, 1990). There are three major types of hearing loss: (1) conductive, (2) sensorineural, and (3) mixed. *Conductive hearing loss* results from any interference with the normal movement of sound vibrations through the external and middle ears. *Sensorineural loss* involves damage to the inner ear, auditory nerve (cranial nerve VII), brainstem, or cortical auditory pathways. *Mixed loss* refers to conductive loss superimposed on sensorineural loss (Nodar, 1990).

Conductive Hearing Loss

This type of mechanical hearing loss, caused by damage to the external auditory canal, the tympanic membrane, or the middle ear ossicles, is the most easily corrected medically or surgically. Damage usually results from accumulated wax, keratoses (impacted skin and hair), chronic eczematoid dermatitis and stenosis, eardrum perforation, otitis media, otosclerosis, or radiation therapy to the head and neck, as well as numerous systemic diseases (Goodhill, 1992).

Individuals with conductive hearing loss have some impairment in hearing for sounds of all frequencies. *Speech discrimination,* or the ability to distinguish and understand sounds, is not impaired, and hearing is better in the presence of extraneous noise than in individuals with normal hearing. Loud noises are tolerated better, but *tinnitus* (ringing in the ears) may occasionally be present. Individuals with conductive hearing loss may speak more softly than normal hearing persons because the sound of their voice to themselves is enhanced by the conductive blockage.

Total blockage of the ear canal with cerumen is a common and treatable cause of conductive hearing loss. Mahoney (1993) reported that more than 25 per cent of nursing home residents have impacted cerumen. Older people should be taught or assisted to clean the ear canal correctly to remove wax accumulations. The ear canal should never be gouged with cotton swabs, bobby pins, or other objects that can harm the external auditory canal or the tympanic membrane. Over-the-counter eardrops, such as Cerumenex or Debrox, can be used as directed, followed by lavage to remove the cerumen and the medication (prolonged instillation of the drugs can cause severe external otitis). Another safe and easy method is instillation of mineral oil into the ear canal for 24 hours, followed by gentle lavage with one part hydrogen peroxide to three parts water at room temperature. A Water-Pik device may be useful in irrigation (Ney, 1993).

Sensorineural Hearing Loss

The primary causes of sensorineural hearing loss are noise damage (acoustic trauma), presbycusis, drugs (ototoxicity), heredity, tumors involving the acoustic nerve, postinflammatory reactions, and complications of arteriosclerosis. Most hearing loss is due to noise exposure (Goodhill, 1992). *Presbycusis* is the most common neurosensory loss among the aged and is a slowly progressive, symmetrical, sensorineural hearing loss that is significantly associated with middle and older age. It is usually bilateral and begins in the third decade and worsens with increasing age, although total deafness rarely occurs. Presbycusis affects 12 million people (60 per cent) older than 65 years and 80 to 90 per cent of nursing home residents; men are affected more frequently than women (Nodar, 1990).

Presbycusis

There are four types of presbycusis: (1) sensory, due to a loss of hair cells at the basal turn; (2) neural, due to a degeneration of the spiral ganglion; (3) metabolic, due to atrophy of the stria vascularis, and (4) mechanical, due to loss of elasticity of the basement membrane (Lichtenstein, 1992). Major symptoms are a progressive bilateral loss of hearing acuity, especially at high frequencies; poor discrimination and comprehension, especially with background noise; and tinnitus, which is especially noticeable in a quiet environment (Nodar, 1990). Loud sounds may become uncomfortably loud, a process called *recruitment,* and this may limit the effectiveness of amplification or the use of hearing aids.

Studies have shown that hearing loss increases with advanced age, particularly at high frequencies (Goodhill, 1992; Lichtenstein, 1992). Adults with normal hearing can perceive sound at a frequency range of 300 to 3500 Hz. With aging, loss begins to affect hearing of sound in the higher frequency ranges (1500 to 4000 Hz) and gradually affects the hearing of lower frequencies (500 to 1500 Hz) (Fig. 13–6). Noise trauma initially affects the ability to hear sound at frequencies of around 4000 Hz, and with continued exposure, the lower frequencies are affected. The loss is greater with louder noise and longer exposure (Goodhill, 1992; Voeks et al., 1993).

Speech discrimination and comprehension are affected by reduced speech perception and high-tone hearing loss. Reduced speech perception results from the increase in time required to process information in the higher auditory centers. Thus, accelerated speech (increase in word rate per minute) is more difficult for the old to understand than it is for the young. High-tone hearing loss, which results from impaired hearing of high frequency sounds, causes poor discrimination of consonants such as "s," "t," "f," and "g," which have high frequencies. The elderly with presbycusis have difficulty in discriminating among phonetically similar words and find it difficult to follow a normal conversation. Background noise exaggerates the problem because the noise tends to mask the weaker speech sounds of the consonants. In a study by Voeks et al. (1993), 198 newly admitted nursing home residents were screened for self-reported hearing difficulty and audiometric thresholds. Fifty-four per cent of the residents were hearing impaired. Table 13–3 reveals difficulties encountered in specific listening situations.

Tinnitus is a disturbing concomitant of both conductive and sensorineural hearing loss that affects over 7 million people, or 10 to 37 per cent of the elderly population. It is a subjective sensation of noise in the ear characterized by hissing, buzzing, or ringing. The sound is generally high pitched with sensorineural loss and low pitched with conductive loss; however, tinnitus may be present with or without hearing loss. The intensity is so low that the sound is heard only during quiet times and is masked by extraneous environmental noises. Tinnitus does not usually awaken afflicted persons, nor does it interfere with pleasurable activity. The cause of the condition when associated with conductive sensorineural hearing loss is not understood; however, other factors leading to tinnitus are otosclerosis; acoustical or mechanical trauma; tumors; ototoxic drugs, such as aspirin, quinidine, furosemide, and gentamicin; metabolic conditions (diabetes mellitus); Meniere's disease; and labyrinthitis. Treatment is often ineffective, but older persons can attempt to alleviate the condition through biofeedback or the use of masking devices that produce a narrow band of noise at the frequency of the tinnitus. Soft music or other competing noises, even radio static, may also be used (*LTC Nurse Rx,* 1993).

Interventions

Simple interventions for both conductive and sensorineural hearing loss can help im-

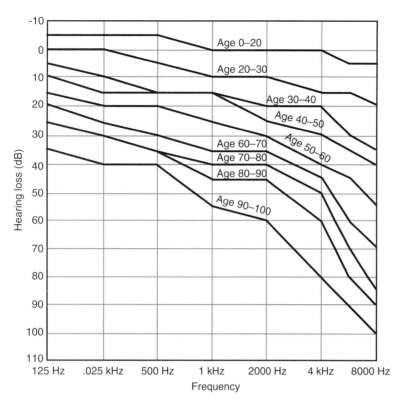

FIGURE 13 - 6

This decade audiogram shows the normal aging patterns in an urban environment. (From Goodhill, V. Evaluation of the aging ear. *Emerg Med* 24(5):166, 1992.)

TABLE 13 - 3

Residents' Responses to Questions Regarding Difficulty in Specific Listening Situations According to Hearing Status and Sensitivity for Each Question

| "DO YOU HAVE DIFFICULTY HEARING WHEN . . . " | ANSWER | HEARING STATUS BASED ON AUDIOMETRY | | SENSITIVITY* |
		Normal, % (n = 91)	Impaired, % (n = 107)	
Talking with several people	No	64	26	73.8
	Equivocal	7	16	
	Yes	30	58	
Watching TV	No	64	38	61.7
	Equivocal	27	31	
	Yes	9	31	
On the telephone	No	64	40	59.8
	Equivocal	27	32	
	Yes	9	28	
No facial cues	No	75	42	57.9
	Equivocal	7	8	
	Yes	19	50	
In the dining room	No	64	50	49.5
	Equivocal	30	31	
	Yes	7	19	
Talking one-to-one	No	92	78	21.5
	Equivocal	3	7	
	Yes	4	15	
With facial cues	No	96	78	21.5
	Equivocal	3	10	
	Yes	1	11	

From Voeks, S.K., Gallagher, C.M., Langer, E.H. and Drinka, P.J. Self-reported hearing difficulty and audiometric thresholds in nursing home residents. *J Fam Pract* 36(1):54–58, 1993.
* Equivocal and "Yes" responses were both considered positive indicators. "No" responses were considered negative indicators.

prove hearing and communication in the elderly. The most dramatic improvement occurs in persons with conductive loss when the external auditory canal is cleared of built-up cerumen. Sensorineural deficits are not as easily "cured," but the nurse can use simple measures to help improve communication with and by elderly patients. The nurse should always face clients directly, so that they may observe lip movement and facial expressions. The use of gestures and body language is also helpful because they give visual clues to the conversation. Speech should be slow and direct, with exaggerated enunciation of consonants. Loudness can be irritating, inducing recruitment of sound; therefore, the nurse should speak in a low voice to enable clients to hear the lower frequencies, which can be heard more easily.

Hearing aids are effective for various kinds of hearing losses, but many older people do not use them. Thinking that deafness is normal and inevitable with aging, they may withdraw from social interaction, rendering hearing aid use less necessary. Thus, many elderly people postpone audiological evaluation until after it is too late for a hearing aid to be effective. Older people may also deny that they have a hearing problem, thereby avoiding any association with older age. The negative social stigma attached to hearing-aid users may be another deterrent. The cost of a hearing aid may be prohibitive for many older people on fixed incomes, especially because there is no Medicare reimbursement for this expense. Hearing aids also may be sources of irritation to the external ear. Hearing aid molds may emit chemicals during use, which can cause contact dermatitis and itching; in addition, increased humidity within the external auditory canal can cause infection, a condition known as otitis externa (Caruso, 1980).

There are several types of hearing aids, including body aids, behind-the-ear (postauricular) aids, eyeglass aids, and in-the-ear aids (Fig. 13–7). Hearing aids may be placed in one or both ears (binaural), according to individual losses and needs. Binaural aids help to improve the speech reception threshold and speech discrimination (especially in a noisy environment) and provide better localization of sound. A trained audiologist is the person best qualified to test and fit older people for hearing aids. A period of adjustment is usually necessary, and all members of the health care team must participate in the education and support of hearing aid users. Problems most frequently encountered include nervousness due to the sudden increase in noise, embarrassment due to appearing with the hearing aid in public, forgetting to turn off or change the batteries in the hearing aid owing to poor memory, and difficulty in manipulating the parts of the hearing aid because of poor vision or lack of manual dexterity. Guidelines for hearing aid users are listed in Box 13–1.

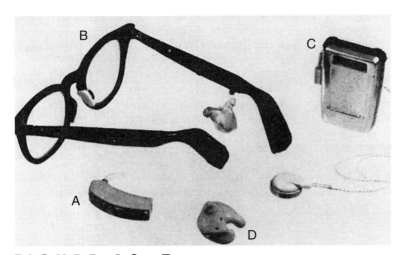
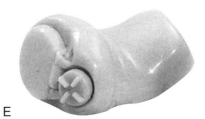

F I G U R E   1 3 – 7

Types of hearing aids. *A,* Postauricular (behind-the-ear) aid. *B,* Eyeglass hearing aid. *C,* Body aid. *D,* All-in-the-ear hearing aid. *E,* Tympanette inserts into the ear canal and contains a tiny class D amplifier microchip. (From Calkins, E., Ford, A.B. and Katz, P.R. *The Practice of Geriatrics.* 2nd ed. Philadelphia: W.B. Saunders, 1992, p. 253; Courtesy of Audio Acoustics Hearing Centers, Odessa, TX.)

BOX 13–1
Guidelines for Hearing Aid Users

1. Practice inserting and removing the hearing aid until you can do these things easily. Put the aid on when relaxed. If you are unable to handle the aid, make sure that your relative or friend can help you.

2. Wear the hearing aid 4 to 5 hours at first. Wear it for a longer period of time the next day. After a week, it should be worn all day.

3. Remove the hearing aid before going to bed, bathing, or showering.

4. Make sure the battery is inserted correctly. Follow + sign for placement of + side of battery. If there is no on-off switch, open the battery case at night to shut the aid off; this will conserve the battery power. If there is an M-T-O (microphone-telephone-off) switch on the aid, turn to O for off at night. Don't forget to turn back to M in the morning to turn the aid on. Store unused batteries in a cool, dry, place.

5. Clean the ear mold daily with a damp cloth. Once a week wipe the mold with a cloth dampened with mild soapy water. Do not immerse the mold in water. If the ear mold gets plugged with wax, clean it out with a toothpick or bent paper clip or wax-removing tool—carefully!

6. Change the batteries every 10 days to 2 weeks. If a whistle (feedback) is *not* heard when the volume control is fully on, change the battery, and the whistle should then be heard. If no whistle is heard despite a new battery, then the problem is in the aid itself.

7. Remember, the aid is a mechanical instrument. Sounds and voices are made louder, not clearer. Expectations should be realistic.

8. Extraneous noises may annoy you at first. Identify the sounds and then forget them. You will get used to hearing background sounds in a short period of time.

9. If the problem persists, the aid should be tested by an audiologist or hearing aid dealer.

Adapted from Margolis, E.M., Levy, B., Sherman, F.T. Hearing disorders. In Libow, L.S. and Sherman, F.T. (eds.). The Core of Geriatric Medicine. St. Louis: C.V. Mosby, 1981, p. 20; Beltone Electronics. The Better Hearing Book. Chicago: Beltone, 1987.

TASTE AND SMELL

The senses of taste and smell are intertwined in a person's appreciation of food, and they provide sensitive responses to the environment. The safety of the environment as well as its pleasantness or unpleasantness can be detected by these senses. The smell of smoke can warn of a dangerous fire, and the scent of a light perfume can provide a delightful background for a romantic interlude. The taste of tainted food or drink can be nauseating, whereas a sip of fine wine can provide a rosy glow to an evening with friends. Changes in the senses of taste and smell with aging are not definitively known, but there is some evidence that they are diminished. If so, this decrease certainly has an effect on the quality of life and on the ability of older people to react safely to the environment.

Taste

The sense of taste is perceived through approximately 9000 taste buds located on the edges and toward the back of the human tongue, the soft palate, the pharynx, and the larynx. The primary taste qualities of sweet, sour, salt, and bitter are associated with particular taste receptors distributed in various parts of the tongue. Generally, sensitivity to sweet taste is located at the tip of the tongue, sourness at the sides, bitterness at the back, and saltiness at the tip and sides of the tongue. Each of the taste buds has 15 to 20 taste cells arranged in a bud-like form on its tip. The taste cells are constantly replacing themselves, and there is a complete turnover for each taste bud every 10 days; however, turnover is generally thought to be more sluggish in the elderly (Calkins, 1992).

It has been found that there is a gradual diminution in the number of taste buds, beginning in females at 40 to 50 years and in males at 50 to 60 years. The taste buds also begin to atrophy around age 40. However, these changes do not affect sensitivity to the four taste qualities until well after 60 years, if at all. Corso (1971) and Engen (1977) reviewed several studies that attempted to determine changes in taste sensitivity with aging. The studies usually involved testing subjects for changes in the primary taste sensations by having them sip mixtures that demonstrated the taste quality—that is, sucrose for sweet, quinine for bitter, hydrochloric acid for sour, and sodium chloride for salty—diluted in water. They measured two types of thresholds: (1) detection threshold—the lowest concentration of a substance that can be distinguished from water and (2) recognition threshold—the lowest concentration of a substance that can be recognized by taste. The studies, even when using the same methodologies, showed conflicting results. Some found no change in sensitivity to all four tastes with age, whereas others found declining sensitivity to particular tastes, such as sweet, bitter, or salty. There were also conflicting data on differences in detection and recognition thresholds in men and women, in smokers, and in persons who wear dentures.

Later studies revealed varying results as well. Weiffenbach et al. (1982) found that detection thresholds increased slightly for salty and bitter tastes with age, but sucrose thresholds did not increase. There was also an increase in the detection threshold for sour tastes in men but not in women. Other studies have found slight increases in sweet thresholds with advancing age (Dye and Koziatek, 1981; Moore et al., 1982), particularly over age 80. Studies examining changes in salt thresholds (Grzegorczyk et al., 1979; Baker et al., 1983) showed slight increases with age, with higher thresholds in smokers and in men (which could be due to the smaller number of women smokers). Baker et al. (1983) found no effect from wearing dentures. Recent studies have shown that decrements in taste sensitivity are not as great as previously thought. However, olfactory loss also affects the sense of taste and clearly contributes to difficulty with food appreciation among elderly persons (Murphy and Davidson, 1992). More research is needed in this area to determine whether and how sense of taste changes with age.

Smell

The sense of smell is perceived through a series of receptors—bipolar nerve cells—located in the mucous membranes high in the nasal cavity. Impulses are relayed to the olfactory bulbs of the brain, which lie just below the frontal lobes, and then to the temporal lobes, the primary olfactory areas of the cortex. With aging, there appears to be a generalized atrophy of the olfactory bulbs and a moderate loss of neurons. Interestingly, the severity of the degeneration is not positively correlated with the age of an individual. It is theorized that damage to the olfactory system may be due to environmental factors, such as smoking, occupational odors, and airborne toxic agents (Corso, 1971).

Regardless of the structural degeneration of the olfactory system, little conclusive evidence exists that shows whether the sense of smell decreases with age. Studies reviewed by Schiffman (1983) tend to support the hypothesis that decrements in odor sensitivity are due to factors other than age, such as disease, accidental poisoning, or smoking. Schiffman and Pasternak (1979) compared ratings of college students and healthy older adults aged 72 to 78 years in distinguishing odors between pairs of food flavors. They found that the ability to discriminate between food odors diminishes considerably with aging. Another study (Schemper et al., 1981) attempted to determine whether aging impairs the ability to process olfactory information by comparing results in college-aged and elderly nonsmoking females. When asked to discriminate among many odors, older people had more difficulty in identifying various smells than young people. In a study published in 1992 and based on a sample of 50 community-dwelling elders, DeVore (1992) discovered that olfactory dysfunction was present in 39 per cent of the subjects, and 18 per cent were unable to detect the smell of smoke. Patients with Alzheimer's or Parkinson's disease, both of which are associated with advancing age, have demonstrated increased loss of olfactory sensory function, presumably because of central neuron loss (Bell et al., 1993).

Conclusions from the results of all studies must be tempered by the fact that there is often considerable bias (older people respond more slowly and carefully to psychomotor testing) in the testing process and that sample sizes are generally small.

At this time, it would not be prudent to conclude that there are any definitive changes in the senses of taste and smell that are specifically related to advancing age. Testing has been uneven and unsystematic, and better psychometric measures are needed to separate the effects of aging from other factors that affect sensory deficits.

TOUCH, VIBRATION, AND PAIN SENSITIVITY

The sensory apparatus of the human body consists of a series of sensory receptors that send signals through the spinal cord, brainstem, thalamus, and cerebral cortex to evoke various types of motor and sensory responses. Sensory receptors are located in the skin, muscles, tendons, joints, and viscera. Receptors in the skin, called exteroceptors, record information about the external environment of the body; specialized receptors, such as Meissner's or Ruffini's corpuscles, detect sensations of touch, heat, or pain. These specialized receptors are distributed throughout the body, but some areas are more sensitive to particular stimuli than others. In addition, different sensory fibers conduct impulses at different rates, so that various sensory modalities (heat, pain, touch) may be perceived differently.

Most somatic sensations evoke affective responses that determine whether the sensation received is pleasant (warmth), unpleasant (pain, excess heat or cold), or neutral (touch). Drugs, brain surgery, or brain lesions may decrease or abolish the affective response while leaving intact the ability to recognize sensory modalities. Thus, individuals can feel and recognize pain, but it no longer bothers them. This phenomenon can be important in the care of elderly clients with delirium or dementia in whom assessment of pain, heat, or cold is extremely difficult.

Proprioceptors are located in muscles, tendons, joints, and visceral organs. They transmit information regarding the position and condition of these deeper organs, although this information does not enter conscious thinking. Many of the responses to proprioceptive stimuli are related to reflex activity that is mediated through the spinal cord or cerebellar areas where posture and movement are controlled.

Changes in Structure and Function

It is difficult to determine whether losses in somesthetic sensitivity can be attributed to aging itself or to the disease states that occur with greater frequency in older age. In a review of the literature related to changes in cutaneous sensitivity (Kenshalo, 1977), most studies were found to demonstrate age-related increases in thresholds for touch, vibration, heat, and pain, particularly in men older than 80 years. However, thresholds were variable among sensory modalities and individuals, so that no uniform conclusions could be made.

Touch and Vibration

Studies related to aging and tactile sense are few, have questionable methodologies, and contain small sample sizes. Increases in thresholds for touch sensitivity have been found in different areas of the body, including the cornea, face, hands, and feet; however, responses to testing are variable and inconclusive (Corso, 1971; Kenshalo, 1977). Thornberry and Minstretta (1981) found increases in tactile thresholds on the pads of index fingers with aging, but they also found that there was wide variation in touch sensitivity among the elderly. Newman (1979) measured palatal sensitivity to touch with the use of air currents in a population aged 20 to 89 years. The study showed that sensitivity diminished progressively with age. Christenson (1990) asserted that this progressive diminution is also mediated by environmental influences. Another study, by Potvin et al. (1980), consisted of a comprehensive series of 128 instrumented tests of neurologic function on 61 normal male subjects aged 20 to 80 years. They found no variance with age in sensitivity to touch of the face and the upper arm.

Vibratory sense is determined by placing a tuning fork on the area to be measured and looking at the frequency threshold. Studies have consistently shown a loss of sensitivity to vibration in a significant proportion of aged subjects who were apparently free of disease or detectable neuropathy (Potvin et al., 1980). They have also shown that the loss begins around age 50 and is more severe in the lower extremities than in the upper limbs (MacLennan, 1980). Change in vibratory sense is of interest because it has been found to be a valuable means of diagnosing disorders of the nervous system. If healthy elderly persons have loss of vibratory sensitivity, diagnosis of abnormalities is more difficult. It is thought that changes with normal aging are due to decreased blood flow to the peripheral structures or spinal cord or to dietary factors, such as thiamin deficiency (Corso, 1971).

Pain

Pain is a complicated phenomenon that is difficult to measure. Data regarding measurement of pain sensitivity are inconsistent and are confounded by variables in the test situation such as the subjects, investigators, and environmental conditions. According to Corso (1975), the level of cutaneous pain sensitivity usually is relatively constant until age 50 and then shows a sharp decline. Sensitivity decreases more in the upper body areas, such as the forehead, upper arm, and forearm, than in the lower limbs, such as the thigh and leg. In a 1990 pilot study of the pain experience of nursing home residents, Ferrell et al. (1990) found that 71 per cent of residents had at least one complaint of intermittent pain. Hamilton, in a 1989 report based on data from semistructured interviews regarding comfort concepts, listed better pain management as the number one need in 30 patients in a long-term geriatric hospital. Kenshalo (1977) differentiated between cutaneous pain and deep pain and concluded that there appear to be higher thresholds for pain perception for both cutaneous and deep pain with aging. It is interesting to note that older persons tend to be more reluctant to report pain than younger persons (Clark and Mehl, 1971), which may influence the results of self-report studies. In a report on age and pain threshold, Vecchi et al. (1983) concluded that there is no relationship between age and pain threshold and that aged persons react in the same way as young persons when they are exposed to painful stimuli of critical intensity. They noted that various ailments can impair the efficiency of the structures and functions that control pain, so that the alteration of pain sensitivity in the elderly should be considered an illness rather than a physiological change due to age.

NURSING DIAGNOSES

1. Activity Intolerance related to pain
2. Pain, Chronic
3. Communication, Impaired Verbal related to hearing impairment
4. Diversional Activity Deficit related to loss of ability to perform usual or favorite activities secondary to sensory losses
5. Home Maintenance Management, Impairment related to sensory losses
6. Mobility, Impaired Physical related to sensory losses
7. Self-Care Deficit: Feeding, Bathing/Hygiene, Dressing/Grooming, Toileting, Instrumental related to sensory losses
8. Sensory-Perceptual Alterations: Visual, Auditory, Kinesthetic, Gustatory, Tactile, Olfactory related to aging processes
9. Social Interactions, Impaired related to sensory losses
10. Thought Processes, Altered related to inability to evaluate reality secondary to sensory losses
11. Violence, Risk for: Directed at Others related to sensory-perceptual alterations
12. Grieving related to sensory losses
13. Knowledge Deficit: Difficulty in Processing Information related to sensory-perceptual alterations

NURSING ASSESSMENT

The elements of a careful nursing assessment of the senses are outlined in Table 13–4.

History

Complaints of visual disturbances, such as diplopia (double vision), inability to focus

T A B L E   1 3 – 4
Nursing Assessment of the Special Senses

History
History of cataracts, glaucoma, diabetes
Symptoms
   Visual problems: diplopia (double vision), inability to focus, tunnel vision, transient blindness, discomfort, headaches, eye fatigue, eye pain
   Hearing loss (sudden or gradual, bilateral or unilateral), ringing in the ears or tinnitus, dizziness, vertigo, pain
   Diminished taste, smell, or touch
Use of aids: glasses, hearing aids

Physical Assessment
Eye/Vision
  Inspection
    External eye, lids, and lacrimal ducts for excess tearing, discharge, ectropion, entropion, swelling
    Conjunctiva and sclera for lesions, redness
    Cornea for opacity, curvature
    Pupils for size, shape, equality, reaction to light
  Funduscopic examination of internal eye
    Optic disc (optic atrophy, papilledema, glaucoma), hemorrhages, exudates, vascular abnormalities
  Intraocular pressure test for glaucoma
  Vision
    Snellen's chart
    Acuity, color, depth perception, peripheral vision, light and dark adaptation, glare, halos
Ear/Hearing
  Inspection
    External ear for lesions, dryness, exudate
    Ear canal for cerumen, scarring, infections
  Measure air and bone conduction
    Weber's test
    Rinne's test
  Hearing
    Tone, frequency, speech discrimination
Smell, taste, and touch
  Identification of odors, food tastes (sweet, sour, bitter, salty), and objects
  Somatic sensations (pinprick, cotton, temperature)

on far or near objects, tunnel vision, and transient blindness, should be noted as well as the onset, duration, and circumstances under which they occur. Intermittent or persistent discomfort related to vision, such as headaches, eye fatigue, or eye pain, should also be noted. Older clients usually wear bifocal or trifocal glasses, so it is important to know the date of the most recent eye examination and the name of the examiner.

Hearing loss, whether sudden or gradual, bilateral or unilateral, should be investigated. Other complaints might be ringing or tinnitus, dizziness or vertigo, and pain. Because family members may be more cognizant of the hearing loss than are older clients, their input is useful.

Complaints of diminished taste and smell are unusual with normal aging. However, older people may experience a blunting of these sensations in the presence of colds or allergies. The impact of sensory losses on activities of daily living should also be explored (Lichtenstein, 1992). In a 1993 study of 1191 community-dwelling elders, Carabellese et al. found significant linkages between sensory impairment and quality of life measures. Changes in somatic sensations should be investigated, especially the occurrence of acute or chronic pain. Chapter 14 presents further discussion of pain assessment.

Physical Assessment

Eye and Vision

The external eye, including the lids and lacrimal ducts, should be inspected for deviations from normal, particularly the presence of excess tearing, discharge, ectropion, entropion, or swelling. The conjunctiva and sclera should be free from lesions or redness. The cornea may have some opacity or abnormal curvature, and an arcus senilis may be seen on the iris surrounding the cornea. The pupils are examined for size, shape, and equality.

The internal eye is observed by funduscopic examination to look for abnormalities of the optic disc (optic atrophy, papilledema, glaucoma), hemorrhages, exudates, and vascular abnormalities. Glaucoma is also identified by measuring intraocular pressure using various types of tonometers (Fig. 13–8).

Vision can be assessed in many ways. Visual acuity is traditionally measured by using the Snellen chart. If this is not available, nurses can ask older clients to read a newspaper aloud, starting with the larger headlines and ending with the finest, smallest print. This provides a gross measure of near vision. Colors can be distinguished by making color charts or by asking clients to identify colors in the environment. Peripheral vision, glare, depth perception, and light and dark adaptation should also be tested. Vision should be assessed with and without glasses. Also, behavioral changes such as bumping into objects, straining to read or watch television, and social withdrawal should be noted (McNeely et al., 1992).

Ear and Hearing

The external ear should be inspected for lesions, dryness, or exudate. The ear canal should be examined for cerumen, scarring, and infections.

Assessment of Hearing Loss

Assessment of hearing loss can be carried out through sophisticated audiometric testing or through cursory examinations in the clinical setting. Older people who find that they have difficulty following conversations or are unable to hear extraneous environmental noises, such as birds singing or the wind blowing, may seek the services of an audiologist to determine the nature and extent of their hearing loss. The audiologist may use screening techniques, including self-estimates of hearing loss by the individual, pure-tone audiometry, and speech perception tests, to facilitate the use of proper rehabilitative techniques. Pure-tone air and bone conduction tests (the Weber and Rinne tuning fork tests) may also be carried out by a nurse in the clinical setting. Air conduction is the measured level of sound transmitted through the ear canal and middle ear ossicles to the inner ear. Bone conduction is measured by placing a vibrator on the mastoid bone behind the auricle, which directly stimulates the inner ear. If air conduction is greater than bone conduction, there is sensorineural loss; if bone conduction is greater than air conduction, there is conductive loss.

Hearing loss can also be determined by a nurse through assessment during a conversation with an older person. The nurse should be alert to discrepancies between questions and answers and to remarks such as, "Would you repeat the question," or "Stop mumbling," or "Please speak louder." Many elderly who are embarrassed, sensitive, or unaware of hearing loss may not acknowledge a hearing difficulty and may merely answer "yes" or smile in reply to questions. The nurse can stand out of the

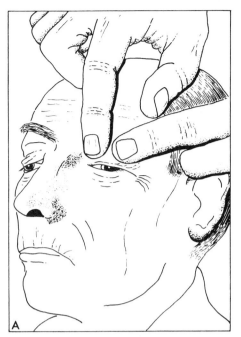

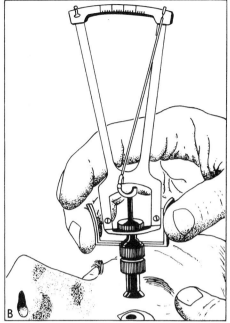

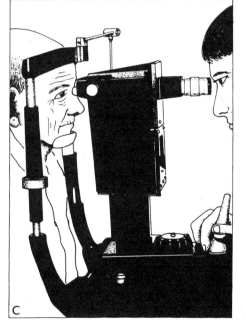

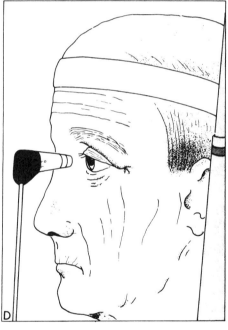

FIGURE 13 – 8

Methods of intraocular pressure estimation. *A,* Finger palpation is useful only when a large difference exists between the intraocular pressure of the two eyes, as in unilateral angle-closure glaucoma. *B,* Schiøtz tonometry can be learned readily, and because the tonometer is relatively inexpensive, it can be used in every physician's office to screen for chronic simple glaucoma. *C,* The air-puff tonometer can be used for screening large numbers of patients but is far more expensive than Schiøtz's tonometer. *D,* Goldmann's applanation tonometer, used with a slit lamp, is the standard instrument for glaucoma diagnosis and management for most ophthalmologists. It is expensive and requires considerable skill. (From Calkins, E., Ford, A.B. and Katz, P.R. *The Practice of Geriatrics.* 2nd ed. Philadelphia: W.B. Saunders, 1992, pp. 238–239.)

range of vision of the client and ask questions that require answers other than "yes" or "no" to determine the hearing loss more accurately. Based on systematic screenings of older adults, O'Rourke et al. (1993) recommended a case history, visual inspection, and pure-tone screening as the most effective hearing assessment protocol. Voeks et al. (1993) recommended assessing hearing while the patient is in a group, watching television, and on the telephone for better sensitivity. Recommendations were based on their work with 198 newly admitted nursing home residents. Walczak et al. (1993) concurred, based on findings from 81 clients in a geriatric day care center.

Smell, Taste, and Touch

Smell, taste, and touch can be assessed by asking the older client to identify odors, food, and objects while blindfolded. Spices can be used for tests of the sense of smell, and foods that are sour, sweet, bitter, and salty may be used to test for the sense of taste. Small objects placed in a paper bag can be used to test the sense of touch; the client can reach in and try to identify the object. Somatic sensations can be measured by using pinpricks or by brushing cotton lightly on the skin.

NURSING INTERVENTIONS AND EVALUATION

Nursing interventions for older persons with any type of sensory deficit aim toward maintaining the highest level of functioning possible and teaching clients and families strategies for maximizing sensory function. For the visually impaired, color contrast, bright lighting, and the use of visual aids, such as eyeglasses and magnifying glasses, should be emphasized. Interventions may also include providing large-print reading material. Safety considerations, including sufficient time to adapt, night lights, color borders on steps, increased caution or even a decrease in night driving, and medication assessment are also important. For hearing-impaired older people, verbal communication by others should be slow and deliberate; the voice should be pitched low, and the speaker should be facing the older person directly. Background noise should be minimized. Rephrasing content and verbal cues when changing subjects may also be helpful nursing actions. Ear irrigations may be indicated as well as monitoring medications that affect hearing. Taste and smells can be enhanced through the liberal use of spices and condiments, attractive food preparation, food served at the appropriate temperature, and regular mouth care. Impaired smell may also have safety implications, making devices such as smoke alarms even more significant (Kee, 1990).

Evaluation is made by ongoing measurement of the ability to see, hear, taste, smell, or touch. The ability to carry out activities of daily living independently can provide a good measure of visual and hearing capacity because visual and hearing deficits frequently impinge on functional abilities. Further losses in sensory capabilities and functional abilities must be investigated to determine whether they are preventable or if further interventions are necessary.

SUMMARY

Sensory changes greatly affect the life of older people and can substantially alter the quality of life and independence once taken for granted. Normal age-related changes in vision include decreases in visual acuity, tol-erance of glare, ability to adapt to dark and light, and peripheral vision. Presbyopia, or the inability to accommodate for far and near vision, is also common. Disorders of the eye that occur frequently in older age include cataracts, glaucoma, senile macular degeneration, diabetic retinopathy, and se-nile entropion and ectropion.

Hearing loss is highly associated with aging. The three types of hearing loss are conductive, sensorineural, and mixed. Hearing loss for high frequencies is especially common, and older people often have difficulty distinguishing words spoken too fast. Presbycusis, which is frequently found in older age, produces bilateral loss of hearing acuity, poor discrimination and comprehension, and tinnitus.

The senses of taste, smell, and touch are thought to diminish with older age; however, more studies are needed in these areas.

Nursing assessment and interventions are geared toward maximizing the ability to see, hear, taste, smell, and touch. Older people and their families should be taught to use more effective methods of communication and to use aids for communication, such as hearing aids, glasses, and so on. These measures help to promote functional independence and well-being in older clients.

REFERENCES

Anderson, B. and Palmore, E. Longitudinal evaluation of ocular function. *In* Palmore, E. (ed.). *Normal Aging II.* Durham, NC: Duke University Press, 1974, pp. 24–32.

Baker, K.A., Didcock, E.A., Kemm, J.R., et al. Effects of age, sex and illness on salt taste detection thresholds. *Age Ageing* 12:159–165, 1983.

Barron, C.R., Foxall, M.J., Von Dollen, K., et al. Loneliness in low-vision older women. *Issues Ment Health Nurs* 13(4):387–401, 1992.

Bell, I.R., Amend, D., Kaszniak, A.W. and Schwartz, G.E. Memory deficits, sensory impairment, and depression in the elderly. *Lancet* 341(8836):62, 1993.

Beltone Electronics. *The Better Hearing Book.* Chicago: Beltone, 1987.

Calkins, E., Ford, A.B. and Katz, P.R. *Practice of Geriatrics.* 2nd ed. Philadelphia: W.B. Saunders, 1992.

Carabellese, C., Appollonio, I., Rozzini, R., et al. Sensory impairment and quality of life in a community elderly population. *J Am Geriatr Soc* 41(4):401–407, 1993.

Caruso, V.G. When the patient has otitis externa. *Geriatrics* 35:35–42, 1980.

Christenson, M.A. Adaptations of the physical environment to compensate for sensory changes. *Phys Occup Ther Geriatr* 8(3/4):3–30, 1990.

Clark, W.C. and Mehl, L. Thermal pain: A sensory decision theory analysis of the effect of age and sex on various response criteria, and 50% pain threshold. *J Abnorm Psychol* 78:202–212, 1971.

Corso, J.F. Sensory processes and age effects in normal adults. *J Gerontol* 26:90–105, 1971.

Corso, J.F. *Aging Sensory Systems and Perception.* New York: Praeger, 1981.

DeVore, P.A. Prevalence of olfactory dysfunction, hearing deficit, and cognitive dysfunction among elderly patients in a suburban family practice. *South Med J* 85(9):894–896, 1992.

Dye, C.J. and Koziatek, D.A. Age and diabetes effects on threshold and hedonic perception of sucrose solutions. *J Gerontol* 36:310–315, 1981.

Eifrig, D.E. and Simons, K.B. An overview of common geriatric ophthalmologic disorders. *Geriatrics* 38:55, 1983.

Eisdorfer, C. and Wilkie I. Auditory changes. *In* Palmore, E. (ed.). *Normal Aging II.* Durham, NC: Duke University Press, 1974, pp. 32–41.

Engen, T. Taste and smell. *In* Birren, J.E. and Schaie, K.W. (eds.). *Handbook of the Psychology of Aging.* New York: Van Nostrand Reinhold, 1977, pp. 554–561.

Ferrell, B.A., Ferrell, B.R. and Osterweil, D. Pain in the nursing home. *J Am Geriatr Soc* 38(4):409, 1990.

Goodhill, V. Evaluation of the aging ear. *Emerg Med* 24(15):165–166, 1992.

Grimes, M.R., Scardino, M.A. and Martone, J.F. Worldwide blindness. *Nurs Clin North Am* 27(3):807–816, 1992.

Grzegorczyk, P.B., Jones, S.W. and Mistretta, C.M. Age-related differences in salt taste acuity. *J Gerontol* 34: 834–840, 1979.

Hall, J.W. Acoustic reflex amplitude: Effect of age and sex. *Audiology* 21:294–309, 1982.

Hamilton, J. Comfort and the hospitalized chronically ill. *J Geriatr Nurs* 15(4):28, 1989.

Kee, C.C. Sensory impairment: Factor X in providing nursing care to the older adult. *J Community Health Nurs* 7(1):45–52, 1990.

Kenshalo, D.R. Age changes in touch, vibration, temperature, kinesthesis and pain sensitivity. *In* Birren, J.E. and Scheie, K.W. (eds.). *Handbook of the Psychology of Aging.* New York: Van Nostrand Reinhold, 1977, pp. 563–570.

Kline, D.W., Ikeda, D.M. and Schieber, F.J. Age and temporal resolution in color vision: When do red and green make yellow? *J Gerontol* 37:705–709, 1982.

Kline, D.W., Kline, T.J., Fozard, J.L., et al. Vision, aging, and driving: The problems of older drivers. *J Gerontol* 47(1):27–34, 1992.

Langston, R.H.S. Sensory and skin problems. *In* Schrier, R.W. (ed.). *Geriatric Medicine.* Philadelphia: W.B. Saunders, 1990.

Lichtenstein, M.J. Hearing and visual impairments. *Clin Geriatr Med* 8(1):173–182, 1992.

Liebowitz, H.M., Krueger, D.E., Maunder, L.R., et al. The Framingham Eye Study Monograph. *Surv Ophthalmol* 24:463, 1980.

LTC Nurse Rx 3(10):1–4, 1993.

MacLennan, W.J., Timothy, J.I. and Hall, M.R.P. Vibration sense, proprioception and ankle reflexes in old age. *J Clin Exp Gerontol* 2:159–171, 1980.

Mahoney, D.F. Cerumen impaction: Prevalence and detection in nursing homes. *J Gerontol Nurs* 19(4):23–30, 1993.

Marmour, M.F. Management of elderly patients with impaired vision. *In* Ebaugh, F.G., Jr. (ed.). *Management of Common Problems in Geriatric Medicine.* Menlo Park, CA: Addison-Wesley, 1981, pp. 17–44.

Marx, M.S., Werner, P., Cohen-Mansfield, J. and Feldman, R. The relationship between low vision and performance of activities of daily living in nursing home residents. *J Am Geriatr Soc* 40(10):1018–1020, 1992.

Mashiah, T. The effect of ageing on colour vision in females. *Age Ageing* 7:114–115, 1978.

McNeely, E., Griffin-Shirley, N. and Hubbard, A. Teaching caregivers to recognize diminished vision among nursing home residents. *Geriatr Nurs* 13(6):332–335, 1992.

Mhoon, E.M. Otology. *In* Cassel, C.K., Riesenberg, D.E., Sorensen, L.B. and Walsh, J.R. (eds.). *Geriatric Medicine,* 2nd ed. New York: Springer-Verlag, 1990, pp. 405–419.

Milne, J.S. Longitudinal studies of vision in older people. *Age Ageing* 8:160–166, 1979.

Moore, L.M., Nielson, C. and Mistretta, C.M. Sucrose taste thresholds: Age-related differences. *J Gerontol* 37: 64–69, 1982.

Murphy, C. and Davidson, T.M. Geriatric issues: Special considerations. *J Head Trauma Rehabil* 7(1):76–82, 1992.

National Eye Institute. Laser treatment found effective in preventing blindness from senile macular degeneration. Prepared by staff of the National Eye Institute, National Institutes of Health, Bethesda, MD. *J Am Geriatr Soc* 31:238–239, 1983.

Netland, P.A., Chaturvedi, N. and Dreyer, E.B. Calcium channel blockers in the management of low-tension and open-angle glaucoma. *Am J Ophthalmol* 115(5):608–613, 1993.

Newman, H.F. Palatal sensitivity to touch: Correlation with age. *J Am Geriatr Soc* 27:319, 1979.

Ney, D.F. Cerumen impaction, ear hygiene practices, and hearing acuity. *Geriatr Nurs* 14(2):70–73, 1993.

Nodar, R.H. Hearing problems. *In* Schrier, R.W. *Geriatric Medicine.* Philadelphia: W.B. Saunders, 1990.

O'Rourke, C.M., Britten, C.F., Gatschet, C.A. and Krien, T.L. Effectiveness of a hearing screening protocol for the elderly. *Geriatr Nurs* 14(2):66–69, 1993.

Pizzarello, L.D. The dimensions of the problem of eye disease among the elderly. *Ophthalmology* 94:1191–1195, 1987.

Potvin, A.R., Syndulko, K., Tourtellotte, W.W., et al. Human neurologic function and the aging process. *J Am Geriatr Soc* 28:1–9, 1980.

Powers, K.L. and Powers, E.A. Hearing problems of elderly persons: Social consequences and prevalence. *Asha* 20:79–83, 1978.

Rai, G.S. and Elias-Jones, A. The corneal reflex in elderly patients. *J Am Geriatr Soc* 27:317–318, 1979.

Rich, L.F. Ophthalmology. *In* Cassel, C.K., Riesenberg, D.E., Sorensen, L.B. and Walsh, J.R. (eds.). *Geriatric Medicine,* 2nd ed. New York: Springer-Verlag, 1990, pp. 394–404.

Salive, M.E., Guralnik, J., Christen, W., et al. Functional blindness and visual impairment in older adults from three communities. *Ophthalmology* 99(12):1840–1847, 1992.

Schemper, T., Voss, S. and Cain, W.S. Odor identification in young and elderly persons: Sensory and cognitive limitations. *J Gerontol* 36:446–452, 1981.

Schiffman, S.S. Taste and smell in disease. *N Engl J Med* 308:1337–1343, 1983.

Schiffman, S. and Pasternak, M. Decreased discrimination of food odors in the elderly. *J Gerontol* 34:73–79, 1979.

Taylor, K.S. Geriatric hearing loss: Management strategies for nurses. *Geriatr Nurs* 14(2):74–76, 1993.

Thomas, P.D., Hunt, W.C., Garry, P.J., et al. Hearing acuity in a healthy elderly population: Effects on emotional, cognitive, and social status. *J Gerontol* 38:321–325, 1983.

Thornberry, J.M. and Minstretta, C.M. Tactile sensitivity as a function of age. *J Gerontol* 36:34–39, 1981.

Vecchi, G.P., Calza, L. and Neri, M. Age and pain threshold. *In* Rizzi, R. and Visentin, M. (eds.). *Pain Therapy.* New York: Elsevier Biomedical, 1983.

Voeks, S.K., Gallagher, C.M., Langer, E.H. and Drinka, P.J. Self-reported hearing difficulty and audiometric thresholds in nursing home residents. *J Fam Pract* 36(1):54–58, 1993.

Walczak, M., Bernstein, A.L., Senzer, C.L. and Mohr, N. Elder hearing aids. Infrared listening device in a geriatric day center. *J Gerontol Nurs* 19(3):5–9, 1993.

Weiffenbach, J.M., Baum, B.J. and Burghauser, R. Taste thresholds: Quality specific variation with human aging. *J Gerontol* 37:372–377, 1982.

Woods, S. Macular degeneration. *Nurs Clin North Am* 27(3):761–775, 1992.

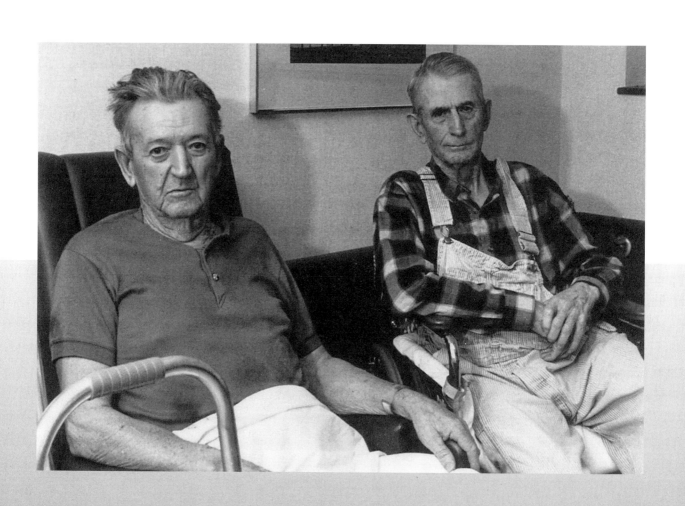

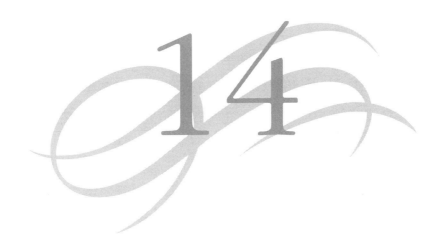

Nursing Diagnoses Related to Physiological Alterations

ELEANOR S. McCONNELL
ANN T. MURPHY

OBJECTIVES

Identify nursing diagnoses that are commonly associated with physiological age-related changes in the elderly.

❖

Discuss the definition and scope of the problem, theoretical issues, and contributing factors for each nursing diagnosis as it relates specifically to the elderly.

❖

Conduct a nursing assessment on an older client related to each nursing diagnosis.

❖

Formulate a plan of care and nursing interventions for older clients for each nursing diagnosis.

❖

Evaluate a plan of care and nursing interventions for older clients for each nursing diagnosis.

ACTIVITY INTOLERANCE

HYPERTHERMIA AND HYPOTHERMIA

BOWEL ELIMINATION ALTERATIONS: COLONIC AND PERCEIVED CONSTIPATION, IMPACTION, AND INCONTINENCE

ALTERATION IN BOWEL ELIMINATION: DIARRHEA

COMFORT ALTERATIONS: ACUTE AND CHRONIC PAIN, FATIGUE, NAUSEA, AND DYSPNEA

COMMUNICATION IMPAIRMENT: VERBAL

FLUID VOLUME DEFICIT

INFECTION, HIGH RISK FOR

PHYSICAL MOBILITY IMPAIRMENT

ORAL MUCOUS MEMBRANE ALTERATION

RESPIRATORY FUNCTION ALTERATIONS: INEFFECTIVE AIRWAY CLEARANCE, INEFFECTIVE BREATHING PATTERN, IMPAIRED GAS EXCHANGE

SELF-CARE DEFICITS: FEEDING, BATHING/ HYGIENE, DRESSING/GROOMING, AND TOILETING

SENSORY-PERCEPTUAL ALTERATIONS: VISUAL, AUDITORY, GUSTATORY, OLFACTORY, TACTILE, KINESTHETIC, AND UNILATERAL NEGLECT

ALTERED SEXUALITY PATTERNS AND SEXUAL DYSFUNCTION

SKIN INTEGRITY IMPAIRMENT

SLEEP PATTERN DISTURBANCE

THOUGHT PROCESS ALTERATION

TISSUE PERFUSION ALTERATIONS: ALTERED PERIPHERAL TISSUE PERFUSION AND HIGH RISK FOR PERIPHERAL NEUROVASCULAR DYSFUNCTION

URINARY ELIMINATION ALTERATIONS: INCONTINENCE (FUNCTIONAL, REFLEX, STRESS, URGE, TOTAL), URINARY RETENTION

Development and classification of nursing diagnoses is in its early stages. Although the concept of nursing diagnosis has been around since the 1950s, the notion of organizing nursing knowledge around a taxonomy of nursing diagnoses remains controversial. Yet increasing numbers of nurses are using the list of diagnoses accepted for testing by the North American Nursing Diagnosis Association (NANDA) (see page 31) and finding the concept to be helpful in organizing their approach to practice (Jaycox, 1994). This chapter describes the current knowl-

edge concerning the various nursing diagnostic categories in the elderly related to physiological problems. Each section describes the scope of the problem in the aged, including the consequences of not treating the problem. Theoretical issues that pertain to diagnostic formulation, natural history of the problem, and interventive strategies are described, followed by guidelines for assessment, planning, intervention, and evaluation.

As more research is done using nursing diagnosis categories as an organizing framework, nurses will be able to streamline their diagnostic reasoning process through knowing the prevalence of the categories in various patient populations. This information has been included where it exists or can be inferred; however, in most cases it is inadequate to inform the diagnostic reasoning process.

Diagnoses with the prefix "High Risk for" have not been included separately, unless that is the only mention of the diagnostic category (e.g., high risk for infection), as much of the assessment and nursing care is similar. When interventions differ for prevention versus treatment of a problem, that is noted in the text.

The diagnoses are arranged alphabetically. Although a taxonomy has been endorsed by NANDA, the language and structure remain controversial and are under revision. Thus, we felt it prudent to use a structure that has been successful in practice settings. As the list of approved diagnoses has developed, there has been a tendency to differentiate further or to subdivide the categories that were initially approved. For example, in addition to altered breathing patterns, there are diagnoses that describe more specific problems, such as difficulty in weaning from a ventilator. To discuss these problems efficiently, the newer diagnoses are clustered with the original, more global categories, and discussed as a group. The alphabetical listing used in the previous edition is retained, and when in doubt about the location of a specific diagnostic label, the index should be consulted.

Finally, a word about diagnostic precision. Many overlaps exist between diagnostic categories at present. This is probably in part due to the nature of nursing as a nonreductionist science and in part due to the youth of the diagnostic classification process in nursing. Nurses should not unduly waste time worrying about whether or not they have found the one correct diagnostic label. As the nursing diagnosis taxonomy is currently constituted, *several* diagnostic categories sometimes apply to one patient situation, when the therapies for the problem are quite similar.

In some instances one etiology may produce several problems, in turn justifying several different diagnostic categories. For example, individuals with hemiplegia often concurrently have the problems of impaired physical mobility, self-care deficit, activity intolerance, and alteration in comfort. Many of the interventions used to correct the impairment in mobility will have beneficial effects on the person's self-care deficits, activity intolerance, and comfort alteration. By focusing on improving self-care skills, the individual performs tasks that will increase physical mobility, improve activity tolerance, and probably reduce pain. Thus, in some cases, the choice of "primary" diagnosis is not important, the nurses should not be discouraged if treatment plans for diagnoses overlap.

The idea of "syndrome" nursing diagnoses has been developed (McCourt, 1991) to facilitate efficient documentation and holistic interventions when clusters of nursing diagnoses commonly occur together (for example, disuse syndrome). This idea is potentially quite useful for gerontological nurses. The presence of multiple chronic diseases and decreased homeostatic reserve in the geriatric population often manifests as multiple and complex responses to a given health problem. For example, the onset of an acute infection is often associated with high risk for altered thought process (delirium), incontinence, and injury (falls). More research is indicated to define better gerontological nursing diagnosis syndromes.

It is interesting that the concept of syndrome appears prominently in the geriatric medicine literature. Rather than being a constellation of medical diagnoses, "geriatric syndromes" in this context are declines in function that are multifactorial in origin, such as falls, confusion, incontinence. In this sense, they are quite similar to nursing diagnoses. This similarity in focus, despite slight differences in terminology, highlights the contribution of a nursing perspective in health care of older adults on both a theoretical and a practical level.

ACTIVITY INTOLERANCE

Definition and Scope of Problem

Activity is the process of exerting energy or accomplishing an effect (O'Toole, 1992). In humans, both threshold amounts of phys-

Patient Phenomena

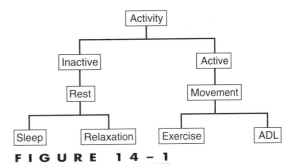

FIGURE 14–1

Classification of activity phenomena in humans. (Adapted from Glick, O.J. Interventions related to activity and movement. *Nurs Clin North Am* 27(2):541–568, 1992.)

ical mobility and sufficient cardiac reserve to generate sustained movement are required. Activity is essential to engaging in human behavior and controlling one's environment and thus has been conceptualized as a basic human need (Glick, 1992). To engage successfully in an activity, individuals must be capable of voluntary motion that is controlled, flexible, coordinated, and strong and can be sustained for a certain period of time. Rating an individual's conduct of activities can be based on the precision, strength, and endurance of the performance.

Activity can be thought of as part of a cyclical process involving both movement and rest. Thus, understanding activity intolerance requires knowledge of normal patterning of movement and rest in humans. Review of the literature on circadian rhythmicity is helpful in this regard. Glick (1992) has proposed a useful heuristic method for classifying activity and rest phenomena in humans (Fig. 14–1).

Activity intolerance is defined as "a state in which an individual has insufficient physiological or psychological energy to endure or complete required or desired daily activities" (NANDA, 1992, p. 55).

The extent to which activity intolerance is a problem for older people can only be inferred, as no epidemiological surveys of the problem in any setting of care exist. However, there are numerous reports of the problems of deconditioning in older people as the result of inactivity and bedrest (Bortz, 1982). Mitchell (1986) observes that fatigue is accepted as "an almost universal symptom of aging." A study by Brody and Kleban (1983) reveals that nearly 70 per cent of all older people surveyed reported fatigue, and of that number, 59 per cent reported feeling fatigued often.

The recent gerontology and geriatrics literature contains many articles on the positive effects of enhancing activity in older patients (Hogue et al., 1993).

Older people suffer disproportionately from cardiorespiratory diseases and musculoskeletal and neurological disorders, all of which contribute to activity intolerance, suggesting that activity intolerance is probably a quite prevalent disorder among the frail elderly. The potential consequences of untreated activity intolerance include disuse atrophy, impaired physical mobility, role change, altered self-esteem, powerlessness, sleep disturbance, and possibly alteration in thought process.

Contributing Factors

Impairments in cardiorespiratory, neurological, musculoskeletal, hepatorenal, or hematopoietic functioning adversely affect activity tolerance.

Age-Related Changes

Many of the physiological changes associated with aging affect the ability to perform activities. Reduced cardiac output, reduced maximal oxygen uptake, and decreased muscle mass and strength all contribute to reduced endurance. Although physical work capacity, as measured by maximal oxygen uptake (VO_2 max) has been shown to decline with age in cross-sectional studies, longitudinal studies of male athletes suggest that declines in physical activity are what causes the age-related reduction in physical work capacity, rather than age alone (Spirduso and McCrae, 1990). Reduced efficiency of thermoregulatory mechanisms, such as perspiration, vasodilation, and decreased ability to concentrate urine, also lead to reduced tolerance for vigorous physical activity. Increased reaction times increase the difficulty of mastering new tasks. In short, the older person's diminished homeostatic capacity leads to decreased ability to tolerate sudden changes in activity level.

In addition to these changes, there is evidence that circadian patterns in activity change with age. In a study of healthy volunteers, the timing and amount of activity differed in younger and older adults. The older adults studied unexpectedly displayed more activity than younger adults. Their peak activity levels occurred earlier in the day (around 1:30 P.M.) than was true for younger volunteers (around 3:15 P.M.), with the older group arising earlier in the morning and having earlier bedtimes at night. Older subjects had more activity at night-

time, consistent with other studies of increased sleep fragmentation with age (Lieberman et al., 1989).

Although this study was carefully conducted, generalization of its results to clinical populations must be made with caution for several reasons. First, only very healthy, community-dwelling older persons were studied in a laboratory setting. Second, the comparison group (many graduate students, adults with time to engage in this laboratory study) may mean that the younger group is not representative of younger adults generally. Furthermore, the effects of various chronic diseases on circadian rhythms have not been studied extensively.

Deconditioning and Cardiovascular and Respiratory Disorders

Intolerance to activity is often a result of deconditioning from prolonged immobility (Siebens, 1992) or pathological cardiorespiratory conditions. Any disorder that reduces tissue oxygenation, such as coronary artery disease, peripheral vascular disease, cardiac arrhythmias, congestive heart failure, chronic pulmonary disease, and pneumonia, will adversely affect activity tolerance.

Neurological and Musculoskeletal Impairments

Frustration from inability to control or coordinate an activity adequately may lead to a psychological intolerance to certain types of activity. For example, individuals with hemiplegia usually have sufficient cardiorespiratory capacity to dress independently. However, some patients encounter such difficulty controlling abnormal synergistic movement patterns (Taylor, 1990) that they lack the endurance to maintain standing balance for the prolonged periods of time that are needed for dressing. As a result, these individuals may cease being independent in dressing and lose an opportunity to engage in a daily living activity that promotes endurance.

Pain, inflexibility, and lack of strength increase the difficulty of completing an activity, also contributing to intolerance. The energy required to perform basic activities of daily living is increased with inefficient movement associated with physical impairments like stroke, hip fracture, or amputation. Table 14–1 shows the relationship between impaired physical mobility and activity tolerance.

In summary, physical impairments may have wide-ranging influences on someone's

TABLE 14-1
Impact of Selected Chronic Diseases on Physical Mobility and Activity Tolerance

Disorders	Impact on Mobility	Impact on Activity Tolerance
CNS PROBLEMS Cerebrovascular accident (CVA)	Lack of cortical inhibitors → spasticity Flaccid muscle tone Impaired kinesthesia	Mobility impairments result in less efficient and slower task completion that requires more patience, ingenuity, equipment, adaptive responses, environmental supports, and energy expenditure
Spinocerebellar pathway degeneration	Uncoordinated movements Impaired kinesthesia	
Parkinson's disease	Rigidity of muscles and joints Tremor Impaired kinesthesia	Little spontaneous initiation of activity
Tardive dyskinesia	Uncoordinated movements	
Dementia	Apraxia of movement Impaired kinesthesia Doesn't know how to move in bed	Etiologies of mobility impairments may be so severe that certain activities are impossible, e.g., bathing
Knowledge deficit		
Pain with movement: e.g., R.A.; DJD; fracture; "frozen joints" s/p CVA; severe edema	Belief that increased movement will cause increased pain	Reduced activity because of fear of pain
SKELETAL PROBLEMS Scoliosis and kyphosis	Limited spinal flexibility, flexion, and truncal rotation	With progression, may reduce intrathoracic space, impairing cardiac and pulmonary function
Vertebral compression fractures	Pain on motion Impingement on spinal nerve roots producing neurological impairments	
Degenerative joint disease (DJD)	Pain on motion Edema and limited function in extremity	Reduced motivation to engage in activities because of pain or fear of pain
Fractures with poor healing	Limited joint mobility: usually extension	
Contractures	Limited joint mobility	
Prostheses		
MUSCULAR PROBLEMS Flaccidity: MD, MS, ALS, and immediate s/p CVA	Decreased grip strength Decreased ability to bear weight Muscle weakness	Increased time required to complete activity
Deconditioning—prolonged inactivity	Muscle atrophy → weakness	Decreased endurance
ENVIRONMENTAL PROBLEMS Restraints, e.g., vests, lap trays, siderails	Prevent voluntary movement	Prevent spontaneous activity
DRUGS Sedatives	Prevent voluntary movement	Reduced activity because of lethargy
Diuretics	Induce muscle weakness Dizziness from orthostasis	
Sedatives	Induce somnolence	Unpredictable performance because of drug effects
Antipsychotics	Produce tardive dyskinesias Produce extrapyramidal SEs Dizziness from orthostasis	
Tricyclic antidepressants	Depression	→ decreased activity tolerance
Beta blockers	CHF	→ decreased activity tolerance
Uninformed caregivers	Discourage movement Improper use of wheelchairs	Discourage activity by: Failure to ambulate with assistance where possible Injudicious use of bedrest Set expectations too high Do not praise enough

activity tolerance. In general, structural abnormalities such as amputation, contracture, and paralysis will result in less efficient activity performance. Some individuals, owing to marginal cardiopulmonary reserve, will become unable to perform the activity in the customary manner. Unless the activity demands are modified or the individual strengthened, the person is likely to stop performing the activity and will be predisposed to further activity intolerance because of a spiraling process of further reduced activity leading to further impairments in strength, range of motion, and endurance.

Indeed, Fried and colleagues (1991) have observed that one pathway to disability in frail older people may be gradual decrease in overall activity level.

Renal, Hepatic, and Hematopoietic Disorders

Renal or hepatic failure results in inefficient removal of wastes from the body, often producing generalized fatigue. These disorders are also commonly associated with fluid accumulation that impedes activity because of the extra weight to be supported, the interference with tissue oxygenation, and, in extreme cases, awkward movement from the edema. Anemia, regardless of the cause, also produces fatigue that may produce activity intolerance.

Nutritional Factors

Both under- and overnutrition have been implicated in the development of activity intolerance. Malnutrition, if sufficiently severe, is associated with anemia, reduced muscle mass, and decreased endurance. Moreover, some studies have associated decreased muscle function with depressed levels of magnesium and vitamin D (Fiatarone et al., 1990; Rosenberg and Miller, 1992). Vitamin deficiency diseases such as pernicious anemia may result in sensory impairment that predisposes individuals to reduced activity levels. Obesity makes engaging in normal functional activities more difficult, because of decreased flexibility and increased energy required to mobilize the individual's excess weight (Astrand, 1992).

Psychological Influences

Engaging in most activities requires an initial act of choice. Overcoming the inertia of rest requires volition, and thus motivation becomes a factor in tolerance of activity. Older people notoriously perform poorly on psychological tests that have little meaning for them. Their responses to requests to perform physical activities that have little meaning are apt to be similarly poor. For example, an exercise regimen, no matter how beneficial or carefully planned, may be poorly tolerated if the older patient does not understand the purpose of the program or believes it to be futile or demeaning.

Assessment

Tolerance of activity should be assessed through direct observation. Key parameters for the assessment of activity tolerance are summarized in Table 14–2. To assess activity tolerance, first determine the patient's customary level of activity and select the activities you will use for assessment accordingly. For example, if the patient has been bedridden for a period of time (more than a few days), begin with assessing tolerance to rolling over in bed or coming to a sitting position. If the individual is chair-bound, begin your assessment with the ability to transfer from one sitting position to another, or activities that require only mild cardiac work (Table 14–3). If the individual is ambulatory, begin with walking as a test activity. Finally, for people known to be living independently, assess first their ability to tolerate walking and then progress to more strenuous activities, such as stairclimbing (see Table 14–3 for other examples of more strenuous activities). Once the test activity is selected, follow this protocol:

1. Obtain resting measures of responses to activity:

- Patient report of symptoms, such as weakness, dyspnea, pain, dizziness, palpitations
- Measurement of pulse (rate and rhythm), blood pressure (lying and standing), respirations
- Observation of skin color, temperature, moistness, postural control, and emotional response to initiation of activity

2. During the activity, observe for changes from baseline. Also note:

- Rate of activity, including use of rest periods
- Degree of coordination, control, and flexibility in performance
- Change in vital signs (blood pressure, respiration, pulse rate or rhythm)
- Change in skin color, temperature, moistness
- Complaints of pain, dyspnea, weakness, dizziness, palpitations
- Emotional response to activity

3. Following the activity, observe:

- Amount of time required for vital signs to return to normal
- Persistence of symptoms or other adverse reactions to activity
- Emotional response to activity completion

The information gleaned from the assess-

TABLE 14-2
Assessing Activity Tolerance

INDEX	EXPECTED OUTCOME	UNEXPECTED OUTCOMES AND ACTIONS
Heart rate (apical or radial pulse)	For patients on bedrest or postcardiac precautions, a 20 beat/minute increase during or immediately after activity. Within 5 minutes postactivity, heart rate should return to baseline	If preactivity tachycardia is present, notify the physician to prescribe a specific expected outcome, e.g., a maximum heart rate permitted or whether exercise is advisable. If the heart rate decreases or exceeds the expected outcome, terminate the activity. If the postactivity recovery extends beyond 5 minutes, the activity was too strenuous or prolonged
Heart rhythm (radial pulse)	Rhythm remains regular	If the rhythm becomes irregular, terminate the activity
Pulse strength	Strength remains similar or increases	If pulse becomes weak, stop the activity
Blood pressure	Slight rise in systolic pressure with strenuous activity; no change with less strenuous activity. Slight increase or no change in diastolic pressure	If systolic pressure *drops* more than 20 mm Hg, cardiac output or vascular dilation is decreased, and termination of the activity is indicated
Respiratory rate, depth, rhythm	Increase in rate and depth; rhythm remains steady	If irregular rhythm, dyspnea, or a decrease in rate occurs, terminate the activity
Skin color	No change or slight flush in cheeks, lips, and nail beds. Light-skinned persons may show marked flushing	If extreme redness, cyanosis, or pallor appears, terminate the activity
Skin temperature and moistness	Increased warmth and perspiration	If the skin becomes cool, this indicates vascular constriction and impending shock; terminate the activity
Posture and equilibrium	No change	If the patient manifests muscle fatigue, by leaning against objects for support, drooping the head and shoulders, or complaining of dizziness or fatigue, this indicates lack of tolerance
Activity rate	Maintenance of performance rate throughout activity. No physical discomfort	If there is progressive slowing, taking frequent rest periods, or reduced dexterity, this indicates lack of tolerance. If tightness, heaviness, or pain occurs in the chest or legs, immediately terminate the activity
Emotional state	No change or positive response	If the patient manifests a worried expression, grimacing, muscle tension or tremors, irritability, or sighing, this indicates anxiety, fear, or boredom

Adapted from Gordon, M. Assessing activity tolerance. *Am J Nurs* 76:72–75, 1976.

ment should provide sufficient data to make a diagnosis of activity intolerance and should point to the relevant contributing factors. Patients who exhibit dyspnea, dizziness, pain, arrhythmia, cyanosis, pallor, diaphoresis, tachypnea, or tachycardia during the exercise, who have a rise in blood pressure of greater than 15 mm Hg diastolic or a drop of greater than 20 mm Hg diastolic, or who require more than 3 minutes following the activity for vital signs to return to normal have activity intolerance (Carpenito, 1993a). Individuals who continually talk about inability to perform the activity or display signs of anxiety during the activity also have activity intolerance (Simko, 1993).

Planning and Intervention

Goals for the individual with activity intolerance depend upon the developmental level of the patient and the specific factors contributing to the activity intolerance. The program for someone with terminal illness will have more limited goals than for individuals with longer life expectancies. Individuals whose activity intolerance is due chiefly to deconditioning have a much better prognosis than those with irreversible pathological conditions, such as chronic pulmonary disease or vascular disease. The specific maneuvers used to increase activity tolerance apply to all etiologies. Three major categories of intervention available are (1) optimizing disease management, (2) exercise programming, and (3) use of energy conservation techniques.

Age Considerations

Advanced age alone is not a contraindication to increasing activity. In fact, increasing activity may have positive effects on the functional ability of older adults. Benefits from exercise have been demonstrated in even the frailest individuals, including those over 90 years of age, living in nursing homes (Fiatarone et al., 1990; Fiatarone et

T A B L E   1 4 - 3
Examples of Activities Requiring Mild, Moderate, and Severe Energy Expenditures

	Position	Cardiac Work (CUBS) or Metabolism (METS)	Cardiac Output (COS)
MILD CARDIAC ACTIVITY			
Eating	Sitting	1.50	—
Sewing	Sitting	1.60	—
Clerical work	Sitting	1.60	—
Setting type	Standing	1.60	1.35
Getting out of and into bed	Bed to chair	1.65	1.45
Leather carving	Sitting on chair	1.70	—
Weaving, table loom	Sitting on stool	1.70	—
Clerical work	Standing	1.80	—
Writing	Sitting	2.00	—
Typing	Sitting on chair	2.00	1.35
Bimanual activity test sanding, 50 strokes/min	Sitting on chair	2.00	1.40
Weaving, floor loom	Sitting on bench	2.10	1.75
Metal work, hammer	Standing	2.15	1.65
Printing, platen press	Standing	2.30	1.75
Bench assembly, moderate	Sitting	2.35	1.70
Hanging clothes on line	Standing–stooping	2.40	1.80
MODERATE CARDIAC ACTIVITY			
Playing piano		2.50	—
Dressing, undressing		2.50–3.50	—
Sawing, jeweler's saw	Sitting	1.90	2.05
Sawing, hack saw	Standing	2.55	2.00
Driving car		2.80	—
Bicycling, slowly		2.90	2.45
Preparing meals		3.00	—
Weight lifting, 10 lb lifted 15″, 46/min	Sitting	2.80	2.00
Walking, 2.0 mph		3.20	—
Handsawing, wood	Standing	3.50	2.35
Warm shower		3.50	—
SEVERE CARDIAC ACTIVITY			
Bowel movement	Toilet	3.60	
Bowel movement	Bedpan	4.70	
Making beds	Standing	3.90	
Hot shower	Standing	4.20	
Walking fast (3.5 mph)		5.00	
Descending stairs		5.20	
Scrubbing floor	Kneeling	5.30	3.00
Master two-step climbing test		5.70	3.00
Weight-lifting, 10–20 lb lifted 36″, 15/min		6.50	3.50
Bicycling, fast		6.90	3.30
Running		7.40	4.00
Mowing lawn		7.70	
Climbing stairs		9.00	

CUBS—cardiac work units, ratio to basal; COS—cardiac output, ratio to basal; METS—metabolism, ratio to basal.
From Kottke, F.J. Therapeutic exercise to maintain mobility. In Kottke, F.J., Stillwell, G.K. and Lehmann, J.F. *Krusen's Handbook of Physical Medicine and Rehabilitation.* 3rd ed. Philadelphia: W.B. Saunders, 1982, pp. 794–795.

al., 1994). The older person should be included in the goal planning and choice of activity to ensure maximal compliance with the exercise prescription. Activities consistent with the older person's lifestyle have a greater likelihood of being carried out than those that are completely new. For example, it is wiser to advise a solitary exercise program for individuals who consider themselves "loners" than to counsel them to join an exercise group at the local health club. The pace of the activity program should be adjusted to the individual's baseline capabilities.

Optimizing Disease Management

Helping individuals modify lifestyle factors that worsen chronic disease is one strategy for enhancing the activity tolerance of the older person with cardiac, respiratory, or vascular disease. For example, if the older person smokes, reduction or cessation of smoking will have beneficial effects on activity tolerance. Reducing or eliminating caffeine consumption may reduce the frequency of intermittent claudication; weight reduction in obese people will increase tolerance for activity.

Manipulation of medications is another strategy for optimizing disease management. There is a tremendous armamentarium of medications to control pathophysiological processes in cardiorespiratory disease and, to a lesser extent, in vascular disease. Nurses should be alert for signs of drug toxicity and adverse side effects that may impair activity tolerance, such as orthostatic hypotension, electrolyte imbalance, dehydration, digitalis, theophylline, or phenytoin toxicity, and intolerance to beta-blockers, to name some common culprits. An individual's chronic disease may be inadequately controlled on a given drug regimen. In patients with chronic obstructive lung disease, teaching proper use of bronchodilators administered with metered-dose inhalants may greatly improve activity tolerance (see Chapter 18). Finally, the older person with claudication may be a candidate for a revascularization procedure, if vascular disease sufficiently interferes with activity. Nurses should be prepared to offer referral or counseling to older people regarding the risks and benefits of such procedures (see Chapter 7).

Exercise Programs

Exercise programs to reduce activity intolerance are based on the principles of aerobic training, in which large muscle groups are used for prolonged periods of time. Cardiac rehabilitation programs have applied these principles to individuals with marginal functional reserve to increase their activity tolerance (Pollock and Wilmore, 1990; Fletcher et al., 1992.) The mode, duration, frequency, and intensity of exercise must be tailored to each individual, based on baseline function, physiological response to exercise, motivation, and preference. Sophisticated exercise testing programs that include electrocardiographic monitoring allow better individualization of the intensity and duration aspects of the exercise prescription.

Careful testing and individualized exercise prescription are important both to enhance safety of exercise in chronically ill individuals and to maximize the likelihood of efficacy. Although the benefits of carefully monitored, multidisciplinary exercise programs for frail older people are increasingly acknowledged, gaining access to such programs remains a problem, owing to cost, attitudinal barriers, and programs that may

not accommodate individuals with functional limitations other than cardiac disease. Notable exceptions are aerobic training programs for those who have physical disabilities (Fletcher and Vassallo, 1992) and arthritis (Fisher and Pendergast, 1992). Until testing programs are available to those with multiple chronic impairments, nurses should be prepared to coordinate exercise regimens in consultation with physicians, rehabilitation specialists, and exercise physiologists. Many excellent guides to exercise programming now exist, including Lewis, 1989; Lewis and Campanelli, 1990; Pollock and Wilmore, 1990; and American College of Sports Medicine's Guidelines for Exercise Programming (1990). Although gradual resumption of independence in basic activities of daily living, such as walking, dressing, and bathing, may reduce activity intolerance in those with severe deconditioning, those with intermediate levels of deconditioning in the community may need a more robust program to enjoy the health protection benefits of exercise.

In the absence of sophisticated exercise testing equipment, a simple guideline for progression of exercise is to determine the activity intensity and duration that produce mild symptoms of intolerance and encourage the individual to exercise at 75 per cent of that level (see Chapter 7 for a more extensive discussion of cardiac rehabilitation principles). Sedentary individuals initially may be able to tolerate only short periods of exercise—for example, 5-minute intervals. Irwin (1986) recommends alternating several brief periods of exercise with rest periods of equal duration, for a total program duration of 20 to 30 minutes. The duration of the exercise phases relative to the rest periods can gradually be increased according to the patient's symptoms, so that eventually a duration and intensity that will allow aerobic training to take place are achieved. Patients who cannot tolerate a long exercise period should exercise more frequently than those who can sustain a full 20 to 30 minutes of high-intensity exercise.

Older people who have experienced prolonged bedrest are likely to need a structured mobilization routine before any systematic program of upright exercises is initiated, because of the likelihood of orthostatic hypotension. Encouraging independence in bed mobility and engaging in other muscular activities while in bed provides some protection against activity intolerance promoted by bedrest (Convertino, 1986). Regimens such as use of tilt tables, use of reverse Trendelenburg's position, and use of the dangling position before allowing the patient to stand are also examples of such pre-exercise programs. Failure to prevent orthostatic hypotension may precipitate cerebrovascular insufficiency, resulting in a variety of adverse outcomes, including greater risk of injury from syncope, increased patient discomfort from dizziness, and, perhaps, reducing the individual's motivation to move because of the associated discomfort.

Memmer (1988) suggests a variety of strategies for reduction of orthostatic hypotension. First, select an optimal time for sitting up for the first time, avoiding the following times: (1) immediately after awakening, because baroceptors may be the most sluggish, (2) immediately after a meal, because of shunting of blood to the gastrointestinal tract, and (3) immediately after administration of drugs that cause vasodilation. She also recommends instructing the patient to arise slowly, and avoids the Valsalva maneuver by instructing the patient to exhale slowly when changing position.

Individuals who have not been on bedrest, but who are quite sedentary may benefit from increased participation in basic ADLs. Suitable activities include walking (or propelling a wheelchair for those who cannot walk), dressing, bathing, and grooming. This approach has the advantage of using familiar activities of mild-to-moderate intensity that are normally repeated several times each day. No special equipment is required. This approach may contribute more directly to the patient's autonomy than a conventional exercise program. Using ADLs as an exercise approach is also advantageous because it takes into account the training specificity effect. Individuals will develop increased endurance primarily for those activities that constitute the exercise stimulus. Therefore, the more people use customary activities as exercises, the more likely they are to experience increased ease and endurance in performing those tasks (Astrand, 1992).

All patients are likely to benefit from a regular exercise habit; however, patients at high risk for developing activity intolerance should receive specific exercise prescriptions. Individuals at high risk are those with chronic cardiac or respiratory disease and those with mobility impairment, including people who are restrained.

Energy Conservation Techniques

Patients who have significant activity intolerance but who still are partially or completely independent in self-care may profit from being taught principles of work simplification or energy conservation. Refer the older person to an occupational therapist when possible, because individualizing these principles takes time and practice. Leslie (1990) has identified some general principles of work simplification:

1. Whenever the condition allows, use both hands in opposite and symmetric motions while working.
2. Lay out work areas within normal reach. Arrange supplies in a semicircle.
3. Slide—do not lift and carry. Use a table with wheels when moving from one work area to another.
4. Use fixed work stations. Have a special place to do each job so that supplies and equipment may be kept ready for immediate use.
5. Use the smallest number of work elements. Select equipment that may be used for more than one job; eliminate unnecessary motions.
6. Avoid the work of holding. Use utensils that rest firmly and are secured by suction cups or clamps. This will free hands for work.
7. Let gravity work. Examples are a laundry chute, refuse chute, and gravity-feed flourbin.
8. Position tools in advance. Store them so that they are placed in position for immediate grasping and use. For example, hang measuring cup and spoons separately within sight.
9. Position machine controls and switches within easy reach. Household appliances should be chosen on the basis of ease of operation.
10. Sit to work whenever possible. Use a comfortable chair and adjust workplace height to the chair, or use an adjustable stool or chair.
11. Use a correct workplace height. The height should be right for the homemaker and the job. There are no standard heights.
12. Good conditions are important—good light and ventilation, comfortable clothing, and ambient temperature.

Evaluation

Criteria for evaluation of nursing care for those with activity intolerance include the following:

1. The patient engages in desired activities and roles.

2. The patient does not experience tachycardia, tachypnea, or anxiety during or after performing desired or necessary customary activities.

3. In the absence of severe paralysis or contractures, unhealed fractures, advanced Parkinson's disease, or muscular dystrophy, the individual can walk 100 feet without distress.

4. In the absence of severe neuromuscular or mental impairments, the patient is able to perform self-care activities.

HYPERTHERMIA AND HYPOTHERMIA

Definition and Scope of Problems

NANDA recognizes the diagnosis "High risk for altered body temperature" as a state in which an individual is at risk of failing to maintain body temperature within the normal range. Clustered within this diagnostic category are *hypothermia,* or "a state in which an individual's body temperature is reduced below normal range" (NANDA, 1992, p. 13) and *hyperthermia,* in which the individual's temperature is elevated above his or her normal range. Both hypo- and hyperthermia are potentially life-threatening disorders. Hypothermia, if sufficiently severe, can cause death through hypoventilation and cardiac dysrhythmia. In addition to the immediate life-threatening consequences of hypothermia, a variety of postsurgical complications may result from postoperative hypothermia, related to increased metabolic demand induced by shivering (Holtzclaw, 1990), and compromised blood flow to the extremities that may result from vasoconstriction to reduce further heat loss. Finally, hypothermia may affect drug clearance and potentiate the effects of muscle relaxants (Burkle, 1988). Hyperthermia can cause death by inducing severe metabolic disturbances and cardiovascular collapse.

Although accurate estimates of the prevalance of altered body temperature are difficult to obtain for reasons discussed later, there can be little doubt that altered thermoregulation is a serious problem for elderly people. According to data compiled by the National Center for Health Statistics, during the period 1979 to 1985, 3326 deaths among those aged 60 years and over could be attributed to excessive cold, and an additional 2077 deaths to excess heat (Macey and Schneider, 1993). Deaths attributed to excessive cold appear to be on the increase: 11.8 per cent of the deaths related to excessive

cold were reported in 1979, compared with 18.8 per cent in 1985. In contrast, the proportion of heat-related deaths seems to be on the decline (57.1 per cent of the deaths during this period were recorded in 1980, compared with 5.5 per cent in 1985).

There is controversy about diagnosis of these conditions in elderly people because of lack of normative data on "normal" temperatures in this population. Hirschmann (1992) points out that normal temperature in an individual is a range of values that depends upon several variables, including time of day, site of measurement, and the person's age. Mean oral temperature is lower in older people, but rectal temperature values are similar to those of younger adults (Weizman et al., 1982). Mean oral temperature is lower, and diurnal variation less, in institutionalized people over age 64 years (Davis and Lentz, 1989).

Darowski and coworkers (1991) attempted to establish norms for temperatures taken with different methods by carefully measuring temperature in hospitalized older patients who were believed to be free of febrile illness. A wide variety of temperature values were obtained in afebrile subjects, and the variability within subjects of temperatures taken at different sites was considerable. Thus, ranges of normal temperature are proposed as follows: rectal temperature: 36.7°C to 37.5°C; auditory canal temperature: 36.4°C to 37.2°C; sublingual temperature: 36.2°C to 37.0°C; and axillary temperature 35.5°C to 37.0°C.

Altered body temperature is a relatively recent addition to the NANDA classification, and thus systematic nursing research into these phenomena, specifically on techniques that are most effective in prevention, is scarce. However, knowledge of the factors underlying altered thermoregulation and aging-related changes that predispose older people to problems of hypo- and hyperthermia should enhance nurses' abilities to recognize those at risk and take appropriate prevention and therapeutic measures to minimize the effects of these potentially devastating disorders.

Contributing Factors

Age-related factors that predispose to altered thermoregulation are best understood by discussing them in the context of how thermoregulation is achieved. Body temperature regulation results from a balance between heat production and heat maintenance or insulation, compared with heat dissipation. Body temperature regulation is accomplished through a combination of behavioral and physiological mechanisms, with behavioral mechanisms usually employed when environmental extremes of temperature are encountered and physiological mechanisms used to perform the "fine-tuning" of thermoregulation (Wakefield et al., 1989). The anterior hypothalamus and higher cortical centers are involved in control of this balance. Autonomic and skeletal muscle responses to thermal stimulation with aging are regulated in the hypothalamus, and voluntary actions to regulate body temperature, such as adjusting clothing, temperature, or location, are cortically determined. Factors that affect higher cortical function, such as the central nervous system (CNS) depressant or judgment-altering side effects of drug or alcohol use, and the presence of dementing illness, will predispose older adults to impaired thermoregulation because they are less able to use active measures to conserve heat (predisposing to hypothermia) or cool the body (predisposing to hyperthermia).

Heat production depends upon basal metabolic rate, muscular activity, the body's response to thyroxine in increasing metabolism, and the effects of catecholamines. Both heat production and insulation may be adversely affected in the aged. Basal metabolic rate is decreased with aging. Older people may be less able to mount a shivering response to cold environments compared with younger adults, but once they begin shivering, they are able to generate heat. Thyroxine is not thought to be a factor in impaired thermoregulation in elderly people, and the effects of age on metabolic response to cold are not well described (Wongsurawat et al., 1990). Metabolic diseases, including hypothyroidism, hypoglycemia, hypoadrenalism, hypopituitarism, and starvation have all been associated with hypothermia.

Insulation is accomplished passively through the protective layer formed by the skin and subcutaneous fat layer and actively through autonomic regulation of blood flow to the skin. Significant age-related changes that contribute to reduced effectiveness of insulation include thinning of the skin, loss of subcutaneous fat, and abnormal peripheral blood flow responses to thermal stimuli, thought secondary to autonomic decline. (Fox et al., 1973; Wagner et al., 1974; Wongsurawat et al., 1990). It is noteworthy that progressive deterioration of blood flow responses to thermal stimulation with aging has been demonstrated in a longitudinal study (Collins et al., 1977).

Heat loss occurs through radiation, conduction, convection, and evaporation. Each of these mechanisms should be considered when assessing for contributors to altered body temperature regulation. All types of heat loss are affected by aging-related changes, which helps account for the increased prevalence of thermoregulatory problems in the aged. Depending upon the type of alteration in body temperature, a different mechanism may be key. Radiation heat loss is likely to be greater in older people with impaired circulatory response to heat and cold and in individuals with baldness or alopecia, predisposing them to hypothermia. In contrast, evaporative heat loss is lessened in older people, as they have both a delayed sweating response and a lower rate of sweating compared with younger adults (Hellon et al., 1956; Wongsurawat et al., 1990). Unfortunately, rather than protecting against hypothermia, this age-related change predisposes older people to another class of thermoregulatory problems: hyperthermia associated with hot weather. Conduction heat losses are also a problem. Dry clothing decreases conductive heat losses, but when clothing is wet, it causes an increased rate of heat transmission. Thus, clothing, which affects radiation and conductive heat loss, can be implicated in both hypo- and hyperthermia. Convection heat losses are most often a problem in older persons exposed to wind and cold in the outdoors but can also be implicated in hypothermia associated with surgery, as the increased laminar flow of air in the operating room used to reduce microbial contamination of wounds may increase heat loss through convection.

Hypothermia: Nosology and Defining Characteristics

Summers (1992) distinguishes three types of hypothermia based on etiology and defining characteristics: accidental, inadvertent, and intentional. Accidental hypothermia is defined as core temperature less than or equal to 35°C, resulting from exposure to cold environments without adequate clothing. Studies in the United Kingdom suggest that up to 10 per cent of community-dwelling older adults have body temperatures close to hypothermic levels. In the United States, the incidence has been estimated at 60,000 cases per year.

Inadvertent and intentional hypothermia are associated with care of hospitalized patients. Inadvertent hypothermia is most commonly seen in surgical patients, resulting from exposure to cool environments like the operating room (OR), in combination with reduced ability to thermoregulate, as in the case of patients receiving anesthetic agents that can both depress hypothalamically mediated temperature regulation and create vasodilatation, promoting increased radiation heat losses. According to Summers (1992), operating room ambient temperature is maintained at cool levels (15.5°C to 17.7°C, or 60°F to 64°F) to retard microbial growth, decrease static electricity, and promote comfort of the operating team. Other factors that may promote heat loss in surgical patients include use of cool intravenous fluids and the presence of open wounds that cause additional radiation losses.

The prevalence of inadvertent hypothermia has been estimated at 12 to 16 million surgical patients per year, and it occurs disproportionately in elderly people (Augustine, 1990). In contrast, intentional hypothermia is purposeful cooling of patients for surgical procedures to induce cardiac dysrhythmia and decrease tissue ischemia. Core body temperatures may be lowered from 26°C to 32°C (80°–90°F). Intentional hypothermia is most commonly used in cardiac surgery (Summers, 1992).

Assessment

Detection of hypothermia requires both a high index of suspicion for the disorder and the availability of accurate thermometers. The key instrument for detecting hypothermia is a low-reading rectal thermometer, as most clinical thermometers record temperatures only as low as 34.5°C (94°F), and the diagnosis can be missed. For this reason, measurement of temperature with a low-reading thermometer has been recommended for all critically ill patients (Wongsurawat et al., 1990).

Robbins (1989) points out that mild-to-moderate hypothermia is often misdiagnosed; with the exception of an abnormally low temperature, the clinical presentation of the disorder is nonspecific, with symptoms such as fatigue, weakness, apathy, gait disturbance, or confusion as common presenting problems. Although other clinical defining characteristics of hypothermia have been delineated, findings of core temperatures below 36°C (95°F) are indicative of hypothermia. Other defining characteristics endorsed by postanesthesia care nurses who commonly see individuals with hypothermia include shivering, cool skin, tachycardia, altered nailbed color, hypotension, and piloerection. Critical defining characteristics include shivering and cool skin. These latter

defining characteristics may help nurses in hospital settings identify those who are developing hypothermia so they can take corrective action before hypothermia develops.

Holtzclaw (1990) recommends identifying those at risk for shivering as part of the nursing assessment for those with altered body temperature, because the shivering experience is distressing to the patient and, if prevented, will eliminate their exposure to the rapid increase in energy requirements associated with shivering. In addition to the risk factors for hypothermia noted earlier, anemia and infection also predispose to shivering. Assessment for prodromal signs of shivering include being alert for subjective complaints of muscle tenseness and palpation for a hum along the lower jaw, near the mandibular angle. The hum results from masseter contractions, which are sometimes detected as electrocardiogram artifact in monitored patients (Holtzclaw, 1992).

Individuals who have accidental hypothermia are most often community-dwelling individuals who are seen in home care, ambulatory care, or emergency department settings. Because use of a low-reading thermometer is not standard procedure in most settings of care, it is particularly important that providers in settings that may see victims of accidental hypothermia be aware that hypothermia is often confused with other common clinical problems in elderly people. Individuals with a high-risk profile for hypothermia include those with cardiovascular and metabolic disorders, and those with pre-existing cognitive impairment; these disorders, singly or in combination, can interfere with heat conservation mechanisms. In addition, those who come from socioeconomically impoverished backgrounds, i.e., those who live alone, who are poor, and who have substandard housing, are particularly at risk.

Identifying those at high risk for unintentional (hospital-associated) hypothermia is less difficult, because the categories of risk factors are fewer and more easily assessed and controlled than is true for accidental hypothermia. Examples of those who are at highest risk include those with impaired peripheral circulation, as in diabetes mellitus, autonomic insufficiency, Parkinson's disease, and peripheral vascular disease. Other patient factors representing greater risk include malnutrition, which results in both decreased adiposity, which predisposes to radiation heat losses, and reduced muscle mass, which diminishes the ability to mount a shivering response to hypothermia. In addition, the type of anesthesia used influences development of hypothermia. Halothane-type anesthetic agents increase surface blood flow and depress hypothalamic function (Burkle, 1988). Thus, older individuals receiving these types of anesthetics are at particularly high risk for hypothermia. Patients receiving regional anesthesia are also at risk because they will lose body heat in regions distal to the level of the block, since vasoconstriction and muscle movement are blocked (Burkle, 1988). Other factors that create a greater risk include the size of the skin area to be prepared for surgery, the size of the wound and use of intraoperative irrigating solutions, and the length of the surgery itself.

Monitoring the individual's temperature during and after surgery should be routine. In addition, monitoring for other signs that may precede the development of hypothermia, such as shivering and mottling, is also indicated. In addition to monitoring temperature, it is important to monitor the patient's responses to warming efforts, because many interventions, such as the use of warming blankets, carry a risk of thermal injury to the skin. Those with delirium and neuropathy are less likely to sense pain from thermal injury.

Planning

The type of hypothermia under consideration has implications for prevention and treatment efforts. Obviously, intentional hypothermia is not to be prevented, but nurses are wise to plan carefully for rewarming older patients placed under intentional hypothermia, because of their reduced homeostatic reserve.

Community health nurses and those who work in home care and ambulatory care settings should be able to identify individuals at risk for accidental hypothermia, and initiate interventions to reduce their risk through counselling or referral. Such interventions are particularly important in areas of the country where the cold weather season is protracted; however, systematic identification and intervention with those at risk in warmer climates is also important. For example, some low-income individuals in Southern states may not have central heat because it is not necessary to use it frequently, yet when a period of cold weather is experienced, they are at greater risk of hypothermia. Nurses involved in health promotion activities should launch awareness campaigns through the use of patient education brochures and posters and one-to-one counseling before the start of cold weather. Information about the risk factors and the

possibilities of preventing hypothermia should be communicated, such as availability of weatherization programs (see Chapter 16), assistance with fuel costs, and the importance of dressing properly (layering clothes) in cooler weather. Programs in which frail individuals have someone to check in with them on a daily basis by telephone or by friendly visit may also help avert episodes of hypothermia. A high-risk profile includes those who live alone; who have low income and/or substandard housing and poor nutritional status; have metabolic or cardiovascular disease or dementia; who take medicines with CNS effects; or who use alcohol. Such patients should be targeted to receive counselling individually as well as through group approaches.

Planning for those at risk for unintentional hypothermia involves identifying those at risk before surgery, so that appropriate preventive measures can be taken, such as raising the temperature of the operating room, warming fluids to be used on the outside or inside of the body, and keeping the patient covered except when exposure is unavoidable, as for preparation of the operative site. Communication between the operating room team and the postanesthesia care team regarding the older person's temperature response to the surgery is also important, as techniques to conserve heat or prevent heat loss can be applied in the recovery room as well. Unintentional hypothermia thus can be prevented in elderly surgical patients if perioperative nurses identify older individuals at particularly high risk for increased heat loss through conduction and radiation mechanisms.

Strategies for prevention of intraoperative hypothermia are all targeted toward reducing the amount of heat lost. Ambient temperature can be increased for individuals who are particularly at risk. Use of warming mattresses on the OR table, keeping the patient covered until the last minute before preparation of the operative site, and use of caps to reduce passive loss from the head are all recommendations that can be implemented readily. In addition, consideration of warming fluids or gases that are used during preparation or conduct of the surgery is indicated. Types of fluids that can be warmed include those used for incisional preparation, irrigation of wounds or organs, and intravenous fluids. In addition, anesthetic agents can be humidified and warmed. Liberal use of warm blankets on body parts not required to be exposed during surgery will prevent heat loss. Reflective blankets and heating lamps are also strategies that have been used effectively to keep the elderly surgical patient warm (Burkle, 1988). Finally, vigilant observation for sources of heat loss, such as wet sheets, should be the rule, and offending agents removed promptly. These techniques can also be applied in the post-anesthesia recovery area.

Intervention

Prevention of hypothermia is infinitely preferable to treatment. Treatment of hypothermia involves gradual rewarming of the individual. Robbins (1989) organizes treatment recommendations according to the severity of the hypothermia. For those with mild hypothermia, defined as those with rectal temperatures of 32.2°C to 35°C (90°C to 95°F), passive rewarming can be used by moving to a room where the ambient temperature is over 21.1°C (70°F), and by insulating against further heat loss through the use of warm clothing or blankets. For those with moderate-to-serve hypothermia (rectal temperature below 32.2°C [90°F]), active rewarming is indicated, but it must be undertaken under carefully controlled circumstances, including continuous monitoring of rectal temperature. Techniques used in core rewarming include inhalation of warm humidified air, use of warmed intravenous solutions, or infusion of warmed fluids into the gastrointestinal tract or through peritoneal dialysis. Augustine (1990) reports on the use of a specialized bed that uses both radiant heat and convection to rewarm actively and recommends its use in postsurgical patients with mild hypothermia, as it is more effective than passive rewarming techniques at normalizing body temperatures. Active rewarming should be conducted in an intensive care unit environment, as patients with such severe hypothermia require careful monitoring for cardiac dysrhythmias and access to definitive treatment of acidosis, shock, pneumonia, and other complications of hypothermia. In addition, once the body is rewarmed, some of the complications such as hypotension and dysrhythmia may spontaneously reverse, so gradual treatment and careful monitoring are essential.

If appropriate preventive measures are taken during surgery, and appropriate monitoring is undertaken perioperatively, core rewarming techniques should not be necessary for the treatment of unintentional hypothermia.

Evaluation

Outcome criteria for evaluation of the patient at risk for hypothermia include (1) maintaining the body temperature within normal limits, (2) gradually regaining body temperature within normal limits without damage to skin, (3) absence of development of complications from hypothermia, such as ischemia, cardiac dysrhythmia, or central nervous system disturbances, and (4) in community settings, at risk patients or their caregivers can identify ways to conserve heat and prevent accidental hypothermia.

Process criteria include (1) assessment of at-risk patients with low-reading thermometers, (2) use of techniques to prevent heat loss in surgical patients identified as at risk of development of hypothermia, and (3) use of systematic educational and referral programs in community care settings prior to the onset of cold weather to prevent accidental hypothermia.

Hyperthermia: Nosology and Defining Characteristics

Hyperthermia can be subdivided into three subtypes: fever, heat injury, and malignant hyperthermia associated with neuroleptic use. Fever is defined as body temperature elevation above 38.3°C (101°F) and is generally considered a sign of a generalized acute response to microbial invasion, tissue injury, or inflammation. In fever, the hypothalmic thermal set point is increased in response to a set of events, including phagocytosis, release of interleukin-1, and stimulation of arachidonic acids, resulting in increased prostaglandin production, which acts to reset the hypothalamic thermal set point. The autonomic and somatic nervous systems are then activated to conserve heat and increase heat production to increase the body temperature. In contrast, hyperthermia is reserved for instances when thermal control mechanisms fail to the point that heat production exceeds heat dissipation.

Hyperthermia is less well defined than hypothermia. Salvage (1991) describes heat-related illness in the elderly as covering a broad spectrum of ailments, including transient heat fatigue, syncope, heat cramps, heat edema, and heat stroke. Body temperatures in excess of 40.5°C (105°F) are life-threatening and can be caused by exposure to extremely high environmental temperatures, such as during "heat waves," or they can be associated with neuroleptic drug use. Each type will be discussed in turn.

Hyperthermia associated with high environmental temperature is more often seen in climates where temperatures exceed 32.2°C (90°F). Epidemiological data show that death rates in elderly people, both community-dwelling and institutionalized, increase because of cardiovascular and cerebrovascular disease during times of extreme heat. According to Wongsurawat and colleagues (1990), changes in the skin and cardiovascular system with aging predispose to heat injury. Inability to mount a sweating response rapidly and effectively and to increase cardiac output and achieve vasodilatation to increase radiant heat loss is thought to be responsible for the increased vulnerability of elderly people to heat injury.

Neuroleptic malignant syndrome is another cause of severe hyperthermia in the aged. It occurs in people who take antipsychotic drugs of the following classes: phenothiazines (such as chlorpromazine), butyrophenones (such as haloperidol), and thioxanthenes (such as thioridazine). Temperatures in people with this disorder may exceed 41°C (105.8°F); accompanying symptoms include muscular rigidity, autonomic instability, and delirium. Severe metabolic disturbance, including rhabdomyolysis and renal failure, can ensue. Although the factors that cause this syndrome, other than neuroleptic use, are not well delineated, dehydration has been implicated in its development. The treatment of choice is bromocriptine. Mortality rate from this disorder has been reported as high as 25 per cent.

Assessment

As is true with hypothermia, symptoms of hyperthermia are nonspecific and can include malaise, dizziness, anorexia, nausea, vomiting, and dyspnea. Thus, accurate determination of body temperature is key in establishing this diagnosis. According to a review by Holtzclaw (1992), oral and axillary temperatures are acceptable for assessment in those with euthermia or low-grade fever. However, in those suspected of hyperthermia, auditory canal or pulmonary artery catheter temperatures are preferred, as oral, axillary, and rectal temperatures may lag behind core temperature readings by as much as 45 minutes. Auditory canal temperatures may be affected by probe placement, so care should be taken to assure that the probe is directly against the tympanic membrane.

Behavioral disturbance is more common as core temperature increases. Temperatures over 41°C (105°F) define heat stroke. Severe hyperthermia will result in cardiogenic shock, cardiac dysrhythmias, pulmonary congestion, bleeding dyscrasias, renal failure, and rhabdomyolysis.

Planning and Prevention

In community-dwelling adults at risk for environmentally induced hyperthermia, prevention is often effective and is certainly preferable to treatment. The same type of educational efforts described for hypothermia should be implemented for those who live in climates with prolonged periods of high temperatures, especially in areas where the humidity is high. Patients should be counselled to wear loose-fitting clothing, drink fluids frequently, and use such cooling techniques as staying in the shade, seeking air-conditioned settings like shopping malls, use of fans, and sponging off with cool water. They should also avoid strenuous activity during the hotter periods of the day. Older people also should be reminded of the importance of increasing their fluid intake during hot weather, as fluid requirements will increase owing to evaporation from sweating and the use of fans. Nurses working in long-term care institutions may need to educate other members of the health team about the risks of heat injury in nursing home patients, counselling modification in the activity schedule and the need to increase vigilance regarding offering fluids and monitoring for dehydration.

Prevention of neuroleptic malignant syndrome can be achieved by using neuroleptics only when there is a clear indication (i.e., psychotic target symptoms that interfere with patient function or safety of patient or caregiver), careful attention to prevention of dehydration in individuals who do use neuroleptic agents, and counselling of patient and caregivers to seek medical attention promptly if fever develops.

Intervention

In medically ill people with fever or hyperthermia, nursing actions to promote comfort and facilitate resolution of medical illness should be based on the following factors: (1) understanding of the basic physiological alteration, (2) a clear nursing therapeutic goal, and (3) understanding of the effects of specific interventions on thermal response (Holtzclaw, 1992). For example, fevers below 39°C (102.2°F) have a few detrimental effects and may enhance immunoregulatory function. In contrast, fevers above 40°C (104°F) do not have benefit and may herald the onset of hyperthermia (Holtzclaw, 1992). Thus, there is little if any rationale for lowering body temperature in those with low-grade fevers. Careful attention to other responses to the febrile state, such as changing linen and bedclothes after an episode of diaphoresis, will not only enhance comfort but reduce the risk of shivering and its associated risks.

In severe hyperthermia, antipyretics such as acetaminophen or aspirin are not effective. The mainstay of treatment, therefore, is use of environmental manipulations to promote heat loss, such as external cooling with fans, cooling blankets, sponge baths, and ice packs. Unfortunately, studies documenting the relative effectiveness of these treatments are lacking (Holtzclaw, 1992). If cooling blankets are used, careful attention should be paid to the rate of cooling, as too rapid cooling will result in a shivering response that may actually increase core body temperature. Holtzclaw recommends lowering temperatures on cooling blankets gradually, so that the temperature is reduced not more than 0.5°C every 30 minutes. Use protective terry-cloth wraps to the extremities and groin prior to placement on a cooling blanket, both to protect skin from thermal injury and to prevent shivering (Caruso et al., 1992). Wongsurawat and colleagues (1990) recommend using vigorous skin massage during external cooling to prevent reflex vasoconstriction. For further details on environmental manipulations to cool patients while minimizing the risk of shivering, see the review by Holtzclaw (1992). External cooling techniques should be used until the temperature reaches 38.8°C (102°F) and reinstituted if the temperature again becomes elevated.

The mortality rate from hyperthermia-associated complications is quite high. Treatment for hyperthermia should be carried out in an intensive care setting, where accurate monitoring of physiological complications of hyperthermia can be assessed and definitive treatment instituted. Particular attention should be paid to fluid and electrolyte balance, as dehydration with sodium excess may adversely influence the temperature set point (Holtzclaw, 1992).

Evaluation

Outcome criteria include maintenance of body temperature within normal limits, without complications associated with heat stress. Process criteria include older persons or caregivers able to express when protection from heat is needed, and what measures should be taken to prevent heat injury. Individuals taking neuroleptic drugs should also be knowledgeable about the possibility of neuroleptic malignant syndrome and should know to seek help emergently should a highly elevated temperature develop.

BOWEL ELIMINATION ALTERATIONS: COLONIC AND PERCEIVED CONSTIPATION, IMPACTION, AND INCONTINENCE

Definition and Scope of Problems

Constipation is "a state in which an individual experiences a change in normal bowel habits characterized by a decrease in frequency and/or passage of hard, dry stools" (NANDA, 1992). Defining the scope of the problem in the aged is made difficult by the fact that constipation is inconsistently defined in the health care literature (Harari et al., 1993). Moreover, it has been shown that elderly people and health care providers may differ markedly in their definitions, with older persons tending to define constipation as straining when defecating, whereas physicians used frequency of defecation as the key criterion (Whitehead et al., 1989). Despite these problems in definition, several statistics suggest that constipation is widespread. First, it has been reported that up to 30 per cent of community-dwelling older people use laxatives on a regular basis (Whitehead et al., 1989), and visits to physicians for the complaint of constipation increase after age 60 years (Sonnenberg and Koch, 1989). A survey of the prevalence of constipation in 838 elderly persons in diverse settings of care in Finland found similar rates of constipation in community-dwelling elders as in the American survey just cited. Also, complaints of constipation and use of laxatives increased dramatically with patient dependency. In geriatric hospital patients, 79 per cent complained of constipation, compared with 59 per cent of those in long-term care facilities, followed by 29 per cent of those in day hospitals. Similar trends were observed for laxative use (Kinnunen, 1991).

The consequences of constipation can be serious: fecal impaction, laxative dependency, and urinary and fecal incontinence. A *fecal impaction* is a hard mass of feces lodged in the colon or rectal vault. This severe form of constipation may result in two major problems: (1) soiling, which may be incorrectly diagnosed as diarrhea, and (2) stercoral ulceration, a pressure necrosis of the large intestine (Fay and Lance, 1992).

Chronic use of stimulant or saline cathartics may result in an atonic colon, sometimes

TABLE 14-4
Components of Normal Bowel Function

COMPONENT	FUNCTION
Food and water	Nothing in—nothing out. Fiber produces bulk in the stool
Central nervous system	Judgment: to take in sufficient quantities of food and fluid
	Control of motor functions: inhibits defecation until socially appropriate time
Intestines	Where nutrients are absorbed and feces are formed (in large intestine or colon). Feces propelled by peristaltic action of intestines
Muscles	Propel fecal matter along intestinal tract
	Allow patient to walk to the toilet and get on the commode
	Abdominal muscles assist peristaltic action
	Sphincter muscles hold feces in rectum until time to defecate
Nerves	Carry messages to the central nervous system about need to defecate. Carry messages to the muscles (sphincters) to relax and defecate
Rectum	Holding area for feces until place to defecate is found

From Snow, T.L. and McConnell, E.S. Bowel and Bladder Management Training Program. Unpublished educational aid, 1985.

referred to as "cathartic colon," or megacolon. Considerable discomfort may result, including bloating, cramping, and inability to defecate without a cathartic or enema (Wald, 1993). Overuse of saline cathartics may result in fluid and electrolyte imbalances.

Fecal incontinence is the involuntary passage of feces, soiling the clothes, bed, chair, or floor. The prevalence of fecal incontinence in long-term care settings is estimated to range from 10 to 23 per cent (Tobin and Brocklehurst, 1986). It is quite rare in community-dwelling older adults. The adverse consequences of fecal incontinence are many, including increased predisposition to skin ulceration and bacteriuria. Additionally, it is a degrading condition.

Constipation is associated with both impaction and incontinence (Kinnunen, 1991). The picture is often one of an immobilized older person who has frequent, small stools in the wheelchair. Until the constipation is addressed, therapies for incontinence and impaction are unlikely to have long-term success. None of these disorders inevitably accompany old age, although age-associated disorders make their prevalence higher in the elderly than among other adults.

Contributing Factors

A psychophysiological approach to bowel problems facilitates their understanding and treatment. For the most effective treatment,

it is important to understand the principles of normal bowel function, psychological influences on bowel function, and cultural beliefs about excretion and bowel habits.

Normal adult bowel function is the result of a complex interplay of many body systems. These include the central nervous system, the peripheral nerves, the autonomic nervous system, the endocrine system, the gastrointestinal tract, and the musculoskeletal system. Table 14–4 is a simplified chart of these complex relationships; it has been used successfully in patient teaching and in instructing families and paraprofessional staff about normal bowel function. Factors that contribute to the development of constipation and fecal incontinence can be considered according to how they affect these essential components of bowel function.

Disease States

People with dementing disorders, such as Alzheimer's disease, multi-infarct dementia, and Parkinson's disease often experience constipation and fecal incontinence. The impairments of judgment, memory, and problem solving associated with dementia can result in an individual who is unable independently to take in proper amounts of fiber and fluid. Inability to find a toilet when the urge to defecate is sensed also contributes to constipation and fecal incontinence.

Endocrinological disorders, such as hypothyroidism and hypercalcemia, can result in constipation, as can depression. Neurological disorders, including demyelinating diseases, autonomic neuropathy, spinal cord injuries, and cerebrovascular accidents, may interfere with the sensation of the urge to defecate or the ability to defecate on command. If a regular toileting regimen is not established, constipation ensues because too much water is reabsorbed in the large intestine, resulting in feces that are hard and difficult to pass. Musculoskeletal disorders, such as severe arthritis, muscular dystrophies, and fractures resulting in prolonged immobility, all may lead to constipation. In these cases, immobility results in diminished activity, which produces decreased peristalsis because voluntary muscles do not assist peristalsis. Kinnunen (1991) found that the risk of being constipated increased dramatically with decreasing mobility. Community-dwellers who walked less than 0.5 kilometer daily had a slightly increased risk, those who required assistance with walking had a threefold increase in risk, those who were chair-bound had a sevenfold increase in risk, and those who were bedbound had a 16-fold increase in risk for constipation. Tumors in either the colon, peritoneal cavity, or rectum may interfere with the peristaltic action required to move fecal material through the colon and out the anus. Hemorrhoids and fistulas may result in pain on defecation that inhibits the normal urge to defecate.

Many pharmacological agents contribute to constipation. Key offenders include anticholinergic drugs, such as many antipsychotics and antidepressants; antacids containing aluminum, bismuth, or calcium; bulk-forming laxatives not taken with sufficient amounts of fluid; any stimulant laxative taken on a regular basis; and some less frequently thought of drugs, such as diuretics and calcium channel blockers.

Inadequate Dietary Fiber Intake

Feces are composed of food which is not absorbed in the stomach or small intestine. A diet which contains primarily highly refined foods and few fruits or vegetables predisposes to constipation, because there is insufficient bulk to stimulate peristaltic movement.

Inadequate Fluid Intake

The large intestine is part of the body's system for maintaining fluid and electrolyte balance. If a person is poorly hydrated, more water will be absorbed in the large intestine in an attempt to maintain homeostasis. This results in dry feces that become hardened and more difficult to pass.

Inadequate Privacy for Toileting

Defecation is a complex process. It involves the autonomic nervous system and the use of voluntary muscles. Both spinal reflexes and cortical control are involved. The process involves simultaneous muscle contraction and relaxation. Inadequate privacy may result in habitual and inappropriate inhibition of the urge to defecate, resulting in constipation.

Improper Positioning

The natural position for defecation allows the assistance of gravity in evacuating the rectum. Attempts to use a bedpan may result in discomfort and less than optimal benefit from the forces of gravity. Discomfort may also lead to the inhibition of the urge to defecate.

Sociocultural Factors

Preoccupation with bowel function as it relates to the excretion of body poisons has been a feature of medical literature since the beginning of written history. As excretion is considered a "private" function, there is ample opportunity for the development of misconceptions and almost mystical beliefs about bowel hygiene. Detailed treatment of these misconceptions is beyond the scope of this book; however, it is important for clinicians to recognize that folklore rather than fact may guide an older person's bowel habits. Nurses should therefore assess the unique beliefs of the client with constipation. Given this high level of misinformation regarding bowel function in the general public, it is essential for nurses to have correct information on normal bowel function and disorders commonly associated with its disruption. It is equally important that nurses be comfortable in explaining normal bowel function in terms easily understood by the general public.

Constipation contributes to incontinence when (1) the patient never completely evacuates the rectum, resulting in frequent, small stools, or (2) the patient oozes liquid stool around an impaction. Other major contributing factors to fecal incontinence are summarized in Table 14–5.

Assessment

Assessment of the individual suspected of having constipation is designed to (1) determine whether the person truly has constipation, (2) identify those persons at high risk for development of constipation, and (3) isolate factors in the individual that contribute to the constipation or high-risk status.

Defining characteristics (NANDA, 1992, p. 16) include

- **Hard-formed stool**
- **Straining at stool**
- **Inability to pass stool**
- Decreased frequency (less than two times per week)
- Decreased activity level
- Palpable abdominal mass
- Reported feeling of pressure in rectum
- Reported feeling of rectal fullness
- Abdominal pain
- Appetite impairment
- Back pain
- Interference with daily living
- Use of laxatives

Characteristics in boldface are diagnostic of constipation; the remaining factors are symptoms or findings that are frequently present in those with constipation.

TABLE 14 – 5
Techniques for Patients with Fecal Incontinence

Etiology	Identifying Characteristics	Intervention
CENTRAL NERVOUS SYSTEM		
Disorientation		
Alzheimer's/dementia	Can't find the right place (early disease)	Establish TOILETING SCHEDULE
Coma	Can't figure out how to get undressed, defe-	Staff must take initiative to prevent "acci-
Stroke	cate, and get dressed again	dents"
Advanced Parkinson's	Can't ask for help	
Acute confusion		
No control over spinal reflexes	Can't control the urge to defecate (late dis-	Establish toileting regimen using patient's
	ease)	habit pattern as a guide
	Can't sense the urge to defecate	
		Behavior Modification
No social awareness	Doesn't care where defecation occurs	Obtain street clothes for patient
	"I'm not worth it"	Explore patient's decreased feeling of self-
		worth
	Never taught that it matters where one defe-	Determine rewards for correct toilet use,
	cates	explain to patient and implement
		Staff Development/Behavior Modification
No positive self-image	No one else cares where defecation occurs	Assess coworkers' actions toward patient
Low energy	"The slows"—it's just too much trouble	Assess for physiological problems and
Too much trouble		treat accordingly
Depressed		Provide structure, reinforce good perform-
Chronically ill		ance
Anemia		Modify the environment to facilitate func-
		tion and equipment
METABOLIC ABNORMALITIES		
Endocrine disorders	Abnormal lab values—diagnosis of hyper-	Medical Diagnosis and Treatment of Etio-
Depression . . . which leads to constipation	calcemia, hyperthyroidism, hypokalemia	logic Disorder
. . . which leads to impaction		During evaluation, resolve constipation,
. . . which leads to fecal incontinence		using medications if necessary
PSYCHOLOGICAL		
Inappropriate expression of anger	Attention getter—"He's just doing that to get	Supportive Counseling/Behavior Modifica-
	attention"	tion
		Positive reinforcement of "good" bowel
		habits
		Look at other ways of giving attention
Misinformed about "normal" bowel habits	"I need to go once a day"	Counsel and Teach
	"I've got to have a BM every day"	Teach and SUPPORT new knowledge re-
	"I drink too much"	garding bowel habits
LACK OF PRIVACY		
Lack of private/comfortable place to defe-	"Habit constipation"	Provision of adequate privacy
cate	Ignoring/suppressing the urge to defecate	Attend to proper equipment and positioning
	Bedpans	
GASTROINTESTINAL SYSTEM		
Reduced peristalsis	Immobility	Start exercise program
	Drug-induced: anticholinergics, narcotics	Consider whether change in drugs is possi-
	Chronic laxative abuse	ble
	Low-fiber diet	Stop laxatives
		Increase bulk and fluid

The assessment should include

- Activity level
- Usual bowel pattern, history of bowel disease
- Characteristics of constipation as just listed
- Medications, including pattern of laxative use
- Rectal examination
- Bowel sounds
- Hydration status (intake and output)
- Diet: amount of fiber; special diets ordered?
- Beliefs about bowel normality, relationship between diet and activity, hydration, scheduling, positioning, bowel function, and hygiene

Development of alterations in fecal elimina-

TABLE 14-5
Techniques for Patients with Fecal Incontinence *Continued*

Etiology	Identifying Characteristics	Intervention
No assistance of peristalsis with voluntary muscles	Muscle inactivity: bedbound/chairbound, cord injury	Start exercise program to increase use of abdominal muscles
Diarrhea in individuals with reduced mobility	Soiling on clothes— "I couldn't get there in time"	Treat diarrhea with medications or diet Protective padding until diarrhea resolved
Not eating fresh vegetables or any fiber	Oral problems: dentures not fitting, edentulous	Refit dentures, or use bulk-forming laxatives
INTAKE PROBLEMS: FLUID AND FIBER		
Not enough intake to form bulk or stimulate peristalsis	Poor appetite Low-fiber diet	Increase bulk and water
Too much bulk for amount of water	Decreased skin tugor Tongue dry/fissured Intake <2000 ml/day	More water—offer small amounts frequently
MUSCULOSKELETAL SYSTEM		
No assist from voluntary muscle action	Neurologic disease Muscular dystrophy ALS Cord injury Inability to sit up in bed voluntarily	ROM—passive sit-ups Assist patients to get upright and sustain upright position while defecating
Reduced assist from voluntary muscles	Neurologic disease leading to decreased activity CVA Alzheimer's	Teach active exercises Support in doing exercises
	Other problems leading to decreased activity Hip fracture with traction Terminal illness	Teach isometric exercises to strengthen abdominal muscles
Can't get to the bathroom	Problems as above	Bedside commode Toileting schedule
Lack of dexterity to wipe and redress	E.g., stroke with hemiplegia, rheumatoid arthritis	Adaptive equipment
PERIPHERAL NERVOUS SYSTEM		
Sphincters that don't work right	Surgical trauma Anorectal disease	Surgical repair
Nerves to the gut don't work properly	Diabetic neuropathy Tertiary syphilis	Enemas
Positioning problems	"I can't use a bedpan" "I can't sit on the pot—I'm afraid I'll fall"	Arrange for bedside commode or toilet use Arrange for SAFE and comfortable restraint system Either stay with the patient or use vest restraint

tion is multifactorial, therefore it is helpful to summarize baseline and ongoing assessment data in a central place. This method aids in evaluating the effectiveness of various interventions. A flow sheet to record this information, developed for use in institutions, is shown in Figure 14–2.

History

The history should include information about lifelong bowel habits, such as use of laxatives, enemas, or suppositories; usual frequency and time of day of bowel movements; beliefs about bowel function; current symptoms of constipation or gastrointestinal distress; previous abdominal surgery; anorectal disease, such as hemorrhoids or rectal prolapse; typical activity patterns; and a 1-week diet history. If patients are unable to give a reliable history, these data may be obtained from family and other caregivers.

Physical Assessment

Maneuvers for physical assessment are evaluation of hydration status, auscultation of bowel sounds, palpation for abdominal masses, and a rectal examination to determine the presence of hemorrhoids, rectal prolapse, or fecal impaction; to evaluate anal sphincter tone; and to test for occult blood.

ASSESSMENT—BASELINE
CIRCLE APPROPRIATE ANSWERS

1. History

Stool Pattern Previously:
>1 time/day
1 time/day
1 time/3 days
1 time/week

Time of Day of Stool:
early AM   late PM
late AM   at night
early PM   variable

2. Laxative Use

Frequency:
never   occasionally
sometimes   weekly   daily

Type of Laxative:
juice   diet   laxative
enema   suppos.   other

3. Medical Diagnoses
CVA
Diabetes
Diverticulitis
Metastatic disease
Colon cancer
Parkinson's disease
Severe arthritis

4. Physical Findings
Fecal impaction   yes/no
Abdominal mass   yes/no
Bowel sounds:
Hypoactive
Normal
Hyperactive

5. Activity Status
a) bedridden
b) bed-to-chair
c) wheelchair-bound
d) exercises
e) wheelchair-mobile
f) walks <25 feet/day
g) walks >25 feet/day
h) in P.T.

6. Medications
C) constipating drugs
opiates
antidiarrheals
psychotropics
iron supplements
antacids
high-dose aspirin
L) laxative-like drugs
stool softeners
antacids

7. Fluid Intake
a) unknown
b) inadequate (<1000 ml)
c) marginal (1000–2000)
d) adequate (>2000 ml)

8. Diet
1) no solid intake
2) no roughage
3) high-fiber diet

KEY TO ABBREVIATIONS:

Y/N = toileted
X = Meds—PRN, or Meds—REG administered
* = episode of incontinence or accidental bowel movement
† = bowel movement in correct location
SUPP = suppository administered
EN = enema administered
LAX = laxative administered

	Day 1			Day 2			Day 3			Day 4			Day 5			Day 6			Day 7		
	D	E	N	D	E	N	D	E	N	D	E	N	D	E	N	D	E	N	D	E	N
Week 1																					
Bowel Movmnt																					
Toileted																					
Diet																					
Fluid Intake				Use codes from baseline assessment on the left, items 5–8																	
Activities																					
LAX SUPP EN																					
Meds—REG																					
Meds—PRN																					
Week 2																					
Bowel Movmnt																					
Toileted																					
Diet																					
Fluid Intake																					
Activities																					
LAX SUPP EN																					
Meds—REG																					
Meds—PRN																					
Week 3																					
Bowel Movmnt																					
Toileted																					
Diet																					
Fluid Intake																					
Activities																					
LAX SUPP EN																					
Meds—REG																					
Meds—PRN																					
Week 4																					
Bowel Movmnt																					
Toileted																					
Diet																					
Fluid Intake																					
Activities																					
LAX SUPP EN																					
Meds—REG																					
Meds—PRN																					
Week 5																					
Bowel Movmnt																					
Toileted																					
Diet																					
Fluid Intake																					
Activities																					
LAX SUPP EN																					
Meds—REG																					
Meds—PRN																					
Week 6																					
Bowel Movmnt																					
Toileted																					
Diet																					
Fluid Intake																					
Activities																					
LAX SUPP EN																					
Meds—REG																					
Meds—PRN																					

FIGURE 14-2

Assessment form to record alteration in bowel elimination. (From Snow, T. and McConnell, E.S. Bowel and Bladder Management Training Program. Unpublished educational aid, 1985.)

Mental Status Examination

Information regarding sensory acuity, short-term memory, judgment, and problem-solving ability is also useful in determining the client's ability to follow through with a bowel management program.

Planning for Prevention

Planning and education are the keys to prevention of constipation; careful planning will save the clinician considerable effort. If the client is ambulatory and living independently, the planning process is greatly simplified. If, however, the client depends upon family or professional caregivers, it is important to include them. Failure to do so may mean that the client receives conflicting messages about the best plan for constipation prevention. This is potentially disastrous given the many products on the market for treatment of constipation. Any of these agents potentially could sabotage a carefully developed prevention program. All caregivers should understand the constipation prevention program: its goals, methods, and scheduled evaluation dates.

A constipation prevention regimen should establish goals in each of these areas:

1. Adequate fluid intake
2. Activity level and specified types of activities
3. Correct amount of fiber in the diet
4. Special equipment needed (such as bedside commode, call buzzer, raised toilet seat)
5. Regular scheduling (e.g., after breakfast or after supper)

Specific goals and approaches for each of these elements should be included in any program but are particularly important for older persons in the hospital or nursing home, as older people have difficulty maintaining accustomed habit structures in institutional settings.

One successful quality improvement project designed to reduce constipation and fecal impaction on a vascular surgery ward used a combination of dietary modification, positioning, and abdominal strengthening exercises to reduce the occurrence of constipation and fecal impaction. The protocol included 4.2 to 5.2 grams of fiber delivered in cookies or muffins, fluid intake of between 1500 and 2000 ml per day, and daily toileting in the upright position with privacy. The prevalence of constipation on this unit dropped from 59 per cent to 9 per cent, the prevalence of fecal impaction dropped from 36 per cent to 0 per cent, and requests for enemas or laxatives declined from 59 per cent to 8 per cent (Hall et al., 1995).

Intervention

Prevention is the key to successful management of constipation, fecal impaction, and fecal incontinence. A protocol for assessment and treatment of alterations in bowel elimination appears in Box 14–1 on pages 430 to 432.

All the elements of a preventive program, listed in "Planning" above should be addressed to treat constipation and fecal impaction properly. Some clients, however, will require selective emphasis on one or more aspects of the general approach. Some will require some pharmacological intervention, although it has been well documented that for most, attention to the aforementioned factors is more than sufficient to achieve normal bowel function in the elderly.

Fecal Impaction

The wisest approach to fecal impaction is prevention. Patients at high risk for impaction should be identified and a preventive bowel regimen established. High-risk individuals are those with a previous history of impaction, immobilized patients, and those taking doses of medicines with constipating properties, such as narcotics and drugs with anticholinergic properties. Unfortunately, many patients develop fecal impaction before a bowel management program is implemented.

Two approaches for treatment of fecal impaction are commonly recommended. The first is the use of an oil-retention enema to soften the stool before manual disimpaction. The second approach is to manually disimpact and then administer a cleansing enema. Tap water enemas should be used rather than soap enemas because of the greater risk of complications associated with soap enemas, including mucosal irritation and necrosis (Harari et al., 1993). No rigorous evaluations of treatment for fecal impaction are reported in the literature. An effective protocol for treatment of fecal impaction appears in the bowel management protocol in Box 14–1.

Constipation

Depending upon the findings of the physical examination, the most appropriate first maneuver may be to assist the patient to the

BOX 14-1
Protocol for Development of Bowel Management Program

DOs AND DON'Ts

DO

1. Make sure the person is well hydrated.
2. Start with the technique that has the fewest side effects.
3. Move to a new technique only after the first approach has had 2 weeks of documented application.
4. Make sure everyone involved in the patient's care (patient, family, volunteers, dietary staff, AND THE NIGHT SHIFT!) knows the goals of the bowel management program, the plan, the reasons for the plan, and when the plan will be re-evaluated.
5. Remember to document your interventions.

DON'T

1. Use negative reinforcement—ever!
2. Do anything before assessing the patient thoroughly.
3. Use medicines when nursing care will work better.
4. Underestimate the power of lifelong habits, both good and bad.

First: Look Before You Leap—Assessment

1. Check for fecal impaction.
   If there is an impaction, GO TO IMPACTION PROTOCOL.
   If there is NO impaction, continue to step 2.
2. Check for diarrhea.
   If there is diarrhea WITHOUT an impaction, GO TO DIARRHEA PROTOCOL.
   If there is NO diarrhea, continue to step 3.
3. Intake and output for 1 week.
4. Identify preadmission and preillness bowel habits.
   Frequency
   Time of day
   Surrounding events: cup of coffee, commode vs. toilet vs. bedpan
   Laxative use
5. Activity patterns
   (Good, fair, and poor is not enough—need to specify type of activity)
6. Diet
   Amount of bulk
   Prune juice?
7. Medications

Second: Start by Doing What Comes Naturally

1. Up, in the bathroom, on the toilet
2. At their usual time
3. With enough privacy
4. Feeling secure
5. For long enough time

Third: Look at the Things You Can Do That Won't Hurt

1. Exercise to increase or assist peristalsis
2. Increase fluid intake
3. Increase fiber content of diet
4. Counsel regarding "need" for daily B.M.

The vast majority of your patient's bowel problems will be resolved using these three steps. However . . .
If you have done these things, given patients sufficient time, and believed in their ability to do the job, with no success,
Then and only then should you turn to medications or enemas for treating constipation.

BOX 14-1
Protocol for Development of Bowel Management Program *Continued*

> ### WARNING
> ### Medications and Enemas
> All have side effects that may be harmful to your patients and may create new and more difficult problems for you and them!

If these things don't work—then look again at your assessments to diagnose the problem.

1. Medications.
2. Undiagnosed medical illness: hypothyroidism, hypokalemia, hypercalcemia.
3. Complication of already-diagnosed illness:
   End-stage diabetes mellitus w/neuropathy.
   End-stage demyelinating diseases.
   Anorectal disease.
4. Psychological problems—adjustment reaction, depression.

IMPACTION PROTOCOL
First: Assessment

1. Perform digital examination.
   If hard stool is present, manual disimpaction is indicated.
   If large amount of soft stool, use either glycerin suppository, oil enema, or hyperosmolar enema.

Second: Intervention

1. Provide privacy.
2. Explain procedure (either manual disimpaction or enema).
3. Ask patient to breathe deeply, slowly, and quietly throughout procedure to promote relaxation.
4. Stop manual disimpaction if patient complains of excessive pain.
5. Do not manipulate impaction beyond the fatigue tolerance of the patient. Allow for a rest period during and following the disimpaction.
6. Follow manual disimpaction with hyperosmotic laxative or enema.

Third: Evaluation

1. Note results of laxative or enema.
2. Check for impaction.
3. Has a bowel management program to prevent recurrent impaction been implemented?

DIARRHEA PROTOCOL
First: Look Before You Leap—Assessment

1. Check for impaction. If impacted, GO TO IMPACTION PROTOCOL.
2. Begin intake and output, including stool count. Elderly patients are at high risk for dehydration and electrolyte imbalance if diarrhea goes untreated.
3. If patient is tube fed, consider possibility of tube feeding as the culprit. Tube feedings administered too fast or hyperosmotic feedings may cause diarrhea.
4. Review medications, especially if a new medication has recently been started. Many drugs have the potential to cause diarrhea as a side effect. Consult with pharmacist.
5. Get diet history. Excessive intake of high-fiber foods may result in diarrhea in some patients.
6. Consider infection (either viral or bacterial) as source of diarrhea. Consult with physician or nurse practitioner.

Second: Intervene

1. Make sure toilet is close by and notify staff of patient's diarrhea and high risk for incontinence. People with diarrhea have a shorter time to respond to the urge to defecate.
2. Match the treatment to the suspected cause of the diarrhea. Bowel rest may be all that is necessary.
3. Remember that antidiarrheals are all strong medications with potential for adverse side effects and drug-drug interactions.

Box continued on following page

BOX 14-1

Protocol for Development of Bowel Management Program *Continued*

Third: Evaluate

1. If a diet modification or drug is prescribed to treat the diarrhea, make sure you establish agreement with the physician or nurse practitioner on criteria to discontinue treatment.
2. Set criteria for discontinuing stool counts and intake and output.
3. If fecal incontinence is prevented or resolved, pat yourself on the back!

(From Snow, T.L. and McConnell, E.S. Bowel and Bladder Management Training Program. Unpublished educational aid, 1985.)

toilet and attempt to facilitate peristalsis. Have the patient bend over from the waist, or press firmly on the lower abdomen. Allow a reasonable amount of time—5 to 10 minutes or longer if patient preference dictates—to facilitate relaxation. These interventions, along with proper positioning on a toilet or bedside commode, with feet supported, sometimes will suffice to resolve the problem. If the maneuvers fail to produce a bowel movement and other defining characteristics of constipation are present, then a laxative is indicated.

The most important consideration in using a laxative is ensuring that a program to prevent future episodes of constipation is implemented. If a good faith effort to prevent further episodes of constipation is established, then the laxative of choice can be either a bulk-forming, saline, hyperosmotic, or stimulant laxative. The choice depends on the patient's other medical problems and preference. In general, bulk-forming laxatives are preferred to other types because of their better side effect profile. Emollient laxatives such as docusate have not been shown to be effective in changing stool water content or frequency of defecation (Chapman et al., 1985), leading some to conclude that they are of limited, if any, value in treating chronic constipation. Mineral oil, another emollient laxative, is contraindicated in debilitated people or those with dysphagia because of the risk of lipid aspiration (Wald, 1993). It is inappropriate to give a saline or hyperosmotic laxative to a dehydrated person, for this will exacerbate the problem.

Fecal Incontinence

Interventions for the treatment of fecal incontinence are summarized in Table 14–5. Many are focused on normalizing bowel function and then scheduling a regular bowel evacuation. Tobin and Brocklehurst (1986) report a cure rate of 87 per cent for fecal incontinence, even in severely demented individuals, through the use of a combination of drug therapies, regular enemas, and toileting. Individuals with fecal incontinence associated with impaction were given lactulose, 10 ml twice daily, plus a weekly enema. Individuals with neurogenic fecal incontinence (inability to suppress the urge to defecate) were given codeine phosphate, 30 to 60 mg daily, to induce constipation, along with twice weekly enemas to produce predictable bowel evacuation. As this regimen involves invasive methods, nurses should attempt simple interventions, such as regular toileting after meals, before considering more extreme interventions. However, the impact of fecal incontinence is so devastating that reasonable medical intervention should be undertaken when more conservative treatment fails. Stone (1991) summarizes research on the use of biofeedback to treat fecal incontinence caused by peripheral and autonomic neuropathies, anal trauma, or surgery. Success rates in selected individuals (those with intact cognition and high motivation) may be as high as 63 per cent.

Evaluation

Criteria for evaluation of the nursing system that is designed depends upon the initial goals established with the patient and caregivers. The more physiological the bowel regimen, the better for the patient. No clear guidelines exist on the amount of time required to establish a bowel program that reliably prevents constipation. Given the pervasiveness of misconceptions regarding bowel function, a several-month course of counseling and alternative treatment seems reasonable before concluding that the problem is either resolved or intractable.

Specific criteria for evaluation include

1. Extent to which laxatives, enemas, or suppositories are requested or used in the bowel regimen.
2. Inclusion of diet and exercise modalities in the bowel regimen.
3. Patient satisfaction with frequency and consistency of bowel movements.
4. Frequency of bowel movements (not less often than every third day).
5. Absence of fecal incontinence.
6. Absence of fecal impaction.

ALTERATION IN BOWEL ELIMINATION: DIARRHEA

Definition and Scope of Problem

Diarrhea is the frequent passage of loose, fluid, unformed stool (NANDA, 1992). Consequences of untreated diarrhea include fluid and electrolyte disturbance, predisposition to fecal incontinence, alteration in comfort, alteration in skin integrity, and altered self-image.

Contributing Factors

The causes of diarrhea in the elderly are the same as causes of diarrhea in anyone: viral or bacterial gastroenteritis, misuse of laxatives, food intolerance, improper hyperosmolar tube feedings, side effects of medications such as antibiotics, side effects of radiation therapy to the abdomen, autonomic neuropathy, inflammatory bowel disease, anxiety, malignancy, malabsorption syndromes, protein-calorie malnutrition, and fecal impaction (Roberts, 1993). Fecal impaction is sometimes mistakenly thought to be diarrhea because liquid stool comes around the impaction and is eliminated frequently.

According to Gangarosa and colleagues (1992), 15 per cent of diarrhea in the aged can be attributed to an infectious source, with 68 per cent caused by viral agents, 19 per cent caused by bacterial infection, and 3 per cent from parasites. Fecal impaction is the culprit in 16 per cent of diarrheas, antibiotic use in 11 per cent, laxative abuse in 6 per cent, and inflammatory bowel disease in 4 per cent (Smith, 1989). Diarrhea can be a serious condition, with associated mortality increasing dramatically in those over age 74 years (Lew et al., 1991).

Protein-calorie malnutrition results in diarrhea when individuals must catabolize their own body proteins to meet their protein and calorie requirements. Tissues that turn over rapidly, including intestinal mucosa, are involved, and flattening of the intestinal villi and decreased amounts of digestive enzymes produce a malabsorption syndrome.

Assessment

Nursing assessment of diarrhea should include stool count, observation of stool consistency, and digital rectal and abdominal examinations for fecal impaction. (See Diarrhea Protocol in Box 14–1.) Fecal impaction and infectious causes must be ruled out before *pro re nata* drugs are administered for diarrhea. The person's usual bowel elimination pattern should be determined, along with the current pattern. Diarrhea that occurs only during the day suggests a functional rather than organic cause. Obtain a drug and diet history, placing particular emphasis on recent changes in medications or dietary habits. Roberts (1993) notes that some medicines in elixir form may contain sorbitol, which may act as an osmotic laxative. Ask specifically about patterns of laxative use. Diarrhea that persists over a 5-day period, diarrhea characterized by bloody stools, or widespread diarrhea in an institutional setting calls for laboratory examination of stool, including Gram stain, presence of fecal leukocytes, culture for ova and parasites, and examination for the presence of the toxin produced by *Clostridium difficile,* an increasingly common cause of diarrhea (Cartmill et al., 1992; Fay and Lance, 1992). Persistent diarrhea requires extensive medical evaluation to determine the cause and definitive treatment.

Assessment of the impact of diarrhea on other aspects of the individual's function is also important. The patient's emotional reaction to the diarrhea and ability to maintain continence, adequate hydration, and skin integrity should be assessed.

Planning and Intervention

The goals of caring for the individual with diarrhea are to identify and treat the causative factor(s), prevent problems associated with diarrhea, such as incontinence and alteration in skin integrity, and promote patient comfort. In addition, if an infectious cause for the diarrhea is suspected, preventing transmission to other people is also a high priority.

ISOLATION. Universal precautions should be used for handling all body fluids, regardless of whether diarrhea is present. However, if an infectious diarrhea outbreak in a long-term care facility is suspected, the following additional steps should be taken. Consider instituting gastroenteritis outbreak management procedures if greater than 3 per cent of all patients in a facility, or more than three patients on one ward, develop diarrhea (Edmond, 1994). Health department and attending physicians should be notified, food service employees should be interviewed regarding recent gastrointestinal illness, and ill employees should be excused from work. If a bacterial pathogen is isolated, culture stool from food service employees, and reassign asymptomatic infected workers until stool cultures are negative. Use enteric precautions for infected patients, reminding paraprofessional staff or family caregivers about the rationale for extra precautions. Strict handwashing between all patients should be observed. Gloves, gowns, and linen should be bagged as close as possible to where they are changed. In some instance, quarantining of patients until infection is resolved is recommended (Edmond, 1994).

MEDICATIONS. Four types of medications are used for symptomatic relief of diarrhea: (1) opiate derivatives, such as paregoric and diphenoxylate (Lomotil); (2) anticholinergics, such as loperamide (Imodium), (3) adsorbent agents, such as kaolin and pectin (Kaopectate) and Metamucil; and (4) demulcents, such as bismuth subsalicylate (Pepto-Bismol). Opiate derivatives are to be avoided where possible, as they have anticholinergic properties and can prolong excretion of toxins in toxin-induced gastroenteritis. Anticholinergics are to be avoided for the same reason. Therefore, neither class of drug should be used to relieve diarrhea until an infectious cause has been excluded. Adsorbent agents usually produce fewer adverse effects, although patients sometimes find the taste objectionable. Medications specific to causes of diarrhea include antibiotics for those with bacterial enteritis and digestive enzyme supplementation for people with malabsorption syndromes. Steroids are sometimes used in individuals with inflammatory bowel disease.

ENTERAL FEEDINGS. Several factors have been implicated in diarrhea associated with enteral feeding, including tube feeding rate, temperature, intermittent versus continuous tube feeding, osmolarity of feeding, and microbial contamination of tube feeding (Vines et al., 1992). In a critical review of this literature, Vines and colleagues concluded that the practice applications best supported by the available research literature included attention to adjustment of feeding osmolarity; adoption of practices to minimize the likelihood of microbial contamination of feeds, such as a maximum 24-hour feeding bag hang time; and careful handwashing technique.

ADAPTIVE EQUIPMENT. Fecal collection bags may prevent alteration in skin integrity for individuals at high risk of skin breakdown who are incontinent with diarrhea. Socially active patients who experience incontinence secondary to diarrhea may also find these devices useful while the diarrhea is being evaluated. Temporary use of a bedside commode for people with immobility problems may prevent diarrhea-induced fecal incontinence.

HYGIENE. Meticulous perineal hygiene should be provided to frail individuals at risk of skin breakdown, after each episode of diarrhea. Use of emollient creams following cleansing may help protect the skin against the caustic effects of fecal material.

Evaluation

The following criteria apply to evaluation of the nursing care for patients with diarrhea:

1. The diarrhea is resolved promptly.
2. A cause for chronic diarrhea is identified, and all treatable causes are addressed.
3. Adverse sequelae of diarrhea are prevented, such as incontinence, alteration in skin integrity, and fluid and electrolyte disturbances.
4. Transmission of infectious diarrhea to others is prevented.

COMFORT ALTERATIONS: ACUTE AND CHRONIC PAIN, FATIGUE, NAUSEA, AND DYSPNEA

Definition and Scope of Problem

Alteration in comfort is often equated with pain. However, nursing care of elderly people involves care of people with a variety of discomforts, in addition to pain, including dyspnea, fatigue, and nausea. These conditions are related for the following reasons:

- They each have a physiological, sensory, and affective component, each of which must be considered for effective treatment (Carrieri-Kohlman, Lindsey, and West, 1993)

- They are all unpleasant, subjective experiences amenable to palliation through nursing care (Hamilton, 1989; Jaycox, 1989)
- Each alteration in comfort is not a predictable function of the underlying physiological stimulus
- The clinical approach to assessment and management of these diagnoses have elements in common, such as the essential nature of the subjective report, importance of measuring symptom severity, and willingness to consider an eclectic treatment approach, rather than relying strictly on pharmacotherapy
- They often overlap in presentation, i.e., pain and fatigue may exist concomitantly, or one may produce the other (Crosby, 1989).

These diagnoses therefore remain clustered here, despite the fact that they are treated separately in NANDA taxonomy, so that the commonalities among the diagnoses can be emphasized and used to promote greater understanding of each category. Where necessary, specific theoretical issues, assessment, and intervention approaches will be outlined for each specific type of alteration in comfort. As noted by Carrieri-Kohlman, Lindsey, and West (1993), scientific study of these phenomena is in an early stage, with pain studies being the most advanced scientifically. Thus, advances in understanding pain and its management will serve as the dominant model for examining other types of alterations in comfort.

Theoretical Approaches

Little conceptual or empirical work exists on the global concept of alterations in comfort. Notable exceptions include Norris' (1982) work on concept clarification in nursing, Hamilton's (1989) qualitative study of comfort in chronically hospitalized elderly patients, and more recently, Kolcaba's (1992) attempt to consider comfort from a holistic perspective. Norris's work advocated clustering of the following phenomena under the rubric of "protection": chronic pruritus, nausea, thirst, fatigue, insomnia, disorientation, and immobilization. Although this work is widely respected for its careful analyses of these problems, little research has followed. Hamilton studied 30 patients in a 284-bed chronic geriatric hospital in Canada. When the patients were asked what comfort meant to them, what barriers to comfort they experienced, and what factors would enhance their comfort, the following do-

mains of comfort were identified: (1) symptom control, including pain, and constipation; (2) freedom from worry about deteriorating function, (3) freedom from worries about caregivers; and (4) environmental factors, such as comfortable positioning that allowed them to carry out desired activities, dependable staff, and access to good food and a variety of social activities, flexibly scheduled. Although this description of comfort may be too global to be useful in targeted clinical situations, it points out the fact that comfort involves more than alleviation of pain, although this is clearly a critical element of promotion of comfort.

Kolcaba's work builds upon Hamilton's studies, proposing a taxonomic structure for comfort. Comfort is viewed as a multidimensional construct, comprising four domains: physical, psychospiritual, environmental, and social. Each domain can be evaluated according to the degree of unmet need experienced by the individual—from relief, to ease, to transcendence. The scope of the discussion that follows will be limited to the physical need/relief portion of Kolcaba's model. However, it is worth noting that in the eyes of many, comfort and its promotion extend well beyond the alleviation of uncomfortable symptoms, to include engaging with one's environment in an autonomous manner, including important psychological variables such as mastery and transcendence of difficult personal experiences.

One promising theoretical approach to alterations in comfort is the use of a nociceptive model, suggested by Steele and Shaver (1992) for use with dyspnea, because of the difficulty of predicting dyspnea severity from the nature of the underlying derangement in physical or physiological function. Nociception is defined as the appreciation of injurious influences (Hensyl, 1990). This appreciation involves cognitive, motivational, and affective dimensions expressed as distress in response to aversive stimuli, in addition to the sensory experience of the phenomenon (Steele and Shaver, 1992). The importance of the nonsensory dimensions of the symptom is that cognitive and affective factors may influence the sensory response. Thus, assessment and treatment of the specific alteration in comfort should include a focus on the underlying injurious factors present and also should examine and treat the sensory, cognitive, and affective response to the discomforting stimuli. This approach suggests that it may be insufficient to treat the sensory component of discomfort without attending to other aspects of the problem, particularly when the discomfort

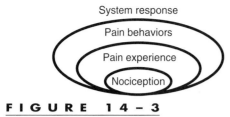

FIGURE 14 – 3

Interactive model of alterations in comfort. (Adapted from Donovan, M.I. Acute pain relief. *Nurs Clin North Am* 25(4):851–861, 1990.)

has the potential to become chronic, or when conditioned responses may develop to stimuli associated with the original noxious stimulus that may potentiate feelings of distress or suffering and may affect function adversely. In other words, if individuals can be helped to increase their tolerance of an unpleasant symptom, then their perception of its intensity may actually change.

In the instance of pain, cultural factors may influence pain perception and response. In the instance of nausea, events surrounding an occasion when an emetigenic drug is given may later stimulate nausea in the absence of administration of the drug. For patients who suffer from dyspnea, it may be possible to dissociate various aspects of the experience, such as separating the sensation of breathing discomfort from breathing effort. According to Carrieri-Kohlman and Janson-Bjerklie (1993), previous experience with and beliefs about dyspnea affect one's tolerance for the symptom.

Figure 14–3 depicts a modification of an interactive pain model (Donovan, 1990) that can be extended to other forms of discomfort, such as dyspnea, nausea, and fatigue. It provides a useful cognitive map for nurses when considering alterations in comfort, because, regardless of the sensation, the nociceptive stimulus will result in a subjective experience, behavioral response, and social system response. Influencing the social system and behavioral responses to alter the patient's subjective experience, as well as intervening to reduce nociceptive stimuli, is the essence of nursing care of those with alterations in comfort.

Fagerhaugh and Strauss (1977) have written the classic work on pain experience in health care settings. According to their view, patients in health care settings have pain "tasks" to accomplish, including pain expression, pain endurance, and pain relief. In elderly people, an additional task is pain recognition, which may be blunted by impairments of the peripheral or central nervous systems, drug therapy, or cognitive impairments. The task of pain recognition is made more difficult in long-term care institutions, as described by Fagerhaugh and Strauss and summarized in Box 14–2. Although other forms of discomfort have not been studied from this framework, there is good reason to think that the so-called "politics of pain management" may extend to management of other distressing symptoms. Thus, it is useful to consider to what extent the observations made about the effects of care routines on pain experience also extend to other distressing symptoms.

Caregivers who work with people who have chronic discomfort must somehow resolve the guilt they experience when they are unable to relieve the patient's discomfort. Failure to address this issue leads either to avoidance of the patient or minimization of the discomfort felt. Neither strategy is helpful or appropriate. People who suffer from discomfort often fear being abandoned, and continuing to work to control or reduce discomfort even when symptoms show little response to treatment is an important therapeutic endeavor.

Specific Alterations in Comfort

Although most would agree that discomforting experiences are numerous for older adults, no reliable estimates of the prevalence of global discomfort exist. Thus, the scope of the problem of alterations in comfort must be inferred by examining data on component diagnoses, such as pain, dyspnea, fatigue, and nausea. Definitions and estimates of prevalence of each problem are discussed next.

Pain

Pain is defined by NANDA (1992) as "a state in which an individual experiences and reports the presence of severe discomfort or an uncomfortable sensation." Pain can be characterized as acute or chronic. Chronic pain is defined by NANDA as that which continues for more than 6 months. Defining characteristics include both subjective complaints of pain and its descriptors, as well as the presence of a variety of pain behaviors, such as guarding, withdrawal from social contact, distraction behavior, and, in acute pain, the presence of autonomic responses such as diaphoresis, increases in blood pressure and pulse, and pupil dilation. A National Institutes of Health (NIH) consensus development conference (1987) suggested three categories of pain based on cause; (1) *acute pain:* pain following acute injury, disease, or surgery, (2) *chronic malignant pain:* pain associated with cancer or other progressive disorders, and (3) *chronic nonmalignant pain:* pain in those whose tissue injury is nonprogressive or healed.

According to a recent review by the Agency for Health Care Policy and Research (AHCPR), the prevalence of pain in community-dwelling people over aged 60 years is twice that of adults under age 60 years (Crook et al., 1984) (250 per thousand versus 125 per thousand, respectively), with the prevalence estimated at over 70 per cent in institutionalized older adults (Acute Pain Management Guideline Panel, 1992; Ferrell, 1991; Sengstaken and King, 1993). Moreover, older adults are more likely to suffer from diseases and conditions associated with pain, such as arthritis, fractures, postherpetic neuralgia, and peripheral vascular disease. It is important to note, however, that the degree of pathology correlates poorly with the amount of pain a person experiences.

Unfortunately, accurate estimates of the prevalence of pain are difficult to obtain for both clinical and methodological reasons. There is no universally accepted approach to measurement of pain in the aged. Clinical observations suggest that pain perception may be altered in elderly people, although the notion that the pain threshold increases with age has lost favor, as this belief was based on studies of experimentally induced pain that may not pertain to clinical situations. Moreover, even the results from these studies do not conclusively demonstrate increased pain threshold in elderly people (Harkins, et al., 1986; McCaffery and Beebe, 1989; Ferrell et al., 1990; Ferrell, 1991). Thus, it is prudent *not* to assume that older adults have a higher pain threshold until more conclusive studies support this belief.

Pain is associated with coronary artery disease, arthritis, peripheral neuropathy, herpes zoster and postherpetic neuralgia, osteomyelitis, peripheral arterial insufficiency, osteoporosis, depression, constipation, chronic pain syndrome from hemiplegia, reflex sympathetic dystrophy, cancer, and amputation. According to Friedman (1990), up to 67 per cent of those with amputations experience phantom pain. Many of the sources of pain in older people are chronic in nature, and thus the range of therapies is somewhat restricted.

Dyspnea

Dyspnea is the "unpleasant sensation of difficult breathing and the human responses to that sensation" (Steele and Shaver, 1992,

---

BOX 14 – 2

Field Notes on the Influences in Long-Term Care Institutions on Pain Experiences of the Elderly

". . . Patients' requests for [pain] relief usually do not get immediate response from the staff because pain and its relief are related to the highly routinized mass work of physical maintenance. For example, a patient may be very uncomfortable from remaining too long in one position or because she was positioned poorly, but staff members, busy with other work, may not immediately attend to pain relief. More often than not a patient must endure her pain until the next prearranged time for moving her arrives, or until she is moved per schedule from wheelchair back to bed for napping, or she must wait until after everyone's feeding time. . . .

"Different assessments of the degree of pain suffered by the patient are made, in accordance with their primary work responsibilities, by both nonprofessional and professional nursing personnel. The former, responsible for much of the physical maintenance, generally tend to assess pains as greater than do the professionals. Understandably, they are the major agents of pain infliction, spending more time at the bedside, so they are more likely to observe grimaces and other pain expressions than the professionals. (Patients' complaints to the researchers were frequently about negligence—an aide or an orderly being too rough in handling them.) Since the professional personnel are responsible for the general administration of the ward, and for doing the more complex treatments—giving medications and assisting the physicians—their assessments of the pain suffered by a given patient are based to a considerable degree on information provided by the nonprofessionals. Because the latters' focus of work is mainly on getting the body work done, they are not likely to report much about pain. Also, since assessment of pain includes observing such cues as groaning, moaning, crying, and requests for drug relief, and since many patients learn to control their expressions of pain tightly, both professional and nonprofessional personnel probably underestimate the pain. . . .

"The major pain task faced by all staff members, then, is pain minimization through a gentle handling of the patients' bodies, allowing them to move at their own speeds, and utilizing comfort measures (such as propping pillows here and there). . . .

"We should add that on these extended-care wards, the patients' main responsibilities concerning pain are, first, to come to terms with living with their chronic pain, even if it is increasing; second, not to be overly expressive about pain (for that might upset the sentimental order of the ward); and third, to learn when and how to ask for drug relief."

(From Fagerhaugh, S. and Strauss, A. Politics of Pain Management: Staff-Patient Interactions. *Menlo Park, CA: Addison-Wesley, 1977.)*

p. 64; Carrieri-Kohlman and Janson-Bjerklie, 1993). It is most commonly associated with individuals who have chronic obstructive pulmonary disease (COPD), asthma, and restrictive airway disease, although other disease states, such as congestive heart failure, lung cancer, and deconditioning can also produce this symptom. Dyspnea is also common in individuals with terminal illness. Dyspnea often can be partially relieved by pharmacotherapy, such as bronchodilator therapy, or sedation (in the case of the terminally ill); however, substantial numbers of patients continue to suffer from unrelieved dyspnea (Gift, 1990). As is true for pain, the severity of dyspnea cannot be predicted from objective tests of pulmonary function (Gift et al., 1992; Carrieri-Kohlman and Janson-Bjerklie, 1993). Components of the dyspnea experience include the sensation, perception, distress, response, and reporting of the symptom. The latter three dimensions are thought to be highly influenced by the affect associated with the dyspnea, which in turn is mediated by personal, health status, and situational variables (Gift, 1990).

Although the prevalence of dyspnea has not been measured nationally, the prevalence of pulmonary and cardiac disorders is quite high among elderly people. According to Carrieri-Kohlman and Janson-Bjerklie (1993), over 5.5 million people over the age of 55 years have COPD, with another 7 million adults suffering from asthma.

Fatigue

Fatigue is defined by NANDA (1992) as "the self-recognized state in which an individual experiences an overwhelming, sustained sense of exhaustion and decreased capacity for physical and mental work that is not relieved by rest" (p. 55). Although fatigue accompanies almost every illness, it becomes a concern when it interferes with function, or when it occurs at inopportune times. Related concepts include tiredness, weakness, and exertion. Many parallels exist in the conceptualization of pain and fatigue. As with pain, fatigue can be classified as chronic or acute (Piper, 1993), with similar ramifications for the ease of identifying the etiology, its responsiveness to treatment, and effects on function. Issues in assessment and measurement of fatigue are similar to those in pain evaluation. Defining the scope and prevalence of fatigue in elderly persons is more difficult, because of a paucity of research and theory development compared with that available for the understanding of pain.

Key issues in understanding the scope of fatigue include (1) poor understanding of how subjective and objective indicators of fatigue are related, (2) complex, poorly understood mechanisms for development of fatigue, and (3) poor understanding of how chronic and acute fatigue interrelate (Piper, 1989). Equally important is understanding the extent to which fatigue is part of larger disease complexes, such as depression, versus to what extent fatigue exists separately as a diagnostic entity. Thus, the scope of fatigue can only be speculated about, based on clinical observations and descriptive studies of fatigue in specific patient populations.

For example, it is known that older adults suffer from many chronic diseases associated with fatigue, such as cancer, renal failure, arthritis, and neurological impairments. One review notes that between 80 and 96 per cent of those receiving chemotherapy experience fatigue, 58 per cent of dialysis patients report moderate-to-severe fatigue, and those undergoing abdominal surgery commonly report fatigue up to 2 months after the surgery (Piper, 1993). It is possible that fatigue is underdiagnosed in elderly people because of a societal expectation that older people should be tired (Hart et al., 1990), or it may be misattributed to a comorbid condition, such as depression. In a recent study of nondemented Parkinson's disease patients, fatigue, while associated with depression, also occurred in nondepressed Parkinson's disease patients, suggesting that fatigue is something other than simply a symptom of depression (Friedman and Friedman, 1993). Potempa (1989) suggests that there may be a disease specificity to fatigue, with the fatigue associated with cancer being qualitatively different from that associated with Epstein-Barr disease and from that associated with end-stage renal disease.

Nausea

Nausea is "a vague, disagreeable, queasy feeling in the stomach, accompanied by tightening sensation in the throat, along with a strong aversion to food and eating" (Carnevali and Reiner, 1990). It is frequently accompanied by vomiting and retching, although these symptoms do not co-occur universally (Hogan, 1990). Nausea has most often been studied in the context of neoplastic disease, although it may also occur with other disorders, such as gastrointestinal disease. Nausea may occur as the result of antineoplastic therapy, as the result of the tumor itself, or from other metabolic disturbances associated with tumors, such as hypercalcemia. In addition, nausea may result from other forms of pharmacotherapy, such as antibiotics, narcotic analgesics, and antiparkinsonian agents. Nausea may also result from other conditions common in those with terminal illness, including pain, constipation, and metabolic dysfunction (Hogan, 1990).

Nausea associated with antineoplastic agents has been described as occurring in three types: anticipatory nausea, acute nausea, and chronic or delayed nausea (Hogan, 1990). Anticipatory nausea is more common in individuals under age 50 years and therefore will not be considered further here. According to Rhodes and colleagues (1989) little is known about the frequency, duration, and severity of distress associated with nausea. Somewhat more is known about the incidence and time of onset after an inciting stimulus. Understanding of nausea is made more complex by its frequent coupling with vomiting: vomiting being more amenable to quantitative, objective assessment. Variability in the patterns of postchemotherapeutic nausea and vomiting suggest that factors other than the toxicity of the chemotherapeutic agent influence symptom severity and duration.

In summary, the number and breadth of disorders experienced by older adults that may precipitate discomfort are great. Consequences of failure to relieve discomfort include decreases in functional independence, affect, and quality of life and increases in suffering and possibly behavioral disturbance. Because altered presentation of disease is so common in the aged (Bender, 1992), nurses should be particularly vigilant in assessing for the presence of alteration in comfort as a contributor to adverse clinical outcomes, such as declines in function or dysphoria in elderly people.

Contributing Factors

Terminal Illness

People who are dying frequently experience a variety of uncomfortable sensations, generally as the result of multiple organ system failure. Sometimes discomfort results from a failure to attend to control of coexistent chronic diseases that are not life-threatening, or sometimes from a failure to attend to basic self-care requirements, such as elimination or position change. Pain may occur from impingement of tumor on nerve, from ischemia from inoperable vascular disease, or from less obvious causes, such as exacerbation of arthritis due to prolonged immobility induced by extreme fatigue or dizziness. Nausea may result from toxic effects of metabolic failure, or from constipation or intestinal obstruction, perhaps induced by attempts to relieve pain using narcotic analgesia. Dyspnea may result from cardiac failure due to severe cardiomyopathy or cor pulmonale associated with end-stage COPD. Pruritus may be due to uremia or to an undiscovered contact dermatitis. Dizziness may result from orthostatic hypotension because of dehydration. Teasing out specific contributing factors may be difficult, even frustrating, for clinicians, but it is often worth the effort, as reversible contributors to the patient's discomfort may be uncovered.

Situational Factors

A variety of situational factors have been noted to increase feelings of distress associated with discomfort from pain, dyspnea, and nausea. Environmental conditions, such as room temperature, noise level, and the presence of noxious stimuli such as cigarette smoke, perfumes, and bodily secretions can increase distress levels (Carrieri-Kohlman et al., 1993). In addition, the presence of individuals with whom the patient has a difficult relationship may also exacerbate symptom distress. Mechanical factors, such as decreased ventilation due to abdominal distention will increase the sense of dyspnea, or increased pressure from positioning the legs in a dependent position in those with leg pain due to edema, will influence severity of discomfort. Body positioning may relieve or exacerbate feelings of discomfort with dyspnea, pain, and possibly nausea. Finally, certain activities may influence discomfort levels. Some people experience worsening of discomfort while stooping or bending, rushing to complete a task, or during episodes of coughing. Careful observation of changes in symptom intensity during various mandatory and optional activities can be used to plan for preventing worsening of symptoms, thus decreasing distress.

Assessment

Assessment of discomforting conditions should first be directed toward determining the seriousness of the problem that underlies the discomfort, and identification of reversible causes. One implication of Norris' (1982) view of discomfort as a form of protection is that discomfort may signal the presence of injury or dysfunction that requires remediation. Thus, pain may signal ischemia, dyspnea may signal hypoxemia, dizziness may

T A B L E   1 4 – 6
Common Misconceptions About Pain in Older Adults

MISCONCEPTION	CORRECTION
Pain is a natural outcome of growing old.	Pain is not an inevitable part of aging. Its presence necessitates assessment, diagnosis, and treatment as in any age group.
Pain perception or sensitivity decreases with age.	Conflicting data exist. This generalization results in failure to note important indicators of pain, resulting in needless suffering and undertreatment.
Potential side effects of narcotics make them too dangerous to use to relieve pain in elderly people.	Narcotics may be used safely in elderly people if the person's response to medication is followed and evaluated closely and the altered pharmacokinetics of narcotics in the elderly recognized.
If the elderly patient appears to be occupied, sleeps, or can be otherwise distracted from pain, then he or she does not have much pain.	The older adult need not show pain behavior actually to feel pain.
If the older person is depressed, especially if there is no known cause for the pain, then depression is causing the pain. Pain is a symptom of depression and will subside if the depression is effectively treated.	Depression may result from chronic pain. It is dangerous to assume that treatment of depression is all that is needed to relieve the pain.
Narcotics are totally inappropriate for all patients with chronic, nonmalignant pain.	Little evidence supports this view; however, several studies show that prolonged narcotic therapy for selected patients with chronic nonmalignant pain can be safe and humane.

Data from McCaffery, M. and Beebe, A. *Pain: Clinical Manual for Nursing Practice.* St. Louis: C.V. Mosby, 1989.

point to inadequate cerebral perfusion, and fatigue may warn of drug intolerance, anemia, or other underlying systemic disease. Nausea and itching may alert the clinician to a toxic or allergic reaction.

The first goal of assessment thus should be to determine whether there is an immediate threat signalled by the discomfort, so that more definitive assessment and treatment may ensue. As this is being established, the nurse should determine what factors exacerbate the discomfort and seek to reduce them. With chronic discomfort, the likelihood that an underlying remediable pathological process that requires immediate attention is lowered. In this instance, the emphasis shifts to describing accurately baseline levels of discomfort and aggravating and alleviating factors, so that a long-term management approach can be developed and evaluated.

Before discussing specific approaches to

assessment of chronic discomfort, it is worthwhile noting that nurses and other health care providers may practice on the basis of misconceptions about pain or treatment of pain. These misconceptions may extend to other forms of discomfort. McCaffery and Beebe (1989) identify common misconceptions about pain in elderly people that impede accurate assessment. These misconceptions and more accurate statements are summarized in Table 14–6. Nurses should examine which of these misconceptions they may subscribe to so that important assessment cues are not overlooked.

Parameters of discomfort to be assessed include

- character of the discomfort
- location
- onset
- severity
- duration
- aggravating factors
- alleviating factors
- impact on daily living, including relationships with others and ability to sleep, eat, work, exercise, and perform sexually

This clinical format is often sufficient to assess the individual's discomfort. However, in some instances, the use of formalized assessment tools is indicated; McCaffery and Beebe (1989) have reviewed several varieties to assess chronic pain. The range of measurement approaches is similar for all types of discomfort. Types of measurement instruments include simple descriptive scales, numeric scales, word scales, graphic rating scales, sensory matching scales, color scales, visual analogue scales, extensive pain questionnaires, and diaries. In addition to these tools for measurement of pain and dyspnea, a number of scales attempt to assess the extent to which the symptom interferes with customary activities (see, for example, Mahler and Harver [1990] on dyspnea measurement and Roland and Morris [1983] for low back pain). It is useful to be familiar with the range of tools available, as individual expression of pain can be quite varied, and choosing the right tool for the right person may be the cornerstone of developing a successful approach to pain management. Specific questions about pain yield more complete and accurate information than open-ended questions. Figure 14–4 displays three different approaches to obtaining ratings of pain.

When selecting an instrument for use in assessment of alterations in comfort, the fol-

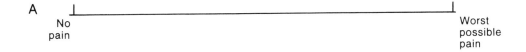

A

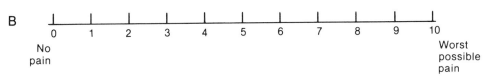

B

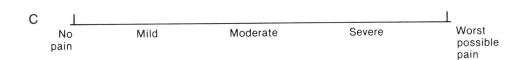

C

FIGURE 14-4

Examples of pain assessment scales. (From Carrieri-Kohlman, V., Lindsey, A.M. and West, C.M. (eds.). *Pathophysiological Phenomena in Nursing: Human Responses to Illness.* 2nd ed. Philadelphia: W.B. Saunders, 1993, p. 315.)

lowing considerations should be met: (1) the instrument should have demonstrated reliability and validity, (2) the instrument should be appropriate for the cognitive level of the patient, and (3) the nurse should be alert to signs that the patient finds the assessment instrument itself burdensome. Many instruments reported in the literature for measurement of specific alterations in comfort were developed initially for research purposes. Such measurement approaches do not always translate easily into clinical settings. Measurement instruments developed for research purposes are frequently lengthy and involve procedures for standardized administration that may prove burdensome for an individual who is uncomfortable. Table 14–7 summarizes many of the widely accepted measurement instruments for dyspnea, pain, fatigue, and nausea.

Planning and Intervention

Planning to prevent or minimize pain in clinical situations in which pain is predictable, such as postoperatively, is now accepted as the standard of care for all patients. The AHCPR Acute Pain Management Guidelines (1992) recommend obtaining a pain history preoperatively when possible; it should include information about (1) significant prior or ongoing episodes of pain and its effect on the person; (2) prior experience with pain control methods, specifying those that did and did not work; (3) the person's attitude toward using opioid and anxiolytic medicines, and determining presence or his-

tory of substance abuse; (4) the person's typical coping responses for stress or pain; (5) family expectations concerning pain, stress, and postoperative course and care; (6) ways in which the person describes or shows pain; and (7) the person's knowledge of, expectations about, and preferences for managing pain.

In addition to these preoperative assessment maneuvers, the AHCPR Acute Pain Guideline panel recommends selecting a pain measurement tool for use prior to the painful procedure or experience, so that the patient can be made familiar with the assessment approach and how it will be used postprocedure. When possible, consider involving the patient in the choice of measurement instrument; many exist, as discussed earlier.

Unfortunately, the opportunities for prevention of dyspnea, fatigue, or nausea are less well-defined in the literature. In the case of nausea associated with cancer chemotherapy, premedication with antiemetics is often advocated. In addition, attempts to reduce pairing of distinctive stimuli with chemotherapy administration are recommended to prevent anticipatory nausea. In prevention of dyspnea, helping patients tune into risk factors or triggers of episodes of dyspnea allows them to manipulate personal situations by avoiding precipitants or to prepare for the dyspnea-inducing stimulus by taking medications or using relaxation techniques. Energy conservation techniques are advocated for prevention of both dyspnea and fatigue (see section on Activity Intolerance).

TABLE 14 - 7
Assessment Options for Alterations in Comfort

ALTERATION	DOMAIN ASSESSED	ASSESSMENT TOOL	SCALE PROPERTIES
Dyspnea	Dyspnea associated with activity	American Thoracic Society Breathlessness Scale (Brooks, 1982)	Ordinal: 0–4 range
		Oxygen-Cost Diagram (OCD) (McGavin et al., 1978)	Visual analogue scale; distance measured along 0–100-mm ruler
		Baseline Dyspnea Index (Mahler and Harver, 1990)	Ordinal rating using specific criteria by interviewer, 0–4 range
	Intensity of dyspnea	Rating of perceived breathlessness (Burdon et al., 1982)	Ordinal rating of adjectives; similar to Borg rating of perceived exertion (RPE)
		Visual analogue scale for breathlessness (Cockcroft et al., 1989)	Distance measured along 0–100-mm ruler
	Behavioral manifestations	Observation for increased respiratory rate, restlessness, diaphoresis, use of accessory respiratory muscles, pursed lip breathing (Carrieri-Kohlman and Janson-Bjerklie, 1993)	No scaling reported—clinical observation only
Pain	Intensity	Visual analogue scale (Scott and Huskisson, 1976)	Distance measured along 0–100-mm ruler
		Numerical rating scale or word graphic scale (Tesler et al., 1991)	0 to 10, or no pain to worst possible pain
	Multidimensional: sensory, affective, evaluative, location, and intensity	McGill/Melzack Pain Questionnaire (Melzack, 1983)	78 descriptors, body diagrams, verbal intensity scale
	Behavioral manifestations	Facial Action Coding System (Ekman and Friesen, 1978)	Codes presence of facial appearances associated with pain
		(Keefe, 1982)	Codes presence/absence of behaviors associated with pain, including position changes, bracing, guarding, rubbing, grimacing

Exercise interventions are increasingly being used as a way to prevent discomfort. Pulmonary rehabilitation has been shown to reduce dyspnea in those with COPD (Carrieri-Kohlman and Janson-Bjerklie, 1993), reduce feelings of fatigue (Piper, 1993), and reduce pain in those with osteoarthritis (Fisher and Pendergast, 1992). Finally, preparing patients with sensory information about the procedure may reduce distress.

When prevention is not possible or fails, interventions should be employed to reduce the specific form of discomfort, remaining alert for new types of discomfort that may arise (Table 14–8). Categories of specific intervention strategies include (1) pharmacotherapy; (2) exercise interventions; (3) other physical modalities, such as positioning, peripheral stimulation, counterirritant application, application of heat and cold; (4) environmental manipulations, such as temperature alteration, use of fans, control of environmental irritants; (5) cognitive strategies, such as relaxation, hypnosis, and interventions to increase perception of control over a symptom; and (6) behavioral changes, such as structuring of activity and rest patterns, avoidance of discomfort-inducing situations, and energy conservation techniques.

Pharmacotherapy

Pharmacological approaches are the mainstay of treatment for both acute and chronic pain. Pharmacological interventions can be directed at various levels of neural and cognitive experience of discomfort, as follows: (1) relieving the initial nociceptive stimulus

T A B L E   1 4 – 7
Assessment Options for Alterations in Comfort *Continued*

ALTERATION	DOMAIN ASSESSED	ASSESSMENT TOOL	SCALE PROPERTIES
	Physiological manifestations	Observation for sympathetic response: increase in heart and respiratory rates, BP, pallor, diaphoresis, pupillary dilation (Puntillo and Tesler, 1993)	No specific metric associated—clinical observation only
Fatigue	Intensity	Visual analogue scale to measure fatigue severity (VAS-F) (Lee et al., 1991)	Distance measured along 0–100-mm ruler
		Likert-type adjective scales (Piper, 1993)	
		Pearson-Byars Fatigue Feeling Tone Checklist (Pearson, 1957)	10-item adjective checklist
		Fatigue Severity Scale (Krupp et al., 1989)	9-item Likert scale rating severity of features of fatigue
	Multidimensional scales: mental fatigue, general fatigue, and specific fatigue	Fatigue Symptom Checklist (Yoshitake, 1978)	30-item checklist
	Four dimensions	Piper Fatigue Scale (PFS) (Piper, 1993)	41-item visual analogue scale
	Behavioral manifestations	Observe for changes in physical appearance, affect, attitude, and in activity and communication patterns (Rhoten, 1982)	No scaling established
Nausea	Intensity	Visual analogue scale for nausea (Kris et al., 1989)	Distance measured along 0–100-mm ruler
	Combines activity level with intensity	Duke Descriptive Scale (Cotanch and Strum, 1988)	Ordinal scale—1–4
	Frequency, severity, and duration of nausea and vomiting	Morrow Assessment of Nausea and Vomiting (MANE) (Morrow, 1984)	Likert scaling
	Duration, frequency, and distress of nausea, vomiting, and retching	Rhodes Index of Nausea and Vomiting (INV-Form 2) (McMillan et al., 1989)	5-point Likert scale

(as in nitrates to relieve angina, or anti-inflammatory agents to reduce tissue destruction in autoimmune disorders); (2) influencing the peripheral receptor site (e.g., nonsteroidal anti-inflammatory agents interfering with prostaglandin synthesis, to prevent sensitization of nociceptors); (3) blocking transmission of the nociceptive stimulus at the peripheral nerve level (nerve blocks); (4) blocking pain perception at the level of the medulla or midbrain (opiate analgesia); and (5) influencing affective response to pain at the cortical level (anxiolytics, antidepressants). Because the experience of discomfort can be modified at so many different sites, most authorities recommend a stepwise approach to pharmacological management, beginning with agents that remove the noxious stimulus, if possible, and then proceeding with agents that have the most acceptable side effect profile.

In severe acute pain, if the underlying stimulus cannot be removed, narcotic analgesia may be used safely and effectively with older adults, as long as altered pharmacokinetics are considered (see Chapter 18). Slowed clearance of these drugs may result in older adults requiring lower total doses to achieve relief. It is interesting that in a comparison of morphine delivered by patient-controlled analgesia (PCA) with intramuscular (IM) injections in 83 men over age 60 years without chronic cognitive impairment who had major elective surgery, the group receiving PCA narcotic had better pain control, less postoperative confusion, and fewer severe pulmonary complications. This finding is particularly noteworthy given

T A B L E   1 4 – 8
Interventions Appropriate for Various Types of Alteration in Comfort

TYPE OF DISCOMFORT	APPLICABLE INTERVENTIONS	TYPE OF DISCOMFORT	APPLICABLE INTERVENTIONS
Pain Secondary to:		Rheumatoid arthritis Continued	Relaxation exercises
Coronary artery disease	Activity modification to include rest periods, energy conservation techniques		Imagery
	Surgical revascularization		Medications: ASA, NSAIDs, antirheumatic drugs (gold, penicillamine), antimalarial drugs, steroids
	Medications: vasodilators		Surgery—joint reconstruction
Peripheral vascular disease	Exercise regimen: gradual increase in walking		Psychotherapy: adjustment to chronic pain
	Modify activity to include rest periods	Constipation	Exercise to increase abdominal muscle tone and peristalsis
	Medications: quinine tablets		Increased fluids to increase amount of fluid in stool
	Surgical revascularization		Positioning: curled in bed to relieve cramping pain, over toilet to facilitate bowel evacuation
Diabetic peripheral neuropathies	Medications: phenytoin and carbamazepine; propranolol (Scadding, 1984)		Medications: laxatives (see section on constipation for hazards)
Metastatic cancer	Hypnosis	Nausea Secondary to:	
	Progressive relaxation	Cancer chemotherapy and radiation therapy	Medications: phenothiazines, tetrahydrocannabinol
	Massage		Progressive relaxation exercises
	Range-of-motion exercises		Imagery
	Distraction		Psychotherapy
	Being with the patient		Reduction of external stimuli
	Medications administered on a regular rather than prn basis		Cool compresses on forehead
	Narcotic and non-narcotic analgesics		Distraction
	Palliative radiation therapy	Ulcer disease	Medications: antacids, H_1 histaminic blockers
Degenerative joint disease	Application of heat to affected joints	Itching Secondary to:	
	Medications: nonsteroidal anti-inflammatory agents, enteric-coated aspirin	Contact dermatitis	Cool compresses
Chronic back pain	Exercises to strengthen abdominal muscles		Topical steroids
	Transcutaneous electrical stimulation		Antihistamines
	Ice massage (Melzack, 1984)		Distraction
Herpes zoster	Medications: steroids during acute phase	Seborrheic dermatitis	Coaltar shampoos
	Cool compresses	Eczema	Cool compresses
	Relaxation exercises		Topical steroids
	Imagery	Neurodermatitis	Emollient creams
Postherpetic neuralgia	Distraction		Distraction
	Counterirritation with cold; vibration	Dry skin	Emollient creams
	Transcutaneous electrical stimulation	Dyspnea Secondary to:	
	Acupuncture	Obstructive lung disease	Position change
	Medications: carbamazepine and antidepressants (Scadding, 1984)	Congestive heart failure	Slow rate of activity
Dependent edema	Positioning to relieve edema: elevate legs	Asthma	Alter breathing pattern
	Use of elastic support stockings		Relaxation techniques
	Ankle-circling exercises while seated		Distraction
	Medications: diuretics		Activity modification
Rheumatoid arthritis	Counterirritant therapy (White, 1973)		Medications: bronchodilators (obstructive disease); diuretics (pulmonary congestion)
	Application of heat		Oxygen
	Splinting		
	Range-of-motion exercises		
	Adaptive equipment to reduce stress on joints		
	Rest periods with joints in extension, body in proper alignment		

that over half the patients had COPD and over 40 per cent had coronary artery disease. The effects were attributed to the more consistent levels of morphine achieved by the PCA group (Egbert et al., 1990).

In chronic pain, most advocate beginning with agents such as acetaminophen, progressing through use of nonsteroidal anti-inflammatory agents, and proceeding to opiate analgesia. In general, use of regular doses of analgesic medicines, rather than a *pro re nata* (prn) dosing schedule is recommended. Note that the mechanisms of opiate and nonopiate analgesics are somewhat different, and therefore there is a rationale for using them in combination. There is evidence that combining opiate and nonopiate analgesia reduces the overall opiate dose required. A role for opiates in controlling chronic nonmalignant pain is increasingly recognized. Although concern about addiction to opiates is frequently expressed by patients and health care providers, little evidence supports the idea that those who take narcotics for chronic pain syndromes become addicted (Puntillo and Tesler, 1993). Withholding of narcotic analgesia for those with chronic malignant pain has resulted in malpractice awards for negligence (Roark, 1991).

Pharmacotherapy for dyspnea generally is focused on reducing the work of breathing through the use of bronchodilators, corticosteroids, and theophylline. Controlled studies have shown inhaled beta$_2$-adrenergic agonists to be effective in reducing dyspnea (Carrieri-Kohlman and Janson-Bjerklie, 1993). Theophylline has been shown to reduce dyspnea without affecting objective pulmonary function tests, but it is often not used because of its potential for toxicity. Benzodiazepines and opiates reduce dyspnea by decreasing the respiratory drive, or by altering central perception of discomfort. Use of nebulized morphine may reduce dyspnea without adversely affecting objective respiratory parameters (Farncombe and Chater, 1993). These medicines are not recommended for routine use in those without terminal illness.

A wide range of drug treatments for nausea are available, most of which are thought to block dopamine receptors in the chemoreceptor trigger zone and histamine and muscarinic cholinergic receptors in the vomiting center (Larson et al., 1993). More recently, a serotonin antagonist (ondansetron) has become an important drug in the management of chemotherapy-induced nausea (Cubeddu et al., 1990). Table 14–9 summarizes commonly prescribed drugs for management of acute nausea and vomiting. The use of these drugs in chronic nausea and vomiting is less well established.

Drug treatments for fatigue are not generally supported by controlled studies. Anecdotal or case studies reports are the primary source of evidence at present. Use of amantadine has been shown in controlled trials to reduce fatigue in patients with multiple sclerosis (Piper, 1993).

Exercise Interventions

Aerobic exercise has been shown to reduce pain in cardiac disease by elevation of

TABLE 14 – 9
Drugs Commonly Used in Treatment of Nausea

DRUG	DOSAGE
Dexamethasone (Decadron)	Oral: 10–40 mg every 3 hr IV: 8–20 mg every 3 hr
Diphenhydramine (Benadryl)	Oral: 25–50 mg IV: 25–50 mg
Droperidol (Inapsine)	IM: 2.5 mg every 4–6 hr IV: 2.5 mg every 3 hr
Haloperidol (Haldol)	Oral: 1–2 mg every 12 hr IM: 1–2 mg every 12 hr
Lorazepam (Ativan)	Oral: 1–2 mg IV: 1–2 mg
Metoclopramide (Reglan)	Oral: 0.5–1 mg/kg every 2 hr IV: 1–2 mg/kg every 2–3 hr for two to six doses
Ondansetron (Zofrin)	Oral: not available IV: 0.15 mg/kg 30 min prior to chemotherapy and every 8 hr for two doses
Prochlorperazine (Compazine)	Oral: 10–20 mg every 4 hr 30 mg spansules every 12 hr p.r.: 25 mg every 4–6 hr IM: 5–10 mg every 4–6 hr IV: 10–30 mg every 4–6 hr
Thiethylperazine (Torecan)	Oral: 10–20 mg every 4 hr p.r.: 10 mg every 4–6 hr IM: 10 mg every 4 hr

IM, intramuscular; IV, intravenous; p.r., per rectum.
Adapted from Fischer, D. and Knobf, M. *The Cancer Chemotherapy Handbook.* 3rd ed. Chicago: Year Book Medical Publishers, 1989, pp. 506–507.

the ischemic threshold (Rechnitzer, 1990), to reduce fatigue in women with breast cancer (Piper, 1993), and to be associated with reduced nausea and vomiting in patients receiving cancer chemotherapy (Larson et al., 1993). Muscle strengthening exercise programs have been shown to decrease pain medication use in those with osteoarthritis (Fisher and Pendergast, 1992), as have fitness walking programs (Kovar et al., 1992), probably by the increased muscle providing better support to the joints. Pulmonary rehabilitation has been shown to reduce dyspnea and fatigue in those with COPD, although the mechanism of the effect is not clear, since pulmonary rehabilitation programs also include a variety of psychoeducational activities as well (Piper, 1993; Carrieri-Kohlman and Janson-Bjerklie, 1993). Inspiratory respiratory muscle training has been demonstrated effective in reducing dyspnea in patients with COPD (Harver et al., 1989), suggesting that exercise may reduce the work of breathing and possibly influence both dyspnea and fatigue in this manner. These exercise programs have not yet been shown to be effective in respiratory muscle fatigue (Ingersoll, 1989).

Physical Modalities

Application of heat and cold has long been used successfully to reduce pain sensations through action on the peripheral nervous system that either removes noxious stimulation or blocks its afferent transmission by providing alternative stimulation. Heat is found to be useful in joint pain associated with degenerative joint disease, muscle soreness, and muscle strain. Heat causes vasodilation, speeding the removal of metabolic byproducts, and can reduce muscle spasm and facilitate relaxation. Methods of delivering heat are quite varied, including heating pads, paraffin baths, heat lamps, whirlpool, steam cabinets, diathermy, and ultrasound. Cold application is more commonly used in acute injury to reduce swelling and inflammation. When both methods are used, the skin should be assessed carefully for injury from application of hot or cold. Another precaution recommended is to limit the time and frequency of treatment to no more than 30 minutes, four times each day (Puntillo and Tesler, 1993). Counterirritant therapies, in the form of topical applications of liniment, or more recently, in the form of capsaicin, have demonstrated efficacy in relieving both joint pain and neuropathic pain, such as that from reflex sympathetic dystrophy.

Other physical modalities used in pain control include cutaneous stimulation, such as tapping, vibration, or rubbing, and transcutaneous electrical nerve stimulation (TENS). TENS stimulation is not effective in treatment of low back pain (Deyo et al., 1990), but it may be effective in various types of neuropathic pain, such as postamputation, or in postherpetic neuralgia (Johnson et al., 1991).

Environmental Manipulations

Monitoring the environment for unpleasant stimuli that may worsen an already uncomfortable person's condition is a routine nursing function. Common areas that require manipulation include room temperature, type of bedcovers, and positioning in bed or chair. Carrieri-Kohlman and Janson-Bjerklie (1993) have noted that some people with dyspnea get immediate relief from a cool fan blowing on the face. Repositioning to facilitate good body alignment or to allow for shifts in body position may help reduce pain or dyspnea. Prompt removal of bodily waste (emptying urinals, suction bottles, and bedside commodes) will remove potential contributors to nausea. Although environmental factors are believed to play a role in control of anticipatory nausea, documentation of the extent of the role environmental triggers play is still needed (Larson et al., 1993). In general, people with alterations in comfort should be given considerable latitude in arranging their physical environment to promote comfort, as reactions to the environment can be highly personalized.

Cognitive Strategies

Relaxation, distraction, and guided imagery are all strategies that have been tried in reducing pain, dyspnea, nausea, and fatigue. In pain, dyspnea, and nausea, the mechanisms by which these work include reduction of anxiety, which is thought to potentiate the reception of noxious stimuli; changing the efferent input to the periphery; and changing the affective experience associated with the symptom. Progressive muscle relaxation, isolated muscle relaxation, deep breathing, and shifting attentional focus have all been demonstrated to reduce either pain intensity or pain distress levels at a minimum, and sometimes indirect measures of pain, such as analgesic use (Puntillo and Tessler, 1993). Gift et al. (1992) found that relaxation tapes were effective in reducing dyspnea and anxiety in COPD patients. The data supporting the use of progressive muscle relaxation in prevention of nausea and vomiting are sparser but suggest that these therapies may be effective (Burish and Lyles, 1981, and Cotanch and Strum, 1987, cited in Larson et al., 1993).

Behavioral Change

A variety of behavioral changes have been used to reduce discomfort. Energy conservation techniques have already been mentioned as possible strategies for management of both dyspnea and fatigue. Dietary modifications are often used in management of nausea, although no controlled studies of their effects are reported. The following examples show how these diverse strategies can be implemented in selected patient situations.

CASE EXAMPLE

Mr. Smith was admitted to the long-term care unit for terminal care, having refused dialysis for chronic renal failure. His other problems included a recent myocardial infarction and balloon angioplasty, left-sided hemiparesis from a cerebrovascular accident 5 years ago, a chronic left-sided pain syndrome thought to be due to the CVA, and a 5-year history of depression. Despite these problems, he was ambulatory with assistance, continent, and able to participate in all activities of daily living. Mr. Smith complained of fatigue and pain whenever he was not asleep. His pain was worse when initiating movement, although once moving the pain intensity seemed to diminish. He was unable to rate the severity of his pain nor describe it precisely. He also had difficulty distinguishing angina from his chronic left body pain.

The goals for this patient were (1) to prevent additional sources of discomfort, such as fatigue from deconditioning, constipation, or discomfort from poor hygiene, (2) to decrease the patient's pain during performance of routine care tasks, and (3) to reduce feelings of fatigue during daytime. The initial evaluation of pain took place during routine A.M. care, when the patient complained of severe chest pain and dizziness while transferring from lying to sitting. An electrocardiogram showed no changes suggesting ischemia, and the pain did not respond to administration of sublingual nitroglycerin. The conclusion was drawn that transfer activities and low-intensity self-care activities did not produce cardiac ischemia, and therefore another source of pain had to be considered.

Attempts to make assignment of staff consistent showed that the patient complained less of pain with familiar staff members whom he trusted to assist him in a predictable manner. A scheduled ambulation program produced no increase in pain complaints and increased the patient's endurance sufficiently so that he could take himself to the toilet and sit up for meals. When breakthrough pain occurred, analgesia was obtained using oral narcotics. As the patient's uremia worsened and he was unable to participate in self-care activities, he complained of pain with bathing. The pain was alleviated by prebath administration of acetaminophen with codeine, and careful attention to keeping him warm during the bath. Fatigue was managed by providing care for energy-consuming tasks, such as bathing and dressing, while providing assistance with transfers to a sitting position for eating and drinking.

Interventions for discomfort may be quite varied, depending upon the source of dis-comfort. One patient had discomfort from dyspnea and chronic lower extremity edema. His dyspnea was better controlled after he was taught energy conservation techniques. He had fewer episodes when he needed supplemental oxygen and a greater feeling of control over his daily routine, because it depended less on assistance from professional staff. Discomfort from lower extremity edema was achieved by assisting him to take a tub bath. The "weightlessness" that his legs felt while he was in the tub was a source of enormous relief.

Consider a third example of care for a patient who has a different source of alteration in comfort, and a different prognosis. Suppose you are caring for a patient with chronic pain following amputation. He frequently requests oxycodone for relief on a regular basis, although his surgery took place over a month ago. The team is concerned about habituation to narcotic analgesics—the patient is concerned about living with unbearable pain if he gives up his narcotics. Figure 14–5 shows an approach to management of pain that is consistent with the suggestions adapted from those made by McCaffery and Beebe (1989) for individualizing pain relief, which are summarized in Box 14–3.

Evaluation

Criteria for evaluation of alteration in comfort include:

1. Is the discomfort relieved?
2. If the discomfort is not resolved permanently, for how long at a time is the patient without discomfort?
3. If the patient always has some discomfort, is the discomfort reduced in intensity?
4. Is an etiology defined for the discomfort?
5. What adverse effect, if any, has the patient experienced from the interventions to relieve discomfort?

COMMUNICATION IMPAIRMENT, VERBAL

Definition and Scope of Problem

Impaired verbal communication is "the state in which the individual experiences a decreased or absent ability to use or understand language in human interaction" (NANDA, 1992, p. 36). Some have suggested broadening this diagnostic category to in-

SYMPTOM	Stump pain r/t disruption in nerve supply, decreased adipose tissue		
DATE/TIME	**MANIFESTATION**	**INTERVENTION**	**RESPONSE**
7/15/94 1440	c/o burning stump pain rated 6/10	Remove prosthesis & elevate leg	c/o little relief—pain now 4/10
	after walking w/prosthesis	Encourage to do rubbing & tapping	Requesting "little red pill"
	No ulceration noted		(narcotic analgesic) for pain
7/15/94 1500	Pain 5/10 after nonpharmacologic	Oxycodone 1 tablet given	Complete relief of pain
	measures attempted	Discussed alternative forms of	Agreed to keep pain diary
		pain control & hazards of oxycodone:	listing activity, intensity of pain
		1) Acetaminophen scheduled q 4 h	
		2) More aggressive stump stim.	
		3) Consider use of TENS unit	
		4) Shorter but more frequent walks	
7/20/94 1700	Pain diary results show:	1) Change major exercise session to AM	Pt. willing to try new approaches
		2) Encourage shorter more frequent sessions	
	1) Baseline pain 2/10 best in AM		Will continue to keep diary
	2) Pain crescendos to max (8/10) q day after PM exercise session		
	3) Pt. only exercises once q/day		
	4) Pt. leaves prosthesis on all day		
	5) Oxycodone use averages tid		
7/23/94 1700	Pain diary results:	1) Encourage continuing current plan	Skeptical @ acetaminophen but
	1) Baseline pain unchanged	2) Try acetaminophen 4 gm per day	willing to try
	2) Pain max now 5/10	in divided doses (pt. to decide when)	Worried @ losing access to oxycodone
	3) Pt. exercises t.i.d.	3) Maintain diary	but understands risks of continued use
	4) Removes prosthesis while in room		
	5) Oxycodone use down to bid		
7/28/94 1730	Pain diary results:	1) Continue current plan	Pt. agrees. Believes he can live with
	1) Baseline pain: 0/10	2) D/c oxycodone	current level of pain
	2) Pain max now 3/10	3) Teach patient to inspect stump	Knows narcotic analgesia can be
	3) Exercise freq. unchanged	& report changes in pain or lesions	reinstituted should need arise.
	4) Greater intensity of exercises		
	5) Oxycodone use down to <1/day		

F I G U R E   1 4 – 5

Sample care plan for patient with Alteration in Comfort: Pain.

clude other forms of communication difficulty, such as incongruent verbal and nonverbal communication and difficulty sending the intended message. However, since these aspects of the diagnosis are only now beginning to be studied (Reimer, 1994), our discussion is limited to problems in verbal communication.

Impairments in verbal communication can be broadly categorized into three groups:

1. Impairments in reception of verbal communication of others—for example, those that occur with severe hearing impairment and altered arousal states;

2. Impairments in central processing of received neural impulses or production of words to be expressed—for example, those in patients with receptive or expressive aphasia or apraxia; and

3. Impairments in the mechanism of

Tips for Individualizing Interventions to Relieve Discomfort

1. Use a variety of discomfort-relieving measures.

2. Implement intervention measures before discomfort becomes severe.

3. Include what the patient believes will be effective.

4. Consider whether the patient is willing or able to be active or passive in application of discomfort-relieving interventions.

5. Select the strength of the discomfort relief measure based on patient behavior indicating severity of discomfort. For example, if the patient complains of severe dyspnea, consider using both oxygen and coached breathing, rather than coached breathing alone.

6. If an intervention is ineffective the first time, encourage the patient to try it a few more times before discarding it.

7. Be open minded about what may relieve discomfort.

8. Don't give up.

9. Do no harm.

speech formation—for example, those in dysarthria and in individuals with laryngectomies or endotracheal tubes.

The consequences of untreated impaired verbal communication include social isolation, being incorrectly diagnosed as cognitively impaired, excess dependency because of inability to express needs and abilities, altered self-concept, decreased self-esteem or powerlessness, and fear and anxiety. Impaired verbal communication may also lead to individual coping problems as well as altered family process and role relationships.

Older people are disproportionately represented among those with communications impairments. Aging-related changes in the respiratory and neuromuscular systems produce changes in speech performance that are hardly noticeable, but certain diseases may produce serious deficits in communication ability when superimposed upon aging changes. For example, chronic lung disease reduces airflow, which may reduce speech

volume to the extent that speech is quite difficult to understand. Parkinson's disease also reduces the intelligibility of speech by reducing the force of airflow and ease of articulation.

Contributing Factors

Communication is "a dynamic, complex, continuous series of reciprocal events through which messages are exchanged, primarily in order to produce a response from a person or a group" (McFarland and Naschinski, 1985, p. 776). Components of communication are sender, message, receiver, and feedback. Impaired communication can occur when any of these elements is disturbed.

The model of verbal communication depicted in Figure 14–6 describes four competencies necessary for formulating and sending a verbal message: language ideation, symbolization, translation, and execution. Impairments in any one of these competencies will produce an impairment in verbal communication. Three of these four competencies require intact neurological and cognitive functioning. Language usage requires the integrated function of the respiratory system and the oral-motor apparatus. One's cultural background greatly influences the processes of symbolization, translation, and execution. Table 14–10 summarizes factors that commonly contribute to impaired verbal communication.

Sensory Impairment

Hearing loss can severely impair an individual's ability to communicate verbally. Messages are incorrectly received and misunderstandings are common. Unlike young people with hearing impairments, older adults are more likely to have concurrent visual impairment, meaning that visual cues useful for younger hearing-impaired persons, like lip reading, are not always available. A review of the impact of hearing and vision loss on a person can be found in Chapter 13 and in the section on Sensory-Perceptual Alterations in this chapter.

Aphasia

Aphasia results from damage to speech and language centers in the dominant cerebral hemisphere, generally caused by cerebrovascular infarction (Brookshire, 1991). Aphasias can be crudely classified into three types, according to the presumed locus of neuronal damage. Broca's aphasia, sometimes called expressive aphasia, results from damage to Broca's area in the third frontal

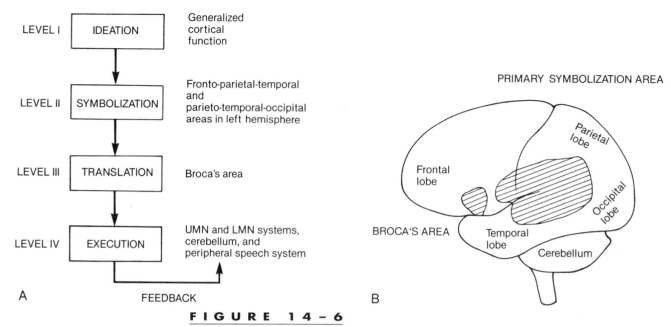

LEVEL I	IDEATION	Generalized cortical function
LEVEL II	SYMBOLIZATION	Fronto-parietal-temporal and parieto-temporal-occipital areas in left hemisphere
LEVEL III	TRANSLATION	Broca's area
LEVEL IV	EXECUTION	UMN and LMN systems, cerebellum, and peripheral speech system

A   FEEDBACK

B

PRIMARY SYMBOLIZATION AREA

BROCA'S AREA   Frontal lobe   Parietal lobe   Occipital lobe   Temporal lobe   Cerebellum

FIGURE 14-6

A, Hierarchical model of human communication. (From Hutchinson, J.M. and Beasley, D.S. Speech and language functioning. *In* Schow, R.L. et al. (eds.). *Communication Disorders of the Aged: A Guide for Health Professionals.* Baltimore: University Park Press, 1978, p. 157.) *B,* The human brain, showing selected communication centers.

convolution of the left hemisphere, the subcortical white matter, extending posteriorly to the inferior motor portion of the precentral gyrus. It is typically characterized by awkward articulation, restricted vocabulary, very simple grammatical structures, and relative preservation of auditory comprehension. In contrast, receptive aphasia (also called sensory aphasia, or posterior aphasia) results from damage to neurons in Wernicke's area, which lies just next to the gyrus of Heschl, where the primary auditory cortext is located. Wernicke's aphasia is characterized by fluent speech, but the speech is often lacking in content or meaning. Conduction aphasia results from damage to the arcuate fasciculus, the pathway connecting

Wernicke's area to Broca's area. Speech quality is more fluent than in Broca's aphasia, and the hallmark is inability to repeat or write what the patient hears (Collins, 1989). Global neuronal degeneration associated with dementing disorders may also produce aphasia, although it usually does not occur until the late stages of the disease.

Aphasia affects the individual's ability to process symbolic materials of all types, including speech, hearing, and written communication. Nonspeech-related problems that often accompany aphasia include facial muscle weakness, visual field deficits, emotional lability, reduced attention span, and impaired short-term memory. The accompanying deficiencies make compensation for

TABLE 14-10

Contributing Factors to Impaired Verbal Communication

RECEPTIVE FACTORS	PERCEPTUAL FACTORS	EXPRESSIVE FACTORS
Hearing loss Disordered arousal states: Coma High anxiety Inadequate time for reception of message or provision of feedback	Unable to interpret foreign language* Delirium or dementia: both may produce a variety of cognitive impairments, such as impaired comprehension, word-finding problems Cerebral infarction	Dysarthria, which may be due to cerebellar dysfunction weakness or paralysis of oral/ facial musculature Destruction of larynx Respiratory disease, resulting in too small an airflow for intelligible speech Cerebral infarction, producing motor sequencing problems (apraxia) or expressive aphasia

* Note that a "foreign" language may be a commonly recognized language, such as English, Spanish, Japanese, and so on, or it may be a less familiar "language," such as medical or nursing jargon.

the lost communications functions more difficult, although not impossible.

Apraxia

Speech apraxia results from a defect in motor speech programming. The lesion responsible involves the left front lobe, but apraxia may result from lesions far away from Broca's area, such as the parietal or temporal lobes. In contrast to the characteristics of aphasic speech, in speech apraxia the amount of articulatory errors depends on the complexity of motor adjustments required. For example, as word length increases, so do errors; high-frequency phonemes are less likely to be the source of errors (Collins, 1989). The deficit is seen in dementing disorders and after cerebral infarction. Hesitancy and reduced rate of speech and problems with speech fluency all may be manifestations of speech apraxia. Apraxia may occur alone or in combination with other speech disorders, such as aphasia or dysarthria.

Dysarthria

Impairments in innervation of speech muscles result in unintelligible speech, known as dysarthria. The various impairments that produce dysarthria include improper breathing patterns and inadequate control of the voice because of muscle weakness, paralysis, or incoordination. Strokes and degenerative neuromuscular diseases are the most common etiologies for dysarthria.

Parkinson's Disease

Individuals with basal ganglia destruction initially have a slowed pace of speech, but gradually the speech becomes inaudible. In addition to the mechanical difficulties experienced by people with Parkinson's disease, neuronal degeneration in the frontal lobes may also affect speech quality. Increasing attention is being paid to subcortical structures and their role in language and speech, but interpretation of findings from these studies is difficult, because the patients studied often have extensive neural lesions, making it difficult to parcel out the contribution of subcortical structures alone (Crosson, 1992).

Cognitive Impairments

Cognitive impairments leave the individual with impaired ability to abstract, an impoverished vocabulary, problems with motor sequencing, and word-finding diffi-

culties. As dementing disorders frequently result from a widespread pattern of neuronal degeneration, predicting the exact nature of the speech or language deficit is difficult. Generally, the more widespread the neuropathological lesions, the greater the communication deficit. See Domenico (1990) for an in-depth review of communication impairments in dementia.

Laryngectomy

Cancer involving the head and neck may require removal of the larynx, requiring the development of compensatory speech mechanisms, such as esophageal speech, or use of an artificial larynx. The resultant speech is often difficult to understand for those unaccustomed to its character, although with patience and increased practice verbal communication is possible. Laryngectomy patients who have not yet had the opportunity to develop verbal compensatory mechanisms must rely on written communication or gestures.

Endotracheal Intubation

Endotracheal intubation is used when short-term ventilatory support is needed. Usually patients are acutely ill and are cared for in an intensive care environment. The inability to communicate verbally can intensify feelings of fear and anxiety. Learning or using an alternative means of communication may be an important intervention to enhance feelings of control and to help conserve the patient's limited energy.

Assessment

Great patience is required to assess the individual with an impairment in verbal communication. Frustration and anxiety from patient or examiner will lead to poor patient performance and an inadequate estimate of the patient's abilities. The examiner should take steps to promote a relaxed, unhurried atmosphere and strive to achieve the characteristics of successful communication listed earlier.

The algorithm in Figure 14–7 summarizes the various strategies for assessment of the person with suspected impairment of verbal communication. Previously obtained clinical information about the probability and nature of the impairment guides the techniques of assessment. However, if the communication status of the patient is completely unknown, then very basic assessment maneuvers apply. First, determine arousability by calling the individual's name. If the person responds appropriately, then hearing and per-

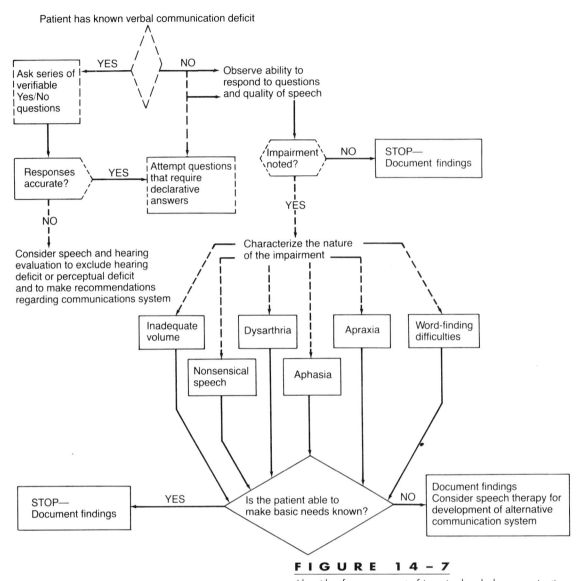

FIGURE 14-7

Algorithm for assessment of impaired verbal communication.

ception are grossly intact. If the individual does not respond appropriately, one of three disorders is present: (1) a severe impairment of arousal, suggesting a delirium or severe dementia, (2) a severe receptive aphasia, or (3) a severe hearing impairment. A fourth, less likely possibility is that severe psychosis, such as a paranoid state, is present, making the patient totally uncooperative. All conditions require prompt further evaluation, because remedying the communication deficit depends upon the underlying etiology.

Next determine whether the person can understand you. Explain that you want to make sure that you are being understood, and so you will be asking some simple questions, requiring only yes/no answers, that are easily verifiable. For example: "Good morning, is your name Mrs. Jones?

Are you from New York City? Is the shirt you are wearing red?" People who are unable to answer two of three questions accurately probably have severe hearing impairment or aphasia or a severe cognitive or emotional disorder. As in the case of people with arousal deficits, further assessment of underlying etiologies by the appropriate health care professional is in order. The order of referral to specialists for evaluation depends upon associated clinical data and the ease of obtaining consultation. For example, medical consultation is generally simple to obtain to assess for easily reversible causes of delirium, such as infection or drug toxicity. However, psychiatric consultation may be more difficult to obtain. Speech and hearing evaluations are available in most care settings and should take place before in-depth mental status testing.

Assessment of patients who can comprehend the examiner is straightforward. The pattern, rate, and content of speech should be observed for the following characteristics:

1. Can the individual make basic needs and desires known? (For example, hunger, pain, thirst, the need to urinate or defecate.)
2. Can other messages be expressed, such as preferred activities, emotions?

If neither is possible, then referral to a speech therapist is indicated, regardless of the precise nature of the speech impairment. One exception is patients with advanced dementing disorders, in which the major communication problem is widespread central nervous system degeneration rather than a more focal deficit in which potential for compensation remains.

Patients who are able to express themselves may still benefit from speech therapy. The speech therapist may be able to provide a less fatiguing, more easily understood system for communicating or may strengthen the patient's remaining capacities to enhance communication.

Planning and Intervention

The primary goal of nursing care for people who have impaired verbal communication is to establish a reliable communication system, readily understood by as many people as possible. In many instances, collaboration with a speech therapist is essential. Secondary goals include promoting normality and assisting the individual to cope with the communication impairment. Difficulty expressing oneself is enormously frustrating for most people. Ironically, that frustration may compound the communication deficit. Four major strategies for intervention exist:

1. Teaching and exercise to treat or compensate for the underlying deficit;
2. Use of alternative communications systems, such as word boards, gestures, yes/no questions;
3. Teaching others in the patient's care and social environment techniques to maximize communication effectiveness; and
4. Counselling to help patients adapt to their altered abilities.

In most cases, consultation with a speech therapist for a specific intervention plan is necessary.

Suggestions for enhancing communication that apply to individuals with communication impairments due to dysarthria, apraxia, and aphasia are adapted from Schow et al., 1978 and Burns and Halper, 1986:

- Provide a quiet, relaxed atmosphere by reducing background noise.
- Show patience by sitting down and controlling nonverbal signs of frustration, such as finger tapping, filling in words for the person, interrupting, or shouting. Tell the person you are not in a hurry.
- Encourage attempts at communication by nodding and providing appropriate feedback, keeping questions and instructions simple and direct.
- **Apraxia:** If a phrase is partially unintelligible, let the person know what part you understood and ask him or her to try again.
- **Dysarthria:** Let the individual know if you are having difficulty understanding. It may be possible for the patient to increase the precision of speech.
- **Aphasia:** Determine which sensory modality is easier for the person to use: auditory or visual, and use that modality preferentially.
- Use a slower rate of speech.
- Use questions that can be answered with "yes" or "no." Encourage the use of gestures.

Selecting an alternative form of communication for intubated patients is based on the patient's cognitive level, ability to form words with the mouth, language, and fine motor skills (Fig. 14–8; Williams, 1992).

Persons whose ability to communicate is impaired because of dementing disorders respond well to a communication style that is concrete, simple, and calm. Specific suggestions listed here are adapted from Lee (1991).

- Establish eye contact before addressing the person.
- Be sure that your body language is consistent with your verbal messages.
- Ask questions that present a choice between two things.
- Break instructions into simple steps and give one step at a time.
- Focus on concrete rather than abstract topics.
- Repeat the name of the object or person in question, thus avoiding the use of pronouns.
- Be direct; avoid the use of analogies.

Evaluation

Criteria for evaluation of care for patients with impaired verbal communication include

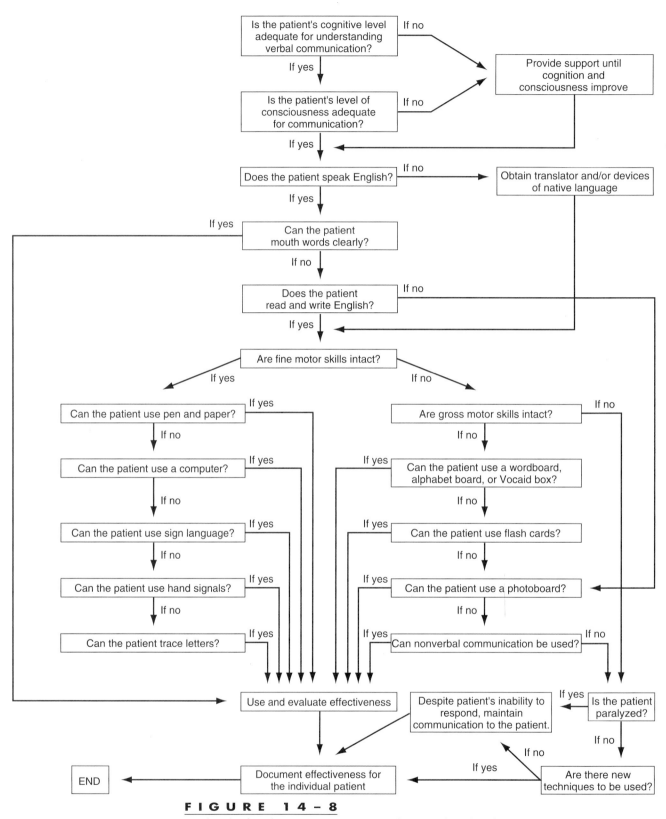

FIGURE 14–8

An algorithm for selecting a communication technique with intubated patients. (From Williams, M.L. An algorithm for selecting a communication technique with intubated patients. *Dimensions Crit Care Nurs* 11:(4):222–223, 1992. Copyright 1992 Hall Johnson Communications, Inc., Lakewood, CO. Reproduced with permission.)

1. Is the patient able to express basic needs?
2. Is the patient able to express a full range of messages, including desires, emotions, opinions, in a widely understood manner?
3. Is the underlying etiology of communication impairment known?
4. Are remedial techniques employed before turning to compensatory techniques?
5. Are patient, family, and other caregivers taught techniques to facilitate verbal communication, such as relaxation techniques, or other tips listed under interventions?
6. Is counselling provided to the patient to facilitate coping with the remaining disability?

FLUID VOLUME DEFICIT

Definition and Scope of Problem

Dehydration, or *fluid volume deficit*, is a common and vexing problem in elderly people. Old people are predisposed to dehydration because of an age-related decline in total body water, a diminished sensation of thirst, a decrease in urine-concentrating ability, and a decrease in the effectiveness of antidiuretic hormone (ADH) (Davis and Minaker, 1990; Rudman and Cohan, 1992). The consequences of fluid volume deficit are serious, including decreased functional ability, predisposition to falls because of orthostatic hypotension, constipation and fecal impaction, cognitive impairment, and predisposition to infection, and could result in death.

Contributing Factors

Decreased blood volume results form one of three factors: inadequate fluid intake, excessive fluid output, and diseases that cause abnormal shifts of fluid into the interstitial space.

Inadequate Fluid Intake

Decreased sensorium, swallowing difficulties, diminished sense of thirst, impaired verbal communication, mobility/dexterity problems, and use of restraints all contribute to difficulty in ingesting sufficient fluid. Many institutionalized patients lack the ability to reach or to manage the water pitcher and thus depend on staff, family, or friends for adequate intake to prevent dehydration. Patients who are physically able to manage their own fluid intake but who are cognitively impaired are also at high risk for inadequate fluid intake (Gaspar, 1988). Un-

fortunately, the answer to this common problem is inadequate in many hospitals and nursing homes. There is often a ritual for passing water pitchers to the bedside, but fluids are not always offered to patients during these rounds. Attempting to provide the daily requirement of fluids with meals is not the best solution, because frail people often have reduced appetites. Ingesting over 800 ml of fluid at each meal is likely to be overwhelming and reduce intake or other nutrients.

Older persons in the hospital may be made "NPO" before diagnostic procedures and have difficulty in "catching up" on fluid intake. Also, the use of thickened liquids to prevent aspiration in persons with impaired swallowing may predispose to an inadequate fluid intake, because patients often dislike the taste of the thickened liquid. Older people with mobility or cognition impairments living at home are also at great risk for inadequate fluid intake, unless fluid intake routines are implemented.

Excessive Fluid Losses

Many diseases cause increased fluid loss, including gastroenteritis with diarrhea or vomiting, uncontrolled diabetes mellitus, diabetes insipidus, fever, severe pulmonary disease with production of copious amounts of sputum, hemorrhage, overzealous diuretic therapy, and use of laxatives or bowel preparations. The ability of the renal system to concentration urine declines with age. Individuals with any of these disorders are at high risk for dehydration and require careful observation and nursing attention to make sure that fluid intake is sufficient to compensate for losses.

Plasma to Interstitial Fluid Shifts

Malignancies, trauma, severe malnutrition, and liver and renal disease may result in disturbances in fluid balance because of severe peripheral edema or ascites. Although this is the least likely cause of dehydration in older people, it should not be overlooked as a contributor.

Assessment

Assessment of fluid volume deficit in older patients is complicated by underlying pathology or age-related changes. For example, skin turgor is difficult to assess in skin that has undergone an age-related decrease in elasticity. Thus, skin turgor, if used at all to assess dehydration in the aged, should be tested on the sternum or forehead. A more useful guide to dehydration is the condition of the tongue and oral mucosa. A furrowed, dry tongue is highly suggestive of dehydration, although the oral mucosa may become dry because of anticholinergic drug use or if the person habitually breathes through the mouth. Likewise, some older people have orthostatic hypotension without dehydration.

According to Wandel (1990), between 10 and 30 per cent of elderly persons may have chronic postural hypotension, although it is unknown what proportion of this is secondary to medication side effects or other factors other than aging processes alone. A wide variety of disorders can produce postural hypotension, including diabetes-induced autonomic neuropathy, Parkinson's disease, chronic alcoholism, cardiovascular accident (CVA), pernicious anemia, and thiamine deficiency. In order to use orthostatic changes in blood pressure and pulse as an indicator of dehydration in the aged, the person's baseline status should be known. For those with baseline orthostatic changes who are at risk of dehydration, monitoring of intake and output may be necessary. Factors known to affect blood pressure and pulse response to postural change in such individuals should be noted, including medication use and prior blood pressure and pulse response to orthostatic challenge. Beta-blockers will depress pulse response and make it an unreliable indicator of volume status. Anticholinergic medications will often induce postural hypotension, but this response may be exaggerated in volume deficit. Wandel (1990) recommends obtaining pulse and BP in the standing rather than sitting position, as studies of orthostatic vital signs in dehydration in younger adults suggest that the sitting position is an inadequate challenge. However, the individual's ability to stand must be assessed carefully before this maneuver is attempted, and when there is any doubt about the individual's balance or ability to remain standing, an assistant should be present during the measurement to prevent fall-related injury.

Planning and Intervention

The primary goal for patients with fluid volume deficit is to restore and preserve adequate plasma volume. Underlying disorders causing fluid losses or shifts must be treated in collaboration with physicians and, in the case of malnutrition, nutritionists. Simultaneously, the patient should receive rehydration, either orally or parenterally if unable to take in sufficient fluids. Parenteral hydration is only a temporary measure, and efforts should begin as soon as possible to encourage the patient to ingest fluids. During intravenous hydration, care should be taken that the older person does not experience fluid overload because of too rapid administration. Subcutaneous administration of fluids is a seldom-used technique that has been shown to be an effective method of fluid replacement and one that may be less likely than intravenous administration to cause fluid overload (Lipschitz et al., 1991; Watt, 1991). If the underlying cause of fluid volume deficit is inadequate intake, then a systematic program for ensuring adequate intake must be implemented.

In hospitals, nurses can actively influence the pace of diagnostic evaluations that include NPO status, including preparations for gastrointestinal studies. A slower trajectory for the diagnostic testing of older adults may be required because of intolerance to fluid shifts. This slower pace can be achieved on an individual patient basis by close monitoring of the older patient's physiological response to fluid restriction and cathartic administration. On an organizational level, the use of care maps that recognize altered homeostatic reserve by lengthening the period of time for bowel preparation, or use of quality improvement indicators that monitor for dehydration in patients undergoing diagnostic testing, may help prevent iatrogenic complications related to fluid deficit.

The importance of offering fluid regularly and with proper technique to patients with mobility or cognitive impairments cannot be overstated. Some patients will refuse water if asked, but will accept it when it is offered. For example, rather than saying "Mrs. Jones, would you care for some water now?" try saying "Mrs. Jones, here is some water for you," or "Drink this water now." The directness of approach depends on the patient's cognitive status and past patterns of accepting or rejecting fluids. Institutions should give thought to incorporating hydration into their routines. For example, when medications are given an extra glass of fluid can be offered. Fluids can be incorporated into social events in the home or at the nursing home. For example, at a holiday party in one nursing home, the activities department had gone to tremendous effort to prepare attractive refreshments, which were placed in the center of the room. The patients were too crowded and immobile to reach the beverages, and so the refreshments remained virtually untouched until a member of the staff was assigned to offer refreshments to all present. Within 30 minutes, all the beverages were consumed. Thus, a minor modification in patient care assignment resulted in enhanced hydration for one afternoon. The pattern of using social events in long-term care facilities to promote hydration should not be difficult to institute. All group activities in nursing homes might include liquid refreshments, at minimal cost if the beverage is ice water.

Evaluation

Unless adequately hydrated, the patient will perform at suboptimal levels and be at higher risk for a host of untoward events. Criteria for evaluation of fluid deficit in the elderly include:

1. Underlying causes of the patient's fluid volume deficit are corrected.
2. No clinical signs of dehydration are present.
3. A plan for adequate daily intake of fluids is evident.

INFECTION, HIGH RISK FOR

Definition and Scope of Problem

Infection, high risk for, is defined by the North American Nursing Diagnosis Association as "the state in which an individual is at increased risk for being invaded by pathogenic organisms" (NANDA, 1992). Infectious disease is widespread among elderly people and has potentially devastating consequences. Infections are a major source of hospitalization for the aged, and old people suffer greater morbidity and mortality from infectious disease than do younger adults. This is especially true for pneumonia, appendicitis, kidney infection, septicemia, endocarditis, meningitis, and tuberculosis (Cantrell and Norman, 1992).

Infections are usually categorized as nosocomial (institutionally acquired) or community-acquired. Nosocomial infections are well studied in the hospital setting, but the data are more limited in nursing homes. The most common sites of nosocomial infection in hospitalized patients in descending order are urinary tract, lower respiratory tract, surgical wounds, and bloodstream. Fifty-four per cent of these infections occurred in patients aged 65 years and older (Emori et al., 1991). In nursing homes, the most common nosocomial infections occur in the respiratory tract, skin, and soft tissues (especially infections in pressure sores); the urinary tract; and with infectious gastroen-

teritis (Smith et al., 1991; Jackson et al., 1992; Toledo et al., 1993).

Healthy elderly individuals living at home have a risk of contracting an infectious disease similar to that of younger adults, with a slightly higher risk of developing respiratory infection, but certain populations of old people carry a higher risk of contracting an infectious disease. Older people at highest risk of infection are those living at home with chronic diseases or functional impairments, and the socially isolated; older people in hospitals; and older people in nursing homes.

Despite the apparent increase in susceptibility to the adverse effects of infection that accompanies old age, clinicians have regarded infectious disease in the aged with some ambivalence, alternately viewing it as a tremendous problem and as a blessing. Even Osler, author of the famous aphorism regarding pneumonia, considered the disease "the special enemy of old age" (1892), as well as the "friend of the aged" (1898).

Contributing Factors

Impact of Aging on Host-Defense Mechanisms

It is generally accepted that age is associated with changes in immunocompetence, but the specific contribution of the aging process compared with chronic diseases is not clear (Phair and Reisberg, 1984; Plewa, 1990). Because an increased production of antibodies to "self" antigens has been noted along with a decreased production of antibodies to foreign antigens, the concept of immune dysregulation rather than immune decline with aging has been suggested (Ben-Yehuda and Weksler, 1992). The majority of the studies of age-related changes in host defense mechanisms have been cross-sectional rather than longitudinal in design. Also, studies tend to describe the changes rather than explain the mechanisms of the changes (Adler and Nagel, 1990). Studies of older people free from chronic disease tend to show little change in immune function. However, elderly people with chronic diseases clearly have a reduced capacity to fight infection, in both nonspecific defenses and cell-mediated immunity. Common age-related changes in each organ system that impair the integrity of defenses against infection are discussed next.

HEMATOPOIETIC SYSTEM. Cell-mediated immunity, responsible for the destruction of foreign tissues like tumors and grafts and for the response to skin testing antigens such as purified protein derivative of tuberculin (PPD) and *Candida,* is diminished with aging (Hirsch and Weksler, 1990). The thymus begins involution early in life, and its ability to produce and differentiate T cells, the agents of cellular immunity, gradually decreases with age (Adler and Nagel, 1990). Increased production of immunoglobulins in elderly people is associated with a higher incidence of monoclonal gammopathies, especially multiple myeloma (Cohen, 1988). The effect of aging on humoral immunity is less well studied than on cell-mediated immunity, but humoral immunity is also found to be depressed in the aged. Studies of the effects of aging on polymorphonuclear leukocyte function are contradictory. However, diseases prevalent in the elderly, such as cancer and diabetes, are associated with leukopenia and therefore reduced immune function.

RESPIRATORY SYSTEM. Ciliary action and coughing are both primary defenses against respiratory infection, and both are impaired in the aged. In addition, IgA, a secretory immunoglobin found in the respiratory tree that helps neutralize viruses, is reduced. Finally, alveolar macrophages often have defective function in the aged.

INTEGUMENTARY SYSTEM. The skin is more prone to injury in the aged because of decreased elasticity, increased dryness, and decreased vascular supply. When the skin is broken, the body's first line of resistance to infection is disrupted. Aging affects other immunologic functions of the skin. The number of epidermal cells responsible for recognizing foreign antigens in the skin is reduced by nearly 50 per cent between early and late adulthood, possibly contributing to decreased immune function in the elderly.

GASTROINTESTINAL SYSTEM. Acidic gastric contents and pancreatic enzymes protect against infection, and both decline with age. The normal flora of the feces are an important protection against pathogens and are unaffected by the aging process but may be destroyed by the use of antibiotics, gastrointestinal surgery, enemas, nasogastric drainage, and enteral feedings. Overgrowth and infection with organisms such as *Clostridium difficile,* with resultant colitis and diarrhea, may result (Carpenter and Zielinski, 1992).

Chronic Diseases

Certain disorders prevalent among elderly people, such as malnutrition, diabetes mellitus, and cancer, are major contributors to the potential for infection. In addition, functional dependence, a nonspecific marker of chronic disease, has been associated with colonization of the oropharynx with gram-negative bacilli. According to Valenti et al. (1978), 19 per cent of older persons living independently, 40 per cent living in skilled nursing facilities, and 60 per cent of those hospitalized were found to be colonized with these bacteria.

Older people with valvular heart disease and implanted prosthetic heart values or joints are at increased risk of infection from bacterial seeding during invasive procedures. Specific guidelines exist and should be followed for antibiotic prophylaxis to prevent bacterial endocarditis for those with valvular heart disease (Friedlander and Yoshikawa, 1990), but they are not currently recommended for those with joint prostheses (Thyne and Ferguson, 1991).

IMMOBILITY. Reduced mobility predisposes to infection through a variety of mechanisms, including promotion of stasis of respiratory secretions, promotion of skin ulceration because of unrelieved pressure, and predisposing to fecal impaction—associated urinary retention.

MALNUTRITION. Malnutrition is associated with a number of defects in primary and secondary immunity (Cantrell and Norman, 1992). In addition, markers of nutritional inadequacy, such as reduced body mass index, have been associated with higher mortality from respiratory infections in nursing homes (Mehr et al., 1992).

CHRONIC OBSTRUCTIVE PULMONARY DISEASE. People with chronic lung disease have enhanced susceptibility to respiratory infections. Difficulty in clearing pulmonary secretions may result in statis, providing an excellent bacterial culture medium. In addition to a disease-related predisposition to infection, drugs may also influence susceptibility to infection. Nicotine impairs ciliary action; steroids suppress inflammatory response.

CANCER. Hematological malignancies interfere with the immune response by altering the production of white blood cells. Other forms of malignancy, including bronchogenic carcinoma, squamous cell carcinoma, and multiple myeloma, are associated with altered polymorphonuclear leukocyte function, depressed cell-mediated immunity, hypogammaglobulinemia, and antibody deficiency. Treatments for cancer, including chemotherapy and radiation therapy, impair immune function through destruction of white blood cells and interference with adequate nutrition.

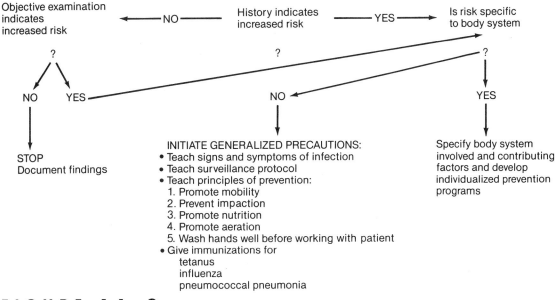

FIGURE 14-9

Overview of nursing process for potential for infection.

DIABETES MELLITUS. Impaired cell-mediated and humoral immunity has been demonstrated in young adults with insulin-dependent diabetes. It is thought that some of these defects, particularly those in neutrophil and T cell function, are influenced by glucose control. Less research has been done on older, noninsulin-dependent diabetic patients. However, the limited work reported suggests that older persons with noninsulin-dependent diabetes are predisposed to infection for reasons similar to those operating in younger diabetics.

NEUROLOGICAL DISORDERS. Patients with dementia have a higher-than-average risk of aspirating oropharyngeal contents, predisposing to pneumonia. This risk exists even when nutrition is supplied through a nasogastric or gastrostomy tube. In addition, these patients often suffer from mobility problems and are thus predisposed to skin and urinary tract infections.

HUMAN IMMUNODEFICIENCY VIRUS (HIV) DISEASE. Infection with HIV affects the immune system directly by decreasing the numbers of CD4+ and T cells and monocytes, leaving the body susceptible to opportunistic infections. Few studies have focused on the nature of HIV infection in older patients. One study of the epidemiological and clinical characteristics of HIV in patients over age 55 years showed that, compared with younger people, older adults were more likely to contract HIV from blood products (21 per cent) versus 67 per cent who had a history of homosexual or bisex-

ual contacts. HIV encephalopathy was more common in the older group, and the older group has a much poorer survival rate (Ferro and Salit, 1992). Although the number of older adults who have HIV disease is quite small in comparison with the HIV-infected population as a whole, the disease does occur in elderly people. The types of opportunistic infections that develop in older persons with AIDS are similar to those experienced by younger persons; they include *Pneumocystis carinii* pneumonia and Kaposi's sarcoma. Once older adults develop an opportunistic infection, they progress more rapidly to end-stage disease or death than do younger persons. Age-related changes in the immune system may contribute to this phenomenon (Kendig and Adler, 1990).

Assessment

The algorithm in Figure 14–9 summarizes the nursing process for those suspected of having a potential for infection.

History

Diseases and drugs commonly associated with altered host-defense mechanisms should be noted. Diabetes mellitus, chronic obstructive pulmonary disease, cancer, dementia, blood dyscrasias, malnutrition, and immobility are of most concern. Drugs to be noted include systemic corticosteroids, sedatives/hypnotics, antibiotics, recent cancer chemotherapy, or immunosuppressive therapy for rheumatic disorders. Determine whether the patient has a history of valvular heart disease or prosthetic valves or joints, and note in the record. Patients with valvular heart disease should receive antibiotic prophylaxis for bacterial endocarditis prior to invasive procedures, including dental work and urologic procedures (Dajani et al., 1990; Friedlander and Yoshikawa, 1990). The role of antibiotic prophylaxis in those with joint replacements is less clear, with some advocating prophylaxis (Calkins, 1992), and others suggesting that, at least for dental work, it is not necessary (Thyne and Ferguson, 1991).

Determine the patient's immunization status. Inquire specifically about the most recent tetanus vaccine, and whether immunization for influenza and pneumococcal pneumonia has been given. Determine beliefs about the usefulness of immunization and the attitude toward influenza vaccine. Note any allergies to chicken eggs or history of untoward reaction to immunizations, including Guillain-Barré syndrome.

Obtain a history of previous infections. Has the individual had recurrent urinary or respiratory tract infections? Has a skin test for TB ever been done? It is reasonable to assume that the factors that have allowed recurrent infections to develop earlier are still at work, unless specific contribution factors have been successfully eliminated.

Objective Assessment

The patient should be assessed for signs of nutritional deficiency (see Chapter 19). Laboratory data that are useful to review include the white blood count for evidence of leukopenia or leukocytosis and the total protein and albumin levels for evidence of malnutrition. Other assessment maneuvers should be keyed to the body system in which infection is suspected.

RESPIRATORY INFECTION. To assess potential for respiratory infection, observe the individual's ability to cough effectively and deep-breathe and determine whether the gag reflex is intact. The presence of bibasilar rales in the absence of congestive heart failure suggests potential for respiratory infection secondary to immobility.

Since the aging population is considered a high-risk group for TB, a PPD skin test should be a routine part of the initial geriatric assessment, unless the individual has a known positive response or a history of TB infection. The use of a control, such as *Candida albicans* or mumps, and a two-step testing (two skin tests placed 1 week apart) increases the accuracy of the test, as there is the possibility of decreased cutaneous delayed hypersensitivity reactions in older persons (Delafuente et al., 1988; Finucane, 1988; Rodysill et al., 1989; Yoshikawa, 1992).

SKIN INFECTION. Assessment for skin infection potential includes inspection for obesity, contractures, or edema (Table 14–11). The first two conditions predispose the skin to fungal infection as well as breakdown, whereas edema interferes with peripheral circulation, predisposing to skin breakdown and subsequent infection. Immobility is also a risk factor for skin infection, as it predisposes to pressure ulceration, and infection commonly ensues.

URINARY TRACT INFECTION. Palpate and percuss the bladder following voiding. If the bladder is identifiable, there is probably residual urine and the potential for infection is high. In this case, a catheterized, postvoid specimen should be obtained to determine residual volume. If an indwelling urinary catheter is chronically used, bacteriuria is nearly inevitable and is related to increased incidence of bacteremia and death. For this reason, many recommend elimination whenever possible of indwelling catheters (Kunin et al., 1992).

Planning and Intervention

Immunizations

Immunization against influenza and pneumococcal pneumonia is advocated for most older persons because of their decreased ability to resist infection and the increased risk of morbidity and mortality. A booster dose of tetanus vaccine is recommended for all older persons at 10-year intervals after the completion of a primary immunization series (Immunization Practices Advisory Committee, 1985), because the incidence of tetanus rises steadily with age, and it has a high mortality (25 per cent).

A review of the efficacy of influenza vaccine indicated that the vaccine was 33 per cent effective in the prevention of clinical illness in institutionalized elderly patients, and 74 per cent effective in reducing mortality (Strassburg et al., 1986). Pneumococcal vaccine is also quite effective, with studies showing a 60 per cent reduction of bacteremia and other life-threatening infections in high-risk older adults (Bolan et al., 1986; Sims et al., 1988). Influenza vaccine must be given annually to be effective. It is contraindicated in those with allergic reactions to

TABLE 14 – 11
Examples of Individualized Infection Prevention Programs

POTENTIAL FOR RESPIRATORY INFECTION RELATED TO:

Difficulty clearing secretions secondary to chronic lung disease	Deep breathing and coughing regimen every 2 hours while awake
	Encourage fluids to >2000 ml every day, unless contraindicated by renal or cardiac disease
	Bronchodilator therapy as prescribed
	Postural drainage with percussion if first three interventions not effective
Depressed cough secondary to use of sedative medications	Deep breathing and coughing regimen every 2 hours while awake
	Encourage fluids to >2000 ml every day, unless contraindicated by renal or cardiac disease
	Implement mobility enhancement program, such as regular walking or other exercise
Risk of aspiration of food secondary to diminished gag reflex	Supervise a mealtime to ensure food is ingested at proper pace and that patient is positioned properly
	Inspect mouth after each meal and clean out as necessary to make sure that no food is left in oral cavity

POTENTIAL FOR SKIN INFECTION RELATED TO:

Intertrigo secondary to obesity and diabetes mellitus	Observe between skin folds daily, or instruct patient or caregivers to do so
	Daily cleansing of skin folds, with moisturized soap and water. Dry thoroughly with towel or hair dryer
	Use cotton undergarments
High pressure sore risk secondary to immobility and incontinence	Institute regular repositioning regimen (at least every 2 hours)
	Use waterproof pressure redistribution mattress and seat cushions
	Use moisturizing lotion after each cleansing of skin
Diabetic peripheral neuropathy	Inspect feet daily for signs of trauma
	Wash feet daily, dry thoroughly, and apply moisturizing lotion
	Avoid shoes that are too tight or produce reddened areas or blisters
	Test water temperature with thermometer or elbow to prevent burns

POTENTIAL FOR URINARY TRACT INFECTION RELATED TO:

Chronic indwelling catheter use	Re-evaluate indications for catheter and remove if possible
	Change catheter only when necessary
	Use aseptic technique when changing catheter
	Maintain closed sterile drainage system
	Maintain unobstructed urine flow
	Secure catheter properly
	Use smallest size catheter possible
	Do not perform meatal care routines with antimicrobials
	Do not irrigate catheter unless specifically indicated to prevent or relieve obstruction
	Emphasize handwashing before and after working with patient
History of chronic urinary tract infections	Encourage toileting at 3- to 4-hour intervals
	Use Credé maneuver to facilitate complete bladder emptying
	If sexually active, encourage toileting shortly after intercourse
	Encourage fluids to >2000 ml per day unless contraindicated by renal or cardiac disorder
	Prevent constipation through use of bowel management program: diet, activity, fluids, and toileting

Source for prevention of catheter-associated infections: Conti, M.T. and Eutropius, L. Preventing UTIs: What works. *Am J Nurs* 87:307–309, 1987.

chicken eggs and in those with a prior history of Guillain-Barré syndrome (Immunization Practices Advisory Committee, 1989b). Although the current recommendation for pneumococcal vaccine is to give it just once in a lifetime, concerns about sustained immunity from the vaccine are leading some to question whether booster shots eventually may not be necessary (Shapiro et al., 1991; Sims et al., 1992).

Individual Patient Considerations

Patients at high risk of developing infection because of reduced immunocompetence secondary to chronic diseases should have a specific plan of care to prevent or foster early detection of infections. Nurses should work to ensure that pneumococcal pneumonia, influenza, and tetanus vaccines are given as recommended. Specific programs to prevent respiratory, skin, and urinary tract infections, such as vigorous pulmonary toilet, special skin care regimens, and bowel management programs should be implemented for susceptible individuals (Table 14–11). The nutritional deficiencies of malnourished individuals should be corrected.

Patients at risk of infection who are able to learn can be taught the early cues signifying infection of the skin, respiratory tract, and urinary tract. Specific preventive regi-

TABLE 14–12
Atypical Presentations of Common Infections

Pneumonia	Blunted fever response; decreased evidence of consolidation in 30% of patients; confusion, disorientation, and changes in behavior common presenting signs and symptoms
Urinary Tract Infection (UTI)	Blunted fever response; anorexia, nausea, vomiting, and abdominal pain; confusion and change in behavior; increased incidence of asymptomatic bacteriuria
Tuberculosis	Cough, weight loss, and weakness may be subtle symptoms and may be attributed to other chronic diseases; chest pain, hemoptysis, and night sweats are seen in later stages of disease
Skin Infections	Decreased inflammatory response may delay diagnosis; peripheral vascular disease will decrease erythema, warmth, and swelling, which are commonly used to determine infection

From Fraser, D. Patient assessment: Infections in the elderly. *J Gerontol Nurs* 19(7):7, 1993.

mens can be learned. Family and paraprofessional caregivers can be taught such information on behalf of patients who are unable to learn. Signs and symptoms of infection differ in older adults, and specific information on these altered presentations (Table 14–12) should be incorporated into the teaching plan. In addition, caregivers should be taught the importance of handwashing in infection prevention.

Community Considerations

Aggressive vaccination programs for influenza, pneumococcal pneumonia, and tetanus should be developed by long-term care institutions and primary care clinics where older adults are treated. Staff should be knowledgeable about the importance of handwashing in preventing cross-infection. Nurses in home care should be aware of their patients' vaccination status and encourage immunization against susceptible disorders.

The value of properly conducted infection control programs in hospitals has been established, and older people benefit from these efforts. Systematic efforts to document and control nosocomial infections in nursing homes are often based on principles of hospital infection control, but the appropriateness of wholesale adoption of hospital methods has been questioned, on the grounds that important differences exist between hos-

pitals and nursing homes (Smith, 1989). Improved guidelines for infection control practices in nursing homes are now emerging, along with enhanced information about the epidemiology of infection in this setting. For guidelines on infection control practice in nursing homes, see Smith (1989) or Levenson (1993). Nurses practicing in nursing homes should encourage infection control practices according to the most recent standards established for long-term care.

Evaluation

Criteria for evaluation of the effectiveness of care for elderly patients with potential for infection include:

1. Rates of nosocomial infection in hospitals and nursing homes: How does the individual institution's rate compare with rates reported in the literature?
2. Death rates from bacteremia compared with national averages.
3. Are programs implemented for prevention and early detection of infection in at-risk patients?
4. Do individuals identified as at risk develop infections?
5. Are infections identified and treated when they are first manifest, or are they only treated when the infection has become life-threatening?
6. Are patients immunized according to prevailing standards?

PHYSICAL MOBILITY IMPAIRMENT

Definition and Scope of Problem

Physical mobility impairment is "a state in which the individual experiences a limitation of ability for independent physical movement" (NANDA, 1992, p. 53). It is a common problem for the elderly with chronic disease. The consequences of impaired physical mobility are significant, including activity intolerance, self-care deficit, incontinence, pressure sores, psychological disturbances, social isolation, decreased muscle strength and endurance, dependent edema, weight loss, osteoporosis, contractures, pain, reduced self-care ability, and increased predisposition to thrombi and respiratory infections (Olson, 1967; Bortz, 1982; Harper and Lyles, 1988). Because impaired physical mobility is associated with so many problems, it deserves serious attention by gerontological nurses.

The extent of physical mobility impairments among the elderly in various care settings remains to be fully described. Epidemiological analyses of mobility problems have only a 20-year history. National surveys tend to report prevalence of diseases or disabilities but not specific impairments. Moreover, national surveys typically assess mobility status through the use of questionnaires rather than by observational methods or direct assessment (Guralnik et al., 1989), leading to potential underestimation of the extent of impairment mobility in elderly people. Although in individual instances dysmobility may be overreported, for the most part individuals do not realize that they have lost reserve joint mobility or strength until it interferes with their function. Buchner and de Lateur (1991) argue that there is a threshold relationship between muscular strength and some functional abilities, such as the ability to climb stairs. This means that normally adults have much more strength than is needed to perform basic daily activities. Thus, if we depend upon people recognizing limitations in function in order to assess reductions in mobility, we are likely to underestimate systematically the amount of impaired mobility in the population as a whole, including in elderly people.

Guralnik and colleagues (1993) reported results from a longitudinal study of changes in mobility in elderly people that used performance measures of mobility—specifically, the ability to climb stairs and walk a half-mile. Over a 4-year period, 6981 subjects from the Established Populations for Epidemiologic Studies of the Elderly (EPESE) in three areas of the country were studied. During this time, 55 per cent of the subjects maintained their baseline mobility status. Thirty-six per cent lost mobility, and 9 per cent died without any change in mobility status detected. Risk factors for decline in mobility were increasing age, lower income, and baseline histories of cardiovascular disease, diabetes, and dyspnea (Guralnik et al., 1993). Although these data are based upon self-report, future EPESE studies will include performance measures of mobility.

Jette and Branch (1984) surveyed musculoskeletal impairment in a probability sample of 825 people living in a community in Massachusetts, all over the age of 70 years. They used trained lay assessors to rate impairments in joint mobility using the maneuvers listed in Table 14–13. *Hand impairments* were observed in 9 to 11 per cent of the population, with women having more impairment than men. Wrist mobility was impaired in 33 per cent with no gender differences ob-

TABLE 14–13

Assessment Maneuvers for Impaired Physical Mobility

Thumb–finger opposition Touch tip of fifth finger with tip of thumb (bilateral)

Fist Bend fingers into palm of hand making a fist (bilateral)

Wrist extension Holding forearms in front of you parallel to the floor, bend elbows 90° and hold at shoulder level; press together palmar surface of your hands, keep fingertips pointed upward

Wrist flexion Holding forearms in front of you parallel to the floor, bend elbows 90° and hold at shoulder level; press backs of hands together, point fingertips downward

Forearm supination Place each hand in front of you with the back of the hand parallel to the floor or table, palms up; bend elbows to 90° and hold at the side of your body (bilateral)

Shoulder abduction; elbow flexion Place each hand on the shoulder of the same side of your body; hold your upper arms parallel to the floor (bilateral)

Shoulder abduction; external rotation While sitting erect, place each hand behind your neck at ear level; hold your upper arms parallel to the floor (bilateral)

Rise from armchair Rise from a standard armchair without using your hands for assistance

Stand on tiptoes Stand on your tiptoes for 15 seconds without using your hands for support

Hip and knee flexion Place the bottom of each foot on the surface of this chair; stand close to the chair, bend your knee, and do not use your hands to lift the leg (bilateral)

From Jette, A.M. and Branch, L.G. Musculoskeletal impairment among the non-institutionalized aged. *Int Rehab Med J* 6:157–161, 1984.

served; however, impairment increased with advanced age. Forearm supination was a problem for less than 10 per cent of the population, without observed gender differences. Of this sample, 19 to 21 per cent had difficulty with shoulder abduction; however, 40 per cent of the oldest subjects (over age 85 years) displayed impairment. *Lower extremity* impairment was more prevalent among women, and the prevalence increased with advancing age. Sixty-five per cent of the sample had difficulty standing on tiptoes, 25 per cent demonstrated impairment rising from an armchair, and 24 per cent had impairments of hip and knee flexion.

Nagi (1976), in a national probability sample of adults aged 18 to 75+ years, discovered that prevalence of physical performance impairments increased linearly with age. It was also noted that physical impairments were highly predictive of need for assistance in maintaining independent living.

More recent surveys of activity limitation in elderly people confirm Nagi's (1976) original findings and provide more insight into factors associated with physical ability. In a study of 1791 community-dwelling people over age 80 years, Harris and coworkers (1989) found that 67 per cent reported no difficulty lifting 10 pounds, 57 per cent had no difficulty climbing up 10 steps, 49 per cent had no problems walking a quarter-mile, and 47 per cent had no problems with stooping, crouching, or kneeling. In a 2-year follow-up survey, 50 per cent of the women and 42 per cent of the men who reported being physically able remained that way. Factors associated with continued ability included never having cardiovascular disease, never having arthritic complaints, being younger, not being obese, and having a higher educational level.

Diagnostic Dilemmas

Overlaps exist among the diagnostic categories of impaired physical mobility, activity intolerance, self-care deficit, and alteration in comfort. The semantic difficulty extends beyond the nursing discipline. The World Health Organization in the ninth revision of the International Classification of Diseases distinguishes between impairment, disability, and handicap in the following way:

- **Impairment** is any loss or abnormality of psychological, physiological, or anatomical structure or function;

- **Disability** is any restriction or lack (resulting from an impairment) of ability to perform an activity in the manner or within the range considered normal for a human being;

- **Handicap** is a disadvantage for a given individual, resulting from impairment or a disability, that limits or prevents the fulfillment of a role that is normal (depending on age, sex, and social and cultural factors) for that individual.

While the WHO classification of terms is gaining acceptance in the rehabilitation field, the classification has not been fully implemented. Part of the difficulty in implementation concerns practical difficulties in measurement and classification (see, for example, Robinson, 1985) and part from what some consider to be conceptual difficulties in this system (Nagi, 1991). Although a variety of approaches to classifying aspects of physical impairment and disability have been proposed, none is universally accepted. There are, however, substantial overlaps in the major theories, and, given the increasing prevalence of disabling disorders, conceptual work on these complex concepts is likely to continue (see, for example, Bury, 1987; Leidy, 1994).

To add to the semantic difficulties, there are complex, incompletely understood interrelationships between impaired physical mobility and the diagnoses just mentioned, as well as among impaired physical mobility and powerlessness, anxiety, potential for injury, and sensory-perceptual alteration. Nurses should not become overly concerned with finding the one right diagnosis for each patient. Multiple diagnoses will often apply in the elderly, and it is wise to consider the differences in intervention strategies suggested by the various diagnostic categories. For example, impaired physical mobility associated with degenerative joint disease may be both a cause and a consequence of alteration in comfort. Deciding which problem is primary is a matter of nursing judgment, based on other assessment data as well as on the resources available for intervention. The individual living at home alone, with no family support, may require analgesics to break the cycle of discomfort and immobility while another individual, with greater social support and access to physical and occupational therapies as well as more intensive nursing intervention, may respond better to nonpharmacological interventions. Other factors that would influence the therapy include the patient's other health problems that affect ability to tolerate medications.

Contributing Factors

Hogue (1985) presents a model of enhancing mobility in the nursing home that helps organize factors contributing to impaired physical mobility. Contributors are numerous, as outlined earlier in Table 14–1. They may be categorized into two major groups: individual factors and environmental factors. Each category is discussed subsequently.

Individual Characteristics

One way to begin considering the specific individual factors that affect physical mobility is to consider mobility from a biomechanical perspective. Biomechanics views mobility as a matter of physical task performance, in which the masses and inertias of the body segments must be supported and moved by the skeletal system through its muscular action (Schultz, 1992). According to this perspective, the effects of neuropathology, disuse, medications, and psychosocial variables are all manifested as changes in the biomechanics of task performance, and thus study of biomechanics is an efficient way to consider mobility.

The first set of age-related changes that can affect mobility are anthropometric changes. Stature and joint range of motion have been shown to decline in cross-sectional studies (Schultz, 1992). People aged 65 to 74 years are approximately 3 per cent shorter than those aged 18 to 24 years, and this is thought to be primarily due to shortening of intervertebral disc spaces and associated kyphosis. Cross-sectional studies of differences in joint range of motion show general decreases with advancing age among healthy elderly people, although the amount of decline varies substantially with the group of individuals studied and the joint measured. For example, a 20 per cent decline in hip rotation between ages 45 and 70 years has been reported, whereas in the same subjects only a 10 per cent decline in wrist and shoulder ROM was noted. Reports of changes in lower extremity range of motion are inconsistent, with reports ranging from none to 57 per cent. Specific reductions in joint range of motion have been associated with functional limitations in persons with arthritis and with community-dwelling elderly people at large. Badley and colleagues (1984) found that the ability to move around in one's environment was related to knee flexion ROM, the ability to perform activities requiring hand and arm use correlated significantly with upper extremity joint range of motion, and the ability to bend down was correlated with hip flexion ROM. In a similar vein, Bergstrom and colleagues (1985) found that knee ROM restriction was associated with reduced use of public transportation. Although it is intuitive that restrictions in joint range of motion should influence the amount of mobility an individual has, the extent to which such impairments are related to reduced function has not been well studied.

Muscular strength is known to decline with age, although how much decrement exists is controversial. Strength measures depend substantially on the conditions under which strength was measured (Schultz, 1992), with joint angle used, type of strength measuring device used, and whether the muscle was lengthening or shortening during the measurement—all factors that can influence the measurement. Moreover, as is the case with joint range of motion, the precise strength requirements for basic activities of daily living have not been well delineated. Thus, it is unclear to what extent impairments in mobility are the result of reduced strength versus a combination of factors that influences an individual's ability to make maximum use of existing strength.

Decreased strength and endurance may occur as the result of prolonged disuse from long-term bedrest or inactivity in a chair, degenerative neuromuscular diseases, severe cardiac disease, and pulmonary disease. Recent studies of strength training in elderly persons suggest that declines in strength that accompany age may be reversed through exercise programs, even in those with moderately severe chronic illness (Shepard, 1990; Hogue et al., 1993).

In addition to age-related changes in anthropometrics, joint range of motion, and strength, age-related declines in postural balance, gait, and ability to transfer from one surface to another may underlie altered physical mobility. Extensive studies of age-related changes in postural balance show age-related decrements in the sensorimotor systems that underlie postural control, even in the absence of awareness of difficulty. Gait disturbances have been documented extensively among older people, including shorter step and stride lengths and decreased ankle extension and pelvic rotation, although it is controversial whether these changes are due to normal aging changes or are pathological changes accompanying old age. Gait speed is related to aerobic capacity (Cunningham et al., 1982); muscle strength (Bassey et al., 1988); presence of other chronic diseases (Bendall et al., 1989); cognition (Visser, 1983); and ability to rise from a chair (Friedman et al., 1988). Reduced mobility may be due to increased effort involved with walking or insecurity about the ability to move about without falling. Associated fatigue can produce the mobility impairment.

Pain or discomfort results from many conditions, including prolonged time in one position, osteoarthritis, rheumatoid arthritis, polymyalgia rheumatica, vertebral compression fractures caused by osteoporosis, osteomalacia, and contractures. Mobility is impaired because the individual fears increased pain with movement. *Perceptual or cognitive impairments* lead to impaired physical mobility by interfering with the drive to move or by generating fear of movement. For example, the individual who is blind may be told not to move without assistance, and so sits for prolonged periods of time. Those with vestibular impairments or visuospatial disturbances may be too frightened or uncomfortable to move because they have lost their sense of position in space.

CONFIDENCE IN MOBILITY. Recently, Tinetti and colleagues (1990) have begun research on the role of confidence in mobility as a factor that may independently affect mobility. Working within a self-efficacy model (Bandura, 1982), a measure of confidence in moving without falling has been constructed (Tinetti et al., 1990). Subjects are asked how confident they are (on a scale of 0 to 10) that they can do a series of tasks, such as cleaning house, getting dressed, preparing simple meals, getting in and out of a chair, hurrying to answer the phone. In a study of 1103 community-dwelling elderly persons, falls efficacy (or confidence in mobility) was associated with both activity level and self-care status, after controlling for the effects of physical performance ability and chronic conditions. This finding suggests that psychological factors, such as how confident a person is in doing a task, may influence overall function.

Memory impairments may reduce the confidence of individuals to the point at which they fear becoming lost or are overwhelmed by the social stimulation or complexity of a movement task. The easiest thing to do is to stay put. *Neuromuscular impairments* include idiopathic Parkinson's disease, drug-induced parkinsonism, hemiplegia, paralysis due to spinal cord injury, spinocerebellar degeneration, and spasticity due to cortical atrophy. Neuromuscular disorders produce impaired movement either because inhibitory neuronal pathways are destroyed or because effector neurons are inactivated through paralysis or through disruptions in motor planning, leading to apraxia. *Musculoskeletal impairments* include degenerative joint disease, rheumatoid arthritis, spinal spondylosis, scoliosis, kyphosis, and amputation. Pain and deformity are the primary causes of impaired mobility related to musculoskeletal disorders. Amputation certainly has the potential to limit mobility; however, in some cases amputation may actually facilitate mobility by relieving pain or by eliminating a contracture that severely restricts mobility.

Environmental Characteristics

Medically prescribed treatments, such as traction, casts, or splints, are designed to produce immobility for a limited period of time. However, targeted immobilization of a specific body part carries the risk that more extensive immobility will occur, caused by muscle atrophy, lost skill in moving a body part, or, in the case of upper extremity immobilization, through adhesive capsulitis. *Physical features of the environment* may result in immobilization. If the old person is always kept in a "geriatric chair," or if the individual is not safely able to get out of a bed that is too high, then a certain amount of immobility is enforced. Improperly prescribed wheelchairs may result in immobilization rather than enhanced mobility. The

old person is placed in the wheelchair and not encouraged or assisted to walk again. Indeed, many of the so-called "standard" wheelchairs, i.e., those with fixed leg rests and sling backs and seats have been shown to contribute to spinal deformity and increase patient discomfort (Harms, 1990; Shaw and Taylor, 1991; Redford, 1993). Although the movement toward restraint-free environment reduces the potentially devastating effects of being placed in a wheelchair to a certain extent, too often the potentially deleterious effects of wheelchair use are overlooked. In addition to spinal deformity, improperly fitted wheelchairs may also contribute to the development of pressure sores and knee flexion contractures and impede independence in wheelchair ambulation. The use of so-called "standard" wheelchairs that collapse easily is to be deplored for individuals whose health and functional status require that they spend substantial amounts of time in a wheelchair.

Policies about mobility where the old person resides dramatically affect mobility, to the extent that pressure sores sometimes develop in patients who can walk independently! The immobility occurs when the old person is judged unsafe to walk alone, is restrained "for safety," and is not given sufficient opportunities to walk with assistance. Over time, the result is muscle weakness and reduced endurance, and all the stigmata of immobility begin to appear. Nursing care patterns have been associated with fostering dependency. One study shows that team rather than primary nursing fosters more patient dependency, which is likely to be related to impaired physical mobility if sustained over any period of time (Hardy et al., 1982). More recent studies support the importance of type and consistency of nursing staff in promoting positive patient outcomes in nursing homes (Spector and Takada, 1991).

Availability of social support may seem at first unrelated to mobility, but consider the patient who experiences pain on motion and the link becomes clear. Many people, if not given sufficient reasons for moving, simply do not. It is too much trouble. Those with social obligations, such as church, family gatherings, or friends who depend on them have much greater motivation for working through discomfort than those who have no "reason" to move about. *Characteristics of others in the environment* have great influences on the attitudes of old people toward mobility. Messages that convey "Be careful, you mustn't do that, you might fall or hurt yourself" are likely to produce more immobility than messages that acknowledge that

T A B L E   1 4 – 1 4
Essential Components for Assessment of Impaired Physical Mobility

Ability to follow verbal commands
Inspection of the joints for deformity and asymmetry
Joint range of motion, both active and passive: note any
  pain on motion
Inspection of the muscles for asymmetry, spasm
Muscle strength testing
Grip strength
Presence of bradykinesia, cogwheeling rigidity
Fine and gross motor coordination
Sensory testing, including proprioception, sensitivity to
  light, touch, pain, hearing, vision
Balance: sitting and standing
Transfer ability
Walking ability
Ability to shift weight while sitting or lying
Toileting ability
Feeding ability
Dressing ability
Mechanical or medically prescribed restrictions of move-
  ments—casts, splints, traction, incisions, restraints
Other devices that promote immobility: intravenous lines,
  indwelling catheters, ventilators

life involves a series of risks. Messages that expect and encourage competent performance from individuals in the immediate environment influence the older person's functional capacity positively, which in turn positively influences mobility.

Assessment

The purpose of assessment of those with impaired physical mobility is to identify treatable causes of the impairment, specify contributors to the impairment, and suggest means to compensate. In addition, mobility assessment can help the clinician identify dysfunctional patterns of coping with reduced mobility that may lead to further decrements in mobility and function. There is an increasing recognition that changes in how people perform tasks, and the frequency with which they perform them, may allow early identification of those at risk for declines in mobility and function (Fried et al., 1991; Fried et al., 1993).

Assessment of impaired physical mobility, therefore, includes individual body systems as well as integrated functioning. Essential components of the assessment are listed in Table 14–14. Note that the emphasis in Table 14–14 is on performance based on observational assessment, rather than on history taking. Although the individual's perception of difficulty and concerns about movement are important, it is critical to obtain direct observation of performance in all older individuals. A variety of techniques are available for quantifying each aspect of the assessment, and, depending upon the specific needs of the individual patient and demands of the setting of care, this information will be more or less detailed. For example, the nursing home minimum data set requires only screening level information about mobility and need for assistive devices. Nurses working to remediate strength or range-of-motion deficits in those with impaired physical mobility will not be satisfied with such crude measures and may collaborate with physical or occupational therapists to obtain more precise measures of physical mobility in selected cases.

Current research on the biomechanics of human performance and on the effects of exercise in very frail elders may also shed light on which assessment maneuvers are the most useful in predicting functional level or in pinpointing needs for intervention to prevent decline. For example, Alexander and colleagues (1992) have developed a "Bed Rise Difficulty Scale" to quantify problems in transferring from bed to sitting. Gerety and colleagues (1993) have developed a more comprehensive Physical Disability Index.

During the assessment, have the patient perform a standardized series of maneuvers, such as those outlined in Tables 14–15 through 14–17. Quantify the amount of assistance required, if any, and note any pain, stiffness, or awkwardness. If impairments are noted, identify the contributors and the conditions that improve mobility. For example, people with Parkinson's disease often have several types of mobility impairments, including bradykinesia, cogwheeling rigidity, and decreased joint range of motion. Frequently, after receiving assistance with an activity such as ambulation, the amount of bradykinesia and rigidity is temporarily lessened. Medications also may lessen the symptoms of impaired mobility. Therefore, documentation should include whether the assessment was conducted before or after exercising and medications currently taken.

When working in settings of care where the patients are bedridden, begin the assessment with bed mobility tasks. Check for medical contraindications to moving in bed, such as an unstable or suspected fracture, unstable vital signs, or increased intracranial pressure. Once any restrictions on movement are understood, try each of the following bed mobility tasks; (1) turning from side to side in bed, (2) flexing the knees bilaterally and raising the hips (bridging), (3) moving from a supine to a sitting position, with legs dangling over the side of the bed, and

T A B L E   1 4 – 1 5
Assessment of Gait in the Elderly*

COMPONENTS†	OBSERVATION	
	Normal	Abnormal
Initiation of gait (patient asked to begin walking down hallway)	Begins walking immediately without observable hesitation; initiation of gait is single, smooth motion	Hesitates; multiple attempts; initiation of gait not a smooth motion
Step height (begin observing after first few steps: observe one foot, then the other; observe from side)	Swing foot completely clears floor but by no more than 1–2 in	Swing foot is not completely raised off floor (may hear scraping) or is raised too high (>1–2 in)‡
Step length (observe distance between toe of stance foot and heel of swing foot; observe from side; do not judge first few or last few steps; observe one side at a time)	At least the length of individual's foot between the stance toe and swing heel (step length usually longer but foot length provides basis for observation)	Step length less than described under normal‡
Step symmetry (observe the middle part of the patch not the first or last steps; observe from side; observe distance between heel of each swing foot and toe of each stance foot)	Step length same or nearly same on both sides for most step cycles	Step length varies between sides or patient advances with same foot with every step
Step continuity	Begins raising heel of one foot (toe off) as heel of other foot touches the floor (heel strike); no breaks or stops in stride; step lengths equal over most cycles	Places entire foot (heel and toe) on floor before beginning to raise other foot; or stops completely between steps; or step length varies over cycles‡
Path deviation (observe from behind; observe one foot over several strides; observe in relation to line on floor [e.g., tiles] if possible; difficult to assess if patient uses a walker)	Foot follows close to straight line as patient advances	Foot deviates from side to side or toward one direction§
Trunk stability (observe from behind; side-to-side motion of trunk may be a normal gait pattern, need to differentiate this from instability)	Trunk does not sway; knees or back are not flexed; arms are not abducted in effort to maintain stability	Any of preceding features present§
Walk stance (observe from behind)	Feet should almost touch as one passes other	Feet apart with stepping‖
Turning while walking	No staggering; turning continuous with walking; and steps are continuous while turning	Staggers; stops before initiating turn; or steps are discontinuous

* The patient stands with examiner at end of obstacle-free hallway, using usual walking aid. Examiner asks patient to walk down hallway at his or her usual pace. Examiner observes one component of gait at a time. For some components the examiner walks behind the patient; for other components, the examiner walks next to patient. May require several trips to complete.

† Also ask patient to walk at a "more rapid than usual" pace and observe whether any walking aid is used correctly.

‡ Abnormal gait finding may reflect a primary neurologic or musculoskeletal problem directly related to the finding or reflect a compensatory maneuver for other, more remote problem.

§ Abnormality may be corrected by walking aid such as cane; observe with and without walking aid if possible.

‖ Abnormal finding is usually a compensatory maneuver rather than a primary problem.

From Tinetti, M. Performance-oriented assessment of mobility problems in elderly patients. *J Am Geriatr Soc* 34:119–126, 1986.

(4) assuming the prone position in bed. Observing performance of each of these tasks can yield considerable information about the patient's muscle strength, joint range of motion, and ability to follow motor commands.

For example, patients who can turn from side to side in bed should be encouraged to participate in that task to the maximum extent possible, as this will help maintain trunk flexibility and strength and possibly upper extremity function. In addition, it allows the individual to maintain control of repositioning schedules. Individuals who cannot perform this task are unlikely to be able to accomplish a supine-to-sit transfer unassisted. Raising the hips 2 to 3 inches into the air requires considerable hip extensor muscle strength. Ability to perform this task suggests sufficient leg strength to stand, although the individual may still need support for balance or assistance in others parts of the sit-to-stand transfer. Absence of the ability to raise the hips in bed may represent motor planning problems rather than an absence of strength, so manual muscle testing is still indicated in patients who cannot complete the bridging task. Moving from a supine to a sitting position is a key movement required for transferring from bed to chair, or from bed to a prewalking position. Retained ability to perform this task is a good sign, as it involves the coordinated

T A B L E   1 4 – 1 6
Assessment of Balance in the Elderly*

| | RESPONSE | | |
MANEUVER	Normal	Adaptive	Abnormal
Sitting balance	Steady, stable	Holds onto chair to keep upright	Leans, slides down in chair
Arising from chair	Able to arise in a single movement without using arms	Uses arms (on chair or walking aid) to pull or push up; and/or moves forward in chair before attempting to arise	Multiple attempts required or unable without human assistance
Immediate standing balance (first 3–5 sec)	Steady without holding onto walking aid or other object for support	Steady, but uses walking aid or other object for support	Any sign of unsteadiness†
Standing balance	Steady, able to stand with feet together without holding object for support	Steady, but cannot put feet together	Any sign of unsteadiness regardless of stance or holds onto object
Balance with eyes closed (with feet as close together as possible)	Steady without holding onto any object with feet together	Steady with feet apart	Any sign of unsteadiness or needs to hold onto an object
Turning balance (360°)	No grabbing or staggering; no need to hold onto any objects; steps are continuous (turn is a flowing movement)	Steps are discontinuous (patient puts one foot completely on floor before raising other foot)	Any sign of unsteadiness or holds onto an object
Nudge on sternum (patient standing with feet as close together as possible, examiner pushes with light even pressure over sternum three times; reflects ability to withstand displacement)	Steady, able to withstand pressure	Needs to move feet, but able to maintain balance	Begins to fall, or examiner has to help maintain balance
Neck turning (patient asked to turn head side to side and look up while standing with feet as close together as possible)	Able to turn head at least half way side to side and be able to bend head back to look at ceiling; no staggering, grabbing, or symptoms of lightheadedness, unsteadiness, or pain	Decreased ability to turn side to side to extend neck, but no staggering, grabbing, or symptoms of lightheadedness, unsteadiness, or pain	Any sign of unsteadiness or symptoms when turning head or extending neck
One leg standing balance	Able to stand on one leg for 5 sec without holding object for support		Unable
Back extension (ask patient to lean back as far as possible, without holding onto object if possible)	Good extension without holding object or staggering	Tries to extend, but decreased range of motion (compared with other patients of same age) or needs to hold object to attempt extension	Will not attempt or no extension seen or staggers
Reaching up (have patient attempt to remove an object from a shelf high enough to require stretching or standing on toes)	Able to take down object without needing to hold onto other object for support and without becoming unsteady	Able to get object but needs to steady self by holding onto something for support	Unable or unsteady
Bending down (patient is asked to pick up small object, such as pen, from the floor)	Able to bend down and pick up object and is able to get up easily in single attempt without needing to pull self up with arms	Able to get object and get upright in single attempt but needs to pull self up with arms or hold onto something for support	Unable to bend down or unable to get upright after bending down or takes multiple attempts to upright
Sitting down	Able to sit down in one smooth movement	Needs to use arms to guide self into chair or not a smooth movement	Falls into chair, misjudges distances (lands off center)

* The patient begins this assessment seated in a hard, straight-backed, armless chair.
† Unsteadiness defined as grabbing at objects for support, staggering, moving feet, or more than minimal trunk sway.
From Tinetti, M. Performance-oriented assessment of mobility problems in the elderly. *J Am Geriatr Soc* 34:119–126, 1986.

movement of many body segments simultaneously.

Once again, inability to perform the task on command may be due to a variety of problems: lack of flexibility or strength, fear, disuse, or an inability to coordinate the ac-

tivities of various body segments in a strange environment. Each of these potential contributors must be assessed individually.

Assessing an individual's ability to assume the prone-lying position is infrequently done, yet it is an important maneu-

TABLE 14–17
Significance of Abnormal Findings in Evaluating Balance and Gait in the Elderly

ABNORMAL MANEUVER	POSSIBLE ETIOLOGIES*	POSSIBLE THERAPEUTIC OR REHABILITATIVE MEASURES†	POSSIBLE PREVENTIVE OR ADAPTIVE MEASURES†
Difficulty arising from chair	Proximal muscle weakness (many causes) Arthritides (especially involving hip, knees) Parkinson's syndrome Hemiparesis or paraparesis Deconditioning	Treatment of specific disease states (e.g., steroids, L-dopa) Hip and quadricep exercises Transfer training	High, firm chair with arms Raised toilet seats Ejection chairs
Instability on first standing	Postural hypotension Cerebellar disease Multisensory deficits Lower extremity weakness or pain Foot pain leading to decreasing weight bearing	Treatment of specific diseases (e.g., adequate salt and fluid status, Fluorinef) Jobst stockings Hip and knee exercises Correct foot problems	Arise slowly Head of bed on blocks Supportive aid (e.g., walker, quadcane)
Instability with nudge on sternum	Parkinson's syndrome Back problems Normal pressure hydrocephalus ? Peripheral neuropathy Deconditioning	Treatment of specific diseases (e.g., L-dopa, shunt) ? Back exercises Analgesia ? Balance exercises (e.g., Frankel's)	Obstacle-free environment Appropriate walking aid (cane, walker) Night lights (more likely to fall if bump into object) Close observation with acute illness (high risk of falling) Avoid slippers
Instability with eyes closed (stable with eyes open)	Multisensory deficits Decreasing proprioception, position sense (e.g., B$_{12}$ deficiency, DM, etc.)	Treatment of specific diseases (e.g., B$_{12}$) Correct visual, hearing problems Remove cerumen ? Balance exercises	Bright lights Night lights Cane
Instability on neck turning or extension	Cervical arthritis Cervical spondylosis Vertebral-basilar insufficiency	? Antiarthritic medication ? Cervical collar ? Neck exercises	Avoid quick turns Turn body, not just head Store objects in home low enough to avoid need to look up
Instability on turning	Cerebellar disease Hemiparesis Visual field cut Decreasing proprioception Mild ataxia	Gait training ? Proprioceptive exercises	Appropriate walking aid Obstacle-free environment Proper-fitting shoes
Unsafe on sitting down (misjudges distance or falls into chair) Decreased step height and length—bilateral (there will often be a flexed posture with all these conditions)	Decreasing vision Proximal myopathies Apraxia Parkinson's syndrome Pseudobulbar palsy Myelopathy (usually spastic gait) Normal pressure hydrocephalus Advanced Alzheimer's disease (frontal lobe gait) Compensation for decreasing vision or proprioception Fear of falling Habit	Treatment of specific diseases ? Coordination training Leg-strengthening exercises Treatment of specific diseases (e.g., L-dopa) Correct vision Gait training (correct problems, suggest compensations, increase confidence)	High, firm chairs with arms, in good repair Transfer training Avoid throw rugs Good lighting Proper footwear (good fit, not too much friction or slip) Appropriate walking aid

* Not an exhaustive list.
† Most of these measures have not been subjected to clinical trials; evidence for effectiveness is usually anecdotal at best.
From Tinetti, M. Performance-oriented assessment of mobility problems in the elderly. *J Am Geriatr Soc* 34:119–126, 1986.

ver for individuals who must spend long periods of time in bed or chair. Hip and knee flexion contractures are common in institutionalized older persons, and they influence the ability to walk and to perform bed-to-chair transfers. Lying in the prone position is increasingly recommended for individuals at risk of these contractures because it is the only bed position that eliminates hip flexion (Siebens, 1992). If the patient is able to lie comfortably in this position, it is another turning position for prevention of skin breakdown.

Gait Assessment

The importance of observing an older person walk cannot be overemphasized. Direct observation of both transfer and walking gives the clinician useful screening data about mental status, muscle strength, joint range of motion, motor planning skills, ability to concentrate, sitting and standing balance, and potential for rehabilitation. Tinetti (1986) offers useful guidelines regarding assessment of gait and balance in the elderly, replicated in Tables 14–15, 14–16, and 14–17. Clinicians sometimes rely on the reports of other caregivers regarding the older person's ability to transfer and ambulate. However, nurses who rely on the observations of others with less skill in assessment risk promoting excess disability. Less sophisticated assessors often assume that an older person who is in a wheelchair or has not walked recently is unable to walk. In time, the assumed impairment becomes a reality, as chair-bound patients are more prone to muscle atrophy, contractures, and reduced endurance than are ambulatory individuals. Many patients in hospitals and nursing homes are confined to wheelchairs when they are able to walk with assistance. Thus, direct assessment of ambulation is essential in the elderly.

History

Historical data, such as patients' and caregivers' perceptions of what activities enhance mobility, are useful to obtain. Determine what adaptations have been made to the mobility impairment, such as environmental modifications, work simplification, and use of adaptive equipment. Finally, determine the extent to which the mobility impairment interferes with the individual's ability to carry out desired roles or attain personal goals.

Planning and Intervention

The goals of nursing care in those with mobility impairments are to (1) prevent the hazards associated with immobility, (2) alleviate the cause(s) of immobility when possible, and (3) help the individual compensate for lost mobility. When considering possible interventions, remember that there are few conditions in the chronically ill that cannot become worse through inattention to preventive measures. For example, the individ-

ual with a pressure sore may develop new and deeper pressure sores, and the person with contractures may develop more pain or new skin problems. Regardless of the extent of the impairment, the opportunity to prevent further impairment is usually present.

The cornerstones of treatment for impaired physical mobility are exercise and mobilization. Depending on the source of the mobility impairment, adjuvant therapy with analgesics, antidepressants, or antiparkinsonian drugs may be indicated. Other therapies, such as massage and psychotherapy, may also be employed. The choice of individual or group exercise program depends on personal preference, sensory and cognitive impairments, accessibility of group programs, and the skill of the exercise leader.

Working with Particular Types of Health Problems

Exercise is "a systematic, planned, structured, repetitive type of physical activity" (Hogue and Cullinan, 1992, p. 60). Exercises can be categorized as those designed to promote joint flexibility, muscular strength, and cardiopulmonary endurance, although some exercise programs accomplish all three simultaneously. Before discussing the characteristics of each type of exercise, it is important to review some general principles of exercise prescription in elderly people. First, there is potential for injury in all forms of exercise, and the individual's risk for sustaining various types of injury should be evaluated. Second, each individual should have an individualized exercise prescription that contains at a minimum (1) the goal of the exercise(s), (2) the type of movement to be performed in each exercise, (3) the intensity of each exercise (often expressed as the number of repetitions of each movement, or the amount of resistance to be used on an ergometer), (4) the frequency with which the exercise should be performed, (5) the duration of the exercise, and (6) any precautions the person should observe. Even in group exercise programs, each individual should have a prescription, even if the prescriptions are quite similar among the members of the group. There is sufficient heterogeneity with advancing age that older people may have individual constraints on certain movements, and such individual differences should be respected. Finally, the risk of injury can be minimized through the use of pre-exercise evaluation, warm-up and cool-down routines, and balanced exercise programs that promote flexibility, strength, and endurance (Pollock and Wilmore, 1990).

The major types of injury associated with exercise include: (1) cardiac events, such as myocardial ischemia, dysrhythmia, blood pressure changes, and sudden death; (2) soft tissue injury, either from muscle strain or tendon damage; (3) joint dislocation from improper handling of body parts; (4) fracture, either from stress to brittle bones or trauma from a fall; (5) exacerbation of underlying chronic diseases, such as joint inflammation and effusion in those with degenerative joint disease, hypoglycemia in individuals with diabetes mellitus, or asthma in those with chronic pulmonary disease.

Prevention of injury begins with pre-exercise evaluation for the presence of conditions that would be contraindications to performing certain types of exercise, or starting an exercise program at all. For example, individuals with unstable medical illness, electrolyte disturbances, previously unevaluated conditions such as anemia, or recent fractures or soft tissue injury should not participate in vigorous exercise programs until their medical conditions have been further evaluated and treated and physician clearance obtained. Individuals with poorly compensated chronic disease should begin exercise in a supervised environment, in which their response to exercise can be monitored and treatment to correct exacerbations of illness can be implemented promptly. Those with specific physical findings such as severe joint disease, osteoporosis, or recent injury may require modification of an exercise program so as not to exacerbate a pre-existing problem. Beyond this type of evaluation, the extent of medical evaluation that is required prior to beginning an exercise program is controversial. Preliminary exercise electrocardiograms are recommended by many (Pollock and Wilmore, 1990) to rule out silent ischemia in individuals without known cardiac disease, although this is not the standard of care in all communities (Siebens, 1992).

A second strategy for minimizing injury is to have available the best prepared professionals possible available to prescribe and monitor exercise. Depending upon the type of exercise planned and the population targeted, a multidisciplinary team may be required to develop an exercise prescription. Team members who consult or directly participate in exercise programs include exercise physiologists, occupational and physical therapists, nurses, physicians, and psychologists. For example, a pulmonary rehabilitation program for patients with moderate-to-severe COPD will call for a different constellation of team members than a flexibility maintenance program in generally fit elderly individuals. Exercise group leaders need to have basic knowledge of exercise physiology and the biomechanics of exercise and the ability to recognize and assess complications of exercise, and obtain prompt treatment of any complications.

A third technique for reducing injury and maximizing benefit during exercise is careful monitoring of participants' performance and symptoms that occur during the exercise. Participants may require physical cues as well as verbal instructions to perform exercises correctly, particularly in the early phases of the program. Siebens (1992) recommends giving specific recommendations to participants and group leaders about how to handle the various types of pain that can accompany exercise: acute pain, temporary soreness, residual soreness, new pain, and chronic pain. Each of these will be described in detail under the section entitled "Pain and Discomfort." Although target heart rate guidelines are often used to keep intensity of exercise within safe limits, older people may have difficulty learning to monitor their pulse during exercise. Use of heart rate monitors is one option; another that is gaining increasing acceptance is the use of Borg's rating of perceived exertion (RPE) (Pollock and Wilmore, 1990, p. 292; American College of Sports Medicine, 1990, cited in Siebens, 1992). Other symptoms that may require advance planning include hypoglycemic episodes in diabetics, respiratory decompensation in individuals with chronic lung disease, and cardiac symptoms, such as angina and syncope. A well-understood standard operating procedure for management of these predictable symptoms and potential emergencies is essential for a smoothly run program. An emergency cart containing basic life-support equipment and ready availability of prn medications for symptom control are basic precautions that will promote prompt treatment of exercise-induced chronic disease symptoms.

If the patient strongly prefers solitary exercise, respect the preference and do not try to force participation in a group. However, the peer support and social interaction available in group settings can be powerful motivators and reinforcers of regular exercise.

People with hearing or visual impairments may perform poorly in a group because of inability to process information or because they are fearful. However, if the visually impaired individual is appropriately paired with a buddy, group exercise may provide more safety and enhance confidence.

Cognitively impaired individuals should not be mixed with unimpaired persons, because they will have difficulty attending and following complex instructions. A special group focusing on those with cognitive impairments may be effective, but such a group will require a much smaller leader-to-participant ratio, and the leader must be skilled in effective communication with the cognitively impaired.

A variety of ways to tailor exercise regimens to individual needs maximize the patient's motivation and commitment. Compliance with physical exercise programs may be problematic in the aged. Failure to adhere to exercise programs may be a problem of motivation, and the traditional structure of supervised exercise programs does not address the highly individualized nature of the older adult.

Stoedefalke (1985) offers the following guidelines for structuring physical exercise programs successfully:

- Meet safety and security needs by providing a clean, well-lighted, aesthetically pleasing environment, with good acoustics. Incorporate information about the beneficial effects of exercise.

- Acknowledge the importance of enhancing personal identity by involving participants in goal setting and selecting rewards for goal attainment. Build in frequent opportunities to recognize success.

- Stimulate the participants' intellectual and physical capabilities through creative approaches to exercise by using music or dance. Verbal cues may enhance the older person's awareness of bodily feelings affected by exercise. For example, "I notice you're breathing more slowly now after walking than when we first started. Can you feel the difference?"

Mobility can be promoted even in the absence of structured exercise programs. Each individual should be encouraged to perform as much of the activities of daily living as is practical. Any individual with the capacity to walk should do so, at least three times daily. People who can use the toilet should be given the opportunity to do so rather than using a bedpan. Simply transferring from a sitting to a standing position, if done using the lower extremities without extensive assistance from the upper extremities or another person, assists in strengthening lower extremity muscles. Standing and bearing weight through long bones retard bone resorption, prevent formation of contractures, and promote return of blood to the heart from the extremities. Encouraging older people to comb their own hair enhances shoulder flexibility and range of motion. Dressing stimulates the older person's fine motor coordination and helps preserve joint mobility. Walking is an excellent general conditioning exercise and should be encouraged within the limits of the individual's cardiorespiratory capacity. Nurses must judge when an individual should not engage in a self-care activity because the energy expenditure is too great or because the activity may actually harm the person. For example, patients in the acute phase of a myocardial infarction require assistance with activities of daily living to reduce the workload on the damaged myocardium. Use of guidelines, such as those outlined under "Activity Tolerance" or in Pollock and Wilmore (1990), can be quite helpful in making these judgments.

Decreased Strength and Endurance

Before an exercise regimen is instituted, resting pulse and respiratory rates, orthostatic blood pressures, and estimates of muscle mass and strength should be obtained. These measures serve as a guide for establishing goals and time schedules for the exercise regimen. People who have been in bed or otherwise immobilized for long periods of time often experience orthostatic hypotension. The dizziness and instability associated with this syndrome may cause fear or discomfort in the older person, with subsequent resistance to increasing activity. People who have a greater than 20 mm Hg drop in diastolic blood pressure or those who experience severe dizziness with change in position should perform "stir-up" movements before attempting more strenuous exercise. A tilt table may be used, or dangling at the bedside several times per day, until a vertical position can be tolerated. Pending the re-establishment of baroreceptor function, the patient may engage in isometric and isotonic in-bed exercises to increase muscle strength and joint flexibility.

An exercise regimen suitable for a bedbound elderly patient includes the following maneuvers:

- Deep breathing (slow inhalation and full exhalation)
- Neck rolls (flex neck forward, lateral flex, and rotate)
- Knee to chest (either supine or side-lying,

bring one knee to chest, wrap arms around, hold and breathe, straighten leg slowly)

- Pelvic tilts (on back, knees bent, feet flat, tuck in abdomen, relax)
- Bridging (on back, feet flat on bed, raise hips, lower slowly)
- Head raising in prone and supine positions
- Unilateral leg lifts
- Ankle circling (or have patient "write" different numbers or letters in the air)
- Rolling from side to side
- Lying prone
- Arms straight over head of bed while lying supine
- Arms out to sides, palms up in supine position
- Hands behind head with elbows bent
- Hands at lower back

The number of repetitions and the pace of an exercise program depend upon the individual's endurance and other health problems. However, the exercises just described are not strenuous and will help promote circulation and prevent contractures.

Resting pulse and respiratory rate are useful indicators of endurance. Most authorities recommend exercising to 70 per cent of the maximum heart rate (calculated as 200 minus the patient's age) for 20 minutes, at least two times each week, to maintain cardiovascular fitness. For an 80-year-old, the target heart rate would be 98 beats per minute. For other means of assessing response to increased activity, consult Table 14–2. An increasing respiratory rate may indicate either anxiety or an ineffective breathing pattern for the new exercise program. The patient may require a slower pace or instruction in deep breathing, as obtaining adequate tissue oxygenation is essential for an effective exercise program.

Muscle mass and strength are useful guides to the strenuousness of the activity that can be tolerated. Patients with extensive muscle wasting or loss of strength will require assistance with walking. The goals and schedules for therapy must be adjusted in light of the patient's baseline performance.

Pain and Discomfort

Pain often serves as a warning signal of tissue damage. Therefore, before beginning an exercise regimen for individuals who have mobility impairments secondary to pain, the location, nature, severity, and etiology of the pain should be described carefully, along with aggravating and alleviating factors. Mobility limitations due to pain from coronary artery disease may be alleviated by establishing the patient on an adequate vasodilator regimen. Activities such as those described under strengthening and endurance are appropriate within the limits of pain.

Those with mobility limitations due to pain from degenerative joint disease, disc disease, contractures, and chronic immobility must learn to distinguish acute pain from chronic pain, because the chronic pain only serves to perpetuate dysfunctional immobility. Analgesics such as nonsteroidal anti-inflammatory agents or acetaminophen may control the pain sufficiently to allow the individual to begin an exercise program. As the individual's mobility improves, pain is likely to diminish, resulting in further gains in mobility.

Siebens (1992) recommends the following approach to assessment and treatment of pain associated with exercise. First, acute pain syndromes can be treated with rest, but if the pain is more chronic, therapeutic exercises as prescribed by a therapist should be performed. Second, temporary soreness lasting only several hours should be treated by lowering the intensity of the exercise during the next session. If soreness persists or increases despite lowering of intensity, medical evaluation should be sought. Residual soreness, which appears later, may last up to 3 to 4 days. Management of this type of pain should be dictated by its location. Pain localized to a muscle will probably resolve spontaneously, and continued exercise is not contraindicated, within the patient's tolerance for discomfort. Pain localized to a joint or to the back may represent injury and should receive medical evaluation. If an individual has pain with a specific exercise, it may be a sign of overuse. The exercise should be stopped, and alternative exercises, such as isometric strengthening exercises, considered to promote strength while the overuse syndrome is treated with rest and medication.

Finally, Siebens notes that chronic pain associated with arthritis or chronic back pain should not be a contraindication to exercise. In these disorders, movement necessary to maintain function often induces pain, but the pain is tolerable and ends when the exercise session is concluded. In these conditions, it is important to maintain muscle strength around the affected joint to prevent joint malalignment during use.

Perceptual or Cognitive Impairment

Cognitive and perceptual impairments make it extremely difficult to teach the older person an exercise regimen. Interventions, therefore, must be highly individualized, capitalizing on the older person's remaining capabilities and support network. For example, some individuals with severe visual impairment will have difficulty following through with an exercise regimen because of difficulty in remembering instructions, or fear of injury. In the first instance, a tape-recorded set of instructions may resolve the problem, or a supportive friend or relative may agree to "coach" the person in the exercise regimen. Fears of injury during an exercise program due to blindness may be alleviated by a "buddy system," in which an individual with sensory impairment is consistently paired with someone who is not impaired. Another strategy to promote confidence in people with sensory impairment is to set up a group exercise session for the visually impaired that is sufficiently supervised to prevent injury. Schwartz (1981) has suggested that nurses become more knowledgeable about the work of "mobility trainers" employed by services to the blind. She contends that assistance in achieving safe mobility in the community applies to navigating safely in nursing home environments as well.

People with hearing deficits also require modifications in exercise regimens. Written instructions and diagrams are more appropriate, with the therapist using touch to guide the person in learning the regimen. Again, supportive family and friends are invaluable in reinforcing exercise programs. Group exercise may be less effective for those with hearing impairments because of the difficulty of communicating in a large and diverse group.

Cognitive impairments present the most special challenge of all to nurses. Some therapists refuse to treat older persons with dementing disorders, with the rationale that they are unteachable or have poor rehabilitation potential. However, when the older person is taught in conjunction with a primary caregiver, the potential for prevention and even restoration of function exists. Dementia does not in itself prevent individuals from walking, nor does it preclude a caregiver from giving repetitive instructions for muscle-strengthening exercises. Designing interventions to prevent or treat mobility impairments in older people with cognitive or perceptual impairments represents a challenge but is not an impossible task.

Neuromuscular Impairment

The specific nature of the neuromuscular impairment influences the exercise regimen prescribed to prevent further loss of mobility and compensate for dysfunction. For example, individuals with hemiplegia secondary to a cerebrovascular accident require forms of exercise and adaptive equipment different from those for individuals with Parkinson's disease. In both instances, encouragement to continue or retain as much independent ADL function as possible is indicated.

Special techniques used to enhance mobility in patients with neuromuscular impairments include drugs, adaptive equipment, and exercise. Drug treatment of Parkinson's disease is discussed in Chapter 9.

Adaptive equipment for patients with impaired physical mobility of neuromuscular origin must be individualized to the patient and the disorder. Splints preserve joint motion and prevent contractures. Slings hold joints in alignment, redistribute weight, and prevent dependent edema formation. Braces stabilize unsteady joints—for example, when muscles are muscle flaccid. Walking aids—canes, walkers, and crutches—assist in maintaining balance and stability. The types of appliances available vary tremendously. Older people should be encouraged to see professionals qualified to prescribe and fit walking aids rather than choosing from their local medical equipment company, so that the most appropriate appliance is selected. Improperly fitted or used adaptive equipment may produce new problems for the older person (Fig. 14–10).

A recent study that compared the traditional four-legged, two-wheeled walker with a new type of three-wheeled walker found the three-wheeled walker superior in terms of stride length, time on an obstacle course, and patient preference (Mahoney et al., 1992). The literature comparing various types of adaptive equipment to improve mobility is likely to continue to increase, and nurses should remain up to date on developments in adaptive equipment to promote mobility.

Wheelchairs are often misused in the elderly. They can be tremendous mobility-enhancers, but too many older people receive a wheelchair prematurely and become its

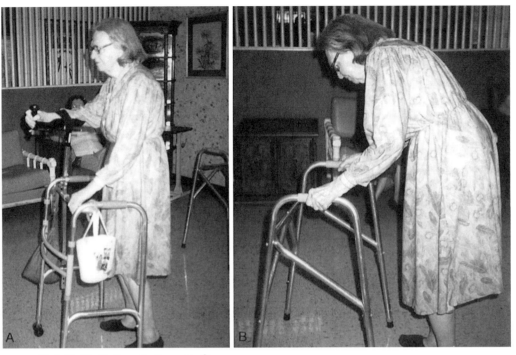

FIGURE 14-10

Note the difference in a person's body alignment when a walker is properly fitted (A), compared with posture when an improperly fitted walker is used (B).

prisoner because they lose their remaining ability to ambulate. Also, wheelchairs must be fitted to the individual; Figure 14–11 shows the effects of poor seating. As with walking aids, wheelchairs come in many dif-

ferent types, and the older person deserves a professional evaluation for the wheelchair. For example, wheelchairs with elevating leg rests and proper back and seat support are essential for people who are inactive and

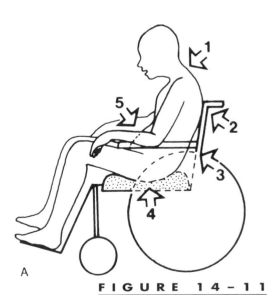

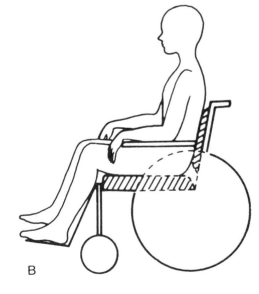

FIGURE 14-11

Lumbar and seat support. Poor lumbar and seat support (A) allows a sacral sitting posture, resulting in (1) neck and upper back strain, (2) excessive scapular pressure, (3) overstretching of lumbar extensors, (4) excessive sacral pressure, and (5) poor ventilation. Proper seat and lumbar support (B) greatly improves function and cosmesis. (From Kottke, F.J. and Lehman, J.F. *Krusen's Handbook of Physical Medicine and Rehabilitation.* 4th ed. Philadelphia: W.B. Saunders, 1990, p. 554.)

spend many hours each day in the wheelchair. Yet elevating leg rests are not "standard" equipment on wheelchairs, and standard seats and backs are of a sling-type fabric that makes proper posture nearly impossible to maintain. Removable arm and foot rests greatly facilitate transfers and access to tabletops for patients with hemiplegia and leg amputations. These features are not standard either. Wheelchairs with one-sided drive mechanisms are available so that people with hemiplegia can propel them with relative ease.

Motorized wheelchairs are more available than in the past, although care must be taken to prescribe the appropriate type to maximize mobility. Redford (1993) recommends classifying people who need wheelchairs into one of four categories to facilitate selection of appropriate design features to promote mobility and safety: (1) nonmobile and dependent, unable to wheel or walk independently, (2) mobile, nonambulatory, (3) ambulatory, but with special wheelchair needs, and (4) ambulatory frail. Wheelchair components that can be customized include seat height, angle, and depth; arm rests, foot rests, and drive (one arm, two arm, motorized). Finally, wheelchair design can be altered to promote safety using antitipping devices for those whose transfer techniques cause them to push back in the chair and risk tipping it backward. Nurses should be aware of the usefulness and misuses of adaptive equipment in mobility enhancement. Occupational and physical therapists are valuable consultants in identifying appropriate equipment and obtaining proper fit.

Range-of-Motion Exercises

General strengthening and conditioning exercises are useful for all patients, but individuals with mobility impairments require specific exercise regimens to prevent contractures and preserve function. Range-of-motion exercises prevent loss of joint motion and, in some instances, help the individual regain lost motion. When possible, older people should be taught how to perform their own range of motion. Experience shows that many individuals who require it are unable to self-range for a variety of reasons, including cognitive impairment, lack of motivation, and impaired mobility. These patients require someone else to construct an exercise program and assist in conducting it. Family members or friends can be taught range-of-motion exercises. Their successful performance by severely impaired

patients requires considerable sophistication. The only way to develop this expertise is to practice the exercises. However, certain do's and don'ts apply:

1. Move in a gentle, circular motion, not in a jerky, rapid motion.
2. Circular motion is more effective in reducing spasticity than direct opposition.
3. When performing range of motion on upper extremities, mobilize the scapulas first to facilitate relaxation in the remainder of the extremity.
4. When working on the lower extremities, mobilize the hips first, to facilitate relaxation in other lower extremity joints.
5. When working on the back, begin with head and neck flexibility (Bobath, 1978; Trombly, 1982).

Musculoskeletal Impairment

Immobility related to musculoskeletal impairments may be divided into three categories: acute inflammatory processes, fracture, and chronic musculoskeletal disorders. Patients with acute inflammatory processes are generally limited by pain, although joint effusion may also be a contributor. Treatment of the immobility depends on accurate diagnosis and treatment of the underlying problem (see Chapter 6). For example, immobility induced by rheumatoid arthritis calls for the use of anti-inflammatory agents, joint rest, and splinting to preserve function until the acute phase is over, followed by gradual mobilization. Polymyalgia rheumatica, causing soft tissue pain, responds to low-dose steroid treatment. Since no joint inflammation is present, joint rest is not required—mobilization to the fullest extent possible is indicated.

Fractures require immobilization of the affected bone, but the rest of the patient is immobilized as little as possible. Lightweight cast materials now allow for greater mobility following a fracture. Adequate analgesia is also important in promoting mobility. People who ache chronically often resist activity. Thus, controlling pain secondary to the injury helps promote activity and mobility. Individuals who must wear casts or who remain in traction for any period of time should be taught isometric exercises to maintain muscle tone and strength in the immobilized body part.

Chronic musculoskeletal impairments include degenerative joint disease and contractures. Degenerative joint disease (DJD) is extremely prevalent in older people; however, its severity varies. Individuals with mild-to-moderate DJD should be evaluated for their response to nonsteroidal anti-inflammatory agents. They should also engage in a daily regimen of flexibility exercises. Decrease in activity in these patients should be evaluated, as reduced activity may precipitate a flare of the arthritis and further impaired mobility. Particular care should be taken with patients who have dementing disorders, for their decline in function may be quite subtle and easily overlooked; regaining lost mobility is especially difficult in these cases.

Contractures are a consequence of immobility, but they also cause further impairment in mobility. They are much easier to prevent than to remedy, and every attempt should be made to prevent them. Contractures occur because inactive muscles eventually shorten, and, with time, tendons and ligaments also shorten. When the contracture involves ligament and tendon shortening, surgical correction is the only available "cure." Flexion contractures of the hips and knees are commonly seen in patients who spend large amounts of time in a wheelchair. However, hip contractures also occur in patients confined to bed, unless the patient spends part of the time in the supine position. Contractures increase the amount of energy that must be expended to maintain an upright position or to walk. They also render the individual much less stable and therefore prone to falls. Range of motion to all joints with three repetitions, two times each day, is recommended to prevent contractures in most patients. Lying in the prone position is a useful technique to promote hip, knee, and back extension for those who are prone to hip and knee flexion contractures (Ellwood, 1990). Although no studies exist about the exact duration and frequency required to prevent contractures, clinical recommendations in the geriatric literature suggest that 10 minutes daily may be sufficient (Siebens, 1992). Patients with acute inflammatory processes in the joints must be handled with particular gentleness, as inflammation reduces the tensile strength of the joint capsule and is likely to be more painful. Gentle stretching over a prolonged period of time is more successful in reducing a muscular contracture than is rapid, vigorous stretching.

Depression and Anxiety

Treatment of psychoemotional disorders that contribute to impaired mobility is essential. Both drugs and psychotherapy are useful. The decision to use medications in either depression or anxiety cannot be made lightly. Both antidepressant medications and anxiolytics are potent drugs, with immobilizing side effects of their own (see Chapter 18). Nurses should therefore be prepared to initiate referrals to appropriate therapists or to provide supportive therapy themselves for these disorders. While appropriate psychotherapy is important, it is also important to include physical rehabilitation strategies, such as exercise and comfort techniques, to prevent further problems and to help the individual compensate for mobility impairments. Successful completion of repetitive tasks may be therapeutic for both depressed and anxious individuals.

Medically Prescribed Treatments

Bedrest, traction, and casts are the three most common prescriptions that result in impaired physical mobility. Nurses should know the hazards of immobility and be assertive in questioning prolonged bedrest orders and in initiating exercise regimens for those who must be immobilized. Individuals on bedrest, with or without traction, should perform isometric and isotonic exercises that have been shown to maintain muscle strength (Kottke, 1990). Individuals who are in casts can and should be taught isometric exercises to prevent loss of muscle mass, tone, and strength.

Environmental Features

PHYSICAL ENVIRONMENT. In the hospital, elderly patients may be intimidated by the numerous tubes, machines, and alarms and become immobilized. Nurses should be aware of this possibility and explain to patients the purpose and hazards of the tubes, encourage mobility as much as possible, and encourage discontinuing tubes and appliances that limit mobility as soon as possible. Most hospitals and nursing homes do not have adequate "wandering" or exercise space, so patients who become restless are sometimes restrained to prevent unsupervised wandering. While in the past physical restraint may have been justified on the grounds of promoting safety, the routine use of physical restraint to treat behavioral disturbance can no longer be considered an acceptable intervention in care of frail elderly people. Physical restraint is accompanied by deleterious physical and psychological sequelae that most clinicians find unacceptable (Evans et al., 1992; Miles and Irvine, 1992; Tinetti et al., 1992). Nurses must plan for adequate exercise and mobilization for individuals who require restraint.

POLICIES. Some institutions still prescribe restraints for patients who require assistance with ambulation. This practice has not been shown to reduce falls (Tinetti et al., 1992), and restraints produce considerable mobility impairment and predispose the older person to further impairment. Institutional policies also may enhance mobility. Consider the difference between facility A, in which all patients, including those who require two-person assistance, walk to every meal each day, and facility B, in which patients are always wheeled to the dining room or fed in their rooms. Which patients do you think have the greatest impairments in mobility?

Characteristics of Caregivers

Attitudes of the caregiver are critical in promoting mobility and in treating mobility disorders. Patience, willingness to persevere and support patients through their pain and boredom, and a belief that promoting mobility is important in the aged are essential characteristics. Most mobility impairments in the elderly are chronic in nature, meaning that it is difficult to sustain enthusiasm for exercise regimens, because the rewards are in what you don't see (the absence of further impairment) rather than in what you do see. Also, it is difficult to notice whether an exercise program is skipped for one day, although failure to be vigilant results in observable declines in function over time.

Evaluation

Criteria for evaluation of patients with impaired physical mobility are as follows:

1. Does the patient have preventable problems associated with immobility, for example: contractures, pressure sores, activity intolerance, self-care deficit(s), emboli, respiratory infections, incontinence?
2. Is there a realistic monitoring plan for identifying preventable problems?
3. Is the person disabled by the mobility impairment or are adequate compensatory mechanisms developed?
4. Does the elderly person pursue meaningful social activities?
5. Are the individual's goals for health met?
6. Are there factors contributing to the mobility impairment that could be alleviated?

ORAL MUCOUS MEMBRANE ALTERATION

Definition and Scope of Problem

Alteration in oral mucosa is defined as "the state in which an individual experiences disruptions in the tissues of the oral cavity" (NANDA, 1992, p. 34). The types of alterations in mucosa commonly experienced by older people include edentulousness and its associated complications, dental caries, stomatitis, xerostomia (dry mouth), and periodontal disease. The risk of oral cancer, which creates changes in the oral mucosa, increases with age.

Consequences of untreated alterations in oral mucosa include alteration in comfort, decreased taste sensation, alteration in nutrition to less than body requirements (Sullivan et al., 1993), increased potential for oral infection, and deformities.

Theoretical Issues

Functions of the Oral Cavity

The oral cavity is a complex organ serving many functions. It is required for normal intake of food, fluids, and air respiration and performs sensory and communication functions. Impairment of the oral mucosa thus has important ramifications for the function of other body systems.

The tissues of the oral mucosa are categorized as (1) freely movable tissue, such as the labial and buccal mucosa, (2) well-keratinized tissue that firmly adheres to underlying bone, such as the mucosa over the gums and the palate, and (3) specialized tissue, such as that on the dorsum of the tongue. The mucosa serves as a lining that protects deeper oral tissues against dehydration, infection, noxious chemicals, and extremes in temperature.

Oral mucous membranes become increasingly thin, smooth, and less elastic and thus are more susceptible to injury with advancing age (Ferguson and Devlin, 1992). The effects, if any, on salivary gland flow rate are unclear. Normal aging changes are probably not clinically significant, but aging is associated with diseases and therapies that cause xerostomia.

Saliva is necessary for the maintenance of dental health, as it performs the following functions: (1) lubricates the oral mucosa, (2) buffers the acid produced by oral bacteria, (3) mediates taste acuity, (4) assists with mechanical cleansing of the teeth, (5) contains the growth of bacteria, and (6) is needed for remineralization of the teeth.

Contributing Factors

Decreased Saliva

The most common adverse effect of medical therapies on the oral mucosa is reduction in the amount of saliva. Common offending agents are drugs with anticholinergic properties (see Chapter 18) and radiation therapy to the head and neck (Atkinson and Fox, 1992). People who habitually breathe through the mouth also have less saliva because it more rapidly evaporates. Tube-fed patients often become mouth breathers and are particularly susceptible to problems in the oral cavity. Persons receiving oxygen, those who are dehydrated, and those who are not allowed to receive food or fluids by mouth (NPO) are also at high risk for dry oral mucous membranes.

Medications

Drugs affect integrity of the oral mucosa in other ways than diminishing the amount of saliva. Broad-spectrum antibiotics may lead to suprainfection with fungi, such as *Candida albicans*. According to Swearingen (1986), 30 per cent of those receiving cancer chemotherapy develop stomatitis. Anticonvulsants, such as phenytoin, can cause gingival hyperplasia.

Trauma

Trauma is another factor implicated in altered oral mucosa. Trauma may result from improperly prepared food, dentures that do not fit properly or are in poor repair, burns from ingestion of food that is too hot, and from oral suctioning injury.

Disease States

Systemic disease may also result in altered oral mucosa (Ship, 1992). Malnutrition is a prime offender, especially vitamin deficiency (Czajka-Narins, 1992). Periodontal disease includes gingivitis, an inflammation of the gums that is usually painless in its initial stages but, if left untreated, causes pyorrhea and tooth loss. The incidence and severity of periodontal disease increase with age. Periodontal disease can be prevented through proper oral hygiene.

Malignant disorders may affect the oral mucosa in one of several ways. Malignant growth in the oral cavity interferes with functioning of the oral mucosa. More often, however, cancer therapies adversely affect oral mucosa. Many chemotherapeutic agents produce stomatitis, and radiation therapy to the head or neck region may also produce uncomfortable lesions in the mouth. The incidence of most cancers, including oral cancer, increases with age. Fifty-eight per cent of all buccal and pharyngeal cancers occur in patients aged 60 years and over (Dellefield, 1986).

Inadequate Oral Hygiene

Proper oral hygiene and preventive dental care practices are often neglected by older persons for several reasons. The high cost of dental care and the lack of third-party reimbursement for dental care for most older people produce an economic barrier to preventive dental care and teaching about proper oral hygiene. Decreased manual dexterity caused by arthritis, stroke, or other neuromuscular disorders can make performing the tasks of oral hygiene quite difficult. Dementing disorders or psychiatric illness often result in impairments in judgment or motivation that lead to inadequate self-care practices, including poor dental hygiene. Finally, the older person may simply not understand the importance of proper oral hygiene. Concepts of preventive dental care have changed in recent times, and the expectation that old people must lose their teeth is no longer valid. Older people who have seen dental care providers only in their youth will not necessarily understand newer concepts of care and thus may be less motivated to perform adequate oral hygiene.

Assessment

Assessment of the oral mucosa involves inspection and palpation primarily. The equipment needed includes a tongue depressor, flashlight, clean glove, and mirror. While examining the oral cavity for signs of pathology, nurses should be alert for conditions that predispose to alterations in oral mucosa, such as dentures and impaired judgment or self-care abilities. The defining characteristics of alterations in oral mucous membranes (NANDA, 1992, p. 34) are

- Oral pain/discomfort
- Coated tongue
- Xerostomia (dry mouth)
- Oral lesions or ulcers
- Lack of or decreased salivation
- Leukoplakia
- Edema
- Hyperemia
- Oral plaque
- Desquamation
- Vesicles
- Hemorrhagic gingivitis

- Carious teeth
- Halitosis

History

Ask the patient about symptoms of pain or discomfort in the mouth. Absence of symptoms does not ensure freedom from problems, but some patients are more bothered than others by xerostomia and are thus more likely to follow through with suggested interventions. Inquire about the person's dental care practices and determine customary habits regarding mouth care. Such questions may highlight knowledge or motivational or physical deficits that will influence oral hygiene. For example, dentures should never be left in the mouth overnight, as this impedes circulation to the palate and predisposes to lesions. Review the patient's medications to identify drugs with anticholinergic properties or other medications that may adversely affect the integrity of the oral mucosa.

Inspection and Palpation

Inspect the teeth; note the number and location of those missing and any carious teeth. For edentulous patients, inspect the dentures for signs of chipping and adequacy of fit. Inquire about dental care practices.

The gums should be inspected for signs of bleeding, plaque, or ulceration. The buccal mucosa and palate and tongue should be inspected for lesions and hyperemia. The lips, the sides and underside of the tongue, the anterior floor of the mouth, the soft palate, and tonsillar region should all be inspected for lesions, as these are prime sites for development of early oral cancer. Early squamous cell carcinomas often appear as red or red and white lesions (Thomas and Faecher, 1992). Any deviations from normal should be noted and referred to a dentist for definitive assessment. Figure 14–12 shows an oral assessment guide that can be used for assessment of the oral cavity and mucosa.

Functional Assessment

The person's ability to perform oral hygiene tasks should be estimated. Manual dexterity, judgment, knowledge, ability to plan tasks, and motivation to carry out adequate dental hygiene must be assessed. Deficiencies in any of these spheres of function suggest potential for alteration in oral mucous membranes. Note whether the patient shows signs of cognitive impairment, as such patients will have special needs for oral

and dental care (Jones et al., 1988; Kiyak et al., 1993).

Planning and Intervention

All individuals require daily attention to oral hygiene, although the frequency of oral hygiene varies according to specific patient conditions and the goals of oral hygiene. These goals include prevention of periodontal disease, prevention of stomatitis, and promotion of comfort. Individuals who cannot perform the necessary tasks independently should be identified, and an alternative caregiving system put into place. Assisting family and nonprofessional caregivers in understanding the correct way to help someone perform oral hygiene and helping the caregiver overcome negative feelings about cleaning another person's mouth are essential. Suggest the use of clean examining gloves as one technique for overcoming reluctance to perform mouth care. Other than toothbrushing after meals and denture cleansing and overnight soaking, specific interventions to treat alterations in oral mucosa depend upon the contributing factors.

General Preventive Oral Care

Individuals who do not have self-care deficits should be encouraged to brush teeth, gums, and tongue with a soft-bristled toothbrush and fluorinated toothpaste after each meal and to floss daily. Older people may still believe that loss of teeth is inevitable with aging and therefore not be motivated to engage in oral hygiene. Those who do have self-care deficits should be evaluated for the need for adaptive equipment, such as enlarged and padded toothbrush handles for arthritic persons or electric toothbrushes for persons with intolerance to upper extremity activity (Danielson, 1988). Patients who are not independent even with adaptive equipment should receive assistance from nursing staff or family caregivers to brush and floss. Dentures should be removed and cleaned after every meal, as the possibility of trauma from food caught between the denture and the palate is high.

Decreased Salivation

Individuals with decreased salivation, regardless of the cause, should receive particularly careful mouth care. Oral lubricants such as artificial saliva, mouth rinses, or sucking on hard candy may be useful (Atkinson and Fox, 1992). Products containing citric acid (lemon swabs) are no longer recommended because they erode enamel and

CATEGORY	TOOLS FOR ASSESSMENT	METHODS OF MEASUREMENT	NUMERICAL AND DESCRIPTIVE RATINGS		
			1	2	3
Voice	Auditory	Converse with patient	Normal	Deeper or raspy	Difficulty talking or painful
Swallow	Observation	Ask patient to swallow. To test gag reflex, gently place blade on back of tongue and depress	Normal swallow	Some pain on swallow	Unable to swallow
Lips	Visual/palpatory	Observe and feel tissue	Smooth and pink and moist	Dry or cracked	Ulcerated or bleeding
Tongue	Visual/palpatory	Feel and observe appearance of tissue	Pink and moist and papillae present	Coated or loss of papillae with a shiny appearance with or without redness	Blistered or cracked
Saliva	Tongue blade	Insert blade into mouth, touching the center of the tongue and the floor of the mouth	Watery	Thick or ropy	Absent
Mucous membranes	Visual	Observe appearance of tissue	Pink and moist	Reddened or coated (increased whiteness) without ulcerations	Ulcerations with or without bleeding
Gingiva	Tongue blade and visual	Gently press tissue with tip of blade	Pink and stippled and firm	Edematous with or without redness	Spontaneous bleeding or bleeding with pressure
Teeth or dentures (or denture bearing area)	Visual	Observe appearance of teeth or denture bearing area	Clean and no debris	Plaque or debris in localized areas (between teeth if present)	Plaque or debris generalized along gum line or denture bearing area

FIGURE 14–12

Oral Assessment Guide. (From Eilers, J., Berger, A.M. and Petersen, M.C. Development, testing and application of the Oral Assessment Guide. *Oncol Nurs Forum* 15(3):325–330, 1988. Reprinted with permission from the University of Nebraska Medical Center.)

may actually dehydrate oral tissues (Roth and Creason, 1986). Some patients with radiation-induced xerostomia may obtain relief by swishing $\frac{1}{16}$ to $\frac{1}{8}$ tsp of butter, margarine, or vegetable oil in the mouth two to three times per day and at bedtime. This remedy, although not tested in a controlled study, appears in the literature as a promising case report (Kusler and Rambur, 1992).

Review the individual's drug regimen. If drugs with anticholinergic properties are being used, it may be possible to substitute a drug with fewer anticholinergic effects, or dosage may be lowered without removing the therapeutic effect.

Stomatitis

An extensive body of nursing research on the efficacy of various mouth care protocols exists. Specific rinses, toothbrushes, and the frequency of mouth care have been studied in both acutely ill and chronically ill patients. No firm conclusions can be drawn about the superiority of one mouth rinse over another. Hydrogen peroxide is criticized as altering the normal oral flora and disrupting granulation tissue (Nieweg et al., 1992). The trend is to use normal saline as a mouth rinse, supplemented by artificial saliva products as needed for xerostomia (National Institutes of Health, 1990; Graham et al., 1993). Similarly, little evidence supports the superiority of a toothbrush versus toothette (foam brush) versus gauze pad. However, studies of the effects of various frequencies suggest that twice weekly thorough oral hygiene (brushing and flossing) may suffice to prevent gingivitis in nonacutely ill elderly patients, but it is doubtful that such infrequent mouth care promotes patient comfort adequately. Patients with acute illness, such as fever, those receiving oxygen, and those with systemic illness affecting the oral mucosa should receive mouth care every 4 hours or more often if the condition of the patient's mouth warrants it.

MEDICATIONS. In patients who develop stomatitis, medications to treat a specific infectious agent, either fungal or bacterial, are used. There is also a place for palliative mouth rinses in patients with extreme discomfort from stomatitis. Care should be taken to use current pain management principles (see Comfort Alterations) with oral pain, including use of systemic analgesics if local intervention is not effective.

Evaluation

Criteria for evaluation of patients with alterations in oral mucosa include the following:

1. The patient is free of oral lesions.
2. The patient is free from discomfort in the mouth.
3. Nutritional deficiencies are corrected.
4. Daily oral hygiene is practiced, either by the older person independently with assistive devices or by a caregiver.
5. Screening for oral cancer is conducted annually.
6. The patient does not have halitosis.
7. The patient's oral cavity is free of debris.

RESPIRATORY FUNCTION ALTERATIONS: INEFFECTIVE AIRWAY CLEARANCE, INEFFECTIVE BREATHING PATTERN, IMPAIRED GAS EXCHANGE

Definition and Scope of Problem

Three diagnostic categories pertaining to respiratory function can be clustered as they are related to each other etiologically and have nursing interventions in common. The categories are ineffective airway clearance, ineffective breathing pattern, and impaired gas exchange (NANDA, 1992). Both ineffective breathing pattern and ineffective airway clearance may contribute to impaired gas exchange, and immobility predisposes to all three problems.

Ineffective airway clearance is "the state in which the individual is unable to clear secretions or obstructions from the respiratory tract to maintain airway patency."

Ineffective breathing pattern is "the state in which an inhalation and/or exhalation pattern does not enable adequate pulmonary inflation or emptying."

Impaired gas exchange is "the state in which the individual experiences decreased passage of oxygen and/or carbon dioxide between the alveoli of the lungs and the vascular system" (NANDA, 1992, p. 25).

The prevalence of chronic pulmonary disease, both obstructive and restrictive, is growing in the United States (Kersten, 1989). In a population study in Arizona, the prevalence of asthma (commonly considered a disease of the young) among elderly people was estimated to be 4 per cent in men and 7 per cent in women (Burrows et al., 1991). Aging-related changes in respiratory function, especially reduced efficiency of host-defense mechanisms, changes in lung compliance, and decreased pulmonary capillary blood flow, predispose older people to alterations in respiratory function. Gerontological nurses thus should be alert for signs of altered respiratory function, particularly when older people's mobility is impaired.

Contributing Factors

Age-Related Changes in the Respiratory System

The effects of the normal aging process predispose the elderly to respiratory problems by diminishing the efficiency of air exchange and by reducing functional reserve. Total lung capacity and vital capacity both decline with age, as do flow rates and efficiency of pulmonary gas exchange. Age-related changes are sufficiently large to lead some to suggest changing reference values for pulmonary function tests based upon normative data in healthy older adults, for prevention of unnecessary introduction of medications with potentially harmful side effects (Enright et al., 1993; Beck, 1994). Disorders common in the aged, such as musculoskeletal deformity, reduced activity, heart disease, and chronic pulmonary disease, put the elderly at even greater risk for respiratory difficulties. Lifestyle factors, such as chronic smoking or exposure to hazardous inhalants in the workplace, also increase the likelihood of respiratory problems. Inadequate hydration is a common problem that places the old person at greater risk of pulmonary problems. The practice of polypharmacy in the elderly also may predispose to respiratory dysfunction. The usual culprits are sedative drugs that depress the older person's mobility, including the drive to take deep breaths and sigh.

Specific Diseases

Neurological impairments such as Parkinson's disease, hemiplegia, and advanced stages of dementing disorders contribute to ineffective airway clearance in different

TABLE 14-18
Defining Characteristics of Alterations in Respiratory Function

INEFFECTIVE AIRWAY CLEARANCE	INEFFECTIVE BREATHING PATTERN	IMPAIRED GAS EXCHANGE
Abnormal breath sounds (rales, rhonchi, wheezes)	Dyspnea	Confusion
	Shortness of breath	Somnolence
	Tachypnea	Restlessness
Changes in rate or depth of respiration	Fremitus	Irritability
	Abnormal arterial blood gas	Inability to move secretions
Tachypnea	Cyanosis	
Cough	Cough	
Cyanosis	Nasal flaring	Hypercapnea
Dyspnea	Respiratory depth changes	Hypoxia
	Assumption of three-point position	
	Pursed-lip breathing/prolonged expiratory phase	
	Increased anterior/posterior diameter	
	Use of accessory muscles	
	Altered chest excursion	

From McLane, A. (ed.). *Classification of Nursing Diagnoses; Proceedings of the Seventh Conference: North American Nursing Diagnosis Association.* St. Louis: C.V. Mosby Company, 1987.

ways. People with Parkinson's disease may be so immobilized that they are unable to cough effectively to clear the airway. They may have associated problems, such as swallowing difficulties predisposing to aspiration pneumonia, that increase the need to clear secretions. Hemiplegia predisposes one to aspiration pneumonia when gag reflexes are impaired; by reducing the patient's mobility, the likelihood that secretions will pool and become more difficult to remove is increased. In the late stages of dementia, individuals may develop ineffective gas exchange and airway clearance because of diminished gag reflexes and mobility.

Congestive heart failure, if uncontrolled, interferes with gaseous exchange in the alveoli. Fluid accumulates where gaseous exchange generally takes place and reduces the lung area available for ventilation. Other cardiac disorders, such as severe coronary artery disease, can predispose to ineffective gas exchange and airway clearance because the patient is immobilized from activity intolerance or pain.

Acute infections, such as pneumonia and influenza, often produce delirium that interferes with the individual's ability to follow directions regarding coughing and deep breathing. Pneumonia may precipitate ineffective airway clearance by producing secretions that are difficult to clear because of pain and fatigue. Older persons with other chronic diseases are particularly likely to have difficulty clearing secretions in pneu-

monia. In chronic respiratory disorders, the airways are often obstructed, making coughing up of secretions more difficult. Individuals with these diseases also produce more secretions than do normal individuals. Chronic obstructive lung disease also contributes to impaired gas exchange because of bronchiolar obstruction in the case of asthma and bronchitis, and because of decreased lung capacity and CO_2 retention in emphysema. Chronic restrictive lung diseases, such as tuberculosis, asbestosis, and coal miner's pneumoconiosis (black lung), contribute to impaired gas exchange by reducing lung capacity. These diseases contribute to ineffective airway clearance by predisposing the patient to respiratory infections.

Assessment

Defining characteristics for the respiratory nursing diagnosis categories are listed in Table 14-18. Assessment aims to identify individuals at risk for these diagnoses as well as those who currently experience such problems. The assessment also should identify significant contributing factors.

Physical assessment techniques of the respiratory system for the elderly do not differ from those used in younger adults. It is important to establish a baseline of "abnormal" findings for each individual, for a significant minority of older people will have chronic abnormalities, such as bibasilar rales or rhonchi from inactive tuberculosis, that do not indicate the presence of acute disorders. Difficulties encountered in assessment include obtaining sufficient cooperation with deep breathing to auscultate the lungs adequately. See Chapter 8 for a detailed review of respiratory assessment techniques.

Planning and Intervention

Older patients with any physical mobility impairment or activity intolerance will benefit from a regimen of pulmonary hygiene. The importance of these interventions increases with the extent of immobility or when overt pulmonary pathology exists. Priority setting may be a difficult task in the patient with many problems. The planning problem may be somewhat alleviated by including deep breathing as a part of each exercise regimen.

Table 14-19 contains a list of nursing interventions that can be used to promote pulmonary hygiene and to treat various alterations in respiratory function. Several nursing interventions to improve respiratory function in those with altered breathing patterns

INTERVENTIONS	EFFECT ON RESPIRATORY FUNCTION	INDICATED FOR TREATMENT OR PREVENTION OF THESE NURSING DIAGNOSES
Deep breathing	Promotes alveolar expansion Enhances O_2–CO_2 exchange Assists in developing effective cough	Ineffective breathing patterns Impaired gas exchange Potential for infection Activity intolerance Alteration in comfort
Encourage effective coughing	Clears respiratory passages of secretions Enhances O_2–CO_2 exchange Prevents bacterial proliferation	Ineffective airway clearance Activity intolerance Potential for infection

Adequate hydration
  2000 ml/day unless on fluid restriction: evaluate for signs of fluid overload
  Frequent offering of fluids or room humidification may be necessary
	Reduces viscosity of secretions
	Reduces energy expenditure required to clear secretions
		Ineffective airway clearance
		Potential for infection
		Potential fluid balance less than body requirements
		Activity intolerance

Encourage and increase activity
  May have to begin with encouraging bed-to-chair rather than bedrest
  Systematically and regularly increase activity
  Consider formal exercise program as adjunct to ADLs
	Improves respiratory rate and depth
	Improves tissue perfusion by increasing cardiac output
	Promotes alveolar expansion by increasing depth of respiration
	Promotes better positioning for coughing
		Impaired physical mobility
		Activity intolerance
		Altered tissue perfusion
		Decreased cardiac output

Positioning
  Discover most comfortable positions for patient
  Develop routine for changing resting positions: sitting, side-lying, prone, supine, semi-Fowler's, etc. and teach rationale to patient and family
	Frequent repositioning prevents pooling of secretions and thus enhances gas exchange and airway clearance, prevents infection
	Maintaining proper body alignment reduces the effort of breathing by not interfering with musculature involved in lung expansion
		Impaired physical mobility
		Alteration in comfort
		Impaired gas exchange
		Ineffective airway clearance

Adequate nutrition Consider small, frequent feedings so as to not compromise ventilatory effort and thus conserve energy	Necessary for adequate lung perfusion Needed for activity tolerance	Decreased tissue perfusion Activity intolerance Alteration in nutrition less than body requirements Ineffective breathing patterns Impaired gas exchange
Look for specific correctable nutritional deficiencies, e.g., iron, protein, vitamins, trace elements, calories	Malnutrition increases fatigue Severe anemia may precipitate CHF, which contributes to impaired gas exchange	

Prevent and identify pulmonary infections
  Control environmental toxins, e.g., cigarette smoke, paint fumes
  Monitor sputum production in those at high risk for infection for changes in color, consistency, amount, odor
	Reduces environmental irritants
	
	Early identification simplifies treatment
		Potential for infection

Suctioning	Stimulates cough Removes some secretions	Ineffective airway clearance
Monitoring of ABGs and vital signs	Assessment data about respiratory patterns, effectiveness of treatment	Impaired gas exchange Ineffective airway clearance
Percussion Postural drainage Pain medication	Helps loosen secretions Helps drain secretions In postsurgical patients or those with pleurisy, enables coughing and deep breathing without severe pain	Ineffective airway clearance Potential for infection Ineffective airway clearance Impaired gas exchange r/t atelectasis Ineffective breathing pattern Ineffective airway clearance Impaired gas exchange r/t CHF
Oxygen	Increases oxygen supply to respiratory system	Impaired gas exchange
Intake and output	Helps monitor adequacy of hydration or overhydration	
Ambulation	Helps mobilize secretions Encourages increased rate and depth of respirations	Ineffective airway clearance Impaired gas exchange
Encouraging self-care	Increases mobility	Ineffective breathing pattern Ineffective airway clearance
Comfort measures	Reduces anxiety, which promotes more effective breathing patterns	Ineffective breathing pattern
Patient/family teaching	Re: work simplification and energy conservation reduce fatigue Re: positioning to facilitate air exchange reduces anxiety	Impaired gas exchange r/t CHF Ineffective breathing pattern

deserve special mention, either because they are controversial, particularly effective, or require special care to achieve maximum benefits. These interventions can be grouped as follows: (1) exercise interventions, (2) positioning, and (3) use of metered-dose inhalers.

EXERCISE INTERVENTIONS. Controversy about exercise interventions for those with pulmonary disease centers on which regimens are effective: because of difficulties in determining the most effective components of the program, and differences in the chosen outcome measure. Reviews by Ingersoll (1989), Wakefield (1991), Saltzman (1992), and Carrieri-Kohlman and Janson-Bjerklie (1993) suggest a role for breathing retraining to improve respiratory muscle strength and endurance (Harver et al., 1989), although its effectiveness in increasing exercise tolerance has not been shown. Breathing retraining is a term that comprises education about COPD, chest wall muscle relaxation and movement synchronization, and pursed lip breathing; the term may also include inspiratory resistance training. Movement synchronization and pursed lip breathing have been shown to increase tidal volume, oxygen saturation, and exercise tolerance, and to decrease respiratory rate and dyspnea in selected patients (Carrieri-Kohlman and Janson-Bjerklie, 1993). Inspiratory resistance training is defined as "normal ventilation with added external loading" (Kersten, 1989, p. 565). The patient breathes at his own rate through the mouthpiece of a trainer, and resistance is increased by reducing the size of the inspiratory opening; it is set just below the patient's fatigue threshold, as signified by clinical parameters demonstrating increased work of breathing, such as tachypnea, asynchronous breathing, or paradoxical chest or abdominal wall movements. Patients are instructed to exercise for 15 to 30 minutes each day, 5 days per week, for 6 to 10 weeks (Kersten, 1989).

Although the research on resistive breathing exercise is promising, more research is clearly needed to define its precise role in care of elderly people. Other approaches to exercise that have improved breathing patterns in patients with chronic lung disease include upper extremity exercise training (Ries et al., 1988; Mahler and O'Donnell, 1991) and relaxation (Gift et al., 1992). Individuals in chronic care settings may derive more benefit from a balanced exercise program than from one targeted only to respiratory muscles (O'Donnell et al., 1993).

POSITIONING. Various strategies of positioning are recommended to increase ventilation and to normalize ventilation/perfusion matching (Ross and Dean, 1989). Positioning can also be helpful in promoting airway clearance, as in the use of postural drainage. Sitting leaning forward is a position commonly used by patients with dyspnea and is thought to improve ventilation by permitting the abdominal organs to drop away from the diaphragm, resulting in better excursion and decreased accessory muscle use (Carrieri-Kohlman and Janson-Bjerklei, 1993). Position change has been shown in laboratory studies to affect pulmonary perfusion; clinical studies on patients with cystic fibrosis and postoperative patients show beneficial effects of position change, but specific clinical guidelines for acutely ill older patients are lacking (Ross and Dean, 1989). However, good evidence shows that for patients with unilateral pulmonary pathology (such as those with pneumonia, neoplasms, pneumothorax, atelectasis, thoracotomy, and lobectomy), positioning with the unaffected side down results in better oxygenation (Yeaw, 1992). The implication of this principle is that rather than turning patients with unilateral disease side to side, avoiding positions that place the diseased side in a dependent status will maximize oxygenation. Increasing attention is being given to the benefits of the prone position to improve ventilation/perfusion. A recent case study suggests that prone or semiprone positioning may be useful in adult respiratory distress syndrome, as well as in the weaning of patients from mechanical ventilation (Schmitz, 1991; Doering, 1993).

METERED-DOSE INHALERS. The ability to deliver medicines via inhalation rather than orally has been a tremendous advance, as it reduces the likelihood of systemic side effects from medicines designed to improve pulmonary function. However, use of metered-dose inhalers requires a technique that places a premium on hand dexterity and coordination, which may be lacking in some older adults. Studies of effectiveness of the performance of older adults in using metered-dose inhalers show that the type of inhaler device and patient factors such as age and cognitive impairment influence the ability to use the inhalers correctly (Armitage and Williams, 1988; Diggory et al., 1991). These studies show that instruction improves performance in over 50 per cent of those studied, but multiple sessions (up to three) may be needed to achieve success.

Use of tube spacers to compensate for poor coordination and cognitive impairment is recommended, as is periodic re-evaluation of patient technique.

Evaluation

Criteria for evaluation of care for the patient with altered respiratory function are as follows:

1. Is the patient comfortable?
2. Does the patient show signs of hypoxia, such as cyanosis, alterations in thought process?
3. Are vital signs within normal limits?
4. Are arterial blood gas levels within normal limits?
5. Are all respiratory irritants removed from the patient's immediate environment?
6. Does the patient follow a regular pulmonary toilet regimen? Is it adequate to mobilize secretions?
7. What is the patient's physical functioning level? Is the patient independent in activities of daily living?
8. Is the patient engaged in any meaningful social activities?
9. Does the patient have any unmet goals?
10. Does the patient use metered-dose inhalers properly?

SELF-CARE DEFICITS: FEEDING, BATHING/HYGIENE, DRESSING/GROOMING, AND TOILETING

Definition and Scope of Problem

Activities of daily living are basic self-care tasks engaged in by adults to maintain health and social acceptability. The North American Nursing Diagnosis Association recognizes the following categories of self-care deficits: feeding, dressing, bathing, grooming, and toileting (NANDA, 1992).

Dependence in basic activities of daily living is widespread among elderly people. National census data estimate that nearly 12 per cent of those over age 65 years who live in the community have limitations in self-care (Administration on Aging, 1994). Those over age 85 years have a higher prevalence. This dependency often results in increased use of formal or informal services. A recent Administration on Aging report of home-based services notes that over 80 per cent of community and home-based services use ADL or IADL deficits as a criterion for re-

ceiving services. In nursing homes, the prevalence of ADL dependence is higher. Between 40 and 91 per cent of those over age 65 years require assistance with basic ADLs, with the breakdown as follows: assistance with eating, 40.3 per cent; assistance with continence, 54.5 per cent; assistance with transferring, 62.6 per cent; assistance with toileting, 63.2 per cent; assistance with dressing, 77.6 per cent; and assistance with bathing, 91 per cent (U.S. Department of Health and Human Services, 1989). The levels of dependency in nursing home patients may be increasing: the average number of ADL dependencies was 3.5 in 1977 compared with 3.9 in 1985. Dependency in hospitalized patients is less well documented, although Hirsch and colleagues (1990) found deterioration in function in two thirds of elderly patients between admission and the second hospital day. Most of these patients did not improve in function at discharge. Thirty-eight per cent of patients in one hospital in Italy were dependent in ADL (Incalzi et al., 1992), and this number was significantly associated with mortality.

It is interesting that although many have predicted an increase in dependence with the increasing life expectancy, Manton and colleagues (1993) recently reported a leveling-off of dependency in community-dwelling older adults, suggesting that some preventive health interventions, such as those to reduce the adverse effects of musculoskeletal and cardiovascular disease and to reduce frailty, may be paying off.

Self-care deficits are important to gerontological nurses because people with functional impairments require considerable nursing assistance to prevent associated problems to compensate for the lost function, and, when possible, to regain the lost abilities.

The consequences of improperly treated self-care deficits include loss of self-esteem, alterations in skin integrity and nutrition, constipation, incontinence, and many other problems, including predisposing to institutionalization. Interviews with next-of-kin of nursing home patients reveal that problems performing basic ADLs were the second most common reason for admission (74 per cent), with the most frequent reason cited (78 per cent) being "required more care than household members could give" (Hing, 1989). Nurses should remember that many self-care deficits in elderly people are reversible; helping older people retain as much independence in self-care as possible should be a high priority.

Theoretical Issues

Meaning of Independence

The ability to perform one's basic personal care tasks is achieved at an early stage in development. Relinquishing control over activities of daily living, therefore, can be devastating to the older person's self-concept as an adult. Inability to perform basic self-care tasks means that the individual must rely on others frequently throughout the day or develop the problems associated with self-neglect.

Dependency Conflicts

Assisting another with self-care tasks generally involves intimate body contact. Both the patient and the caregiver must resolve feelings of shame, guilt, and anxiety that may be aroused by such intimate contact. Health care professionals are assisted with the identification and resolution of these feelings during their educational preparation. Paraprofessional and lay caregivers have no formal means of working through feelings aroused by provision of intimate care. Unresolved negative feelings about providing personal care assistance may adversely affect the care rendered.

Complexity of Self-Care Tasks

Most adults perform self-care tasks automatically. The activities of daily living are habitual and routine and require minimal thought or energy expenditure. However, analysis of each activity of daily living reveals that the tasks are actually quite complex, requiring intact, integrated function of several body systems. The systems most involved include the central and peripheral nervous systems, the special senses, the musculoskeletal system, the cardiorespiratory system, and the psyche. Impairments in any of these systems make performance of basic activities of daily living considerably more complex. Severe impairments in any of the systems may make independent self-care impossible.

Influence of Environment on Self-Care Task Performance

A growing body of literature documents the effects of environmental factors on human performance (Faletti, 1984; Lawton, 1985; Czaja et al., 1993), often known as "human factors" research (Charness and Bosman, 1990). Nurses should be aware of the potential contributions of this type of investigation to generating interventions for those with self-care deficits.

Human factors research is based in an engineering perspective. One major tenet of this framework is the notion that functional independence of older adults can be improved by changing the designed physical environment to be more congruent with the capabilities of older adults. A second major principle is the belief that activities such as ADLs can be analyzed systematically for their task demands in a given environment, and the environment modified to lessen task demand. For example, the average hand grip strength of an older adult has been estimated to be 15 pounds. Although the force required to operate sink controls is less than this average (approximately 8 pounds), human factors research has demonstrated that if the controls are at an awkward height, or if the individual has difficulty grasping owing to joint deformity, then the required amount of force may not be delivered.

Other examples of human/environmental interactions that may affect functional performance include the amount of reach to clothing in closets and the amount of bending to get into or out of a bathtub or shower. Human factors research delineates many of the anthropometric and biomechanical demands of tasks. Future studies are likely to be helpful in describing the sensory and cognitive demands of everyday tasks. More clinically oriented investigators are beginning to describe aspects of everyday environments that older adults encounter outside their homes, and their implications for everyday function. For example, it is known that chair height affects the likelihood of a frail older person's being able to rise from a chair successfully. Weiner and colleagues (1993) measured chair heights in a cross-section of primary care physicians' offices and noted that many were of a height that made a successful transfer difficult for older adults.

Contributing Factors

Both physiological and psychological impairments may result in self-care deficits. Environmental factors may also produce or exacerbate a self-care handicap.

Intolerance to Activity

Activity intolerance leads to a self-care deficit, because the individual lacks the stamina to perform the necessary tasks. According to epidemiological and laboratory data, many older adults have reduced stamina, including the ability to balance or maintain posture in one position for an extended period of time (Kovar and LaCroix, 1987; Spirduso, 1990). Those who perform activities of daily living independently despite severe activity intolerance are often left with a socially impoverished existence, because they lack the time or resources to engage in other activities, work, or leisure.

Pain

Alterations in comfort predispose individuals to self-care deficit. Pain due to coronary artery disease, arthritis, fracture, or other pathological conditions may so overwhelm the patient that self-care becomes difficult, if not impossible. Pain also may restrict mobility, so that performance is impaired. Finally, the compensations made by individuals attempting to minimize pain during activity may make performance of the most basic activities of daily living extremely time- or energy-consuming. For example, Mrs. Wells has a painful left arm from severe lymphedema. Although technically she is able to dress herself independently (that is, she has the motor skill), she is totally dependent in dressing because the pain in her arm when performing the task unassisted is much greater.

Perceptual or Cognitive Impairment

Activities of daily living are usually considered routine or automatic behaviors, but perceptual and cognitive impairments may still impair function. Typically, the more complex tasks, such as toileting, grooming, and dressing are first affected, followed by bathing and feeding.

In a large-scale longitudinal study, visual impairment, as measured by endorsing the presence of glaucoma, cataracts, retinal disorder, blindness in one or both eyes, or having difficulty seeing even with glasses, was predictive of disability at 4 years' follow-up, even after controlling for baseline disability and chronic disease status (Rudberg et al., 1993).

Sensory-perceptual impairments affect self-care ability in several ways. First, they interfere with the individual's ability to receive signals that prompt them to perform a self-care task. For example, people with visual impairment lack visual cues to tell them when it is time to comb their hair or when they have put their clothes on properly, thus potentially developing two impairments in self-care: grooming and dressing. Sensory impairments also affect the ability to execute selected tasks. For example, people with severe visual impairment have difficulty locating toilets in strange surroundings, interfering with their ability to self-toilet. They also have difficulty finding the food on a plate, relying on the sense of touch and smell unless guided by another. Finally, visual impairment may result in disturbances in balance, owing to the multisensory nature of the balance mechanism (Woollacott, 1993). Disturbances in balance make the individual more prone to fall-related injury and thus may make some self-care tasks, such as bathing or dressing, unsafe if carried out in the standing position.

Cognitive impairments also affect self-care abilities in many ways. People with cognitive disorders may lose the social awareness that it is important to perform activities of daily living and omit these tasks unless prompted to perform. Cognitive impairments also interfere with the reasoning ability needed to perform self-care tasks in new environments. Thus, a demented person may be independent in self-care tasks in the home environment, but become unable to perform the tasks when relocated to a hospital or relative's home. Those with severe cognitive impairment actually may forget how to perform even the most familiar tasks, become apraxic, and because of their impaired cognition they are unable to relearn the task.

A wide variety of studies confirms the relationship between cognitive impairment and self-care deficit, in both dementia and delirium. Freels and colleagues (1992) studied 240 patients with Alzheimer's disease from six different clinics. Forty-two per cent of subjects had no impairment in basic ADLs, and 4.6 per cent had impairment in all ADLs. Most had impairments in dressing, bathing, and transferring (37 per cent, 33 per cent, and 33 per cent, respectively), followed by dependency in toileting (22 per cent), walking (15 per cent), and eating (14 per cent). Mental status factors that were most highly associated with ADL dependencies included apathy and behavior problems. Murray and colleagues (1993) studied the long-term effects of delirium on function in 291 elderly patients from the EPESE study site in Boston who were admitted to medical-surgical units and who did not have delirium on admission. Patients were admitted from both the community and from a nursing home. Thirty-one per cent of these subjects developed delirium while in the hospital. Their functional status was compared with matched control subjects who did not develop delirium. The number of ADL dependencies was associated with a higher incidence of delirium in community-dwelling patients. At the 3- and 6-month follow-up, patients who were delirious in the hospital had more dependency in ADLs than patients who did not develop delirium.

Neuromuscular Impairment

Impaired physical mobility due to neuromuscular impairment is likely to affect self-care abilities. Hemiplegia is a classic example of a neuromuscular disorder common among the elderly that dramatically affects self-care ability. With the use of only one half of the body, all aspects of self-care become extraordinarily complex. Hemiplegia is often associated with other disorders that affect self-care abilities, such as unilateral neglect, a condition in which the individual is unaware of or does not attend to one side of the body, chronic pain syndromes, and sensory impairments. Other neuromuscular dysfunctions associated with self-care deficits include Parkinson's disease and the demyelinating disorders, such as amyotrophic lateral sclerosis, multiple sclerosis, and degenerative cerebellar disorders.

Musculoskeletal Impairment

Arthritis, contractures, scoliosis, kyphosis, and decreased muscle mass and strength all contribute to self-care deficits in the aged. In a study of 541 community-dwelling elders aged 60 years and older, 98 per cent had impairment in at least one joint, based upon physical examination by a rheumatologist. Fifty-seven per cent of these subjects had mild disability, and 21 per cent had moderate-to-severe disability. The presence of joint impairment was significantly associated with disability; however, self-reported joint pain was also found to be an important predictor of disability. These disorders contribute primarily by inducing impaired mobility, endurance, strength, or coordination.

Depression

Performance of self-care activities requires that individuals value themselves sufficiently to invest the time and energy in performing ADLs. People who are depressed may lose interest in self-care and thus either become dependent upon others or suffer the effects of neglect. In grooming and hygiene, the effects are not life threatening but certainly reinforce a cycle of negative self-

worth. The individual feels too poorly to bathe or dress properly and, in turn, begins to feel worse and lose social contacts because of a socially unacceptable appearance. Going without food or toileting is a more life-threatening lapse that calls for definitive intervention to resolve the depression and the associated self-care deficits.

Assessment

All elderly individuals should be assessed for their ability to perform activities of daily living. Options for assessing ADL function include direct observation, patient report, and proxy report (usually a family member or paid caregiver). Although direct observation is probably the most valid data, reported function is more commonly used because it is quicker and, in many instances, correlates highly with performance-based assessments (Myers et al., 1993). However, there is growing recognition that performance-based measures of function and reported function provide complementary data (Reuben et al., 1992; Guralnik et al., 1994), and therefore both approaches should be used, as indicated by the patient's condition and clinician's purpose.

Direct observation is the most objective and richest source of information about ADL capability. Elam and colleagues (1991) compared direct observation of ADL performance with ratings of patients, family members, and physicians for 73 patients aged 60 years and over who had just been admitted to a rehabilitation facility. Patients were 85 to 90 per cent correct in rating their ability to walk; patients, families, and physicians were no more than 80 per cent accurate in ratings of ability to complete ADLs. Similarly, discrepancies between direct observation and reported function were found in 3 to 6.5 per cent of community-dwelling elderly, with elders tending to overreport disability. Discrepancies were more common in those with cognitive impairment (Kelly-Hayes et al., 1992). The application of direct observation is limited in some settings of care, however, because of time constraints or lack of appropriate evaluative resources. For example, in the ambulatory care setting, it is impractical to obtain performance evaluation of bathing, as typically no bathtubs or showers are readily accessible. Even in the hospital, the shower or bathtub may be different enough from that used at home that a misleading notion of the individual's capability may be obtained. This has led to the development of physical performance test batteries that select aspects of performance common to many ADLs; see for example the Physical Performance Test (PPT) of Reuben and Siu (1990), or the Performance Activities of Daily Living (PADL) by Kuriansky and Gurland (1976).

Self-report or proxy report of function provides a different type of information about self-care deficit. It is worthwhile determining whether there is a gap between performance of ADLs and self-perceived abilities or caregiver-perceived abilities. If an individual performs at a higher level than is reported, the person may suffer from excess disability, deserving of further assessment and intervention. If the individual functions at a level lower than that reported, unmet needs may be present, or there may be medical or environmental reasons for fluctuation in performance level that deserve further evaluation.

In some instances, self- or proxy-reported ADL status may provide an adequate substitute for direct observation. Some clinicians, recognizing that basic and instrumental activities of daily living are hierarchically arranged in complexity, use self-report of basic ADLs for those individuals whom they know to be IADL independent. In addition, on some measures of function, such as the Barthel index of ADL, self-report ratings and those based on direct observation are highly correlated; however, bias toward underestimating function may occur if proxy respondents are used (Dorevitch et al., 1992).

Nurses have unique opportunities to assess performance unobtrusively. For example, in outpatient care, older people are often assisted with undressing to save time. However, this wastes an excellent assessment opportunity. In the hospital, similar dependency-reinforcing behavior often takes place. In the nursing home, nurses often rely on reports from nursing assistants about self-care ability rather than taking the time to assess directly.

When older adults have reported deficits in ADLs, direct observation of performance by a professional skilled in assessment of ADL deficits is mandatory. In this instance, relying only on reports of observers untrained in assessment and treatment of self-care deficits as the sole measure of capacity to perform activities of daily living is completely unacceptable.

During observation of the self-care task, the nurse should consider the following questions:

1. Does the person perform the task independently and with evidence of functional reserve? That is, if this person were in a different environment, or becomes fatigued because of acute illness, could he or she still manage independently?
2. Is the activity done with precision? Does the patient require frequent rest periods or are there other signs of fatigue?
3. What special equipment or cues are needed to perform the task?
4. What assistance does the individual require from others?

The defining characteristics listed next are a useful guide for deciding whether a self-care deficit is present and its extent (NANDA, 1992).

A. Self-feeding deficit
   Defining characteristics
   Inability to bring food from a receptacle to the mouth
B. Self-bathing/hygiene deficit
   Defining characteristics
   Inability to wash body or body parts
   Inability to obtain or get to water source
   Inability to regulate temperature or flow
C. Self-dressing/grooming deficits
   Defining characteristics
   Impaired ability to put on or take off necessary items of clothing
   Impaired ability to obtain or replace articles of clothing
   Impaired ability to fasten clothing
   Inability to maintain appearance at a satisfactory level
D. Self-toileting deficit
   Defining characteristics
   Unable to get to toilet or commode
   Unable to sit on or rise from toilet or commode
   Unable to manipulate clothing or toileting
   Unable to carry out proper toilet hygiene
   Unable to flush toilet or empty commode

The individual's performance can be recorded according to the following scale:

0 = Completely independent

1 = Requires use of equipment or device

2 = Requires help from another person for assistance, supervision, or teaching

3 = Requires help from another person and equipment or device

4 = Dependent, does not participate in activity

A wide variety of other numerical schemes are available for rating dependence in ADLs. For example, the nursing home Minimum Data Set uses a five-level rating scheme that emphasizes assistance from others rather than the use of adaptive equipment. It distinguishes assistance from others as follows: 1=supervision only, 2=limited physical assistance, 3=extensive physical assistance, and 4=total dependence (Morris et al., 1990). Another rating system is the Functional Independence Measure (FIM) developed by Hamilton and colleagues (Heinemann et al., 1993). The FIM has several advantages as a rating instrument. First, it was developed by an interdisciplinary group of rehabilitation professionals. Second, it acknowledges that environmental factors influence ADL performance, as it rates separately bathing, toileting, and simple bed-to-chair transfers. Finally, in bathing and dressing, it rates lower and upper extremity tasks separately, acknowledging that different tasks are associated with different aspects of dressing and bathing. This distinction allows for a more fine-grained assessment of function that should more accurately reflect changes in patient status than cruder rating systems. The drawback to the use of instruments like the FIM is that the more fine-grained the instrument, the more training and time are required to use the tool accurately.

Planning and Intervention

Goals for those with self-care deficits are to *regain lost function, compensate for lost function, prevent further disability, and maintain physiological integrity.* One or all of these goals may be pursued, depending upon the other problems and strengths of the patient and the resources and priorities of the treatment. For example, in many long-term care settings, it is difficult to assist patients to regain or compensate for lost function, because the level of staffing does not allow the time for restorative approaches to care. Initially it takes more time to encourage and supervise someone to perform a task than to do the task for them. In addition, nursing home staff may not have adequate training in restorative care techniques. In contrast, rehabilitation center staff are highly motivated and well-trained to assist patients in regaining lost function or in compensating for impairments.

Interventions for self-care deficits include positioning, teaching, providing adaptive equipment, modifying the environment, supervising or assisting, and/or doing for the patient. Each of these approaches is discussed in the context of specific self-care deficits.

Self-Feeding Deficit

Self-feeding deficits generally fall into three categories: (1) an inability to ingest sufficient food, (2) an inability to ingest food in a socially acceptable manner, and (3) an inability to ingest food safely. The etiologies of self-feeding deficits include upper extremity sensorimotor impairments, visual impairments, apraxia, and oral-motor dysfunctions.

POSITIONING. Proper positioning is essential for safe and comfortable eating. Individuals with difficulty maintaining postural control are at high risk for aspiration of food during a meal or for weight loss and malnutrition because of discomfort during a meal (Donahue, 1990). Some patients require repositioning more than once during a meal. Two frequently observed errors in positioning are (1) patients slumped in wheelchairs and (2) patients who do not have heads upright, with chins tucked in.

ADAPTIVE EQUIPMENT. Patients with upper extremity impairments that interfere with self-feeding are often candidates for adaptive equipment. The variety of tools available ranges from simple, easily obtained equipment, such as a drinking straw, to complex apparatus, including motor-driven orthoses. A midrange of equipment in widespread use includes specialized handles on cutlery for individuals with grasp problems and plate guards for people with poor coordination. Most adaptive equipment requires individualization and instruction, which are best done by an occupational therapist. It is most important that caregivers be instructed in the proper use of adaptive equipment, because misuse of the equipment can aggravate the patient's self-feeding problem. For example, a plate guard if improperly placed on the plate obscures the patient's view of the plate, making eye-hand-mouth coordination more difficult.

TEACHING. Feeding problems caused by visual impairment may be partly resolved by teaching. The individual is taught to approach the meal place setting as though it were the face of a clock. The meal server can then assist the patient to locate food through a verbal description. Individuals with impaired sensation in the mouth can be taught to sweep the affected side of their mouths with their tongues to dislodge any pocketed food particles, thus reducing the danger of aspiration.

ENVIRONMENTAL MODIFICATION. Modification of the diet consistency is a common intervention for those who have oral-motor dysfunction. A softer diet is often easier to handle, because the need for extensive manipulation of the food during chewing is eliminated. In extreme cases a puréed or liquid diet may be indicated, although these should be avoided unless absolutely necessary. Food in puréed or liquid form lacks varied texture, an important ingredient in the enjoyment of food.

A useful diet modification for people with upper extremity impairments is a "finger food" menu. Individuals with coordination problems find utensils difficult to control and often messy to eat with.

SUPERVISION AND ASSISTANCE WITH EATING. When the patient has swallowing difficulties, apraxia, oral-motor dysfunction, or incomplete compensation for upper extremity and sensory impairments, supervision of eating is indicated. Supervision may be as unobtrusive as observing the intake of blind patients and reminding them if food is overlooked. Supervision of a meal may require substantial assistance—for example, placing the food on the patient's spoon and telling the person to put the food in the mouth. Many patients do well with verbal prompting ("Mr. Jones, take another bite of food"), whereas others require physical as well as verbal prompts ("Miss Smith, put your spoon down." The nurse then uses touch to guide the patient's hand to put the spoon down on the plate. "Swallow the food in your mouth"). Providing extensive verbal and physical prompting to eat a meal is a laborious process but is vastly superior to feeding the patient, because it preserves the patient's control over the act of eating and avoids atrophy of hand-mouth coordination.

Some institutional facilities manage the labor intensiveness of supervision during meals by placing those who require supervision in one dining area and assigning one staff member to provide assistance as needed during the meal. This type of group arrangement can also be used to assess patients with new onset of dysphagia or self-care deficit in eating. Staff members assigned to supervise this area should be knowledgeable about positioning techniques, correct use of adaptive equipment, and use of physical and verbal cues to enhance independence. In addition, staff members should be skilled in providing first aid for choking and aspiration (Shemansky, 1991).

FEEDING. Feeding another person is an intervention that requires great sensitivity on the part of the caregiver. When people are fed, they have no control over the pace of feeding, the type of food ingested, or the order of solid and liquid foods. Few if any people enjoy being fed. Every attempt, therefore, should be made to make the meal as normal as possible. The pace of feeding should be unhurried, and the mixing of dissimilar foods, such as oatmeal and scrambled eggs, should be discouraged. Syringes should never be used to instill food or fluid into people's mouths, as the force from the fluids may cause aspiration or choking (Price and DiIorio, 1990). Conversing with the patient, even if the patient does not seem to hear, is encouraged. The older person should be assisted with oral hygiene following the meal, to promote comfort and to ensure that no food is pocketed in the mouth where it might later be aspirated into the respiratory tract. See Chapter 19 for a more detailed discussion of feeding techniques.

Self-Bathing Deficit

Bathing and hygiene difficulties can result from environmental barriers to safe hygiene, activity intolerance and reduced endurance, mobility impairments—specifically, lack of flexibility, coordination, or strength—lack of awareness of poor hygiene, and poor self-esteem.

POSITIONING. Environmental resources control the position used for bathing. Some people do not have running water in the home or accessible bathrooms. A sponge bath is the only alternative. People with activity intolerance should be "set up" for their bath, so that the bath is taken in an energy-conserving position—seated, with feet well supported. All necessary toilet items should be within easy reach.

TEACHING. Principles of energy conservation and work simplification identified earlier apply to those whose self-bathing deficit is due to activity intolerance. Hemiplegic patients can be taught positioning techniques that make self-bathing feasible.

ADAPTIVE EQUIPMENT. Long-handled bath sponges help those with reduced flexibility reach distal parts of the lower extremities and the back without assistance from another person. Special shower chairs and bathtub benches facilitate independent transfer to the shower or tub. The chairs also reduce energy expenditure and risk of falling for those with limited activity tolerance. Suitably placed grab rails in the bathroom greatly enhance independence and safety of transfers. A hand-held shower attachment that can also be fixed to the wall increases the number of bathing options. All equipment should have nonskid grips or bases to prevent unexpected slippage in the wet bathroom environment.

SUPERVISION. Apraxic individuals find bathing a formidable task. The complexity of such activities as undressing, running wash water, getting into the shower or tub, washing, and drying may be completely overwhelming. Caregivers can assist greatly by breaking down the massive, complex task into smaller, easier-to-manage tasks, rather than taking over and bathing the patient. People with sensory impairments may require "stand-by" assistance only, in case of a fall or slip. Some patients require extensive verbal and physical prompting to bathe but are then able to perform the task.

BATHING THE PATIENT. Bathing patients is another self-care task that requires great sensitivity. Naked people feel extremely vulnerable. Baths that are given with attention to pace, with communication inherent in touch, and with privacy respected can be comforting and soothing. Baths characterized by rough handling and indifference can become an anxiety-provoking nightmare for both patient and caregiver (Wagnild and Manning, 1985).

Self-Dressing and Grooming Deficit

Deficits in the ability to dress and groom are precipitated by the same conditions that cause bathing and feeding deficits: apraxia, reduced self-esteem, activity intolerance, impaired mobility, and pain.

ADAPTIVE EQUIPMENT. A wealth of adaptive equipment and adapted clothing exists for people who have difficulty dressing themselves. Velcro closures instead of zippers, buttons, and shoelaces, dresses that open down the back for wheelchair-bound women, and oversized buttons all facilitate dressing in the face of impaired mobility. Consultation with an occupational therapist is extremely helpful in selecting and individualizing the many possible options for the patient. Other adaptive equipment sometimes employed includes long-handled shoehorns and combs, zipper pulls, and button hooks. Unfortunately, the cost of most of this equipment is not reimbursed by third-party payers. However, patients and families can be counseled to use birthdays and other celebrations for the giving of needed adapted clothing, and volunteers may be employed to adapt already-purchased clothing.

TEACHING. Patients with mobility impairments can benefit greatly from simple teaching about the simplest methods of dressing. For example, individuals with hemiplegia will find it is easier to dress if they begin with their affected side. Larger sizes of clothing will also simplify the task. If adapted clothing or new equipment is introduced, the older person and caregivers will probably require some instruction in its proper use.

SUPERVISION. A key approach to providing supervision and assistance to people with self-dressing deficits is manipulating the environment. Important considerations include positioning the patient near a grab rail or other secure device to facilitate standing, and placing clothing within easy reach. Simplifying the task of dressing to this extent may be all the supervision that some patients require. The principles of verbal and physical prompting described in bathing and feeding deficits apply to supervision of dressing. As the risk of the impaired individual being hurt because of inadequate supervision is less with dressing and grooming than with the other self-care tasks, caregivers have more latitude to provide supervision rather than doing for, without fearing adverse consequences. Particularly in institutions, patients have considerable time on their hands, and there is no sound rationale for insisting that patients be finished with dressing by an early hour. Caregivers can perform other tasks while supervising dressing, such as making beds, tidying the room, or assisting the patient's roommate.

Beck and colleagues (1992), working with older adults who have dementia in long-term care facilities, developed a sophisticated system for characterizing the type of assistance required for dressing (Table 14–20). Note that seven different levels of assistance are possible, depending upon the demented person's cognitive level. Beck also recommends using both interactional and environmental strategies to support dressing performance. Table 14–21 shows examples of both general and specific interventions to promote self-dressing in patients with dementia (Beck et al., 1992).

DRESSING. Nurses must make a judgment about when supervision only is too time consuming, energy consuming, or demoralizing for the patient and dressing the patient becomes the preferred alternative. If dressing the patient is chosen, the challenge is to find ways in which the patient can participate in the task, such as choosing clothing for the day or helping with a small part, such as fastening buttons or combing hair.

Self-Toileting Deficit

Patients with self-toileting deficits run the risk of skin breakdown and social stigma if they are unable to compensate for or regain the lost function. Impaired mobility and sen-

T A B L E 1 4 – 2 0

Definition of Levels of Caregiver Assistance and Scoring for the Beck Dressing Performance Scale (BDPS)

SCORE	LEVELS OF ASSISTANCE
0	No Assistance: The subject is able to perform the component of dressing without assistance from a caregiver. The caregiver may be present but does not speak or have any contact with the subject or clothing items.
1	Stimulus Control: The subject is able to perform the component of the dressing task if the caregiver controls the environment—for example, laying clothes out in the correct order.
2	Initial Verbal Prompt: The subject is able to perform the component of the dressing task if the caregiver gives an initial one-step command—for example, "Pull up your pants."
3	Repeated Verbal Prompts: The subject is able to perform the component of the dressing task if he or she is verbally prompted more than once to initiate or complete the behavior.
4	Gestures or Modeling: The subject is able to complete the component of the dressing task if the caregiver points out significant parts of the correct behavior or demonstrates how to perform the behavior.
5	Occasional Physical Guidance: The subject is able to complete the component of the dressing task if the caregiver provides occasional touching, physical prompting, or guiding—for example, guiding the subject's arm into a sleeve and releasing the arm to permit the subject to complete the action.
6	Complete Physical Guidance: The subject is able to complete the component of the dressing task if the caregiver provides constant touch and guidance.
7	Complete Assistance: The caregiver completes the component of the dressing task. The subject does not use his hands or complete any actions that would assist with the component of the dressing task.

From Beck, C., Heacock, P., Mercer, M. and Walton, C. Decreasing caregiver assistance with older adults with dementia. *In* Funk, S.G., Tornquist, E.M., Champagne, M.T. and Wiese, R.A. (eds.). *Key Aspects of Elder Care: Managing Falls, Incontinence and Cognitive Impairment.* New York: Springer, 1992, p. 312. Copyright Springer Publishing Company, Inc., New York. Used by permission.

sory impairment can present tremendous barriers to self-toileting. The chief interventions include toileting schedules and adaptive equipment.

ADAPTIVE EQUIPMENT. Raised toilet seats and properly placed grab rails in the toilet stall are essential items for most patients with mobility problems, including those with arthritis, hemiplegia, and neurological impairments. Long-handled toilet paper holders can be obtained for those who have flexibility problems that impair the ability to perform perineal hygiene after toi-

T A B L E 1 4 – 2 1

Behavioral Strategies for Dressing

SPECIFIC BEHAVIORAL STRATEGIES
I. Interactional
  A. Verbal
    1. Use one-step verbal commands. Keep sentences simple; use one or two words if possible.
    2. Ask yes/no questions.
    3. Be concrete; tell the resident exactly what you want him or her to do.
    4. Give verbal praise after completing each step.
    5. Give praise regarding appearance after completion of dressing.
  B. Nonverbal
    1. Dress bottom half, then top half of body. (This eliminates the confusion of moving back and forth from the upper to lower body.)
    2. Hand clothing items to the resident in the correct position.
    3. Place shoes beside the foot the resident will put them on.
    4. Use gestures to indicate what you want the resident to do (i.e., point to the item of clothing you want the resident to put on).
    5. Use modeling to indicate what you want the resident to do (i.e., show the resident how to pull up pants by making the motion of pulling up pants).
    6. Use physical touch to indicate to the resident which body part you want moved or used.
    7. Use physical guidance to start the resident's movement, then allow the resident to complete the action without help.
    8. Use reverse chaining (graduated physical guidance) by allowing the resident to finish the dressing step, and decrease assistance as the resident is able to do more.
    9. Stop perseveration and replace with dressing activity.
    10. Use touch by giving the resident a pat on the back or a hug after completing each dressing step.
II. Environmental
  A. Prepare a consistent environment
    1. Use a dark-color bedspread to contrast with clothing.
    2. Lay clothes face down in the order they will be put on.
    3. Cluster matching outfits on hangers.
    4. Introduce clothing one item at a time.
    5. Reduce the number of clothing options. (Let the resident choose from only two clothing items.)
    6. Provide an incentive for completing dressing.
  B. Reduce external stimuli
    1. Turn off radio or TV.
    2. Reduce number of people in room.
    3. Provide privacy.

GENERAL BEHAVIORAL STRATEGIES
I. Interactional
    1. Restrict conversation to dressing.
    2. Speak in a calm voice.
    3. Keep pitch of voice low.
    4. Speak clearly.
    5. Call resident by name.
    6. Keep sentences simple, using one or two words when possible.
    7. Consistently use the same word for the same thing (shirt/blouse).
II. Environmental
    1. Make up the bed.
    2. Minimize clutter of nonclothing items in the area.
    3. Put other clothing out of resident's sight (range of vision).
    4. Increase lighting.
    5. Eliminate improper clothing options (i.e., place dirty clothes in hamper).

From Beck, C., Heacock, P., Mercer, M. and Walton, C. Decreasing caregiver assistance with older adults with dementia. *In* Funk, S.G., Tornquist, E.M., Champagne, M.T. and Wiese, R.A. (eds.) *Key Aspects of Elder Care: Managing Falls, Incontinence and Cognitive Impairment.* New York: Springer, 1992, pp. 317–318. Copyright Springer Publishing Company, Inc., New York. Used by permission.

leting. If the patient is wheelchair bound, removable leg rests on the wheelchair often make transfers easier. Bedside commodes are indicated when the toilet cannot be suitably modified. Bedside commodes, like any other piece of adaptive equipment, should be tailored to the individual's situation. Bedside commodes come in adjustable heights, and some are available with arm rests that drop down easily to facilitate transfers.

SUPERVISION AND ASSISTANCE. Toileting schedules are useful for people who have difficulty sensing a need to go to the toilet. In more independent patients, a watch or clock and a written schedule may be all that is needed. Other patients will require verbal prompting. Finally, some patients will require physical assistance in toileting. A toileting schedule remains a useful adjunct for those who require physical assistance, as it provides some reassurance that the patient does not have to ask for help at each toileting episode. Toileting schedules also send a message that continence is valued. Unfortunately, many long-term care facilities and hospitals do not incorporate toileting into their routines. The routinization of toileting in child day care centers, where there is tremendous emphasis on toileting, could profitably be applied to institutional settings of care. In many child day care centers, before each major activity change (that is, approximately every 2 hours), time is blocked in for toileting. Unfortunately, in many long-term care facilities, the emphasis is on "changing" rounds, rather than on "toileting" rounds. A change in this emphasis would do a great deal to reduce incontinence in institutions.

Evaluation

Evaluation of the effectiveness of nursing care for those with self-care deficits can be conducted according to the following criteria:

1. Does the independence of the individual in self-care change over time?
2. Has the person regained the lost self-care ability? If not, has the person developed successful compensatory mechanisms for the self-care deficit?
3. Does the patient experience alterations in physiological integrity because of the self-care deficit (such as malnutrition, aspiration pneumonia, alteration in skin integrity)? Specify.
4. Does the patient experience disturbance in self-esteem because of the self-care deficit or the compensatory response?
5. Is adaptive equipment appropriate for the patient obtained, and are caregivers knowledgeable about its use and misuse?

SENSORY-PERCEPTUAL ALTERATIONS: VISUAL, AUDITORY, GUSTATORY, OLFACTORY, TACTILE, KINESTHETIC, AND UNILATERAL NEGLECT

Definition and Scope of Problem

Sensory-perceptual alterations are defined as "a state in which the individual experiences a change in the amount of patterning, or interpretation of incoming stimuli, accompanied by a diminished, exaggerated, distorted, or impaired response to such stimuli" (NANDA, 1992, p. 65). Sensory-perceptual alterations include sensory deprivation, sensory overload, and sensory distortion.

Aging is accompanied by many changes in the sensory apparatus (Table 14–22), leading to a high prevalence of sensory impairment. For example, blinding eye diseases affect as many as 10 per cent of the aged (see Chapter 14). The prevalence of visual impairment in community-dwelling people over age 65 years is 9 per cent, and it continues to rise with age. In those aged 75 to 84 years, the prevalence is 12.5 per cent, and 18 per cent of those aged 85 years and over who have visual impairment (Mermelstein et al., 1993). The prevalence of hearing impairment is estimated to be 38 per cent (Mermelstein et al., 1993) in those over age 65 years living in the community. In institutionalized elderly, the prevalence of mild hearing loss, as determined by audiometric techniques, is estimated at 77 per cent, and moderate hearing loss was present in 51 per cent of those studied (Garahan et al., 1992). A subpopulation (approximately 3 per cent) of hearing-impaired older adults has been deaf since early childhood (Walsh and Eldredge, 1989) (see Chapter 13).

The consequences of sensory-perceptual alteration can be quite serious, including delirium, anxiety, fear, social isolation, reduced confidence in self, reduced mobility, alteration in comfort, impaired verbal communication, and self-care deficit.

Sensory impairments are often classified according to sensory modality. Although this is a useful classification, it provides an incomplete view of the problem. Some alterations in sensory perception can easily be related to dysfunction in one sensory organ (for example, glaucoma), but older people also suffer from disorders that produce less specific alterations in sensory processing. In patients with dementing disorders, cerebrovascular disease, and degenerative central nervous system diseases, simultaneous alterations in the function of several sensory modalities predominate, because of deficits in central processing of sensory input (DiFabio and Badke, 1991). Unilateral neglect is an example of impaired central processing of afferent stimuli. Although it is considered as a diagnosis separate from sensory perceptual alterations by NANDA, it is included in this section.

Difficulty in accurately processing sensory stimuli is further compounded if the patient is cared for in a place where environmental stimulation is minimal, because hypostimulation may lead to further deterioration of central processing abilities.

Disturbances in one sensory modality also affect function of other modalities. For example, vision plays a role in kinesthesia because of central connections between the visual apparatus and the vestibular system. In visual impairment, the sense of balance and position in space is affected, and adaptations must be made for safe locomotion to take place. Older people are at high risk for both sensory deprivation and distortion because of the high prevalence of disorders that influence sensory function in old age.

Diagnostic Dilemmas

The nursing literature lacks clarity as to when the diagnostic category of altered thought process applies to a patient exhibiting confused behavior and when the category of sensory-perceptual alteration is more appropriate. Because of overlap between the defining characteristics, the diagnostic dilemma will remain until further precision in the defining characteristics is achieved. It has been recognized for a long time in the nursing literature that sensory deprivation can result in disturbed thought process (Wolanin and Phillips, 1981). A more recent observation is that conditions that result in alterations in thought process, such as cerebrovascular accidents, dementing disorders, and Parkinson's disease, may cause sensory-perceptual alterations. The working distinction between the two categories used here is to reserve the diagnosis of sensory-perceptual alteration for when there is a fairly direct link between a documented sensory or perceptual impairment and a behavior disturbance. The less precise diagnosis of alteration in thought process is used for an

TABLE 14 – 22
Common Age-Related Sensory Changes

TYPE OF CHANGE	IMPACT ON FUNCTION
Vision	
Lens thickens, yellows, is less pliable, and develops opacities	Less light enters the eye
	Color discrimination is impaired
	Images are blurred
	Sensitivity to glare is increased
	Ability to see small objects at close range is impaired
Pupil diameter decreases	Less light enters the eye
Pupillary accommodation is slower	Adaptation from dark to light is slower
Retina has fewer cones	Color vision is impaired
Hearing	
Outer ear	
Predisposition to cerumen impaction, especially in men	Conductive hearing loss, may be superimposed upon sensorineural loss
Middle ear	
Scar tissue on eardrum from recurrent middle ear infections with rupture of tympanic membrane	
Inner ear	Impaired ability to hear high-pitched sounds
Aging-related changes in cochlea, including loss of neurons and stiffening of basilar membrane	Difficulty with speech discrimination
Taste	
Number of taste receptors diminishes	Enjoyment of food reduced
Threshold for stimulation of taste sensation increased	Appetite sometimes reduced
Reduced salivation inhibits taste receptor function	Use of taste "enhancers," such as salt or sugar, increased
Kinesthesia	
Vestibular system: Reduction in numbers of myelinated vestibular nerve fibers with aging*	Decreased ability to maintain balance relative to younger adults; increased predisposition to falls
Reduction in numbers of hair cells in inner ear†	Increased use of wheelchairs to "prevent" falls, resulting in further impairment of balance

   * Data from Bergstrom, B. Morphology of the vestibular nerve. II. The number of myelinated vestibular nerve fibers in man at various ages. *Acta Otolaryngol* 76:173, 1973.
   † Data from Rosenhall, U. Degenerative patterns in the aging human vestibular neuroepithelia. *Acta Otolaryngol* 76:208, 1973.

instance of thought disorder and behavioral disturbance that has less clear-cut linkages to sensory or perceptual impairment.

Contributing Factors

Model of Sensory Alteration

Phillips (1981) proposes a useful model of sensory alteration in the aged. It is based upon theories of sensoristasis, which state that individuals have a basic drive to maintain "an optimal range and variety of external stimulation to maintain awareness" (p. 173) and that individual differences exist in the optimal level of stimulation. At the neurological level, she contends, the reticular activating system is programmed with expectations about acceptable levels of stimuli. The reticular activating system is stimulated by both internal and external sources; if stimulation from either source becomes excessive, disturbances of awareness and attention result. Under conditions of external stimulus deprivation, uncontrolled input from internal stimuli may produce cognitive disturbances.

For example, Holroyd and colleagues (1992) found that 13 of 100 consecutively reviewed patients with macular degeneration experienced visual hallucinations. Factors associated with hallucinations included living alone, lower cognition, history of stroke, and worse bilateral visual acuity, but they were unrelated to psychiatric disorders like depression, suggesting that sensory deprivation, or decreased cortical inhibition of internally generated sensory stimuli, may be responsible for the hallucinations.

Sensory distortion results from both overload and deprivation. *Sensory deprivation* occurs as the result of too little intensity or variation in the patterning or complexity of sensory stimulation while the relevance of stimuli is also low. *Sensory overload* occurs when the intensity or variation of patterns and complexity of stimuli is high and relevance is low.

Aging Process

Age-related changes in sensory receptors and central processing of sensory information predispose older people to sensory-perceptual alteration. The concept of reduced homeostatic reserve is pertinent. Cross-sectional research shows a diminished number of functional neurons in most sensory modalities. However, most people do not experience functional impairment or sensory-perceptual alterations because of aging changes alone. The diminished reserve of the aged makes them extremely vulnerable to sensory-perceptual alteration when disease states or environmental deprivation occurs.

Disease States

Many disease states potentially interfere with sensory function, either because they induce altered neuronal function or because the treatment of the disease results in sensory deprivation or interference with neuronal function. For example, the aminoglycoside antibiotics are ototoxic drugs. Treatment of infectious diseases thus can predispose to altered sensory perception. Individuals with Parkinson's disease, dementing disorders, and cerebrovascular accidents may develop

severe sensory-perceptual alteration because of several factors, including disrupted central processing of afferent messages, immobility resulting in reduced stimulation of afferent fibers, and social isolation (Koller, 1992; Rizzo et al., 1992). Diabetes mellitus may produce dizziness because of inadequate input from mechanoreceptors in the joints and muscles, among other sensory disturbances such as retinopathy and peripheral neuropathy (see Chapter 13). Diseases or drug treatment producing xerostomia can result in reduced taste acuity.

Inattention to Remediable Problems

Many diseases that cause sensory impairment in the elderly are remediable. Table 14–23 lists some diseases implicated in sensory-perceptual alterations; treatable or partially treatable disorders are starred. Failure to treat such disorders further predisposes older people to sensory-perceptual alterations, especially sensory deprivation.

Environmental Characteristics

Hospital and nursing home environments contain many unfamiliar sensory experiences for the elderly. Odors, noises, sights, textures, routines, and activity patterns are all different from those experienced at home. This applies especially to persons with a pre-existing dementing disorder or perceptual deficit, who will have increased difficulty interpreting new stimuli. There is great potential for reduced relevance of stimulation, predisposing to sensory-perceptual alteration. In addition, the intensity of stimulation in hospitals is typically quite high: many caregivers, around-the-clock noise, many questions and procedures, and disruptions in habit patterns, resulting in a high likelihood of sensory overload and associated adverse outcomes (Schnelle et al., 1993b). In the nursing home and at home, sensory deprivation is more likely to be the predominant problem. The pace of activity is slower and more routine, and stimulation may be less varied, producing monotony. All predispose to sensory deprivation.

Assessment

Determination of sensory-perceptual alteration requires synthesis of sensory acuity information with other measures of function. The defining major characteristics of sensory-perceptual alteration are disorientation in time, in place, or with persons; altered abstraction; altered conceptualization; change in problem-solving abilities; reported or measured change in sensory acuity;

change in behavior pattern; anxiety; apathy; change in usual response to stimuli; indication of body-image alteration; restlessness; irritability; and altered communication patterns. The minor characteristics are complaint of fatigue; alteration in posture; change in muscular tension; inappropriate responses; and hallucinations. Begin assessment for this disorder by carefully assessing sensory acuity.

Assessment of sensory abilities in the elderly is one of the most important parts of a generalized health assessment, because inability to accurately receive and process sensory information seriously impedes any assessment maneuver that depends on interpretation of patient responses to questions or directions. For example, the results of a mental status examination are unreliable and invalid if the patient cannot hear the questions being asked. Similarly, historical information about a specific complaint is not very reliable if the patient has poor comprehension of the examiner's questions but is eager to please. Choice of interventions is also influenced by the person's sensory abilities. If the individual is severely impaired, the amount of patient education that can be done without a significant other present is quite limited.

Vision

Minimal vision assessment includes evaluation of acuity and delineation of visual field deficits. Visual acuity should be measured using a standardized tool, such as a Snellen chart. Hand-held Snellen charts are available when a standard chart is not feasible. Visual fields should be evaluated using the confrontation method. The use of Schiøtz tonometry in screening for glaucoma in the elderly is controversial. Although some advocate annual screening for adults over age 40 years (Kollarits, 1992), a high rate of false-positive results occurs.

An approximation of the ability to function in the environment also should be obtained. Can the older person find a number in the telephone directory? Can the person read medicine labels and differentiate pills based on color and shape? Does the older person appear clumsy and bump into furniture? In institutional settings, can the menu or patient education materials be read? Is the person bothered by the visual impairments experienced? The Activities of Daily Vision Scale is a questionnaire that measures the amount of functional deficit associated with vision loss (Mangione et al., 1992). High reliability and good validity have been demonstrated in elderly patients before and

TABLE 14-23

Common Disorders That Result in Sensory Impairment in Elderly People

DISEASE	IMPACT ON SENSORY ABILITY
Vision	
Cataracts*	Opacities in the lens interfere with light focusing on the retina, also interfere with entry of light into the eye
Glaucoma* (2% of persons over age 40)	Increased intraocular pressure impinges on optic nerve (and/or artery?) and causes permanent blindness, beginning with peripheral vision
Macular degeneration*	Destruction of rods and cones in the central portion of the retina leads to loss of central vision. Peripheral vision initially may be preserved
CVA	Homonymous hemianopia or other visual field disturbance
Hearing	
Drug-induced hearing loss	Auditory nerve damaged by drugs, resulting in sensorineural hearing loss
Meniere's disease*	Episodic attacks of tinnitus and sensorineural hearing loss
Tertiary syphilis*	Bilateral sensorineural hearing loss often associated with vestibular disturbance
Paget's disease*	Slowly progressive sensorineural and conductive hearing losses, with losses most prominent in high-frequency ranges
Hypothyroidism*	Slowly progressive sensorineural hearing loss affecting all frequencies
Otosclerosis*	Immobility of stapes results in profound conductive hearing loss, but patient has normal speech modulation, something not characteristic of those with profound sensorineural loss
Taste	
Rhinorrhea*	Interferes with olfaction, which influences taste; also produces secretions that may mask taste of foods
Dentures	Cover taste receptors on palate
Stomatitis*	Interferes with reception by taste receptors on tongue
CVA	May impair hypoglossal nerve, which carries some afferent signals from the tongue
Smell	
Rhinorrhea*	Secretions interfere with function of smell receptors
Injury to olfactory nerve	Destroys pathway that allows central reception of afferent signals
Touch	
Diabetes mellitus	Peripheral neuropathies result in inability to sense light touch in distal portions of extremities, may also produce paresthetic sensation
CVA	Interferes with central reception of afferent signals
Arterial insufficiency	Peripheral ischemia may destroy peripheral nerve endings, resulting in inability to perceive light or deep touch
Toxin-induced peripheral neuropathy	Peripheral nerve endings and pathways destroyed by toxin, resulting in inability to perceive touch
Kinesthesia	
Vestibular dysfunction induced by CVA, Meniere's disease; dementia	Interferes with sense of balance, righting reflexes, proprioception, and visual function

* Treatable diseases.

after cataract surgery; however, its use in other populations has not been reported. The instrument is composed of 20 visual activities, representing the following five areas of visual function: distance vision, near vision, glare disability, night driving, and daytime driving. Each subscale is rated from 0 to 100, ranging from inability to perform an activity because of visual difficulty to no visual difficulty. Individuals with significant deficits but without an explanatory medical diagnosis should be referred to an ophthalmologist for further evaluation.

Hearing

Hearing assessment includes inspection of the ear canal for impacted cerumen, questioning regarding any recent changes in hearing, estimation of functional hearing loss, audiometric evaluation, and estimation of the hearing handicap. Simple clinical tests of hearing include asking the person to perform a task in a conversational tone, or asking the individual to repeat a word list—first facing the examiner and then with the examiner facing away from the patient—and testing for the ability to hear a whispered word at a distance of 2 feet, with the other ear plugged and the eyes closed (Macphee et al., 1988). If a hearing loss is demonstrated, the Weber and Rinne tests determine whether the hearing loss is symmetrical or unilateral and whether a conductive component is present. The person's ability to function with the current level of hearing should be assessed.

More sophisticated bedside assessment technology is also available. The audioscope is a device available to screen for hearing deficits in the aged. It combines the visualization capabilities of an otoscope with the ability to test for hearing loss at four different frequencies, from 500 to 4000 Hz at 20, 25, and 40 decibels. A setting of 40 is recommended for use with geriatric patients (Ney, 1993). Findings from audioscope screening compare favorably with standard audiometric testing results. The Speech-in-Noise test is a technique for identifying those with hearing-induced communication deficits. It holds promise as a functionally oriented screening test for older persons who may profit from more comprehensive hearing evaluation (Davignon and Leshowitz, 1986).

The American Speech and Hearing Association (1989) advocates the use of the screening version of the "Hearing Handicap Inventory" (Ventry and Weinstein, 1982) to identify the impact of a hearing loss on the patient's function. Determine whether the individual has ever used a hearing aid in the past and what that experience was like. Behaviors that mask the impact of the hearing loss should be noted. For example, many people are embarrassed by having to ask a speaker to repeat—instead they will simply smile and nod as if they understood. Ask questions that test comprehension, to ensure that the message has been understood despite a hearing impairment.

Ney (1993) found an efficient and accurate screening method in four "case history" questions along with visual inspection of the ear canals and pure tone hearing testing with an audioscope. All these measures could be performed in the time it took to administer the screening version of the Hearing Handicap Inventory for the Elderly (HHIE). A small number (approximately 3 to 5 per cent) of persons identified as at risk by the HHIE would have been missed by the case history, inspection, and audioscope protocol alone.

Mahoney (1992) also recommends against the use of only self-assessed hearing loss in the nursing home population; she found that residents were often unaware of their deficits.

Persons who have a hearing aid require additional assessment. First, examine the hearing aid for adequacy of functioning. Next, observe for difficulties with manual dexterity as the person manipulates the aid, during battery changing or insertion. Knowledge of care and maintenance of the aid should also be assessed (Val Palumbo, 1990).

Olfaction

The sense of smell is often omitted in routine assessments, although it can easily be tested and may provide clues to patients who are at risk for malnutrition. Information about the olfactory abilities also may help explain "bizarre" behaviors, such as inattention to bathing or not noticing that food in the refrigerator has spoiled. All that is needed for testing olfaction is a variety of different stimuli, such as cloves, cinnamon, oranges, ammonia, coffee. Results of the testing are useful as baseline data and may indicate a need for patient teaching regarding alterations in smelling.

Taste

Testing for taste sensation is also frequently omitted during routine assessment. It should never be omitted in the assessment of anorexia or feeding problems. The procedure is simple, involving only a variety of tastes and the opportunity between tastes to clear the palate. Patients close their eyes, and the stimulus is administered. Mint oil, sugar water, salt water, quinine, and lemon juice suffice to test the range of sensation.

Touch

The person's ability to accurately report light touch, pinprick, deep pressure, vibration, hot and cold, and proprioception of distal portions of the extremities should be assessed, using standard sensory testing methods. Such information guides development of individualized self-care programs, such as regular foot inspection for injury and use of appropriate footwear, and testing of bathwater with a thermometer instead of relying on inadequate temperature sensitivity to prevent accidental burns.

Kinesthesia

The sense of where the body is in space requires information from the vestibular apparatus, proprioceptors, and the visual system. Minimal testing of kinesthesia involves observation of the person's ability to maintain a sitting and standing balance, the ability to recover from a disequilibrating force, such as a gentle shove on one shoulder, and observation for nystagmus. During the testing, attention should be paid to the patient's emotional response and complaints of symptoms. For example, an impaired kinesthetic sense may underlie the older person's fear of falling. This fear or diffuse anxiety may be elicited during the testing, and the nurse should be prepared to provide reassurance by describing the safety precautions incorporated into the testing procedures.

Unilateral Neglect

Unilateral neglect is "a state in which an individual is perceptually unaware of and inattentive to one side of the body" (NANDA, 1992, p. 68). Its major defining characteristic is consistent inattention to stimuli on an affected side. Neglect is more than a primary motor or sensory loss; it represents a defect in the central processing of sensory information. When present, it is a predictor of poorer outcome after stroke. It is more common with damage to the non-dominant hemisphere (usually the right hemisphere). It also occurs with left hemispheric, dominant-sided strokes (Stone et al., 1993). The focus of the nursing assessment includes the practical consequences of neglect for performance of ADLs and IADLs, the safety of the patient in the environment, and body image changes. Specifically, the nurse should observe for:

- pocketing of food in the affected side of the mouth
- eating food on one side of the plate or tray
- bathing, grooming, or dressing only on the unaffected side
- bumping or injuring limbs on the affected side
- compensatory mechanisms employed by the patient

Integrated Functioning

Consider how the individual functions in the current environment. Are there deficits in self-care, mobility, or arousal that are out of proportion to the individual's disease state? What is the individual's customary lifestyle? How is a typical day spent? If there is reduced awareness, hypervigilance, or hyperactivity, sensory alteration may be the problem.

Planning and Intervention

The following goals apply to individuals with sensory alterations (Phillips, 1981):

- Provide a sense of control for the client
- Provide a sense of organization
- Help the client focus thoughts and determine purpose for activities
- Help the client achieve an optimal level of stimulation

Helping the individual organize, control, and determine the meaning of sensory stimuli may increase the relevance of incoming stimuli, reducing distortion.

Sensory Overload

General interventions for overload include attempts to help affected individuals master their environments. When the patient is in extreme distress or immobilized by the sensory-perceptual alteration, the nurse must act to limit the amount, intensity, and complexity of stimulation, as well as strive to enhance the relevance of stimulation. Such interventions are likely to be most successful if the patient can be enlisted in identifying the particular elements of the environment that are most disturbing. If the patient is not sufficiently communicative, then trial and error, as well as interpreting historical data from family, must suffice. Help the patient take control over small bits of the environment as appropriate—for example, choosing when self-care routines will take place or selecting items from a menu.

Other techniques advocated by Phillips include:

1. Explore with patients their perception of the environment, and help them interpret unfamiliar experiences;
2. Encourage the use of structured activities, to reduce the complexity of environmental stimuli and enhance the patient's feeling of control;
3. Provide anticipatory sensory information about procedures; and
4. Develop a mutually acceptable system for calling for help (patients unfamiliar with institutional environments may use "inappropriate" means of summoning help, resulting in unexpected outcomes for the patient, further complicating the pattern of stimulation).

Be prepared to teach family and nursing personnel about the potentially devastating impact of sensory-perceptual alterations in order to achieve consistent follow-through with recommendations.

Sensory Deprivation

Interventions to reduce sensory deprivation are of two types: generalized approaches and modality-specific approaches. An example of a generalized approach is movement therapy. Generalized approaches emphasize stimulation of several sensory modalities simultaneously. Rigorous evaluation of these methods is lacking, but preliminary studies show promising results in their effectiveness in increasing arousal and environmental awareness.

Specific interventions for sensory-perceptual alterations vary according to the impaired sensory modality and the motivation of patient and family to obtain assistance. Most types of sensory impairment are managed by prevention, referral for further assessment and treatment, use of adaptive equipment, and modification of the environment.

Vision

Visual impairments occur as the result of many treatable diseases. Treatment of diseases of the eye that were previously thought to be irreversible is increasingly available and successful—for example, laser surgery for those with diabetic retinopathy and macular degeneration (see Chapter 13). Early identification of these disorders is essential for optimal results. It is important, therefore, that older people have ready access to eye care professionals to obtain routine assessment for glaucoma, cataracts, and the diverse other eye diseases that affect older persons. Teaching older people and their family members about the possibilities for treatment of visual disorders is an important nursing function, along with coordinating referrals. Unfortunately, reimbursement for routine eye examinations and refraction to fit eyeglasses is not currently available under Medicare. However, treatment for diseases of the eye is reimbursed under Medicare; therefore, treatment of pathological conditions is affordable by many. Nurses should be prepared to function in an advocacy role for demented individuals. The fact that an older person has a cognitive impairment should not preclude treatment of visual disturbance. Sensory-perceptual alterations are likely to exacerbate the patient's confusion and therefore should be treated as aggressively as in any other patient.

Adaptive equipment used by individuals with visual disturbance includes eyeglasses, contact lenses, and artificial eyes. Eyeglasses and contact lenses can provide dramatic improvements in visual acuity, particularly for aphakic patients. However, they are of no use unless they are worn as prescribed. Unfortunately, it is commonplace to find eyeglasses in the bedside tables of elderly patients in hospitals or nursing homes. Nurses should be knowledgeable about which patients require eyeglasses and be vigilant in making sure they are regularly cleaned and used.

Contact lenses are being used more often in people of all ages. Two types are currently in use: daily wear and extended wear. Daily wear lenses are removed, cleaned, and disinfected daily. Extended wear lenses may stay in the eye for between 2 and 4 months (Hall, 1984). Nurses should know how to insert, remove, and care for contact lenses, so that if the patient lacks the manual dexterity or mental ability to care for the lenses properly the problem can be identified and a compensatory system developed. Good handwashing is essential before handling the lenses. Follow the specific instructions for lens removal, insertion, cleaning, and disinfection recommended by the patient's eye care professional. Eye prostheses usually require removal once each day to cleanse the eye socket and then can be replaced immediately.

Modification of the environment requires creativity and familiarity with available resources (for example, the Lighthouse Inc. 1991–92 catalogue). Two basic principles facilitate visual perception for all people and should be incorporated when possible into the physical environments of older people: use of adequate lighting intensity and use of color.

People over age 60 years require twice the illumination for close tasks as people aged 20 years. However, in increasing lighting intensity the problem of glare should be considered. Glare occurs when the peripheral field is much darker than the central field, or when the eyes pass from a darkened area to a greatly illuminated area. Factors that create glare include shiny surfaces, such as floors, magazine paper, or walls, and lighting that is not diffuse. Older people and health care administrators should be counseled on the need for bright, indirect environmental lighting.

Color contrast can be used quite effectively to provide cues for people with low vision and to reduce the monotony of the environment. Monochromatic color schemes are to be avoided, such as white plates on a white placemat or gray chairs on gray carpeting, as the older person may have difficulty discriminating the borders of the plate or the chair, leading to embarrassment or injury. Use of black borders or of contrasting colors, such as red and yellow, will enhance the visual capacity of the older person.

For individuals with some intact visual function, large-print materials—books, periodicals, patient education materials, clocks, calendars, and telephone dials—are examples of useful environmental modifications. Regardless of the extent of the visual impairment, caregivers should be cautioned not to move objects in the visually impaired person's environment without warning; to do so impairs the older person's independent function and may precipitate an accident. Individuals who are completely without vision should have the opportunity to receive the services of specialists in visual rehabilitation. Sometimes blind people will need to develop a relationship with others who can assist with tasks such as grocery shopping, bill paying, and transportation. If the individual has disabilities in addition to blindness and demonstrates difficulty in managing simple self-care tasks, use of a paid companion or institutionalization may be warranted.

Hearing

Referral for evaluation of treatable disorders that cause hearing impairment is essential. Institutional protocols for removal of impacted cerumen by nurses should be developed. This intervention in affected indi-

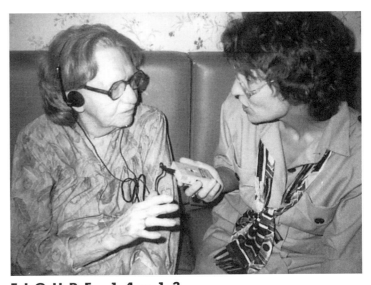

FIGURE 14–13

A hand-held voice amplifier increases the nurse's ability to communicate with hearing-impaired individuals.

viduals has been shown to improve the hearing of 75 per cent of hospitalized elderly people (Lewis-Cullinan and Janken, 1990). Evaluation for a hearing aid is a complex process, requiring a sensitive audiologist who must consider not only the older person's audiologic profile but also the finances, motivation, manual dexterity, and ability to learn the skill of using a hearing aid. If a hearing aid is obtained, the older person may need considerable support and encouragement in using it, for there are disadvantages to the increased volume, such as increased background noise, new problems with speech discrimination, and new tasks to learn. A nationally affiliated hearing-impaired support group, called "Shh," is located in many communities, another avenue of support for the person learning to cope with hearing impairment.

Other adaptive equipment for the hearing impaired includes hand-held assistive hearing devices that can be used for many patients within a facility or a clinic (Fig. 14–13), and visual cues that substitute for auditory cues, such as lights that signal the telephone ringing or someone at the door. Some programs have been developed to train dogs to respond to certain auditory cues, and in turn alert the hearing-impaired person (Burnside, 1981). The use of cochlear implants for correction of sensorineural hearing loss has been approved by the Food and Drug Administration, and there are promising reports in the literature about their impact on the function of older persons.

Modification of the environment to promote hearing ability in those with presbycusis or other hearing impairments has many possibilities. Eliminate background noise as much as possible before trying to communicate. Focus on the most common sources, such as the television set, radio, air conditioners, fans, people talking in the next room, or rattling of cutlery at a meal. It may be necessary to go to a different room to eliminate the background noise, an intervention well worth the trouble if the message to be communicated is important. The rate of speech should be moderate, and the volume should be even throughout each sentence. Take care to articulate words clearly, especially consonants. Do not shout but consider lowering the pitch of your voice. Speak with your mouth clearly visible to the older person. Many people lipread without realizing it. If the older person expresses difficulty in understanding a sentence, try rephrasing it rather than repeating the same words. Some people may have such severe hearing impairments that verbal communication becomes nearly impossible. Written communication may be the only alternative.

Managers of institutions where elderly persons live who have been deaf since early childhood (prelingual deafness) should consider light-signal devices for fire alarms, smoke detectors, room doorbells, telephones, and alarm clocks. A telecaption decoder for the television is helpful. A communication board for basic needs or a staff member fluent in American Sign Language for interpretation of more complex information is also indicated (Walsh and Eldredge, 1989; Andrews and Wilson, 1991).

Olfaction and Taste

Social interactions can include varied scents, such as cosmetic-sharing parties, thematic food tastings, flower arranging, and wheelchair gardening. The clinician or volunteer should draw attention to the scent or taste during the activity. Varying the smells and tastes available in both institutional settings and home care settings should be a conscious effort. Although much of the sensory stimulation literature emphasizes group intervention, nurses have many opportunities to focus an older patient's attention on a taste or smell that may help stimulate further sensory exploration or reminiscence. For example, when serving a cognitively impaired patient medication with juice, the conversation might touch on the flavor of the juice and whether the taste evokes any special memories.

Touch

Nurses have many opportunities to touch elderly patients, yet are not always sensitive to the messages conveyed through touch. Simple acts, such as taking a blood pressure or giving a bath, may be reassuring or uncomfortable, depending upon the type of touch used. Firm, steady pressure is perceived as more calming than a light, intermittent touch. Individual assessment is required to determine what level of tactile stimulation the older person prefers, but nurses should observe patient care practices in their work setting to determine the ways in which tactile stimulation may be varied or increased.

Kinesthesia

Immobilized patients are at most risk from kinesthetic deprivation and distortion. Regular exercise that carries the body parts through various planes stimulates proprioceptive and vestibular function. People who have been immobilized for long periods of time may find such activity very anxiety provoking, because their position sense is impaired and they fear injury. Gradual introduction of exercise is therefore important, along with explanations regarding the rationale for the exercise, and reassurance about safety measures being employed during the exercise session.

Unilateral Neglect

Nursing interventions should focus on enabling the patient to develop compensatory mechanisms so that injury to the affected side is prevented and independent function is maximized. Physical and occupational therapies are critical. Interventions should be customized and aimed first at increasing awareness of the neglected side through strategies such as the use of full-length mirrors and placement of a neglected arm at midline on a lapboard. Adaptation to the deficit can be encouraged by teaching and reminding the patient to scan the full visual field for objects, or, when reading, to use a brightly colored cue card to encourage visual search across the entire page. Labels on clothing to denote right and left may also be helpful (Carpenito, 1993b).

Evaluation

Specific criteria for evaluation of nursing care for patients with sensory overload or sensory deprivation are difficult to identify because the measures of these syndromes are primitive. However, criteria such as the ability to function independently, the presence of a normal state of arousability, and awareness of the environment are relevant. Does the individual feel in control of the environment? Does the individual report illusions or hallucinations?

The environments of individual patients can be assessed for the presence of obvious hypo- or hyperstimulation qualities. For example:

1. Is the lighting intensity adequate for an elderly population?
2. Is excessive glare present?
3. What is the level of background noise? Does it interfere with clear verbal communication?
4. Is a monochromatic color scheme used, or is color contrast used effectively?

Further research is needed into the impact of sensory-perceptual alterations before more specific criteria can be derived.

ALTERED SEXUALITY PATTERNS AND SEXUAL DYSFUNCTION

Definition and Scope of Problem

Altered sexuality patterns refers to "the state in which an individual expresses concern regarding his/her sexuality" (NANDA, 1992, p. 45). This condition is closely related to the diagnosis of sexual dysfunction, or "the state in which an individual experiences a change in sexual function that is viewed as unsatisfying, unrewarding, inadequate" (NANDA, 1992, p. 40). Sexual dysfunction in elderly people is a largely hidden problem because of social stereotypes of them as sexually inactive and because of clinicians' reluctance to inquire about sexual function. When sexual histories are obtained, sexual dysfunction is discovered as often as 50 per cent of the time (Gill and Ducharme, 1992; Keil et al., 1992).

Sexuality is "the behavioral expression of sexual identity. It may involve, but is not limited to, sexual relationships with a partner" (Gordon, 1982, p. 93).

Many studies have documented that older people retain interest in sex and remain sexually active, although there are physiological alterations in sexual response with aging (Gill and Ducharme, 1992). In a recent study of sexual activity among a random sample of elderly married couples, the majority of those over age 60 years reported having had sexual relations in the past month (53 per cent). The proportion of reports of sexual activity decreased with increasing age, with only 24 per cent of those aged 76 years and

older reporting sexual relations during the previous month. Factors predictive of sex in the past month included the older person's sense of self-worth, the spouse's health status, satisfaction with the marital relationship, amount of shared activities, and length of marriage (Marsiglio and Donnelly, 1991). Another study also confirms that sexual function is an important aspect of the lives of elders. From a cross-sectional national survey of 2765 people, including 441 people over age 65 years (212 men and 221 women), the following information about sexual activity is pertinent. Fifty-three per cent of men and 41 per cent of women reported engaging in sexual activity either daily or a few times weekly. Forty per cent reported decreased sexual activity in the past 3 years, but a similar number (39 per cent) reported increased sexual activity. These figures were not dramatically different for younger adults who answered the questionnaire: in those aged 27 to 38 years, 60 per cent of men and 49 per cent of women reported having sex daily or a few times weekly (Janus and Janus, 1993). It is important to bear in mind several key aspects of the study design. First, masturbation as well as coital sexual activity was included, unlike many studies of sexual activity. Second, the responses were tabulated from mailed questionnaire results. Thus, it is possible that those who are most interested in sexual activity responded, resulting in inflated sexual activity rates for the aged. Nonetheless, these figures point to sexual function remaining important to the elderly.

The consequences of sexual dysfunction in the aged include altered self-image, failure to reach fullest human potential, alterations in family process, behavior problems, and social isolation.

Age-Related Changes

Research on age-related changes in sexual function is sparse, and existing studies do not always study the same variables, making comparisons between studies difficult (Bancroft, 1989). However, frequency of intercourse, masturbation, and sexual dreams leading to orgasm declines with age for both men and women, regardless of marital status. The factors most commonly associated with the level of sexual function in women are marital status, age, and past sexual enjoyment. In men, factors associated with a high level of sexual function include level of sexual functioning earlier in life, age, present health status, social class, present life satisfaction, and physical function rating (Bancroft, 1989). Age-related changes in the sex response noted by Masters and Johnson are summarized in Chapter 9. It is emphasized that none of these changes in themselves preclude intercourse leading to orgasm.

Contributing Factors

Friedeman (1978) offers a useful model that summarizes factors influencing sexual behavior in the aged (Fig. 14–14). The model is used to organize a discussion of etiology of altered sexuality in the aged.

Demographic Variables

Increased age is shown consistently to be correlated with decreased intercourse. The data on noncoital sex remain extremely limited. In one report, masturbation frequency shows age differences in both men and women, with 17 per cent of men over age 65 years masturbating at least several times weekly, and 50 per cent of men reporting masturbating at least monthly. This rate is slightly decreased in comparison with younger men, among whom 23 to 32 per cent reported masturbating at least several times weekly, and between 47 and 58 per cent at least monthly. Both older and younger women report lower rates of masturbation, with between 8 and 14 per cent of younger women reporting masturbating at least several times weekly, compared with 2 per cent of women over age 65 years. Rates of women reporting masturbating at least monthly were more similar, with between 27 and 47 per cent of younger women endorsing this item, compared with 27 per cent of women over age 65 years (Janus and Janus, 1993). While there is tremendous interindividual variability in sexual activity, age remains a useful general marker of coital activity. Other demographic variables associated with sexual function include gender, marital status, and race. Men consistently report higher sexual activity than women, and data show that marital status does not affect sexual activity in men. Women consistently report absence of a partner as a major barrier to sexual activity.

Demographic variables are relatively easy to measure and have been widely reported as covariates of sexual function. Demographic variables reflect other factors in the conceptual model, such as the individual's belief system and social resources. However, demographic variables may prove to be useful as predictors of individuals at risk for sexual dysfunction. For example, individuals who are likely to be sexually active can be identified based on demographic characteristics, when coupled with a brief sexual history. When these people are institutionalized abruptly, they probably are at risk for sexual dysfunction because of an abrupt alteration in their pattern of sexual functioning; they are, therefore, candidates for intervention. Similarly, sexually active individuals experience greater disruption in their well-being when placed on drugs that interfere with potency and libido, and attempts should be made to identify those individuals prospectively. Demographics are thus helpful as a rough screen for individuals at risk for sexual dysfunction.

Belief System

Friedeman (1978) believes that Western social norms regarding sexual activity in old age are largely proscriptive. She cites the following erroneous stereotypes and attitudes: old people are too unattractive to be sexually appealing, the elderly are too fatigued, sick, or "feeble-minded" to engage in sexual activity, and "children" of all ages have difficulty accepting their parents as sexual beings because of oedipal conflicts.

Societal norms are often influenced by religious beliefs. Although systematic studies of the influence of religious belief on sexuality are few in number, some work suggests that strong religious beliefs are related to attitudes about sexuality (Adams et al., 1990; Hillman and Stricker, 1994). If one's religion teaches that the purpose of sex is procreation, then interest in sexual relationships in old age probably will be greatly diminished. Those who believe that sexual expression is appropriate only between spouses will not seek a sexual relationship if they are widowed and remain unmarried.

Although religious beliefs may narrow or eliminate the circumstances that allow for "appropriate" sexual expression, the older person's desire or need for sexual expression may remain strong. Conflict between beliefs about the propriety of sexual expression thus may result in sexual dysfunction.

KNOWLEDGE OF SEXUALITY IN OLD AGE. Information about age-related changes in sexual response has been available since 1966, yet it has not been widely disseminated. Few older people have had specific training in the changes in sex response that accompany aging. Ignorance of these changes may lead to anxiety, depression, or fear of inadequate performance—all pre-

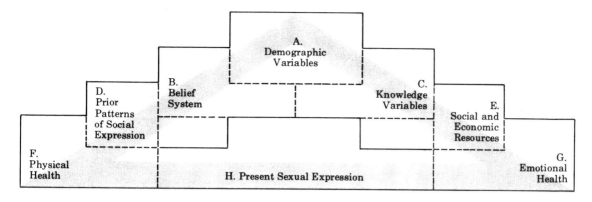

A. Demographic Factors
  Age
  Gender
  Marital Status
  Religion
  Church Attendance
  Education
  Occupation/Previous Occupation if Retired
  Income
  Lifestyle
  Ethnic Background

B. Belief System
  Desire the Conformity to System
  Religiosity, Values, Norms
  Variations with Age Cohorts

C. Knowledge Variables
  Information on Physiology of Aging
    and Sexuality

D. Prior Patterns of Sexual Expression
  Sexually Active
  Sexuality Expressed in Other Ways
  Sexual Deviance

E. Social and Economic Resources
  Availability of Partner
  Extent of Social Participation

F. Physical Health
  Physical Changes

G. Emotional Health
  Psychological Adaptations with Aging
  Specific Emotional Disorders

H. Present Sexual Expression
  Sexually Active
  Sexually Expressed in Other Ways
  Sexual Deviance

FIGURE 14–14

Variables influencing sexual expression in old people. (From Friedeman, J.S. Factors influencing sexual expression in aging persons: A review of the literature. *J Psych Nurs Mental Health Serv*, July 1978, p. 35.)

ventable with adequate information regarding the effects of normal aging on sexual function. It is possible that routine sex education for the aged could prevent some forms of sexual dysfunction, although this has not been studied. No systematic studies of older persons' knowledge regarding sexuality have been reported; however, anecdotes about elderly men assuming they are impotent because it takes them longer to achieve an erection are commonplace. Similarly, some women believe that sexual function will be impaired after menopause or hysterectomy. Several investigators point to the need for increased educational opportunities for older people about the sexual response in old age (Bancroft, 1989; Gamel et al., 1993; Goldstein and Runyon, 1993); however, one small-scale study showed that although knowledge of sexual changes can be increased in an educational intervention, other measures of sexual dysfunction did not change (Steinke, 1988).

Prior Patterns of Sexual Behavior

Sexual function in late life correlates highly with earlier patterns of sexual behavior (Bancroft, 1989). Individuals who had high sexual interest and activity in their youth retain these in old age. Heterosexual patterns are generally maintained in old age. A sudden loss of opportunity for sexual expression in sexually active individuals may occur through loss of partner, change in health status, or change in living arrangements. A sudden loss may precipitate sexual dysfunction in the older person.

Social and Economic Resources

Interesting and interested partners are a key variable in sexual expression. Social isolation depresses sexual expression; social activity can be influenced by economic resources, as transportation and admission to social events often cost money.

Another important social variable influencing sexual expression is the ability to achieve privacy. Old people living with younger family members and institutionalized older people may not find the privacy to develop or maintain a sexual relationship.

Physical Health

According to Bancroft (1989), few medical conditions lack sexual implications. He classifies the effects of medical diseases on sexual function into three categories: (1) the direct physical effects of the disorder, both specific and nonspecific; (2) the psychological effects of the condition, both on the individual and on the relationship, as well as concerns about the effects of sexual activity on the condition; and (3) the effects of treatment on sexual function: either drug effects, surgical treatment, or the psychological effects of treatment, especially surgery.

Examples of direct effects of medical disorders common in older adults include neurological impairments affecting sexual response, as can be seen in diabetes and peripheral vascular disease. Nonspecific effects of the medical disorders include reduced exercise tolerance in severe cardiac or pulmonary disease and pain due to arthritis or spasticity making assumption of customary sexual positions difficult. Lipe and colleagues (1990) found that 81 per cent of men studied with Parkinson's disease reported decreased sexual function. Levels of sexual dysfunction in men with Parkinson's disease and with arthritis were similar, as were frequency and satisfaction of spouses, suggesting that the role of physical impairments is important. Psychological contributors to sexual dysfunction from medical disorders include embarrassment about the effects of a disorder, or fear of inability to please a partner. Some people worry about the effects of sexual activity on chronic disorders, such as angina, hypertension, or stroke. Finally, treatment of many medical disorders may influence sexual function. Many antihypertensive agents have been associated with erectile dysfunction in men. Drug treatment for Parkinson's disease has been associated with hypersexuality, thought secondary to stimulation of the dopaminergic system (Cummings, 1991). Prostatectomy may also result in erectile dysfunction, for physical or psychological reasons. Finally, disfiguring effects of surgery, as in creation of an ostomy or mastectomy, may affect sexual desire, performance, or satisfaction.

A consensus statement of the National Institutes of Health (NIH) on impotence suggests that the term "erectile dysfunction" be substituted for the less precise and more pejorative term "impotence." The statement underscores the importance of not attributing erectile dysfunction to the aging process and highlights the important role of chronic disease effects in interfering with penile erection. Physical disorders that are most likely to interfere with penile erection include diseases that interfere with arterial blood supply and diseases affecting autonomic nervous system function. Specific diseases identified as risk factors for erectile dysfunction by the NIH consensus panel include diabetes mellitus, hypogonadism, hypertension, vascular disease, hypercholesterolemia, depression, and renal failure (National Institutes of Health, 1992).

Emotional Health

Most erectile dysfunction in men is believed to have a psychological component. In addition, emotional factors such as fatigue, anxiety, and use of alcohol and other central nervous system depressants have all been implicated in male erectile dysfunction. Although the knowledge base concerning emotional contributors to sexual dysfunction in men is scarce, even less is known about factors diminishing libido or sexual arousal in women.

Present Sexual Expression

Little is known about the various patterns of sexual expression engaged in by older persons and the extent to which the prevalent patterns of expression are satisfying. Homosexuality is reported in the literature, but the relationship between this pattern of sexual expression and other variables has not been studied. Masturbation is a form of sexual expression recommended by some experts for those without available partners. Deviant forms of sexual expression among the aged, such as pedophilia and exhibitionism, are much talked about, but elderly people commit these offenses less often than do younger adults.

Assessment

Nurses interested in promoting sexual health in the elderly must become comfortable in obtaining a sexual history. The social norms that conspire to portray old people as sexless affect clinicians as well. Older people are often quite ready to talk about sexuality with a clinician if the clinician can project ease and openness in discussing sexuality. Clinicians should examine their own values regarding sexual expression to avoid imposing them on the elderly person, as well as to gain comfort with assessing and intervening in sexual matters.

Every general health examination, therefore, should include a sexual history and provide an opportunity for the older person to voice concerns or raise questions about sexual function. The opportunity should be provided regardless of the setting, for it cannot be assumed that providers in other settings will conduct an assessment of sexual function or provide counseling regarding aging and chronic disease effects on sexual functioning.

Assessment should include a description of the older person's past patterns of sexual expression, recent changes in the pattern of sexual activity, knowledge of aging and disease-related changes in sexual function, beliefs about sexual expression, and perceived difficulties in sexual expression. The nurse should also be alert for covert signs of sexual dysfunction, such as repeated references to sex; repeated, socially inappropriate attempts to touch the nurse; or reports of sexually deviant behavior from staff or family.

Staff education concerning sexuality in the aged has been recommended by many investigators to increase the comfort of health care providers in working with older adults to prevent or treat sexual dysfunction (Aletkey, 1980; Goldstein and Runyon, 1993). It is important to note, however, that the relationship between knowledge about sexuality and permissive attitudes toward sexual expression is not always positive (Hillman and Stricker, 1994). Thus, when designing training programs, teachers should consider carefully the outcomes desired and whether the design will achieve those outcomes. Teachers may want to include not only factual information about changes in sexuality with aging but also should allow for individual values assessment and clarification regarding sexuality, although these approaches have not been tested rigorously. An increasing variety of high-quality audiovisual aids are available for those interested in increasing knowledge of sexual patterns in the aged, including homosexuality, and in helping health care professionals explore attitudes. For descriptive reviews of some of these aids, see Almvig, 1994; East, 1994; and Vining, 1994. Such educational opportunities promote more realistic policy setting regarding privacy and sexual expression and better handling of inappropriate sexual behavior. It

seems likely that nursing staff in all settings of care would benefit from such education, as sexual expression in the aged is a typically neglected part of sex education generally.

Planning and Intervention

Successful intervention depends upon careful identification of the contributing factors. Therefore we discuss interventions according to common contributing factors to sexual dysfunction in the aged.

Teaching About Sexuality in Late Life

Guarino and Knowlton (1980) describe a group training program for independently living older adults that combines information about sexual response with information on relationship building and intimacy in old age. Based on their experiences, they make the following recommendations about education in sexuality for the aged:

- Teachers should have formal training in sexuality.
- The group should be a closed group.
- The meeting room should be small, quiet, and comfortable.
- The administrative unit sponsoring the course should be truly supportive of the program, to avoid subtle sabotaging maneuvers.
- The group should meet for at least six sessions, with previously announced topics.
- Teaching strategies should include opportunities for touch.
- Follow-up procedures, such as the instructors remaining after class, should be part of the program.

Counseling

Widowhood and social isolation pose problems in sexual expression for many older people. Possible interventions include addressing the problem of social isolation, exploring the individual's beliefs and conflicts about resuming sexual activity following death of a spouse, and exploring the individual's views about masturbation as a form of sexual expression. Chronic diseases, such as angina, atrophic vaginitis, and degenerative joint disease, may result in painful intercourse. Thoughtful medical intervention, such as use of nitrates prior to sexual intercourse for patients with coronary artery disease, may restore sexual enjoyment. Estrogen replacement therapy is often successful in treating dyspareunia, although use of a water-soluble lubricant like K-Y jelly may suffice. Adjustments of analgesics or positions in patients with arthritis may make resumption of preferred patterns of sexual activity possible.

In addition, a variety of medical treatment options are available for male erectile dysfunction, over and above treatment of potentially reversible medical causes. Options include androgen therapy for those with low serum testosterone levels and no contraindications to this therapy, injections of vasodilators into the corpora of the penis, vacuum constrictive devices, vascular surgery, and implantation of penile prostheses. As each of these treatment options involves risks as well as benefits, treatment should be approached in a staged manner, after a careful evaluation of physical and psychological contributors to erectile dysfunction (Bancroft, 1989; National Institutes of Health, 1992).

Loss of a sexual partner is most commonly thought of as occurring through death of a spouse; however, physical and mental illness also may result in loss of a sexual partner. Pain, disfigurement, impotence, and mental dysfunction all may affect one spouse but not the other, effectively removing the able spouse's sex partner. Helping someone whose spouse is not a viable sex partner requires considerable sophistication and understanding on the part of the nurse. The nurse's role is to guide the couple in establishing realistic, mutually acceptable goals and developing an outlet for both to air their feelings safely.

Environmental Modification

Lack of privacy for sexual activity is a difficult problem to overcome in health care settings. In nursing homes, not all married patients are guaranteed conjugal visitation and privacy, and double beds are seldom found in institutions. Nursing home staff must consider the issue of competence to consent to sexual activity when cognitively impaired patients are involved in a sexual relationship. When competence is not an issue, patients must still contend with the long-term care facility community's values about sexual behavior. The sexually active older person must often bear the burden of a deviant label, because of lingering societal views of sexual expression among the elderly. Nurses can lead in considering the sexual expression needs of each client and

help arrange for privacy where possible and appropriate. Nurses may also help other staff members understand the problems of sexual expression in an institutional environment, focusing on the normality of sexual feelings and expression.

If the older person lives at home with other family members—children or extended kin—obtaining privacy may also be a problem.

Evaluation

Criteria to apply to the evaluation of nursing care for patients with sexual dysfunction are

1. The older person verbalizes satisfaction with the current level of sexual activity and type of sexual expression.
2. The older person is knowledgeable about the impact of drug therapy on sexual response.
3. The older person has confronted the impact of recent life changes on sexual response.
4. There is no evidence of inappropriate sexual behavior, such as unwanted touching of staff or others.

SKIN INTEGRITY IMPAIRMENT

Definition and Scope of Problem

Impairments in skin integrity have many manifestations that can be broadly categorized as either rashes or dermal ulcers. Dermal ulcers include pressure sores, ulcers due to venous stasis or arterial insufficiency, and ulcers from trauma. Adverse consequences from untreated skin problems in the aged include altered comfort, disfigurement, systemic infection, and loss of limbs and subsequent functional impairment. Older people are at high risk for impaired skin integrity and the associated adverse effects for a variety of reasons, summarized in Table 14–24.

The integumentary system performs a variety of functions that are often overlooked by clinicians and lay persons alike. These include

1. providing a protective barrier for the body against trauma, infection, temperature fluctuations, chemical irritants, and excessive losses of body fluids;
2. producing vitamin D when exposed to sunlight or ultraviolet light;
3. protecting sensory receptors; and

4. covering body tissues, individualizing appearance.

When skin integrity is impaired, one or more of these functions may be affected.

Foot Problems

Skin problems affecting the feet are numerous in older persons and therefore deserve special mention. The range of problems includes dry skin, onychogryphosis, diminished sensation, deformities of feet and nails, inadequate hygiene from reduced ability to reach or see feet, and improperly fitting footwear (Lagana, 1992). Foot ulcers and infections are particularly devastating, because if vascular supply is compromised then wound healing and prevention of infection become much more difficult. Nonhealing ulcers of the foot are a significant source of dysfunction in the elderly, for they may later necessitate amputation because of osteomyelitis or gangrene. The older person then experiences pain and disability associated with the loss of a lower extremity. Nurses, therefore, should pay particular attention to the integrity of skin on the feet of older people.

Contributing Factors

Age-Related Changes in Skin

Age-related skin changes that result in increased risk of injury and prolonged healing times include a tendency toward thickening of the epidermis, thinning of the dermal layer, decreased and less well-organized collagen, reduced elasticity and strength of the skin, reduced vascularity and density of hair follicles, and decreased production from sebaceous glands. Aged skin is more prone to injury and slower to heal.

DERMAL ULCERS. The three major contributors to dermal ulcers are arterial insufficiency, venous insufficiency, and chronic unrelieved pressure. In all three categories, the pathophysiological process is the same: ischemia produces cellular necrosis and ulceration. Patients with arterial insufficiency have ischemia because of inadequate arterial circulation to the affected body part—usually a distal part of a lower extremity. Venous insufficiency interferes with blood flow to the extremities by producing chronic peripheral edema, which interferes with exchange of nutrients at the cellular level. Chronic unrelieved pressure occludes capillaries and produces a local edema and hemorrhage that disrupts nutrient exchange and

TABLE 14 – 24
Risk Factors for Impaired Skin Integrity in Elderly People

FACTOR	IMPLICATION
Dermal Ulcers	
Increased likelihood of immobility	Increased potential for injury and trauma
	Increased likelihood of pressure sores
Increased incidence of peripheral vascular disease	Increased potential for ischemic ulcers (e.g., arterial ulcers)
	Increased potential for venous insufficiency
Increased prevalence of nutritional deficiency	Prolonged wound healing
	Reduced immunocompetence
Increased prevalence of peripheral neuropathy	Increased potential for injury/trauma
Increased prevalence of cerebellar dysfunction	Same
Rashes	
Increased drug use	Increased potential for allergic or toxic drug reactions
Increased incidence of herpes zoster	
Decreased immunocompetence	Increased potential for superinfection of rash
Increased prevalence of dry skin	Decreased protection against chemical irritants
Increased incidence of incontinence	Increased exposure to chemical irritants, e.g., urine

removal of toxic metabolites (Goode and Allman, 1989).

RASHES. Rashes are a common manifestation of altered skin integrity, with a variety of contributors, including infections, allergic responses, chemical irritations, psychological stressors, and poor hygiene. The pathogenesis and treatment of these disorders are summarized in Chapter 6.

Rashes associated with poor hygiene are commonly seen in elderly persons who are not independent in bathing. Often other underlying factors predispose to fungal infection, including immunosuppressant drug use, diabetes mellitus, and antibiotic therapy (DeWitt, 1990). The most common sites for these rashes are underneath the breasts in women and in the groin for both men and women. Several contributors are generally present:

1. Adductor spasticity of the lower extremities, making perineal hygiene difficult to achieve, leaving a chronically moist environment ideal for the growth of fungal organisms;

2. Incontinence, providing both a chemical irritant to the skin and a chronically moist environment that supports the growth of fungi;

NORTON SCORE CHART

Name of Patient _____ Room No. _____

			Dates		
General physical condition:	Good	4			
	Fair	3			
	Poor	2			
	Bad	1			
Mental state:	Alert	4			
	Apathetic	3			
	Confused	2			
	Stuporous	1			
Activity:	Ambulant	4			
	Ambulant with help	3			
	Chair-bound	2			
	Confined to bed	1			
Mobility:	Full	4			
	Slightly limited	3			
	Very limited	2			
	Immobile	1			
Incontinence:	Not incontinent	4			
	Occasionally incontinent	3			
	Usually incontinent of urine	2			
	Doubly incontinent	1			
		Totals			

F I G U R E 1 4 – 1 5

The Norton Score for measuring the risk of pressure sore formation. Rate the patient for each of the categories. Patients scoring 15 to 20 have little risk of pressure sore development, whereas patients with scores between 12 and 15 have a moderately high risk of developing a pressure sore, and patients scoring below 12 are at high risk. Pressure sore prevention methods should be instituted for those with scores less than 15. (From Norton, D., McLaren, R.S. and Exton-Smith, A.N. Pressure sores. *In Investigation of Geriatric Nursing Problems in Hospitals.* London: The National Corporation for the Care of Old People, 1962.)

3. Low energy or motivation, leading to inadequate drying under breasts or in the perineal area during baths;

4. Staff or family members with inadequate training or motivation to adequately dry patients under breasts or in the perineum.

Assessment

See Chapter 5 for a generalized approach to assessment of the older person's skin. Here we discuss in depth some maneuvers to assess the risk for impaired skin integrity as well as existing dermal ulcers and rashes.

Risk Assessment

Assessment of the older adult with a high potential for dermal ulcers should include the following elements:

• Interview of the patient or caregiver

about self-care practices such as bathing, foot soaking, and nail clipping.

• Inspection of the extremities for edema, erythema, cyanosis, pallor, hair distribution, dry skin, abnormalities of the nails, presence of bony deformities, adequacy of fit of footwear.

• Palpation of edema, peripheral pulses, and warmth of extremities.

• Testing sensation in lower extremities.

Individuals with any abnormalities, such as absent dorsalis pedis pulses; reduced sensitivity to light touch, pressure, pain, and temperature; greater than 2+ edema in feet; cyanosis, erythema, or pallor; and bony deformities, are at high risk for impaired skin integrity related to vascular insufficiency (Levine, 1990). Those with reduced sensation are at high risk for impaired skin integrity related to sensory impairment. Functional and environmental factors such as poorly fitting shoes, hazardous foot care practices, and inability to cut own toenails may interact with vascular and sensory factors to further increase risk.

PRESSURE SORE RISK. Pressure sores are the second major type of dermal ulcer. The primary etiology is chronic unrelieved pressure, resulting in localized ischemia, edema, necrosis, and ulceration. Other factors correlated with increased pressure sore incidence include immobility, incontinence, impaired nutritional status, and altered level of consciousness (Agency for Health Care Policy and Research, 1992).

Two instruments to assess severity of pressure sore risk have been endorsed by the AHCPR multidisciplinary panel on prediction and prevention of pressure sores: the Norton Scale (Norton et al., 1962) and the Braden Scale (Bergstrom et al., 1988). Dependent elderly patients should be assessed with one of the risk assessment tools on a regular basis for risk of pressure sore development (Figs. 14–15 and 14–16). Frequency should be determined by the same criteria nurses use for routine periodic assessment of patients generally. Patients with Norton scores of less than 15 or Braden scores less than 16 should have in place a specific, individualized plan for pressure sore prevention.

ASSESSMENT OF EXISTING ULCERS. The prerequisite for treatment of impaired skin integrity is an accurate description of the lesion.

Dermal ulcers should be carefully described, including location, size, depth, presence of granulation or necrotic tissue, char-

Client's Name _____		Evaluator's Name _____		Date of Assessment
Sensory perception Ability to respond meaningfully to pressure-related discomfort	**1. Completely limited** Unresponsive (does not moan, flinch, or grasp) to painful stimuli because of diminished level of consciousness or sedation OR limited ability to feel pain over most of body surface	**2. Very limited** Responds only to painful stimuli; cannot communicate discomfort except by moaning or restlessness OR has a sensory impairment that limits the ability to feel pain or discomfort over 1/2 of the body	**3. Slightly limited** Responds to verbal commands but cannot always communicate discomfort or need to be turned OR has some sensory impairment that limits ability to feel pain or discomfort in 1 or 2 extremities	**4. No impairment** Responds to verbal commands; has no sensory deficit that would limit ability to feel or voice pain or discomfort
Moisture Degree to which skin is exposed to moisture	**1. Completely moist** Skin is kept moist almost constantly by perspiration, urine; dampness is detected every time the client is moved or turned	**2. Moist** Skin is often but not always moist; linen must be changed at least once a shift	**3. Occasionally moist** Skin is occasionally moist, requiring an extra linen change approximately once a day	**4. Rarely moist** Skin is usually dry; linen requires changing only at routine intervals
Activity Degree of physical activity	**1. Bedfast** Confined to bed	**2. Chairfast** Ability to walk severely limited or nonexistent; cannot bear own weight and must be assisted into chair or wheelchair	**3. Walks occasionally** Walks occasionally during the day but for very short distances, with or without assistance; spends the majority of each shift in bed or chair	**4. Walks frequently** Walks outside the room at least twice a day and inside the room at least once every 2 hours during walking hours
Mobility Ability to change or control body position	**1. Completely immobile** Does not make even slight changes in body or extremity position without assistance	**2. Very limited** Makes occasional slight changes in body or extremity position but unable to make frequent or significant changes independently	**3. Slightly limited** Makes frequent though slight changes in body or extremity position independently	**4. No limitations** Makes major and frequent changes in position without assistance
Nutrition Usual food intake pattern	**1. Very poor** Never eats a complete meal; rarely eats more than 1/3 of any food offered; eats 2 servings or less of protein (meat or dairy products) per day; takes fluids poorly; does not take a liquid dietary supplement OR is NPO or maintained on clear liquids or IV for more than 5 days	**2. Probably inadequate** Rarely eats a complete meal and generally eats only about 1/2 of any food offered; protein intake includes only 3 servings of meat or dairy products per day; occasionally will take a dietary supplement OR receives less than optimal amount of liquid diet or tube feeding	**3. Adequate** Eats over half of most meals; eats a total of 4 servings of protein (meat, dairy products) each day; occasionally will refuse a meal, but will usually take a supplement if offered OR is receiving tube feeding or total parenteral nutrition, which probably meets most nutritional needs	**4. Excellent** Eats most of every meal; never refuses a meal; usually eats a total of 4 or more servings of meat and dairy products; occasionally eats between meals; does not require supplementation
Friction and shear	**1. Problem** Requires moderate to maximum assistance in moving; complete lifting without sliding against sheets is impossible; frequently slides down in bed or chair, requiring frequent repositioning with maximum assistance; spasticity, contractures, or agitation leads to almost constant friction	**2. Potential problem** Moves feebly or requires minimum assistance; during a move, skin probably slides to some extent against sheets, chair, restraints, or other devices; maintains relatively good position in chair or bed most of the time but occasionally slides down	**3. No apparent problem** Moves in bed and in chair independently and has sufficient muscle strength to lift up completely during move; maintains good position in bed or chair at all times	
				Total score

F I G U R E 1 4 – 1 6

The Braden Scale. (Source: Barbara Braden and Nancy Bergstrom. Copyright, 1988. Reprinted with permission.)

Stage I

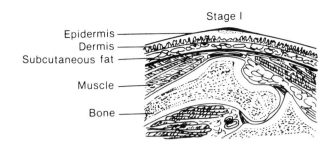

Non-blanching erythema of intact skin; the heralding lesion of skin ulceration.

Stage II

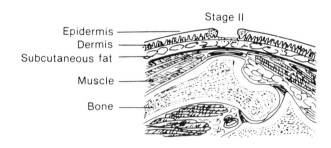

Partial-thickness skin loss involving epidermis and/or dermis. The ulcer is superficial and presents clinically as an abrasion, blister, or shallow crater.

Stage III

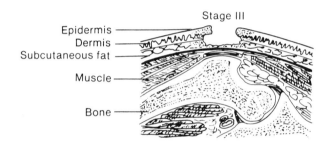

Full-thickness skin loss involving damage or necrosis of subcutaneous tissue, which may extend down to, but not through, underlying fascia. The ulcer presents clinically as a deep crater with or without undermining of adjacent tissue.

Stage IV

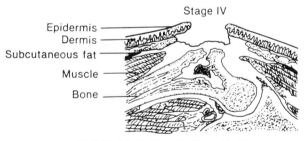

Full-thickness skin loss with extensive destruction, tissue necrosis, or damage to muscle, bone, or supporting structures (e.g., tendon, joint capsule, etc.).

FIGURE 14-17

Classification of pressure ulcers. (From Chenitz, W.C., Stone, J.T. and Salisbury, S.A. *Clinical Gerontological Nursing.* Philadelphia: W.B. Saunders, 1991, p. 254. [Based on the National Pressure Ulcer Advisory Panel, 1989.])

acteristics of drainage, odor, presence of inflammation, extent of undermining, and aggravating factors.

Pressure sores should be classified, using the staging system described in Figure 14–17. If necrotic tissue or eschar is extensive, it is impossible to stage the ulcer because the depth of the lesion cannot be determined until the eschar is removed. After the initial assessment, documentation of changes in the ulcer should be made at least every 3 days. An assessment form like that in Figure 14–18 greatly assists in standard-

izing the assessment and evaluation of pressure sores when several caregivers are involved.

ASSESSMENT OF RASHES. Assessment of rashes includes inspection of the entire body for distribution and careful description. The color, configuration, and symptoms associated with the rash should be described (DeWitt, 1990). Drug reactions are commonly distributed over the trunk and face, whereas cellulitis is generally confined to the locale of prior ulceration, although erysipelas may involve an entire extremity and not

WOUND DOCUMENTATION

Report on _____

or

Continuation of S.F. _____

(Strike one line)   *(Specify type of examination or data)*

Patient's name - Social Security No. - Date

Lesion	#1	#2	#3
Location			
Stage			
Appearance			
Size (LxW in cm)			
Shape			
Drainage			
Odor			
Surrounding skin			
Pain			
Consults			
Treatment			
Evaluation			
Signature/Title			

Stage I   Nonblanchable erythema
Stage II   Blister, skin break
Stage III   Skin break, exposing subcutaneous tissue
Stage IV   Skin break, exposing muscle and bone

Appearance:
  P = Pink
  SL = Slough
  ES = Eschar
  U = Undermining

Shape:
  B = Butterfly
  R = Round
  OV = Oval
  OB = Oblong

Drainage:
  P = Purulent
  S = Serosanguineous

Odor:
  O = None
  M = Mild
  F = Foul

Surrounding Skin:
  H = Healthy
  P = Pink
  E = Edema
  I = Indurated
  D = Dry
  M = Macerated

Evaluation:
  U = Unchanged
  I = Improving
  D = Deteriorating
  H = Healed

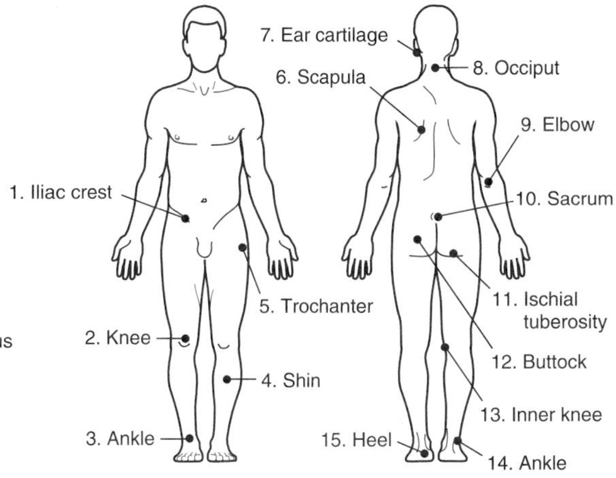

7. Ear cartilage
6. Scapula
8. Occiput
9. Elbow
10. Sacrum
1. Iliac crest
11. Ischial tuberosity
12. Buttock
5. Trochanter
2. Knee
13. Inner knee
4. Shin
3. Ankle
15. Heel
14. Ankle

FIGURE 14–18

Flow sheet for impaired skin documentation. (Source: Mary Kay Wooten, RN, ET Clinical Nurse Specialist, Durham Veterans Affairs Medical Center, Durham, NC.)

have continuous distribution. Refer to Chapter 5 for a depiction of common skin lesions and descriptive terms. Other important parts of the assessment include historical information, such as:

- recent changes in drug regimen
- recent skin trauma or ulceration
- history of chronic skin problems, such as eczema or seborrheic dermatitis
- associated symptoms, such as itching, pain
- ability to perform skin hygiene routines independently
- patient's perception of the problem and its impact

It is important to distinguish potentially life-threatening rashes, such as those from drug reactions and cellulitis, from those with more benign courses, as physicians often rely on nursing judgment regarding the urgency of treating a rash.

Planning and Intervention

COLLABORATIVE PRACTICE ISSUES. Nurses have long had a prominent role in the treatment of skin problems in patients. However, some ambiguity regarding the responsibilities of nurses and physicians in treating some skin conditions is also present, particularly in the case of pressure sores and foot problems.

Nursing care plays a critical role in prevention of pressure sores, yet in some institutions nurses may not independently order pressure-relieving devices, such as foam mattresses. In contrast, in practice settings where old people predominate, physicians often consider the patient's skin the nurse's domain of practice, unless a specific pathological lesion is present other than pressure or irritation from urine. Nurses should clarify their responsibilities regarding prevention and treatment of skin disorders where they work.

The goals of intervention in patients with

impaired skin integrity are to prevent and treat associated problems, such as infection, pruritus, and body image disturbance, and to heal the wound.

Dermal Ulcers

To heal dermal ulcers, two categories of intervention must be applied with equal zeal: prevention and wound care. AHCPR-recommended pressure ulcer prevention protocols include activities that maintain and improve tissue tolerance of pressure and those that protect against the adverse effects of the external mechanical forces of pressure, friction, and shear (Agency for Health Care Policy and Research, 1992). An algorithm for pressure sore prediction, as well as specific intervention strategies, appears in Figure 14–19.

In addition to ongoing preventive measures, wound care of existing ulcers should consist of the following components:

- *Assessment*, including that described above, plus wound culture if the patient shows signs of infection such as fever, increased white blood count, inflammation or edema around the ulcer, or purulent drainage. The procedure for obtaining a wound culture varies according to the amount of exudate and the type of wound. In general, excess pus should be removed with normal saline prior to obtaining the culture (see Cuzzell [1993] for a review of procedures).

- *Debridement* to remove necrotic tissue, such as slough and eschar. The most rapid and effective technique for debridement is sharp debridement, using scalpel and scissors, followed by enzymatic debridement. Other methods of debridement include whirlpool and wet-to-dry dressings. When the ulcer bed is pink with granulation tissue, debridement should be discontinued.

- Gentle *cleansing* with tepid normal saline. Antiseptic solutions such as povidone-iodine and hypochlorite have been shown to be cytotoxic to healthy tissue as well as bacteria and are no longer routinely recommended. Antiseptic solutions may be indicated for infected wounds, but they should always be followed by a normal saline irrigation (Young and Dobranski, 1992).

- The *dressing* chosen for the ulcer should provide an environment that supports healing. Research on wound healing suggests that a clean, moist wound environment is more conducive to healing than a dry environment, because epithelial cells proliferate and migrate more readily. Dressings that produce a moist healing environment include occlusive dressings (like Duoderm) and the semipermeable transparent films (like Opsite). In deep wounds that have a large amount of exudate, absorptive gels, such as karaya powder, Debrisan, and Bard absorptive dressings are useful in absorbing the excess drainage and necrotic tissue without overly drying the wound. Occlusive dressings should not be used if wound infection is present, as vapor-impermeable dressings may promote growth of anaerobic organisms.

- Intensified *pressure relief* efforts for stage III and stage IV pressure sores. Air fluidized beds, although costly, have been shown to be effective in the few randomized clinical trials published to date (Allman et al., 1987; Ferrell et al., 1993; Inman et al., 1993). Because none of these trials were limited to older adults and just one involved persons with stage II to stage IV ulcers, further studies are needed. Lovell and Anderson (1990) and Ceccio (1990) provide a thorough review of existing specialty beds.

- *New treatments* such as use of growth factors to stimulate angiogenesis, epithelial cell migration, and fibroblast activity are available in selected centers with physician supervision. Growth factors hold promise for improving the treatment of chronic dermal ulcers (Braden and Bryant, 1990). Young and Dorbranski (1992) provide an excellent review of pressure sore treatment.

Prevention and treatment for venous stasis ulcers and arterial insufficiency ulcers differ from treatment of pressure sores in only a few respects (Tam and Moschella, 1991). Arterial ulcers require loose dressings so that circulation is not further impaired, whereas in venous stasis ulcers, compressive dressings, such as an Unna boot, may be used to decrease edema. Both groups of patients should be instructed in prevention of and surveillance for ulcers.

Rashes

Treatment of the various rashes experienced by older people depends on the causative agent. Once the definitive therapy has been instituted, preventing and alleviating associated problems like discomfort and in-

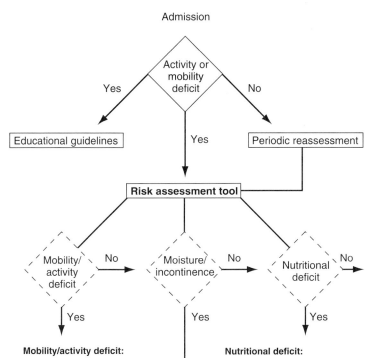

Admission

Activity or mobility deficit

Yes

Educational guidelines

Yes

Risk assessment tool

No

Periodic reassessment

Mobility/ activity deficit

No

Moisture/ incontinence

No

Nutritional deficit

No

Yes

Yes

Yes

Mobility/activity deficit:

Mechanical loading and support surface guideline

For bed-bound individuals:
• Reposition at least every 2 hours.
• Use pillows or foam wedges to keep bony prominences from direct contact.
• Use devices that totally relieve pressure on the heels.
• Avoid positioning directly on the trochanter.
• Elevate the head of the bed as little and for as short a time as possible.
• Use lifting devices to move rather than drag individuals during transfers and position changes.
• Place at-risk individuals on a pressure reducing mattress. **Do not use donut-type devices.**

For chair-bound individuals:
• Reposition at least every hour.
• Have patient shift weight every 15 minutes if able.
• Use pressure-reducing devices for seating for seating surfaces. **Do not use donut-type devices.**

Skin care and early treatment guideline

• Inspect skin at least once a day.
• Individualize bathing schedule. Avoid hot water. Use mild cleansing agent.
• Minimize environmental factors such as low humidity and cold air. Use moisturizers for dry skin.
• Avoid massage over bony prominences.
• Use proper positioning, transferring, and turning techniques.
• Use lubricants to reduce friction injuries.
• Institute a rehabilitation program.
• Monitor and document interventions and outcomes.
• Consider postural alignment, distribution of weight, balance and stability, and pressure relief when positioning individuals in chairs or wheelchairs.
• Use a written plan.

Nutritional deficit:

Skin care and early treatment guideline

• Investigate factors that compromise an apparently well-nourished individual's dietary intake (especially protein or calories) and offer him or her support with eating.
• Plan and implement a nutritional support and/or supplementation program for nutritionally compromised individuals.

Moisture/incontinence:

Skin care and early treatment guideline

• Cleanse skin at time of soiling.
• Minimize skin exposure to moisture. Assess and treat urinary incontinence. When moisture cannot be controlled, use underpads or briefs that are absorbent and present a quick-drying surface to the skin.

F I G U R E   1 4 – 1 9

Pressure ulcer prediction and prevention algorithm. (Adapted from Agency for Health Care Policy and Research [AHCPR] Panel for the Prediction and Prevention of Pressure Ulcers in Adults. *Pressure Ulcers in Adults: Prediction and Prevention.* Clinical Practical Guideline No. 3, AHCPR Publication No. 92-0047. Rockville, MD: AHCPR, Public Health Services, 1992, pp. 16–17.)

fection is the concern. Proper hygiene of rashes includes gentle cleansing to remove exudate and gentle drying to prevent further skin trauma. Tender skin can be dried either by patting gently with a towel or using a hair drier on cool or warm setting after washing and rinsing. When the patient's rash is related to dry skin, moisturizing agents should be applied to the skin immediately after a bath, while the skin is still damp to seal water within the hydrated epidermis (DeWitt, 1990). Efforts to ensure adequate systemic hydration should also be made.

Undergarments and positioning have a role in treatment and prevention of fungal infections. For breast candidiasis, a well-fitting cotton brassiere will help absorb moisture and reduce chafing. In perineal candidiasis, an adductor block pillow may improve air circulation to the affected area, reducing moisture accumulation. Appropriate treatment of the rash with antifungal agents and good hygiene often reduce the discomfort and anxiety associated with rashes. However, itching sometimes persists as a major source of discomfort. Local counterirritation, such as massage, or the use of cool compresses is sometimes effective. If the discomfort is severe, short-term use of antihistaminic drugs or topical corticosteroids is warranted, but attention should be paid to other drugs the patient is taking—to establish the correct dosage and prevent adverse drug interactions.

Evaluation

Timing of the evaluation in skin conditions deserves special note. The evaluation of responses to therapy for acute skin conditions that produce discomfort or threaten life is done much more frequently than evaluation of chronic, basically clean skin ulcers. Frequent evaluation of treatment regimens for chronic ulcers may lead to the patient's becoming frustrated and inappropriately changing treatments before an adequate trial. Although observation for a sudden increase in the amount of wound drainage or a sudden change in appearance should be done daily, evaluation of treatment regimens should be less frequent—for example, weekly.

Criteria for evaluation of patients with impaired skin integrity include

1. The wound or rash is resolved.
2. The patient does not develop preventable consequences such as infection from impaired skin integrity.

3. If discomfort accompanies the skin problem, appropriate measures are taken to relieve the discomfort.
4. The patient is counseled regarding the meaning of the skin problem, including appropriate preventive measures.
5. Measures to prevent skin breakdown in at-risk individuals are taught to caregivers and implemented.

SLEEP PATTERN DISTURBANCE

Definition and Scope of Problem

Sleep pattern disturbance is an alteration in the individual's habitual pattern of sleep and wakefulness that causes discomfort or interferes with a desired lifestyle (NANDA, 1992). The disturbance may be the result of too much sleep, or too little. It is present when an individual complains of sleep difficulties or when observable signs of diminished function are present, combined with observation of a sleep pattern that deviates from the norm for the age group. Functional problems associated with sleep deprivation in people of all ages include difficulty with memory, concentration ability, and motor skills; increased aggressiveness and irritability; and neurological disturbances, including nystagmus, hand tremor, ptosis, and reduced facial expressions (Hammer, 1991; Robinson, 1993). The defining characteristics as recognized by NANDA are

- Verbal complaints of difficulty falling asleep
- Awakening earlier or later than desired
- Interrupted sleep
- Verbal complaints of not feeling well rested
- Changes in behavior and performance:
  Increasing irritability
  Restlessness
  Disorientation
  Lethargy
  Listlessness
- Physical signs:
  Mild, fleeting nystagmus
  Slight hand tremor
  Ptosis of eyelid
  Expressionless face
  Dark circles under eyes
- Thick speech with mispronunciation and incorrect words
- Frequent yawning
- Changes in posture

Sleep complaints are highly prevalent in elderly people. Many studies show that older adults frequently experience nighttime waking and between 10 and 15 per cent of older adults routinely use sedative-hypnotic agents to induce sleep. Whether the aged have a greater prevalence of increased sleep latency is more controversial, although difficulty falling asleep is a common complaint (Bliwise, 1993). The increased frequency of sleep complaints is probably due to the co-occurrence of chronic diseases and the effects of the aging process. Some sleep disorders, such as sleep apnea and periodic leg movements, are more common in the aged. Ancoli-Israel and colleagues (1991) have shown prevalence of sleep apnea to be quite high in community-dwelling elders (24 per cent) and even higher in those hospitalized (33 per cent), with the highest rate of all (42 per cent) in older adults in a nursing home. Although periodic leg movements are less well studied, their prevalence in community-dwelling adults has been estimated at 45 per cent (Bliwise, 1993).

In addition to clinical manifestations of sleep disturbance, the aging process is accompanied by changes in the duration of the various stages of sleep, as identified by polysomnograms. As noted earlier, nocturnal sleep efficiency is 70 to 80 per cent less than that of younger adults. The percentage of time spent in light sleep (stages 1 and 2) is greater in older adults, with substantially less time spent in deep sleep (stages 3 and 4). Also with aging, the amount of rapid eye movement sleep (REM) is reduced (Ancoli-Israel and Kripke, 1992; Bliwise, 1993).

Some elderly individuals perceive little difficulty with sleep, despite objective age-related changes in pattern. To quote one noted sleep expert, "Whether an aged individual views his or her 75 per cent sleep efficiency as insomnia or merely accepts this as a normal part of aging may depend largely on that individual's perspective on growing old and what that means to him or her" (Bliwise, 1993, p. 40).

Contributing Factors

The *internal factors* that contribute to sleep disturbance in the elderly, and their mechanisms of action, are

1. Aging process: Degenerative CNS changes result in decreased amounts of deep sleep and in conditions that promote frequent awakenings and disturbed circadian rhythms.
2. Aging process: Sensory impairments make it more difficult to use environmental cues, such as time of day and activity level in the environment, to guide activity/rest patterns.
3. Illness: Symptoms of disease that interfere with uninterrupted sleep, including paroxysmal nocturnal dyspnea, orthopnea, anxiety, pain, sleep apnea, and nocturia.
4. Psychological stress: Ineffective individual coping may result in decreased sleep, because the individual worries about problems at night. Nightmares, unresolved grief, and depression all may interfere with sleep, either by causing difficulty getting to sleep or early morning awakening.

Factors external to the patient that may contribute to sleep disturbance are

1. Environmental changes: Changes in the environment result in changes in habits, which may interfere with sleep. The physical properties of the sleeping quarters may differ, as may the rules determining bedtime. Additionally, the noise level, particularly in institutional settings, may interfere with sleep. A cross-sectional study of sleep patterns and factors associated with interrupted sleep in 118 incontinent nursing home residents from four different nursing homes showed that on average, patients slept only 66 per cent of the time they were in bed and that sleep was very fragmented (Schnelle et al., 1993a). Average duration of each bout of sleep was 20 minutes, with the peak duration 83 minutes. Moreover, when noise and light levels and nursing care practices at night were examined in relationship to the sleep measures, 50 per cent of nocturnal waking episodes were associated with nursing care activities and 35 per cent of all waking episodes of 2 minutes or shorter (Schnelle et al., 1993b). Although these parameters have not been studied in hospital settings, it is likely, given the need for frequent medical interventions, that care routines involve even more disruptions in sleep.
2. Drugs: Side effects of many agents used in chronic disease management affect sleep, including nightmares, periodic leg movements, hallucinations, confusion, obstructive sleep apnea, daytime sleepiness, and other disruptions in sleep phasing.

Degenerative aging changes in the central nervous system can affect the regulation of circadian rhythms and may result in difficulty maintaining synchronous rhythms. They may also result in a decreased amplitude of circadian rhythm (Bliwise, 1993). Age-related sensory impairment is also implicated in sleep disturbance. Visual impairment may reduce sensitivity to external cues, such as light and dark, that are used to prompt sleep patterns. Changed sleep patterns may also influence the quality of sleep. If the older person takes frequent daytime naps because of decreased endurance or boredom, biorhythms may be influenced by altering the mix of rapid eye movements (REM sleep) and slow-wave sleep. REM sleep is more prominent in morning napping and slow-wave sleep is more prevalent in afternoon naps.

Physical diseases interfering with sleep include nocturnal angina associated with cardiac disease, pain from undiagnosed peptic ulcer disease, and hypoxia associated with chronic obstructive lung disease. Withdrawal from sleep medications or alcohol also may precipitate insomnia.

Emotional contributors to sleep disturbance in the elderly include anxiety and depression. The mechanism for the disturbance in sleep is not fully understood.

Drugs are typically thought of as interventions for sleep disturbance, but they are also implicated as contributors to the problem. For example, in individuals whose sleep disorder is related to nocturnal hypoxia, sedative drugs that depress respirations will aggravate rather than alleviate the problem (Ancoli-Israel and Kripke, 1992). Rebound insomnia from long-term use of benzodiazepine sedatives may occur. Withdrawal from sedatives such as alcohol, benzodiazepines, or barbiturates frequently causes sleep disturbances. Other drugs, such as antiparkinsonian agents, tricyclic antidepressants, and antihypertensives, have been implicated in sleep disturbances. Drugs are infrequently tested in the elderly population for their effects on sleep patterns, and therefore clinicians must be particularly alert for adverse effects.

Assessment

Nurses who fail to use a systematic approach when assessing sleep disorders in elderly people are likely to overestimate the prevalence of sleep disorders. Assessment begins with a detailed history of the client's perception of the disturbance, symptoms of disease that occur during the client's usual sleep time (such as dyspnea, chest pain, or anxiety), and a history of any environmental changes. A detailed record of activity and rest patterns throughout a 24-hour period helps identify contributors to sleep difficulties. Patterns of nap taking or inactivity may

reveal that the individual is unrealistic about the amount of sleep required in a 24-hour period when balanced with a sedentary lifestyle.

Obtain a detailed drug history, because many drugs may interfere with sleep, most notably the antianxiety agents, narcotics, and alcohol. The history should guide the remainder of the assessment.

Physical examination is indicated for individuals who report symptoms of disease that may interfere with sleep (such as pain, dyspnea, a recent change in voiding patterns) to identify remediable symptoms. In institutions, have staff note their observations of the amount of sleep obtained by the individual. Sometimes clients report that they have not slept at all, when direct observations demonstrate that sleep is obtained. If the patient can be observed while sleeping, pay particular attention to signs that may indicate sleep apnea, such as periods of no respirations, or snoring. Monitoring oxygen saturation with a pulse oximeter while the person is sleeping may also help diagnose probable sleep apnea and can help justify referral to a sleep center for further evaluation. When one does not feel rested despite sleep, the nature of the problem is more likely to be a coping difficulty rather than a sleep disturbance, although the two problems are not always mutually exclusive.

Parameters to be included in the assessment of a person with disturbed sleep patterns are:

- Daytime activity–work pattern: Individuals who are extremely sedentary may have difficulty sleeping at night. Increasing activity during the day or teaching about the relationship between activity and need for sleep may resolve the sleep disturbance.

- Time client usually retires: May reveal unrealistic expectations regarding the amount of sleep required. May also reveal excessive amounts of time spent in bed, which may interfere with sleep.

- Problems in falling asleep: May reveal symptomatology of other diseases that contributes to sleep disturbance, which may in turn suggest interventions. For example, people with anxiety at bedtime may respond well to progressive relaxation exercises or some type of bedtime routine, such as warm milk or focusing on pleasant images or fantasies.

- Problems in staying asleep: May indicate symptoms of disease contributing to the problem—for example, poorly controlled congestive heart failure that results in paroxysmal nocturnal dyspnea, or an inadequate pain control regimen. May also indicate a new problem, such as nocturia associated with benign prostatic hypertrophy.

- Early morning awakening: Most often associated with depression. Indicates need for further evaluation for depression. May also point to unrealistic expectations about sleep.

- Quality of sleep: Impaired quality of sleep suggests aging-related phenomenon. Teaching about changes in sleep patterns with age may be beneficial.

- Dreams, nightmares: May precipitate more frequent awakenings. Dream material also may provide insights into coping with problems.

- Sleeping environment: Environmental factors may influence sleep greatly. Specific factors include change in habit pattern; changes in noise level; changes in social cues that stimulate sleep; and changes in availability of alcohol, drugs, or warm milk. Temperature control, the "feel" of the bed, and the presence or absence of a roommate or bedpartner may interfere with sleep. In institutional settings, observe care routines at nighttime, to get a sense for how disruptive nursing care routines are to sleep.

- Activities associated with sleep: Activities may interfere with sleep, as in the case of someone who works on a particularly difficult or vexing problem just before retiring. Additionally, if environmental changes interfere with the conduct of rituals surrounding sleep, such as bath time or certain foods, drink, or medications, the ability to fall asleep may suffer.

- Personal beliefs about sleep: Individuals may place excessive importance on the value of getting some arbitrary amount of sleep each night. Additionally, an unwillingness to alter one's patterns of obtaining sleep (several shorter periods day and night rather than one long period of sleep at night) may result in problems of not feeling rested or in being overtired.

Planning

Sleep patterns are a type of habit, and habits typically require a substantial time period to change. Both client and nurse, therefore, should be prepared for slow changes. There are no specific guidelines for the timing of evaluation; however, drug withdrawal may take many months. It is self-defeating to set overly ambitious schedules for treatment.

Interventions

Strategies for treating sleep pattern disturbances in elderly people fall into four categories: (1) teaching about aging-related sleep changes, (2) environmental modification, (3) changes in activity patterns, and (4) medical therapies. Most recommendations for interventions to treat sleep pattern disturbance are based on clinical experience rather than rigorous evaluation in controlled studies, as only recently have sophisticated measurements of sleep been possible outside the sleep laboratory. Studies that support an intervention are cited in the text.

Bliwise (1993) warns against judging the sleep patterns of older adults according to norms for younger people. Nurses as well as older persons do this, and it may lead to undue concerns about health problems for the older person. Explaining common age-related changes in sleep patterns may be reassuring to older people.

Environmental modifications include developing a specific routine for sleep, altering behavior patterns to allow only sleep-related activities in the bedroom, and using interventions such as engaging in monotonous activities after experiencing an awakening. In institutional settings, every effort should be made to consolidate care activities (such as medication administration, dressing changes, observation of vital signs, other procedures) so that a minimum number of interruptions of sleep occur. In addition, it is worthwhile to question whether certain care routines are necessary. For example, Schnelle and colleagues suggest an alternative to waking incontinent, dysmobile patients every 2 hours for changing and turning. They propose hourly nursing assistant rounds: if the patient is already awake, incontinence care and repositioning are given. If asleep, the patient is left undisturbed until the next scheduled round. Only if the patient is asleep on three consecutive rounds is the patient awakened for care. They reason that given the high prevalence of sleep fragmentation in nursing home patients, it is unlikely that patients will be asleep on all rounds. Increasing the frequency to hourly (instead of two hourly, as is a common practice) increases the probability that a resident will be found spontaneously awake, rather than having to be awakened (Schnelle et al.,

T A B L E   1 4 – 2 5
Normative Data for Sleep Patterns in Elderly

SLEEP BEHAVIOR	RANGE (n = 212)	MEAN
Time for going to bed	8:00 P.M.–2:00 A.M.	11:00 P.M.
Sleep latency	Less than 15 min to over 2 hr	35 min
Amount of wake time after sleep onset	0 to over 2 hr	30 min
Number of wake times after sleep onset	0 to 7 times	1.5 times
Time awake before arising	Less than 15 min to over 2 hr	20 min
Time for arising	4:00 A.M.–11:00 A.M.	7:30 A.M.
Amount of sleep during daytime naps	0 to over 4 hr	30 min
Number of daytime naps	0 to 4 naps*	.7 naps
Total time in bed, including naps	5.5–14.5 hr	9.1 hr
Total time in bed, excluding naps	4.5–12.5 hr	8.6 hr
Total time asleep, including naps	Less than 4 hr to 12.5 hr	7.5 hr
Total time asleep, excluding naps	Less than 4 hr to 10.5 hr	7.2 hr

* An additional 25 subjects reported that they doze involuntarily when they had not intended to take a nap.
From Hayter, J. Sleep behaviors of older persons. *Nurs Res* 32(4):242–246, 1983.

1993a). This suggestion applies equally well to hospital settings of care.

There is growing interest in the effects of phototherapy on sleep disturbance. Satlin and colleagues (1992) studied the effects of bright light treatment for sleep disturbance in 10 patients with Alzheimer's disease. All subjects had a history of fragmented sleep-wake cycles and associated evening behavioral disturbance. Subjects were given 2 hours per day of exposure to a lighting intensity of 1500 to 2000 lux of light from 7:00 to 9:00 P.M. Compared with their control condition, eight of the subjects improved according to nurse ratings of sleep-wake disturbance, and daytime activity monitor data suggested an increased stability of circadian rhythmicity.

Interventions involving modification of activity patterns should be undertaken only after careful analysis of the person's 24-hour activity pattern. Interventions range from reducing the time spent in bed, reducing the number or frequency of naps, increasing the structure and vigor of daytime activities, relaxation techniques, or a combination of these.

Sleep restriction therapy (establish a sleep schedule with set bedtimes and awakenings, no naps) and muscle relaxation exercises were evaluated in 22 community-dwelling older adults with insomnia. In both groups, self-reported sleep latency and the number of nocturnal wakings were decreased during the trial. Reduced sleep latency and increased total sleep time were found at 3-month follow-up. Sleep restriction therapy was superior to relaxation in increasing total sleep time and sleep efficiency (Friedman et al., 1991). Similar results were reported for a cognitive-behavioral intervention that was designed to improve poor sleep habits and change dysfunctional beliefs and attitudes about sleep. A 53 per cent improvement in sleep latency was found in the intervention group, compared with only 10 per cent in controls. Other positive outcomes included discontinuation of sedative-hypnotic medicines, and improvement on polysomnographic measurements. Therapeutic outcomes were maintained at 3- and 12-month follow-up assessments (Morin et al., 1993).

Medications are a frequent response to sleep disturbance in both community and institutional populations. Studies show that rates of hypnotic drug use in the community range from 5.9 to 33 per cent in Great Britain and 6.6 to 18.3 per cent in the United States. In institutions, the use of hypnotics is more frequent, ranging from 22.6 to 54.0 per cent. The frequent use of hypnotics is unfortunate, because of the increased vulnerability of the elderly to the adverse side effects. The most common adverse effects include confusional states, decline in psychomotor performance, and daytime sedation. When sedatives or hypnotics are used for sleep, shorter-acting benzodiazepines are preferred over the longer-acting ones because of older persons' tendencies to accumulate these drugs. The geriatric prescription caveat "Start low and go slow" certainly applies here. Benzodiazepines are recommended for short-term rather than long-term use, as there is great potential for habituation to these drugs and withdrawal is a lengthy, painful process.

Evaluation

Evaluation of the effectiveness of interventions for sleep disturbance should be based upon normative data for sleep patterns of the aged. Normative data on sleep behaviors for older persons living in the community, as well as a smaller sample of those in homes for the aged, are summarized in Table 14–25. While it is important to follow the individual's report of adequacy of sleep, it is equally important that the older person understand how sleep patterns change with age. Documentation should reflect the frequency of occurrence of offending symptoms and the progress toward restoration of the client's sleep pattern. Information regarding the client's quality and quantity of rest and sleep should be recorded.

THOUGHT PROCESS ALTERATION

Definition and Scope of Problem

Alteration in thought processes is "a state in which an individual experiences a disruption in cognitive operations and activities" (NANDA, 1992, p. 70). The defining characteristics identified by NANDA are sparse and include distractibility, memory deficit/problems, inappropriate nonreality-based thinking, egocentricity, cognitive dissonance, hyper- or hypovigilance, and inaccurate interpretation of the environment.

Other writers (Hall, 1991; Carpenito, 1993a) discuss an expanded list of defining characteristics that includes

- Disorientation to time, place, or person
- Altered ability to think abstractly
- Disorders of memory
- Misinterpretation of environmental stimuli
- Changes in problem-solving abilities
- Changes in behavior patterns, including regression
- Irritability
- Distractibility
- Hallucinations
- Delusional thought
- Inappropriate responses to commands

Although there is controversy among nursing diagnosis theorists as to how the syndrome of delirium fits into this diagnostic category, delirious patients clearly fit most diagnostic criteria for alterations in thought processes. Therefore, it is worth considering whether it might be more useful to include the American Psychiatric Association's *Diagnostic and Statistical Manual (DSM-IIIR)* criteria for delirium under defining characteristics for alterations in thought processes (see Rockwood [1993] for a summary of *DSM-IIIR* criteria and their prevalence among hospitalized older persons).

Alteration in thought processes may be related to a wide variety of metabolic and environmental disturbances. Although the effects of these disturbances are mediated through the neurological system, the typical combination of factors involved in creating an alteration in thought process means that the assessment needed to make this diagnosis is complex. Data from neurological, functional, emotional, and mental status examinations must be considered before such a diagnosis can be made with confidence. It is important to consider alteration in sensory processes as a competing diagnosis, for the treatment of these two entities is quite different.

People with acute confusional states are an important group who experience alterations in thought processes. Foreman (1992) notes that many older adults experience acute confusion while in the hospital. Estimates of the incidence of acute confusion vary widely, from 20 to 80 per cent depending upon the specific subgroup of elderly people studied, and the criteria and methods used for diagnosing acute confusion. It is estimated that between 37 and 72 per cent of those who experience acute confusion are not identified by their nurses or physicians as being confused (Foreman, 1992).

A second key group of individuals who suffer from alterations in thought processes are those who have a dementing illness. Although accurate prevalence figures are not available for hospitalized older people, it is estimated that 3 per cent of community-dwelling elderly between ages 65 and 74 have Alzheimer's disease, with the proportion of the elderly population with dementia increasing steadily with age. An estimated 19 per cent of people aged 75 to 84 years have Alzheimer's disease, and for those aged 85 years and over, the rate may be as high as 50 per cent (Evans et al., 1989; Reichman and Cummings, 1992). An estimated 60 per cent of nursing home patients meet diagnostic criteria for alterations in thought processes (Hing, 1989).

Contributing Factors

The major categories of contributors to alteration in thought processes in elderly people are:

- Imbalance between oxygen supply and demand in the central nervous system (CNS)
- Imbalance between glucose supply and demand in the CNS
- Accumulation of toxic metabolites affecting CNS function

- Structural abnormalities of the CNS, such as neoplasm or infarct
- Drug intoxication or adverse reaction
- Psychiatric disorders
- Dementing disorders
- Sensory-perceptual alterations
- Environmental challenge

It is important to specify the etiology of alteration in thought processes in the elderly, because many causes are reversible. This notion runs counter to the erroneous stereotype held by many lay and professional persons—that "confusion" or "senility" is a part of normal aging. Additionally, alteration in thought process may be the only presenting symptom in an individual with serious underlying medical problems that are amenable to treatment. Examples abound, including hypothyroidism, infection, "silent" myocardial infarction, and subdural hematoma. These disorders frequently present in elderly people only with confusion rather than with the classic symptomatology exhibited in younger persons.

Assessment

Assessment includes a general observation of the client's level of consciousness, ability to communicate with others and to follow commands, and a mental status examination. Figure 14–20 is a flow diagram outlining the neurological assessment of clients suspected of having altered thought processes.

Level of Consciousness

Levels of consciousness and communicative ability generally fall into three categories: (1) comatose or unable to interact verbally, (2) alert but unable to interact verbally, and (3) alert and able to interact verbally. Assessment of older persons in comatose states should be obtained through a history and physical examination to determine the etiology and nature of the condition. The Glasgow Coma Scale is commonly used to document level of arousal (Teasdale and Jennett, 1974). Assessment includes cranial nerve testing, reflex testing, and testing responses to stimuli such as pain and loud noises. Laboratory data are useful for determining metabolic abnormalities.

Older individuals who are alert but unable to interact may have conditions such as aphasia, laryngectomy, language barriers, extreme hearing loss, or psychiatric disorders. In such individuals, alternative means

for assessing thought processes may be used. Consultation with a speech therapist can be helpful when an organic disorder is present to develop alternative communication methods, such as a word board or "yes-no" system. Schow et al. (1978, pp. 394–397) offer helpful suggestions for communicating with individuals with speech or hearing disorders. Behavioral observation is also useful for validating information from significant others and when communication is minimal.

If older clients are alert and able to communicate, a mental status examination should be attempted. Before such examination is carried out, it is prudent to assess the client's ability to follow commands. The nurse should begin with a simple one-stage command, such as "Tell me your name," or "Squeeze my hand." Having established the client's ability to follow a simple command, the nurse follows with more complex commands, such as "Pick up the pencil and write your name at the top of this form." Finally, the nurse goes on to multistage commands, which require simple problem-solving skills, such as "Fill in the rest of the information on the form." Information is gained about the client's ability to perform complex cognitive functions that rely on the integration of several body systems, including the special senses, the musculoskeletal system, and both the central and peripheral nervous systems. Remember that physical constraints and environmental conditions may influence ability to perform with pencil and paper testing. The client's educational level and baseline ability to read and write will also affect test results and should therefore be determined when possible.

The assessment situation should be nonthreatening, and the environment should be modified to provide optimal pace, volume and pitch of voice, level of background noise, light intensity, and complexity of commands.

If the older person is able to follow commands, a formal mental status examination should be performed to assess reasoning, orientation, memory (both short-term and long-term), abstraction, judgment, and emotionality. Several tests are available for carrying out a screening mental status examination; these are useful for comparing results with the extant norms and for measuring change over time.

Many tests and approaches are available for assessment of cognition. The major distinctions among them include how structured an assessment is provided, and how broadly cognition is assessed. For example,

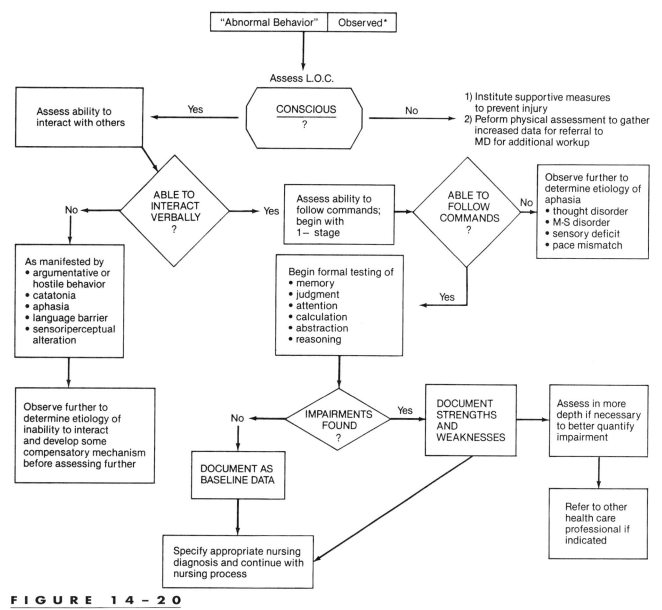

FIGURE 14-20

Algorithm for assessing patients suspected of having alteration in thought process.
*If abnormal behavior is *reported* before the nurse observes the patient, it is *very* useful to obtain a detailed history of the abnormal behavior, if time permits. Historical data that are particularly helpful include onset of behavior, duration, fluctuations, aggravating factors, alleviating factors, severity, recent life changes, and alterations in medications.

the FROMAJE (Libow, 1981) and the JAAMCO (Burnside, 1981) are frameworks for assessing function rather than cognitive tests with established psychometric properties. In contrast, the remainder of the tests and measures described next have established reliability and validity for evaluating different aspects of cognition. Before adopting one of these instruments, it is vital that the clinician understand what the measures are designed to assess, and choose an instrument based on the instrument's validity for

the clinician's purposes. The Short Portable Mental Status Questionnaire (SPMSQ) of Pfeiffer (1975) assesses orientation, short-term memory, and long-term memory. As its name implies, it is highly portable, as no specialized equipment is needed. Additional advantages include (1) rapid administration, (2) three domains of cognition, and (3) published norms adjusted for educational level and race. In contrast, instruments such as the Mini-mental State Examination (Folstein et al., 1975; Crum et al., 1992) and the Neurobehavioral Cognitive Screening Examination (NCSE), developed by Kiernan and colleagues (1987), assess progressively broader aspects of function. The trade-off for the additional information is that they require more time and equipment to administer and are more prone to educational bias.

In addition to these screening tests of cognitive function, a growing number of instruments are available for the assessment of acute confusion, such as the confusion assessment method instrument (Inouye, 1990), the Neecham Scale (Neelon et al., 1992), and the Clinical Assessment of Confusion Scale (Vermeesch, 1992). These confusion scales tend to focus on cognitive and behavioral factors that are sensitive to delirium, including altered motor function, rather than emphasizing aspects of thinking affected by chronic cognitive impairment alone. All three instruments were developed for research purposes, and have a relatively short history. Their utility for clinical practice, although promising, remains to be established.

Finally, two newer measures of cognitive function have recently appeared that help assess cognition as it relates to everyday functioning. Algase (1992) has developed the Everyday Indicators of Cognition Scale, and Dawson and colleagues (1992) have also developed an approach to evaluating cognitive abilities that may be preserved despite severe cognitive impairment.

Although these mental status tests are useful for obtaining objective baseline data, they have several drawbacks:

1. They are not appropriate for all elderly clients.
2. Their use may not be completely understood by each client, leading to inaccurate scores and misleading conclusions.
3. Their use may not fit the style of the assessor, resulting in a stilted atmosphere and inaccurate conclusions.
4. Time for administration may be longer than the nurse has available.
5. Staff may use the numerical scores derived from these instruments to stereotype clients, hindering the development of individualized plans of care.

It is difficult to recommend one test over another. They were originally developed for different purposes, and fine distinctions exist among them with regard to the spheres of function measured. Each nurse should develop a repertoire of screening and assessment techniques to be used in a variety of situations. Any of these tests are suitable for screening for gross mental abnormality; however, they may have to be modified for the geriatric client's cultural and educational levels and possible deficits in other body systems.

Planning

The plan of care should seek to

1. Correct reversible physiological deficits.
2. Support the individual's remaining functional abilities.
3. Prevent further injury or dysfunction.
4. Resolve feelings of stress, related to altered thought process, in the client and family members.

Planning should involve all those who are responsible for the client's care, including family and other caregivers. Families are a valuable resource in planning care as they have the best knowledge of the personality and history of the client. They can help interpret aberrant behavior and can be excellent allies in helping a patient process stimuli accurately, by explaining matters in familiar and easily understood terms. They often have suggestions for increasing the client's comfort and decreasing anxiety.

Although a multidisciplinary approach is desirable, consistency is important to avoid exacerbation of the thought disorder. The team should establish a realistic, explicitly stated plan of care, as well as criteria for evaluation, to be carried out within a given time frame. Thought disorders are often difficult to manage and produce feelings of frustration if planning is not realistic.

Hall (1991) has proposed a model for understanding, preventing, and treating behavioral disturbance in those with altered thought processes. The model, called the Progressively Lowered Stress Threshold (PLST) model, is based on the concept that individuals with altered thought processes have a lower tolerance for environmental stressors and, when overwhelmed, respond with anxious and subsequently dysfunctional behavior. The key to planning care for these individuals is to be alert for cues of anxious and escalating behavior and to plan routines for these patients that are not over-stimulating. The PLST model suggests that lowered tolerance to stressors results from decreased cortical abilities to integrate new information and to interpret stimuli. Thus, attention to keeping the environment of the patient with altered thought processes simple and predictable, and introducing novel experiences in short periods interspersed with periods when familiar and unchallenging events occur, may be key in maximizing coping responses and function.

Interventions

Specific interventions for the various contributing factors to altered thought process depend upon the underlying contributors to alterations in thought processes. Interventions such as supplemental oxygen, nutritional support, drug re-evaluation, and antibiotic therapy may each be used successfully for alterations in thought processes induced by hypoxemia, nutritional deficit, drug toxicity, and infection, respectively. Counseling and family support are nonspecific interventions that may benefit all patients with alterations in thought processes. One of the nurse's most important roles is to optimize the environment to compensate for diminished abilities and to provide support for diminished general function, reasoning, orientation, memory, abstraction, judgment, and emotions.

GENERAL FUNCTION. Typically, in alteration in thought process, the ability of the individual to function as an integrated whole is altered. This means that any human function that depends upon several body systems operating together on a conscious level is likely to be affected. For example, an individual with this condition may forget to eat or lack the judgment to make the effort to attend to personal hygiene.

In a study of 158 elders hospitalized on a general medical ward, patients with alterations in thought processes (as measured by low scores on the Neecham confusion scale) generally did not meet basal energy requirements during their hospital stay and were more likely not to take in adequate amounts of protein, compared with those without cognitive impairments (McConnell et al., 1990). Such individuals are likely to have difficulty in learning new skills (such as turn, cough, deep breathe regimens, or using a call light) because of impaired reasoning and memory. Careful assessment of each aspect of mental functioning should indicate which aspects of more global function will require support. Be alert for the client's need for assistance in many areas of function but try to avoid taking over activities the individual can do without help.

Beck (1992) developed a scale describing levels of assistance for dressing needed by cognitively impaired persons. The invasiveness of interventions progressed from controlling the environment to verbal instructions, to modeling of behavior, and, finally, to physical guidance and assistance. This is an excellent example of graded interventions that maximize independent functioning (see Tables 14–20 and 14–21 for the scale and examples of associated interventions).

REASONING. The ability to solve problems involves the ability to perceive and interpret external stimuli and relate these to past experience. The person with alteration in thought process may have mild-to-severe deficits in reasoning ability. This should be tested with real-life here-and-now problems, starting with the simplest tasks first. Patients with severe deficiencies need frequent checks to see whether they need assistance to perform such functions as toileting, bathing, or making a phone call.

Nurses should assume that because of patients' diminished reasoning abilities, they will need to anticipate problems for the patient with alterations in thought processes and generate solutions in advance. For example, if such a person undergoes a painful procedure like a tooth extraction, the person may lack the ability to figure out that prn pain medication is available. Anticipating the need for pain relief and offering analgesics without waiting for the patient to ask is a way to substitute for decreased reasoning.

ORIENTATION. Disorientation is a frightening experience for clients and their families. The usual sequence in which disorientation develops is time, then place, then person. Use of consistent nursing staff, therefore, is effective with disoriented persons because orientation to person is preserved until very late in the process of cognitive decline.

Disoriented individuals respond best to short, simple interactions. They may derive comfort and security from reorienting information that has meaning for their current situation. They rarely need information about the day, month, or year on a frequent basis, but they can utilize information about time of day (morning, afternoon, evening) and who their nurses are and their functions. Validating disoriented patients' feeling states is more important than rigidly insisting that they share the nurse's reality (Bleatman and Morton, 1992). Some individuals may panic or suffer extreme anxiety; others may be mildly annoyed or apathetic. Although some individuals are disoriented because they have not received orienting information, the majority of patients experience processing difficulties and require comfort and understanding rather than repetitive reality orientation (Dietch et al., 1989).

Disorientation sometimes occurs because the patient does not have access to orienting information. Environmental deprivation and sensory impairment are the two chief causes of this type of disorientation. Fortunately, it is easily prevented and remedied if nurses are conscientious about assessing for sensory impairment and then supplying orienting cues individualized to their elderly patients' sensory impairments and lifestyle. The precise mechanisms available for giving the client the opportunity to be oriented varies with the environment. In the hospital, orienting cues are least available and therefore present the greatest challenge. In the nursing home, because of less frequent patient turnover, it may be simpler to devise reliable orienting devices.

The emergence of "special care units" (Maas et al., 1992) for those with dementing disorders has resulted in a broader array of strategies for conveying useful orienting information. For example, some units post the resident's picture on the door of the room. Others use familiar, distinctive door decorations to help patients identify their rooms, or post the resident's name in a clearly visible location as the resident walks down the hallway (Peppard, 1991). In the community, special difficulties with economic resources and diminished staff support may be encountered that make use of orienting devices difficult.

Specific methods for promoting orientation to time, place, and person are discussed next.

Orientation to Time. In the *hospital* or *nursing home,* it may be possible to hang large wall calendars and cross off the days as they pass. Many hospitals and nursing homes now have selective menus for patients to choose foods for their meals. These frequently have the date printed on them. The nurse can draw attention to the date when helping the client make choices. In many hospitals it is possible to purchase newspapers on the floor. Encouraging your patient to do so, if this fits the lifestyle, provides another source of orienting information. Encouraging family and friends to discuss the events of the day or season with the client and bring newspapers or magazines is good. For clients without adequate support from family or friends, volunteers may provide this type of input. The changes of shifts are another opportunity to provide information about time. For example, "Mr. Jones, it is eleven o'clock in the evening and I will be leaving shortly. Ms. Smith will be your nurse from now until seven o'clock tomorrow morning."

Some patients who are disoriented to time

experience considerable distress because they cannot adequately keep track of the day's activities. They become agitated because they've been waiting all morning for lunch, or for a bath, or for a pill, when they have actually only waited a short period of time. Alternatively, some individuals feel as though things are moving too fast for them. This type of situation, while not the most common, is probably under-recognized and may be related to sensory overload. Few solutions apply to all persons, but the principle of treatment is to listen actively, modify the schedule of activities as possible, and provide the individual with feedback regarding your perception of time passing. Sometimes written schedules of activities may be of use.

For clients in the *community,* promoting orientation to time is more challenging. Certainly friends and family can be taught the aforementioned strategies. Additionally, calls from a telephone reassurance program may add structure to the client's day. For those receiving home health services, staff can provide the stimulations just mentioned.

Orientation to Place. In institutions, this may be difficult to achieve. Hospitals or nursing homes that have the institution's name printed on meal trays, napkins, blankets, or other equipment clearly have an easier time in this regard. Often such environmental supports are all that is necessary. Fortunately, most clients are less troubled by this type of disorientation.

In the community disorientation to place is more worrisome, as the client who wanders in addition to being disoriented to place represents a significant safety problem. In this situation, clients should either have constant companionship or be treated in an institution.

Promoting Orientation to Person. Professionals working in either institutions or the community should wear easy-to-read name tags. This, coupled with a brief introduction of self at the beginning of each encounter with a patient—particularly in the early phases of establishing a relationship—provides ample opportunity for orientation to new persons. Such introductions may be necessary for clients with alteration in thought process whose distant or infrequently seen relatives visit. Family anxieties about prognosis will be relieved by explanations of the nature of altered thought process and its effect on orientation to person.

MEMORY. Both short-term and long-term memory may be affected by alteration in thought processes, but usually short-term memory is most seriously impaired. The implication is that any new information given to the client is apt to be quickly forgotten. Written reminders may facilitate short-term remembering—e.g., posting a note on the wall: "Mr. Jones, every quarter hour you should do the deep-breathing exercises below," centered beneath a clock, with a simple picture of the exercise. However, the effectiveness of written reminders must be evaluated carefully, as individuals with memory deficits may have impairment in other domains of function, such as interpreting written information, or attention deficits that preclude the effectiveness of written reminders.

Frequent verbal reminders are also effective if the staff is diligent in implementation. For example, each time the nurse sees Mr. J., she offers him a cup of water because he is apt to *forget* the importance of increasing his oral intake. Family, friends, and volunteers may also provide useful support for memory impairment. For example, Mr. Jones forgets that it takes him a long time to get to the toilet, and therefore he is sometimes incontinent. Visitors help him remember to toilet on a regular basis by suggesting that he go to the toilet at prearranged intervals posted at his bedside. Mr. J. loves to watch golf on television but would forget to turn on the television without a friend to suggest it (or if at home to call and remind him).

Helping people remember important events using alarms or other audible reminders has not been shown to be especially effective. As with any form of adaptive equipment, such items should be individualized to the patient's strengths and deficits. The use of technical memory aids for people with extensive memory impairments is at present quite limited. However, proper use of memory supplementation techniques may prove to be an important therapy in maintaining function and therefore preventing some of the contributors to altered thought process, such as nutritional deficits or improper medication.

ABSTRACTION. Abstraction is likely to be impaired; the nurse can do little to compensate for this dysfunction. It is useful to quantify the extent of the problem so that the nature of the client's deficit can be explained to family and other staff. Dysfunction in this domain has important implications for the ability of the client to give informed consent for various procedures. While not certifiably incompetent, the client may not be able to understand fully the implications of a procedure. The nurse then has an ethical responsibility to alert other staff and family or significant others to this information. Such action may result in a more detailed evaluation of the client's ability to give informed consent (usually done by psychiatric specialists). A temporary guardian may be appointed, or family or friends may participate in the decision-making process. Raising these questions may result in a durable power of attorney, health care power of attorney, or living will being discovered or activated (see Chapter 3).

It is particularly important to raise such questions when data suggest that consent to a procedure would violate a spiritual belief system (i.e., result in spiritual distress for the client) or that the procedure carries a high risk of complications that would result in a lifestyle the client would find unacceptable.

Another important implication of diminished ability to abstract is that learning is much more difficult. If possible, postpone major teaching or learning activities until the altered thought process has resolved. If this is not possible, include a family member, friend, or neighbor in the teaching, for opportunity for reinforcement or support later. Be sure to obtain a return demonstration to make sure the needed skill or information has been learned. If none of these options is viable, document your concerns about the adequacy of client teaching because of the altered thought process and communicate this information to those responsible for making discharge plans for the client.

JUDGMENT. The ability to select an appropriate course of action depends upon memory, abstraction, and reasoning abilities. Thus, impairment in these other domains may be manifest as poor judgment. Nursing care for those with impaired judgment requires careful planning and implementation. The goal is to prevent injury without providing too many restrictions. Overly restricting a client's activity is harmful. First, it is a violation of a basic human right: the right to autonomy. Second, it may result in further disability, either through disuse atrophy or rebellion. Finally, undue restriction inhibits growth.

Risks to the client with impaired judgment include the potential for injury because of falls, wandering, ingestion of toxic substances, overdose of medicines, failure to recognize activity limitations or dietary restrictions, and traumatic removal of intravenous lines, catheters, and other tubes. The client with impaired judgment may suffer from social isolation, as the ability to perform appropriately in diverse social situations is impaired. Interventions to supplement impaired judgment depend highly upon the environment of the client.

In hospitals and nursing homes, patients are sometimes restrained, using devices such as hand or vest restraints, bedside rails, and chairs with tables across them that restrict patients' mobility (so-called "geri-chairs"). The belief that restraints prevent more injuries than they promote is not supported by the literature (Evans and Strumpf, 1990; Tinetti et al., 1991). The specific indication for restraints should be evaluated on at least a shift-by-shift basis for each individual. If restraints must be used, it is essential that adequate supervision to prevent injury is provided and that regular supervised activity without the restraint also be provided. It is interesting that when this standard of care is adhered to, the nursing care time becomes greater for those in restraints than for those who are not restrained.

The same principles apply to the use of restraints in community settings. The nurses' role here is to teach other caregivers about these principles and to monitor compliance with them. Failure to follow such principles constitutes abuse of the client.

EMOTIONS. Depression may also present as slowed thinking, memory loss, and disorientation in elderly persons (Emery and Oxman, 1992). Individuals with alteration in thought processes may demonstrate emotional lability, crying one minute over an apparently trivial matter and then laughing a few moments later. The lability can be frightening and mysterious to family and paraprofessional caregivers, who benefit from explanations about the source of the emotional aberration and reassurance that whatever inappropriate affect is displayed will probably subside quickly.

Evaluation

Criteria for evaluation of the patient with altered thought processes are somewhat complex because of the broad impact of the disorder.

1. Does the patient complain of feeling confused at present?
2. Are preventable problems associated with altered thought processes present, such as evidence of malnourishment, poor hygiene, injury, immobility?
3. Are all potential causes of alteration in thought process identified and treated when possible?
4. Are all sensory deficits identified and treated?
5. Is the patient cared for in the least restrictive manner possible?
6. Does the family receive teaching and counseling regarding the nature of the patient's alteration in thought processes, and options for treatment and management?
7. Is the family included in the care of the patient—specifically, in the assessment, goal setting, choice of interventions, and evaluation process?
8. If psychotropic drugs are used, is there a clear indication, goal for therapy, and monitoring system for adverse effects?
9. Are physical needs anticipated and attended to in a timely manner?

TISSUE PERFUSION ALTERATIONS: ALTERED PERIPHERAL TISSUE PERFUSION AND HIGH RISK FOR PERIPHERAL NEUROVASCULAR DYSFUNCTION

Definition and Scope of Problem

Alterations in peripheral tissue perfusion exist when an individual has decreased nutrition and respiration at the cellular level because of decreased capillary blood supply (NANDA, 1992). Clustered with this diagnosis is "High risk for neurovascular dysfunction," defined as "a state when an individual is at risk of experiencing a disruption in circulation, sensation, or motion of an extremity" (Carroll-Johnson and Paquette, 1994). If not detected and treated, peripheral neurovascular dysfunction progresses to the medical diagnosis of compartment syndrome (Carpenito, 1993a). Because older adults frequently undergo joint replacement therapy and are at higher risk of traumatic injury, their risk for this diagnosis is increased. In addition, older adults often suffer from chronic diseases that blunt warning signs of neurovascular dysfunction, such as diminished peripheral sensation due to peripheral neuropathy associated with diabetes mellitus. Older people are at particular risk for altered tissue perfusion because of decreases in cardiac output associated with aging, and because many of the chronic diseases associated with aging disrupt microcirculation. The consequence of untreated reduced tissue perfusion is ultimately necrosis and death of the involved tissue. Nurses are in an excellent position to identify those at risk for alterations in peripheral tissue perfusion and take preventive action.

Contributing Factors

Age-Related Changes

Physiological changes in the myocardium and vasculature predispose to reduced peripheral tissue perfusion. Maximal heart rate, cardiac output, and stroke volume all decrease with age. The vasculature becomes less elastic with age, providing more resistance to the pumping action of the heart. The basement membrane of the capillaries thickens, resulting in slowed exchange of nutrients between blood and tissue.

Disease-Related Factors

Older persons are more prone to immobility, which predisposes to thrombus formation. They are thus predisposed to reduced tissue perfusion from an obstruction in the venous or arterial vasculature. The prevalence of peripheral vascular disease rises with age, as does the prevalence of diabetes mellitus, which disrupts microcirculation. Therapies for bone fractures, including knee and hip replacement surgery, may cause restriction of peripheral circulation and increase the risk of peripheral neurovascular dysfunction.

Assessment

The history should determine whether the patient has any pain in the extremities, either at rest or with activity. The patient should be questioned regarding tobacco habits, as nicotine adversely affects peripheral circulation. Finally, a history of recurrent leg ulcers is highly suggestive of chronic alterations in tissue perfusion.

Physical examination should begin with observation of the older person's footwear and ability to reach the lower extremities. Ill-fitting footwear and inability to reach the lower extremities with ease in the presence of alterations in tissue perfusion greatly predispose the older person to injury. The nurse should also note any medically prescribed devices that may interfere with peripheral tissue perfusion, such as circumferential dressings, nonpatent wound drainage systems, casts, splints, braces, and bandages. Palpate the peripheral pulses and note the temperature of the extremities. Observe the skin for dependent rubor, pallor, cyanosis, capillary refill, distribution of hair, and edema. Note the extent of the edema by measuring the circumference of the extremities in millimeters. Sensation in the extremities should be tested, with particular emphasis on the ability to perceive light touch, pain, and temperature. Finally, if the patient is bedridden, test for Homans' sign (Kuhn and McGovern, 1992).

Planning and Intervention

Nursing care for those with alteration in tissue perfusion centers on preventing tissue necrosis. The care of people with chronic vascular impairment differs from the care of people with acute interruptions in tissue perfusion. Acute threats to tissue perfusion require immediate treatment to alleviate the underlying cause, usually in collaboration with physicians. If peripheral tissue perfusion is severely impaired by a dressing, cast, or splint, as evidenced by impaired neurovascular responses, the appliance must be removed. The individual can then be reevaluated for refitting and reapplication of the appliance or dressing. Individuals with chronically decreased tissue perfusion require a lifelong plan for assessment and prevention of tissue necrosis and promotion of adequate perfusion.

PERIPHERAL VASCULAR DISEASE. Patients suffering from venous insufficiency and associated edema should wear support garments to control edema. Elevation of extremities when sitting for prolonged periods is also indicated. Positioning for patients with arterial insufficiency depends on the severity of the disease. They should avoid standing in one position for long periods of time, avoid crossing their legs when seated, and use comfort as a guide to positioning. They should engage in exercise programs to promote increased cardiac output and develop collateral circulation (see section on Activity Intolerance). Individuals with peripheral vascular disease should inspect their extremities daily for minor trauma and ulceration of the skin. Regular foot care is also necessary, with meticulous attention to toenail trimming by a professional if the patient is unable to reach and see the toenails, or if onychogryphosis of the toenails is present. If ulceration occurs, treatment should be instituted to promote healing and prevent infection (see section on Skin Integrity Impairment).

DEEP VENOUS THROMBOSIS. Patients suspected of having this condition should be referred immediately for further medical evaluation and treatment. For a detailed discussion of treatment of deep venous thrombosis, see Chapter 7.

ACUTE COMPARTMENT SYNDROME. Compartments are areas where muscle, nerve, and blood vessels are enclosed within inflexible boundaries of skin, fascia, or bone. There are 46 compartments in the body. Acute compartment syndrome occurs when the pressure in a compartment exceeds 30 mm Hg, causing ischemia of the muscles and nerves within the compressed area (Ross, 1991). Older people who require orthotic devices, casts, or dressings must be observed carefully for signs of reduced peripheral tissue perfusion. A period of edema often immediately follows casting of a fracture, during which time the older person is particularly vulnerable. Elevation of the affected extremity may be sufficient to prevent trauma, but if elevation is not sufficient, the case will require revision. Elevation is contraindicated if sensory or motor impairments have already developed. Regular neurovascular checks (every 2 hours for the first 48 hours) are essential to identify altered tissue perfusion in a timely manner. Figure 14–21 illustrates some of the nerves commonly affected by acute compartment syndrome.

Braces and splints that have been used for extended periods of time still may be culprits in reducing peripheral tissue perfusion. The older person may gain weight or develop mild peripheral edema, resulting in a constricting action from the orthosis. Reduction of the amount of time the orthosis is worn may suffice to preserve tissue integrity, but, again, revision of the orthosis may be required.

Bandages applied to the lower extremities while the patient is in bed may later impede peripheral circulation, if the patient spends extensive periods of time with the lower extremities dependent. Nurses should check circumferential dressings to the lower extremities at least two times per shift to ensure that a tourniquet-like effect does not occur.

Evaluation

Criteria for evaluation of alteration in peripheral tissue perfusion and neurovascular dysfunction include:

1. Is skin integrity preserved?
2. Does the individual complain of pain?
3. Is a routine surveillance regimen in place to detect alterations in peripheral tissue perfusion in at-risk individuals?
4. Are patients with signs of deep venous thrombosis referred promptly for further evaluation and definitive treatment?
5. Are individuals with signs of acute obstruction referred and treated promptly?

URINARY ELIMINATION ALTERATIONS: INCONTINENCE (FUNCTIONAL, REFLEX, STRESS, URGE, TOTAL), URINARY RETENTION

Definition and Scope of Problem

Alterations in urinary elimination are defined by NANDA as a state in which the individual experiences a disturbance in urine elimination (NANDA, 1992). Disorders such as dysuria, urinary frequency, urgency and hesitancy, urinary retention, and incontinence fall into this diagnostic category. Consequences of altered urinary patterns include restricted social activity, altered self-concept, decreased self-esteem, and alteration in skin integrity.

Nocturia

Nocturia is so common among older people that it is not considered a symptom of underlying urinary pathology. According to Stewart and colleagues (1992), the community prevalence of nocturia among the elderly may be as high as 80 per cent. The reasons for an increased prevalence of nocturia in older people include decreased ability to concentrate urine, increased use of diuretics, better perfusion of kidneys in a supine position, and altered sleep patterns in the elderly that result in easier arousal during sleep.

Urinary Retention

Urinary retention is another alteration in urinary elimination patterns commonly found in old people, but it is not a normal finding. Urinary retention predisposes to urinary tract infection, incontinence, and, if sufficiently severe, renal failure. Urinary retention is caused by anatomical obstructions, such as prostatic hypertrophy and fecal impaction, and by drugs with anticholinergic side effects that interfere with urinary sphincter relaxation and detrusor action.

Dysuria

Dysuria is a much less common symptom, with a reported prevalence of 6 to 22 per cent in community-dwelling elderly. Hesitancy and urgency are much more common in men, whereas women are more likely to suffer from pain on urination.

Nerve	Assessing Sensation	Assessing Motion
Peroneal nerve	Prick web space between great toe and second toe 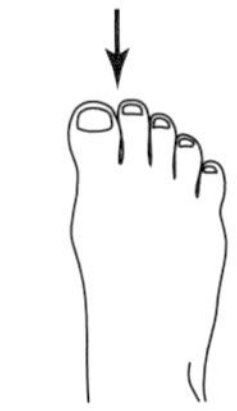	Have patient dorsiflex ankle and extend toes at metatarsophalangeal joints 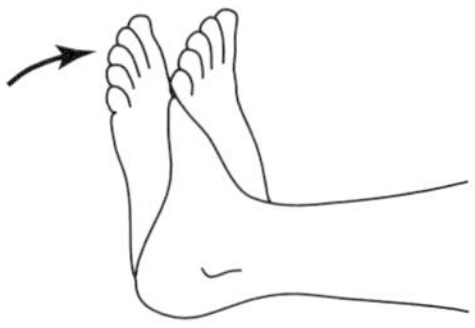
Tibial nerve	Prick medial and lateral surfaces of sole 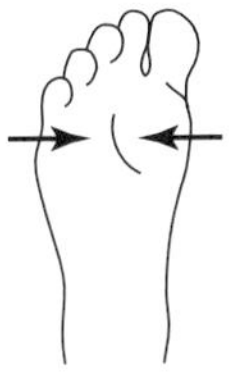	Have patient plantar flex ankle and toes 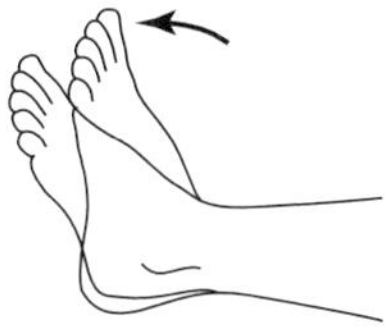
Radial nerve	Prick web space between thumb and index finger 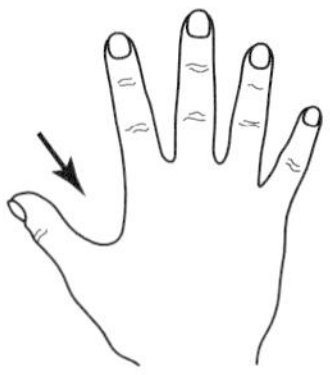	Have patient hyperextend thumb, then wrist, and hyperextend four fingers at metacarpophalangeal joints 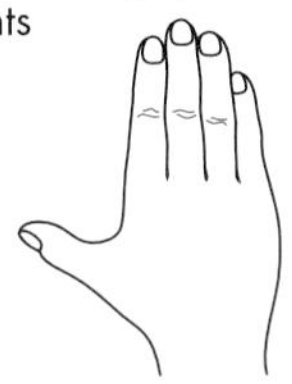
Ulnar nerve	Prick distal fat pad of little finger 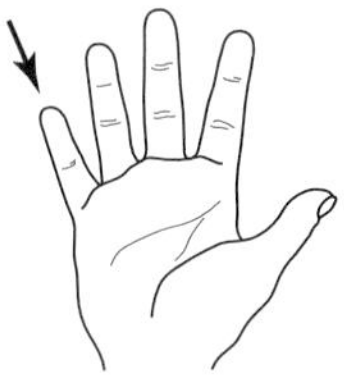	Have patient abduct all fingers 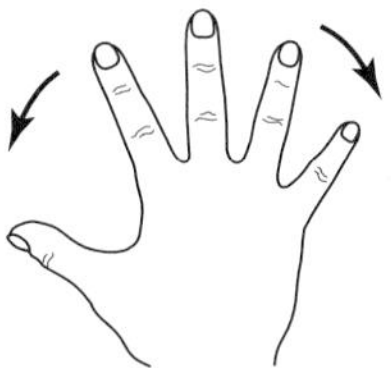
Median nerve	Prick distal surface of index finger 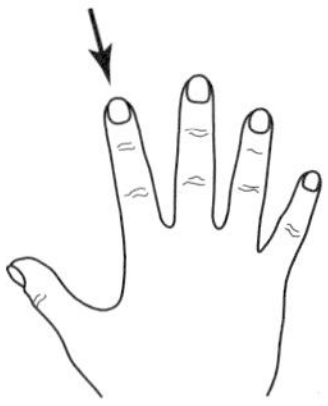	Have patient oppose thumb and little finger; note whether patient can flex wrist 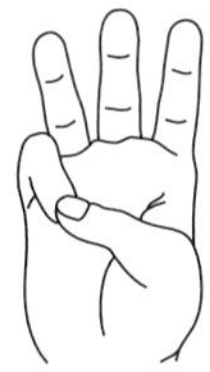

FIGURE 14–21

Assessing nerves commonly affected by acute compartment syndrome. (Adapted from Stearns, E., and Brunner, N.A. *OpCare,* Vol. 1. Rutherford, NJ: Howmedica, Inc., 1987, p. 89. Illustrations courtesy of Howmedica, Inc.)

TABLE 14-26
Requirements for Normal Adult Urination

COMPONENT	FUNCTION
Central nervous system	Receives messages that bladder is filling, and sends inhibiting signals
	Remembers social sanctions if inappropriate voiding occurs
	Remembers how to dress and undress, wipe, and flush
Eyes and CNS	Identify location of "appropriate places to urinate"
Fluid	Substrate for urine production
Circulatory system	Kidneys must be adequately perfused to make urine from waste products transported in the blood
Hormones	
Adrenal corticosteroids	Influence amount of urine produced
Estrogen	Influences function of external urinary sphincter
Kidneys	Make the urine
Ureters	Carry the urine from the kidney to the bladder
Bladder	Stores urine until socially acceptable place is found for elimination, then bladder helps expel urine from the body
Nerves	Notice that bladder is distending
	Send message to CNS that bladder is filling
	Keep the sphincter from releasing until the proper moment
	Allow the sphincter to relax and tell the bladder muscle (detrusor) to contract at the appropriate time
Musculoskeletal system	Allows movement and transfer to the toilet
	Allows dressing, undressing, and perineal hygiene
Sphincters	Help hold the urine in the bladder until the proper moment
Detrusor	Holds the urine until time to go, then pushes the urine out
Urethra	Carries the urine from the bladder to outside the body

From Snow, T. and McConnell, E. Bowel and Bladder Management Training Program. Unpublished educational aid, 1985.

Urinary Incontinence

Urinary incontinence is an extreme form of alteration in urinary elimination but one that is highly prevalent and particularly troublesome for older persons and their caregivers. According to the Urinary Incontinence Guideline Panel (1992) of the Agency for Health Care Policy and Research, between 15 and 30 per cent of community-dwelling elders over the age of 60 years suffer from urinary incontinence, as do roughly half the 1.5 million nursing home residents. Urinary incontinence is the involuntary leakage of urine, regardless of the amount. A variety of overlapping categories of incontinence are described in the literature. The International Continence Society defines four types:

Stress incontinence: Involuntary loss of urine that occurs with increased abdominal pressure but in the absence of a detrusor contraction or an overdistended bladder (International Continence Society, 1990)

Urge incontinence: Involuntary loss of urine associated with an abrupt and strong desire to void (Urinary Incontinence Guideline Panel, 1992)

Overflow incontinence: Involuntary loss of urine when the intravesical pressure exceeds the maximum urethral pressure associated with bladder distention but in the absence of detrusor activity (Urinary Incontinence Guideline Panel, 1992)

Reflex incontinence: The involuntary loss of urine caused by abnormal activity in the spinal cord in the absence of sensation usually associated with the desire to micturate

Additional categories of interest to gerontological nurses include

Mixed incontinence: Involuntary loss of urine due to a combination of the aforementioned factors (Fantl, Wyman, McClish et al., 1990)

Functional incontinence: Involuntary loss of urine because of a functional limitation of either neurological, musculoskeletal, or psychiatric origin

Other terms are used to describe urinary incontinence, but these categories are consistent with categories used by NANDA (1992), although providing more specificity than is true for NANDA urinary incontinence terminology. In addition to the terms just defined, urinary incontinence is often classified as either "transient" or "established." Transient incontinence is generally reserved for incontinence of abrupt onset, generally associated with a specific precipitant, such as delirium, a drug side effect, or presence of infection.

Social Impact of Altered Urine Elimination

Control over elimination, like many other self-care tasks, is achieved early in life and is an essential aspect of self-concept as an adult. Difficulties with urination are not typically discussed in ordinary social conversation. The subject is in many ways taboo. Changes in urinary elimination patterns may be worrisome to people of all ages because of the threat of eventual loss of control, resulting in social ostracism. The fearfulness is compounded by the fact that little information is generally available for the lay public about the normal and abnormal changes in patterns of urinary elimination that occur with age, and the meanings of those changes.

In addition to social withdrawal and emotional reactions to urinary incontinence, economic costs can also be documented. According to Hu (1990), the direct costs of urinary incontinence care exceed 10 billion dollars annually.

Contributing Factors

Alterations in urine elimination can be caused by a variety of factors, including drugs, environmental changes, psychological factors, anatomical obstruction, and physiological disturbances. Pain on urination is usually associated with infection. Difficulty in urinating is often seen with prostatic hypertrophy in men or as a side effect of drugs with anticholinergic properties. Table 14–26 is a simplified description of the necessary components of normal adult urination. Impairments in one or more of these systems predispose to alterations in urinary elimination patterns.

Table 14–27 summarizes common causes of *transient* urinary incontinence. The causes of *established* urinary incontinence are complex. Interference with any of the requirements for normal adult urination, as described in Table 14–26, may precipitate incontinence. Often more than one factor is implicated. Table 14–28 summarizes various contributors to established urinary incontinence.

Assessment

Screening

Initial assessment for alterations in urinary elimination patterns includes the following:

- History of urinary symptoms: nocturia, dysuria, frequency, urgency, incontinence. Clinicians should ask specifically about urine leakage or wetting, otherwise this important symptom may be minimized or overlooked
- Physical examination: observation for smell of urine on clothes, evidence of poor perineal hygiene, ability to urinate on demand, presence of difficulty starting or stopping a stream of urine, palpable or percussable bladder postvoiding, rectal examination for size of prostate, presence of fecal impaction, vaginal examination for atrophic vaginitis, cystocele, or rectocele

- Laboratory: urinalysis if symptoms of urinary tract infection are present, e.g., dysuria, frequency, urgency, incontinence

This assessment protocol is sufficient to identify alterations and likely causes and provides a base for counseling older patients about age-related changes in their urinary elimination patterns. Patients with urinary retention, prostate abnormalities, or symptoms of urinary tract infection should be referred for medical evaluation and treatment. Individuals who show signs of incontinence require more detailed assessment to determine the type of incontinence and likely contributors.

In-Depth Assessment

There is widespread consensus that individuals who have urinary incontinence should have at least a basic evaluation (1) to confirm the presence of urinary incontinence objectively, (2) to identify factors associated with urinary incontinence, and (3) to identify patients who need more in-depth evaluation before treatment should begin. Components of the basic evaluation include a detailed history, physical examination, urinalysis, and simple tests of lower urinary tract function. Before beginning the evaluation, assessment of mental function and mobility is worthwhile, as these domains of function may influence the individual's ability to cooperate with some aspects of urinary incontinence evaluation and may of themselves be contributors to urinary incontinence.

MENTAL STATUS TESTING. Mental status testing includes evaluation of cognitive function, presence of delusions or hallucinations, and affect. In addition, the impact of incontinence on the life of the individual should be estimated. The ability to follow simple commands is key to participating in any continence treatment plan (Schnelle et al., 1990).

MOBILITY ASSESSMENT. Elements include the ability to transfer out of chairs of various heights, ability to transfer on and off the toilet, ability to dress and undress, and length of time required to travel to the toilet in customary environs. For men who are wheelchair bound, the ability to manipulate buttons, zippers, and underclothes and to place a urinal are important aspects of performance to observe directly. For women, toileting is dependent not only on transferring on and off a toilet, but also upon sufficient standing balance to manipulate waistbands or pull up clothing prior to toileting.

TABLE 14-27
Factors Contributing to Transient Urinary Incontinence

POTENTIAL CAUSES	COMMENT
Delirium (confusional state)	In the delirious patient, incontinence is usually an associated symptom that will abate with proper diagnosis and treatment of the underlying cause of confusion.
Infection (symptomatic urinary tract infection)	Dysuria and urgency from symptomatic infection may defeat the older person's ability to reach the toilet in time. Asymptomatic infection, although more common than symptomatic infection, is rarely a cause of incontinence.
Atrophic urethritis or vaginitis	Atrophic urethritis or vaginitis may present as dysuria, dyspareunia, burning on urination, urgency, agitation (in demented patients), and occasionally as incontinence. Both disorders are readily treated by conjugated estrogen administered either orally (0.3–1.25 mg/day) or locally (2 mg or fraction/day).
Pharmaceuticals Sedatives-hypnotics	Benzodiazepines, especially long-acting agents such as flurazepam and diazepam, may accumulate in elderly patients and cause confusion and secondary incontinence. Alcohol, frequently used as a sedative, can cloud the sensorium, impair mobility, and induce a diuresis, resulting in incontinence.
Diuretics	A brisk diuresis induced by loop diuretics can overwhelm bladder capacity and lead to polyuria, frequency, and urgency, thereby precipitating incontinence in a frail older person. The loop diuretics include furosemide, ethacrynic acid, and bumetanide.
Anticholinergic agents Antihistamines Antidepressants Antipsychotics Opiates Antispasmodics (dicyclomine and Donnatal) Antiparkinsonian agents (trihexyphenidyl and benztropine mesylate)	Nonprescription (over-the-counter) agents with anticholinergic properties are taken commonly by older patients for insomnia, coryza, pruritus, and vertigo, and many prescription medications also have anticholinergic properties. Anticholinergic side effects include urinary retention with associated urinary frequency and overflow incontinence. Besides anticholinergic actions, antipsychotics such as thioridazine and haloperidol may cause sedation, rigidity, and immobility.
Alpha-adrenergic agents Sympathomimetics (decongestants) Sympatholytics (e.g., prazosin, terazosin, and doxazosin)	Sphincter tone in the proximal urethra can be decreased by alpha-antagonists and increased by alpha-agonists. An older woman, whose urethra is shortened and weakened with age, may develop stress incontinence when taking an alpha-antagonist for hypertension. An older man with prostate enlargement may develop acute urinary retention and overflow incontinence when taking multicomponent "cold" capsules that contain alpha-agonists and anticholinergic agents, especially if a nasal decongestant and a nonprescription hypnotic antihistamine are added.
Calcium channel blockers	Calcium channel blockers can reduce smooth muscle contractility in the bladder and occasionally can cause urinary retention and overflow incontinence.
Psychological	Severe depression may occasionally be associated with incontinence but is probably less frequently a cause in older patients.
Excessive urine production	Excess intake, endocrine conditions that cloud the sensorium and induce a diuresis (e.g., hypercalcemia, hyperglycemia, and diabetes insipidus), and expanded volume states such as congestive heart failure, lower extremity venous insufficiency, drug-induced ankle edema (e.g., nifedipine, indomethacin) and low albumin states cause polyuria and can lead to incontinence.
Restricted mobility	Limited mobility is an aggravating or precipitating cause of incontinence that can frequently be corrected or improved by treating the underlying condition (e.g., arthritis, poor eyesight, Parkinson's disease, or orthostatic hypotension). A urinal or bedside commode and scheduled toileting often help resolve the incontinence that results from hospitalization and its environmental barriers (e.g., bed rails, restraints, and poor lighting).
Stool impaction	Patients with stool impaction present with either urge or overflow incontinence and may have fecal incontinence as well. Disimpaction restores continence.

Urinary Incontinence Guideline Panel. *Urinary Incontinence in Adults: Clinical Practice Guideline.* AHCPR Pub. No. 92-0038. Rockville, MD. Agency for Health Care Policy & Research, Public Health Service, US Department of Health & Human Services, March, 1992. Table 1, pp. 7–9.

DOCUMENTATION OF PATTERN OF INCONTINENCE. The purpose of documenting the incontinence is to determine the pattern in terms of frequency and amount and to determine the environmental circumstances surrounding episodes of incontinence. Describing incontinence over time requires the use of some form of diary. Checklists such as the one detailed in Figure 14–22 are very helpful. However, the tool must be tailored to the abilities of the individual completing the record. If the older person is too impaired cognitively to keep a diary, enlist the aid of a family member, friend, or caregiver.

Stress incontinence is often characterized by dribbling of urine associated with increases in intra-abdominal pressure. Urge and reflex incontinence is suggested by a pattern of periodic "floods" of urine, often en route to the toilet. Overflow incontinence is also characterized by dribbling, but a large postvoid residual is typically found on physical examination, allowing differentiation from stress incontinence. Mixed incontinence is likely to produce a pattern of both dribbling and flooding. No particular pattern is associated with functional incontinence, as the underlying contributors are not urological but cognitive, musculoskeletal, or psychological. However, the record may still provide cues about possible interventions.

HISTORY. The history should include information about the onset, duration, and characteristics of urinary incontinence. Based on that information, a medical history should be obtained and reviewed for possible causes of transient incontinence (see Table 14–27), with an emphasis on medications, recent functional and cognitive changes, and other contributing medical problems such as diabetes or cardiac disease. In addition, information about the individual's fluid intake, caffeine use, bowel habits, sexual function, use of pads or briefs, and other attempts to treat the urinary incontinence should be elicited (Urinary Incontinence Guideline Panel, 1992).

PHYSICAL EXAMINATION. Abdominal examination may reveal masses or suprapubic fullness or tenderness. Genital examination in men should focus on identifying abnormalities of the foreskin, penis, and perineal skin. Pelvic examination in women may reveal atrophic vaginitis, pelvic prolapse, or mass. Experienced clinicians may be able to assess for urethral and bladder neck hypermobility. Rectal examination is performed to assess for perineal sensation, sphincter tone, and the bulbocavernosus reflex, and to determine whether fecal impaction or rectal mass is present. Prostate examination is not helpful in determining whether bladder outlet obstruction is present (Urinary Incontinence Guideline Panel, 1992).

Other assessments of bladder function are also commonly recommended. Postvoid residual (PVR) volume may be estimated using palpation and percussion during physical examination; it can be determined more

TABLE 14 – 28

Contributing Factors to Established Urinary Incontinence in the Aged

	IMPACT ON CONTINENCE
CNS disturbance—e.g., delirium, dementia, CVA	Difficulty finding the toilet
	Destruction of ability to inhibit detrusor action
	Inability to sense urge to void
	Apraxia, resulting in difficulty with transfer, dressing, and hygiene tasks associated with toileting
	Loss of social inhibitions that make toileting important
Depression	Loss of self-esteem, combined with fatigue, makes maintaining continence too costly
Drugs	CNS depressants may interfere with ability to sense the urge to void or to act on the sensation
	Anticholinergic drugs may induce urinary retention, resulting in overflow incontinence

Psychological impairments
  Learned helplessness
  Inappropriate expression of anger
  Attention-getting device
	Reduced motivation to use toilet to urinate

Vision impairment	Difficulty finding the toilet
Fluid	Dehydration predisposes to fecal impaction and urinary tract infection: both contribute to incontinence by serving as irritants to detrusor and obstructing bladder outlet, respectively
Hormones: Estrogen	Influences function of external urinary sphincter in women
Kidneys	Diuretics stimulate increased production of urine, which may overwhelm patient's usual routines for maintaining continence
Bladder	Hyperreflexia produces urge incontinence—hyperreflexia, or detrusor instability, is precipitated by foreign bodies in bladder, such as catheter balloons, stones, and tumors
Nerves	Loss of bladder innervation because of spinal cord lesions, autonomic neuropathies, or demyelinating neurological disorders results in inability to sense urge to void or inability to adequately contract detrusor, resulting in overflow incontinence
Musculoskeletal system	Pain or limited mobility may limit patient's ability to get to the toilet in a timely manner or to perform associated dressing and hygiene tasks
Sphincters	Weak sphincter muscles result in reduced ability to resist detrusor hyperreflexia or dribbling from distended bladder

From Snow, T. and McConnell, E. Bowel and Bladder Management Training Program. Unpublished educational aid, 1985.

accurately by urinary catheterization or ultrasound (Ireton et al., 1990). Care must be taken in interpreting the PVR volume, as it may be influenced by situational factors,

INCONTINENCE MONITORING RECORD

INSTRUCTIONS: EACH TIME THE PATIENT IS CHECKED:
1) Mark *one* of the circles in the BLADDER section at the hour closest to the time the patient is checked.
2) Make an X in the BOWEL section if the patient has had an incontinent or normal bowel movement.

🖋 = Incontinent, small amount	Ø = Dry	X = Incontinent BOWEL
● = Incontinent, large amount	⊘ = Voided correctly	X = Normal BOWEL

PATIENT NAME _____ ROOM # _____ DATE _____

	BLADDER			BOWEL			
	INCONTINENT OF URINE	DRY	VOIDED CORRECTLY	INCONTINENT X	NORMAL X	INITIALS	COMMENTS
12 am	● ●	O	△ cc ___				
1	● ●	O	△ cc ___				
2	● ●	O	△ cc ___				
3	● ●	O	△ cc ___				
4	● ●	O	△ cc ___				
5	● ●	O	△ cc ___				
6	● ●	O	△ cc ___				
7	● ●	O	△ cc ___				
8	● ●	O	△ cc ___				
9	● ●	O	△ cc ___				
10	● ●	O	△ cc ___				
11	● ●	O	△ cc ___				
12 pm	● ●	O	△ cc ___				
1	● ●	O	△ cc ___				
2	● ●	O	△ cc ___				
3	● ●	O	△ cc ___				
4	● ●	O	△ cc ___				
5	● ●	O	△ cc ___				
6	● ●	O	△ cc ___				
7	● ●	O	△ cc ___				
8	● ●	O	△ cc ___				
9	● ●	O	△ cc ___				
10	● ●	O	△ cc ___				
11	● ●	O	△ cc ___				
TOTALS:							

c1984

FIGURE 14-22

Form for monitoring incontinence. (From Greengold, B.A. and Ouslander, J. Bladder retraining. *J Gerontol Nurs* 12(6):31–35, 1986.)

such as inability of the patient to void upon request. Provocative stress testing is also commonly recommended. The patient is asked to cough vigorously while being observed for urine loss. Urine loss that occurs immediately after coughing is considered indicative of stress incontinence. If urine loss is delayed or persists after the cough, urge incontinence is the more likely diagnosis (Urinary Incontinence Guideline Panel, 1992).

Urinalysis is performed to detect the presence of conditions contributing to urinary incontinence, such as hematuria, pyuria, bacteriuria, glycosuria, and proteinuria. Positive findings mandate referral for further evaluation and management of the associated medical conditions.

In addition to these elements of the assessment, several supplementary assessment maneuvers are often helpful, including specialized diagnostic tests of the urinary tract, voiding records or diaries, and assessment of mental status and mobility.

SPECIALIZED TESTS OF URINARY FUNCTION. A variety of specialized tests may be used to better characterize the nature of the urinary incontinence or voiding dysfunction, in order to more precisely guide treatment.

Uroflowmetry measures the urine flow rate and may help in detecting abnormal voiding patterns, although it is not helpful in distinguishing among various types of urinary incontinence in women and cannot differentiate bladder outlet obstruction from detrusor weakness. *Cystometry* allows the testing of detrusor function. Simple cystometry may be performed at the bedside by using a sterile catheter and filling the bladder with sterile saline. Bladder sensation and capacity can be assessed, along with the presence and strength of involuntary detrusor contractions. More sophisticated cystometrograms can be obtained using pressure transducers to allow measurement of intra-abdominal pressures and intravesicular pressure, but they must be done in specialized clinics. Cystometry results can be affected by patient cooperation and therefore must be interpreted within the context of the patient's behavior during the test. Both false-positives and false-negatives can result.

Electromyography of the urethral sphincter can be obtained when attempting to diagnose detrusor sphincter dyssynergia (Blaivas, 1990). *Cystoscopy* is used to help identify bladder lesions and foreign bodies, as well as urethral diverticula, fistulas, strictures, or intrinsic urethral sphincter deficiency due to radiation injury, trauma, or congenital malformations.

Planning and Intervention

The first step in treatment and management of urinary incontinence is to obtain treatment for existing conditions known to contribute to incontinence—for example, urinary tract infection, fecal impaction, atrophic vaginitis, metabolic disturbances such as poorly controlled diabetes mellitus, and modification of drug regimens. If incontinence remains a problem, then the intervention depends on the type of incontinence diagnosed. The interventions suggested for various alterations in urinary elimination are summarized in Table 14–29.

The major intervention modalities for urinary incontinence in the elderly include

1. Treating conditions predisposing to incontinence, such as metabolic derangements, urinary tract infection, dehydration, fecal impaction, immobility (all forms of urinary incontinence)
2. Implementation of individualized toileting schedules (functional incontinence and possibly urge incontinence)
3. Exercises and biofeedback (urge and stress incontinence)
4. Drug therapy (for urge, stress, and overflow incontinence)
5. Catheterization (overflow incontinence and other forms if they are completely refractory to other treatments and alteration in skin integrity is present)
6. Use of adult diapers or underpads

Behavioral treatments for functional, urge, and stress incontinence have demonstrated success in controlled trials (Urinary Incontinence Guideline Panel, 1992). Schnelle and colleagues have demonstrated that prompted voiding is an effective behavioral intervention for nursing home patients, including those with substantial cognitive impairments, over extended periods of time (Schnelle, 1990; Schnelle et al., 1990). In prompted voiding, the staff attempts to teach the incontinent person to become more aware of the incontinent status and to ask for help from caregivers. The implementation protocol calls for staff to monitor the patient on a regular basis and to ask patients if they are wet or dry. Patients are then asked to try to use the toilet. Patients are praised for trying to use the toilet, and for times when monitoring shows them to be dry.

Habit training, or adapting toileting schedules to a patient's natural voiding pattern, has also been shown to be effective, although this intervention is less well studied than prompted voiding (Hu et al., 1989; Colling et al., 1992). It can be contrasted with a technique called bladder training, in which scheduled voiding, distraction techniques, and positive reinforcement are combined as a therapy for urge or stress incontinence. The general goal is to reduce the number of incontinent episodes and to increase the time between scheduled voids. Success with this technique has been reported in community-dwelling elders (Fantl, Wyman, Harkins et al., 1990, 1991; Rose et al., 1990). For details about its implementation, the reader is referred to a book by Jeter and colleagues (1990).

Pelvic muscle exercises (sometimes known

TABLE 14-29

Treatment Approaches to Alterations in Urinary Elimination in Elderly People

ALTERATION	APPROACHES
Nocturia	Explain that this pattern is normal in older persons. Explore whether the patient experiences associated difficulties, such as difficulty falling asleep
Dysuria	Evaluate for urinary tract infection and other causes and treat as indicated
	If no cause is evident or the cause is not remediable, consider pyridium as a urinary tract anesthetic
Urinary frequency	Evaluate for urinary tract infection or atrophic vaginitis in women and obtain treatment as indicated
	Obtain postvoid residual: if present, evaluate for possible causes of urinary retention and treat. If not treatable, teach patient Credé maneuver or bending over from waist while on toilet to see if more urine can be expelled
	Obtain record of toileting frequency and amount over 3 days
	Try a toileting schedule, based on previous records of voiding frequency and amount, setting goal of an increase in intervals by 30 minutes progressively, until q 2–3 hr voiding pattern is reached. Document toileting pattern, including amounts voided at each toileting
	Teach relaxation exercises as a form of distraction and anxiety alleviation, which may decrease the sense of urgency
	Teach Kegel exercises to raise patient's confidence in competence of urinary sphincter
Hesitancy	Evaluate for obstructive process: e.g., prostatic hypertrophy, fecal impaction, and treat as indicated
	Teach deep breathing and relaxation exercises, to assist in relaxation of sphincters during urination
Urinary retention	Obtain postvoid residual
	Determine cause of retention: anatomical obstruction, side effect of drug therapy, autonomic neuropathy, and treat as indicated
Stress incontinence	Kegel exercises
	Biofeedback
	Medications: anticholinergics, estrogen replacement (if atrophic vaginitis diagnosed)
	Padding
	Surgery
Overflow incontinence	Toileting schedule
	Positioning and Credé maneuver
	Medications: parasympathomimetics, such as bethanechol
	Catheterization: intermittent, clean self-catheterization; indwelling
Urge incontinence (detrusor instability; reflex bladder)	Toilet schedule
	Biofeedback
	Medications: anticholinergics and adrenergic antagonists
Functional incontinence	Toilet schedule
Mobility problems	Bedside commode to reduce distance to toilet
	Kegel exercises
	Intervene to optimize mobility
Learned helplessness	Help patient resume control over decisions in life in small ways: e.g., choice of clothing, food, then set expectations that patient control bodily functions and positively reinforce expected outcomes
Inappropriate expression of anger	Explore anger with patient. Help find more appropriate means of expressing anger
Attention-getting maneuver	Respond to incontinent episodes with as little attention or fuss as possible. Find positive behaviors in patient; pay attention, reward those behaviors

as Kegel exercises) have also been demonstrated to be efficacious in treatment of stress incontinence, in both men (Burgio et al., 1989) and women (Burns et al., 1990). In one study, pelvic floor muscle exercises compared favorably with phenylpropanolamine in percentage cured (Wells et al., 1991).

Electrical stimulation of the pelvic viscera, muscles, or nerves has also been used with varying degrees of success in different types of urinary incontinence. Stimulation of afferent nerve fibers is thought to facilitate storage of urine, and stimulation of efferent fibers is believed to facilitate emptying. Electrical stimulation has been associated with pain and discomfort. Evaluation of it is made difficult by the variability in protocols, including differences in type and placement of electrodes and differences in methods of delivering the electricity; therefore, its use should be restricted until more definitive studies are available (Urinary Incontinence Guideline Panel, 1992).

A variety of drug treatments have been shown to be efficacious in both stress and urge incontinence. For urge incontinence, the per cent of individuals cured with oxybutynin ranges from 28 to 44, with a 9 to 56 per cent reduction in urinary incontinence. In trials using imipramine, approximately one third were cured, with a 20 to 77 per cent reduction of urinary incontinence. Success rates are somewhat less in treatment of stress incontinence, with only 0 to 14 per cent achieving total remission with phenylpropanolamine, but 30 to 60 per cent receiving improvement in symptoms over placebo (Urinary Incontinence Guideline Panel, 1992).

Individuals with overflow incontinence for whom medical therapies and surgical intervention are not possible must receive some form of regular bladder drainage, either in the form of intermittent or indwelling catheterization. Clean intermittent catheterization (CIC) is the preferred treatment for those with overflow incontinence due to inoperable obstruction, underactive detrusors, or detrusor hyperreflexia with sphincter dyssynergia (Urinary Incontinence Guideline Panel, 1992). Complications of CIC include urethritis, urinary tract infection, difficulty with inserting the catheter, urethral stricture, epididymitis, and bladder stones. Although complication rates have been reported as high as 20 per cent, the range of complications is less than with indwelling catheters, and the likelihood of urinary tract infection and death from sepsis is higher in those with indwelling catheters (Kunin et al., 1992).

External catheters have also been associated with higher rates of urinary tract infections (Urinary Incontinence Guideline Panel, 1992). Every attempt, therefore, should be made to manage urinary incontinence without the use of indwelling catheters. When urinary catheters are used, nurses should pay particular attention to infection control procedures, so that other patients are not infected from the colonized patient. Procedures like meatal care have been found to increase the incidence of symptomatic urinary tract infections. Vigilant handwashing between emptying catheter bags and taping of the catheter to prevent traction are recommended. Table 14–30 lists the various containment options in incontinence, along with the advantages and disadvantages of each type.

Evaluation

Criteria for evaluation of the patient with alterations in urinary elimination are

TABLE 14 – 30

Advantages and Disadvantages of Various Forms of Management of Urinary Incontinence

METHOD OF MANAGEMENT	ADVANTAGES	DISADVANTAGES
Incontinence pads	Nonintrusive Can be managed easily by patients and caregivers Removable for toileting	Cost ($6–8/dozen) "Diapers" Odor Visible under most clothing Medicare does not pay as medical supply Not available for women
Condom catheters	Nonintrusive Easier to manage than indwelling Leg bags are available Covered as a medical expense	Risk of infections Adhesives irritate genitals Need frequent replacements
Intermittent catheterization	Limited intrusion Self-done/private Limited expense Lower infection risk than Foley	Some skill needed to do task Scheduling necessary for effectiveness Not thought of for OLD patients
Indwelling catheterization	Limited leakage No retention Covered as a medical supply Entitles patient to RN home health	Risk of infection greater Independent mobility less Risk of trauma greater Risk of skin breakdown greater Need for medical supervision greater

Adapted from Giduz, B.H. et al. *A Geriatric First Aid Kit.* Chapel Hill, N.C.: University of North Carolina School of Medicine, 1986, p. 24.

1. Does the patient have unanswered questions about any changes in urinary elimination, or urinary symptoms?
2. Are patients with symptoms of genitourinary pathology referred for medical evaluation and treatment appropriately?

For patients with incontinence:

3. How often is the patient wet?
4. Does the patient suffer the adverse effects of incontinence, such as social isolation, alterations in skin integrity?
5. Is drug therapy chosen to minimize adverse effects on urinary function?

REFERENCES

Acute Pain Management Guideline Panel. *Acute Pain Management: Operative or Medical Procedures and Trauma.* Clinical Practice Guideline. AHCPR Publication No. 92-0032. Rockville, MD: Agency for Health Care Policy and Research, Public Health Service, U.S. Department of Health and Human Services, 1992.

Adams, M.A., Rojas-Camero, C. and Clayton, K. A small-group sex education/intervention model for the well elderly: A challenge for educators. *Educ Gerontol* 16:601–608, 1990.

Adler, W.H. and Nagel, J.E. Clinical immunology. *In*

Hazzard, W.R., Andres, R., Bierman, E.C. and Blass, J.P. (eds.). *Principles of Geriatriac Medicine and Gerontology.* 2nd ed. New York: McGraw-Hall, 1990, pp. 60–71.

Administration on Aging. U.S. Department of Health and Human Services. *Infrastructure of Home and Community Based Services for the Functionally Impaired Elderly.* State Source Book, 1994.

Agency for Health Care Policy and Research Panel for the Prediction and Prevention of Pressure Ulcers in Adults. *Pressure Ulcers in Adults: Prediction and Prevention.* Clinical Practice Guideline No. 3. AHCPR Publication No. 92-0047. Rockville, MD: AHCPR, Public Health Services, USDHHS, May 1992.

Alessi, C.A., Henderson, C.T. and Linderborn, K.M. A review of research on common bowel problems in the nursing home. *In* Rubenstein, L.Z. and Wieland, D. (eds.). *Improving Care in the Nursing Home: Comprehensive Reviews of Clinical Research.* Newbury Park, CA: Sage Publications, 1993, Chap. 6.

Aletkey, P.J. Human sexuality: Sexuality of the nursing home resident. *Topics Clin Nurs* 1:53–60, 1980.

Alexander, N.B., Fry-Welch, D.K., Ward, M.E. and Folkmier, L.C. Quantitative assessment of bed rise difficulty in young and elderly women. *J Am Geriatr Soc* 4: 685–691, 1992.

Algase, D. Cognitive discriminants of wandering among nursing home residents. *Nurs Res* 41:78–81, 1992.

Allman, R.M., Walker, J.M., Hart, M.K. et al. Air fluidized beds or conventional therapy for pressure sores: A randomized trial. *Ann Intern Med* 107:641–648, 1987.

Almvig, C. Reviews of "Forbidden love: The unashamed stories of lesbian lives" and "Women like us." *Gerontologist* 34:281, 1994.

Alvarez, O.M., Mertz, P.M. and Eaglstein, W.H. The effect of occlusive dressings on re-epithelialization and collagen synthesis. *J Surg Res* 35:142–148, 1983.

American College of Sports Medicine. *The Recommended Quantity and Quality of Exercise for Developing and Maintaining Cardiorespiratory and Muscular Fitness in Healthy Adults.* Position Stand, 1990.

American Speech and Hearing Association. Guidelines for the identification of hearing impairment and handicap in adults/elderly persons. *ASHA* 31(8):59–63, 1989.

Ancoli-Israel, S. Epidemiology of sleep disorders. *Clin Geriatr Med* 5:347–362, 1989.

Ancoli-Israel, S. and Kripke, D.F. Sleep and aging. *In* Calkins, E., Ford, A.B. and Katz, P. (eds.). *Practice of Geriatrics.* 2nd ed. Philadelphia: W. B. Saunders, 1992.

Ancoli-Israel, S., Kripke, D.F., Klauber, M.R. et al. Sleep disordered breathing in community-dwelling elderly. *Sleep* 14:486–495, 1991, Chap. 36.

Andrews, J.F. and Wilson, H.F. The deaf adult in the nursing home. *Geriatr Nurs* Nov/Dec:279–283, 1991.

Armitage, J.M. and Williams, S.J. Inhaler technique in the elderly. *Age Ageing* 17:275–278, 1988.

Astrand, P.O. Physical activity and fitness. *Am J Clin Nutr* 55:1231S–1236S, 1992.

Atkinson, J.C. and Fox, F.C. Salivary gland dysfunction. *Clin Geriatr Med* 8(3):499–511, 1992.

Augustine, S.D. Hypothermia therapy in the post-anesthesia care unit: A review. *J Post-Anest Nurs* 5:254–263, 1990.

Avorn, J. and Langer, E. Induced disability in nursing home patients: A controlled trial. *J Am Geriatr Soc* 30(6):397–400, 1982.

Badley, E.M., Wagstaff, S. and Wood, P.H.N. Measures of functional ability (disability) in arthritis in relation to impairment of range of joint movement. *Ann Rheum Dis* 43:563–569, 1984.

Bancroft, J. *Human Sexuality and Its Problems.* Edinburgh: Churchill Livingstone, 1989.

Bandura, A. Self-efficacy mechanism in human agency. *Am Psychol* 37:122–147, 1982.

Bassey, E.J., Bendall, M.J. and Pearson, M. Muscle strength in the triceps surae and objectively measured customary walking activity in men and women over 65 years of age. *Clin Sci* 74:85–89, 1988.

Beck, C., Heacock, P., Mercer, M. and Walton, C. Decreasing caregiver assistance with older adults with dementia. *In* Funk, S.G., Tornquist, E.M., Champagne, M.T. and Wiese, R.A. (eds.). *Key Aspects of Elder Care: Managing Falls, Incontinence and Cognitive Impairment.* New York: Springer, 1992, pp. 309–319.

Beck, J.C. Commentary, p. 93 in Beck, J., Burton, J., Goldstein, S. et al. (eds.). *Yearbook of Gerontology & Geriatrics.* St. Louis: Mosby-Year Book, 1994.

Bendall, M.J., Bassey, E.J. and Pearson, M.B. Factors affecting walking speed of elderly people. *Age Ageing* 18: 327–332, 1989.

Bender, P. Deceptive distress in the elderly. *Am J Nurs* 92:29–33, 1992.

Ben-Yehuda, A. and Weksler, M. Host resistance and the immune system. *Clin Geriatr Med* 8(4):701–711, 1992.

Bergstrom, G., Aniansson, A., Bajelle, A. et al. Functional consequences of joint impairment at age 79. *Scand J Rehab Med* 17:183–190, 1985.

Bergstrom, N., Braden, B.J., Laguzza, A. and Holman, V. The Braden scale for predicting pressure sore risk. *Nurs Res* 36:205–210, 1988.

Blaivas, J.G. Diagnostic evaluation of incontinence in patients with neurologic disorders. *J Am Geriatr Soc* 38: 306–310, 1990.

Bleatman, C. and Morton, I. Validation therapy: Extracts from 20 groups with dementia sufferers. *J Adv Nurs* 17:658–666, 1992.

Bliwise, D.L. Review: Sleep in normal aging and dementia. *Sleep* 16(1):40–81, 1993.

Bobath, B. *Adult Hemiplegia: Evaluation and Treatment.* 2nd ed. London: William Heineman Books, 1978, p. 86.

Bolan, G., Broome, C.V., Facklam, R.R. et al. Pneumococcal vaccine efficacy in selected populations in the US. *Ann Intern Med* 104:1–6, 1986.

Bortz, W.M. Disuse and aging. *JAMA* 248:1203–1205, 1982.

Braden, B.J. and Bergstrom, N. Utility of the Braden Scale for predicting pressure sore risk. *Decubitus* 2(3): 44–51, 1982.

Braden, B.J. and Bryant, R. Innovations to prevent and treat pressure ulcers. *Geriatr Nurs* 11:182–186, 1990.

Britell, C.W. Wheelchair prescription. *In* Kottke, F.J. and Lehmann, P. (eds.). *Krusen's Handbook of Physical Medicine and Rehabilitation.* 4th ed. Philadelphia: W. B. Saunders, 1990, Chap. 23.

Brody, E. and Kleban, M. Day to day mental and physical health symptoms of older people: A report on health logs. *Gerontologist* 23(1):75–86, 1983.

Brooks, S.M. Task group on surveillance for respiratory hazards in the occupational setting. *ATS News* 8:12–16, 1982.

Brookshire, R.H. *An Introduction to Neurogenic Communication Disorders.* St. Louis: Mosby-Year Book, 1991.

Buchner, D.M. and de Lateur, B.J. The importance of skeletal muscle strength to physical function in older adults. *Ann Behav Med* 13(3):91–98, 1991.

Burdon, J., Juniper, E., Killian, K. et al. The perception of breathlessness in asthma. *Am Rev Respir Dis* 126: 282–285, 1982.

Burgio, K.L., Stutzman, R.E., and Bengel, B.T. Behavioral training for post-prostatectomy urinary incontinence. *J Urol* 141(2):303–306, 1989.

Burish, T.G. and Lyles, J.N. Effectiveness of relaxation training in reducing adverse reactions to cancer chemotherapy. *J Behav Med* 4:65–78, 1981.

Burkle, N.L. Inadvertent hypothermia. *J Gerontol Nurs* 14(6):26–30, 1988.

Burns, M.S. and Halper, A.S. Language disorders associated with aging. *Topics Geriatr Rehab* 1(4):15–28, 1986.

Burns, P.A., Pranikoff, K., Nochasjski, T. et al. Treatment of stress incontinence with pelvic floor exercises and biofeedback. *J Am Geriatr Soc* 38(3):341–344, 1990.

Burnside, I.M. The senses. *In* Burnside, I.M. (ed.). *Nursing Care of the Aged.* 2nd ed. New York: McGraw-Hill, 1981, pp. 468–491.

Burrows, B., Barbee, R.A., Cline, M.G. et al. Characteristics of asthma among elderly adults in a sample of the general population. *Chest* 100:935–942, 1991.

Bury, M.R. The ICIDH: A review of research and prospects. *Intl Disabil Studies* 9:118–128, 1987.

Calkins, E. Musculoskeletal diseases in the elderly. *In* Calkins, E., Ford, A.B. and Katz, P. (eds.). *Practice of Geriatrics.* 2nd ed. Philadelphia: W. B. Saunders, 1992, p. 387.

Calvani, D. How well do your clients cope with hearing loss: Hearing Handicap Inventory. *J Gerontol Nurs* 11(7):16–20, 1985.

Campbell, S.D. The audioscope: A valuable hearing assessment tool. *J Gerontol Nurs* 12(12):28–32, 1986.

Cantrell, M. and Norman, D. Infections. *In* Calkins, E., Ford, A.B. and Katz, P. (eds.). *Practice of Geriatrics.* 2nd ed. Philadelphia: W. B. Saunders, 1992, pp. 554–564.

Carnevali, D.L. and Reiner, A.C. *The Cancer Experience: Nursing Diagnosis and Management.* Phildelphia: J. B. Lippincott, 1990.

Carpenito, L.J. *Handbook of Nursing Diagnosis.* Philadelphia: J. B. Lippincott, 1993a.

Carpenito, L.J. *Nursing Diagnosis: Application to Clinical Practice.* 5th ed. Philadelphia: J. B. Lippincott, 1993b.

Carpenter, D.R. and Zielinski, D.A. How do you treat and control *C. difficile* infection? *Am J Nurs* 92:(9):22–24, 1992.

Carrieri, V.K. and Janson-Bjerklie, S. Strategies patients use to manage the sensation of dyspnea. *West J Nurs Res* 8(3):304–305, 1986.

Carrieri-Kohlman, V. and Janson-Bjerklie, S. Dyspnea. *In* Carrieri-Kohlman, V., Lindsey, A.M. and West, C.M. (eds.). *Pathophysiological Phenomena in Nursing.* 2nd ed. Philadelphia: W. B. Saunders, 1993, Chap. 11.

Carrieri-Kohlman, V., Lindsey, A.M. and West, C.M. (eds.). *Pathophysiological Phenomena in Nursing.* 2nd ed. Philadelphia: W. B. Saunders, 1993.

Carroll-Johnson, R.M. and Paquette, M. High risk for peripheral neurovascular dysfunction. *In* Carroll-Johnson, R.M. and Paquette, M. (eds.). *Classification of Nursing Diagnoses: Proceedings of the Tenth Conference.* Philadelphia: J. B. Lippincott, 1994, p. 414.

Cartmill, T.D.I., Shrimpton, S.B., Panigrahi, H. et al. Nosocomial diarrhoea due to a single strain of *Clostridium difficile*: A prolonged outbreak in elderly patients. *Age Aging* 21:245–249, 1992.

Caruso, C.C., Hadley, B.J., Shukla, R. et al. Cooling effects and comfort of four cooling blanket temperatures in humans with fever. *Nurs Res* 41:68–72, 1992.

Ceccio, C.M. Understanding therapeutic beds. *Orthop Nurs* 9(3):57–70, 1990.

Chapman, R.U., Sillery, J., Fontana, D.D. et al. Effect of oral dioctyl sodium sulfonsuccinate on intake-output studies of human small and large intestine. *Gastroenterology* 9:489–493, 1985.

Charness, N. and Bosman, E.S. Human factors and design for older adults. *In* Birren, J. E. and Schaie, K. W. (eds.). *Handbook of the Psychology of Aging.* 3rd ed. San Diego: Academic Press, 1990.

Cockcroft, A., Adams, L. and Guz, A. Assessment of breathlessness. *Q J Med* 72:669–676, 1989.

Cohen, H.J. Monoclonal gammopathies and again. *Hosp Pract* 23(3A):75–80, 82, 85–89, 1988.

Colling, J., Ouslander, J., Hadley, B.J. et al. The effects of patterned urge-response toileting (PURT) on urinary incontinence among nursing home residents. *J Am Geriatr Soc* 39:135–141, 1992.

Collins, K.J., Exton-Smith, A.N., Fox, R.H. et al. Accidental hyperemia and impaired temperature homeostasis in the elderly. *Br Med J* 1:353, 1977.

Collins, M.J. Differential diagnosis of aphasic syndromes and apraxia of speech. *In* Square-Storer, P. (ed.). *Acquired Apraxia of Speech in Aphasic Adults: Theoretical and Clinical Issues.* Hillsdale, N.J.: Lawrence Erlbaum Associates, 1989, Chap. 4.

Convertino, V.A. Exercise responses after inactivity. *In* Sandler, H. and Vernikos, J. (eds.). Inactivity: Physiological Effects. New York: Academic Press—Harcourt Brace Jovanovich, 1986, pp. 149–191.

Cotanch, P. and Strum, S. Progressive muscle relaxation as antiemetic therapy for cancer patients. *Oncol Nurs Forum* 14:33–37, 1987.

Crook, J., Rideout, E. and Browne, G. The prevalence of pain complaints among a general population. *Pain* 18:299–314, 1984.

Crosby, L.J. Fatigue, pain, depression and sleep disturbance in rheumatoid arthritis patients. *In* Funk, S.G., Tornquist, E.M., Champagne, M.T. et al. (eds.). *Key Aspects of Comfort: Management of Pain, Fatigue, and Nausea.* New York: Springer Publishing Company, 1989, pp. 299–302.

Crosson, B. *Subcortical Functions in Language and Memory.* New York: Guildford Press, 1992.

Crum, R.M., Anthony, J.C., Bassett, S.S. and Folstein, M.F. Population-based norms for the mini-mental state examination by age and educational level. *JAMA* 269:2386–2391, 1992.

Cubeddu, L.S., Hoffman, I.S., Fuenmayor, N.T. and Finn, A.L. Efficacy of ondansetron (GR38032F) and the role of serotonin in cisplatin-induced nausea and vomiting. *N Engl J Med* 322:810–816, 1990.

Cummings, J. Behavioral complications of drug treatment of Parkinson's disease. *J Am Geriatr Soc* 39:708–716, 1991.

Cunningham, D.A., Rechnitzer, P.A., Pearce, M.E. and Donner, A.P. Determinants of self-selected walking pace across ages 19 to 66. *J Gerontol* 37:560–564, 1982.

Cuzzell, J.Z. The right way to culture a wound. *Am J Nurs* 93:(5)43–50, 1993.

Czaja, S.J., Weber, R.A. and Nair, S.N. A human factors analysis of ADL activities: A capability-demand approach. *J Gerontol* 48(Special Issue):44–48, 1993.

Czajka-Narins, D.M. The assessment of nutritional status. *In* Mahan, L.K. and Arlin, M.T. (eds.). *Krause's Food, Nutrition and Diet Therapy.* Philadelphia: W. B. Saunders, 1992, Chap. 17.

Dagon, E.M. Aging and sexuality. *In* Nadleson, C.C. and Marcotte, D.B. (eds.). *Treatment and Interventions in Human Sexuality.* New York: Plenum Press, 1983.

Dajani, A.S., Bisno, A.L., Chung, K.J. et al. Prevention of bacterial endocarditis: Recommendations by the American Heart Association. *JAMA* 264:2919, 1990.

Danielson, K.H. Oral care and older adults. *J Gerontol Nurs* 14(11):6–10, 1988.

Darowski, A., Weinberg, J.R. and Guz A. Normal rectal, auditory canal, sublingual and axillary temperatures in elderly afebrile patients in a warm environment. *Age Ageing* 20:113–119, 1991.

Davignon, D.D. and Leshowitz, B.H. The speech in noise test: A new approach to the assessment of communication capability of older persons. *Intl J Aging Human Dev* 23(2):149–160, 1986.

Davis, C. and Lentz, M.J. Charting oral temperatures: Circadian rhythms to spot abnormalities. *J Gerontol Nurs* 15(4):34–39, 1989.

Davis, K.M. and Minaker, K.L. Disorders of fluid and electrolyte balance. *In* Hazzard, W.R., Andres, R., Bierman, E.C. and Blass, J.P. (eds.). *Principles of Geriatric*

Medicine and Gerontology. 2nd ed. New York: McGraw-Hill, 1990, pp. 1079–1083.

Dawson, P., Wells, D.L. and Kline, K. *Enhancing the Abilities of Persons with Alzheimer's and Related Dementias: A Nursing Perspective.* New York: Springer Publishing Company, 1992, pp. 139–154.

Delafuente, J.C., Meuleman, J.R. and Nelson, R.C. Anergy testing in nursing home residents. *J Am Geriatr Soc* 36:733–735, 1988.

Dellefield, M.E. Caring for the elderly patient with cancer. *Oncol Nurs Forum* 13(3):19–27, 1986.

DeWitt, S. Nursing assessment of the skin and dermatologic lesions. *Nurs Clin North Am* 25(1):235–245, 1990.

Deyo, R.A., Walsh, N.E., Martin, D.C. et al. A controlled trial of transcutaneous electrical nerve stimulation (TENS) and exercise for low back pain. *N Eng J Med* 322:1627–1634, 1990.

Dietch, J.T., Hewett, L.J. and Jones, S. Adverse effects of reality orientation. *J Am Geriatr Soc* 37:974–976, 1989.

DiFabio, R.P. and Badke, M.B. Stance duration under sensory conflict conditions in patients with hemiplegia. *Arch Phys Med Rehabil* 72:292–295, 1991.

Diggory, P., Bailey, R. and Vallon, A. Effectiveness of inhaled bronchodilator delivery systems for elderly patients. *Age Ageing* 20:379–382, 1991.

Doering, L.V. The effect of positioning on hemodynamics and gas exchange in the critically ill: A review. *Am J Crit Care* 2(3):208–216, 1993.

Domenico, R.A. Verbal communication impairment in dementia: Research frontiers in language cognition. *In* Zandi, T. and Ham, R.J. (eds.). *New Directions in Understanding Dementia and Alzheimer's Disease.* New York: Plenum Press, 1990, pp. 79–88.

Donahue, P.A. When it's hard to swallow: Feeding techniques for dysphagia management. *J Gerontol Nurs* 16(4):6–9, 1990.

Donovan, M.I. Acute pain relief. *Nurs Clin North Am* 25(4):851–861, 1990.

Dorevitch, M.I., Cossar, R.M., Bailey, F.J. et al. The accuracy of self- and informant ratings of physical functional capacity in the elderly. *J Clin Epidemiol* 45:791–798, 1992.

Dunlevy, J. Hearing before the subcommittee on public assistance and employment compensation of the House Committee on Ways and Means, Ninety-sixth Congress, 1979, pp. 52–59.

East, M.B. Review of "Sexuality and Aging." *Gerontologist* 34:283–284, 1994.

Edmond, M. *Enteric Infections in the Nursing Home.* Paper presented at 17th Midwestern Conference on Health Care in the Elderly, University of Iowa, Iowa City, 1994.

Egbert, A.M., Parks, L.H., Short, L.M. and Burnett, M.L. Randomized trial of postoperative patient-controlled analgesia v. intramuscular narcotics in frail elderly men. *Arch Intern Med* 150:1897–1903, 1990.

Eilers, J., Berger, A. and Person, M.C. Development, testing and application of the oral assessment guide. *Oncol Nurs Forum* 15(3):325–330, 1988.

Ekman, P. and Friesen, W.V. *Facial Action Coding System.* Palo Alto, CA: Consulting Psychologist Press, 1978.

Elam, J.T., Graney, M.J. et al. Comparison of subjective ratings of function with observed functional ability of frail older persons. *Am J Public Health* 81:1127–1130, 1991.

Ellwood, P. Bed positioning. *In* Kottke, F.J. and Lehmann, P. (eds.). *Krusen's Handbook of Physical Medicine and Rehabilitation.* 4th ed. Philadelphia: W. B. Saunders, 1990, Chap. 21.

Emery, V.O. and Oxman, T.E. Update on the dementia spectrum of depression. *Am J Psychiatry* 149:3, 1992.

Emori, T.G., Banerjee, S.N., Culver, D.H. et al. The National Nosocomial Infections Surveillance System: Nosocomial infections in elderly patients in the United States, 1986–1990. *Am J Med* 91(Suppl 3B):289–293, 1991.

Enright, P.L., Kronmal, R.A., Higgins, M. et al. Spirometry reference values for women and men 65 to 85 years of age: Cardiovascular health study. *Am Rev Resp Dis* 147:125–133, 1993.

Epstein, C.F. Wheelchair management: Developing a system for long-term care facilities. *J Long-Term Care Admin* 8:1–12, 1990.

Evans, D.A., Finenstein, H.H., Albert, M.S. et al. Prevalence of Alzheimer's disease in a community population of older persons: Higher than previously reported. *JAMA* 268:2551, 1989.

Evans, L.K. and Strumpf, N.E. Myths about elder restraint. *Image* 22(2):124–128, 1990.

Evans, L.K., Strumpf, N.E. and Williams, C.C. Limiting use of physical restraints: A prerequisite for independent functioning. *In* Calkins, E., Ford, A.B. and Katz, P. (eds.). *Practice of Geriatrics.* 2nd ed. Philadelphia: W. B. Saunders, 1992, Chap. 22.

Fagerhaugh, S. and Strauss, A. *Politics of Pain Management: Staff-Patient Interactions.* Menlo Park, CA: Addison-Wesley, 1977.

Faletti, M.V. Human factors research and functional environments for the aged. *In* Altman, I., Lawton, M.P. and Wolwill, J.F. (eds.). *Elderly People and the Environment.* New York: Plenum Press, 1984, pp. 191–237.

Fantl, J.A., Wyman, J.F., Harkins, S.W. and Hadley, E.C. Bladder training in the management of lower urinary tract dysfunction in women: A review. *J Am Geriatr Soc* 38(3):329–332, 1990.

Fantl, J.A., Wyman, J.F., McClish, D.K. and Bump, R.C. Urinary incontinence in community-dwelling women: Clinical, urodynamic and severity characteristics. *Am J Obstet Gynecol* 162(4):946–951, 1990.

Fantl, J.A., Wyman, J.F., McClish, D.K. et al. Efficacy of bladder training in older women with urinary incontinence. *JAMA* 265(5):609–613, 1991.

Farncombe, M. and Chater, S. Case studies outlining use of nebulized morphine for patients with end-stage chronic lung and cardiac disease. *J Pain Symptom Management* 8:221–225, 1993.

Fay, D.E. and Lance, P. Disorders of the alimentary tract. *In* Calkins, E., Ford, A.B. and Katz, P.R. (eds.). *Practice of Geriatrics.* 2nd ed. Philadelphia: W. B. Saunders, 1992, Chap. 54.

Ferguson, M.W. and Devlin, H. Aging and the orofacial tissues. *In* Brocklehurst, J.C., Tallis, R.C. and Fillit, H.M. (eds.). *Textbook of Geriatric Medicine and Gerontology.* Edinburgh: Churchill Livingstone, 1992, pp. 494–506.

Ferrell, B.A. Pain management in elderly people. *J Am Geriatr Soc* 39:64–73, 1991.

Ferrell, B.A., Ferrell, B.R. and Osterweil, D. Pain in the nursing home. *J Am Geriatr Soc* 38:409–414, 1990.

Ferrell, B.A., Osterwein, D. and Christenson, P. A randomized controlled trial of low-air-loss beds for treatment of pressure ulcers. *JAMA* 269(4):494–497, 1993.

Ferro, S. and Salit, I.E. HIV infection in patients over 55 years of age. *J Acquir Immune Defic Syndr* 5:348–355, 1992.

Fiatarone, M.A., Marks, E.C., Ryan, D.N. et al. High-intensity strength training in nonogenarians. *JAMA* 263:3029–3034, 1990.

Fiatarone, M.A., O'Neill, E.F., Ryan, N.D. et al. Exercise training and nutritional supplementation for physical frailty in very elderly people. *New Engl J Med* 330:1769–1775, 1994.

Fink, M., Green, M. and Bender, M.B. The face-hand test as a diagnostic sign of organic mental syndrome. *Neurology* 2:46–59, 1952.

Finucane, T.E. The American Geriatrics Society statement on two-step PPD testing for nursing home patients on admission. *J Am Geriatr Soc* 36:77–78, 1988.

Fisher, N.M. and Pendergast, D.R. Quantitative Progressive Exercise Rehabilitation (QPER): Rehabilitation of patients with osteoarthritis. *In* Funk, S.G., Tornquist, E.M., Champagne, M.T. and Wiese, R.A. (eds.). *Key Aspects of Caring for the Chronically Ill: Hospital and Home.* New York: Springer Publishing Company, 1992, pp. 178–189.

Fletcher, B.J. and Vassallo, L.M. Exercise testing and training in physically disabled subjects with coronary artery disease. *In* Funk, S.G., Tornquist, E.M., Champagne, M.T. and Wiese, R.A. (eds.). *Key Aspects of Caring for the Chronically Ill: Hospital and Home.* New York: Springer Publishing Company, 1992, pp. 189–201.

Fletcher, G., Blair, S., Blumenthal, J. et al. American Heart Association medical/scientific statement on exercise. *Circulation* 86:340–344, 1992.

Folstein, M.S., Folstein, S. and McHugh, P.R. Mini-mental state: A practical method for grading the cognitive state of patients for the clinician. *J Psychiatr Res* 12: 189–198, 1975.

Foreman, M. Acute confusional states in the hospitalized elderly. *In* Funk, S.G., Tornquist, E.M., Champagne, M.T. and Wiese, R.A. (eds.). *Key Aspects of Elder Care: Managing Falls, Incontinence and Cognitive Impairment.* New York: Springer, 1992, pp. 262–277.

Fox, R.H., Woodward, P.M., Exton-Smith, A.N. et al. Body temperatures in the elderly: A national study of physiological, social and environmental conditions. *Br Med J* 1:200, 1973.

Fraser, D. Patient assessment: Infections in the elderly. *J Gerontol Nurs* 19(7):5–11, 1993.

Freels, S., Cohen, D., Eisdorfer, C. et al. Functional status and clinical findings in patients with Alzheimer's disease. *J Gerontol Med Sci* 47:M177–182, 1992.

Fried, L.P., Bandeen-Roche, K., Chee, E. and Rubin, G. Is preclinical disability a transitional state of physical function? *Gerontologist* 33(Spec Ed I):174, 1993.

Fried, L.P., Herdman, S.J., Kuhn, K.E. et al. Preclinical disability: Hypotheses about the bottom of the iceberg. *J Aging Health* 3:285–300, 1991.

Friedeman, J.S. Factors influencing sexual expression in aging persons: A review of the literature. *J Psych Nurs Mental Health Serv* 16:34–47, 1978.

Friedlander, A.H. and Yoshikawa, T.T. Pathogenesis, management and prevention of infective endocarditis in the elderly dental patient. *Oral Surg Oral Med Oral Pathol* 69:177–181, 1990.

Friedman, J. and Friedman, H. Fatigue in Parkinson's disease. *Neurology* 43:2016–2018, 1993.

Friedman, L.W. Rehabilitation of the lower extremity amputee. *In* Kottke, F.J. and Lehmann, P. (eds.). *Krusen's Handbook of Physical Medicine and Rehabilitation.* 4th ed. Philadelphia: W. B. Saunders, 1990, Chap. 49.

Friedman, L., Bliwise, D.L., Yesavage, J.A. and Salom, S.R. A preliminary study comparing sleep restriction and relaxation treatments for insomnia in older adults. *J Gerontol Psych Sci* 46:P1–P8, 1991.

Friedman, P.J., Richmond, D.E. and Baskett, J.J. A prospective trial of serial gait speed as a measure of rehabilitation in the elderly. *Age Ageing* 17:227–235, 1988.

Gamel, C., Davis, B.D. and Hengeveld, M. Nurses' provision of teaching and counseling on sexuality: Review of the literature. *J Adv Nurs* 18:1219–1227, 1993.

Gangarosa, R.E., Glass, R.I., Lew, J.F. et al. Hospitalizations involving gastroenteritis in the United States, 1985: The special burden of the disease among the elderly. *Am J Epidemiol* 135:281–290, 1992.

Garahan, M.B., Waller, J.A., Houghton, M. et al. Hearing loss prevalence and management in nursing home residents. *J Am Geriatr Soc* 40:130–134, 1992.

Gaspar, P.M. What determines how much patients drink? *Geriatr Nurs* July/Aug:221–224, 1988.

Gerety, M.B., Mulrow, C.D., Tuley, M.R. et al. Development & validation of a physical performance instrument for the functionally impaired elderly: The Physical Disability Index (PDI). *J Gerontol* 48:M33–M38, 1993.

Giduz, B., Snow, T. et al. *A Geriatric First Aid Kit.* Chapel Hill, NC: University of North Carolina, 1986.

Gift, A. Dyspnea. *Nurs Clin North Am* 25:955–965, 1990.

Gift, A.G., Moore, T. and Soeken, K. Relaxation to reduce dyspnea and anxiety in COPD patients. *Nurs Res* 41:242–246, 1992.

Gill, K.M. and Ducharme, S. Sexual concerns of the elderly. *In* Calkins, E., Ford, A.B. and Katz, P. (eds.). *Practice of Geriatrics.* 2nd ed. Philadelphia: W. B. Saunders, 1992, pp. 276–281.

Glick, O.J. Interventions related to activity and movement. *Nurs Clin North Am* 27(2):541–568, 1992.

Goldstein, H. and Runyon, C. An occupational therapy educational module to increase sensitivity about geriatric sexuality. *Phys Occup Ther Geriatr* 11(2):57–76, 1993.

Goode, P.S. and Allman, R.M. The prevention and management of pressure ulcers. *Med Clin North Am* 73(6): 1511–1524, 1989.

Gordon, M. *Nursing Diagnosis.* New York: McGraw-Hill, 1982.

Graham, K.M., Percoraro, D.A., Ventural, M. and Meyer, C.C. Reducing the incidence of stomatitis using a quality assessment and improvement approach. *Cancer Nurs* 16(2):117–122, 1993.

Greengold, B.A. and Ouslander, J.G. Bladder retraining. *J Gerontol Nurs* 12(6):31–35, 1986.

Guarino, S.C. and Knowlton, C.N. Planning and implementing a group health program on sexuality for the elderly. *J Geriatr Nurs* 6(1):600–603, 1980.

Guralnik, J.M., Branch, L.G., Cummings, S.R. and Curb, J.D. Review: Physical performance measures in aging research. *J Gerontol* 44:M141–M146, 1989.

Guralnik, J.M. et al. A short physical performance battery assessing lower extremity function: Association with self-reported disability and prediction of mortality and nursing home admission. *J Gerontol Med Sci* 49: M85–94, 1994.

Guralnik, J.M., LaCroix, A.Z., Abbot, R.D. et al. Maintaining mobility in late life I: Demographic characteristics and chronic conditions. *Am J Epidemiol* 137:845–857, 1993.

Hall, G.R. Altered thought processes: Dementia. *In* Maas, M., Buckwalter, K.C. and Hardy, M. (eds.). *Nursing Diagnoses and Interventions for the Elderly.* Menlo Park, CA: Addison-Wesley, 1991, Chap. 29.

Hall, G.R., Karstens, M., Rakey, B. et al. Managing constipation in elderly postoperative vascular surgery patients using a research-based protocol. *Med Surg Nurs* 4(1):11–18, 1995.

Hall, S.S. Extended-wear contact lenses. *J Gerontol Nurs* 10(6):28–33, 1984.

Hamilton, J. Comfort and the hospitalized chronically ill. *J Gerontol Nurs* 15(4):28–33, 1989.

Hammer, B. Sleep pattern disturbance. *In* Maas, M., Buckwalter, K.C. and Hardy, M. (eds.). *Nursing Diagnoses and Interventions for the Elderly.* Menlo Park, CA: Addison-Wesley, 1991, Chap. 27.

Harari, D., Gurwitz, J.H. and Minaker, K.L. Constipation in the elderly. *J Am Geriatr Soc* 41:1130–1140, 1993.

Hardy, V.M., Capuano, E.F. and Worsam, B. The effect of care programmes on dependency status of elderly residents in extended care facilities. *Adv Nurs* 7:295–300, 1982.

Harkins, S.W., Price, D.D. and Martelli, M. Effects of age on pain perception: Thermonociception. *J Gerontol* 41:58–63, 1986.

Harms, M. Effect of wheelchair design on posture and comfort of users. *Physiotherapy* 76:266–271, 1990.

Harper, C.M. and Lyles, Y.M. Physiology and complications of bed rest. *J Am Geriatr Soc* 36:1047–1054, 1988.

Harris, T., Kovar, M.G., Suzman, R. et al. Longitudinal study of physical ability in the oldest-old. *Am J Public Health* 79:698–702, 1989.

Hart, L.K., Freel, M.I. and Milde, F.K. Fatigue. *Nurs Clin North Am* 25(4):967–975, 1990.

Harver, A., Mahler, D.A. and Daubenspeck, J.A. Targeted inspiratory muscle training improves respiratory muscle function and reduces dyspnea in patients with chronic obstructive pulmonary disease. *Ann Intern Med* 111:117–124, 1989.

Hayter, J. Sleep behaviors of older persons. *Nurs Res* 32(4):242–246, 1983.

Heinemann, A.W., Linacre, J.M., Wright, B.D. et al. Relationships between impairment and physical disability as measured by the functional independence measure. *Arch Phys Med Rehab* 74:566–573, 1993.

Hellon, R.F., Lind, A.R. and Weiner, J.S. The physiological reactions of men of two age groups to a hot environment. *J Physiol* 133:118, 1956.

Hensyl, W. *Stedman's Medical Dictionary.* 25th ed. Baltimore: Williams & Wilkins, 1990.

Hillman, J.L. and Stricker, G. A linkage of knowledge and attitudes toward elderly sexuality: Not necessarily a uniform relationship. *Gerontologist* 34:256–260, 1994.

Hing, E. Nursing home utilization by current residents: US, 1985. *Vital and Health Statistics,* Series 13: Data from the National Health Survey, No. 102, 1989.

Hirsch, B.E. and Weksler, M.E. Normal changes in host defense. *In* Abrams, W.B. and Berkow, W. (eds.). *Merck Manual of Geriatrics.* Rahway, NJ: Merck and Company, 1990.

Hirsch, C.H., Sommers, L., Olsen, A. et al. The natural history of functional morbidity in hospitalized older patients. *J Am Geriatr Soc* 38:1296–1303, 1990.

Hirsh, D.D., Fainstein, V. and Musher, D.M. Do condom catheter collecting systems cause urinary tract infection? *JAMA* 242:340–341, 1979.

Hirschmann, J.V. Normal body temperature. *JAMA* 267:414, 1992.

Hogan, C.M. Advances in the management of nausea and vomiting. *Nurs Clin North Am* 25(2):475–497, 1990.

Hogue, C.C. Mobility. *In* Schneider, E.L. et al. (eds.). *The Teaching Nursing Home: A New Approach to Geriatric Research, Education, and Clinical Care.* New York: Raven Press, 1985.

Hogue, C.C. and Cullinan, S. Exercise training for frail rural elderly: A pilot study. *In* Funk, S.G., Tornquist, E.M., Champagne, M.T. and Wiese, R.A. (eds.). *Key Aspects of Caring for the Chronically Ill: Hospital and Home.* New York: Springer Publishing Company, 1992, pp. 202–211.

Hogue, C.C., Cullinan, S. and McConnell, E.S. Exercise interventions for the chronically ill: Review and prospects. *In* Funk, S.G., Tornquist, E.M., Champagne, M.T. and Wiese, R.A. (eds.). *Key Aspects of Caring for the Chronically Ill: Hospital and Home.* New York: Springer Publishing Company, 1993, pp. 59–78.

Holroyd, S., Rabins, P.V., Finkelstein, D. et al. Visual hallucinations in patients with macular degeneration. *Am J Psychiatry* 149:1701–1706, 1992.

Holtzclaw, B.J. Shivering: A clinical nursing problem. *Nurs Clin North Am* 25(4):977–987, 1990.

Holtzclaw, B.J. The febrile response in critical care: State of the science. *Heart Lung* 21(5):482–501, 1992.

Hu, T.W. Impact of urinary incontinence on health-care costs. *J Am Geriatr Soc* 38(3):292–295, 1990.

Hu, T.W., Igou, J.F., Kaltreider, D.L. et al. A clinical trial of a behavioral therapy to reduce urinary incontinence in nursing homes. Outcome and implications. *JAMA* 261:2656–2662, 1989.

Immunization Practices Advisory Committee. Diphtheria, tetanus, and pertussis: Guidelines for vaccine prophylaxis and other preventative measures. *Morbid Mortal Weekly Rep* 34:405–414, 419–426, 1985.

Immunization Practices Advisory Committee. Pneumococcal polysaccharide vaccine. *Morbid Mortal Weekly Rep* 38:64–76, 1989a.

Immunization Practices Advisory Committee. Prevention and control of influenza. *Morbid Mortal Weekly Rep* 38:297–311, 1989b.

Incalzi, R.A., Gemma, A., Capparella, O. et al. Predicting mortality and length of stay of geriatric patients in an acute care general hospital. *J Gerontol* 47:M35–M39, 1992.

Ingersoll, G.L. Respiratory muscle fatigue research: Implications for clinical practice. *Appl Nurs Res* 2(1):6–15, 1989.

Inman, K.J., Sibbald, W.J., Rutledge, F.S. et al. Clinical utility and cost effectiveness of an air-suspension bed in the prevention of pressure ulcers. *JAMA* 269(9): 1139–1143, 1993.

Inouye, S.K. Clarifying confusion: The confusion assessment method. *Ann Intern Med* 113(12):941–947, 1990.

International Continence Society. Report of the Committee for the Standardization of Terminology of Lower Urinary Tract Function. *Br J Obstet Gynaecol* (Suppl) 6: 1–16, 1990.

Ireton, R.C., Krieger, J.N., Cardenas, D.D. et al. Bladder volume determination using a dedicated, portable ultrasound scanner. *J Urol* 143(5):909–911, 1990.

Irwin, S.C. Cardiac rehabilitation for the geriatric patient. *Topics Geriatr Rehab* 2(1):44–54, 1986.

Issacs, B. and Kennie, A.T. The set test as an aid to the detection of dementia in old people. *Br J Psychiatry* 123:467–470, 1973.

Jackson, M.M., Fierer, J., Barrett-Connor, E. et al. Intensive surveillance for infections in a three-year study of nursing home patients. *Am J Epidemiol* 135:685–696, 1992.

Jacobs, J.W., Bernhard, M.R., Delgado, A. and Strain, J.J. Screening for organic mental syndromes in the medically ill. *Ann Intern Med* 86:40–46, 1977.

Janus, S.S. and Janus, C.L. *The Janus Report on Sexual Behavior.* New York: John Wiley & Sons, 1993.

Jaycox, A. Key aspects of comfort. *In* Funk, S.G., Tornquist, E.M., Champagne, M.T. et al. (eds.). *Key Aspects of Comfort: Management of Pain, Fatigue, and Nausea.* New York: Springer Publishing Company, 1989, pp. 8–22.

Jaycox, A. Toward inclusiveness of scope in nursing diagnosis. *In* Carroll-Johnson, R.M. and Paquette, M. (eds.). *Classification of Nursing Diagnoses: Proceedings of the Tenth Conference.* Philadelphia: J. B. Lippincott, 1994, pp. 17–26.

Jeter, K., Faller, N. and Norton, C. *Nursing for Continence.* Philadelphia: W. B. Saunders, 1990.

Jette, A.M. and Branch, L.G. Musculoskeletal impairment among the non-institutionalized aged. *Int Rehab Med* 6:157–161, 1984.

Johnson, M.I., Ashton, C.H. and Thompson, J.W. An in-depth study of long-term users of transcutaneous electrical nerve stimulation (TENS): Implications for clinical use of TENS. *Pain* 44:221–229, 1991.

Jones, J.A., Niessen, L.C., Hobbins, M.J. and Zocchi, M.C. Oral health care for patients with Alzheimer's disease. *In* Volicer, L., Fabiszewski, K.J., Rheaume, Y.L. and Lasch, K.E. (eds.). *Clinical Management of Alzheimer's Disease.* Rockville, MD: Aspen Publishers, 1988.

Kahn, R.L., Goldfarb, A.I., Pollack, M. and Peck, A. Brief objective measures for the determination of mental status in the aged. *Am J Psychiatr* 117:326–328, 1960.

Keefe, F.J. Behavioral assessment and treatment of chronic pain: Current status and future directions. *J Consult Clin Psychol* 50:896–911, 1982.

Keil, J.E. et al. Self-reported sexual functioning in elderly blacks and whites: The Charleston Heart Study experience. *J Aging Health* 4(1):112–125, 1992.

Kelly-Hayes, M., Jette, A.M., Wolf, P.A. et al. Functional limitations and disability among elders in the Framingham Study. *Am J Public Health* 82:841–845, 1992.

Kendig, N.E. and Adler, W. The implications of the acquired immunodeficiency syndrome for gerontology research and geriatric medicine. *J Gerontol Med Sci* 45: M77–M81, 1990.

Kersten, L.D. *Comprehensive Respiratory Nursing: A Decision-Making Approach*. Philadelphia: W. B. Saunders, 1989.

Kiernan, R.J., Mueller, J., Langston, W. and Van Dyke, C. The neurobehavioral cognitive screening examination: A brief but differentiated approach to cognitive assessment. *Ann Intern Med* 107:481–485, 1987.

Kinnunen, O. Study of constipation in a geriatric hospital, day hospital, old people's home and at home. *Aging* 3:161–170, 1991.

Kiyak, H.A., Grayston, M.N. and Crinean, C.L. Oral health problems and needs of nursing home residents. *Commun Dent Oral Epidemiol* 21:49–52, 1993.

Kollarits, C.R. The aging eye. *In* Calkins, E., Ford, A.B. and Katz, P. (eds.). *Practice of Geriatrics*. 2nd ed. Philadelphia: W. B. Saunders, 1992, Chap. 26.

Kolcaba, K.Y. Holistic comfort: Operationalizing the construct as a nurse-sensitive outcome. *Adv Nurs Sci* 15(1):1–10, 1992.

Koller, W.C. How accurately can Parkinson's disease be diagnosed? *Neurology* 42:S6–S16, 1992.

Kottke, F.J. Therapeutic exercise to maintain mobility. *In* Kottke, F.J. and Lehmann, P. (eds.). *Krusen's Handbook of Physical Medicine and Rehabilitation*. 4th ed. Philadelphia: W. B. Saunders, 1990, Chap. 18.

Kovar, M.G. and LaCroix, A.Z. Aging in the eighties: Ability to perform work-related activities. *Nat Center Health Statistics Adv Data* 136:1–2, 1987.

Kovar, P.A., Allegrante, J.P., MacKenzie, C.R. et al. Supervised fitness walking in patients with osteoarthritis of the knee: A randomized, controlled trial. *Ann Intern Med* 116:529–534, 1992.

Kris, M., Gralla, R., Tyson, L. et al. Controlling delayed vomiting: Double-blind, randomized trial comparing placebo, dexamethasone alone, and metoclopramide plus dexamethasone in patients receiving cisplatin. *J Clin Oncol* 3:1379–1384, 1989.

Krupp, L.B., LaRocca, N.G., Muir-Nash, J. and Stinberg, A. The fatigue severity scale: Application to patients with multiple sclerosis and systemic lupus erythematosus. *Arch Neurol* 46:1121–1123, 1989.

Kuhn, J.K. and McGovern, M. Peripheral vascular assessment of the elderly client. *J Gerontol Nurs* 18(12): 35–38, 1992.

Kunin, C.M., Douthitt, S., Dancing, J. et al. The association between the use of urinary catheters and morbidity and mortality among elderly patients in nursing homes. *Am J Epidemiol* 135:291–301, 1992.

Kuriansky, J. and Gurland, B. The performance test of activities of daily living. *Int J Aging Hum Dev* 7:343–352, 1976.

Kusler, D.L. and Rambur, B.A. Treatment for radiation-induced xerostomia: An innovative remedy. *Cancer Nurs* 15(3):191–195, 1992.

Lagana, F.J. Dermatologic pedal manifestations in the elderly. *Topics Geriatr Rehab* 7(3):14–23, 1992.

Larson, P., Halliburton, P. and DiJulio, J. Nausea, vomiting and retching. *In* Carrieri-Kohlman, V., Lindsey, A.M. and West, C.M. (eds.). *Pathophysiological Phenomena in Nursing*. 2nd ed. Philadelphia: W. B. Saunders, 1993, Chap. 15.

Lawton, M.P. The impact of the environment on aging and behavior. *In* Birren, J.E. and Schaie, K.L.W. (eds.). *Handbook of the Psychology of Aging*. New York: Van Nostrand Reinhold, 1985, pp. 703–724.

Lee, K.A., Hicks, G. and Nino-Murcia, G. Validity and reliability of a scale to assess fatigue. *Psychiatry Res* 36: 291–298, 1991.

Lee, V.K. Language changes in Alzheimer's disease: A literature review. *J Gerontol Nurs* 17(1):16–20, 1991.

Leidy, N.K. Functional status and the forward progress of merry-go-rounds: Toward a coherent analytical framework. *Nurs Res* 43:196–202, 1994.

Lentz, M. Selected aspects of deconditioning secondary to immobilization. *Nurs Clin North Am* 16:729, 1981.

Lerune, J.M. Leg ulcers: Differential Diagnosis in the elderly. *Geriatrics* 45(6):32–34, 39–42, 1990.

Leslie, L.R. Training in homemaking activities. *In* Kottke, F.J. and Lehmann, P. (eds.). *Krusen's Handbook of Physical Medicine and Rehabilitation*. 4th ed. Philadelphia: W. B. Saunders, 1990, Chap. 25.

Levenson, S.A. Infection control roles and responsibilities. *In* Levenson, S.A. (ed.). *Medical Direction in Long-Term Care*. 2nd ed. Durham, N.C.: Carolina Academic Press, 1993, pp. 305–319.

Levine, J.M. Leg ulcers: differential diagnosis in the elderly. *Geriatrics* 45(6):32–34, 39–42, 1990.

Lew, J.F., Glass, R.I., Gangarosa, R.E. et al. Diarrheal deaths in the US, 1979–1987. *JAMA* 265:3280–3284, 1991.

Lewis, C.B. *Improving Mobility in Older Persons: A Manual for Geriatric Specialists*. Rockville, MD: Aspen Publishing, 1989.

Lewis, C.B. and Campanelli, L.C. *Health Promotion and Exercise for Older Adults: An Instructors' Guide*. Rockville, MD: Aspen Publishers, 1990.

Lewis-Cullinan, C. and Janken, J.K. Effect of cerumen removal on the hearing ability of geriatric patients. *J Adv Nurs* 15:594–600, 1990.

Libow, L. A rapidly administered, easily remembered mental status evaluation: FROMAJE. *In* Libow, L. and Sherman, F. (eds.). *The Core of Geriatric Medicine*. St. Louis: C.V. Mosby, 1981, pp. 85–91.

Lieberman, H.R., Wurtman, J.J. and Teicher, M.H. Circadian rhythms of activity in healthy young and elderly humans. *Neurobiol Aging* 10:259–265, 1989.

Lighthouse, Inc. *The Lighthouse Low Vision Products Consumer Catalog*. New York: Lighthouse, Inc., 800 Second Ave, New York, N.Y. 10017, 1991–92.

Lipe, H., Longstreth, W.T., Jr., Bird, T.D. and Linde, M. Sexual function in married men with Parkinson's disease compared to married men with arthritis. *Neurology* 40:1347–1349, 1990.

Lipschitz, S., Campbell, A.J., Roberts, M.S. et al. Subcutaneous fluid administration in elderly subjects: Validation of an underused technique. *J. Amer. Ger. Soc.* 39:6–9, 1991.

Lovell, H. and Anderson, C. Put your patient on the right bed. *RN* May:66–72, 1990.

Maas, M.L., Hall, G.R., Specht, J.P. and Buckwalter, K.C. Dedicated, not isolated: Development of long-term care Alzheimer's units. *In* Buckwalter, K.C. (ed.). *Geriatric Mental Health Nursing: Current and Future Challenges*. Thorofare, N.J.: Slack, Inc., 1992, Chap. 4.

Macey, S.M. and Schneider, D.F. Deaths from excessive heat and excessive cold among the elderly. *Gerontologist* 33:497–500, 1993.

Macphee, G.J., Crother, J.A. and McAlpine, C.H. A simple screening test for hearing impairment in elderly persons. *Age Aging* 17:347–351, 1988.

Mahler, D.A. and Harver, A. Clinical measurement of dypnea. *In* Mahler, D.A. (ed.). *Dyspnea*. Mt. Kisco, N.Y.: Futura Publishing, 1990, pp. 75–126.

Mahler, D.A. and O'Donnell, D.E. Alternative modes of

exercise training for pulmonary patients. *J Cardiopulm Rehab* 11:58–63, 1991.

Mahoney, D.F. Hearing loss among nursing home residents. *Clin Nurs Res* 1(4):317–332, 1992.

Mahoney, J., Euhardy, R. and Carnes, M. A comparison of a two-wheeled walker and three-wheeled walker in a geriatric population. *J Am Geriatr Soc* 40:208–212, 1992.

Mangione, C.M., Phillips, R.S., Seddon, J.M. et al. Development of the "Activities of Daily Vision Scale:" A measure of visual functional status. *Med Care* 30:111–126, 1992.

Manton, K.G., Corder, L.S. and Stallard, E. Estimates of change in chronic disability and institutional incidence and prevalence rates in the U.S. elderly population from the 1982, 1984, and 1989 national long-term care surveys. *J Gerontol Soc Sci* 48:S153, 1993.

Marsiglio, W. and Donnelly, D. Sexual relations in later life: A national study of married persons. *J Gerontol Soc Sci* 46:S338–S344, 1991.

McCaffery, M. and Beebe, A. *Pain: Clinical Manual for Nursing Practice*. St. Louis, C.V. Mosby, 1989.

McConnell, E.S., Neelon, V.J. and Champagne, M.T. The relationship between nutritional status and cognitive status in the hospitalized elderly. *In* Funk, S.G., Tornquist, E.M., Champagne, M.T. et al. (eds.). *Key Aspects of Recovery: Nutrition, Mobility and Sleep*. New York: Springer Publishing Company, 1990, pp. 8–22.

McCourt, A.E. Syndromes in nursing: A continuing concern. *In* Carroll-Johnson, R.M. (ed.). *Classification of Nursing Diagnoses: Proceedings of the Ninth Conference*. Philadelphia: J. B. Lippincott, 1991.

McFarland, G.K. and Nashinski, C.E. Impaired communication. *Nurs Clin North Am* 20:775–785, 1985.

McGavin, C.R., Artvinli, M., Naoe, H. and McHardy, G.J.R. Dyspnea, disability and distance walked: Comparison of estimates of exercise performance in respiratory disease. *Br Med J* 2:241–243, 1978.

McMillan, S., Johnston, L., Tedford, K. and Harley, C. Measurement of chemotherapy-induced nausea and vomiting. *Appl Nurs Res* 2:93–95, 1989.

Mehr, D.R., Foxman, B. and Colombo, P. Risk factors for mortality from lower respiratory tract infections in nursing home patients. *J Fam Prac* 34:585–592, 1992.

Melzack, R. The McGill Pain Questionnaire. *In* Melzack, R. (eds.). *Pain Measurement and Assessment*. New York: Raven Press, 1983, pp. 41–47.

Memmer, M.K. Acute orthostatic hypotension. *Heart Lung* 17:134–141, 1988.

Mermelstein, R., Miller, B., Prohaska, T. et al. Measures of health. *In* Van Nostrand, J.F., Furner, S.E. and Suzman, R. (eds.). *Vital and Health Statistics: Health Data on Older Americans: U.S., 1992*. Series 3: Analytic and Epidemiological Studies No. 27. Hyattsville, MD: U.S. Department of Health and Human Services Publication No. PHS 93-1411, 1993.

Miles, S.H. and Irvine, P. Deaths caused by physical restraints. *Gerontologist* 32:762–766, 1992.

Mitchell, C.A. Generalized chronic fatigue in the elderly: Assessment and intervention. *J Gerontol Nurs* 12(4):19–23, 1986.

Mito, M.J. Aging and motor speech production. *Topics Geriatr Rehab* 1(4):29–44, 1986.

Molenbroek, J.F.M. Anthropometry of the elderly people in the Netherlands: Research and applications. *Appl Ergonomics* 18:187–199, 1987.

Morin, C.M., Kowatch, R.A., Barry, T. and Walton, E. Cognitive-behavior therapy for late-life insomnia. *J Consult Clin Psychol* 61:137–146, 1993.

Morris, J.N., Hawes, C., Fries, B.E. et al. Designing the national resident assessment instrument for nursing homes. *Gerontologist* 30:293–307, 1990.

Morrow, G. The assessment of nausea and vomiting:

Past problems, current issues and suggestions for future research. *Cancer* 53:51–62, 1984.

Murray, A.M., Levkoff, S.E., Welte, T.T. et al. Acute delirium and functional decline in the hospitalized elderly patient. *J Gerontol Med Sci* 48:M181–M186, 1993.

Myers, A.M., Holliday, P.J., Harvey, K.A. and Hutchinson, K.S. Functional performance measures: Are they superior to self-assessments? *J Gerontol Med Sci* 48:M196–M206, 1993.

Nagi, S. Disability concepts revisited: Implications for prevention. *In* Pope, A.M. and Tarlov, A.R. (eds.). *Disability in America: Toward a National Agenda for Prevention*. Washington, DC: National Academy Press, 1991, pp. 309–327.

Nagi, S. An epidemiology of disability among adults in the United States. *Milbank Mem Fund Q*, Fall, 1976.

National Institutes of Health. NIH Consensus Development Conference Statement: The treatment of sleep disorders of older people. *Assoc Prof Sleep Soc* 14:169–177, 1990.

National Institutes of Health. *NIH Consensus Statement: Impotence*. 10(4):1–31, 1992.

National Institutes of Health Consensus Development Conference. The Integrated Approach to the Management of Pain. *J Pain Sympt Manage* 2:35–44, 1987.

National Institutes of Health Consensus Development Panel. *Consensus Statement: Oral Complications of Cancer Therapies*. National Cancer Institute Monographs No. 9, 1990, pp. 1–8.

Neelon, V.J., Champagne, M.T., McConnell, E. et al. Use of the Neecham Confusion Scale to assess acute confusional states of hospitalized older patients. *In* Funk, S.G., Tornquist, E.M., Champagne, M.T. and Wiese, R.A. (eds.). *Key Aspects of Elder Care: Managing Falls, Incontinence and Cognitive Impairment*. New York: Springer, 1992, pp. 278–288.

Newman, D.K., Lynch, K., Smith, D.A. et al. Restoring urinary continence. *Am J Nurs* 91:28–34, 1991.

Ney, D.F. Cerumen impaction, ear hygiene practices and hearing acuity. *Geriatr Nurs* Mar/April, 1993.

Nieweg, R., Tinteren, J., Poelhuis, E.K. and Abraham-Inpija, L. Nursing care for oral complications associated with chemotherapy. *Cancer Nurs* 15(5):313–321, 1992.

Norris, C.M. *Concept Clarification in Nursing*. Rockville, MD: Aspen Publishers, 1982.

North American Nursing Diagnosis Association. *NANDA Nursing Diagnoses: Definitions and Classification 1992–1993*. Philadelphia: J. B. Lippincott, 1992.

Norton, D., McLaren, R.S., Exton-Smith, A.N. Pressure sores. *In Investigation of Geriatric Nursing Problems in Hospitals*. London: The National Corporation for the Care of Old People, 1962.

O'Donnell, D.E., Webb, K.A. and McGuire, M.A. Older patients with COPD: Benefits of exercise training. 48(1):59–66, 1993.

Olson, E.V. The hazards of immobility. *Am J Nurs* 67:779–793, 1967.

Osler, W. *The Principles and Practice of Medicine*. New York: D. Appleton and Company, 1892, p. 511.

Osler, W. *The Principles and Practice of Medicine*. 3rd ed. New York: D. Appleton and Company, 1898, p. 109.

O'Sullivan, S.B. Motor control assessment. *In* O'Sullivan, S.B. and Schmitz, T.J. (eds.). *Physical Rehabilitation: Assessment and Treatment*. 2nd ed. Philadelphia: F. A. Davis, 1988, Chap. 9.

O'Toole, M. (ed.). *Miller-Keane Encyclopedia and Dictionary of Medicine, Nursing and Allied Health*. 5th ed. Philadelphia: W. B. Saunders, 1992.

Parmalee, P.A., Katz, I.R. and Lawton, M.P. The relation of pain to depression among institutionalized aged. *J Gerontol Psychol Sci* 46:P155, 1991.

Pearson, R.G. Scale analysis of a fatigue checklist. *J Appl Psychol* 41:186–191, 1957.

Peck, S.A. Crush syndrome: Pathophysiology and management. *Ortho Nurs* 9(3):33–38, 1990.

Peppard, N.R. *Special Needs Dementia Units: Design, Development and Operations.* New York: Springer Publishing Company, 1991, p. 76.

Pfeiffer, E. A short portable mental status questionnaire for the assessment of organic brain deficits in elderly patients. *J Am Geriatr Soc* 23:433–441, 1975.

Phair, J. and Reisberg, B. Nosocomial infections. *In* Fox, R.A. (ed.). *Immunology and Infection in the Elderly.* New York: Churchill Livingstone, 1984, Chap. 4.

Phair, J., Reising, K.S. and Metzger, E. Bacteremic infection and malnutrition in patients with solid tumors: Investigation of host defense mechanisms. *Cancer* 45: 2702, 1980.

Phillips, L.R.F. Care of the client with sensoriperceptual problems. *In* Wolanin, M.O. and Phillips, L.R.F. *Confusion: Prevention and Care.* St. Louis: C.V. Mosby, 1981, Chap. 10.

Phillips, P.A., Bretherton, M., Johnston, C.I. and Gray, L. Reduced osmotic thirst in healthy elderly men. *Am J Physiol* 261:R166–R171, 1991.

Piper, B.F. Fatigue: Current bases for practice. *In* Funk, S.G., Tornquist, E.M., Champagne, M.T. et al. (eds.). *Key Aspects of Comfort: Management of Pain, Fatigue, and Nausea.* New York: Springer Publishing Company, 1989, pp. 187–198.

Piper, B.F. Fatigue. *In* Carrieri-Kohlman, V., Lindsey, A.M. and West, C.M. (eds.). *Pathophysiological Phenomena in Nursing.* 2nd ed. Philadelphia: W. B. Saunders, 1993, Chap. 12.

Plewa, M.C. Altered host response and special infections in the elderly. *Emerg Med Clin North Am* 8(2): 193–206, 1990.

Pollock, M.L. and Wilmore, J.H. *Exercise in Health and Disease.* 2nd ed. Philadelphia: W. B. Saunders, 1990.

Potempa, K. Chronic Fatigue: Directions for research and practice. *In* Funk, S.G., Tornquist, E., Champagne, M.T., Copp, L.A., and Wise, R.A. (eds.). *Key Aspects of Comfort: Management of Pain, Fatigue, and Nausea.* New York: Springer, 1989, pp. 229–233.

Price, M.E. and DiIorio, C. Swallowing: A practice guide. *Am J Nurs* 90(7):43–46, 1990.

Puntillo, K. and Tesler, M.D. Pain. *In* Carrieri-Kohlman, V., Lindsey, A.M. and West, C.M. (eds.). *Pathophysiological Phenomena in Nursing.* 2nd ed. Philadelphia: W. B. Saunders 1993, Chap. 13.

Rechnitzer, P.A. Exercise, fitness and coronary heart disease. *In* Bouchard, C., Shepard, R.J., Stephens, T. et al. (eds.). *Exercise, Fitness and Health: A Consensus of Current Knowledge.* Champaign, Ill.: Human Kinetics Books, 1990, pp. 451–453.

Redford, J. Seating and wheeled mobility. *Arch Phys Med Rehabil* 74:877–885, 1993.

Reich, N. and Otten, P. What to wear: A challenge for disabled elders. *Am J Nurs* 87:207–210, 1987.

Reichman, W.E. and Cummings, J.L. Dementia. *In* Calkins, E., Ford, A.B. and Katz, P. (eds.). *Practice of Geriatrics.* 2nd ed. Philadelphia: W. B. Saunders, 1992, pp. 294–304.

Reimer, M. Impaired nonverbal communication: A photo investigation. *In* Carroll-Johnson, R.M. (ed.). *Classification of Nursing Diagnoses: Proceedings of the Ninth Conference.* Philadelphia: J. B. Lippincott, 1994, p. 331.

Reuben, D.B. and Siu, A. An objective measure of physical function of elderly outpatients: The physical performance test. *J Am Geriatr Soc* 38:1105–1112, 1990.

Reuben, D.B., Siu, A. and Kimpau, S. The predictive validity of self-report and performance-based measures of function and health. *J Gerontol Med Sci* 47:M106–M110, 1992.

Rhodes, V.A., Watson, P.M., Johnson, M.H. et al. Post-chemotherapy nausea and vomiting. *In* Funk et al. (eds.). *Key Aspects of Comfort: Management of Pain, Fatigue and Nausea.* New York: Springer, 1989, pp. 248–258.

Rhoten, D. Fatigue and the post-surgical patient. *In* Norris, C.M. (ed.). *Concept Clarification in Nursing.* Rockville, MD: Aspen Systems, 1982, pp. 277–300.

Ries, A.L., Ellis, B. and Hawkins, R.W. Upper extremity exercise training in chronic obstructive pulmonary disease. *Chest* 93:688–692, 1988.

Rizzo III, J.F., Cronin-Golumb, A., Growdon, J.H. et al. Retinocalcarine function in Alzheimer's disease: A clinical and electrophysiological study. *Arch Neurol* 49:93–101, 1992.

Roark, A.C. One man's pain brings verdict on nursing home. *News and Observer,* Raleigh, N.C., Dec. 12, 1991, p. 10B.

Robbins, A.S. Hypothermia and heat stroke: Protecting the elderly patient. *Geriatrics* 44(1):73–80, 1989.

Roberts, M.F. Diarrhea: A symptom. *Holistic Nurse Pract* 7(2):73–80, 1993.

Robinson, C.R. Impaired sleep. *In* Carrieri-Kohlman, V., Lindsey, A.M. and West, C.M. (eds.). *Pathophysiological Phenomena in Nursing: Human Responses to Illness.* Philadelphia: W. B. Saunders, 1993, Chap. 20.

Robinson, D. A collection of papers concerning application of the International Classification of Impairments, Disabilities and Handicaps. *Intl Rehabil Med* 7:60, 1985.

Rockwood, K. The occurrence and duration of symptoms in elderly patients with delirium. *J Gerontol* 48: M162–M166, 1993.

Rodysill, R.J., Hansen, L. and O'Leary, J.J. Cutaneous delayed hypersensitivity in nursing homes and geriatric clinic patients. Implications for the tuberculin test. *J Am Geriatr Soc* 37:435–443, 1989.

Roland, M. and Morris, R. A study of the natural history of back pain—part I: Development of a reliability and sensitive measure of disability in low-back pain. *Spine* 8(2):141–144, 1983.

Rose, M.A., Baigis-Smith, J., Smith, D. and Newman, D. Behavioral management of urinary incontinence in homebound older adults. *Home Healthcare Nurse* 8(5): 10–15, 1990.

Rosenberg, I.H. and Miller, J.W. Nutritional factors in physical and cognitive functions of elderly people. *Am J Clin Nutr* 55:1237S–1243S, 1992.

Ross, D. Acute compartment syndrome: *Ortho Nurs* 10(2):33–38, 1991.

Ross, J. and Dean, E. Integrating physiological principles into the comprehensive management of cardiopulmonary dysfunction. *Phys Ther* 69:255–259, 1989.

Roth, P.T. and Creason, N.S. Nurse-administered oral hygiene: Is there a scientific basis? *J Adv Nurs* 11:323–331, 1986.

Rudberg, M.A., Furner, S.E., Dunn, J.E. and Cassel, C.K. The relationship of visual and hearing impairments to disability: An analysis using the longitudinal study of aging. *J Gerontol Med Sci* 48:M261–M265, 1993.

Rudman, D. and Cohan, M.E. Nutrition in the elderly. *In* Calkins, E., Ford, A.B., and Katz, P. (eds.). *Practice of Geriatrics.* 2nd ed. Philadelphia: W. B. Saunders, 1992, pp. 19–32.

Saltzman, A.R. Pulmonary disorders. *In* Calkins, E., Ford, A.B. and Katz, P. (eds.). *Practice of Geriatrics.* 2nd ed. Philadelphia: W. B. Saunders, 1992, pp. 429–435.

Salvage, A. Old people in hot weather: Commentary. *Age Ageing* 20:233–235, 1991.

Satlin, A., Volicer, L., Ross, V. et al. Bright light treatment of behavioral and sleep disturbances in patients with Alzheimer's disease. *Am J Psychiatry* 149:1028–1032, 1992.

Schmitt, R. Double meanings: The patient with Alzheimer's. *Am J Nurs* October, 1992, p. 33.

Schmitz, T.M. The semi-prone position in ARDS: Five case studies. *Crit Care Nurs* 11(5):22–33, 1991.

Schnelle, J.F. Treatment of urinary incontinence nursing home patients by prompted voiding. *J Am Geriatr Soc* 38(3):356–360, 1990.

Schnelle, J.F., Newman, D.R. and Fogarty, T.E. Management of patient continence in long-term care nursing facilities. *Gerontologist* 30(3):373–376, 1990.

Schnelle, J.F., Ouslander, J.G., Simmons, S.F. et al. Nighttime sleep and bed mobility among incontinent nursing home residents. *J Am Geriatr Soc* 41:903–909, 1993a.

Schnelle, J.F., Ouslander, J.G., Simmons, S.F. et al. The nighttime environment, incontinence care, and sleep disruption in nursing homes. *J Am Geriatr Soc* 41:910–914, 1993b.

Schow, R.L., Christensen, J.M. et al. (eds.). *Communication Disorders of the Aged.* Baltimore, University Park Press, 1978.

Schultz, A.B. Mobility impairment in the elderly: Challenges for biomechanics research. *J Biomechanics* 25:519–528, 1992.

Schwartz, D. Remarks made at University of Pennsylvania School of Nursing, Robert Wood Johnson Foundation Conference on Development of Teaching Nursing Home Proposals, Aug. 31, 1981.

Scott, J. and Huskisson, E.C. Graphic representation of pain. *Pain* 2:175–184, 1976.

Sengstaken, E.A. and King, S.A. The problems of pain and its detection among geriatric nursing home residents. *J Am Geriatr Soc* 41:541–544, 1993.

Shapiro, E.D., Berg, A.T., Austrian, R. et al. The protective efficacy of polyvalent polysaccharide vaccine. *N Engl J Med* 325:1453–1460, 1991.

Shaw, G. and Taylor, S.J. A survey of seating problems of the institutionalized elderly. *Assistive Technol* 3:5–10, 1991.

Shemansky, C.A. Choking: Clear and present danger for elders. *Geriatr Nurs* Mar/Apr: 68–71, 1991.

Shepard, R.J. The scientific basis of exercise prescribing for the very old. *J Am Geriatr Soc* 38:62–70, 1990.

Ship, J.A. Oral sequelae of common geriatric disease, disorders and impairments. *Clin Geriatr Med* 8(3):483–497, 1992.

Siebens, H. Practical issues in physical medicine, rehabilitation and pain management. *In* Calkins, E., Ford, A.B. and Katz, P. (eds.). *Practice of Geriatrics.* 2nd ed. Philadelphia: W. B. Saunders, 1992.

Simko, L.C. Cardiac rehabilitation in the long-term care setting. *In* Glickstein, J. (ed.) *Focus on Geriatric Care and Rehabilitation.* 6(8):1–9, 1993, pp. 1–9.

Sims, R.V., Boyko, E.J., Maislin, G. et al. The role of age in susceptibility to pneumococcal infections. *Age Ageing* 21:357–361, 1992.

Sims, R.V., Steinmann, W.C., McConville, J.H. et al. The clinical effectiveness of pneumococcal vaccine in the elderly. *Ann Intern Med* 108(5):653–657, 1988.

Sloane, P.D., Hartman, M. and Mitchell, C.M. Psychological factors associated with chronic dizziness in patients aged 60 and older. *J Am Geriatr Soc* 42:847–852, 1994.

Smith, P.W. (ed.). *Infection Control in Long-Term Care Facilities.* New York: John Wiley & Sons, 1989.

Smith, P.W., Daly, P.B. and Roccaforte, J.E. Current status of nosocomial infection control in extended care facilities. *Am J Med* 91(Suppl 3B):281S–285S, 1991.

Snow, T.L. and McConnell, E.S. Bowel and Bladder Management Protocols. Unpublished educational aids for workshops on bowel and bladder management. Chapel Hill, N.C.: University of North Carolina, 1985.

Sonnenberg, A. and Koch, T.R. Physician visits in the U.S. for constipation: 1958 to 1986. *Dig Dis Sci* 34:606–611, 1989.

Spector, W. and Takada, H.A. Characteristics of nursing homes that affect resident outcomes. *J Aging Health* 3(4):427–453, 1991.

Spirduso, W.W. and McCrae, P.G. Motor performance and aging. *In* Birren, J.E. and Schaie, K.W. (eds.). *Handbook of the Psychology of Aging.* 3rd ed. San Diego: Academic Press, 1990.

Steele, B. and Shaver, J. The dyspnea experience: Nociceptive properties and a model for research and practice. *Adv Nurs Sci* 15(1):64–76, 1992.

Steinke, E. Older adults' knowledge and attitudes about sexuality and aging. *Image* 20(2):93–95, 1988.

Stewart, R.B., Moore, M.T., May, F.E. et al. Nocturia: A risk factor for falls in the elderly. *J Am Geriatr Soc* 40:1217–1220, 1992.

Stoedefalke, K.G. Motivating and sustaining the older adult in an exercise program. *Topics Geriatr Rehab* 1(1):31–39, 1985.

Stone, J.T. Managing bowel function. *In* Chenitz, W.C., Stone, J.T. and Salisbury, S.A. (eds.). *Clinical Gerontological Nursing: A Guide to Advanced Practice.* Philadelphia: W. B. Saunders, 1991.

Stone, S.P., Halligan, P.W. and Greenwood, R.J. The incidence of neglect phenomena and related disorders in patients with an acute right or left hemispheric stroke. *Age Ageing* 22:46–52, 1993.

Strassburg, M.A., Greenland, S., Sorviollo, F.J. et al. Influenza in the elderly: Report of an outbreak and a review of vaccine effectiveness reports. *Vaccine* 4:38–44, 1986.

Strumpf, N. and Evans, L. Physical restraint of the hospitalized elderly: Perceptions of nurses and patients. *Nurs Res* 37:132, 1988.

Sullivan, D.H., Martin, W., Flaxman, N. and Hagen, J. Oral health problems and involuntary weight loss in a population of frail elderly. *J Am Geriatr Soc* 41:725–731, 1993.

Summers, S. Hypothermia: One nursing diagnosis or three? *Nurs Diagn* 3(1):2–11, 1992.

Swearingen, P. *Manual of Nursing Therapeutics: Applying Nursing Diagnoses to Medical Disorders.* Reading, MA: Addison-Wesley, 1986.

Tam, M. and Moschella, S.C. Vascular skin ulcers of limbs. *Cardiol Clin* 9(3):555–563, 1991.

Taylor, L.P. *Taylor's Manual of Physical Evaluation and Treatment.* Thorofare, N.J.: Slack, Inc., 1990, pp. 688–690.

Teasdale, G. and Jennett, B. Assessment of coma and impaired consciousness: A practical scale. *Lancet* 2:81–84, 1974.

Tesler, M.D., Savedra, M.C., Holzemer, W.L. et al. The word graphic rating scale as a measure of children's and adolescents' pain intensity. *Res Nurs Health* 14:361–371, 1991.

Thomas, J.E. and Faecher, R.S. A physician's guide to early detection of oral cancer. *Geriatrics* 47(1):58–63, 1992.

Thyne, G.M. and Ferguson, J.W. Antibiotic prophylaxis during dental treatment in patients with prosthetic joints. *J Bone Joint Surg* 73B:191–194, 1991.

Tinetti, M.E. Performance-oriented assessment of mobility problems in elderly patients. *J Am Geriatr Soc* 34:119–126, 1986.

Tinetti, M.E., Liu, W.-L. and Ginter, S.F. Mechanical restraint use and fall-related injuries among residents of skilled nursing facilities. *Ann Intern Med* 116:369–374, 1992.

Tinetti, M.E., Liu, W.L., Marottoli, R.A. and Ginter, S.F. Mechanical restraint use among residents of skilled nursing facilities: Prevalence, patterns and predictors. *JAMA* 265:468–471, 1991.

Tinetti, M.E., Mendes de Leon, D. and Baker, D.I. Fear of falling, and fall-related efficacy in relationship to functioning among community-living elders. *J Gerontol Med Sci* 49:M140–M147, 1994.

Tinetti, M.E., Richman, D. and Powell, L. Falls efficacy as a measure of fear of falling. *J Gerontol Psych Sci* 45: P239–P243, 1990.

Tobin, G.W. and Brocklehurst, J.C. Faecal incontinence in residential homes for the elderly: Prevalence, aetiology and management. *Age Ageing* 15:41–46, 1986.

Toledo, S.D., An, A., Takemoto, F. and Norman, D.C. Infections and infection control. *In* Rubenstein, L.Z. and Wieland, D. (eds.). *Improving Care in the Nursing Home: Comprehensive Reviews of Clinical Research.* Newbury Park, CA: Sage Publications, 1993, Chap. 3.

Trombly, C.A. *Occupational Therapy for Physical Dysfunction.* 2nd ed. Baltimore: Williams & Wilkins, 1982.

Urinary Incontinence Guideline Panel. *Urinary Incontinence in Adults: Clinical Practice Guideline.* AHCPR Publication No. 92-0038. Rockville, MD: Agency for Health Care Policy and Research, Public Health Service, U.S. Department of Health and Human Services, 1992.

U.S. Department of Health and Human Services. *Vital and Health Statistics:* Nursing Home Utilization by Current Residents: U.S., 1985. Series 13: Data from the National Health Survey, No. 102. Hyattsville, MD: DHHS Publication No. (PHS) 89-1763, 1989.

Valenti, W.M., Trudell, R.G. and Bentley, D.W. Factors predisposing to oropharyngeal colonization with gram-negative bacilli in the aged. *N Engl J Med* 298:1108–1111, 1978.

Val Palumbo, M. Hearing Access 2000: Increasing awareness of the hearing impaired. *J Gerontol Nurs* 16(9):26–31, 1990.

Ventry, I.M. and Weinstein, B.E. The Hearing Handicap Inventory for the elderly: A new tool. *Ear Hearing* 3(3): 128–134, 1982.

Vermeesch, P.E.H. Clinical assessment of confusion. *In* Funk, S.G., Tornquist, E.M., Champagne, M.T. and Wiese, R.A. (eds.). *Key Aspects of Elder Care: Managing Falls, Incontinence and Cognitive Impairment.* 1992, pp. 251–261.

Vines, S.W., Arnstein, P., Shaw, A. et al. Research utilization: An evaluation of the research related to causes of diarrhea in tube-fed patients. *Appl Nurs Res* 5(4): 164–173, 1992.

Vining, D. Review of "Turnabout: Gays in their Nineties." *Gerontologist* 34:282, 1994.

Visser, H. Gait and balance in senile dementia of the Alzheimer's type. *Age Ageing* 12:296–301, 1983.

Wagner, J.A., Robinson, S. and Marino, R.P. Age and temperature regulation of humans in neutral and cold regulation. *J Appl Physiol* 37:562, 1974.

Wagnild, G. and Manning, R.W. Convey respect during bathing procedures. *J Gerontol Nurs* 11(12):6–10, 1985.

Wakefield, B.M. Ineffective breathing pattern. *In* Maas, M., Buckwalter, K.C. and Hardy, M. (eds.). *Nursing Diagnoses and Interventions for the Elderly.* Menlo Park, CA: Addison-Wesley, 1991, Chap. 21.

Wakefield, K.M., Henderson, S.T. and Streit, J.G. Fever of unknown origin in the elderly. *Primary Care* 16(2): 501–513, 1989.

Wald, A. Constipation in elderly patients: Pathogenesis and management. *Drugs Aging* 3(3):220–231, 1993.

Walsh, C. and Eldredge, N. When deaf people become elderly: Counteracting a lifetime of difficulties. *J Gerontol Nurs* 15(12):27–31, 1989.

Wandel, J.C. The use of postural vital signs in the assessment of fluid volume status. *J Prof Nurs* 6(1):46–54, 1990.

Watt, S. Quenching the body's thirst. *N. Z. Nurs J*, Nov. 1991, pp. 18–19.

Weiner, D.K., Long, R., Hughes, M.A. et al. When older adults face the chair rise challenge: A study of chair height availability and height modified chair rise in the elderly. *J Am Geriatr Soc* 41:6–10, 1993.

Weizman, E.D., Moline, M.L., Czeiler, C.A. and Zimmerman, J.C. Chronobiology of aging: Temperature, sleep-wake rhythms, and intrainment. *Neurobiol Aging* 3:299–309, 1982.

Wells, T.J., Brink, C.A., Diokno, A.C. et al. Pelvic muscle exercise for stress urinary incontinence in elderly women. *J Am Geriatr Soc* 39:785–791, 1991.

Whitehead, W.E., Drinkwater, D., Cheskin, L.J. et al. Constipation in the elderly living at home: Definition, prevalence and relationship to life style and health status. *J Am Geriatr Soc* 37:423–429, 1989.

Williams, M.L. An algorithm for selecting a communication technique with intubated patients. *Dimensions Crit Care Nurs* 11(4):222–233, 1992.

Wolanin, M.O. and Phillips, L. *Confusion.* St. Louis: C.V. Mosby, 1981.

Wongsurawat, N., Davis, B.B. and Morely, J.E. Thermoregulatory failure in the elderly. *J Am Geriatr Soc* 38: 899–906, 1990.

Woollacott, M.H. Age-related changes in posture and movement. *J Gerontol* 48:(Special Issue): 56–60, 1993.

Wrenn, K. Fecal impaction. *N Engl J Med* 321:658–662, 1989.

Yeaw, E.M.J. Good lung down? How position affects oxygenation. *Am J Nurs* 92(5):27–29, 1992.

Yoshikawa, T.T. Tuberculosis in aging adults. *J Am Geriatr Soc* 40:178–187, 1992.

Yoshitake, H. Three characteristic patterns of subjective fatigue symptoms. *Ergonomics* 21:231–233, 1978.

Young, J.B. and Dobranski, S. Pressure sores: Epidemiology and curent management concepts. *Drugs Aging* 2(1):42–57, 1992.

Psychosocial Aging Changes

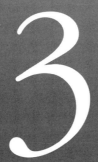
3

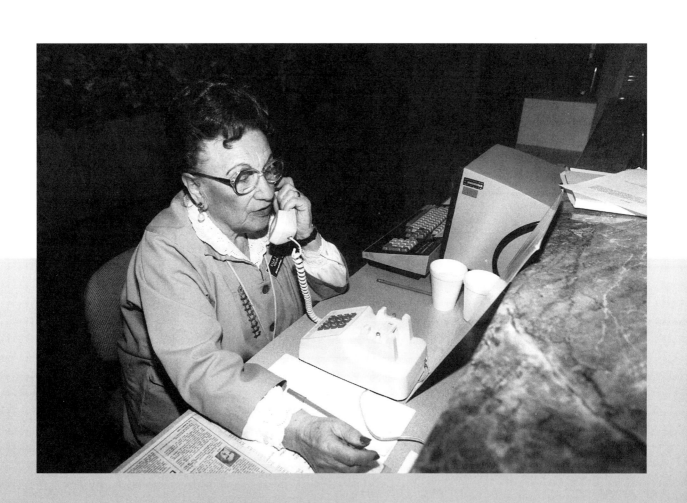

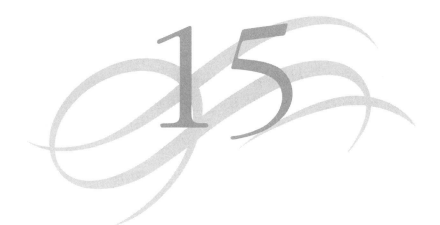

Psychosocial Aging Changes

MARY ANN MATTESON

OBJECTIVES

Identify demographic patterns associated with the older population, including gender, racial differences, marital status, living arrangements, educational levels, work and leisure, and health.

❖

Discuss age-related changes in intelligence, cognition, learning, and memory.

❖

Describe the effect of the aging process on personality, attitudes, and self-concept.

❖

Compare and contrast sociocultural influences on older persons in relation to social support networks and attitudes and relationships.

❖

Differentiate the various developmental theories of aging.

STATISTICAL PROFILE
Demographic Patterns
Educational Level
Employment
Health Indices

PSYCHOLOGICAL AGING CHANGES
Cognition, Memory, Learning, and Attention
Intelligence
Personality and Self-Concept
Life Satisfaction and Morale
Attitudes

SOCIOCULTURAL INFLUENCES ON AGING
Cultural Influences
Social Support Networks

DEVELOPMENTAL THEORIES OF AGING
Developmental Tasks
Activity Theory
Disengagement Theory
Continuity Theory

Figure 15–1 depicts the relevant structures of interest to gerontological nurses as they study the impact of social structure and process on the health of aged individuals.

Behavior patterns are influenced by attributes of the social environment and characteristics of the individual. Eventually, individual characteristics may influence attributes of the social environment, and, eventually, attributes of the social environment may influence the characteristics of individuals.

The essential questions for nurses to answer from the extant social gerontology literature are as follows:

1. How do individual characteristics influence patterns of behavior and the social context?

2. How do patterns of behavior influence individual characteristics and attributes of the social environment?

3. How do attributes of the social environment influence patterns of individual behavior and characteristics of elderly individuals?

In the answers to these questions lies the rationale for nursing interventions to promote self-esteem, optimal role performance, social interaction, and activity.

This section of the text reviews the relevant social science literature in an attempt to answer these important questions, beginning

Psychological functioning and social opportunity are inextricably linked in the elderly. Behavior and feelings about self depend on physiological and cultural factors. Distinguishing cause and effect is therefore extremely difficult, and no one theory exists to explain psychosocial aspects of functioning in the aged.

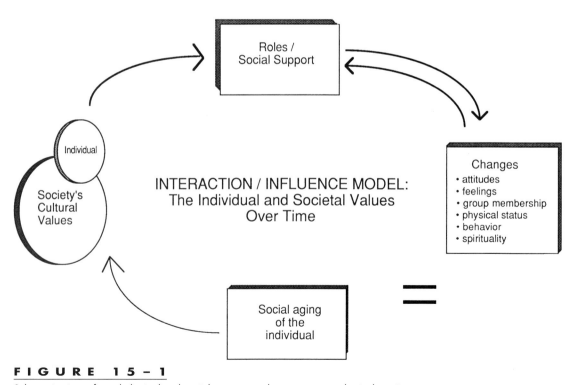

FIGURE 15–1

Schematic view of psychological and social structures relevant to gerontological nursing.

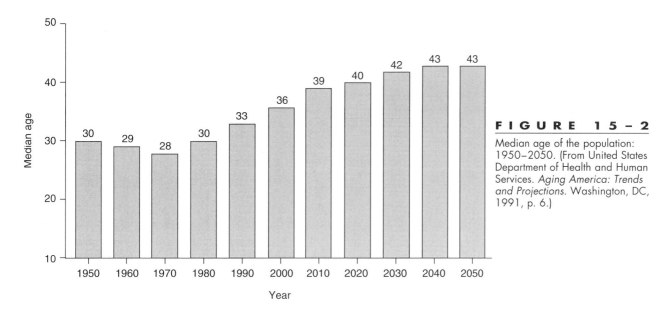

FIGURE 15–2

Median age of the population: 1950–2050. (From United States Department of Health and Human Services. *Aging America: Trends and Projections.* Washington, DC, 1991, p. 6.)

with a statistical overview of the elderly in the United States.

STATISTICAL PROFILE

Demographic Patterns

The population of the United States is growing older, and the number of people over age 65 has increased far more rapidly than any other segment of the population. In 1989, approximately 31 million Americans were age 65 and older, representing 12 per cent of the total population. In 1900, only one in 25 Americans was over age 65; in 1989, the number rose to one in eight. The graying of America will continue well into the next century with the aging of the baby boom.

The projected growth in the older population is expected to raise the median age of the United States population. From 1950 to 1970, the median age declined from 30 to 28 years and then rose again to 33 years in 1990. It is expected to rise to 40 years in the year 2020 and 43 years in 2050 (Fig. 15–2).

The oldest old age group (age 85 and older) is a growing segment of the older population. Between 1989 and 2050, the population aged 85 years and older is expected to climb from about 1 to 5 per cent of the total population (Fig. 15–3). In 1990, 10 per cent of people aged 65 years and older were older than 85. That number is expected to rise to 20 per cent in 2050 (United States Department of Health and Human Services, 1991).

Gender

Women generally outlive men, and, with advancing age, women constitute a greater proportion of the population. In 1989, there were 18.3 million women and only 12.6 men aged 65 years and older. Older women now outnumber older men by three to two as opposed to six to five in 1960. Figure 15–4 shows the number of men per 100 women by age group. Because women live longer than men, they average a longer period of retirement and are more likely to be living alone in late life (United States Department of Health and Human Services, 1991).

Racial Differences

The proportion of older people is higher in the white population than in minority populations. In Americans 65 years or older, approximately 90 per cent are white, 8 per cent are African-American, 3 per cent are Hispanic (of any race), and 2 per cent are of other races (Native Americans, Asian or Pacific Islanders). For each race or color group, the approximate percentages of persons 65 years or older among the respective populations are as follows: whites, 13 per cent; African-Americans, 8 per cent; Hispanics (of any race), 5 per cent; and other races (Native Americans and Asians or Pacific Islanders), 7 per cent. These figures show an overall growth trend in the proportions of elderly Americans who are members of minority groups (Fig. 15–5). It is expected that this trend will continue into the next century, leading to greater ethnic diversity among the aged.

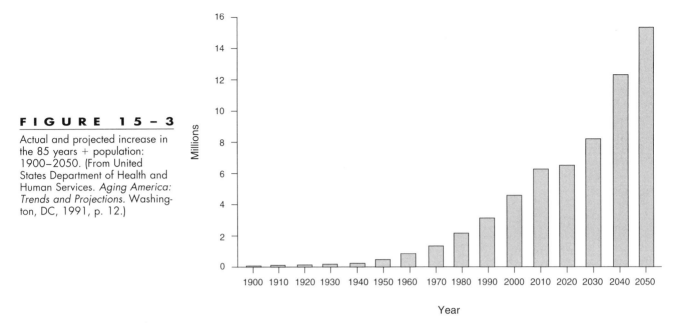

FIGURE 15-3

Actual and projected increase in the 85 years + population: 1900–2050. (From United States Department of Health and Human Services. *Aging America: Trends and Projections*. Washington, DC, 1991, p. 12.)

Marital Status

The proportion of widowed persons grows steadily with age in both sexes, whereas the proportion of married persons drops. Women are much more likely than men to be widowed, as evidenced by the fact that between ages 65 and 74, 37 per cent of women and only 9 per cent of men are widowed. Between ages 75 and 84, the incidence increases, with 62 per cent of women and 20 per cent of men being widowed. Widowhood in people aged 85 years and older increases even further to 82 per cent in women and 42 per cent in men. Only about 9 per cent of all people aged 65 years and older are either never married or divorced, and the proportion diminishes somewhat for divorced people as they age, to about 2 per cent aged 85 years and older (United States Bureau of the Census, 1990).

African-Americans have higher rates of widowhood than either whites or Hispanics. White men and women aged 65 years and older are more likely to be married and living with a spouse than are African-Americans (41 per cent of white women versus 28 per cent of African-American women; 76 per cent of white men versus 56 per cent of African-American men). Thirty-eight per cent of women and 66 per cent of men of Hispanic origin aged 65 and older are married with a spouse present. The reasons for the disparity in marital status between older men and women is thought to be the fact that men tend to marry women younger than themselves and have a shorter life expectancy; thus, they tend to predecease their wives. In addition, men who lose a spouse through divorce or widowhood are eight times more likely to remarry than women in the same situation (National Center for Health Statistics, 1990).

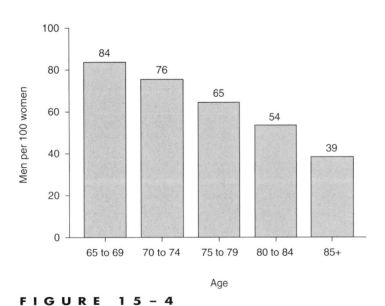

FIGURE 15-4

Number of men per 100 women by age group in 1989. (From United States Department of Health and Human Services. *Aging America: Trends and Projections*. Washington, DC, 1991, p. 17.)

Living Arrangements

Only about 5 per cent of people over 65 years of age are in institutions such as nursing homes at any given time; however, an estimated 43 per cent of people who were age 65 in 1990 will use nursing homes at some time during their remaining years (Murtaugh et al., 1990). The rate of nursing home use has almost doubled since the introduction of Medicare and Medicaid in 1966, from 2.5 to 5 per cent of the population aged 65 years and older. Older women are twice as likely to spend time in a nursing home than are older men. About 45 per cent of older nursing home residents stay less than 3 months, about 10 per cent stay for 6 months to a year, 17 per cent stay for 1 to 3 years, and 9 per cent stay for 5 or more years. Typically, a nursing home resident is an 80-year-old white widow with several chronic conditions. On average, she is in the nursing home 18 months after having been a patient in a hospital or other health care facility (Spence and Wiener, 1990; United States Department of Health and Human Services, 1991).

Of those living in the community, 31 per cent live alone. Approximately 54 per cent are married and live with their spouses, and the remaining reside with others, including children, relatives, and friends. Women are more likely to live alone than men, and men are more likely to live with a spouse than alone. The proportion of older people living alone increases with age, from about 25 (ages 65 to 74) to 38 per cent (ages 75 to 84) to 47 per cent (ages 85 and older) (Fig. 15–6, United States Department of Health and Human Services, 1991). The number of people living alone is expected to increase dramatically, from 9.2 million in 1990 to 15.2 million by the year 2020 (United States Department of Health and Human Services, 1991; Schick and Schick, 1994).

Differences in living arrangements also exist among ethnic groups. Older whites and African-Americans are about equally likely to live alone (31 versus 33 per cent), whereas a smaller proportion of Hispanics live alone (22 per cent). Although the proportion of older African-Americans living alone is about equal to older whites, the numbers are somewhat different. The number of older white people living alone is approximately 8 million, whereas the number of both African-Americans and Hispanics living alone is relatively small—813,000 African-Americans and 221,000 Hispanics. The minority older population is expected to increase more rapidly than the older white population, so that by the year 2020, the number of African-Americans living alone is expected to triple, and the number of Hispanics living alone is expected to quadruple (United States Department of Health and Human Services, 1991).

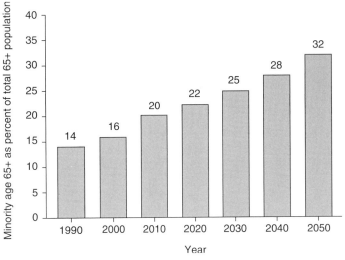

FIGURE 15 – 5

Growth of the minority population: 1990–2050. (From United States Department of Health and Human Services. *Aging America: Trends and Projections.* Washington, DC, 1991, p. 16.)

HOUSING. A majority of older Americans own their own homes. Of all households, 22 per cent are headed by someone aged 65 and older; 76 per cent of older persons own a home, and 24 per cent pay rent. Of older people living alone, 62 per cent own a home, and 38 per cent rent. Of those in rented dwellings, 29 per cent receive some governmental subsidy. Even higher percentages of older African-Americans (47 per cent) and Hispanics (40 per cent) receive rent subsidies. Older adults are more likely to live in older houses and homes with less

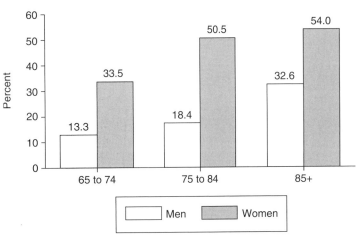

FIGURE 15 – 6

Older people living alone by age and sex in 1989. (From United States Department of Health and Human Services. *Aging America: Trends and Projections.* Washington, DC, 1991, p. 214.

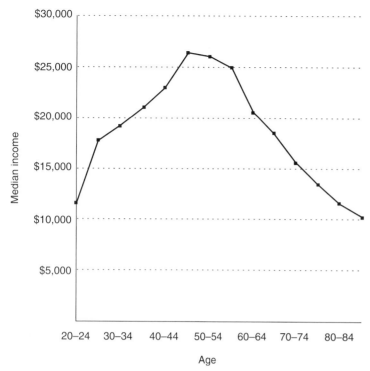

FIGURE 15-7

Median family unit income, by age of head of household in 1990. (From U.S. Bureau of the Census. In Schick, F.L., and Schick, R. *Statistical Handbook on Aging Americans*. Phoenix, AZ: Orynx Press, 1994, p. 215.)

value than younger adults. The median value of homes belonging to older African-Americans is considerably less than that of homes owned by all older people ($39,700 versus $58,900), but the median value of homes belonging to older Hispanics is higher ($65,300) (United States Bureau of the Census, 1989, 1990).

GEOGRAPHICAL DISTRIBUTION AND MOBILITY. Over half of the country's older population live in nine states: California, New York, Florida, Pennsylvania, Texas, Illinois, Ohio, Michigan, and New Jersey. States with the highest percentage of older residents are Florida (18 per cent), Pennsylvania (15 per cent), Iowa (15 per cent), Rhode Island (14.8 per cent), Arkansas (14.8 per cent), West Virginia (14.6 per cent), and South Dakota (14.4 per cent). It is predicted that by the year 2010, California's elderly population will increase and continue to have the largest number, followed by Florida and New York.

Older adults change residences less often than younger people, reflecting the high percentages of elderly persons in states, particularly agricultural states, where younger people have moved out. Elderly people who move tend to relocate to the sunbelt, and

during the past several decades, the increase in the older population has been more rapid in the South and the West. Interestingly, countermigration is occurring, which is the trend toward moving back home or to a state where family members live. The average age of countermigrants is 73, and they are more likely to have incomes below the poverty level, to have disabilities, and to live in nursing homes. Retirement communities also are attracting large numbers of older people in nonmetropolitan areas in all sections of the country.

Of the population aged 65 years and older, 23 million reside in metropolitan areas (including the suburbs), and 8.3 million reside in nonmetropolitan areas. In 1980, the number of older people living in the suburbs outnumbered those living in central cities (10 million versus 8 million) for the first time in history. They generally reside in suburbs that were established before or just after World War II, where incomes and the cost of living are lower and the population density is higher (United States Department of Health and Human Services, 1991).

Income

The elderly are disproportionately represented in the lower income brackets. The median income is approximately one half of the median income of younger age groups. Figure 15-7 shows the income distribution of households headed by people aged 20 to 84 years (Schick and Schick, 1994). Several factors are associated with decreased income in the elderly, including sex (women have, on the average, smaller incomes than men), race (minorities have, on the average, smaller incomes than whites), and living arrangements (people living alone have smaller average incomes than those living with a family).

Legislation passed in the 1974 amendments to the Social Security Act mandated cost of living increases in Social Security benefits. This has resulted in modest gains in economic status for some older persons; however, significant numbers of older persons (11.4 per cent in 1989) still live below the poverty level. In addition, people aged 65 years and older are more likely to have incomes just above the poverty level (15.8 per cent) than those under the age of 65 (8.3 per cent). Fortunately, the poverty rate has declined by about 3.5 per cent since 1979.

Minority groups and women have lower incomes than do whites and men. In 1989, the poverty rate among African-American

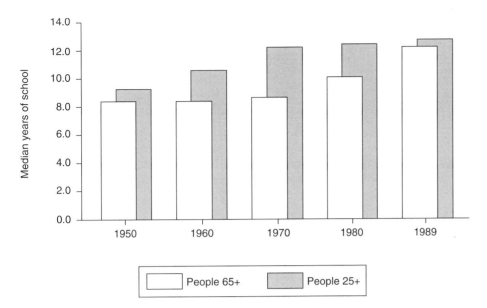

Median years of school for people aged at least 25 years and for those aged at least 65 years: 1950–1989. (From United States Department of Health and Human Services. *Aging America: Trends and Projections.* Washington, DC, 1991, p. 190.)

elderly persons was 30.8 per cent in comparison with Hispanic elderly persons (20.6 per cent) and white elderly persons (9.6 per cent). Sixty-one per cent of African-American women living alone had incomes below the poverty level. Hispanic women had the lowest median incomes ($4992), and white men had the highest ($13,391) (United States Department of Health and Human Services, 1991).

Over 90 per cent of the elderly receive Social Security benefits; however, this represents only 38 per cent of their aggregate income. The majority of Social Security recipients have other sources of income, including earnings from paid employment, income from assets, other governmental pensions, private pensions, and public assistance. Social security is the sole source of income for 20 per cent of the older population. Income from assets is the second most important income for older adults (25 per cent). Private pension plans are receiving increasing attention as a means of preventing poverty in old age. Pensions now account for 18 per cent of total earnings (United States Department of Health and Human Services, 1991).

Educational Level

Another characteristic that distinguishes today's elderly from previous generations of old people is degree of educational attainment. Figure 15–8 shows the educational attainment of older and younger persons for the past five decades. The proportion of older adults who have had a high school education has increased to 55 per cent, and

future cohorts of elderly people will have higher educational levels as the percentage of the population graduating from high school steadily increases. Among minorities, only 25 per cent of African-Americans and 28 per cent of Hispanics aged 65 years and older have completed high school. Although the percentage of minority individuals under the age of 65 who have completed high school is lower than that of whites, the proportion has significantly increased, so that future cohorts of older African-Americans and Hispanics will be more highly educated (Schick and Schick, 1994).

Employment

Currently, the elderly constitute an increasingly *smaller* proportion of the paid work force in the United States. Figure 15–9 shows this gradual decline over the past 40 years, especially in older men. The rate of women aged 65 and older in the work force has held relatively steady; however, participation in the work force has increased in the 55- to 64-year age group. Projections for the future indicate that the rate will continue to rise for women in the 55- to 64-year age group. Of those in the work force, 59 per cent of women and 48 per cent of men are employed part time. The percentage of older people in part-time rather than full-time employment is increasing. It has been found that many older adults prefer part-time work with flexible hours after retirement.

The United States economy is shifting from agricultural and heavy industry to service and light industry. Therefore, jobs are

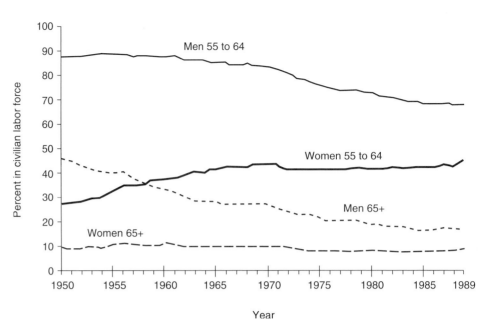

FIGURE 15-9

Annual averages of labor force participation of older men and women, by age: 1950–1989. (From United States Department of Health and Human Services. *Aging America: Trends and Projections.* Washington, DC, 1991, p. 95.)

likely to be found in white-collar and service occupations. Most workers aged 65 years and older are employed in the following occupational categories: managerial and professional; technical, sales, and administrative support; and service occupations. The shift from physically demanding or hazardous jobs to those that require knowledge and skills may increase the potential for

older workers to remain in the work force longer.

Since 1950, there has been a trend toward early retirement. Because most private pension plans provide benefits to eligible employees at ages below 65 (the present Social Security retirement age for men), workers are electing to retire at an earlier age. The pension plans incorporate strong incentives to exit the labor force at age 60 or earlier, so that the proportion of male pension recipients aged 50 to 64 has increased markedly over the past two decades. Therefore, the policy change raising the age from 65 to 67 by the year 2022 for eligibility for full Social Security benefits is not expected to have a significant impact on the work force (United States Department of Health and Human Services, 1991).

Health Indices

Life Expectancy and Functional Impairment

There is a clear trend toward increased life expectancy over the last century for men and women, both whites and nonwhites. Chronic conditions are prevalent in older age, including arthritis, hypertension, heart disease, diabetes, and visual and hearing impairments (Fig. 15–10). Chronic illness can influence an older person's ability to carry out activities of daily living (ADLs). Fewer than 25 per cent of all people aged 65 to 74 years are unable to carry out normal ADLs because of chronic illness. With each decade

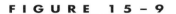

Condition	Rate per 1000 people
Arthritis	483.0
Hypertension	380.6
Hearing impairment	286.5
Heart disease	278.9
Cataracts	156.8
Deformity/orthopedic	155.2
Chronic sinusitis	153.4
Diabetes	88.2
Visual impairment	81.9
Varicose veins	78.1

Rate per 1000 people

FIGURE 15-10

The top 10 chronic conditions for people 65 years of age or older in 1989. (From United States Department of Health and Human Services. *Aging America: Trends and Projections.* Washington, DC, 1991, p. 95.)

after the age of 65, the proportion of individuals experiencing difficulty with at least one physical or instrumental ADL grows, so that approximately 40 per cent of those 75 to 84 years and 60 per cent of those older than 85 need some assistance (Table 15-1) (United States Department of Health and Human Services, 1991).

Self-Rated Health

Despite the reported impairments in daily functioning for many people over age 65, the majority (71 per cent) of the elderly rate their health as good to excellent. There are no sex differences in the ratings, but differences exist according to race and income level. African-American men and women report their health to be good or excellent less often than do white men and women (65 and 53 per cent versus 70 and 71 per cent). Of those having incomes of $35,000 or greater, 83 per cent report good or excellent health, versus 59 per cent of those with incomes of under $10,000 (United States Department of Health and Human Services, 1991).

Utilization of Health Care Professionals and Services

The elderly have a higher average number of visits to physicians than younger persons, and the number increases with advancing age. People aged 45 to 64 years average 6.1 visits to the physician per year, whereas the 65 to 74 and the over-75 age groups average 8.2 and 9.9 visits per year, respectively. Men tend to visit physicians more than women in late life (ages 85 and older), and, as expected, all older adults who rate their overall health as fair or poor have significantly more physician visits than those who rate their health as excellent or good.

Utilization of hospital care and length of hospitalization increase with older age. In 1987, the hospital discharge rate (number of discharges per 1000 population) for people aged 85 years and older was 90 per cent higher than for those aged 65 to 74 years. The average hospital stay for people aged 65 to 74 years was 8.2 days, compared with 9.5 days for those aged 85 years and older. During the past three decades, the average length of stay has been declining until recently. In 1968, the average stay was 14.2 days, compared with 8.5 days in 1986. In 1988, the number rose to 8.9 days (Fig. 15-11).

Most (78 per cent) of older persons are

TABLE 15-1

Percent Distribution of Persons with Difficulty in Activities of Daily Living and Instrumental Activities of Daily Living, by Sex and Age

SEX AND AGE	DIFFICULTIES IN ADLs AND IADLs			
	None	ADL Difficulty Only	IADL Difficulty Only	Both
Total	66.6	5.2	10.9	17.3
Sex				
Male	74.7	6.6	7.4	11.3
Female	60.9	4.3	13.4	21.5
Age				
65–74 years	74.1	4.7	9.2	12.0
75–84 years	58.7	6.5	12.5	22.4
85 years or over	37.1	4.8	18.3	39.8

From Schick and Schick, 1994. ADL = activities of daily living; IADL = instrumental activities of daily living.

discharged from the hospital to their home; however, as people age, they are more likely to be discharged to a nursing home. Of the older adults discharged from the hospital to a nursing home, 3.9 per cent are ages 65 to 74, whereas 15.9 per cent are age 75 and over.

Dental care frequently is difficult to obtain for the elderly. Routine care is not covered by federal insurance programs, and private insurance provides minimal coverage. In 1989, 41 per cent of older adults in nonmetropolitan areas and 33 per cent living in metropolitan areas were edentulous. Of those living in nonmetropolitan areas, 58 per cent had made no visits to the dentist in the

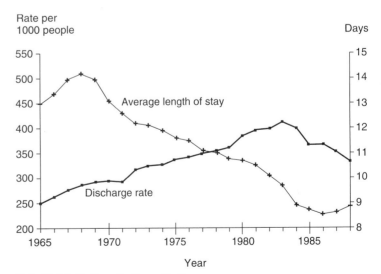

FIGURE 15-11

Trends in hospital use by people 65 years of age or older: 1965–1988. (From United States Department of Health and Human Services. *Aging America: Trends and Projections.* Washington, DC, 1991, p. 125.)

previous year, compared with 52 per cent living in metropolitan areas (United States Department of Health and Human Services, 1991; National Institute for Dental Research, 1989; Schick and Schick, 1994).

PSYCHOLOGICAL AGING CHANGES

Disagreement exists among psychologists regarding how essential personality attributes are conceptualized. However, three key areas of the psychology of aging with relevance to nursing have been well researched: cognition, morale, and self-concept. Numerous cross-sectional studies on personality traits exist but have limited applicability because cohort differences and life events are more powerful influences on personality than the aging process.

Cognition, Memory, Learning, and Attention

Memory, learning, and attention are all aspects of cognition that have complex relationships. Cognition is the process by which sensory input is transformed, reduced, elaborated, stored, and retrieved. Memory is essential to cognition and also involves the mental processes of retaining information for later use and retrieving such information. Learning is defined as the acquisition of information, skills, and knowledge measured by an improvement in some overt response. Learning depends on memory, and both memory and learning depend on attention. Attention is defined as the mechanisms by which we prepare to process stimuli, focus on what to process, and determine how far it will be processed and whether it should call us to action (Sugar and McDowd, 1992; Whitbourne and Sperbeck, 1981).

Information processing models of learning and memory (Atkinson and Shiffrin, 1968; Gagńe, 1974; Greeno and Bjork, 1973) postulated a number of internal structures in the human brain and some corresponding processes to illustrate the cognitive process. These models view the sequence of operations and transformations involved in cognitive activity as a complex system with many interacting stages.

The major stages of the information processing models are *registration*, (the input of information), *storage* (retention for subsequent use), and *retrieval* (the process of obtaining information from storage information essential to the production of an overt response). Some components of the cognitive processes are perception, thinking, memory, and problem solving (Arenberg and Robertson, 1973). Cognition, learning, memory, and attention involve all of these processes and components, and all can be affected by age-associated changes.

Attention

During the registration phase of the information processing model, the learner receives stimulation from the environment that activates his receptors and is transformed to neural information (Gagńe, 1974). Attention is an integral component of registration in that an individual must focus on stimuli and decide what to process. Deficits in attention may affect learning and memory (Birren and McDowd, 1990; Sugar and McDowd, 1992). How the older learner perceives the information can be affected by environmental influences, age-related sensoriperceptual changes, and pacing of instruction.

ENVIRONMENTAL INFLUENCES. The majority of learning situations in which the elderly have been involved during research investigations have been conducted in laboratory settings. It has been found that the present generation of older people feel uncomfortable in learning situations that are not related to real life situations or that are carried out in unfamiliar environments. Therefore, one should proceed cautiously when interpreting findings from laboratory studies about learning and cognition. Older people often feel less motivated to learn and more threatened in a setting in which declining cognitive abilities may be publicly demonstrated. It is therefore difficult for them to maintain the attention and interest necessary for perception and registration of information to be learned (Kausler, 1990).

Interfering factors can also jeopardize the perceptual capabilities of the elderly. Older people have difficulty attending to more than one task or input at a time, and it is difficult to ignore extraneous stimuli. Thus, selective attention processes and the capacity to disregard irrelevant information decrease with age (McDowd and Birren, 1990; Giambra, 1989; Allen et al., 1993).

SENSORIPERCEPTUAL FACTORS. Older people frequently experience deficits in vision and hearing that can interfere with perception (Matteson, 1979). Visual changes include presbyopia (inability to focus the lens at various distances), altered color perception (difficulty in distinguishing blues and greens due to a yellowing of the lens), diminished depth perception, decreased peripheral vision, slowed adaptation to dark and light, and poor tolerance for glare.* In a large classroom or lecture hall, older learners may have difficulty seeing writing on a blackboard or visual illustrations; they may also have difficulty reading small print in handouts. This may account for their minimal use of imagery as a learning strategy (Fullerton, 1983).

Sensorineural hearing loss, or presbycusis, affects mainly high frequencies and is often a barrier to communication in the elderly. Problems with hearing consonants or high-pitched voices are a special concern, especially when unfamiliar material is presented. Background noises also interfere with hearing in a group setting, so that perception and registration of information are virtually impossible.

PACING OF INSTRUCTION. With aging, there is a normal tendency toward slowing of both physiological and psychological responses. Reaction time increases, making perception of fast-paced (including rate of presentation and amount of material presented) instruction difficult (Cerella, 1991; Madden, 1992; Spirduso and MacRae, 1990; Norris and West, 1991). In addition, many of the reported age deficits in learning are attributable to overarousal of older individuals in laboratory learning tasks. They respond less frequently and perform less effectively at a fast pace (Eisdorfer, 1968). Studies have shown that the elderly appear to learn more efficiently (need fewer trials and make fewer errors) when they are allowed to determine their own pace when learning the material or when preparing their response (Arenberg, 1974; Hulicka and Grossman, 1967; Monge and Hultsch, 1971; Canestrari, 1963).

Storage

The storage phase involves short-term and long-term memory processes. Short-term memory includes primary memory, which represents a store of limited capacity in which contents are subject to displacement, and secondary memory, which represents a rehearsal-dependent store of a relatively large capacity. In long-term memory, information is semantically fully encoded and stored in a conceptual or meaningful mode. Studies have shown that whereas deficits seem small or nonexistent on tasks requiring only primary memory abilities, older persons do relatively poorly on almost all laboratory tasks involving secondary memory (Earles and Coon, 1994; Salthouse, 1992; Wiegersma and Meertse, 1990; Belsky, 1990). Secondary memory deficits are thought to be due to a general deficiency in the spontaneous use of either organizational or mediational memory strategies (Rabinowitz et al., 1982; Hulicka and Grossman, 1967). According to Bower (1972), the amount of information that can be stored and retrieved from memory, especially secondary memory, is determined by organizational processes. Older persons generally do not attend to organizational characteristics of information (Craik, 1968; Rabbitt, 1968; Hulicka and Grossman, 1967; Kausler and Lichty, 1988), and it has been shown that proper instruction in the use of mediators leads to clear improvements in memory processing and problem solving. Programs should be tailored to the individual because some people and age groups prefer different techniques. A favorite memory aid for older adults is writing things down (Willis and Schaie, 1986; Siegler and Poon, 1989; Hultsch and Dixon, 1990; Karuza, 1992; Sugar and McDowd, 1992).

Such findings underpin the optimism behind memory-enhancement programs for the aged. Although some studies have shown that older people report more memory "failures," such as missed appointments and forgotten names, than do younger adults (Cavanaugh et al., 1983; Lowenthal, 1967), recent studies have found that older adults' everyday memories are often at least equal to younger adults' memories (Sinnott, 1986) and are sometimes better than younger adults' memories (Martin, 1986; Moscovitch, 1982; Poon and Schaffer, 1982). Unfortunately, the elderly are more distressed about their perception of memory loss than the young (Sugar and McDowd, 1992; Zarit et al., 1981). They may, therefore, derive both subjective and objective benefit from memory-training programs.

According to Salthouse (1980), the speed-loss mechanism, based on the age-related slowing of the central and peripheral nervous system, accounts for age differences in memory performance. Because all time-dependent memory processes decline with age, the speed and efficiency with which mental operations are performed are responsible for declines in memory skill. Related to the issue of general slowing with age is the fatigue factor in memory processing. Many older persons have physical impairments and chronic illnesses that increase the rate of fatigue in learning situations. Several studies also have noted that impaired nutritional

---

*For an in-depth discussion of the sensoriperceptual changes seen with aging, see Chapters 13 and 14.

status may elicit poor memory performance in older adults (Cherkin, 1984; Goodwin et al., 1983). Fatigue hinders motivation to carry out the processes necessary to store new information.

Retrieval

Storage and retrieval are so closely related, especially in terms of research investigation, that it is difficult to separate the two. Most memory studies involve some type of recall, thus clouding the issue of learning versus performance. Studies generally show an age-related slowing in the rate of retrieval from secondary memory. Lorsbach and Simpson (1984) found that older subjects were slower to respond under all experimental conditions, but, in particular, they required more time to search through secondary memory than through primary memory.

In addition, older people frequently commit omission errors in laboratory learning tasks. They have a tendency to not respond or to say, "I don't know," in performance testing situations related to recall. Omission errors are thought to be due to a valuation of accuracy, a fear of making a mistake, a need for certainty, or some other "noncognitive" reason that keeps older individuals from taking the risk of giving an answer when less than absolutely sure (Botwinick, 1978; Erber et al., 1980).

Intelligence

Controversies exist regarding whether intelligence declines with aging. In standard intelligence (IQ) testing using the Wechsler Adult Intelligence Scale (WAIS) developed in 1955 and recently revised (WAIS-R), both longitudinal and cross-sectional studies have demonstrated mild-to-moderate decrements in IQ scores with age. Most abilities tend to peak in early midlife, plateau until the late 50s or early 60s, and then show decline, initially at a slow rate but accelerating as the late 70s are reached. The largest decrements have been in the subtests related to performance (Schaie and Willis, 1993; Schaie, 1990; Poon et al., 1992). However, major problems in validity and reliability associated with the testing procedure tend to color the research findings. Issues such as defining intelligence, the types of tests used, sampling procedures, research methods, testing procedures, and extraneous influences interfere with the ability to draw clear inferences from test scores.

The first issue relates to the definition of intelligence, i.e., what is it that is actually being tested, and the types of tests used.

Wechsler (1971) has defined intelligence as the "ability to perceive relationships between things, regardless of substance; to recognize and recall what has been perceived; to think logically and to plan." In addition, intelligence has been further defined as either fluid intelligence, that is, the integration of neuroanatomical functioning, or crystallized intelligence, that is, the assimilation of learning and experience (Cattel, 1963). Fluid intelligence has been correlated with performance subtests on the WAIS-R, and crystallized intelligence has been associated with verbal subtests. Studies have found that fluid intelligence tends to decrease with age and that crystallized intelligence is usually maintained until very late in life (Horn and Cattell, 1967; Hayslip and Sterns, 1979; Belsky, 1990).

The validity problem here is whether these definitions of intelligence are appropriate for the aged and whether the conclusions drawn from the test scores are accurate. The WAIS test was originally developed as an aid in placing children in appropriate academic settings and measuring skills emphasized in educational settings (Watson, 1982). The items on the test are not relevant to the everyday functioning of average older adults and, therefore, have little value in predicting the success with which they can manipulate their environment. Demming and Pressey (1957) attempted to overcome this validity problem by measuring intellectual functioning according to the ease of using telephone directories, understanding common paralegal concepts, and securing essential social services. It was found that middle-aged and older adults scored higher on tests measuring everyday tasks but continued to score lower on standard IQ tests.

Another issue relates to the sampling procedures and research methods used for intelligence testing. Critics of both cross-sectional and longitudinal studies claim that sample selection limits generalizability of findings to other populations. In cross-sectional studies, aged cohorts are compared with younger cohort groups, who have had different educational opportunities, life experiences, and environmental influences. Studies have shown that educational levels are positively correlated with IQ test scores and, because the elderly have had less education than the young, the comparisons among scores are not valid. The elderly are also far removed from the type of test-taking experience required in intelligence testing, whereas the young maintain their skills every day in their educational settings (Birren and Morrison, 1961). Other correlates include intact marriages, exposure to stimulating environments, and use of cultural and educational resources throughout childhood (Belsky, 1990; Rowe and Raker, 1987; Schaie, 1990; Birren and Morrison, 1961).

Longitudinal studies, although appearing to be more valid measurements of intellectual decline, also have methodological and sampling problems. These studies generally demonstrate fewer decrements in intellectual functioning of elderly subjects; however, subjects in the sample are frequently volunteers who are deemed most healthy and most able to participate in the studies over a long period of time. Retrospective examinations of longitudinal studies have revealed that test scores decrease up to 5 years before death (Siegler and Botwinick, 1979; Botwinick et al., 1978; Jarvik and Falek, 1963); thus, the survivors tend to maintain higher and more consistent scores, biasing the sample.

Finally, testing procedures and extraneous influences can affect the outcome of IQ tests. Many older persons do not see or hear well enough to read adequately and respond appropriately to the test items. The increase in reaction time, ubiquitous in the normal aging process, has a profound influence on the performance test and timed test scores (Grant et al., 1978; Gottsdanker, 1982; Belsky, 1990; Anstey et al., 1993). As noted earlier, the greatest decrements in IQ associated with age are related to fluid intelligence and performance scores. A study by Christensen and MacKinnon (1993) found that physical activity was associated with higher performance on fluid tasks in older subjects.

Health also plays an important role in influencing IQ test scores. Older people afflicted with one or more chronic illnesses either tire easily or may not feel well on the testing day. Variability of test scores tends to increase with age, so that one set of test scores may be extremely unreliable. In addition, persons with health problems, such as cardiovascular disease and hypertension, have decrements in cognitive functioning that affect WAIS-R scores (Belsky, 1990; Schaie, 1990; Busse and Maddox, 1985; Sands and Meridith, 1992; Poon et al., 1992.)

Conclusions from intelligence test scores of older adults should be drawn cautiously and thoughtfully owing to the highly suspect nature of test validity and reliability. It is not certain that the WAIS or WAIS-R test actually measures intelligence, and the appropriateness of the content is questionable. Because content is not related to cognitive tasks in everyday life, it is difficult to predict performance outside of the testing laboratory. In addition, older people who are asked to take intelligence tests that have been constructed for their younger counterparts tend to view the questions as meaningless or silly, and they have little motivation or interest in completing the testing tasks. When tests relevant to everyday functioning of older adults are used, results usually show that intelligence does not decrease with age.

Personality and Self-Concept

Personality is characterized by individual differences in emotional, interpersonal, experiential, attitudinal, and motivational styles. Ways of viewing personality have changed in recent years, mainly from a developmental approach to a trait approach. According to the developmental approach, each stage of life presents a developmental task that must be accomplished to attain personal growth and self-actualization. An example of the developmental approach is Erikson's psychosocial stages of personality development (Erikson, 1963). The developmental approach has fallen into disfavor, chiefly because of lack of empirical support and poor design of research studies (Kogan, 1990).

Other theories that have been proposed and studied in the past have described three personality changes that appear to occur with aging. First, there is a change from focus on the outer world to focus on the inner world, or "introversion" (Chown, 1968; Neugarten, 1977). Second, there is a movement from active mastery to passive mastery of the environment (Neugarten, 1977; Gutmann, 1975; Shanan and Sharon, 1965), that is, older persons are more likely to accommodate to a set of circumstances, whereas younger persons are more likely to try to change the environment. Finally, increased cautiousness with age has been observed. Although these theories often conflict with one another, they all suggest that adulthood is not a plateau but a period of dynamic growth and change in personality (Costa and McCrae, 1988).

The trait approach to personality is presently favored and focuses on certain traits that characterize an individual personality. According to several theorists and findings of research studies (Goldberg, 1990; McCrae and Costa, 1987; Costa and McRae, 1988), there are five major personality domains: (1) neuroticism, (2) extroversion-introversion, (3) openness to experience, (4) sociability-agreeableness, and (5) conscientiousness. Each domain contains characteristic traits (Table 15–2). Both cross-sectional and longitudinal studies confirm that although individuals may vary, there is general stability in personality throughout the lifespan (Costa and

TABLE 15 – 2
Examples of Traits from the Five Personality Factors

FACTOR	CHARACTERISTIC	
	Low Scorer	High Scorer
Neuroticism	Calm	Worrying
	Even-tempered	Temperamental
	Self-satisfied	Self-pitying
	Comfortable	Self-conscious
	Unemotional	Emotional
	Hardy	Vulnerable
Extraversion	Reserved	Affectionate
	Loner	Joiner
	Quiet	Talkative
	Passive	Active
	Sober	Fun-loving
	Unfeeling	Passionate
Openness	Down-to-earth	Imaginative
	Uncreative	Creative
	Conventional	Original
	Prefers routine	Prefers variety
	Uncurious	Curious
	Conservative	Liberal
Agreeableness	Ruthless	Softhearted
	Suspicious	Trusting
	Stingy	Generous
	Antagonistic	Acquiescent
	Critical	Lenient
	Irritable	Good-natured
Conscientiousness	Negligent	Conscientious
	Lazy	Hard-working
	Disorganized	Well-organized
	Late	Punctual
	Aimless	Ambitious
	Quitting	Persevering

From Costa, P.T. Jr., and McCrae, R.R. Personality stability and its implications for clinical psychology. *Clin Psychol Rev* 6:407, 1986. Copyright 1986, with kind permission from Elsevier Science Ltd., The Boulevard, Langton Lane, Kidlington, U.K.

McCrae, 1988, 1993; Karuza, 1992; Busse and Maddox, 1985). Although earlier studies found changes between adolescence and adulthood (Mortimer et al., 1982) and occasional changes, such as declines in activity, in late adulthood (Douglas and Arenberg, 1978), most studies report little or no change in personality traits after about age 30 (Costa and McCrae, 1993; Thomae, 1992; Kogan, 1990; Field and Millsap, 1991; Hagberg et al., 1991). In addition, studies have found that personality traits are more predictive than age is of attitudes and behaviors in late life (Peterson and Maiden, 1992; Toner and Morris, 1992).

Self-concept is a component of personality that can be viewed as an attitude toward the self. Personality type appears to influence self-concept and adaptation to role transitions, such as widowhood or retirement. Research supports the notion of a relatively stable self-concept through the lifespan, with life events more than the aging process itself affecting self-concept. A study of twins aged 27 to 86 years supported the conclusion that self-concept crystallizes early in adulthood and reflects genetically influenced psychological characteristics (McGue et al., 1993).

Research related to personality traits and self-concept indicates that individuals can maintain continuity and coherence in the course of adult life. People do not necessarily become depressed, isolated, and rigid with older age, and well-adjusted and happy individuals are likely to remain so in later life. Those who are less happy with themselves can take steps such as professional counseling to change their lives at any age (Costa and McCrae, 1994).

Life Satisfaction and Morale

Life satisfaction is an attitude toward one's own life; it may be defined as a reflection of feelings about the past, present, and future. Life satisfaction and morale are closely related to well-being. According to George (1981), life satisfaction is the cognitive assessment of well-being, and happiness is the affective assessment. The two major components of well-being—affect (happiness) and satisfaction (realized expectations)—may reflect a changing balance with age. Thus, age-related declines in positive affect may be countered by increases in the sense of satisfaction with life accomplishments (Maddox, 1994).

Although results of studies on life satisfaction and morale are often inconsistent, longitudinal analyses tend to show that levels of well-being remain stable throughout life (Costa et al., 1987; Siegler and Poon, 1989). Most older people say that they are happy, and very few claim that older age is "the dreariest time of my life." Fewer than one third of older people report feelings of boredom or loneliness, and they express more life satisfaction when their social networks include friends as well as relatives (Grundy and Bowling, 1991).

Some studies have found a relationship between personality characteristics, well-being, and quality of life (Grembowski et al., 1993; Heidrich and Ryff, 1993; Smits and Kee, 1992); other studies have shown a relationship between health or perceived health and well-being (Pinquart, 1991; Stolar et al., 1992; Moore et al., 1993). Roberts et al. (1994) assessed the attenuating effects of physical, psychological, and social resources on the relationship between stress and mental health in the oldest old (aged 85 years and older). They found that greater independence in instrumental ADLs and greater perceived control of events significantly attenuated the adverse effects of stress on psychological well-being.

In a study investigating the relationship between feelings of dependency and well-being, investigators found that dependent attitudes were correlated negatively with well-being (Eddington et al., 1990). Krause (1993) also found a relationship between lower levels of life satisfaction and economic dependence. Other studies have linked parenthood (Connidis and McMullin, 1993) and goal achievement (Hooker and Siegler, 1993) with subjective well-being and life satisfaction. Studies have failed to provide evidence that aging per se decreases life satisfaction.

Attitudes

Attitudes are important determinants of behavior (Kiesler et al., 1981). Research on attitude change across the lifespan suggests that most attitudes are remarkably stable over the course of adulthood, and the older the individual, the more firmly attitudes are held. Not only are attitudes of older people more likely to be stable, but their attitudes are more stable in the face of systematic pressures to change. The pressures may come from life cycle events, self-interest, mass communication, relocation, or other status changes or discrepancies that might influence attitudes (Sears, 1981).

There are more similarities than differences between young and old people with regard to their attitudes about most topics (Keith, 1982; Harris et al., 1982). Studies have shown that older and younger Americans share many attitudes and stereotypes about old age. In addition, many older people maintain attitudes about other "old people" that they do not apply to themselves. For example, only 33 per cent of the elderly surveyed thought that *other* old people were "very bright and alert," but 68 per cent thought *themselves* to be "very bright and alert." This figure differs little from the 73 per cent of the 18- to 64-year-old population who considered themselves "bright and alert." It has also been found that many of the "problems of old age," such as loneliness, shrinking job opportunities, not enough to do to keep busy, and not enough medical care, occur in the same proportions in older people as in younger people. Two exceptions are poor health and fear of crime, which are more evident in the aged.

Work and Retirement

Ample evidence suggests that older people work in a competent manner, despite the prevailing stereotype that older workers are less competent, efficient, or capable. Older workers perform at steadier rates and have less job turnover and absenteeism than younger workers. They also have fewer accidents, and their output tends to be more consistent. In addition, older workers are able to compensate for productivity declines by taking advantage of improved skills and knowledge gained through experience (Sterns et al., 1990).

Past research has shown that the performance of older workers depends on the nature of the work being undertaken (Welford, 1984). In jobs with low physical demand, such as clerical work, older workers are more accurate and have steadier work output patterns; however, productivity can decline when jobs require significant physical exertion, such as manufacturing positions (Kelleher and Quirk, 1973).

There is an increasing awareness of the importance of postretirement work as a component of the transition from "career jobs" to permanent retirement (Hayward et al., 1994; Jacobs et al., 1991; Myers, 1991; Ruhm, 1990). Older workers frequently engage in other labor market activity before withdrawing completely from the labor market; however, the number of workers diminishes with advancing age. Data from the National Longitudinal Surveys of Older Men show that 20 per cent of men aged 69 to 74 years and 12.5 per cent of those aged 75 to 84 years remain economically active on a part-time or full-time basis. Good health, a strong psychological commitment to work, and a corresponding distaste for retirement were characteristics related to continued employment into older age (Parnes and Sommers, 1994).

In a study of older women in the labor market, Pienta et al. (1994) examined the effect of early work and family experiences on women's labor force participation in later life. They found that approximately 25 per cent of the women in the sample worked continuously throughout their lives, whereas 60 per cent had taken time out for family obligations. Their findings indicate that women who were the most work oriented throughout their life course were more likely to work either part time or full time in later life than were women who experienced family-related spells of non–labor-marked activity.

Apparently, both men and women who participate in the labor force either part or full time in later life have had stronger life-long work identities than those who do not. Social interactions at work and health also

TABLE 15–3
Historical Events Shaping Attitudes Toward Retirement and Work

YEAR	EVENT	IMPACT
1889	Germany: Old Age and Survivors Benefits Act	First nationalized pension plan, set 65 as retirement age
1908	Great Britain: Similar	Set pensionable age at 70
1935	United States: Social Security Act	First nationalized pension system in the United States, pensionable age at 65
1967	Age Discrimination in Employment Act	Made age discrimination in places of employment illegal
1978	Amendments to Age Discrimination in Employment Act	Mandatory retirement age raised to 70

appear to be related to employment in the retirement years (Mor-Barak et al., 1992; Herzog et al., 1991; Erdner and Guy, 1990).

Retirement from work is a relatively modern concept. Kart and Manard (1981) noted that the idea of retirement as something to be anticipated as a just reward rather than something to be feared or looked on with suspicion is as recent as the 1960s. Table 15–3 summarizes historical events affecting work and retirement in the elderly. Retirement does not result inevitably in a crisis for older persons (Atchley, 1971). Although a strong work orientation is often found in retired people, there is no evidence of widespread maladjustment. The concept of retirement has been increasingly incorporated into American culture, so that more people view work as a temporary part of life.

Attitudes toward retirement and adjustment to retirement are influenced by preretirement lifestyles and values. Those with leisure pursuits during their work life seem to adjust better to retirement than those whose lives are dominated by work. However, for many of today's older people, work has provided a central purpose in life because of the profound influence of the Great Depression (Glick, 1982). Not only did work dominate the lives and shape the identities of today's elderly, but it became an end in itself, deeply ingrained in the pattern of living. When work is gone, a profound loss is felt, and something must be substituted.

Death

Attitudes toward death in the elderly are difficult to measure, chiefly because older people may be reluctant to divulge their true fears of death and because different methods of measuring the concept can uncover different degrees of fear. In addition, fear of death may have different facets. For example, some people may fear being dead, whereas others may fear the dying process (Belsky, 1990; Fry, 1990).

Most studies have shown that attitudes about death, preferred styles of dying, and the experience of dying vary with age. The elderly tend to think and talk about death more than younger people, but they find the prospect of death less frightening (Kalish and Reynolds, 1976; Cameron et al., 1973). According to Kalish (1977), there is a three-part explanation for this phenomenon: (1) there is a diminished social value placed on the life of those of advanced age; (2) the "life expectancy" for people in industrialized countries is known to be approximately 70 years, so those who live longer feel they have received more than their entitlement; and (3) older people have the opportunity to become "socialized" to death. That is, by the time they reach advanced age, they have experienced the death of family members and close friends, thus having many chances to work through this stressful life event.

Older people appear to give considerable thought to the end of their lives, including planning for their death (Courage et al., 1993), and they welcome the opportunity to participate in decision making for life-sustaining interventions (Kellogg et al., 1992; Moore et al., 1993). Recent studies have indicated that older people prefer death to living with dementia or in a comatose state (Patrick et al., 1994; Robertson, 1993), and the expressed wish to die is often a predictor of mortality (Dewey et al., 1993).

Religiosity appears to have an effect on attitudes toward death. Religious people are less fearful of death than people who are not religious, and an acceptance of personal transcendence or transcendent meaning to life makes dying easier (Fishman, 1992; Cartwright, 1991; Thorson and Powell, 1990). Some studies report that irregular churchgoers have more death anxiety than either confirmed agnostics or atheists or regular churchgoers (Kalish, 1963; Nelson and Nelson, 1973).

Religion

Religion is a multidimensional and complex phenomenon. Some dimensions of religion include the ritualistic (praying, attending services), the ideological (religious beliefs), the intellectual (knowledge of scripture, creeds), the experiential (religious feelings, sensations, emotions), and the consequential (effects of the other four dimensions on daily life) (Glock, 1962). Religiousness may include institutional religious participation or an individual religion or personal faith. In addition, a spiritual component of religion cuts across and infuses all of the other dimensions (Moberg, 1967). All of these concepts overlap with one another in complex combinations, so that it is difficult to characterize an individual as simply "religious" or "nonreligious."

Religion appears to be an important part of life for many older people. The elderly are more likely to attend church and participate in bible study or prayer groups than the young, and most receive comfort and support from their religious beliefs. Approximately 75 per cent of the older population belong to religious organizations. The highest church attendance occurs among the younger old (ages 65 to 75), with a subsequent decline among the older old as infirmities bring problems of mobility, vision, and hearing (Moberg, 1990; Schick and Schick, 1994). Older women participate in religious activities more than older men, and older African-Americans participate more than older whites (Levin et al., 1994).

Some gerontologists have proposed that the age-period-cohort issue may be responsible for higher religiosity among the old. For example, the older generation may have had more religious training during their early socialization, or they may have had different kinds of experiences during periods such as the world wars or the Great Depression during their life cycle. If that were true, then the pattern of higher religiosity among the old would be expected to change over time. However, this pattern of change has not been observed, and cross-sectional data have shown higher religiosity in later life with each successive generation (Moberg, 1990).

Several explanations have been put forth for the higher levels of religiousness among the old. One is that older people may be disengaged from other activities and hence have more time to devote to religion than do younger people. Each person has a desire for unity with God that is squelched by the pressures of life during youth and middle age but is released by freedom from social constraints in older age. Another explanation is that in later life, people are closer to death and thus depend on religion to resolve the existential fear of death. Highly religious people tend to have a sense of serenity and peace that may be related to a resolution of the existential problems that everyone must face.

One intriguing explanation for the higher levels of religiosity in the oldest generation arises out of studies showing that religious people tend to live longer. They have personal habits more conducive to physical and mental health and are less likely to indulge in behaviors such as smoking or alcohol abuse that are conducive to higher morbidity and mortality rates. Colantonio et al. (1992) found an association between more frequent attendance at religious services and lower incidence of stroke. In addition, religion has been found to be a source of strength for older adults who are medically ill. Studies have found that elderly people who are more religious recover from acute illnesses quicker, require fewer medications to control pain, and benefit from prayer and other religious devotions that seem to speed up the natural recuperative forces of the body (Zukerman et al., 1984; Koenig et al., 1988; Johnson et al., 1986; McNutt, 1977). Thus, the higher proportion of religiously committed people in later life may result from their outliving those who are not as committed (Moberg, 1990).

"Inner religion" more than ritualistic practices becomes increasingly important in later life as spiritual growth and maturity are achieved. Institutional religious participation serves both spiritual and social needs, including counseling, transportation, education, and recreation, and the church often acts as a family surrogate. The clergy and other representatives of the church provide comfort to the bereaved, counsel to the distressed, and material aid during emergencies. Most people turn first to their clergy when they have a social service need (McClellan, 1977; Ellor et al., 1987; Veroff et al., 1981; Moberg, 1990).

Problems that elderly persons have with organized religion include physical and social barriers that prevent participation in church activities. Physical barriers are related to access to the church buildings and activities and include steps, heavy doors, dull acoustics, and slippery or sloping floors. Social barriers are related to the alienation older people sometimes feel when programs appear to be geared to younger audiences. Some elderly people have felt that they were pushed aside from meaningful jobs within the organization, were not able to make sufficient financial contributions, were slighted or ignored, or were not able to dress well enough to fit into the congregation. In some cases, changes in the worship styles or music to appeal to younger members of the congregation were disturbing. In addition, some clergy lack knowledge of the aging process and have been insensitive to the needs of older adults in their congregations (Moberg, 1990).

Religion has been strongly correlated with well-being and life satisfaction in later life. Several studies have found that older people with high levels of religious activities and

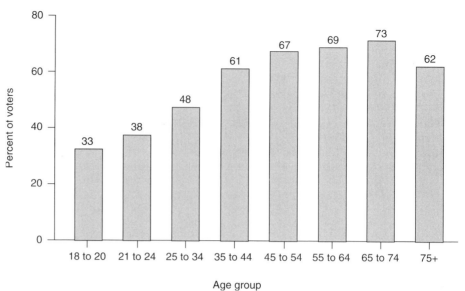

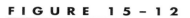

FIGURE 15-12

Percentage of people who reported voting in 1988, by age group. (From United States Department of Health and Human Services. *Aging America: Trends and Projections.* Washington, DC, 1991, p. 202.)

beliefs are psychologically healthier and have a higher morale than those with low levels (Coke, 1992; Morse and Wisocki, 1987; Koenig et al., 1988; Witter et al., 1985).

Spirituality is closely related to religion. Human nature has a spiritual component, and it is thought that everyone is a spiritual being. According to the National Interfaith Coalition on Aging (NICA), spiritual well-being is central to all concerns of the religious sector. The NICA working definition of spiritual well-being is "the affirmation of life in a relationship with God, self, community and environment that nurtures and celebrates wholeness" (Thorson and Cook, 1980, pp. xiii–xiv). Accumulating evidence suggests that spiritual well-being is one of the most significant sources, if not the central core, of life satisfaction, psychological health, and holistic well-being. All valid indicators of spiritual wellness correlate positively with measures of mental, physical, and social wellness (Moberg, 1990).

Hobbies and Leisure Pursuits

Most older people enjoy the retirement years, and two-thirds of the younger old who are recently retired are in good-to-excellent health and are very satisfied with their lives. Patterns of leisure activity are correlated with sex, personality, past experience, opportunity to pursue various types of activities, socioeconomic status, and health status. Leisure activities may continue into late life, although as people become more frail, some activities are may be more difficult to carry out (Grundy and Bowling, 1991; Schick and Schick, 1994).

Approximately 50 per cent of persons aged 65 years and older enjoy travel activities. Other favored leisure activities are mainly related to the creative arts, including performing needlework, weaving, and handiwork; performing photography; playing a musical instrument; singing in a choir; painting or drawing; writing; making pottery or ceramics; and folk dancing. It is interesting to note that elderly people either continue or develop new involvement in the creative arts because most studies support the notion that creativity is one intellectual function that does not decline with older age (Schick and Schick, 1994; Belsky, 1990).

Nearly half of all older people engage in some type of volunteer work, and over 6.3 million Americans aged 75 years and older are actively engaged in volunteerism. Many provide direct help to children or grandchildren, and 23 per cent give care to the sick or disabled. Twenty-two per cent volunteer through organizations, most frequently through religious organizations. The median amount of volunteer hours per week is approximately 5 hours, and the median number of weeks per year is approximately 35 (United States Department of Labor, Bureau of Labor Statistics, 1990).

Politics

The elderly maintain a strong interest in the elective process and have a high voting record (Fig. 15–12). During the 1990 congressional elections, 77 per cent of the population aged 65 years and older were registered, and more than 60 per cent voted, compared with 40 per cent registered and 20 per cent voting among the 18 to 24-year age group. Older men are more likely to vote than older women, and older whites are more likely to vote than older African-Americans and Hispanics (Schick and Schick, 1994; United States Department of Health and Human Services, 1991). Older people are a politically diverse group and generally do not vote as a bloc or as a special interest group.

Health Care

Older people today were born before the advent of many of the miracles of modern health care, such as antibiotics, vaccines, and coronary bypass operations. In general, the elderly appear to have a greater acceptance of physician authority than the young (Haug, 1982); however, this generalization is dependent on factors such as previous experiences with the health care world and general attitudes toward authority. Future cohorts of elderly are likely to be similar to the population at large regarding questioning the authority of physicians and other health professionals. This apparent acceptance of physician authority by the elderly should not be construed to mean that older persons are not accepting of health care provided by other disciplines. Research to evaluate the impact of nonphysician primary care providers on the health care of older persons and their health outcomes has shown widespread acceptance of nurse practitioners where they are in practice (Romeis et al., 1985; Panicucci et al., 1985).

SOCIOCULTURAL INFLUENCES ON AGING

Age-related changes in behavior may alter an individual's relationships with others. The aging of large numbers of people may also precipitate changes in social structures or processes. Characteristics of the social environment have been implicated in how individuals respond to biological aging changes and disease states.

Two major observable changes in the social environment occur with aging. First, the opportunities for social interaction change, resulting in altered role structures. The key mechanisms for the alteration in opportunities include health status changes and altered societal expectations based on age. At the same time that role expectations are in a state of flux, the social support available to the older person is changing. Financial support from governmental sources increases, whereas salary income decreases. The older person may initially give more support to younger members of the family than is re-

ceived, but with increasing frailty this dynamic usually changes. Patterns of mutual aid among friends change with changes in residence, dependency, and morality. A simplified view of those changes that affect role enactment is provided in Figure 15–1.

Individuals are seldom consciously aware that these changes in roles and social support are occurring. Therefore, there is ample opportunity for role conflict, overload, or rolelessness depending on the individual's life situation. Similarly, the adequacy of basic physical and emotional resources for coping with daily living vary with each individual.

The dynamics of age-related changes in role opportunities, expectations, and performance levels occur against a backdrop of cultural elements, including values, rituals, and conceptions of the life course and its meaning. Thus, a review of cultural influences on aging facilitates an understanding of various solutions and opportunities available to individuals as they confront age-related social stressors.

Cultural Influences

The study of cultural influences on the aging process and treatment of the elderly is considerably sparser than in other fields of gerontology (Keith, 1985; Holzberg, 1982). Cultural gerontology offers insights about (1) age grading in society, (2) status and treatment of the elderly, (3) social change and its effects on older people, and (4) ethnicity as a means of coping with problems engendered by age-related change.

The synthesis of research findings into a coherent theory of cultural influences on aging has been hampered by limited numbers of studies and oversimplification of concepts, such as status and treatment of the aged; failure to distinguish the effects of social variables, such as sex, social class, and economic status within cultural groups; and an overemphasis on the study of the problems of disadvantaged minority groups in the United States rather than the study of all ethnic groups (Keith, 1985; Holzberg, 1982). Despite the limitations of the research base, cultural factors undoubtedly influence the experience of aging, and it is therefore worthwhile to consider the available research findings.

Age Grading

Most cultures have some system of organization based on age groupings (Keith, 1982; Riley, 1976). How age is defined, graded, and marked varies among cultures.

For example, a range of two to eight age groupings has been noted in one study of 60 preindustrial societies (Glascock and Feinman, 1981). In most of these societies, the age gradations are more elaborate for men than for women. Markers frequently used for delineating age groups include chronological age and membership in age groups according to functions served. Glascock and Feinman (1981) found that the most common definition of old age is a change in social role, such as altered work responsibilities, or a change in the status of children. Chronological age is the next most commonly used marker, followed by changes in physical capabilities.

In the United States, there is little consensus on age gradations, and the complexity of age grades described is related to the life stage of the individual doing the categorization. In one study, individuals between the ages of 46 and 65 made the fewest categories, whereas older and younger individuals made more categories. One interpretation of these variations in defining age categories is that when other means of categorizing people, such as through work or other social roles, exist, age categorization has less meaning (Fry, 1976).

A birth cohort is a type of age grouping. One significance of birth cohort in working with aged clients is that society uses birth cohort to designate or label people as old. Insofar as the "old people" accept this designation, they become a social group subject to certain previously established social norms concerning appropriate behavior for old people. These norms may severely restrict social opportunity for the elderly.

Effects on Attitudes and Behaviors of the Individual

Each age stratum has its own life course dimension and historical (or cohort) dimension, both of which come together to form a unique type of subculture for each age group at a given point in history (Riley et al., 1979). This subculture can be characterized by such variables as labor force participation, consumer behavior, leisure activities, religious activities, education, and values and attitudes toward health, illness, and death. Specifically, previous cohorts of elderly persons have been shown to be more cautious, more religious, more accepting of death, and more politically active than younger cohorts. The existence of these differences along with other factors, such as observations concerning role loss associated with old age, has led some sociologists to consider the aged as a subcultural group in

society (Rose, 1965), although the theory is by no means universally held.

The concept of "social clocks" has been used to summarize the observation that Americans seem to agree about proper timing for various life events, such as retirement, child rearing, marriage, and education (Neugarten and Hagestad, 1976). When a major life event occurs at a different time than the social norm would suggest, the event is perceived as more stressful. Neugarten et al. (1965) also found that norms regarding age-appropriate dress existed and that such norms were emotionally charged. The norms that currently exist for "old age" may not be entirely satisfactory to the present or future occupants of that group, and thus behavioral expectations for "old people" may change with future cohorts of old people.

Clinicians should develop an appreciation for age-related differences in the attitudes, values, and behaviors of clients. Because attitudes, values, and beliefs are shaped by the unique interaction of the aging process, cohort factors, and the environment, it is difficult to draw generalizations about groups of old people. Thus, it is particularly important that clinicians working with the elderly update their concepts of these attitudes as they work with successive cohorts of older persons. For example, some of the formality that is currently important to observe between health care providers and the elderly may not be necessary or appropriate 20 years from now.

Effects on Intergenerational Relationships

Age grading also leads to expectations regarding treatment of one age group by another. For example, most Americans traditionally have shared the expectation that younger generations should care for their elders in times of need (McCullough et al., 1993; Wolfson et al., 1993; Stevens et al., 1993). Although such values have been widely shared, sufficient social proximity must exist for these norms to be enforced (Keith, 1982). In a study of the treatment of old people in an Appalachian community where most families have lived in the same community for many generations, children who did not treat their elders properly were judged negatively. Lozier and Althouse (1974) pointed out that the old people are treated well by the youth because of concern about how others will judge them, not because older people control important resources. Other examples of close cultural or geographical ties contributing to the well-being of frail elderly in urban settings have been documented (Hendel-Sebestyen, 1979; Moore, 1978; Tennstedt et al., 1993). The fact that most American elderly have children living in geographical proximity bodes well for the enforcement of the norms of filial piety. However, socially isolated or recently relocated old people may be more vulnerable than those who remain in their home communities.

Effects on Transitions Between Age Categories

Few clear rites of passage exist in modern industrialized society to mark the boundary between one adult chronological age group and the next. Exceptions to this include age 18 (the voting age), age 21 (the age of full legal maturity as an adult), and age 65 (the age at which one usually becomes eligible for Social Security and Medicare benefits). Increasingly society is recognizing that chronological age categories have limited usefulness; indeed, they can sometimes be detrimental to the interests of the public at large. Therefore, in considering the effects of age-related transitions, there is more meaning in discussing transitions between functional age categories, such as the transition between worker and nonworker or between an individual with generally good health and one with generally poor health, than in the transition from age 59 to 60 or age 69 to 70. The range of responses to these functional transitions is discussed later in this chapter.

Research on role transitions accompanying the passage into old age such as widowhood, retirement, and institutionalization, and dying has shown that the majority of people achieve these life transitions without extreme difficulty (Butler et al., 1991). However, clinicians are more likely to see individuals who are experiencing difficulty with these transitions, so it is important to consider the dynamics involved. These transitions are discussed in detail later in this chapter.

Not all social gerontologists agree with the notion that role transitions are not problematic for the aged. Rosow (1973) observed that age-related changes in roles and statuses are all marked by successive social growth in number and importance of roles until old age. At that point, the changes in roles are primarily decremental, that is, the elderly give up roles or engage in roles that are increasingly marginal. He further contended that old people are not properly socialized for their role loss, leading to a socially unstructured life in which there are few responsibilities, expectations, or standards by which to judge themselves. This he termed "direct, sustained attack on the ego," as social roles are the essence of self-concept and self-esteem (Rosow, 1985). Thus, the net effect of transition from middle adulthood to old age is viewed as progressive loss of roles and social importance.

Most difficulties encountered in age-related transitions can be directly related to the role changes that occur. Role change at any age is generally considered to be stressful, but role change for those of advanced age may be particularly difficult because of diminished social opportunity. Additionally, the role changes that accompany old age, unlike those in younger years, may represent a discontinuity with prior roles (Rosow, 1974), which makes adjustment more difficult.

Status and Treatment of the Elderly

Preindustrial Societies

Cross-cultural studies suggest that the aged have a higher status in society when they control vital information, have accumulated more wealth or property relative to younger adults, or have great political control (Keith, 1985; Maxwell and Silverman, 1970). Despite high status, old people may receive nonsupportive treatment from their society. Abandonment and killing of the aged have been documented in preindustrial societies where the climate is harsh and where the economy is subsistence level. The popularized notion that old people universally received better treatment in the "good old days" is not supported by cross-cultural studies or historical data (Keith, 1985).

Impact of Social Change

Extrapolations from cross-cultural studies have led to concern about the effects of modernization and rapid social change on the status of old people in industrial and postindustrial societies. The fear has been that urbanization destroys extended kin networks, and industrialization and the development of high technology reduce the dependence on oral traditions and the old ways, leaving the elder members of society without economically vital information stores. Finally, traditional sources of wealth, such as property and control of manufacturing enterprises, may be replaced in importance by service industry and new product development activities, and old people may therefore lose economic and political control. The theory of the impact of modernization on the status of the aged was described by

Cowgill and Holmes (1972) and was later refined (Cowgill, 1974).

Although social change related to modernization may cause the status of older people to decline relative to that of younger adults (Gilleard and Gurkan, 1987), improvements in the society's standard of living generally are likely to have a positive influence on the old people also. Development of strong social welfare programs is more likely in industrialized societies, and the old may achieve special status under such circumstances. Finally, when revivalist change occurs and past customs and values become revered, old people enjoy increased status because they once again control vital information about the past (Keith, 1985). Modernization theory has been tempered by studies that show that rapid industrialization may evoke a temporary drop in status for the elderly, followed by a gradual increase in status and positive treatment as the society enters a postindustrial phase (Palmore and Manton, 1974; Keith, 1985; Grundy and Bowling, 1991).

Social Responses to Growth in the Elderly Population

Societal responses to the pressures generated by increasing numbers of people living into advanced years include the following:

- Development of special aging interest groups to advocate on behalf of the elderly

- Increase in the bureaucracy necessary to deal with rapidly increasing numbers of dependent older adults

- Changing attitudes toward work and leisure

- Increased pressure on women as concurrent demands for their energies from both the workplace and dependent elderly conflict

Special Interest Groups

The aged and gerontological professionals are organized into several key special interest groups, which have gained recognition as powerful forces for social change. Some of the groups include the American Association of Retired Persons (AARP), the National Council on the Aging (NCOA), the Gray Panthers Network, and the Gerontological Society of America (GSA). These groups have been in the forefront of lobbying for maintaining services currently available to older people, increasing community-based options for long-term care, and improving access to specialized training in gerontology and geriatrics for health care providers. Finally, the special interest groups have led the fight against outmoded stereotypes of the elderly and ageist public policy through demonstration projects, research, public education, and lobbying efforts. Some examples of the specific activities of these special interest groups will help to further define their range and potential.

NCOA is involved in such diverse projects as developing standards for senior centers and adult day care, stimulating medical student interest in geriatrics through funding of small-scale predoctoral fellowships, producing publications for individuals working in the field of gerontology, and sponsoring national meetings to provide a communications network for service innovations that contribute to well-being in old age.

AARP is the largest organization for older people in the country. Among other activities, it produces a variety of widely read publications for older adults; operates an economical, high-volume pharmaceutical service; and does extensive lobbying at the federal level. It also sponsors small-scale research projects designed to enhance the quality of life for the aged.

The Gray Panther network is a loosely confederated, intergenerational group that is more responsive to local issues, where strong networks are in place. The organization is interested in a fairly broad social agenda that includes concerns of older people.

The GSA is a multidisciplinary professional and scientific organization for those working in the field of gerontology. It produces research publications, holds scientific meetings, publishes compilations of relevant research, and is a resource of experts in the field of gerontology. Annual scientific meetings are held to enhance communication among researchers and practitioners. The GSA also sponsors a postdoctoral fellowship program in applied gerontology to help link academics with practical problems of aging service delivery or policy formulation.

Growth of Bureaucracy

The population explosion of elderly persons has occurred at a time when Americans have increasingly turned to government for assistance with social problems. Additionally, because American families have never had a legal responsibility to care for their elders, only a moral one, there has been an increased need for solutions generated by formal organizations. These two factors have contributed to the plethora of bureaucratic "solutions" to some of the problems associated with aging. The Social Security system is perhaps the largest and most visible example. Others include the Medicaid program (which funds approximately 75 per cent of nursing home care in the United States), various programs sponsored under the Older Americans Act, and local bureaucracies established to disburse private sector philanthropy. The nature of the problems of dependent older persons has not changed fundamentally over the past century, but the numbers of persons who need care have, and the mechanisms for addressing those needs are in tremendous flux. The problems associated with the increasing bureaucratization of human services are discussed later in this chapter.

Changes in Attitudes Toward Work and Leisure

Attitudes concerning basic social structures and values are undergoing major revision. As individuals begin to plan for a lifespan that includes old age, alternative views of the balance between work and leisure are emerging. There is a gradually increasing interest in flexible work patterns, from early retirement, to delayed retirement, to no retirement at all.

Concern about the long-range effects of lifestyle and health practices is growing. There is an increased social awareness of the problems of dependent older persons, with an increased focus on alternatives to institutional solutions to these problems. The high cost of medical care for older persons has helped fuel a national discussion on the high cost and appropriateness of high-technology medical care.

Conflicts in Women's Roles

Women traditionally have been the caregivers of dependent elders in modern society. Over the past several decades, women have been entering the work force in unprecedented numbers. Various factors foster this development, including changing opportunities in the workplace for women, the women's movement, and economic necessity.

There is a serious tension between the woman's role as a wage earner and the woman's role as caregiver for dependent older family members. Employers typically have not been sympathetic toward some of the special circumstances that surround caring for dependent elderly individuals. At present, this conflict is manifested primarily within the lives of the women affected. It remains to be seen what societal remedies will be applied to help resolve this conflict, which is likely to affect many women in the decades ahead. Rapidly increasing numbers of women in the work force highlight the

conflict many women face between their work role expectations and their traditional role as caregiver for the dependent elderly family (Lue et al., 1993; Pollock, 1994; Denton et al., 1990; Moen et al., 1994).

Ethnicity and Aging

American culture is highly pluralistic, meaning that it is composed of many subcultures. However, a set of cultural values do predominate, including (1) an emphasis on self-reliance and independence, (2) an appreciation for accomplishments and productivity over longevity, and (3) a higher value placed on "new and improved" than "old and trusted."

Whereas Americans have a fairly well-developed social welfare system, European countries have clearly superior models. The predominant American cultural values lead to ambivalence about the importance of a strong social welfare system and the degree to which services should be provided (Maddox, 1994).

Elderly people experience special hardships in a culture with these ambivalent values, including decreased role opportunities because work for the young is valued over work for the old, and decreased access to health care because curing diseases is valued over humane dependent care. Holzberg (1982) suggested that greater identification with ethnic groups is one means of buffering the negative effects of the predominant American cultural values regarding the status and treatment of the aged.

Holzberg defined ethnicity as . . . social differentiation based on such cultural criteria as a sense of peoplehood, shared history, a common place of origin, language, dress, food preferences and participation in particular clubs or voluntary associations [which] engenders a sense of exclusiveness and self-awareness that one is a member of a distinct and bounded social group. . . . Ethnic ideologies tend to pursue cultural norms not shared by others in society. What ethnic membership thus implies for the elderly is the opportunity for individuals to *sustain continuity in their repertoires of already familiar lifestyles and culturally stylized patterns of social involvement* (1982, pp. 252–253, emphasis added).

Strong identification with an ethnic group can enhance role opportunities and status for the elderly. In addition, certain ethnic groups, such as African-Americans, Hispanics, and Asians, are believed to provide greater emotional and material support to their elders, although the research base on ethnicity and aging often rests on a weak empirical base (Silverstein and Waite, 1993; Burr and Meitchler, 1993).

Double Jeopardy Hypothesis

Minority groups experience aging differently from white males (the dominant cultural group) for several reasons, including institutionalized victimization of minority groups and systematic discrimination against minority groups. Life circumstances and negative environmental, social, and economic conditions early in the life course of ethnic minorities can have significant influences on the quality of life in the latter stages. This has led to the suggestion that there is a "multiple jeopardy" effect of age and minority status that has particular significance in the variability in responses to aging.

There are currently two contradictory perspectives on the effect of minority group membership on aging. The first perspective suggests that minority aged are in a position of double jeopardy, that is, they suffer from diminished status and opportunities because of their ethnic status and their age. The opposing perspective contends that increasing age tends to diminish the effects of inequality based on ethnic background because of reduced social status associated with old age (Grundy and Bowling, 1991; Jackson et al., 1990).

It is important for clinicians to realize that most social gerontology research and aging policies in the United States have ignored cultural variables. It is a significant limitation of the gerontological literature that the majority of the research has been done on white, male, urban individuals. This is expected to change with time, as researchers systematically include minority and rural populations in study samples.

Implications for Practice

Three caveats should be remembered when considering the effects of ethnicity on aging:

1. Ethnicity appears to be an important dimension of social stratification among the aged.
2. Norms and values of the predominant cultural group of the older person should be considered in working with the elderly.
3. Although membership in an ethnic group may represent unique problems for that group of aged individuals, it is likely that membership in that subcultural group also brings important resources in coping with age-related adjustments (Bengtson, 1979).

Social Support Networks

Social support ranges from the occasional unexpected letter or telephone call from a distant relative, through daily responses to role performances, to financial and physical assistance with essential ADLs for those with severe physical or cognitive impairments.

A support system is an enduring pattern of attachment among individuals and groups that helps the individual cope with short-term crises, life transitions, and long-term problems (Caplan and Killilea, 1976). Support systems work by providing guidance in dealing with problems at hand; offering feedback to the individual, which fosters improved performance; and promoting a sense of control over the situation.

Support networks are important to the elderly in several ways. Support systems are key in helping individuals maintain physical and psychological health, maintain self-concept, and obtain material assistance with mental or physical impairments (Roberts et al., 1994).

Social support comes from a variety of sources, ranging from family and friends to neighbors, bureaucratic organizations such as health care agencies and religious and voluntary organizations (Felton and Berry, 1992). Cantor (1977) proposed a model of social support for the elderly that was com-

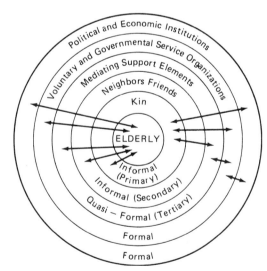

F I G U R E   1 5 – 1 3

Schematic model of the social support system of the elderly. (From Cantor, M. Neighbors and friends: An overlooked resource in the informal support system. Paper presented at the 30th Annual Meeting of the Gerontological Society, San Francisco, 1977. Reprinted in Cantor, M. and Little, V. Aging and Social Care. *In* Binstock, R. and Shanas, E. (eds.). *Handbook of Aging and the Social Sciences.* 2nd ed. New York: Van Nostrand Reinhold, 1985, p. 748.)

TABLE 15–4

Major Tasks Performed by Informal and Mediating and Formal Systems According to Level of Functional Impairment of the Elderly

		INFORMAL SYSTEM	MEDIATING AND FORMAL SYSTEMS
Frail impaired, 10%	Low ↑	Co-residence Total money management Assistance in home—extensive, light and heavy housekeeping, meals, shopping, etc. Personal care—washing, bathing, supervising of medical regimen, etc.	Institutional care Protective service Case management Counseling—older person and/or families, self-help groups Respite service—day hospital, day care, special set-aside beds Homemaker service Home health aides, visiting nurse Meals on wheels
Moderately impaired, 30%	Level of Competency	System negotiation Help with financial management Accompanying to medical appointments Assistance in home—more frequent, wider array of tasks, i.e., shopping, occasional meal preparation, light housekeeping	Linkage to services, counseling older person Escort, transportation Friendly visiting Congregate housing Chore service—limited in time and amount
Well elderly, 60% of population	↓ High	Assistance when ill—short term Assistance in home—short term Escort, transportation Advice Gifts, money Visiting, providing affective support	Reduced-fare programs on public transportation Information and referral Assistance with entitlements Cultural and spiritual enrichment programs Socialization, recreation opportunities, i.e., senior center, nutrition, parks

From Cantor, M. and Little, V. Aging and social care. In Binstock, R. and Shanas, E. (eds.). *Handbook of Aging and the Social Sciences.* 2nd ed. New York: Van Nostrand Reinhold, 1985, p. 750.

Note: The services shown are cumulative, and it is assumed that any services shown in a prior level will continue to be available if appropriate.

posed of many interacting systems (Fig. 15–13). In general, the closer to the center of the figure, the more flexible the source of support. Most older persons receive support from more than one of these sources. It is important for clinicians to consider how these various groups work together in providing support for the elderly individual.

Cantor and Little (1985) contended that the end of the life cycle is characterized by an increased dependence on others because of waning physical strength, mobility, and economic resources, resulting in individual conflicts between personal needs and the Western cultural values of self-reliance and independence in adulthood. The use of informal helping networks, such as family, neighbors, and friends, reduces the psychological damage of dependency because older people tend to view members of informal support networks as extensions of themselves. However, informal support systems are not always sufficient to meet the needs of older people, particularly the frail elderly. Table 15–4 lists the varying tasks typically provided by informal and formal support systems for older people according to their level of functional ability. Older people most often turn for assistance to family first, followed by friends, neighbors, and formal organizations (Cantor, 1980; Stoller and Earl, 1983; Logan and Spitze, 1994).

The Family

The family is the cornerstone of the social support network of most people, playing a key role in providing material support and serving as an important source of socialization and value transmission. The early literature on family relationships in late life emphasized theories about gradual weakening of ties between generations despite empirical evidence of close intergenerational relationships. There has been a tendency for researchers and practitioners to idealize the past, resulting in a mythology surrounding family relationships in advanced age. Early theorists failed to note the tremendous adaptability of family systems to societal changes, such as modernization and migration. To quote (Shanas et al., 1968, p. 180):

The traditional assumptions about the changes in the family and the disintegration of relations between the generations in modern societies have never been supported by empirical evidence. On the contrary, a number of studies have demonstrated that the generations, although preferring to live apart, maintain contact and exchange mutual services. What is found between the generations is "intimacy at a distance" rather than isolation.

Many studies confirm that older people in Western societies are well connected with their families and are active participants in the exchange of social support (Silverstein and Beugtson, 1994; Perry and Johnson, 1994; Beach, 1993; Tennstedt et al., 1993).

Family Structure and Aging

The structure of the American family has changed in recent years. At the present time, an older person generally is part of a four- or five-generation family that is made up of fewer members per generation than a family would have been earlier in this century. In addition, as a result of shifts in mortality and fertility, families have more older members than younger members. Fewer children in the family and longer lifespans have increased the time individuals spend within the intergenerational family, and older persons may spend up to 50 years with their children, as compared with 20 or 30 years in the 1880s. Grandparenthood also has become an expanded and clearly delineated role that is separate from parenthood. People who become grandparents at the median age of 45 and who live to the current life expectancy of 75 years can expect to be a grandparent for nearly half of their lives (Intrieri and Rapp, 1994).

Most older people have a small immediate family but are likely to belong to an extended kin network. Thus, children have the opportunity to interact on a regular basis with elders in their families, suggesting that the elderly continue to have the potential to form a viable role in the kinship network. For the majority of elderly, aging serves to reduce the size of the household but increases the number and complexity of role relationships within the kinship network, as subsequent generations produce more kinspeople. One notable exception is the case of individuals who as younger adults had limited kin networks and no children. In this case, increased death rates of aged members obviously reduces the size of the network.

Intergenerational Family Relationships

Support within families flows in all directions, so that chronological age is not useful in distinguishing providers from recipients. Intergenerational support takes many forms, including the giving and receiving of money and material resources, care, household assistance, and companionship and advice. The configuration of the family has a significant effect on family support. For example, it is not uncommon to find siblings caring for one another if no spouses or children are present. Another growing phenomenon is younger old people who are in their late sixties caring for older-old relatives in their eighties or nineties. This may occur in mother-daughter relationships or some other kin combinations.

Mutran and Reitzes (1990) summarized major research findings from research on intergenerational relationships. The overriding finding is that intergenerational relationships between elderly parents and their adult children are both extensive and important to both parties. Although children provide satisfaction and well-being to older parents, contact with friends and neighbors appears to be more closely associated with well-being than are contacts with children. Thus, family and nonfamily interactions can be viewed as complementary, so that when relationships with friends and neighbors are satisfying, there is more satisfaction from attention from children. Other findings emphasize the influence of past experiences on intergenerational interactions and expectations and the effect of socioeconomic status on the exchange and type of support provided. Women have greater intergenerational family roles than men, and female-linked kin networks have greater interaction, more emotional exchanges, and more frequent patterns of mutual aid.

Most discussions of family support and the aged center on the support received by older persons, but older people often serve as standard bearers of family values, provide emotional support to children and grandchildren, and care for dependents, their children or their dependent elders. Through these activities, they assist in coping with age-related losses and carry out linkage functions with bureaucracies. In short, the elderly can and do fulfill all available support functions within families (Hogan et al., 1993).

The Marital Relationship

Over half of all persons aged 65 years and older are married (Schick and Schick, 1994). Couples who have been married for many years find that their marriage is different from that in their earlier years. Expectations in older marriages include care during illness, household management, and emotional gratification. Women are more likely to be named confidants by their husbands than they are to name their husbands as confidants. Women also are less likely to report receiving social support from their spouses. Marital satisfaction appears to be higher among older adults who confide in their spouses, and men report higher satisfaction with marriage than do women (Anderson and McCulloch, 1993).

Kelley (1981) characterized the nature of

marital relationships in late life in terms of interdependence. He described two types of interdependence between spouses: (1) interdependence in specific behaviors and (2) interdependence of attitudes and values. Shifts in the nature of these interdependencies as a result of aging may cause marital stress. For example, retirement can cause an increased interdependence between spouses and can precipitate marital stress. Szinovacz and Harpster (1994) found in a subsample of the National Survey of Families and Households that the employment or retirement status of both partners in a marriage affected the division of household tasks. The retired spouse usually had the heaviest responsibility for carrying out both "male" and "fe-male" household tasks if the other spouse was working.

Atchley and Miller (1983) identified three age-related changes for couples that have potential impact on the quality of the marital relationship: (1) retirement, (2) changes in the health of one spouse, and (3) changes in residence. The impact of changes in marital relationships accompanying retirement seems to depend on how rigidly the couple defined their roles before retirement. Those with more rigid definitions experienced more adjustment problems than those who define their roles more flexibly.

The following case example depicts one pattern of marital interdependence and its change across the lifespan.

CASE

Mr. and Mrs. H. have been married for 65 years. Consider the changes in interdependence in their relationship over the years.

Mr. and Mrs. H. met in college, where Mr. H. was an engineering student. He successfully completed his degree, and they were married.

Mr. H. worked for the next 40 years for a national engineering firm. During this time, the family moved to two different locales and raised two children. Mrs. H. never worked outside the home but was active in civic and church work in each locale. Mr. H., in addition to his work activities, was active in civic organizations. Both of the children went to college, pursued advanced degrees, moved away from the family home, and married and have nine children between them.

When Mr. H. retired, they moved to the southeast, near Mrs. H.'s original home, and built a house approximately 50 miles from their son's residence. They developed a new circle of friends and activities. Mr. H. was an avid swimmer. He continued to make the major financial decisions in the household, and Mrs. H. kept the social calendar for the household.

They both enjoyed excellent health until 20 years after Mr. H.'s retirement, at which time he developed Parkinson's disease and an associated major depression. Mrs. H. has assumed increasing responsibility for managing the household finances and making decisions about moving to a retirement community.

- Shift from courtship to marriage relationship
- Shift from major financial responsibility for oneself to responsibility to wife and family
- Expansion of family roles to include parenting responsibilities
- Alteration in parent roles due to maturation of children
- Assumption of grandparent role
- Change in daily activities with Mr. H.'s retirement
- Maintenance of traditional responsibilities despite role change with retirement
- Health status decline forcing major realignment of household responsibilities

---

SEXUALITY. Attitudes toward sexuality in later life vary among both young and old adults. For example, many individuals believe that sexual behavior in older age is a private matter not to be discussed. Others find the subject distasteful and view sex in old people as ugly and inappropriate. Conversely, recent positive attitudes toward elderly people as sexual beings have developed based on information about the realities of sex in old age. Finally, some people narrowly view sexuality in later life in relation to the act itself that occurs between heterosexual partners rather than in the context of the wider range of sexual expressions among various types of partners (Oppenheimer, 1991).

These attitudes can have an effect on research regarding sexuality in older age. However, despite methodological problems in many studies, most findings support the notion that many elderly persons continue to carry out a sexual component to their spouse role. In a survey of married people 60 years of age and older, 53 per cent of the entire sample and 24 per cent of those over age 75 reported having had sexual relations at least once in the previous month (Marsiglio and Donnelly, 1991). In another national survey, it was found that nearly one third of persons older than 70 years had engaged in at least one act of sexual intercourse over the previous year (Smith, 1991).

There is a gradual decline in sexual activity, interest, and quality with older age. The Duke Longitudinal Study (Busse and Maddox, 1985) found a 50 per cent decline in sexual activity in men aged 68 years and older during a 10-year period, and a 1989 general social survey conducted by the National Opinion Research Center found that the amount of abstinence from sexual activity increased from 13 per cent among respondents under age 30 to 68 per cent at age 70 or older (Smith, 1991).

Although the decline in sexual activity in the elderly is generally universal, there is marked variability in interest and capacity within the older population. Some older spouses are celibate, whereas others maintain the same level of activity as during their younger years. Continuity appears to be the best predictor of sexual activity in later life, so that people who were sexually active in their youth are more likely to be active in older age (Levy, 1994).

Social factors that affect sexual interest and behavior include self-perceptions of being sexually attractive, access to a sexually functional partner, and access to a conducive environment (Levy, 1994; Marsiglio and Donnelly, 1991). In older age, men are more likely to view themselves as desirable than women because they tend to have more positive views of their aging bodies (Byers, 1983). Women are more likely than men to be without a sexual partner in later life because of their greater longevity. In addition, studies conducted during the past 30 years

report that in older married and cohabiting couples, male sexual dysfunction is the prime reason for not engaging in sexual intercourse (Masters and Johnson, 1966; Starr and Weiner, 1981; White, 1982).

Social environment also plays a part in sexual activity. Although most older couples live by themselves, many reside in joint household arrangements with children or others or in nursing homes. These environments often interfere with privacy, and negative attitudes of others may hinder sexual activity (Levy, 1994).

Research findings on sexuality and the aged are significant because many health care professionals erroneously conclude that loss of sexual drive or potency is not a matter of concern for the elderly. Thus, the impact of medications that may decrease libido or result in impotence is frequently not discussed with older adults or considered in the selection of a drug or treatment regimen. Similarly, elderly people are sometimes not adequately assessed for sexual dysfunction related to diseases, such as myocardial infarction; treatment of diseases, such as mastectomy or prostatectomy; or pharmacotherapy for hypertension.

WIDOWHOOD. Loss of a spouse is a highly significant life event that can have negative implications for the surviver; however, most widows and widowers cope remarkably well. The bereavement process involves three distinct tasks: (1) the loss is accepted intellectually, (2) the loss is accepted emotionally, and (3) the person's model of self and outer world is changed to match the new reality. Theoretically, the process should be near completion approximately 2 years after the death of a spouse (Gallagher and Thompson, 1989). However, it has been found that the grief process in older adults is frequently unpredictable, and at the end of 2 years, people may still be actively grieving. Furthermore, along with signs of recovery, some even have symptoms supposedly typical of the earliest weeks—shock, disbelief, and avoidance of the fact (Belsky, 1990).

Many factors may affect the depth of bereavement and the ease of recovery, including antecedent factors; mode of death; concurrent factors, such as sex and age; and subsequent factors, such as social support or secondary stressors (Table 15–5). Older people seem to handle the death of a spouse better and have less intense levels of distress during the first few months than do younger people (Zisook et al., 1993). In addition, older women appear to handle the trauma of widowhood best of any age or

TABLE 15-5
Hypothetical Factors Determining the Outcome of Mourning

ANTECEDENT FACTORS	MODE OF DEATH	CONCURRENT FACTORS	SUBSEQUENT FACTORS
Childhood experiences (especially losses of significant persons) Later experiences (especially losses of significant persons) Previous mental illness (especially depressive illness) Life crises prior to bereavement Relationship with deceased: kinship, strength of attachment, security of attachment, degree of reliance, intensity of reliance, intensity of ambivalence (love/hate)	Timeliness Previous warning Preparation for bereavement Need to hide feelings	Sex Age Personality Socioeconomic status Nationality Religion Cultural factors Familial factors	Social support or isolation Secondary stresses Emergent life opportunities

From Parkes, C. Bereavement: Studies of Grief in Adult Life. New York: International Universities Press, 1972.

gender category, and they are least likely to develop emotional and physical problems after their spouse dies. The myth that older men have more intense periods of grief and prolonged adjustment difficulties is largely unfounded, however. Most researchers have found few differences in the grief experience of older men and women (Belsky, 1990).

Parent-Child Relationship

For most adults, the parent-child bond persists throughout life and does not weaken appreciably over the years. The relationship is based on affection and is characterized by closeness and caring. Contrary to popular opinion, the frequency of contact between older parents and their grown children does not diminish. In addition, although few older adults live with their children, many live nearby. In a series of classical cross-sectional studies over a period of 20 years, Shanes (1979a, 1979b) found that there was little change in the patterns of interactions. Over 75 per cent lived within a 30-minute drive of a child, and more than half had seen a child either that day or the day before; about 80 per cent had seen a child in the past week.

The quality of the contacts appears to be more important than the quantity. Field et al. (1993) observed stability in family contacts and family feelings over 14 years of advanced old age. Older adults who were in better health had more contact with family and had more feelings of closeness than those in poorer health. However, frequent or increased contacts may arise out of a negative emotion and indicate a need by either the parent (such as an illness) or the child (such as a divorce). The quality of the rela-

tionship appears to diminish when either the parent or child needs excessive help (Belsky, 1990).

The number of older parents living with adult children has markedly decreased since 1900. In 1900, more than 60 per cent of all people aged 65 years and older lived with an adult child, and in 1975, the figure dropped to 16 per cent. In 1990, fewer than 8 per cent of men and 16 per cent of women over age 65 lived with children; the percentage increases with age to approximately 21 per cent in men and 28 per cent in women over age 85 (Schick and Schick, 1994).

The relationship between older parents and their children appears to be healthier when some distance is between them (Cohler and Grunebaum, 1981; Hagestad, 1985). The myth that the close extended family living under one roof was more caring than today's family living in separate quarters has perpetuated. However, Shanas (1979b) found that the ideal arrangement is one called "intimacy at a distance," that is, not living together but very close by. And, it is the parent generation that prefers the separate living arrangement; most elderly vigorously reject the idea of moving in with a child.

Parents continue to maintain the role of advisor to children in later life. Most advising occurs when older parents are vigorous and healthy, and the role of advisor shifts to the children when parents become frail or needy (Belsky, 1990). Aged parents also may serve as caregivers to grandchildren and transmitters of family culture and values. Most elderly people in the community feel close to their children, and, for the most part, the feelings are mutual (Cicirelli, 1981).

Grandparent Relationship

Grandparenting is frequently a joyous reward in older age. Neugarten and Weinstein (1964) developed a typology of grandparenting styles, including

Formal: in which the grandparents have rigid role expectations for themselves and their grandchildren, with interaction being somewhat constrained and characterized as fairly authoritarian

Fun seekers: in which the grandparents tend to interact with grandchildren around pleasurable, leisure activities

Surrogate parents: in which the grandparents assume caregiving responsibilities for the grandchildren on a regular basis

Reservoirs of family wisdom: in which the primary role is to pass down information about family culture and heritage

Distant: in which interactions are infrequent and limited to holidays

These styles tend to change according to the age of the grandchild. For example, Cherlin and Furstenberg (1985) found that the fun-seeking style did not appear when grandparents interacted with teenage grandchildren. They observed that it was easy for grandparents to treat toddlers as sources of leisure time fun, but "a grandmother doesn't bounce a teenaged grandchild on her knee" (p. 100).

The styles can also change according to the age of the grandparent. Younger grandparents are more likely to be highly active and involved, whereas older grandparents (over age 65) tend to be more removed and peripherally involved (Belsky, 1990).

Access to grandchildren often depends on factors related to the parents. Matthews and Sprey (1985) found that young adults feel closest to grandparents whom they saw most often during childhood, and these were the ones that the parents had the closest relationships with. Divorce of the parents also can affect the grandparent-grandchild relationship. Jaskowski and Dellasega (1993) noted a significant decline in the quality of grandparent-grandchild relationship after parents divorced, and the relationship was influenced by custodial arrangements rather than by distance.

Most people view the grandparent role as having vital meaning in their life. Grandparents are valued and loved for just "being there" and are looked on as a stabilizing force in the family. In a time of crisis, they often step in to keep the family afloat and provide emotional support and other types of help. They also can be family mediators and can keep the family close (Belsky, 1990).

Sibling Relationship

Sibling relationships in later life can be very meaningful and enriching. It is often the longest lasting of any family relationship and may be the most egalitarian of any kin tie (Cicirelli, 1983). This, plus the blood ties and shared history that exists between siblings, makes the sibling relationship unique in the family (Gold, 1987). According to Bedford (1989), social losses due to retirement, relocation, and death can be better filled by siblings, because of their peer status, than by adult children.

Cicirelli (1980) found that elders with frequent contact with siblings had a greater sense of control in life than adults with infrequent interaction. It has also been found that the loss of a sibling or lack of interaction contributes to loneliness among older persons (Gold, 1987; Dugan and Kivett, 1994). Sibling ties are particularly close and active in women and in elders who are single, divorced, widowed, and childless (Connidis, 1994).

Currently, there is an inadequate research base to make generalizations about intergenerational support in minorities. Data from the 1987–1988 National Survey of Family and Households (Hogan et al., 1993) refuted earlier findings that would suggest stronger patterns of support in African-American and Hispanic families than in white Americans. Results of the survey indicate that routine intergenerational support occurs about as often in African-Americans as in whites. However, taking racial differences in family structure, needs, and resources into account, African-American families are less involved in intergenerational assistance than are white families. Multigenerational African-American families in need often lack the financial, human, and capital resources to meet the needs of all generations adequately. In a study of oldest-old African-Americans, Perry and Johnson (1994) found that females receive more help from relatives and friends, and males receive more help from immediate family members. Overall, fewer family members were available to assist the oldest-old with community living, although many were able to increase the number of helpers available to assist them. Thus, a pattern of substitution for intergenerational help emerged, particularly in older African-Americans who were childless and female.

Mexican-Americans are less involved in giving and receiving assistance than are whites and African-Americans, and only 23 per cent of other Hispanic groups are involved in intergenerational assistance. The lower participation in intergenerational exchange for Mexican-Americans may be accounted for by greater distance from relatives who remained in Mexico (Hogan et al., 1993).

In minority elderly, as in whites, the strength and quality of the relationships between older people and their kin are highly dependent on the lifelong quality and strengths of the relationships. Problems may arise when a caregiver feels unduly burdened with instrumental tasks and is unable to provide for the affective needs of the elder.

Family Functions

It is common to view family functions from a family life cycle perspective. Although this perspective provides some useful specificity regarding tasks that confront families with elderly members, it is useful to remember that all families share some very basic functions, regardless of the age of their members. These include socialization and support for role performance, providing affection and emotional support, caring for dependent members when needed, and providing linkages with other social institutions.

SOCIALIZATION AND ROLE SUPPORT. Socialization that occurs within the family is a two-way process, involving mutual influence between generations. The old may teach and indoctrinate the young regarding norms, traditions, and skills, but the young also teach their elders as society changes over time. The following example illustrates the two-way nature of adult socialization within the family.

An elderly man visits his daughter for an extended period of time after the death of his wife. The man describes himself as being in "a poor mental and physical state" after having cared for his wife for the previous 5 years. He seriously considers his daughter's invitation to move in with her. When he tells his daughter that he really does not want to move in with her, she says to him, "Dad, you need to get on with your life!" and suggests that he join the local senior volunteer program. He contacts the Retired Senior Volunteer Program with the assistance of his daughter and becomes involved in helping organize a neighborhood watch program. Without his daughter's assistance, this individual would have experienced a very different self-image and quality of life.

The family, through its functions of socialization and role support, is an important force in shaping the older person's self-image. Family members share experiences over time, and through these shared experiences, family relationship histories, made up of shared oral traditions regarding family events, relationship patterns, and behavioral expectations, evolve. Such processes generate family role identities and interaction styles that continue over the lifetime of family members. Thus, socialization and previous family relationships can have an effect on the affection and emotional support given to aging family members (Whitbeck et al., 1994).

AFFECTION AND EMOTIONAL SUPPORT. Older people obtain emotional support from their spouses, siblings, children, and other kin. According to Mutran and Reitzes (1994), well-being is closely related to the quality of the relationship between older parents and adult children. In addition, the parent-child relationship affects well-being in the older adult more when the parent is widowed.

Relationships between siblings are most important for elderly people without spouses, children, or grandchildren. The nature of the helping relationship between siblings is more egalitarian than are the helping relationships across generations. The unique attributes of the sibling relationship underscore the importance of considering siblings when assessing the older adult's kin network.

CAREGIVING. Informal caregiving refers to activities and experiences involved in providing help and assistance to relatives or friends who are unable to provide for themselves. Caring is the *affective* component of one's commitment to the welfare of another, and caregiving is the *behavioral* expression of this commitment. Caregiving is the extension of caring about someone, and caring and caregiving are intrinsic to any close relationship (Pearlin et al., 1990).

Despite myths to the contrary, family members remain the primary providers of care to disabled or dependent older adults, and formal services, such home and day care, tend to be used as adjuncts rather than substitutes (Belsky, 1990). Older persons who have regular contact with kin have a lower risk of institutionalization than do those without kin, especially when the caregiver is a spouse (Freedman et al., 1994; Montgomery and Kosloski, 1994). Current trends in federal, state, and local policy formation suggest an increasing emphasis on the family as appropriate caregivers (Barnes et al., 1992; Thompson et al., 1993).

People in their middle and later years are very likely to have dependent elderly family members. On average, the family caregiver spends 4 hours a day, 7 days a week providing care (Stone et al., 1987). Assisting frail, elderly parents increases distress in both men and women, but men are more affected than women by the multiplicity of roles associated with the demands of the "middle generation" and caregiving (Spitze et al., 1994). Regardless of gender, caregivers readily relinquish personal activities to perform caregiving tasks (Beach, 1993).

Women consistently have been found to be primarily responsible for caregiving, and recent increases in their labor force participation do not appear to alter their caregiving responsibilities (Moen et al., 1994; Beach, 1993; King, 1993). Many women have been forced to drop out of the labor force to become unpaid caregivers because of lack of support systems. Brody et al. (1994) found that never married and widowed daughters provide larger portions of care than do those who are married, remarried, or separated or divorced. Married daughters have the most informal helpers, such as other relatives, and those who were never married are more often their parents' sole helpers. There are also gender differences in spousal caregiving: wives provide approximately twice the number of hours of care than husbands provide (Allen, 1994).

Research on the nature of caregiving and its effects on family members has increased in recent years. Caregiving can be transformed from the ordinary exchange of assistance to an extraordinary and unequally distributed burden, which can cause a profound restructuring of the established relationship (Pearlin et al., 1990).

Caregiver burden appears to increase with decreased levels of functioning and increased levels of dysphoria or depression in the elderly person (Satoh et al., 1993). Many studies have found that children caring for ailing parents have relatively high rates of depression and anxiety and low levels of morale (Cantor, 1983; Fischer, 1985; George and Gwyther, 1986). Adult children may feel guilty because they think they should feel more loving or should be doing more. There is potential for poor family relationships and conflict between dependent older parents and their children (Belsky, 1990).

Caring for elders with dementia presents unique problems. According to Browning and Schwirian (1994), mental impairment has the most significant negative impact on caregiver burden. Pearlin et al. (1990) developed a conceptual model of Alzheimer's caregivers' stress based on information derived from over 500 caregivers (Fig. 15–14). Caregiver stress is conceptualized as a process that includes four domains: (1) the

background and context of stress, (2) the stressors, (3) the mediators of stress, and (4) the outcomes or manifestations of stress. The model focuses on the relationships between conditions or variables that lead to personal stress, how these conditions arise, how the conditions are related to one another, and how the relationships change over time. Caregiver stress is thought of not as an event or as a unitary phenomenon; rather, it is a mix of ever-changing circumstances, experiences, responses, and resources that vary among caregivers and in their impact on caregivers' health and behavior. The model provides useful guidelines for research on family caregiving of noninstitutionalized older adults with dementia.

Several scales have been developed to measure and assess burden in caregivers (Morycz, 1985; Robinson, 1983; Zarit et al., 1980; Zarit and Zarit, 1982). The measures focus on caregivers' feelings and experiences and are largely unidimensional, providing an overall score of caregiver burden. Novak and Guest (1989) developed a Caregiver Burden Inventory that purports to be a diagnostic tool to measure the many dimensions of caregiver burden. The instrument consists of five factors: (1) *time-dependence burden,* or burden related to restrictions on the caregiver's time; (2) *developmental burden,* or the caregivers' feelings of being "off-time" in their development with respect to their peers; (3) *physical burden,* or the caregivers' feelings of chronic fatigue and damage to physical health; (4) *social burden,* or the caregivers' feelings of role conflict; and (5) *emotional burden,* or the caregivers' negative feelings toward their care receivers. The instrument may be useful for identifying different patterns of burden, social and psychological needs, and interventions for caregivers.

Guerriero Austrom and Hendrie (1992) found that the strength of the existing relationship and the presence of a social support system strongly affect the caregiving experience. Suitor and Pillemer (1993) identified family members and friends as important sources of social support for married daughters caring for parents with dementia; however, siblings, although important sources of support, were also the most important source of interpersonal stress. In a study of male caregivers of Alzheimer's disease victims, the following common themes emerged: commitment, social isolation, loss of companionship, control, sense of accomplishment, a problem-solving approach, burden lessening with years of caregiving, and limited expectations of children (Harris,

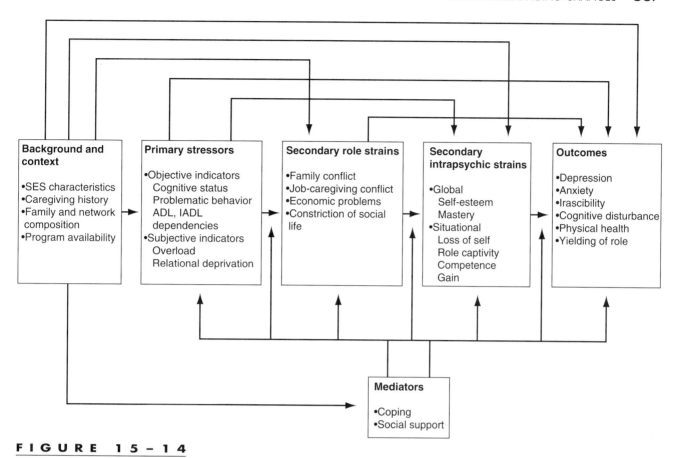

FIGURE 15 – 14

A conceptual model of Alzheimer's caregivers' stress. The stress process is made up of four domains: the background and context of stress, the stressors, the mediators of stress, and the outcomes or manifestations of stress. ADL = activities of daily living; IADL = instrumental activities of daily living. (From Pearlin, L.I., Mullan, J.T., Semple, S.J. and Skaff, M.M. Caregiving and the stress process: An overview of concepts and their measures. *Gerontologist* 30:586, 1990. Copyright © The Gerontological Society of America.)

1993). Grief and bereavement accompany the caregiving experience and exist both before and after the death of the Alzheimer's victim (Jones and Martinson, 1992; Liken and Collins, 1993).

It has been found that engaging in social interaction for fun and recreation can diminish the burden of caregiving (Thompson et al., 1993). Support programs that provide emotional and informational assistance for families of dependent older people have gained popularity in the United States. The Alzheimer's Disease and Related Disorders Association exemplifies this type of support at both the national and the local levels. Its members have worked to highlight the unique problems of caring for elderly persons with dementia and have stimulated and facilitated research on dementing disorders. In addition, local support groups provide support and education for caregivers.

Because more working Americans, especially women, are caring for elderly relatives, employers are challenged to provide

support. Most employed elderly caregivers want support from their companies, especially regarding information about community resources, flex-time, fewer hours without reduced benefits, cafeteria benefits, senior day centers, respite care, and job sharing. Unfortunately, although employers appreciate the burdens of workers with elder care responsibilities, most have not developed policies to address the problems and needs of these workers. Employers, employees, and government need to contribute collectively to the development of an elder care policy that meets these needs (Denton et al., 1990).

An understanding of the caregiver stress process can enhance the clinician's ability to meet the needs of caregivers. A variety of caregiver interventions, including teaching interventions to manage behavioral symptoms associated with chronic impairment and supporting the family caregivers' coping resources to reduce the impact of caregiver stress, can help strengthen families and support the functional capacity and quality of life of chronically impaired elderly people in the community (Stevens et al., 1993).

Natural Helping Networks

Natural helping networks are informal support systems found in most communities. The term encompasses friends, neighbors, and individuals from community groups. There is no such thing as a "typical" natural helping network for the elderly. Such networks are the result of a lifetime of interactions in such settings as work, church, service organizations, and neighborhoods. Categories of individuals and organizations that form natural helping networks include church- or synagogue-related groups; grass roots support groups, such as those formed for new widows or groups for those with chronic diseases or impairments such as Reach to Recovery (for postmastectomy patients) and Shhhh (for those with chronic hearing impairment); fraternal organizations, such as Kiwanis and Masons; and neighborhood organizations, such as homeowners' groups, community watch organizations, hobby or special interest groups, or senior citizens clubs. The number of individuals or groups in such a network is highly individualized. The pattern of interaction is also diverse. Most older persons have some connection with a natural helping network. The older person who has recently relocated to a new community or an institution is often isolated from a natural helping network. Part of the vulnerability of newly relocated individuals may be related to the paucity of social support available.

Most natural helping networks provide assistance on an infrequent, irregular basis. The assistance received is often similar to that provided by family, but, either because no family exists or because the older person prefers to receive such assistance outside the family, this network is activated. The degree to which this network provides instrumental or affective assistance is highly variable. Some examples illustrate this diversity.

Mrs. A. has lived in her neighborhood for the past 73 years. She has attended church in this community and is an honorary member of the Ladies Circle, although she is no longer able to attend their meetings owing to severe arthritis. When he was living, her husband was active in the Sertoma Club, and the members of this group drop by regularly to check on things around the house. Although she is no longer able to keep a garden, her neighbors keep her well supplied with produce from their gardens throughout the summer.

Ms. B. has children who live outside the state. She has recently been diagnosed as having cancer of the soft palate. While she is undergoing radiation therapy, she receives help with housekeeping and meals from her neighbor, despite her daughter's offer to come stay with her during the course of radiation.

Mr. C. has lived in his neighborhood for the past three years. His lifestyle for most of his adult life was that of a drifter. He lives in an urban subsidized housing project. His neighbor across the street looks for him to come out and get his paper each day and says she would call the housing manager if she did not see him for several days. Prior to becoming debilitated from an inoperable brain cancer, he played checkers with a group of men at the local convenience store. He no longer sees these friends because he says he would not enjoy their company if he could not keep pace with the game.

These three people derive quite different types and amounts of support from their natural helping networks. Mrs. A. and Mr. C. use nonfamily sources of support because they have no family. In contrast, Ms. B. elects to use an alternative source of support. Mrs. A. receives support from friends and neighbors of a lifetime, whereas Ms. B. and Mr. C. tap into more recently developed networks. All three individuals receive both instrumental and expressive assistance. Mr. C. receives assistance on a daily basis for an indefinite period of time. Ms. B. receives daily assistance on a time-limited basis. Mrs. A. obtains periodic assistance on an indefinite basis.

One positive attribute of natural helping networks is that the nature of the support is usually highly individualized. Another positive aspect is that the support often comes from a member of the same subcultural group as the older person, in contrast to that provided by bureaucratic organizations. Although this is not always the case, there is a greater likelihood that the individual's lifestyle and preferences will be respected than when bureaucratic uniform procedures and regulations are applied to care of the older person.

Natural helping networks are fueled primarily by goodwill, friendship, or a sense of community, not by a sense of filial responsibility. As such, they are free of many of the emotional conflicts characteristic of family interactions, although the emotional attachments involved in natural helping networks may be quite strong. Usually, the dependability of the network is influenced by the nature and the number of demands placed on it. Natural helping networks are useful for fulfilling such roles as confidante and friendly visitor and for occasional services, such as transportation or other instrumental tasks for a short period. These networks are generally less successful at providing intensive or repetitive help (such as personal care, meal preparation, housekeeping) for an extended period of time, although exceptions do exist.

Conflict or problems may occur in natural helping networks for several reasons, including demands exceeding the network's capacity, breaches in privacy, and depletion of the network through death or relocation. Requests for help may be too frequent, interfering with the helper's other role responsibilities, or the help recipient may become too deviant, as may be the case with individuals who have advanced Alzheimer's disease and related functional impairments (e.g., incontinence or bizarre behavior). Because there are no formal rules surrounding helping behaviors in informal networks, individuals may reject help because they fear becoming the object of community gossip. Finally, the loss of key network members without replacement as a result of illness, relocation, or death may result in a system that is inadequate to support the needs of its members.

FRIENDS AND NEIGHBORS. Friends are believed to be important determinants of physical, psychological, and social well-being (Bleiszner and Adams, 1992). The major change in friendship patterns is an increasing loss of lifelong friends through death or relocation. The loss of friends or decreased contact with friends can lead to loneliness in the elderly (Dugan and Kivett, 1994; Mullins and Duncan, 1991). Although there is no evidence to support the idea that older people are less able than younger people to make friends, it is clear that for some, mobility difficulties and financial considerations limit their opportunity to make new friends.

Patterns of friendship among members of the same age cohort are determined by age, sex, class, race, and ethnicity. However, most older adults have friends who are near their own age, and the friendships are based on shared interests, experiences, and concerns. Friends often are like family to older adults, and the friendships may contribute as much or more to feelings of well-being as contacts with family members. Female friendships generally are more intimate and emotionally self-disclosing, whereas male friendships tend to be more superficial; thus, men are more likely to turn to their spouse for emotional intimacy (Butler et al., 1991).

Studies from the past 30 years indicate that housing arrangements may not affect friendships in older adults (Hess, 1979; Rosow, 1967). For example, urban elderly persons have greater access to transportation, and the population density is conducive to interactions with friends; however, rural elderly persons have as much contact with friends as their urban counterparts. In a National Health Interview Survey, it was found that only 3 per cent of both metropolitan and nonmetropolitan elderly persons had had no contact with friends in the previous month, whereas more than half had had contact with one to five friends. Moreover, 39 per cent of the metropolitan elderly and 44 per cent of the nonmetropolitan elderly had had contacts with more than five friends in the previous month. In addition, approximately one third of both the metropolitan and the nonmetropolitan elderly said that they had one to three friends they could call on for help (Schick and Schick, 1994).

Hess (1972) reported that older people in age-segregated settings have more friends than those in age-integrated settings. One explanation is that older people who have a more restricted set of roles than their younger counterparts have a more narrow basis on which to build friendships with people outside their age cohort than do younger individuals. The popularity of retirement communities may be in part related to this phenomenon.

Bureaucratic Organizations

A wide variety of formal organizations provide supportive services to older persons. Formal organizations are a part of the life of every older American. Some of these organizations could be classified as part of either the natural helping network or the formal support network. Organizations such as religious institutions, as opposed to church-related social groups discussed earlier, or the United States Postal Service, although bureaucratically organized, have manifest functions other than support of the elderly. However, it is commonplace for agents of these bureaucracies (and other bureaucracies) to provide considerable support for older persons. For example, many churches and synagogues have programs designed to reach "shut-ins." These people are often older persons, and they may derive considerable instrumental or affective benefit from such programs. In the case of the Postal Service, in some communities, the mail carrier provides an informal checking service for frail older persons who live alone. Important though these functions are for the individuals who receive them, this discussion is lim-

TABLE 15-6
Typology of the Development of Closed and Open Care in 24 Selected Countries

CLOSED CARE			OPEN CARE		
Stage of Development	Characteristics	Example	Stage of Development	Characteristics	Example
Stage 1	One or more privately sponsored old age homes, often by church/religious groups	Western Samoa	Stage 1	Embryonic, essentially unorganized, no public assistance, no or few private agencies	Western Samoa
Stage 2	Beginning regulation and nationalization of private homes	Singapore Hong Kong	Stage 2	Emergent, largely private sector, limited public funding to private sector	Hong Kong
Stage 3	Establishment of model old age homes	Burma	Stage 3	Rapid transition and expansion of services emanating from public welfare offices	Japan
	Semipublic auspices				
	Public	Philippines			
	In national capital	Thailand			
	In different regions				
Stage 4	Public reimbursements to private institutions and attendant regulation	United States	Stage 4	A highly developed public system with services extended to entire country, including rural areas	Sweden
Stage 5	A mix of public and private-for-pay institutions	Japan			
Stage 6	A highly developed public system of institutions of specialized types and varying levels of care	Great Britain Sweden			

From Cantor, M. and Little, V. Aging and social care. In Binstock, R. and Shanas, E. (eds.). *Handbook of Aging and the Social Sciences*. 2nd ed. New York: Van Nostrand Reinhold, 1985, p. 765.
Countries studied: Afghanistan, Indonesia, Western Samoa, Burma, Pakistan, Kenya, Iran, India, Philippines, Greece, Singapore, Hong Kong, New Zealand, Australia, Austria, Germany, Netherlands, United States, Japan, Israel, Canada, Great Britain, Denmark, Sweden.

ited to those organizations with some legal mandate for serving the aged.

Currently in the United States, bureaucratic organizations provide a whole range of support services to dependent older persons (see Table 15–4). Specific descriptions of the myriad services potentially available are contained in Chapter 20. The point to be remembered is that in most communities, the spectrum of services is often incomplete. Most communities may have the rudiments of a care continuum, but there frequently are gaps in that continuum as a result of problems with adequate funding that lead to waiting lists or poor quality of care and associated underutilization.

Cantor and Little (1985) categorized support services provided by formal organizations as either closed or open, with closed care referring to traditional, institution-based care and open care referring to community-based long-term care. They noted that in most countries, closed care develops prior to open care, with open care developing in response to two factors: (1) increased personal expectations for independent living and (2) escalating costs of medical care. Little (1982) constructed a typology of development of open versus closed care based on studies of 24 countries (Table 15–6). She contended

that progression through the typology is not necessarily orderly or linear.

Bureaucracies are large, formal organizations with interactions that are far less individualized than in other social groups. Bureaucracies perform best when specialized knowledge or impartiality is required or when there is a large volume of repetitive tasks to be accomplished. Examples of problems handled well by bureaucracies include open heart surgery, crime investigation, and processing of Social Security checks. Unfortunately, many of the social problems that befall the elderly are more individualized in nature than the issuance of monthly income checks. Therefore, bureaucratic institutions are imperfect organizations to deal with the problems of older persons. Critics of bureaucracies argue that this type of organization stifles creativity, fosters fragmentation of services and individuals' lives, and treats individuals inhumanely.

Despite longstanding criticisms of the hazards of bureaucratization, formal organizations continue to develop as the modernization of Western society progresses. As work becomes increasingly specialized, with larger numbers of traditional caregivers in the work force, tasks that in preindustrial societies were performed within the family group have increasingly become the province of formal organizations. So, despite their shortcomings, bureaucracies are here to stay for the foreseeable future.

Litwak (1965) contended that in modern societies, families and bureaucracies share functions in all aspects of life. Society and individuals are best served when functions are shared, because these two social groups use different but complementary means of achieving the same goals. It is important for formal organizations and primary groups to develop linkages that facilitate working together in a coordinated manner to achieve the most good. For example, individuals with advanced-stage dementia can benefit from services offered by formal organizations as well as by family members. A formal organization, the nursing home, provides staff who are expert in caring for those with behavioral disturbances and providing for routine, repetitive tasks, such as physical care and supervision, to prevent wandering or unsafe behavior. The family continues to provide the majority of affective care through visiting, controlling personal finances, monitoring care provided by the nursing home, and negotiating with the nursing home staff for as individualized a plan of care as is possible.

The effect of a bureaucracy on a specific individual depends on several factors, including the individual's residence, the extent of informal support available, the personal financial resources, and the previous experience with bureaucracies. For example, someone living in a nursing home has a different bureaucratic support network to negotiate than a person of similar dependency living alone in the community. People with large, supportive extended kin networks are far less dependent on bureaucratic structures than single persons who have no ties with a geographical community. People who depend on Social Security as their sole source of income are much more affected by errors in the Social Security system or political manipulation of this system than are those who have alternative sources of income. Although all formal organizations have idiosyncrasies, the broad ways in which they differ from other social groups remain constant. Thus, those who have learned in earlier years to deal successfully with bureaucracies may have a greater likelihood of positive outcomes with bureaucracy in later life.

The United States is currently in considerable conflict regarding the proper role of federal, state, and local governments in providing support for the elderly. This political climate makes understanding bureaucracy and the aged even more complex. However, the increasing modernization of Western society and the changing demographic picture (increasing proportion of dependent elderly as a result of increased longevity and decreased fertility) suggest that bureaucracy will become an increasingly important aspect of the daily lives of the elderly.

DEVELOPMENTAL THEORIES OF AGING

What is successful aging? There are those who pessimistically regard aging as a process of inevitable decline with no positive features. Others acknowledge decline in some domains of function but note gains in other aspects of function. Those who regard aging as a purely deteriorative process tend to view the aged as inferior, handicapped, less able, and likely to be dependent (Riley et al., 1979). Those who regard aging as a developmental process, with both positive and negative aspects, are more likely to regard the aged as valued members of society. Successful aging is demonstrated by an ability to adjust to the decremental changes while continuing to grow and contribute to society.

Developmental Tasks

As with other age groups, the elderly must perform certain developmental tasks to successfully master the process of aging. Clark and Anderson (1967) differentiated the concepts of developmental and adaptive tasks in relation to aging. They defined development as learning to live with oneself as one changes, whereas adaptation is learning to live in a particular way according to a particular set of values as one or as one's culture changes. They identified five adaptive tasks associated with aging:

1. Recognition of aging and definition of instrumental limitations
2. Redefinition of physical and social life space
3. Substitution of alternate sources of need satisfaction
4. Reassessment of criteria for evaluation of the self
5. Reintegration of values and life goals

These tasks require older individuals to be aware of and accept changes in physical and mental capabilities, relinquish certain roles while constructing a new network of social relationships, substitute feasible interests and activities for those that can no longer be pursued successfully, reconsider the ideas used as a basis for self-concept, and revise life goals and values to give coherence, integration, and social meaning to new lifestyles. Most older people adapt to aging successfully. Those who do not have difficulty in finding substitutes for the things that satisfy their needs.

According to Vaillant (1977), several "adaptive strategies" have been found to be effective in adjusting to aging. Adaptive strategies serve to resolve conflict, and the success of adaptation depends on an interplay between the choice of adaptive strategies and sustained relationships with other people. The best adaptive strategies are *altruism,* a type of unselfishness that allows people to see their own needs in a context that includes the needs of others; *humor,* which allows people to defuse the anger of the moment by focusing on its comical elements; *sublimation,* which involves directing the energies produced by conflict into constructive and socially acceptable channels; *anticipation,* which is the capacity to perceive future danger clearly and thus minimize its effects; and *suppression,* which is the ability to cope with conflict by putting it out of one's consciousness temporarily. These adaptive strategies involve learning how to adapt to life without denying or distorting the nature of oneself or the situation within one is trying to adapt.

Erikson (1963) has described the developmental task for older adulthood as "ego-integrity versus despair." Ego-integrity is the acceptance of one's own life as inevitable and meaningful. It is the process of working through one's own life in relation to humanity and one's place in history. It reduces the fear of death and enables one to look ahead to the last years with equanimity (Erikson et al., 1986). Lack or loss of ego-integrity results in despair. This signifies a nonacceptance of one's lifestyle and a fear of death. Time appears too short to attempt to start another life and to try out alternate roads to integrity. Despair may be manifested through decreased life satisfaction, depression, or apathy.

Activity Theory

According to the activity theory, older persons who are more socially active are more likely to adjust well to aging (Lemon et al., 1972). This theory is based on the following propositions: (1) social activity is necessary for continued role enactment, (2) role enactment is essential for maintenance of a positive self-concept, (3) people who have a wide range of roles have many op-

portunities to reaffirm this positive self-concept, and (4) people with increased social opportunity have more chances for role enactment, which is the substance of self-concept. Studies have shown that those with higher social involvement have higher morale and better life satisfaction, personal adjustment, and mental health than those who are less involved. These propositions are based on, among others, the following findings:

- A greater amount of time spent in social and voluntary organizations is characteristic of subjects with high personal adjustment (Burgess, 1954; Lebo, 1953).
- There is a direct relationship between high levels of activity and high degrees of morale (Kutner et al., 1956; Reichard et al., 1962).
- With advancing age, activity is an increasingly important predictor of life satisfaction (Tobin and Neugarten, 1961).
- High morale is not found among highly disengaged persons (Tallmer and Kutner, 1970).
- Interpersonal and noninterpersonal activities are related to morale (Maddox, 1963).
- A relationship with a close confidante is positively associated with mental health and morale. The emphasis is on a stable, intimate relationship rather than on the amount of social interaction or the maintenance of all social roles (Lowenthal and Haven, 1968).
- There is a substantial positive association between total activity in 12 social roles and general life satisfaction (six different national-cultural groups were used in the study) (Havighurst et al., 1969).
- A positive association has been demonstrated between total activity in 12 social roles held across two separate occupational groups (Bengtson et al., 1969).
- High degrees of role loss are associated with low morale (Rosow, 1967).
- Role changes are inversely related to morale (Phillips, 1957).

It is important for older adults to be active in a wide variety of pursuits, using activity levels from middle age as a norm. If activities or roles are given up, replacements should be found. Failure to do so results in a "roleless role," or a situation in which an older person has no social function (Burgess, 1960).

Both the number and the quality of activities are important. Activities that involve close personal contact are of special value. According to Lemon et al. (1972), activity

. . . provides various role supports necessary for reaffirming one's self-concept. The more intimate and the more frequent the activity, the more reinforcing and the more specific will be the role supports. Role supports are necessary for the maintenance of a positive self-concept, which in turn is associated with high life satisfaction.

Critics of the activity theory argue that the aging process is too complex to be characterized by such a simplistic formulation. It has also been noted that there is insufficient research data to support the theory in its current form. Some studies have produced little evidence to support a relationship between life satisfaction and social activity; in addition, a relationship has not been found between role losses, such as widowhood or retirement, and decreased life satisfaction. Critics conclude that other intervening variables are needed to explain responses to aging.

Disengagement Theory

The disengagement theory states that there is a "mutual withdrawal or 'disengagement' between the aging person and others in the social system to which he belongs—a withdrawal initiated by the individual himself, or by others in the system" (Cumming and Henry, 1961). Such a withdrawal keeps the elderly from being frustrated in roles that they are no longer able to competently fulfill, while making a place in society for younger members to fulfill important roles. This is characterized as a normal, intrinsic, inevitable, and universal process.

There are several major criticisms of the disengagement theory:

1. It does not account for the many active, highly engaged elderly who are well adjusted (Maddox, 1963).
2. It is not seen in all cultural groups and therefore is not a universal process (Gutmann, 1977).
3. Logical flaws exist in the initial proposition of the disengagement theory that make it difficult to disprove. An example is Cumming and Henry's conclusion that people who have not disengaged are merely demonstrating an alternative pattern of disengagement (Hoschild, 1976).
4. What is normative is not necessarily normal. Although disengagement patterns may have existed in some urban older Americans in the late 1950s, these patterns may not predict what is normal for future cohorts or for people of other cultural backgrounds.
5. There is a paucity of confirming research. This theory is based on one study, that of Cumming and Henry (1961), and has received little validation.

Continuity Theory

Some theorists believe that personality and lifestyle are important factors to consider in adjustment to aging. According to Havighurst et al. (1969), the critical factor in adjustment to old age is previously acquired coping abilities and the ability to maintain continuity with previous roles and activities. Four patterns of personality and coping have been identified:

Integrated personalities: those who are mature and happy but have varied activity levels from highly active to disengaged

Defended personalities: those who maintain middle-age values and norms and who are distressed by the losses that accompany old age

Passive-dependent personalities: those who have high dependency needs or who are apathetic

Unintegrated personalities: those who exhibit mental illness

Knowledge of individuals' personality types is thought to be helpful in predicting their response to the aging process (Neugarten and Datan, 1973). Thus, according to the continuity theorists, individuals who were never highly involved with society adjust best to old age if they are able to maintain the same level of involvement. Their adjustment is *not* facilitated by encouraging them to become more socially active. Conversely, individuals who have been highly active socially should not endeavor to disengage from such pursuits but should maintain the same level of activity. Thus, adjustment to aging is optimized by maintaining the same level of social activity achieved in younger adulthood.

Continuity theorists also contend that individuals strive to maintain a role orientation in late life similar to that developed in early adulthood. This implies that those who develop interests and roles that can be continued despite physical infirmity and are compatible with societal expectations of appropriate roles for older people will have the easiest adjustment to old age.

Critics of the continuity theory argue that

it is too simplistic and does not take into account the myriad of variables that affect people's adjustment to aging.

SUMMARY

The influences of culture, social institutions, and age-related psychological changes on individual behavior and feelings of well-being are complex. The research base in social gerontology is far from complete. However, some caveats for use in clinical nursing practice can be distilled.

1. *The psychological and sociocultural diversity of older people calls for more comprehensive assessment of the aged, rather than assumptions based on chronological age.* The few safe assumptions about changes in cognition and personality can be summarized as follows:

- Learning is possible in the absence of severe dementing disease, but the pace of teaching should be slower and should accommodate common age-related sensory changes.
- There is no typical personality of old age; rather, there is a continuity with past patterns.
- Morale in old age is influenced by many of the same factors that affect morale in younger persons: socioeconomic status and health status.

Behavior of the aged is influenced by cultural factors such as identification with an ethnic group, demographic factors such as gender, living arrangements, socioeconomic status, educational level, and age-related role changes. Assessment of each individual's life situation is important in assisting that person to develop, prioritize, and actualize goals concerning health.

2. *There is high potential for role change in late life, which may affect self-perception, behavior, and availability of social support.* Nurses should therefore be alert to signs of role strain, such as social isolation, decreased self-esteem, altered self-concept, and coping difficulties, and should be knowledgeable about the treatment of these problems.

3. *Family and natural helping networks are essential sources of social support for the aged.* There are no safe assumptions to be made about the nature of social support in old age. The number and type of supporters vary tremendously, and there is no substitute for careful assessment of the social networks that are salient for the older individual. Assessment should include identification of the key support persons and the nature of support derived from the networks. Such assessment may point to gaps or weak points in the individual's support systems, which in turn may suggest the need for intervention to promote social and emotional health.

4. *Ethnic group identification may provide important sources of social support for the aged client.* Nurses should be aware of the extent to which the older person identifies with a particular ethnic group and strive to respect the values held by that group.

5. *Society is affected by the increasing proportion of people living into advanced old age.* Nurses should expect to be involved in conflicts surrounding the changing role of women in terms of traditional caregiving roles and the workplace and the expectations of formal organizations in providing solutions to problems of the aged.

6. *Health status is an important determinant of morale in old age.* Nurses should remain cognizant of the powerful psychological impact of disease and work toward minimizing the negative psychological effects of disease and dysfunction.

REFERENCES

Allen, P.A., Groth, K.E., Weber, T.A. and Madden, D.J. Influence of response selection and noise similarity on age differences in the redundancy gain. *J Gerontol* 48(4):P189–P198, 1993.

Allen, P.A., Patterson, M.B. and Propper, R.E. Influence of letter size on age differences in letter matching. *J Gerontol* 49(1):P24–P28, 1994.

Allen, S.M. Gender differences in spousal caregiving and unmet need for care. *J Gerontol* 49(4):S187–S195, 1994.

Anderson, T.B. and McCulloch, B.J. Conjugal support: Factor structure for older husbands and wives. *J Gerontol* 48(3):S133–S142, 1993.

Anstey, K., Stankov, L. and Lord, S. Primary aging, secondary aging, and intelligence. *Psychol Aging* 8(4):562–570, 1993.

Arenberg, D. A longitudinal study of problem solving in adults. *J Gerontol* 29:560–568, 1974.

Arenberg, D. and Robertson, E. The older individual as learner. *In* Grabowski, S.M. and Mason, W.D. (eds.). *Education for the Aging.* Compiled by ERIC Clearinghouse on Adult Education. Washington, D.C.: Education Resources Division, Capitol Publications, 1973, pp. 2–40.

Atchley, R.C. Retirement and leisure participation: Continuity or crisis. *Gerontologist.* 11:13–17, 1971.

Atchley, R.C. and Miller, S.J. Types of elderly couples. *In* Brubaker, T.H. (ed.). *Family Relationships in Later Life.* Beverly Hills, CA: Sage Publications, 1983.

Atkinson, R.C. and Shiffrin, R.M. Human memory: A proposed system and its control processes. *In* Spence, K.W. and Spence, J.T. (eds.). *The Psychology of Learning and Motivation.* Vol. 2. New York: Academic Press, 1968.

Barnes, C.L., Given, B.A. and Given, C.W. Caregivers of elderly relatives: Spouses and adult children. *Health Soc Work* 17(4):282–289, 1992.

Beach, D.L. Gerontological caregiving: Analysis of family experience. *J Gerontol Nurs* 19(12):35–41, 1993.

Bedford, V.H. Understanding the value of siblings in old age: A proposed model. *Am Behav Sci* 33:33–44, 1989.

Belsky, J.K. *The Psychology of Aging.* 2nd ed. Pacific Grove, CA: Brooks/Cole Publishing Company, 1990.

Bengtson, V.L. Ethnicity and aging: Problems and issues in current social science inquiry. *In* Gelfand, D.E. and Kutzik, A.J. (eds.). *Ethnicity and Aging.* New York: Springer Publishing Company, 1979.

Bengtson, V.L., Chiriboga, D. and Keller, A.W. Occupational differences in retirement: Patterns of life-outlook and role activity among Chicago teachers and steelworkers. *In* Havighurst, R.J., et al. (eds.). *Adjustment to Retirement: A Cross-National Study.* Netherlands: Van Gorkum, 1969.

Birren, J.E. and Morrison, D.F. Analysis of the WAIS subtests in relation to age and education. *J Gerontol* 16:363–369, 1961.

Blieszner, R. and Adams, R.G. *Adult Friendship.* Newbury Park, CA: Sage Publications, 1992.

Botwinick, J. *Aging and Behavior.* 2nd ed. New York: Springer Publishing Company, 1978.

Botwinick, J., West, R. and Stornadt, M. Predicting death from behavioral test performance. *J Gerontol* 33:755–762, 1978.

Bower, G.H. A selective review of organization factors in memory. *In* Tulving, E. and Donaldson, W. (eds.). *Organization of Memory.* New York: Academic Press, 1972, pp. 93–137.

Brody, E.M., Litvin, S.J., Albert, S.M. and Hoffman, C.J. Marital status of daughters and patterns of parent care. *J Gerontol* 49(2):S95–S103, 1994.

Browning, J.S. and Schwirian, P.M. Spousal caregivers' burden: Impact of care recipient health problems and mental status. *J Gerontol Nurs* 20(3):17–22, 1994.

Bureau of the Census. Current Population survey, unpublished tabulations. Marital Status and Living Arrangements: March 1990. *Current Population Reports,* Series P-20, No. 450, Appendix B, 1990.

Burgess, E.W. Social relations, activities and personal adjustment. *Am J Sociol* 59:352–360, 1954.

Burgess, E.W. (ed.). *Aging in Western Societies.* Chicago: University of Chicago Press, 1960.

Burr, J.A. and Mutchler, J.E. Nativity, acculturation, and economic status: Explanations of Asian American living arrangements in later life. *J Gerontol* 48(2):S55–S63, 1993.

Busse, E.W. The myth, history, and science of aging. *In* Busse, E.W. and Blazer, D.G. (eds.). *Geriatric Psychiatry.* Washington, D.C.: American Psychiatric Press, 1989, pp. 3–34.

Busse, E.W. and Maddox, G.L. (eds.). *The Duke Longitudinal Studies of Normal Aging 1955–1980.* New York: Springer Publishing Company, 1985, pp. 77–132.

Butler, R.N., Lewis, M.I. and Sunderland, T. (eds.). *Aging and Mental Health: Positive Psychosocial and Biomedical Approaches.* New York: Macmillan Publishing Company, 1991, pp. 3–115.

Byers, J.P. Sexuality and the elderly. *Geriatr Nurs* 4:1293, 1983.

Cameron, P., Stewart, L. and Biber, H. Consciousness of death across the lifespan. *J Gerontol* 28:92–95, 1973.

Canestrari, R.E. Paced and self-paced learning in elderly and young adults. *J Gerontol* 18:156–168, 1963.

Cantor, M. Neighbors and friends: An overlooked resource in the information support system. Paper presented at the 30th Annual Meeting of the Gerontological Society, San Francisco, CA, 1977.

Cantor, M. The informal support system: Its relevance in the lives of the elderly. *In* Borogotta, E. and McCluskey, N. (eds.). *Aging and Society.* Beverly Hills, CA: Sage Publications, 1980.

Cantor, M. and Little, V. Aging and social care. *In* Binstock, R. and Shanas, E. (eds.). *Handbook of Aging and the Social Sciences.* 2nd ed. New York: Van Nostrand Reinhold, 1985.

Cantor, M.H. Strain among caregivers: A study of the experience in the United States. *Gerontologist* 23:597–604, 1983.

Caplan, G. and Killilea, M. *Support Systems and Mutual Help.* New York: Grune & Stratton, 1976.

Cartwright, A. Is religion a help around the time of death? *Public Health* 105(1):79–87, 1991.

Cattell, R.B. Theory of fluid and crystallized intelligence: A critical experiment. *J Educ Psychol* 54:1–22, 1963.

Cavanaugh, J.C., Grady, J.G. and Perlmutter, M.P. Forgetting and use of memory aids in 20- and 70 year-old's everyday life. *Int J Aging Hum Dev* 17:113, 1983.

Cerella, J. Age effects may be global, not local. Comment on Fisk and Rogers (1991). *J Exp Psychol Gen* 120:215–223, 1990.

Charness, N. and Bosman, E.A. Human factors and age. *In* Craik, F.I.M. and Salthouse, T.A. (eds.). *The Handbook of Aging and Cognition.* Hilldale, NJ: Lawrence Erlbaum Association, 1992, pp. 495–503.

Cherkin, A. Effects of nutritional factors on memory function. *In* Armbrecht, H.J., Prendergast, J.M. and Coe, R.M. (eds.). *Nutritional Intervention in the Aging Process.* New York: Springer-Verlag, 1984, pp. 229–249.

Cherlin, A. and Furstenberg, F. Styles and strategies of grandparenting. *In* Bengtson, V.L. and Robertson, J.R. (eds.). *Grandparenthood.* Beverly Hills, CA: Sage Publications, 1985.

Chown, S.M. Personality and aging. *In* Schaie, K.W. (ed.). *Theory and Methods of Research on Aging.* Morgantown, WV: West Virginia University Library, 1968.

Christensen, H. and MacKinnon, A. The association between mental, social and physical activity and cognitive performance in young and old subjects. *Age Ageing* 22(3):175–182, 1993.

Cicirelli, V.G. Sibling relationships in adulthood: A lifespan perspective. *In* Poon, L. (ed.). *Aging in the Eighties: Psychological Issues.* Washington, D.C.: American Psychological Association, 1980.

Cicirelli, V.G. *Helping Elderly Parents: Role of Adult Children.* Boston: Auburn House, 1981.

Cicirelli, V.G. Adult children and their elderly parents. *In* Brubaker, T.H. (ed.). *Family Relationships in Later Life.* Beverly Hills, CA: Sage Publications, 1983.

Clark, M. and Anderson, P.B. *Culture and Aging.* Springfield, IL: Charles C Thomas, 1967.

Clarkson-Smith, L. and Hartley, A.A. Structural equation models of relationships between exercise and cognitive abilities. *Psychol Aging* 5(3):437–446, 1990.

Clingempeel, W.G., Colyar, J.J., Brand, E. and Hetherington, E.M. Children's relationships with maternal grandparents: A longitudinal study of family structure and pubertal status effects. *Child Dev* 63(6):1404–1422, 1992.

Cogwill, D.O. Aging and modernization: A revision of the theory. *In* Gubrium, D. (ed.). *Late Life.* Springfield, IL: Charles C Thomas, 1974.

Cogwill, D.O. and Holmes, L. (eds.). *Aging and Modernization.* New York: Appleton-Century-Crofts, 1972.

Cohler, B.J. and Grunebaum, H.V. *Mothers, grandmothers and daughters: Personality and childcare in three-generation families.* New York: Wiley, 1981.

Coke, M.M. Correlates of life satisfaction among elderly African Americans. *J Gerontol* 47(5):P316–P320, 1992.

Colantonio, A., Kasi, S.V. and Ostfeld, A.M. Depressive symptoms and other psychosocial factors as predictors of stroke in the elderly. *Am J Epidemiol* 136(7):884–894, 1992.

Connidis, I.A. Sibling support in older age. *J Gerontol* 49(6):S309–S317, 1994.

Connidis, I.A. and McMullin, J.A. To have or have not: Parent status and the subjective well-being of older men and women. *Gerontologist* 33(5):630–636, 1993.

Costa, P. and McCrae, R. Personality in adulthood: A six-year longitudinal study of self reports and spouse ratings on the NEO personality inventory. *J Pers Soc Psychol* 54:853, 1988.

Costa, P.T., Jr. and McCrae, R.R. Psychology research in the Baltimore longitudinal study of aging. *Gerontologist* 26:138–141, 1993.

Costa, P.T. Jr., McCrae, R.R. and Zonderman, A.B. Environmental and dispositional influences on well-being: longitudinal follow-up of an American national sample. *Br J Psychol* 78:299–306, 1987.

Courage, M.M., Godbey, K.L., Ingram, D.A. et al. Suicide in the elderly: staying in control. *J Psychosoc Nurs Mental Health* 31:26–31, 1993.

Cowgill, D.O. Aging and modernization: A revision of the theory. *In* Gubrium, D. (ed.). *Late Life.* Springfield: Charles C Thomas, 1974.

Cowgill, D.O. and Holmes, L. (eds.). *Aging and Modernization.* New York: Appleton-Century-Crofts, 1972.

Craik, F.I.M. Two components in free recall. *J Verbal Learning Verbal Behav* 7:996–1004, 1968.

Cumming, E. and Henry, W. *Growing Old: The Process of Disengagement.* New York: Basic Books, 1961.

Demming, J.A. and Pressey, S.L. Tests "indigenous" to the adult and older years. *J Counsel Psychol* 4:144–148, 1957.

Denton, K., Love, L.T. and Slate, R. Eldercare in the '90s: Employee responsibility, employer challenge. *J Contemp Hum Serv* pp. 349–359, 1990.

Dewey, M.E., Davidson, I.A. and Copeland, J.R. Expressed wish to die and mortality in older people: A community replication. *Age Ageing* 22(2):109–113, 1993.

Douglas, K. and Arenberg, D. Age changes, cohort differences, and cultural change on the Guilford-Zimmerman Temperament Survey. *J Gerontol* 33:737, 1978.

Dugan, E. and Kivett, V.R. The importance of emotional and social isolation to loneliness among very old rural adults. *Gerontologist* 34(3):340–346, 1994.

Earles, J.L. and Coon, V.E. Adult age differences in long-term memory for performed activities. *J Gerontol* 49(1):P32–P34, 1994.

Eddington, C., Piper, J., Tanna, B. et al. Relationships between happiness, behavioral status and dependency on others in elderly patients. *Br J Clin Psychol* 29(Pt 1):43–50, 1990.

Eisdorfer, C. Arousal and performance: Experiments in verbal learning and a tentative theory. *In* Talland, G.A. (ed.). *Human Aging and Behavior.* New York: Academic Press, 1968, pp. 189–216.

Elder, G.H., Jr. and Pavalko, E.K. Work careers in men's later years: Transitions, trajectories, and historical change. *J Gerontol* 48(4):S180–S191, 1993.

Ellor, J.W., Stettner, J. and Spath, H. Ministry with the confused elderly. *J Religion Aging* 4(2):21–33, 1987.

Erber, J., Freely, B.A. and Botwinick, J. Reward conditions and socioeconomic status in the learning of older adults. *J Gerontol* 35:565–570, 1980.

Erdner, R.A. and Guy, R.F. Career identification and women's attitudes toward retirement. *Int J Aging Hum Dev* 30(2):129–139, 1990.

Erikson, E.H., Erickson, J.M. and Kivnick, H.Q. *Vital Involvement in Old Age.* New York: W.W. Norton, 1986.

Erikson, E. *Childhood and Society.* New York: W.W. Norton, 1963.

Felton, B.J. and Berry, C.A. Do the sources of the urban elderly's social support determine its psychological consequences? *Psychol Aging* 7(1):89–97, 1992.

Field, D. and Millsap, R.E. Personality in advanced old age: Continuity or change? *J Gerontol* 46(6):P299–P308, 1991.

Field, D., Minkler, M., Falk, R.F. and Leino, E.V. The influence of health on family contracts and family feelings in advanced old age: A longitudinal study. *J Gerontol* 48(1):P18–P28, 1993.

Fischer, L.R. Elderly parents and the caregiving role: an asymmetrical transition. *In* Peterson, W.A. and Quadango J. (eds.). *Social Bonds in Later Life: Aging and Interdependence.* Beverly Hills, CA: Sage, 1985.

Fishman, S. Relationships among an older adult's life review, ego integrity, and death anxiety. *Int Psychogeriatr* 4(suppl 2):267–277, 1992.

Freedman, J.A., Berkman, L.F., Rapp, S.R. and Ostfeld, A.M. Family networks: Predictors of nursing home entry. *Am J Public Health* 84(5):843–845, 1994.

Fry, C. The ages of adulthood: A question of numbers. *J Gerontol* 31:170–177, 1976.

Fry, P.S. A factor analytic investigation of home-bound elderly individuals' concerns about death and dying, and their coping responses. *J Clin Psychol* 46(6):737–748, 1990.

Fullerton, A.M. Age differences in the use of imagery in integrating new and old information in memory. *J Gerontol* 38:326–332, 1983.

Gagne, R.M. *Essentials of Learning and Instruction.* Hinsdale, IL: Dryden Press, 1974.

Gallagher, D. and Thompson, L.W. Bereavement and adjustment disorders. *In* Busse, E.W. and Blazer, D.G. (eds.). *Geriatric Psychiatry.* Washington, D.C.: American Psychiatric Press, 1989, pp. 459–473.

George, L. and Gwyther, L. Caregiver well-being: A multidimensional examination of family caregivers of demented adults. *Gerontologist* 26:253–259, 1986.

George, L.K. Subjective well-being: Conceptual and methodological issues. *In* Eisdorfer, C. (ed.). *Annual Review of Gerontology and Geriatrics.* Vol. 2. New York: Springer, 1981, pp. 346–382.

Giambra, L.M. Task-unrelated-thought frequency as a function of age: A laboratory study. *Psychol Aging* 4:136–143, 1989.

Gilleard, C.J. and Gurkan, A.A. Socioeconomic development and the status of elderly men in Turkey: A test of modernization theory. *J Gerontol* 42:353–357, 1987.

Glascock, A. and Feinman, S. Social asset or social burden: An analysis of treatment of the aged in nonindustrial societies. *In* Fry, C.L. (ed.). *Dimensions: Aging, Culture and Health.* New York: Prager, 1981.

Glick, R. Assessing the quality of life. *Perspect Aging* 11(3):11–16, 1982.

Glock, C.Y. On the study of religious commitment. *Religious Educ* 57 (res suppl):S98–S110, 1962.

Gold, D.T. Siblings in old age: Something special. *Can J Aging* 6:199–215, 1987.

Gold, D.T., Woodbury, M.A. and George, L.K. Relationship classification using grade of membership analysis: A typology of sibling relationships in later life. *J Gerontol* 45:S43–S51, 1990.

Goldberg, L.R. An alternative "description of personality": The big-five factor structure. *J Pers Soc Psychol* 59:1216, 1990.

Goodwin, J.S., Goodwin, J.M. and Garry, P.J. Association between nutritional status and cognitive functioning in a healthy elderly population. *JAMA* 249:2917–2921, 1983.

Gottsdanker, R. Age and simple reaction time. *J Gerontol* 37:342–348, 1982.

Grant, E., Storandt, M. and Botwinick, J. Incentive and practice in the psychometric performances of the elderly. *J Gerontol* 33:413–415, 1978.

Greeno, J.G. and Bjork, R.A. Mathematic learning theory and the new "mental forestry." *Annu Rev Psychol* 24:81–116, 1973.

Grembowski, D., Patrick, D., Diehr, P. et al. Self-efficacy and health behavior among older adults. *J Health Soc Behav* 34(2):89–104, 1993.

Grundy, E. and Bowling, A. The sociology of ageing. *In* Jacoby, R. and Oppenheimer, C. (eds.). *Psychiatry in the Elderly*. New York: Oxford University Press, 1991, pp. 35–57.

Guerriero Austrom, M. and Hendrie, H.C. Quality of life: The family and Alzheimer's disease. *J Palliat Care* 8(3):56–60, 1992.

Gutman, D.L. Parenthood: A key to the comparative study of the life cycle. *In* Datan, N. and Ginsberg, L.H. (eds.). *Lifespan Developmental Psychology: Normative Life Crises*. New York: Academic Press, 1975.

Gutman, D.L. The cross-cultural perspective: Notes toward a comparative psychology of aging. *In* Birren, J.E. and Schaie, K.W. (eds.). *Handbook of the Psychology of Aging*. New York: Van Nostrand Reinhold, 1977.

Gutmann, D. *Reclaimed Powers: Toward a New Psychology of Men and Women in Later Life*. New York: Basic Books, 1987.

Hadjistavropoulos, T., Taylor, S., Tuokko, H. and Beattie, B.L. Neuropsychological deficits, caregivers' perception of deficits and caregiver burden. *J Am Geriatr Soc* 42(3):308–314, 1994.

Hagberg, B., Samuelsson, G., Lindberg, B. and Dehlin, O. Stability and change of personality in old age and its relation to survival. *J Gerontol* 46(6):P285–P291, 1991.

Hagestad, G. Continuity and connectedness. *In* Bengtson, V.L. and Robertson, J. (eds.). *Grandparenthood*. Beverly Hills, CA: Sage Publications, 1985.

Harris, L. et al. *The Myth and Reality of Aging*. Washington, D.C.: National Council on Aging, 1982.

Harris, P.B. The misunderstood caregiver: A qualitative study of the male caregiver of Alzheimer's disease victims. *Gerontologist* 33(4):551–556, 1993.

Haug, M. *Elderly Patients and Their Doctors*. New York: Springer Publishers, 1982.

Havighurst, R.J., Neugarten, B.L., Munichs, J.M.A. and Thomae, H. (eds.). *Adjustment to Retirement: A Cross-National Study*. Netherlands: Van Gorkum, 1969.

Hayslip, B. and Sterns, H. Age differences in relationships between crystallized and fluid intelligences and problem solving. *J Gerontol* 34:404–414, 1979.

Hayward, M.D., Crimmins, E.M. and Wray, L.A. The relationship between retirement life cycle changes and older men's labor force participation rates. *J Gerontol* 49(5):S219–S230, 1994.

Hazzard, W.R., Bierman, E.L., Blass, J.P. et al. *Principles of Geriatric Medicine and Gerontology*. 3rd ed. New York: McGraw-Hill, 1994.

Heidrich, S.M. and Ryff, C.D. Physical and mental health in later life: The self-system as mediator. *Psychol Aging* 8(3):327–338, 1993.

Hendel-Sebestyen, G. Role diversity: Toward the development of community in a total institutional setting. *Anthropol Q* 52(special issue):19–28, 1979.

Herzog, A.R., House, J.S. and Morgan, J.N. Relation of work and retirement to health and well-being in older age. *Psychol Aging* 6(2):202–211, 1991.

Hess, B. Friendship. *In* Riley, M.W., Johnson, M. and Foner, A. (eds.). *Aging and Society: A Sociology of Age Stratification*. Vol. II. New York: Russell Sage Foundation, 1972, pp. 357–393.

Hess, B. Sex roles, friendship, and the life course. *Res Aging* 1:494–515, 1979.

Hirshorn, B.A. and Hoyer, D.T. Private sector hiring and use of retirees: The firm's perspective. *Gerontologist* 34(1):50–58, 1994.

Hogan, D.P., Eggebeen, D.J. and Clogg, C.C. The structure of intergenerational exchanges in American families. *Am J Sociol* 98(6):1428–1458, 1993.

Holzberg, C.S. Ethnicity and aging: Anthropological perspectives on more than just the minority elderly. *Gerontologist* 22(3):249–257, 1982.

Hong, L.K. and Duff, R.W. Widows in retirement communities: The social context of subjective well-being. *Gerontologist* 34(3):347–352, 1994.

Hooker, K. and Siegler, I.C. Life goals, satisfaction, and self-rated health: Preliminary findings. *Exp Aging Res* 19(1):97–110, 1993.

Horn, J.L. and Cattell, R.B. Age difference in fluid and crystallized intelligence. *Acta Psychol* (Amst) 26:107–129, 1967.

Hoschild, A. Disengagement theory: A logical empirical, and phenomenological critique. *In* Gubrium, J.F. (ed.). *Time, Self, and Roles in Old Age*. New York: Human Sciences Press, 1976.

Hu, Y. and Goldman, N. Mortality differences by marital status: An international comparison. *Demography* 27(2):233–250, 1990.

Hulicka, I.M. and Grossman, J.L. Age group comparisons for the use of mediators in paired-associated learning. *J Gerontol* 22:46–51, 1967.

Hultsch, D.F. and Dixon, R.A. Learning and memory in aging. *In* Birren, J.E. and Schaie, K.W. (eds.). *Handbook of the Psychology of Aging*. 3rd. ed. New York: Academic Press, 1990, pp. 258–274.

Intrieri, R.C. and Rapp, S.R. Caring for the older adult: The role of the family. *In* Hazzard, W.R., Bierman, E.D., Blass, J.P., et al. (eds.). *Principles of Geriatric Medicine and Gerontology*. 3rd ed. New York: McGraw-Hill, 1994, pp. 229–234.

Jackson, J.S., Antonucci, T.C. and Gibson, R.C. Cultural, racial, and ethnic minority influences on aging. *In* Birren, J.E. and Schaie, K.W. (eds.). *Handbook of the Psychology of Aging*. 3rd ed. New York: Academic Press, 1990, pp. 103–123.

Jacobs, K., Kohli, M. and Rein, M. The evolution of early exit: A comparative analysis of labor force participation patterns. *In* Kohli, M., Rein, M., Guillemard, A.M. and Van Gunsteren, H. (eds.). *Time for Retirement*. New York: Cambridge University Press, 1991.

Jarvik, L.F. and Falek, A. Intellectual stability and survival in the aged. *J Gerontol* 18:173–176, 1963.

Jaskowski, S.K. and Dellasega, C. Effects of divorce on the grandparent-grandchild relationship. *Issues Compr Pediatr Nurs* 16(3):125–133, 1993.

Johnson, D.M., Williams, J.S. and Bromley, D.G. Religion, health and healing: Findings from a southern city. *Sociol Anal* 47:66–73, 1986.

Jones, P.S. and Martinson, I.M. The experience of bereavement in caregivers of family members with Alzheimer's disease. *Image: J Nurs Scholarship* 24(3):172–176, 1992.

Kalish, R.A. An approach to the study of death attitudes. *Am Behav Sci* 6:68–80, 1963.

Kalish, R.A. Death and dying in a social context. *In* Birren, J.E. and Schaie, K.W. (eds.). *Handbook of the Psychology of Aging*. New York: Van Nostrand Reinhold, 1977.

Kalish, R.A. and Reynolds, D.K. *Death and Ethnicity: A Psychocultural Study*. Los Angeles: University of Southern California Press, 1976.

Kart, C.S. and Manard, B.B. *Aging in America: Readings in Social Gerontology*. 2nd ed. Palo Alto, CA: Mayfield Publishing Company, 1981.

Karuza, J. Psychological aspects of aging. *In* Calkins, E., Ford, A.B. and Katz, P.R. (eds.). *Practice of Geriatrics*. 2nd ed. Philadelphia: W.B. Saunders, 1992, pp. 149–153.

Kausler, D.H. Motivation, human aging, and cognitive performance. *In* Birren, J.E. and Schaie, K.W. (eds.). *Handbook of the Psychology of Aging.* 3rd ed. New York: Academic Press, 1990, pp. 171–182.

Keith, J. *Old People as People: Social and Cultural Influences on Aging and Old Age.* Boston: Little, Brown, 1982.

Keith, J. Aging and culture. *In* Binstock, R. and Shanas, E. (eds.). *Handbook of Aging and the Social Sciences.* 2nd ed. New York: Van Nostrand Reinhold, 1985.

Kelleher, C.H. and Quirk, D.A. Age, functional capacity and work: An annotated bibliography. *Industr Gerontol* 19(Fall):80–98, 1973.

Kelley, H.H. Marriage relationships and aging. *In* Fogel, R.W., Hatfield, E., Kiesler, S.B. and Shanas, E. (eds.). *Aging: Stability and Change in the Family: Generational Relations.* Englewood Cliffs, NJ: Prentice-Hall, 1965.

Kellogg, F.R., Crain, M., Corwin, J. and Brickner, P.W. Life-sustaining interventions in frail elderly persons: Talking about choices. *Arch Intern Med* 152(11):2317–2320, 1992.

Kemper, S. Language and aging. *In* Craik, F.I.M. and Salthouse, T.A. (eds.). *The Handbook of Aging and Cognition.* Hilldale, NJ: Lawrence Erlbaum Association, 1992, pp. 213–263.

Kiesler, S.B. et al. *Aging: Social Change.* New York: Academic Press, 1981.

King, T. The experiences of midlife daughters who are caregivers for their mothers. *Health Care Women Int* 14(5):419–426, 1993.

Koenig, H.G., Kvale, J.N. and Ferrel, C. Religion and well-being in later life. *Gerontologist* 28:18–28, 1988.

Koenig, H.G., Smiley, M. and Gonzales, J.P. *Religion, Health and Aging: A Review and Theoretical Integration.* Westport, CT: Greenwood, 1988.

Kogan, N. Personality and aging. *In* Birren, J.E. and Schaie, K.W. (eds.). *Handbook of the Psychology of Aging.* 3rd ed. New York: Academic Press, 1990, pp. 330–346.

Krause, N. Race differences in life satisfaction among aged men and women. *J Gerontol* 48(5):S235–S244, 1993.

Kutner, B., Fanshel, D., Togo, A. and Langer, S.W. *Five Hundred Over Sixty.* New York: Russell Sage Foundation, 1956.

Lebo, D. Some factors said to make for happiness in old age. *J Clin Psychol* 9:384–390, 1953.

Lee, G.R., Dwyer, J.W. and Coward, R.T. Gender differences in parent care: Demographic factors and same-gender preferences. *J Gerontol* 48(1):S9–S16, 1993.

Lemon, B.W., Bengtson, V.L. and Peterson, J.A. An exploration of the activity theory of aging: Activity types and life satisfaction among in-movers to a retirement community. *J Gerontol* 27:511–523, 1972.

Levin, J.S. (ed.). *Religion in Aging and Health: Theoretical Foundations and Methodological Frontiers.* Thousand Oaks, CA: Sage Publications, 1994.

Levin, J.S., Taylor, R.J. and Chatters, L.M. Race and gender differences in religiosity among older adults: Findings from four national surveys. *J Gerontol* 49(3):S137–S145, 1994.

Levy, J.A. Sexuality and aging. *In* Hazzard, W.R., Bierman, E.D., Blass, J.P., et al. (eds.). *Principles of Geriatric Medicine and Gerontology.* 3rd ed. New York: McGraw-Hill, 1994, pp. 115–124.

Light, L.L. Interactions between memory and language in old age. *In* Birren, J.E. and Schaie, K.W. (eds.). *Handbook of the Psychology of Aging.* 3rd ed. New York: Academic Press, 1990, pp. 275–289.

Liken, M.A. and Collins, C.E. Grieving: Facilitating the process for dementia caregivers. *J Psychosoc Nurs Ment Health Serv* 31(1):21–26, 1993.

Little, V. *Open Care for the Aging: Comparative International Approaches.* New York: Springer Publishers, 1982.

Litwak, E. Extended kin relations in an industrial democratic society. *In* Shanas, E. and Strieb, G. (eds.). *Social Structures and the Family Generational Relations.* Englewood Cliffs, NJ: Prentice-Hall, 1965.

Logan, J.R. and Spitze, G. Informal support and the use of formal services by older Americans. *J Gerontol* 49(1):S25–S34, 1994.

Lorsbach, T.C. and Simpson, G.B. Age differences in the rate of processing in short-term memory. *J Gerontol* 39(3):315–321, 1984.

Lowenthal, M.F. and Haven, C. Interaction and adaptation: Intimacy as a critical variable. *Am Soc Rev* 33:20–30, 1968.

Lowenthal, M.F. et al. *Aging and Mental Disorder in San Francisco.* San Francisco: Jossey Bass, 1967.

Lozier, J. and Althouse, R. Social enforcement of behavior toward elders in an Appalachian Mountain settlement. *Gerontologist* 14:69–80, 1974.

Mackinnon, C.A. The association between mental, social and physical activity and cognitive performance in young and old subjects. *Age Ageing* 22:175–182, 1993.

MacNutt, F. *The Power to Heal.* Notre Dame, IN: Ave Maria Press, 1977.

Madden, D.J. Four to ten milliseconds per year: Age-related slowing of visual word identification. *J Gerontol* 47:P59–P68, 1992.

Maddox, G. Activity and morale: A longitudinal study of selected elderly subjects. *J Soc Forces* 42:195–204, 1963.

Maddox, G.L. Sociology of aging. *In* Hazzard, W.R., Bierman, E.D., Blass, J.P., et al. (eds.). *Principles of Geriatric Medicine and Gerontology.* 3rd ed. New York: McGraw-Hill, 1994, pp. 125–133.

Marsiglio, W. and Donnelly, D. Sexual relations in later life: A national study of married persons. *J Gerontol* 46(6):S338–S344, 1991.

Martin, M. Ageing and patterns of change in everyday memory and cognition. *Hum Learning* 5:63–74, 1986.

Masters, W.H. and Johnson, V.E. *Human Sexual Response.* Boston: Little, Brown, 1966, p. 233.

Mathison, J.A. A cross-cultural view of widowhood. *Omega* 1(3):201–217, 1970.

Matteson, M.A. A report of sensory assessment in a senior citizen's center. *J Gerontol Nurs* 5:34–37, 1979.

Matthews, S.H. and Sprey, J. Adolescents' relationships with grandparents: An empirical contribution to conceptual clarification. *J Gerontol* 40:621–626, 1985.

Maxwell, R. and Silverman, P. Information and esteem. *Aging Hum Dev* 1:361–392, 1970.

McClellan, R.W. *Claiming a Frontier: Ministry and Older People.* Los Angeles: University of Southern California Press, 1977.

McCrae, R.R. and Costa, P.T. Jr. Validation of the five-factor model across instruments and observers. *J Pers Soc Psychol* 52:81, 1987.

McCullough, L.B., Wilson, N.L., Teasdale, T.A. et al. Mapping personal, familial, and professional values in long-term care decisions. *Gerontologist* 33(3):324–332, 1993.

McDowd, J.M. and Birren, J.E. Aging and attentional processes. *In* Birren, J.E. and Schaie, K.W. (eds.). *Handbook of the Psychology of Aging.* 3rd ed. New York: Academic Press, 1990, pp. 222–233.

McGue, M., Hirsch, B. and Lykken, D.T. Age and the self-perception of ability: A twin study analysis. *Psychol Aging* 8(1):72–80, 1993.

McNutt, F. *The Power to Heal.* Notre Dame, IN: Ave Maria Press, 1977.

Meyers, D.A. Work after cessation of career job. *J Gerontol* 46:S93–S102, 1991.

Moberg, D.O. The encounter of scientific and religious values pertinent to man's spiritual nature. *Sociol Anal* 28:22–23, 1967.

Moberg, D.O. Religion and aging. *In* Ferraro, K.F. (ed.). *Gerontology: Perspectives and Issues.* New York: Springer Publishing Company, 1990, pp. 179–205.

Moen, P., Robinson, J. and Fields, V. Women's work and caregiving roles: A life course approach. *J Gerontol* 49(4):S176–S186, 1994.

Monge, R. and Hultsch, D. Paired-associate learning as a function of paced and self-paced associations and response time. *J Gerontol* 26:157–162, 1971.

Montgomery, R.J. and Kosloski, K. A longitudinal analysis of nursing home placement for dependent elders cared for by spouses vs adult children. *J Gerontol* 49(2): S62–S74, 1994.

Moore, B.S., Newsome, J.A., Payne, P.L. and Tiansawad, S. Nursing research: Quality of life and perceived health in the elderly. *J Gerontol Nurs* 19(11):7–14, 1993.

Moore, J.S. Old age in a life-term social arena. *In* Myerhoff, B. and Simic, A. (eds.). *Life's Career-Aging: Cultural Variations on Growing Old.* Beverly Hills, CA: Sage Publications, 1978.

Mor-Barak, M.E., Scharlach, A.E., Birba, L. and Sokolov, J. Employment, social networks, and health in the retirement years. *Int J Aging Hum Dev* 35(2):145–159, 1992.

Morris, R.G. Cognition and ageing. *In* Jacoby, R. and Oppenheimer, C. (eds.). *Psychiatry in the Elderly.* New York: Oxford University Press, 1991, pp. 58–88.

Morse, C.K. and Wisocki, P.A. Importance of religiosity to elderly adjustment. *J Religion Aging* 4(1):15–26, 1987.

Mortimer, J.T., et al. Persistence and change in development: The multi-dimensional self-concept. *In* Baltes, P.B. and Brim, O.G., Jr. (eds.). *Life-Span Development and Behavior.* Vol. 4. New York: Academic Press, 1982, pp. 264–315.

Morycz, R.K. Caregiving strain and the desire to institutionalize family members with Alzheimer's disease. *Res Aging* 7:329–361, 1985.

Moscovitch, M. A neuropsychological approach to memory and perception in normal and pathological aging. *In* Craik, F.I.M. and Treuhub, S. (eds.). *Aging and Cognitive Processes.* New York: Plenum Press, 1982, pp. 55–78.

Mullins, L.C. and Dugan, E. Elderly social relationships with adult children and close friends and depression. *J Soc Behav Pers* 6:315–328, 1991.

Murtaugh, C., Kemper, P. and Spillman, B. The risk of nursing home use in later life. *Med Care* 28(10):952–962, 1990.

Mutran, E. and Reitzes, D.C. Intergenerational exchange relationships in the aging family. *In* Ferraro, K.F. (ed.). *Gerontology: Perspectives and Issues.* New York: Springer Publishing Company, 1990, pp. 149–162.

Myers, D.A. Work after cessation of career job. *J Gerontol* 46:S93–S102, 1991.

National Center for Health Statistics. Current Estimates from the National Health Interview Survey, 1989. *Vital and Health Statistics.* Series 10, No. 176, October 1990.

National Center for Health Statistics. Advance Report of Final Marriage Statistics, 1987. *Monthly Vital Statistics Report* Vol. 38, No. 12, Supplement, April 1990.

National Institute of Dental Research, National Institutes of Health. *National Health Interview Survey—1989 Dental Supplement.* National Center for Health Statistics.

Nelson, L.P. and Nelson, V. Religion and death anxiety. Presentation at the Annual Joint Meeting of the Society for the Scientific Study of Religion and the Religious Research Association, San Francisco, 1973.

Neugarten, B. Personality and aging. *In* Birren, J.E. and Schaie, K.W. (eds.). *Handbook of the Psychology of Aging.* New York: Van Nostrand Reinhold, 1977.

Neugarten, B. and Datan, N. Sociological perspectives on the life cycle. *In* Baltes, P. and Schaie, K. (eds.). *Lifespan Developmental Psychology: Personality and Socialization.* New York: Academic Press, 1973.

Neugarten, B. and Hagestad, G. Age and the life course. *In* Binstock, R. and Shanas, E. (eds.). *Handbook of Aging and the Social Sciences.* New York: Van Nostrand Reinhold, 1976.

Neugarten, B., Moore, J. and Lowe, J. Age norms, age constraints, and adult socialization. *Am J Sociol* 70(6): 710–717, 1965.

Neugarten, B.L. and Weinstein, K. The changing American grandparent. *J Marriage Fam* 26:199–204, 1964.

Norris, M.P. and West, R.L. Age differences in the recall of actions and cognitive activities: The effects of presentation rate and object cues. *Psychol Res* 53(3):188–194, 1991.

Novak, M. and Guest, C. Application of a multidimensional caregiver burden inventory. *Gerontologist* 29: 798–803, 1989.

Oppenheimer, C. Sexuality in old age. *In* Jacoby, R. and Oppenheimer, C. (eds.). *Psychiatry in the Elderly.* New York: Oxford University Press, 1991, pp. 872–900.

O'Reilly, E. and Morrison, M.L. Grandparent-headed families: New therapeutic challenges. *Child Psychiatry Hum Dev* 23(3):147–159, 1993.

Palmore, E. and Manton, K. Modernization and status of the aged: International correlations. *J Gerontol* 29(2): 205–210, 1974.

Panicucci, C., Ingman, S. and Alyea, B. The nurse practitioner-physician team in nursing home practice. *Gerontol Geriatr Educ* 5(2):55–64, 1985.

Parnes, H.S. and Sommers, D.G. Shunning retirement: Work experience of men in their seventies and early eighties. *J Gerontol* 49(3):S117–S124, 1994.

Parsons, T. Definitions of health and illness in light of American values and social structure. *In* Jaco, E.G. (ed.). *Patients, Physicians, and Illness.* New York: Free Press, 1972.

Patrick, D.L., Starks, H.E., Cain, K.C. et al. Measuring preferences for health states worse than death. *Med Decis Making* 14(1):9–18, 1994.

Pearlin, L.I., Mullan, J.T., Semple, S.J. and Skaff, M.M. Caregiving and the stress process: An overview of concepts and their measures. *Gerontologist* 30:583–591, 1990.

Perry, C.M. and Johnson, C.L. Families and support networks among African American oldest-old. *Int J Aging Hum Dev* 38(1):41–50, 1994.

Peterson, S.A. and Maiden, R. Personality and politics among older Americans: A rural case study. *Int J Aging Hum Dev* 36(2):157–169, 1992.

Pfeiffer, E. and Davis, D.C. The use of leisure time in middle life. *Gerontologist* 11:187–195, 1971.

Pfeiffer, E. et al. Sexual behavior in aged men and women. *Arch Gen Psychiatry* 19:753, 1988.

Phillips, B.S. A role theory approach to adjustment in old age. *Am Soc Rev* 22:212–217, 1957.

Pienta, A.M., Burr, J.A. and Mutchler, J.E. Women's labor force participation in later life: The effects of early work and family experiences. *J Gerontol Sci* 49(5):S231–S239, 1994.

Pinquart, M. Analysis of the self concept on independently living senior citizens [German]. *Z Gerontol* 24(2): 98–104, 1991.

Pollock, A. Carers' literature review. *Nurs Times* 90(25): 31–33, 1994.

Poon, L.W. and Schaffer, G. Prospective memory in young and elderly adults. Presented at the American Psychology Association Meeting, Washington, D.C., August 1982.

Poon, L.W., Martin, P., Clayton, G.M. et al. The influences of cognitive resources on adaptation and old age. *Int J Aging Hum Dev* 34(1):31–46, 1992.

Powers, E.A., Keith, P. and Goudy, W.J. Family relationships and friendships among the rural aged. *In* Byerts, T.O., Howell, S.C. and Pastalan, L.A. (eds.). *Environmental Context of Aging: Life-styles, Environmental Quality and Living Arrangements.* New York: Garland STPM Press, 1979.

Rabbit, P. Age and the use of structure in transmitted information. *In* Talland, G.A. (ed.). *Human Aging and Behavior.* New York: Academic Press, 1968, pp. 75–92.

Rabinowitz, J.C., Ackerman, B.P., Craik, F.I.M. and Hinchley, J.L. Aging and metamemory: The roles of relatedness and imagery. *J Gerontol* 37:638–692, 1982.

Reichard, S., Livson, F. and Peterson, P.G. *Aging and Personality: A Study of 87 Older Men.* New York: John Wiley & Sons, 1962.

Riley, M.W. Age strata in social systems. *In* Binstock, R.H. and Shanas, E. (eds.). *Handbook of Aging and the Social Sciences.* New York: Van Nostrand Reinhold, 1976.

Riley, M.W., Abeles, R.P. and Teitelbaum, M.S. *Aging from Birth to Death. Vol. II. Sociotemporal Perspectives.* Boulder, CO: Westview Press, 1979.

Roberts, B.L., Dunkle, R. and Haug, M. Physical, psychological, and social resources as moderators of the relationship of stress to mental health of the very old. *J Gerontol* 49(1):S35–S43, 1994.

Robertson, G.S. Resuscitation and senility: A study of patients' opinions. *J Med Ethics,* 19(2):104–107, 1993.

Robinson, B.C. Validation of a caregiver strain index. *Gerontologist* 38:344–348, 1983.

Romeis, J.C., Schey, H.M., Marion, G.S., and Keith, J.F., Jr. et al. Extending the extenders. Compromise for the geriatric specialization-manpower debate. *J Am Geriatr Soc* 33:559–565, 1985.

Rose, A. The subculture of the aging: A framework for research in social gerontology. *In* Rose, A. and Peterson, P.G. (eds.). *Older People and Their Social Worlds.* Philadelphia: F.A. Davis, 1965.

Rosow, I. *Social Integration of the Aged.* New York: Free Press, 1967.

Rosow, I. The social context of the aging self. *Gerontologist* 13:83–87, 1973.

Rosow, I. *Socialization to Old Age.* Berkeley, CA: University of California Press, 1974.

Rosow, I. Status and role change through the life cycle. *In* Binstock, R. and Shanas, E. (eds.). *Handbook of Aging and the Social Sciences.* 2nd ed. New York: Van Nostrand Reinhold, 1985.

Rowe, J. and Kahn, R. Human aging: Usual and successful. *Science* 237:143, 1987.

Ruhm, C.J. Bridge jobs and partial retirement. *J Labor Econ* 8:482–501, 1990.

Salthouse, T.A. Age and memory: Strategies for localizing the loss. *In* Poon, L.W. et al. (eds.). *New Directions in Memory and Aging.* Hillside, NJ: Erlbaum Associates, 1980.

Sands, L.P. and Meredith, W. Blood pressure and intellectual functioning in late midlife. *J Gerontol* 47(2):P81–P84, 1992.

Satoh, S., Morita, N., Kusumoto, K. et al. Mental health in family members living with elders. *Jpn J Psychiatry Neurol* 47(4):801–809, 1993.

Schaie, K.W. Intellectual development in adulthood. *In* Birren, J.E. and Schaie, K.W. (eds.). *Handbook of the Psychology of Aging.* 3rd ed. New York: Academic Press, 1990a, pp. 291–309.

Schaie, K.W. The optimization of cognitive functioning in old age prediction based on cohort-sequential and longitudinal data. *In* Baltes, P.B. and Baltes, M.M. (eds.). *Longitudinal Research and the Study of Successful (Optimal) Aging.* Cambridge, England: Cambridge University Press, 1990b, pp. 94–117.

Schaie, K.W. and Willis, S.L. Age difference patterns of psychometric intelligence in adulthood: Generalizability within and across ability domains. *Psychol Aging* 8(1):44–55, 1993.

Schaie, K.W., Willis, S.L. and O'Hanlon, A.M. Perceived intellectual performance change over seven years. *J Gerontol* 49(3):P108–P118, 1994.

Schick, F.L. and Schick, R. *Statistical Handbook on Aging Americans.* Phoenix, AZ: Orynx Press, 1994.

Sears, D.L. Life stage effects on attitude change, especially among the elderly. *In* Kiesler, S.B., et al. (eds.). *Aging: Social Change.* New York: Academic Press, 1981.

Shanan, J. and Sharon, M. Personality and cognitive functioning of Israeli males during the middle years. *Hum Dev* 8:2–15, 1965.

Shanas, E. The family as a social support system in old age. *Gerontologist* 19:169–174, 1979a.

Shanas, E. Social myth as hypothesis: The case of the family relations of old people. *Gerontologist* 19:3–9, 1979b.

Shanas, E., Townsend, P., Wedderburn, D., et al. *Old People in Three Industrial Societies.* New York: Atherton Press, 1968.

Siegler, I.C. and Botwinick, J. A long-term longitudinal study of intellectual ability of older adults: The matter of selective subject attrition. *J Gerontol* 34:242–245, 1979.

Siegler, I.C. and Poon, L.W. The psychology of aging. *In* Busse, E.W. and Blazer, D.G. (eds.). *Geriatric Psychiatry.* Washington, D.C.: American Psychiatric Press, 1989, pp. 163–201.

Silverstein, M. and Bengtson, V.L. Does intergenerational social support influence the psychological well-being of older parents: The contingencies of declining health and widowhood. *Soc Sci Med* 38(7):943–957, 1994.

Silverstein, M. and Waite, J. Are blacks more likely than whites to receive and provide social support in middle and old age? Yes, no, and maybe so. *J Gerontol* 48(4):S212–S222, 1993.

Sinnot, J.D. Prospective/intentional and incidental memory: Effects of age and passage of time. *Psychol Aging* I:101–116, 1986.

Smith, R.W. Adult sexual behavior in 1989: Number of partners, frequency of intercourse and risk of AIDS. *Fam Plann Perspect* 3:102, 1991.

Smits, M.W. and Kee, C.C. Correlates of self-care among the independent elderly: Self-concept affects well-being. *J Gerontol Nurs* 18(9):13–18, 1992.

Spence, D.A. and Wiener, J.M. Nursing home length of stay patterns: Results from the 1985 National Nursing Home Survey. *Gerontologist* 30(1):16–20, 1990.

Spirduso, W.W. and MacRae, P.G. Motor performance and aging. *In* Birren, J.E. and Schaie, K.W. (eds.). *Handbook of the Psychology of Aging.* 3rd ed. New York: Academic Press, 1990, pp. 183–199.

Spitze, G., Logan, J.R., Joseph, G. and Lee, E. Middle generation roles and the well-being of men and women. *J Gerontol* 49(3):S107–S116, 1994.

Starr, B.D. and Weiner, M.B. *The Starr-Weiner Report on Sex and Sexuality in the Mature Years.* New York: Briarcliff Manor, 1981.

Steinitz, L.Y. The local church as support for the elderly. *J Gerontol Soc Work* 4(2):43–53, 1981.

Sterns, H.L., Matheson, N.K. and Schwartz, L.S. Work and retirement. *In* Ferraro, K.F. (ed.). *Gerontology: Perspectives and Issues.* New York: Springer Publishing Company, 1990, pp. 163–178.

Stevens, G.L., Walsh, R.A. and Baldwin, B.A. Family caregivers of institutionalized and noninstitutionalized elderly individuals. *Nurs Clin North Am* 28(2):349–362, 1993.

Stolar, G.E., MacEntee, M.I. and Hill, P. Seniors' assessment of their health and life satisfaction: The case for contextual evaluation. *Int J Aging Hum Dev* 35(4):305–317, 1992.

Stoller, E. and Earl, L. Help with activities of everyday life: Sources of support for the noninstitutionalized elderly. *Gerontologist* 23:64–70, 1983.

Stone, R., Cafferata, G.L. and Sangl, J. Caregivers of the

frail elderly: A national profile. *Gerontologist* 27:616–626, 1987.

Sugar, J.A. and McDowd, J.M. Memory, learning, and attention. *In* Birren, J.E., Sloane, R.B. and Cohen, G.D. (eds.). *Handbook of Mental Health and Aging.* 2nd ed. New York: Academic Press, 1992, pp. 307–337.

Suitor, J.J. and Pillemer, K. Support and interpersonal stress in the social networks of married daughters caring for parents with dementia. *J Gerontol* 48:S1–S8, 1993.

Szinovacz, M. and Harpster, P. Couples' employment/retirement status and the division of household tasks. *J Gerontol* 49(3):S125–S136, 1994.

Tallmer, M. and Kutner, B. Disengagement and morale. *Gerontologist* 10:317–320, 1970.

Tennstedt, S.L., Crawford, S. and McKinlay, J.B. Determining the pattern of community care: Is coresidence more important than caregiver relationship? *J Gerontol* 48(2):S74–S83, 1993a.

Tennstedt, S.L., Crawford, S.L. and McKinlay, J.B. Is family care on the decline? A longitudinal investigation of the substitution of formal long-term care services for informal care. *Milbank Q* 71(4):601–624, 1993b.

Thomae, H. Emotion and personality. *In* Birren, J.E., Sloane, R.B. and Cohen, G.D. (eds.). *Handbook of Mental Health and Aging.* 2nd ed. New York: Academic Press, 1992, pp. 355–375.

Thompson, E.H., Jr., Futterman, A.M., Gallagher-Thompson, D. et al. Social support and caregiving burden in family caregivers of frail elders. *J Gerontol* 48(5):S245–S254, 1993.

Thorson, J.A. and Cook, T.C. (eds.). *Spiritual Well-Being of the Elderly.* Springfield, IL: Charles C Thomas, 1980.

Thorson, J.A. and Powell, F.C. Meanings of death and intrinsic religiosity. *J Clin Psychol* 46(4):379–391, 1990.

Tobin, S.S. and Neugarten, B.L. Life satisfaction and social interaction in the aging. *J Gerontol* 16:344–346, 1961.

Toner, H.M. and Morris, J.D. A social-psychological perspective of dietary quality in later adulthood. *J Nutr Elderly* 11(4):35–53, 1992.

United States Bureau of the Census and United States Department of Housing and Urban Development. American Housing Survey for the United States in 1987. *Current Housing Reports* Series H-150-87, December 1989.

United States Bureau of the Census. Homeownership Trends in the 1980's. *Current Housing Reports* Series H-121, No. 2, December 1990.

United States Bureau of the Census. Marital Status and Living Arrangements: March 1989. *Current Population Reports* Series P-20, No. 445, June 1990.

United States Department of Health and Human Services. *Aging America: Trends and Projections.* Washington, D.C., 1991.

United States Department of Labor, Bureau of Labor Statistics. Thirty-Eight Million Persons Do Volunteer Work. Press Release USDL 90-154. Data are from May 1989 Current Population Survey, March 29, 1990.

Vaillant, G. *Adaptation to Life.* Boston: Little, Brown, 1977.

Veroff, J., Kulka, R.A. and Douvan, E. *Mental Health in America.* New York: Basic Books, 1981.

Watson, W. *Aging and Social Behavior.* Monterey, CA: Wadsworth Health Sciences Division, 1982.

Wechsler, D. Intelligence: Definition, the IQ. *In* Caucio, R. (ed.). *Intelligences: Genetic and Environmental Influences.* New York: Grune & Stratton, 1971, pp. 50–55.

Welford, A.T. Psychomotor performance. *In* Eisdorfer, C. (ed.). *Annual Review of Gerontology and Geriatrics.* Vol. 4. 1984, pp. 237–274.

Whitbeck, L., Hoyt, D.R. and Huck, S.M. Early family relationships, intergenerational solidarity, and support provided to parents by their adult children. *J Gerontol* 49(2):S85–S94, 1994.

Whitbourne, S.K. and Sperbeck, D.J. Health care maintenance for the elderly. *Fam Community Health* 3(4):11–27, 1981.

White, C.B. Sexual interest, attitudes, knowledge, and sexual history in relation to sexual behavior in the institutionalized aged. *Arch Sex Behav* 11(1):11, 1982.

Wiegersma, S. and Meertse, K. Subjective ordering, working memory, and aging. *Exp Aging Res* 16(1–2):73–77, 1990.

Willis, S.L. and Schaie, K.W. Training the elderly on ability factors of spatial orientation and inductive reasoning. *Psychol Aging* 1:239–247, 1986.

Witter, R.A., Stock, W.A., Okun, M.A. and Haring, M.J. Religion and subjective well-being in adulthood: A quantitative synthesis. *Rev Religious Res* 26:332–342, 1985.

Wolfson, C., Handfield-Jones, R., Glass, K.C. et al. Adult children's perceptions of their responsibility to provide care for dependent elderly parents. *Gerontologist* 33(3):315–323, 1993.

Youmans, E. The rural aged. *Ann Am Acad Polit Soc Sci* 429:81–90, 1977.

Zarit, J.M. and Zarit, S.H. Measuring burden and support in families with Alzheimer's disease elders. Presented at the 35th Annual Scientific Meeting of the Gerontological Society of America. Boston, MA, 1982.

Zarit, S.H., Cole, K.D. and Guider, R.L. Memory training strategies and subjective complaints of memory in the aged. *Gerontologist* 21:158–164, 1981.

Zarit, S.H., Reever, K. and Bach-Peterson, J. Relatives of the impaired elderly: Correlates of feelings of burden. *Gerontologist* 20:649–655, 1980.

Zisook, S., Shuchter, S.R., Sledge, P. and Mulvihill, M. Aging and bereavement. *J Geriatr Psychiatry Neurol* 6(3):137–143, 1993.

Zukerman, D.M., Kasl, S.V. and Ostfeld, A.M. Psychosocial predictors of mortality among the elderly poor. *Am J Epidemiol* 119:410–423, 1984.

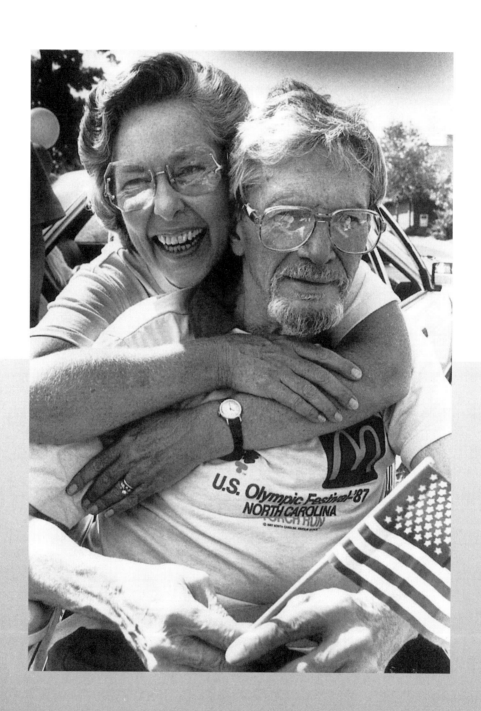

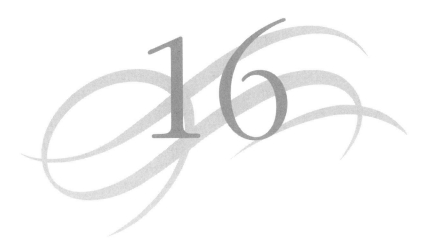

Psychosocial Problems Associated with Aging

MARY ANN MATTESON
LUCILLE B. BEARON
ELEANOR S. McCONNELL

OBJECTIVES

Define ageism and describe its effect on the elderly population.

❖

Discuss the relationship between poverty and housing problems among the elderly.

❖

Identify problems associated with public policy and its effect on the dependent elderly.

❖

Recognize and describe elder abuse and explain its ramifications for older people, families, and health care providers.

❖

Analyze the issues involving older women in the United States.

❖

Compare and contrast symptoms and treatments of common mental disorders among older people, including depression, suicide ideation, anxiety and somatoform disorders, schizophrenia, and delusional disorders.

❖

Conduct a psychosocial assessment of an older adult.

❖

The diversity of the older adult population provides us with the knowledge that there are "many ways of aging." Gerontologists now know that later life is a healthy and satisfying time for many adults. For a minority, however, including those seen most frequently by health care providers, old age may be a time of serious psychosocial problems, including economic hardships, strained social relationships, and poor psychological adjustment.

The focus of this chapter is on a number of problems encountered by older adults, including ageism, poverty, housing problems, dependency, abuse and neglect, women's issues, depression, substance abuse, suicide ideation, anxiety and somatoform disorders, schizophrenia, and delusional disorders. Although these problems occur in other age groups, the impact on older adults may be particularly stressful when they are experienced along with physical frailty and diminished adaptive reserves.

A full understanding of these complex problems requires recognition that they occur in a social context and may be induced or worsened by social factors. Some problems originate in societal attitudes and public policies that disempower older adults; other problems are influenced by community, institutional, or family approaches to dependency.

Failure to acknowledge the sociogenic component of these problems may result in nurses' taking a "blame-the-victim" approach, which can render them virtually incapable of assisting clients with serious psychosocial problems. Also, nurses must recognize the consequences of psychosocial problems on an individual's response to health and illness. Without an understanding of the dynamic relationship between psychosocial problems and physical health, nurses may have unrealistic expectations of clients, leading to frustration on the part of both client and nurse.

One positive benefit of acknowledging the influence of social factors in later life is that many of these problems can be eliminated or improved through social interventions, e.g., aggressive attempts to change public opinion or public policy. Other problems can be addressed through interventions in the immediate social context, e.g., accessing appropriate community-based services and providing family therapy in addition to individual counseling.

AGEISM

Definition

Ageism refers to prejudice or discrimination toward people based on their chronological age or on symbols of old age such as gray hair or a slow gait. The term was coined by Robert Butler in 1969 to explain neighbors' strong resistance to the construction nearby of housing for older people (Butler, 1993).

Butler first defined ageism as "a systematic stereotyping of and discrimination against people because they are old. . . . Ageism allows the younger generations to see older people as different from themselves; thus they subtly cease to identify with their elders as human beings" (Butler, 1975, p. 12).

The definition of ageism was expanded by Binstock (1983, p. 136) as "the attribution of the same characteristics, status, and just desserts to a heterogeneous group that has been artificially homogenized, packaged, labeled, and marketed as the aged."

Ageism has been compared with racism and sexism by those who seek to understand its causes and impact. It is characterized by simplistic beliefs or stereotypes, usually negative, perpetuated under conditions in which older persons have decreased social status and diminished contact with younger individuals. This physical and psychological distance (implied in the term "generation gap") also leads some older people to hold negative stereotypes about younger people, simply because of their age.

Ageist beliefs and attitudes often cause older people to receive differential treatment or to be excluded from opportunities. Ageism affects the health care of older people by influencing the attitudes of health care professionals and policy makers toward aggressiveness in diagnosis and treatment of the elderly. These attitudes are often based on erroneous assumptions regarding the utility of chronological age as a marker of function or ability to contribute to society. The tragedy of ageism is that it robs society of the fullest contributions of its older members, and it denies people fulfillment of their potential as human beings throughout the life course.

Some scholarly papers and political commentaries have pointed to a disturbing trend regarding ageism in public perceptions of the elderly. Because of the improved health and well-being of large segments of today's older population, negative stereotypes of older people have been partially replaced by *overly positive* stereotypes of older people.

One major consequence has been a backlash in public opinion; some people argue that older people are no longer deserving of "entitlement" programs or other social programs designed to enhance quality of life. As with negative ageism, this "positive ageism" uses simplistic characterizations to obscure the diversity within the older adult population and to ignore those with real needs.

Scope of the Problem

Stereotypical beliefs about older persons have been demonstrated in many different groups of people, including children, college students, health care professionals, and even older people themselves. The stereotypes are both positive and negative but are consistent among all age groups. Health professionals hold essentially the same ageist stereotypes of older people as the rest of society does (Palmore, 1990). Some negative stereotypes include beliefs that older people are dependent, asexual, pessimistic toward the future, insecure, meddlesome, lonely, not valued by their families, and in poor physical and mental condition. Many older people themselves subscribe to a stereotyped view of the elderly and have negative beliefs about the aging process.

Some analysts have suggested that negative stereotypes are disappearing, reflecting the improving and heterogeneous circumstances of today's older people. Butler (1993, p. 76) noted, "I believe that the last decade has witnessed a steady improvement in the attitudes toward the aged; in part a consequence of general public education; increased media attention; the expansion of education in the community, colleges and universities; and the continuing growth of gerontology." He added, however, that "success has been uneven. Residual pockets of negativism toward the aged still exist, most occurring subtly, covertly, and even unconsciously; like racism and sexism, ageism remains recalcitrant, even if below the surface."

Negative stereotypes frequently are being replaced with positive ones. A study by Bell (1992, p. 305) of images of aging in prime-time television programs found that "earlier television stereotypes of the elderly as more comical, stubborn, eccentric, and foolish than other characters have been replaced by more positive stereotypes of them as powerful, affluent, active, admired and sexy." Shenk and Achenbaum (1993, p. 6) assert, however, that even if negative stereotyping is on the decline, "vivid images have staying power in large part because they are so ambiguous. Even when they become obsolete they maintain a niche in popular culture, serving as a caricature of the world view that once sustained them."

Contributors to Ageism

Attitudes, Values, and Beliefs

From a social psychological point of view, ageism is a complex phenomenon, encompassing at least three interrelated elements: (1) erroneous or simplistic beliefs (stereotypes) that are based on lack of knowledge, misinformation, or selective perception; (2) biased attitudes (opinions or dispositions imbued with negative feelings); and (3) discriminatory behavior (active or passive). There is considerable evidence that erroneous and simplistic beliefs about older people pervade all segments of our society. There is also evidence that many people have attitudes biased against the elderly. Often, the source of bias could be negative beliefs about older people; some would say that beliefs are one category of attitude. Other factors shape attitudes, however, such as authoritarian personality, anger, hostility or projection provoked by personal experience, and need to scapegoat. Attitudes are shaped by family experiences and adult socialization. In addition, it has been shown that later learning, through the media or through other sources such as formal training, can modify attitudes.

Gerontologists have documented many examples of individual and institutional discriminatory behavior. Evidence of individual discrimination against older people has been found in medical decision making, surgical intervention, provider-patient interaction, decreased autonomy, choice, autocratic policies, infantilization, and communication (Jones, 1993; Schmid, 1991; Ryan et al., 1991; McDonald and Bridge, 1991; Derby, 1991). Efforts are under way to teach physicians new ways to act; epistudies point out injustices, corrective action, and advocacy.

Theory and research on the relationship between attitudes and behavior suggest that attitudes toward the aged (framed broadly to include beliefs) are probably key determinants of people's behavior toward the elderly. For example, if a nurse believes that old people are unable to learn new skills, then the nurse is unlikely to teach an older person to use a sphygmomanometer to monitor blood pressure. This means that the older person is dependent on others to monitor blood pressure, reinforcing a stereotype that old people are dependent.

There is little question that attitudes are shaped by both family experiences and adult socialization. In addition, it has been shown that later learning, through the media or through other sources such as formal training, can modify attitudes. Attitudes toward older persons develop in the same way as other attitudes and can be modified in a similar manner.

Stereotyping

A stereotype is "the holding in common by the members of a group of a standardized mental picture representing an oversimplified and uncritical judgment of another group" (Solomon and Vickers, 1979). Barrow and Smith (1979) suggested that stereotyping and labeling fulfill a human need to decrease ambiguity and clarify where an individual stands relative to another person or group. As noted earlier, stereotyping of older persons by health care professionals and gerontologists of nearly every discipline is widespread.

At first glance, this seems paradoxical; those who regularly encounter the elderly should be most aware of the diversity among the aged. This apparent paradox can be explained as follows: because the elderly are *so* diverse, professionals apply stereotypes to simplify an already complex interaction. Unfortunately, this oversimplification often results in suboptimal care for the older person. In the example of the nurse and the elderly hypertensive patient, it is simpler for the nurse to assume that all older persons cannot learn new skills than to assess each older person for the ability and readiness to learn and adapt teaching approaches accordingly. Although this approach simplifies the nurse's work, the dependency reinforced in this situation is not the desired outcome for most older persons. Indeed, this lack of control over one's illness may predispose to noncompliance and further complicate the patient's situation at a later date. Stereotyping thus provides a false economy of time.

Another possible consequence of stereotyping is scapegoating. Scapegoating is when one group, individual, or thing is blamed for the problems of another individual or group. This generally involves some oversimplification of the issues or problems at hand. Scapegoating is of concern because it may lead to a situation in which health professionals depersonalize their clients and adopt a blame-the-victim attitude.

Blaming the victim is a phenomenon whereby the problems of a disadvantaged group are attributed to the behavior or values of the victimized group rather than to external conditions (Ryan, 1971). The effects of a blaming-the-victim mentality include distracting attention from the basic cause of the social injustice, rationalizing current social conditions, and, ultimately, internalizing the blaming mentality so that the victimized group also believes that "they only have themselves to blame." The most extreme consequence of this practice can be "internalized oppression" or "self-hate" in which a member of a persecuted group becomes ashamed of or hostile toward other members or suffers low self-esteem because of membership in the group.

The term *crock* is familiar to many in the health care field. It generally refers to someone who is uncooperative or unable to give a concise or accurate medical history or who has multiple medical complaints. The aging process and its associated illnesses may result in patients who *through no fault of their own* may fit this description. Such patients are generally regarded negatively, as if the individual did have some control over memory loss, diffuseness of pain, or multiplicity of illnesses. The older person becomes a scapegoat for the clinician's feelings of inadequacy. This is a common example of both scapegoating and blaming the victim.

Another example is the incontinent patient. The older person has one episode of incontinence and is quickly padded with incontinence pads. The nurses note in the change of shift report that Mrs. J. is incontinent and therefore they do not offer her the opportunity to go to the bathroom. One week later when Mrs. J. wets the bed in the presence of a nurse, she is chastised for not calling for help. The nurse warns that the patient may end up with a Foley catheter if she cannot call for help with the bedpan.

A final example is the complaining patient. Ms. S. believes that a good hot meal once a day is essential to maintain good nutrition. In the nursing home, there are two staff members to serve and feed 30 patients. Ms. S. frequently receives a cold dinner. Each time this happens, she asks to have her tray warmed. The staff now refer to Ms. S. as the crotchety lady in Room 15. Once again, the "victim" who receives the cold meal is blamed as the problem, despite the fact that the patient has no control over the problem.

Labeling

Labeling is an important concept in understanding the causes and impact of ageism. This concept draws upon a symbolic interactionist principle, i.e., individuals use symbols that have shared meanings. The meanings of symbols are influenced by culture and may change over time. It is possible for individuals to have widely disparate perceptions of the same symbol, therefore, and one individual's meaning may be forced on another. In the example of incontinence cited previously, the wet bed that, in the patient's eyes, was "one episode of involuntary urinary leakage in a high-stress situation" became "incontinence" in the eyes of her caregivers. The two labels have different implications for care.

Another example of the impact of negative labeling in the elderly is demonstrated in the following familiar joke:

An 81-year-old woman visits her doctor because she has pain in her left knee. After briefly examining her, the doctor pats the patient on the head and says, "Now Mildred, you're 81 years old—what else can you expect at your age?" To which the patient replies, "Doctor, my right knee is as old as my left knee, and it does not hurt."

What the patient understands far better than the physician is that aging is not an illness. Therefore, it is inaccurate and harmful to attribute symptoms of disease to normal development or aging. Attributing symptoms to untreatable causes without thorough examination would not be accepted by people in their 20s or 30s, yet for a long time this type of response has been accepted by old people or accepted on their behalf.

One phenomenon closely related to labeling is the infantilization of older adults in professional and personal interactions (Learman et al., 1990). An example of this is referring to elders with undue familiarity using "pet" names such as "sweetie" or "dearie." The message given to older people is that they are children and expected to be docile, unquestioning, and compliant.

Some old people may live in a state of triple jeopardy, in which negative labels associated with race, sex, and age may have been internalized. It is important for professionals to recognize the degree to which they practice such labeling, thus contributing to further stereotyping and adverse outcomes for those in the labeled or scapegoated group.

Cultural Factors

MODERNIZATION AND CHANGING VALUES. The rapid technological and social changes of the 20th century have had a significant impact on how Americans view and value older adults. In traditional societies and in earlier periods of American history, older people were valued, respected, and obeyed for skills and wisdom acquired and refined over a lifetime. Older people were important members of extended families, assisting with farming, child rearing, housekeeping, and the transmission of family history and values.

In modern societies, however, people are valued for their technical knowledge, efficiency, productivity, and movement on "the fast track." Older people frequently live apart from their children and grandchildren, who may know their elders only impressionistically. The diminished importance of older adults' work and family roles has encouraged people to label the skills and knowledge of the old as obsolete and to see older people as less productive and therefore less valuable members of our society. The ensuing generational tensions have provided a fertile environment for the birth and growth of ageist stereotypes and of public policies that create or reinforce social inequalities.

STEREOTYPE-BASED POLICY DEVELOPMENT. To some extent, our public policy has institutionalized ageism by making chronological age a criterion for eligibility for a wide range of public benefits. Binstock (1983) suggested that "compassionate stereotypes" of older people deeply influenced the establishment and continuation of many social programs in operation today. In the 1930s, when Social Security was introduced, the aged were perceived as (1) poor, frail, and in need of collective assistance and positive image-building; (2) an impotent political force, in need of assistance developing "senior power"; and (3) "the deserving poor" forced out of work by mandatory retirement, the frailties and disabilities of old age, and the prejudices of a youth-oriented society. Palmore (1990) has stated that the social programs and other privileges granted to older people are also examples of positive ageism.

In today's harsh economic climate, citizens no longer take for granted the entitlement of elders to be beneficiaries of public funds. With improvements in health and longevity and the political strength of older people, compassionate stereotypes have been replaced by stereotypes of affluent, leisure-oriented, manipulative freeloaders ("greedy geezers") or of people who may be needy but are perhaps unworthy of aid because they did not take enough initiative to plan years ago for all possible contingencies of old age. These new ageist stereotypes, widely cited by opinion leaders and interest groups, have created a backlash of public opinion against the elderly that makes it difficult to protect the interests of the truly needy segments of the older adult population. With intense competition for limited resources, our earlier social contract to protect "the tired, the poor" has been challenged by a new ideology that places the locus of control and responsibility back in the hands of each individual, even those who can now do little to help themselves.

Consequences of Ageism

All types of ageism have negative consequences for older persons, and its effects are felt at the individual, family, small group, and community levels. The social breakdown theory (Kuypers and Bengtson, 1973) provides a framework for understanding how ageism affects older persons.

Social Breakdown Syndrome

Kuypers and Bengtson (1973) build on Zusman's work (1966) with the mentally ill and suggest that psychosocial pathology may occur in a downward spiral. The key events contributing to that spiral include an initial *vulnerability* to dysfunction, which leads to *dependency*, which results in *negative labeling*, followed by *helplessness*, leading to *atrophy* of social and interpersonal skills, resulting in a *negative self-image*. This cascade of events leads to further vulnerability to psychosocial stressors, and the cycle begins anew.

Evidence of social breakdown syndrome may be seen in different settings, such as in the workplace and in long-term care. For example, negative comments from younger workers about higher paid older workers who are "dead wood" or not "pulling their weight" may lead older workers to think of themselves in negative terms. Thus, they may become more vulnerable to poor performance on the job.

In a nursing home setting, frail elders may be temporarily dependent on staff and friends to assist with basic functions while they are in rehabilitation. They may be negatively labeled as helpless old people who cannot do anything for themselves. After a while, the older person, rather than becoming more independent, may begin to feel helpless and lose any self-care abilities that remain.

Interestingly, some research that has been conducted on the social breakdown syndrome or other psychological effects of stereotyping has raised doubts about the extent to which the syndrome actually has an impact on elders' self-concept or self-esteem. There is some evidence that many older people (as do members of minority groups) adopt a defensive perspective about their own group known as "pluralistic ignorance." They believe the stereotypes to be true of other people but see themselves as exceptions to the rule (O'Gorman, 1980; George, 1991; Ferraro, 1992). Some even use the negative stereotypes to gain a sense of relative advantage and well-being (Kearl, 1981–82; Bearon, 1989). The presence of effective defense mechanisms among some elderly individuals does not excuse the injustice of stereotyping or the toxic environment created by aging, however.

Age Differentiation and Age Integration

Ageism promotes "age differentiation," a phenomenon that is based on the mistaken belief in a universal and inevitable decline with aging. Age-differentiated structures divide societal roles into three parts: (1) educational roles for the young, (2) work roles for the middle-aged, and (3) leisure roles for the old (Henrichs et al., 1991). These differentiated roles are held fast today, even though people are living longer and in better health. Older people spend nearly one third of their life in retirement, even though they are comparatively "robust" and capable of making contributions to society (Riley and Riley, 1994).

According to Riley and Riley (1994), our society should remove the barriers of age-differentiated structures and move toward age-integrated structures (Fig. 16–1). Age-integrated structures would provide role opportunities in all structures (education, work, and leisure) to people of every age. Therefore, individuals of all ages would be brought together or "integrated." The change in societal roles would benefit the young and old alike because opportunities for leisure would be available to the young and opportunities for education and work would be available to the old. In addition, these structures would broaden the economic base for support of people at any age who are frail and needy.

An age-integrated society would address the needs of a widely heterogeneous older population. Some may choose to teach or go to school; others may choose to combine leisure time with part-time work or volunteerism. The key is to allow older people to participate in roles in which they are not disregarded, denigrated, or dependent (Riley and Riley, 1994).

Implications for Nursing Care of the Aged

Informed nurses should be aware of the generalized nature of ageism in American

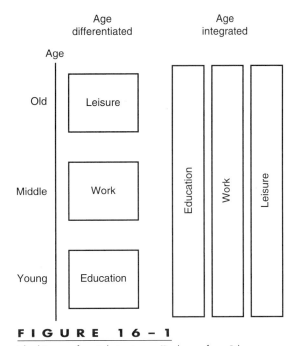

FIGURE 16–1

Ideal types of social structures. (Redrawn from Riley, M.W. and Riley, J.W., Jr. Age integration and the lives of older people. *Gerontologist* 34:111, 1994. Copyright © The Gerontological Society of America.)

society and alert to the likelihood that fellow health care providers often subscribe to ageist stereotypes. Negative stereotypes can profoundly influence an older person's behavior as well as the opportunities available to that older person for rehabilitation, treatment, and self-actualization. An example helps to illustrate the influence of ageism on health outcomes.

An 86-year-old man was admitted to the hospital after an acute embolic left-sided cerebrovascular accident (CVA). His condition stabilized and he was referred to rehabilitation for evaluation and possible transfer. He was refused because his fluctuating mental status would not allow cooperation with the rehabilitation program. He was referred for nursing home placement.

Further assessment revealed that this patient had lived alone and was functionally independent before this hospitalization. Three days before the CVA, he had hosted a Halloween party for the neighborhood children. Physical examination showed mild right-sided weakness and dysphagia, but the patient was able to feed himself if cued. Despite these findings, the nursing staff was performing all activities of daily living for the patient. When the high prevalence of depression accompanying stroke was pointed out to the ward team, the patient received care from a different perspective. The patient was ultimately accepted into a rehabilitation program in another hospital.

Initially, the attitudes and approaches of the ward team were guided almost entirely by one piece of data: the patient's chronological age. This resulted in a custodial approach to care. When additional data regarding the patient's functional status were considered in care planning, the care was more aggressive and the goals more rehabilitative. Failure to recognize the ageism in the first approach would have sentenced this patient to premature institutionalization and dependency.

Thus, through awareness of the pervasiveness of ageism and astute clinical assessment, nurses can help their elderly clients combat the opportunity-narrowing effects of ageism.

POVERTY

Although the economic status of older Americans is far more varied than that of any other age group, the elderly are more likely than other adults to be poor. One fourth of the older population have incomes and other economic resources below or just barely above the poverty level. In addition, people who are age 85 and older (oldest-old) have significantly lower incomes than those who are age 65 to 74 (young-old) or age 75 to 84 (old-old) (U.S. Department of Health and Human Services, 1991).

Health care providers need to be aware of the extent of poverty in their clientele, for it significantly affects the availability of care options and the prognosis for restoration and maintenance of health. In addition, members of the older population who are poor tend to have higher mortality rates than those who have adequate incomes (Najman, 1993).

Definition and Scope of the Problem

Poverty is officially defined in the United States as an annual income of $6532 or less (1991 dollars) for a single person older than 65 or $8241 (1991 dollars) or less for a two-person household headed by someone older than 65 (American Association of Retired Persons [AARP], 1993). The poverty threshold is adjusted each year to reflect changes in the Consumer Price Index (Clark et al., 1988). Many impoverished persons are excluded from this definition because income is only one determinant of financial adequacy to meet basic needs. The other determinant is the cost of daily living, which fluctuates according to locality; ability to obtain certain types of goods and services

without money; and special needs, such as adaptive equipment, drugs, or therapeutic diets. National survey data that describe the poor are limited to those who meet the official income criteria, thus excluding from analysis those who are "near-poor" and those who have inadequate income to meet their expenses.

In 1991, 12.4 per cent of persons aged 65 and older, 3.8 million people, had incomes below the poverty line. The near-poor, with incomes between poverty level and 125 per cent of this level, constitute another 7 per cent or 2.3 million elderly persons (AARP, 1993). The aged poor are disproportionately represented among older women, the oldest-old, African-Americans, Hispanics, those living alone, and those living in rural areas (McLaughlin and Jensen, 1993).

MINORITY GROUP MEMBERSHIP. Non-whites are overrepresented among the elderly poor; 10 per cent of elderly whites are poor, 34 per cent of elderly African-Americans live in poverty, and 21 per cent of Hispanic older persons live below the poverty level (AARP, 1993).

LIVING ARRANGEMENTS. The income of individuals living alone tends to be lower than that of those living with family (either spouse or extended family members). Of those living with family, only 9.7 per cent were below the poverty level, compared with nearly 30 per cent of those living alone or with unrelated individuals (Jackson, 1980).

RURAL AND URBAN DIFFERENCES. Older adults in nonmetropolitan areas are more likely to be poor than are older city dwellers. In 1990, 16.1 per cent of nonmetropolitan elders were poor, compared with 10.8 per cent of metropolitan residents. Nonmetropolitan elders are also more likely than urban adults to be near-poor (Glasgow, 1993). Whereas some have suggested that these differences in poverty rates reflect the fact that rural elders are older and less educated, a study has found these differences even after controlling for age, sex, race, education, disability status, marital status, and living arrangements (McLaughlin and Jensen, 1993). One study pinpointed characteristics of the rural community that put older residents at a disadvantage: "small size, dispersed population, geographic isolation, limited public sector capacity, and economic concentration in a relatively small number of industrial sectors. These rural-community attributes constrain lifelong opportunities for individual economic accumulation; limit effective public sector responses to the elderly's social and economic needs; and in certain instances, reduce elders' access to informal helper networks that can provide social, economic and psychological support" (Glasgow, 1993, pp. 309–310).

Economics of Old Age

Households headed by people older than 65 have lower per person consumer expenditures than households headed by people 35 to 64 years. Older people consume less than younger people do because they have less income to spend, fewer people in the household to support, and needs different from those of younger people. Households headed by a person age 65 and older spent $18,967, and those headed by a person age 75 and older spent $15,919, compared with $30,191 spent by households headed by younger persons. Elderly people spend more on utilities, health care, and cash contributions than younger people do. Older and younger households spend about the same proportion on food and housing.

Health care costs are the greatest threat to economic security among the elderly. High out-of-pocket expenses consume a large share of the reduced budget of the average older household. Because the total budget of older people is smaller, the share they spend on health care is substantially higher than the share spent by younger people. In addition, older households spent more than twice as much as younger counterparts did on health insurance and more than twice as much on prescription drugs and medical supplies (U.S. Department of Health and Human Services, 1991).

Generally, employment ceases, and income from salary is lost. Pensions usually provide less income than the wages earned when the person was working, and increases in income are less for retirees than for employed persons. Those who have not planned for adequate retirement income use savings or investment monies to help pay for day-to-day needs so that the income from investments gradually declines over time. If pension and investment income does not keep pace with expenses, then the older person must either find a job or depend on government or private assistance to make up the difference. In a society that considers work a role for people younger than 65, employment is seldom a realistic option, explaining why older people are disproportionately represented among the poor. Because of discrimination and health-related barriers to employment, finding work is often an unrealistic option.

Contributors to Poverty in the Elderly

Two groups of poor elderly persons can be distinguished: (1) those who have lived in poverty all their lives and (2) those who have become impoverished in late life. Individuals who have lived in poverty all their lives are unlikely to improve their economic status with advanced age. As Social Security recipients, they may be hurt less severely by inflation than younger adults are, because Social Security benefits are currently indexed to the cost of living. However, old people are less likely to own their homes and therefore are vulnerable to the effects of rising housing costs. These individuals may have better developed skills for coping with the problems of poverty than those who are newly impoverished. They are less likely to experience the loss associated with lifestyle change seen in those who experience poverty for the first time in late life. With this exception, however, the problems that all poor elderly experience are essentially similar.

Impoverishment in old age may result through a number of mechanisms, operating singly or in combination. These include inadequate retirement income, extended illness and the added burden of high medical bills, discrimination against women in pension benefits, and financial exploitation and victimization.

Inadequate Retirement Income

The trend in the 20th century in the United States has been toward decreased work force participation by the elderly and, thus, diminished income. Older persons who relied on savings from earlier working years as retirement income often found that inflationary factors in the cost of living severely diminished buying power. People who expected to be able to live comfortably on their Social Security income or a small pension may find this income inadequate to maintain their current lifestyle. Indeed, for most, Social Security income is barely enough to keep an individual or couple above the poverty line.

High Cost of Medical Care

A significant source of impoverishment for older Americans is the high cost of medical care. Individuals older than 65 (12 percent of the population) account for more than one third of the country's total personal health care expenditures. In the 10-year period between 1977 and 1987, the average annual growth rate of per capita spending for health care for the elderly was 14 per cent. Per capita spending reached $5360, one third of which was paid by the older individuals through direct payments to providers or insurance premiums. Spending on prescription drugs continues to constitute a substantial out-of-pocket cost for older adults. Thus, medical costs figure significantly in the budget of older persons (U.S. Department of Health and Human Services, 1991).

The scenario of late-life impoverishment due to high medical care costs runs something like this:

An elderly husband and wife live alone in a small bungalow that they own in a declining neighborhood in a small urban center. He is retired, and they live on his Social Security check and a small pension. She has four chronic illnesses and requires quarterly physician visits and takes four medicines each day. Her monthly drug bill is around $150. His health status is similar.

One day after breakfast he slumps over at the table, no longer able to speak or move his right side. He is taken to the hospital, where a diagnosis of acute embolic CVA with dense right hemiplegia and aphasia is made. After a 12-day stay, he is referred to a nursing home for convalescent care. Medicare pays for his stay for the first two weeks, after which time it is decided that he is no longer making progress in rehabilitation and will not be able to return home. The family must pay $3000 to $4000 per month for the nursing home until all their resources are consumed. The wife is allowed to keep the home but may have no more than $12,000 in liquid assets. After this time, she must pay all of his Social Security check ($461) to the nursing home, and Medicaid pays the remainder of the bill. She is left with $230 per month (her dependent's benefit from his Social Security work credits). The adjustment in lifestyle from a household income of $661 per month to one of $230 per month will be tremendous.

This example is not unusual. With more than 1 million older persons in nursing homes and approximately 70 per cent of nursing home care paid for by Medicaid, this scenario is all too common. The causes of disability may vary, but the net effect on older individuals is the same—impoverishment, loss of control, and diminished potential to maintain health because of insufficient resources to meet basic daily needs.

Women's Pensions

Although most women are employed today, the majority of the women older than 65 did not have an extended time in the work force. Therefore, most older women receive survivor's benefits from either Social Security or other pension plans rather than benefits based on their own work record. The amount of survivor's benefits is generally lower than a worker's pension.

Women who have earned pension benefits also receive a lower amount than men who have worked the same amount of time. The median income for nonmarried women age 65 and older is approximately $2000 less annually than for nonmarried men (Schick and Schick, 1994). The fact that women have been in the work force for shorter times, receive lower pay, and are in lower paying occupations accounts for the discrepancy in income in older age. This discrepancy may gradually diminish as the gains of the women's movement for equal opportunity in the work force are realized.

Financial Exploitation and Criminal Victimization

Although it is rare, some older people face financial hardship in later life because of financial exploitation by other people. Some forms of exploitation, such as selling unnecessary insurance policies or television church solicitations, may not be criminal but may result in diminished income and could be regarded as victimization. The impact of victimization on an older person may be greater than on a younger person because of decreased earning capacity to compensate for the loss. However, criminal victimization may be underreported among the elderly because of several factors, including dependency, physical and mental disability, and failure to recognize that a crime has been committed (Schick and Schick, 1994).

Consequences of Poverty in Late Life

Diminished Well-Being

In many ways, the impact of poverty on the well-being of the elderly is no different from that for younger persons. Basic human needs for food, clothing, shelter, and medical attention may go unmet. Poor people have diminished social status, reduced social opportunity (many social activities require money for participation, e.g., travel, entrance fees, dues), fewer choices among products or providers of services, and diminished control over their lives. Trying to make ends meet is a continual challenge, and the anxiety of not being able to handle new problems effectively because of diminished financial resources is ever present.

In American society, poor people must interact regularly with large bureaucracies if they are to take advantage of governmental benefits designed to help them. This results in command appearances before agency examiners or interviewers on a regular, periodic basis, often waiting in line for long periods. Dealing with such bureaucracies typically requires the ability to read and write and to interpret bureaucratic instructions. Failure to follow bureaucratic directives results in reduction or termination of benefits. Poor people are also subject to rules within bureaucracies, which can change on little notice and are sometimes more responsive to political cycles than individual needs. There is also the problem of diminished self-esteem that often accompanies dependence on a large bureaucracy.

Some find receiving help from governmental bureaucracy too difficult or unpleasant and seek assistance from friends, family, or church. Although these groups are important in support of the poor, the financial resources of these groups are far more limited than governmental resources. The result sometimes is that elderly persons simply do without income or services to which they are entitled, because the process of obtaining help is too difficult or because they are too proud to accept help that is grudgingly offered.

The impact of poverty on elderly persons in the absence of a responsive and effective bureaucracy is highly individualized and dependent on the extent of informal resources and coping skills available. For those who live in rental housing, the impact of poverty may be eviction or living in a substandard dwelling. Older persons who have a diminished ability to adapt to temperature changes may find their health adversely affected by such living conditions. Other older persons may feel the impact of poverty at the dinner table. For those who do not raise their own produce, poverty may mean an inability to obtain adequate nutrients for body requirements. Still others may experience the effects of poverty as the inability to control chronic cardiopulmonary disease because they cannot afford a month's supply of medicine or the surcharge for in-home oxygen.

Impact on Health Care

Poverty has a significant impact on the health care of older people. Those living in poverty have higher rates of mortality, poorer health, and lower health-related quality of life than those in higher socioeconomic classes (Najman, 1993; Thorslund and Lundberg, 1994; Grembowski et al., 1993). In addition, older adults who are poor are less likely to participate in health screening (Mandelblatt et al., 1993) and more likely to use the emergency room as a pathway to admission to the hospital (Stern et al., 1991).

Although Medicaid has helped to relieve the health care burdens of the poor and the elderly, it continues to fall short of its charge to provide the poor and indigent with access to quality health care (Staebler, 1991). Medicare has also fallen short of providing medical costs for the elderly. Although Medicare has historically covered acute medical care costs, the coverage for primary care and chronic disease care is extremely limited. For example, Medicare does not pay for medicines taken on an outpatient basis. Yet it is not uncommon for older clients to be taking several medications simultaneously, with monthly bills of more than $100.

The high prevalence of poverty among the elderly makes economic data an important part of any comprehensive health assessment. Without this information, clinicians make incorrect assumptions about the resources available for treatment follow-through. Patients may be incorrectly labeled noncompliant when the correct diagnosis is poverty.

For example, a 68-year-old woman with chronic obstructive pulmonary disease was a monthly visitor to the emergency room of the community hospital. Careful assessment of this patient's social situation revealed inadequate finances to meet her most basic needs. To stretch her income to the end of the month, she would take her medicines less often than prescribed "to make them last," with the result that her pulmonary status became compromised. Noncompliant? No. Yet how easy it is to ascribe this patient's problems to noncompliance.

Willingness to discuss financial issues is vital if the older person is to make informed choices regarding health care expenditures. Acknowledging that poverty is a potential outcome of chronic illness for all but the most wealthy people may help open a frank discussion of financial issues in maintaining health.

Consider the woman with multiple chronic diseases who required minimal assistance with meal preparation and bathing. Without counseling regarding the costs and benefits of hiring a homemaker on a daily basis versus nursing home care, this person would have gone to a nursing home because her friend considered the homemaker an extravagance. Compared with the cost of nursing home care, which the patient did not want, the finances available allowed the patient to stay at home until those resources were exhausted. Lack of this type of counseling would have resulted in premature nursing home admission.

Awareness that financial issues affect chronic disease management for most clients increases the probability that realistic management plans will be developed and carried through. Knowledge of the resources for poor people in the community, along with how referrals are made, may enhance the older person's support network and thus improve health and opportunity for follow-through with plans for disease management and health promotion.

Attempts to Resolve Poverty in Late Life

Supplemental Security Income

Since 1972, elderly persons with the lowest incomes have been eligible for a monthly check from Social Security under the Supplemental Security Income (SSI) program. This program for people 65 years and older (as well as blind and disabled persons) was designed to supplement the income of those who do not qualify for standard Social Security benefits or whose Social Security benefits are not adequate for subsistence (U.S. Senate, 1993). Eligibility is determined by a means test based on income and assets of the individual. In 1992, 1.5 million adults age 65 and older received SSI payments averaging $229 per month (Schick and Schick, 1994).

Although SSI has resulted in a guaranteed source of income for many older persons, some have criticized the program because the benefit levels still leave many older people as much as 25 per cent below the poverty level (U.S. Senate, 1993). Also, several independent studies have shown that only about half of all older persons eligible for SSI actually receive program benefits (U.S. Senate, 1993). Many people surveyed had never heard of the program, did not know how to apply for assistance, thought the benefits were lower than they are, encountered language barriers, felt it was associated with the stigma of being on welfare, or thought it would result in a loss of privacy.

Although SSI is tied into the Medicaid program, few respondents realized that being under SSI would entitle them to gain health care benefits under Medicaid. Because of the high degree of unfamiliarity with or confusion about the SSI program, nurses may encounter older persons who are eligible for this type of assistance but not receiving it.

Older Americans Act Programs

The Older Americans Act (OAA) was first enacted in 1965. The mission of the OAA is "to foster maximum independence by providing a wide array of social and community services to those older persons in greatest economic and social need. The key philosophy of the program has been to help maintain and support older persons in their homes and communities to avoid unnecessary and costly institutionalization" (U.S. Senate, 1993, p. 313). Designed to address a number of the problems of older persons without regard to income, its programs have nonetheless addressed some of the problems of poor older persons. Three specific programs are worthy of note: nutrition programs, senior employment programs, and transportation programs.

Nutrition programs offered under the auspices of the OAA include both home-delivered meals and congregate meal programs. Both provide one third of the minimum daily requirements for anyone aged 60 and older regardless of income. This partially helps to address the problem of inadequate nutrition related to poverty, without the embarrassment or ordeal of a means test or eligibility determination. These programs have been helpful in averting institutionalization by providing meals to the homebound who are unable or unwilling to prepare meals for themselves and a source of socialization as well as nutrition for those who are able to get out of the house.

Senior employment services under OAA are designed to help develop employment opportunities for those aged 55 and older who wish to work. These services include job training, job placement, and demonstration of the effectiveness of older workers. Workers are placed in part-time minimum wage positions in community service organizations. The program targets people with incomes no higher than 125 per cent of the poverty level. This type of service attacks the problem of poverty among those who are capable of employment.

Transportation programs are also aimed at resolving one of the problems associated with poverty. Although older adults who are not impoverished cite transportation as a major problem, it is clear that without adequate income to purchase or maintain a car or to pay cab or bus fare, transportation is a serious problem. OAA funds have been used in diverse ways to address this problem, from funding "dial-a-ride"–type services using volunteers to providing bus or van transportation for grocery shopping or medical appointments.

OAA funds have also been applied to the development of senior centers, which, in many communities, serve as an important source for information about available services as well as a place where diverse services may be obtained. OAA monies have additionally been applied to the development of health-related services such as adult day care and in-home health care.

Title XX of the Social Security Act

Title XX of the Social Security Act is a "block grant" to the states that provides funding for a wide array of social services to people of low income. Although this money is not specifically targeted for the elderly, services such as homemakers for disabled older people, home-delivered meals, and adult day care are provided through this funding in some communities. Decisions about allocation of these scarce dollars are made at the local level, so the services available to older persons vary from community to community. The eligibility guidelines for recipients of these services are much less stringent than those for Medicaid. The problem most communities face is a greater need among potential recipients than can be met through available funding. This results in long waiting lists for services in many communities.

Medicaid

Medicaid is a program that funds medical care for poor older persons, disabled people, and families with dependent children. The program deserves special mention because of the major role it plays in the financing of nursing home care. Medicaid is a federal program that is administered at the state level. Its financing is a combination of federal, state, and local funds. For this reason, there is considerable variability from state to state as to the type of services provided under Medicaid. Criteria and procedures for eligibility also vary by state.

Medicaid is designed so that those who cannot afford to pay for medical care will not be denied this care regardless of their living arrangement. Owing to the complexities of eligibility and coverage, the reality is that the majority of elderly Medicaid recipients are in nursing homes, although Medicaid will pay for some non–institution-based services. Three fourths of nursing home care is paid for by Medicaid.

Eligibility for Medicaid benefits requires the older person to exhaust nearly all savings and income on medical expenses. Stiff penalties exist for those who try to defraud the system by giving away property or other assets in an attempt to become eligible for Medicaid. Determination of eligibility is a long and somewhat arduous process, generally carried out through a local department of social services. The process involves extensive financial disclosure and repeated recertification. For those without other means to pay for medical care, it is an important resource. Some older persons are reluctant to apply for Medicaid for various reasons including pride or refusal to accept charity, fear of losing their home, assumption that they would not qualify for welfare, and inability to withstand or understand complex bureaucratic processes. It takes considerable sensitivity to help elderly clients and their families understand the benefits to which they may be entitled. Assistance may be needed in going through the necessary bureaucratic processes to obtain such benefits.

Senior Citizen Discount Programs

One example of a public-private sector joint initiative in reducing the economic burden on older people is the existence of senior citizen discount programs for goods and services including hot meals, retail merchandise, hotels, and transportation.

Prevention of Late-Life Poverty

Although the prospects for preventing poverty in old age for those who have always been poor are not good, there does seem to be some potential for preventing late-life impoverishment. Although no easy solutions exist, it is clear that those who plan carefully for their retirement years will probably fare better than those who do not. Taking economic needs in retirement seriously is an important factor in having adequate income in retirement. Recent laws encouraging investment in private pension plans may reduce dependence on the federal government for income in retirement.

HOUSING PROBLEMS

Definition and Scope of the Problem

For most older adults, finding and maintaining adequate and affordable housing presents few problems. Many continue to live in accommodations purchased or rented over decades. Others use their retirement nest egg to find scaled-down housing, to purchase a living arrangement in a continuing care retirement community, or to migrate to more favorable climates and geographical settings.

For a sizable minority, however, living arrangements made earlier in life become unsatisfactory in later life. As people live longer and experience longer periods of frailty, many older persons find it difficult to "age in place." In some cases, older adults watch their homes and neighborhoods deteriorate over time and become unsafe living environments. In other cases, elders are no longer able to live alone without an array of supportive, in-home services. Attempts to move to upgraded dwellings or congregate/assisted living facilities may be impractical because of high costs or limited availability of affordable housing.

The psychosocial and health implications of inadequate housing (and of relocation in some cases) are potentially significant, especially for the poor, the frail, the isolated, and the cognitively impaired. According to one analyst (Pynoos, 1985, p. 26):

Housing is intimately tied to the quality of life for all age groups because it consumes a large proportion of income and its location affects status and available services. But housing has a special relevance for older persons because they frequently spend a great deal of time in it and are highly reliant on their immediate neighborhood for services and support.

Redfoot and Gaberlavage (1991, p. 35) addressed a similar theme: "Housing . . . provides a secure and meaningful old age or magnifies the disability and isolation that too often accompany advanced years."

Although the specific problems of housing inadequacy differ for homeowners and renters, for urban and suburban or rural residents, and for people with varying impairments, the primary housing-related problem for older adults is inadequacy of housing for an individual's needs. Kendig (1990) reported that in 1983, 1 million households headed by older persons lived in physically deficient housing. Although the majority of older persons own their own homes (75 per cent), more than 80 per cent of those mort-gage free (U.S. Senate, 1993), one study showed that 26 per cent of homeowners with a mortgage and 17 per cent of homeowners with no mortgage experienced excessive housing cost burden (mortgage, utility costs, real estate taxes, and insurance) (U.S. Bureau of the Census and U.S. Department of Housing and Urban Development, 1989). Taking homeowners and renters together, approximately 4 million elderly households spend more than 35 per cent of their incomes on housing (U.S. Senate, 1993). An uncounted number of elderly people live in neighborhoods that are inadequate or unsafe.

Historically, the federal government has played a major role in subsidizing housing, through construction of rental units, rent subsidies for low-income people, or substantial tax deductions for those holding home mortgages. Observers contend that the demographics and epidemiology of aging will require changes in future public housing policies for the aged. Because shelter is a basic human need, housing problems may significantly affect the older individual's health status.

Theoretical Issues

Person-Environment Interaction

Adequacy of housing can be evaluated by many criteria. At one extreme, there are localities where there is *no* housing code. This means that in the eyes of public officials, there is no such officially recognized entity as inadequate housing. At the other end of the spectrum is the notion of person-environment fit. Persons who consider housing adequacy from this perspective operate on the belief that environmental considerations greatly influence functional ability. It is therefore possible to have environmental conditions that detract from a person's ability to function independently as well as environments that compensate for an individual's deficits. The concept of environmental press (Lawton and Nahemow, 1973) suggests that it is insufficient to evaluate adequacy of housing without simultaneously considering the individual who will live in that environment. Although such an individualized view of housing adequacy complicates the mass development of housing for older persons, it does provide a useful framework for those seeking criteria by which to evaluate the older person's life situation, with an eye toward maximizing function and health.

Studies have found that the majority of

older Americans are satisfied with their housing even if it is substandard (Rabushka and Jacobs, 1980). Analysts suggest that favorable self-reports of housing hardship or inadequacy could be misleading because many older people have low expectations (Lawton, 1985) or have other, higher priorities for spending or saving hypothetical income increases (Stoller and Stoller, 1987). A study by Carp (1976) found that the high satisfaction people express with their housing may reflect their perceptions of available housing options. When applicants were actually offered new apartments, they re-evaluated their current housing unfavorably, whereas those who were not offered the option to move had stable evaluations of current housing.

Neighborhood

Housing considerations are inevitably tied to the concept of neighborhood. Neighborhood social contacts often serve as environmental supports that influence the older person's ability to live in the community (Lawton, 1979; Carp, 1979; Cantor, 1979; Cullinane, 1992). Clinicians should bear in mind the importance of such supports when evaluating the suitability of a neighborhood for an older individual. Popularly held notions regarding criminal victimization of older people are significantly overstated (U.S. Bureau of the Census, 1991), and therefore older persons should not be encouraged to move merely because they live in a deteriorating neighborhood.

Meaning of Home

A final theoretical issue of some importance in considering housing and the elderly is the psychological meaning of home. According to Fogel (1992, p. 15), "Economic studies of housing wealth in the elderly suggest that homes are not treated as mere economic assets but as objects of emotional attachments." He asserts that renters also experience similar psychological attachments. He added, "Some people feel attached to their homes much as they would feel attached to a significant person—their love transcends any rational calculation of benefit. They can enumerate reasons why a move would be wise, but then conclude that the only way they would leave their home would be in a box" (p. 16).

In a review of the literature on the meaning of home, Fogel (1992) enumerated six benefits of home: (1) independence, privacy, and control over the physical environment; (2) familiarity; (3) neighborhood and social network; (4) meaningfulness of home maintenance activities; (5) a place to entertain and pursue activities; and (6) a source of memories of past events.

These observations help to explain the complexity of housing decisions for the elderly. They also provide a framework for analysis of conditions that promote a comfortable change in housing arrangements for the elderly. Howell (1985) summarizes five situations in which elderly persons make changes in housing arrangements voluntarily: (1) retirement to a resort community, (2) a move to be closer to children or grandchildren, (3) a return to the community of their childhood or early adulthood, (4) a move to a planned retirement community, and (5) a move from a suburban to an urban locale to be closer to cultural activities and social services. She notes that all of these situations involve planned rather than forced change, whereby the older people have the opportunity to invest in a new place based on a gradually changing self-identity. The situation for those in forced housing changes is considerably different and more likely to provoke some of the relocation stress phenomena described by Tobin and Lieberman (1976).

Adequacy of Housing

Although the majority of older persons own their homes, adequate housing may still present a problem. Home ownership does not guarantee that the dwelling is suited to any physical infirmities the individual might have, nor does it ensure that the home is in good repair. The money necessary to perform even routine maintenance on older dwellings may not be available on the retiree's or widow's income. An elderly owner may lack the physical ability to perform needed repairs or maintenance, and the community may not have local workers to provide such a service. Redfoot and Gaberlavage (1991) stated that housing quality problems are most frequent among four subgroups of older homeowners: (1) minority elders (particularly the old-old), (2) single-person households, (3) rural elders, and (4) central-city dwellers.

For some older persons, however, apartment living may have distinct advantages over home ownership because residents have the security of nearby neighbors and the availability of maintenance services (Mutschler, 1992). Elderly renters, however, are older than elderly homeowners and more likely to spend a greater proportion of their income on housing. Older African-Americans and Hispanics are much more likely to live in moderately to severely inadequate housing than are whites (Mikelsons and Turner, 1991). Renters may be troubled by indifferent landlords, uncontrolled increases in rent, problems with security, and a declining stock of affordable rental units. Skinner (1992, p. 51) commented on the special problems of the inner-city elderly: "With few options available to them, they are not only aging in place, they are stuck in place, prisoners in their own homes, without the ability to move to appropriate housing."

SANITATION. Proper sanitation has been noted as a problem in some houses where older persons reside. The problem may be a result of physical or mental impairment of the older person, or it may be related to the neighborhood or community. Because some communities do not have minimum housing standards, it is still possible to encounter houses without running water or those with pests.

CRIMINAL VICTIMIZATION. Neighborhoods change with time. Many older persons reside in a house bought many years ago. The neighborhood may have changed considerably during that time. Those in urban areas may be in communities with high crime rates. With limited economic reserves and diminished property values, the older person may be forced to remain in a neighborhood where a serious risk of crime exists simply because of the paucity of affordable housing alternatives.

INCREASED ECONOMIC BURDEN. Home ownership may represent a significant economic burden. Although the security of owning a home is important, characteristics of the home may present difficulties. For example, many older homes may be poorly insulated or otherwise energy inefficient. The net result is that the cost of heating the home is prohibitive. Older houses may be expensive or difficult to maintain because older materials require more upkeep. Vital structures of the home, such as plumbing, heating, or roofing, may need replacement. Finally, paying taxes on a home, for someone with a limited income, may stretch the individual's budget beyond its limits.

SAFETY PROBLEMS. Some housing situations present specific safety problems to older people if they have functional disabilities. For example, the presence of stairs may make a house or apartment unsuitable for an older person with severe cardiopulmonary disease. Bathrooms frequently require modification to be used safely.

Housing arrangements place different amounts and types of demands on individuals, depending on the older person's functional status. A change in functional capacity because of new onset of illness or exacerbation of chronic illness may render a previously satisfactory housing arrangement inadequate. The concept of environmental press is useful in evaluating the suitability of the older person's housing arrangement to his or her needs. Something as simple as the location of the toilet may make the difference between continence and incontinence in an elderly individual. Similarly, kitchen and bedroom placement and access to the outside may become problems in a house owned by an older person but designed for younger individuals.

Consequences of Inadequate Housing

Adequate shelter is something that many Americans take for granted. It is a basic human need, yet some elderly clients make do with substandard housing. Ecological field theorists remind us of the dynamism between the individual's environment and the demands made on the individual. Thus, those in substandard housing are presumably at higher risk for poor outcomes in rehabilitation, have higher demands placed on a functional reserve that is already marginal, and thus perhaps may be at higher risk for institutionalization. For example, inadequate cooling systems in the summer may cause heat-induced illness such as dehydration or hyperthermia. Similarly, in cooler parts of the country, hypothermia is a serious acute medical problem among those older persons with inadequately heated homes.

Further, housing situations may affect discharge plans for hospitalized patients. It is not acceptable to discharge a patient with a new disability such as hemiplegia to a home where the only bathroom is on the second floor, unless sufficient compensation for toilet and bathing facilities can be made. In this way, housing conditions may be a determinant of institution versus community living for disabled older persons.

The economic requirements of maintaining a home may compete with other basic needs, such as food, medicine, and clothing. Inadequate/substandard housing may contribute to health problems, such as falls, incontinence, hypothermia, hyperthermia, social isolation, and poverty, thus affecting the maintenance of health and well-being.

Clinicians working with older persons should have an appreciation for the housing conditions of their clients. Chapter 21 includes a section on impaired home maintenance management, which details assessment of the home environment. This information is needed to plan realistically for the long-term care needs of dependent clients. Such information is also useful in counseling for or assisting with environmental modifications that may reduce the risk of accidental injury. It is also important for clinicians to be aware of the psychological importance of a housing arrangement for older persons. It is not reasonable to assume that simply because one housing environment is unsuited to older persons' needs, they will find it easy to move, even if alternative arrangements are available.

Attempts to Resolve Housing Problems

Attempts to resolve housing dilemmas of older people vary according to the concept of housing adequacy. Indecision about criteria for housing adequacy is evident in the variety of housing programs. Some programs address only the physical attributes of housing. More commonly, there is an attempt to consider service availability in conjunction with housing adequacy. Alternatives include development of new housing and relocation of the elderly, enhancing older housing through home improvements, increasing services available to older persons in their existing homes, and shared housing arrangements.

Initiatives from the public and private sectors have had distinctly different emphases, although the problems addressed are similar. Public initiatives have focused on upgrading existing housing and providing rent subsidies. Public programs have also tended to explicitly consider enhancing social support. Private-sector initiatives have focused on the more affluent older person and development of increased leisure opportunities and medical services. Programs for those of more modest incomes include such strategies as reverse annuity mortgages, which attempt to use the equity in the older person's home to finance needed social and medical services (Belling et al., 1985; Redfoot and Gaberlavage, 1991).

Governmental Initiatives

Attempts by the federal government to address the housing problems of the elderly date back more than 20 years. One reason for particular interest in housing and the elderly is the thought that congregate housing for the elderly, based on European models for service delivery to the elderly, holds promise for preventing or postponing institutionalization for those who need social

support primarily. The concept of congregate housing is that by housing large numbers of older persons in one location, it is cost effective to locate supportive health and social services close by, forestalling institutionalization for more frail individuals. Pynoos (1985) noted that the development of congregate housing projects has lagged far behind other federal initiatives in housing, despite considerable demonstration project experience to support the positive outcomes of such housing.

The government assists the elderly to obtain adequate and appropriate housing in two basic ways: (1) provision of rent subsidies for individuals to use in renting in the private rental market (Section 8 Housing) and (2) development of low-income housing for the elderly and handicapped (Section 202).

In recent years, the government has also assisted elderly homeowners with home repairs to improve housing adequacy. Repair programs may include basic maintenance work, improving energy efficiency through weatherization projects, and modification to improve safety and mobility of the residents.

Box 16–1 details the history of the federal government's involvement in housing for the elderly. During the 1980s, the federal role in housing for older people decreased dramatically. Some states established their own initiatives to fill the gaps, and private developers have shown increased interest in the development of congregate housing. Federal policy has recently taken a positive turn toward meeting the special needs of older adults. The National Affordable Housing Act of 1990 authorized major revisions in federally supported projects to provide services to frail residents. In addition, the Housing and Community Development Act of 1992 helped provide the means for residents who can continue to live in their homes with modest forms of supportive services or with appropriate modifications to their apartment, such as handrails or grab bars.

Retirement Communities

Retirement communities are relatively recent responses to meeting the housing and service needs of older adults. Few such communities existed before 1960. Pastalan (1985) categorized retirement communities as follows:

New towns are self-contained communities for the elderly with a wide range of recreational, social, and medical services. The populations may be large (up to 47,500 in

---

BOX 16-1

History of Governmental Initiatives in Housing for the Elderly

1937: Fair Housing Act: federal government involved in housing as a basic right for all Americans.

1949: Congress adopted a national housing policy calling for a decent home and suitable living environment for every American family.

1950: First National Conference on Aging recommended greater federal emphasis on the housing needs of older persons.

1959: Housing Act creates Section 202, which provides low-cost construction loans to nonprofit groups for building housing for the elderly and handicapped.

1960: Victoria Plaza, San Antonio, Texas; first public housing for the elderly opens.

1962: President Kennedy's message to Congress on housing needs of the elderly and concept of group residences or congregate housing resulted in five experimental projects under the low-rent program of the Public Housing Administration.

1974: Section 8 housing assistance program established to provide subsidized housing to families with low incomes to obtain decent housing in the private market.

1978: Congregate housing services demonstration project passed.

1980: Reagan administration begins to cut back federal role in housing projects by turning emphasis to private-sector initiatives, cutting back on HUD budget, and changing eligibility requirements for receiving housing assistance.

1990: National Affordable Housing Act authorized changes in Section 202 and Section 8 programs to facilitate coordination of housing and services.

1992: Housing and Community Development Act authorized supportive services and modifications to enable people to "age in place."

Sun City, Arizona). They are built for healthy middle- and upper-income couples looking for a leisurely, active lifestyle.

Retirement villages, smaller communities, are not self-contained but designed for a population similar to the new town population. There is considerable variation as to shopping facilities, medical care, and security arrangements.

Retirement subdivisions are designed for the less affluent and are typically located in relatively service-rich communities. There are few, if any, specialized services for residents.

Retirement residences are targeted to older, widowed, or single populations with modest incomes. These are often sponsored by nonprofit groups, such as religious organizations, unions, or benevolent organizations. Services such as laundry, transportation, and dining facilities may be available, although the residences have all the necessary equipment for independent living. Social activities may be organized, but there typically are no health or medical services provided.

Continuing care communities provide both independent living arrangements and health care within one setting and are targeted toward the more affluent older person. Such communities are designed to serve both the well and the frail elderly. The chief attraction of this type of living arrangement is that the older person lives independently with the assurance that supportive or medical care is readily available should it be needed.

There is considerable variability among retirement communities in the types of services offered and the way in which those services are paid for. Pynoos (1985) defined continuing care communities as having, at the very least, (1) independent living and congregate, nursing care units; (2) a contract lasting more than 1 year that guarantees access to various health care services, including nursing care whenever needed; and (3) an arrangement whereby the financial risk for health care is spread over the community and whereby at least some of the fees are prepaid.

Entry fees vary considerably (from $40,000 to $200,000 or more), as do the monthly maintenance fees, which range from $150 to $3000 per month, depending on number of services used. The pioneers in this field have been organizations affiliated with church groups, although many nonsectarian organizations now sponsor retirement communities.

Most people move to retirement communities because they want to regain the sense of "community" lost when they left their families, neighborhoods, and community networks. These organizations can offer residents this feeling of belonging (Forschner, 1992). According to a survey of elders living independently in two retirement communities (MacDowell and Clawson, 1992), the factors that influenced facility selection were mental and physical activities, comfort and security, personal services, conveniences, and independence-promoting features. The appeal of continuing care retirement centers appears to be the security of independent living and the prospect of assistance with declining capabilities (Paul, 1993; Crowley, 1992).

Whereas retirement residences were once thought to be an option only for the well-to-do, such living arrangements are increasingly being thought of as within the financial means of the middle class.

Cooperative housing arrangements are another alternative developed in recent years. Such arrangements are gaining in visibility and popularity. Although implementation of the concept varies from community to community, it is essentially an older person's communal living arrangement whereby the residents of the house pay rent but usually employ a housekeeper and someone to perform maintenance on the property. Residents are generally expected to be capable of independent living; however, some cooperative housing arrangements have been designed specifically with less functional people in mind. In some locales, such arrangements have developed with church or other nonprofit group sponsorship. There is room for considerable creativity. However, there are risks associated with such cooperative arrangements. Specifically, it is important for the older person to clarify to what extent the living arrangement provides housing only versus housing with supportive services.

DEALING WITH DEPENDENCY: PUBLIC POLICY FAILURE

Americans place a high value on independence. Contributions of adults to society are often evaluated in economic terms. Those who are dependent are least likely to make a positive economic contribution. Provisions for care of dependent members of society have historically been based on a welfare mentality tempered by the vision that some poor or disadvantaged persons are more "deserving" than others. Treatment of the handicapped in recent times has ranged from isolation or segregation of the less able to mainstreaming or integration of those with handicaps into society at large. These trends in dealing with handicapped members of society both influence and reflect the ways we regard dependency and handicaps in the elderly.

Definition and Scope of the Problem

Dependency can be defined as requiring assistance with one or more activities of daily living (ADLs) because of mental or physical infirmity. ADLs can be character-ized as basic or instrumental. The basic ADLs include feeding, bathing, dressing, toileting, ambulating, and transferring. Instrumental ADLs (IADLs) include housekeeping, grocery shopping, laundry, meal preparation, telephone use, correspondence, financial management, medication taking, and use of transportation. It is estimated that 5.2 per cent of adults age 65 and older have difficulty with ADLs, and 10.9 per cent have difficulty with IADLs. More men than women (6.6 versus 4.3 per cent) have difficulty with ADLs, but more women than men (13.4 versus 7.4 per cent) have difficulty with IADLs. In older women, impaired function is associated with a combination of many factors, including medical conditions (especially musculoskeletal problems); health habits, such as obesity, smoking, and alcohol abuse; and physical inactivity (Ensrud et al., 1994).

Impairments in both ADLs and IADLs increase in people older than 65 and triple in those 85 years or older (Schick and Schick, 1994). African-Americans experience more functional limitations than either whites or Hispanics do. In noninstitutionalized elderly, the most frequently experienced ADL limitations are bathing and walking (Fig. 16–2), and IADL limitations are the ability to get around in the community and to go shopping (U.S. Department of Health and Human Services, 1991).

Older people who reside in the community function more independently than those who are in institutional care. However, many older adults living in their own homes are unable to function without help and depend on family members for informal care. It has been found that relatives represent 84 per cent of all caregivers for older men and 79 per cent for older women. Daughters provide the greatest amount of care (29 per cent), followed by wives (23 per cent), other women (20 per cent), husbands (13 per cent), sons (8 per cent), and other men (7 per cent). The majority of assistance is with IADLs (shopping, transportation, household tasks) followed by personal care (one or more of feeding, bathing, dressing, toileting). The more limitations people have, the more likely they are to have paid help. People who live alone are at greatest risk for institutionalization, presumably because of the lack of unpaid assistance from family members and friends. The need for formal and informal services is expected to increase as the elderly population increases (U.S. Department of Health and Human Services, 1991).

Despite the widespread prevalence of de-

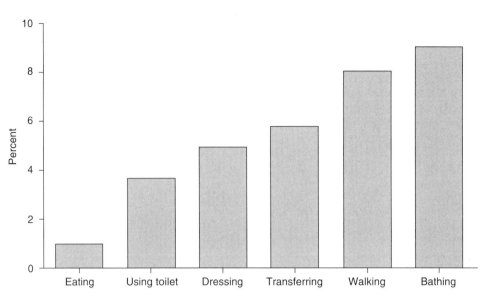

FIGURE 16-2

People age 65+ with limitations in the activities of daily living, by type of limitation: 1987. (Redrawn from United States Department of Health and Human Services. *Aging America: Trends and Projections.* Washington, DC, 1991.)

pendent older adults, there is little consistent national policy for dealing with the problem associated with long-term dependency. Although long-term care recipients generally require assistance from both medical and social service systems, neither takes consistent responsibility for those in need of long-term care. Thus, it is important to consider the interaction of problems in long-term care with problems of dependency.

Theoretical Issues

Historical Perspectives

Policy regarding dependency has been in a state of flux in 20th century America. Before the 20th century, most severely dependent people did not live long. Those who did were cared for in one of two places: at home with their family or in an institution (an orphanage, almshouse, or mental asylum). At that point in history, the economy was primarily agrarian. Children were not required to attend school, and once they reached the age of maturity, they worked in local farms or small factories.

Rehabilitative approaches to those with chronic diseases are fairly recent. The need to deal with casualties from two world wars brought the young specialty of rehabilitation into being. Care of the war heroes (a new kind of dependent adult) heightened the need for new technologies to assist injured persons in living with their disabilities. The development of phenothiazines and other psychotropic drugs in the 1950s meant that large numbers of people who formerly resided in institutions had the potential to live more normal lives in the community. This sparked the development of community care centers for those with chronic mental illness.

The rethinking of national policy and local philosophies regarding the care and treatment of dependent people has been gradual. The most prominent public debate has occurred over care for children with various disabilities. A shift has been made from segregated, institution-based programs to normalization or mainstreaming of children so that they will have the greatest opportunity to participate in society. This approach is considered more humane and more cost effective than earlier segregationist approaches. Provisions for the special needs of handicapped children are made within the structure of public schools and recreational programs.

The concept of normalization next affected the workplace, where barriers to employment of handicapped adults have gradually been removed. Treatment of adults with various types of dependencies has changed dramatically in the past two decades. Achievements range from elimination of legalized discrimination in hiring practices to implementation of barrier-free environments.

The enlightened treatment of elderly persons with dependencies remains a frontier. Increased longevity is a phenomenon that has only recently resulted in rapid growth in the proportion of the population with chronic illnesses hindering ability to function. Approaches to dependent older people remain primarily institution-based and segregated according to disability. Community-based programs with demonstrated efficacy, such as adult day care and respite programs, remain underdeveloped and underfunded. However, community services are expected to increase in the future. During 1990, about 1.5 million impaired older adults used some type of community service at least once. By the year 2020, the number is expected to increase to 2.4 million. Approximately 5.2 million unimpaired older adults used community services in 1990; the number is expected to increase to 8.6 million by the year 2020.

Semantics and Self-Perception

Semantic difficulties abound in discussions of handicap and dependency. This reflects the fear most people have of becoming disabled, disfigured, or dependent. To avoid such difficulties, the definitions of impairment, disability, and handicap, published by the World Health Organization in 1980, are reviewed.

Impairment: any loss or abnormality of psychological, physiological, or anatomical structure or function.

Disability: any restriction or lack of ability to perform an activity in the manner or within the range considered normal for a human being (resulting from an impairment).

Handicap: a disadvantage for a given individual, resulting from an impairment or disability, that limits or prevents the fulfillment of a role that is normal (depending on age, sex, and social and cultural factors) for that individual (World Health Organization, 1980).

The three terms distinguish simple abnormalities of structure or function of body systems from limitation of desired activities and inability to carry out accustomed roles. Impairment does not inevitably lead to disability or handicap. For example, blindness is a visual impairment that is fairly common among the elderly. The impairment may result in an inability to perform self-care activities, such as dressing, walking independently, or cooking. However, if the older person with the visual impairment receives proper counseling, training, and environmental modifications, it is entirely possible that he or she can learn to perform all self-care activities independently within the home environment and even cook safely. This older person now has an impairment, not a disability.

The handicap associated with visual impairment may be loss of work role or of opportunities to carry out certain leisure roles. Again, with proper counseling and environmental supports, the development of a handicap due to visual impairment can be prevented.

Segregation Versus Normalization

One tenth of the world's population has a physical or mental handicap. Under conditions of segregation or institutionalization, handicapped people are unable to participate in society in a meaningful way because they are denied maximal self-expression and development. Concerns about the adverse effects of segregating handicapped persons have led to the principle of "normalization" developed by Wolfensberger (1972). According to this concept, programming for disabled individuals is organized to promote functioning in a manner as similar as possible to that of the society at large. For example, normalization advocates would argue that it is important for residents in nursing homes to administer their own medications (unless this is impossible because of cognitive incapacity), because this is a responsibility held by all "normal" adults in American society.

Institutionalization of disabled individuals is no longer considered by most thoughtful observers to be the optimal societal response to disability. At one time, institutionalization and segregation were the only alternatives to home care for the disabled because no community-based programs to support or treat those with handicaps existed. Now such programs are commonplace for children and younger adults, but the disabilities of older people are not always dealt with in the same manner. Although it has been shown in other populations that institutionalization is a costly means of providing care for those with disabilities, this line of thinking has not yet penetrated policies about care for the elderly.

Cohen (1994) has argued that it is unfair to make the assumption that increased health care costs are determined solely by the growing numbers of older people in our society. It has long been assumed that the increase in the older population will bring an equal rise in the prevalence of disability. However, according to data from the National Long Term Care Surveys, between 1982 and 1989, the number of people who were chronically disabled and institutionalized rose by only 9.2 per cent; this is in contrast to the total population of older people (age 65 and older), which grew by 14.7 per cent (Manton et al., 1993). In addition, disability is not primarily a problem of the elderly because most seriously disabled adults living in the community are younger than 65 (Gornick et al., 1985).

Enthusiasm for community-based long-term care continues to be tempered by the following assumptions: (1) the aging of the general population is likely to raise the costs of long-term care; (2) the quality of long-term care needs to be improved, and measures to improve quality are likely to increase cost; and (3) there are few (if any) accurate estimates of the potential cost savings from more efficient use of existing services or reduced institutionalization.

O'Shea and Blackwell (1993) found that although it may be better for some dependent elders to live at home, it is not necessarily cheaper. The overall cost of care in the community increases with dependency, and if older people living in the community are attending a day hospital or have occasional inpatient stays in acute care hospitals, the cost rises accordingly. The desire for community-based care for the disabled, coupled with increasing activism on the part of older persons regarding health care delivery, suggests that the wave of deinstitutionalization and integration of disabled persons into society at large may eventually extend to programming for disabled older persons. Elderly advocacy groups are promoting long-term care as a problem that affects all age groups, not just older people, to counter arguments about generational equity. They have joined with nonelderly advocacy groups to promote policy for a single program based on new-found political strength. The strategy has thus far been successful in influencing health care reform in the 1990s, which includes a large new home care plan for the severely disabled of all ages and all income groups.

LEAST RESTRICTIVE ENVIRONMENT. Although deinstitutionalization and integration of the disabled into the mainstream of society is humane and cost effective in many cases, a tension remains between providing services in the least restrictive environment and maximizing cost efficiency. It is generally easier for health care professionals to function in an institutional setting. Services and patients are conveniently located, and it is easier to maintain control over patients on the professional's "turf." Such convenience makes a powerful argument regarding cost effectiveness of the institutional setting. More restrictive environments additionally offer a sense of increased safety. That aura of increased security in institutions is not always well founded. An example serves to illustrate.

Ms. J., who has vertebrobasilar insufficiency, falls and fractures her hip. She lives alone. While in the hospital, her physician and niece begin to make plans for her discharge. Both are concerned that she may fall again, and therefore make arrangements for nursing home placement. Ms. J. does not wish to live in the nursing home because she sees little benefit of this plan regarding fall prevention.

In this case, there is little reason to expect that Ms. J. would benefit from institutionalization. If Ms. J. were to fall, she perhaps would be discovered sooner in the nursing home than at home, but there is no evidence to support the theory that a fall would be prevented by nursing home admission. Yet this reason for institutionalization is familiar to many.

It is always possible to cite examples in which it is more costly to support an individual in the community than at home. The example is often given of an individual who is severely impaired and who requires services that could more easily be provided in the more centralized, institutional setting. Such arguments ignore two key points. First, the majority of handicapped persons do not have such extensive disability. Second, such arguments place a dollar value on the quality of human life. Quality of health services, regardless of the source, is notoriously difficult to measure. It is clear, however, that in a community setting, the individual generally has more control over matters than in an institutional setting. Such control does not guarantee high-quality service, but it may reduce vulnerability to undue control from health care providers. The value judgments regarding the amount of control disabled older persons should retain over their lives are for society to make explicitly. In the case of older persons, the debate has not been a public one.

SOCIETAL VERSUS FAMILIAL RESPONSIBILITY. For providing care to dependent elders, gerontologists have increasingly recognized the existing partnership between *informal* support systems, which include the networks of relationships among family members, friends, and neighbors; and *formal* support systems, which include hospitals, nursing homes, senior centers, home health agencies, and long-term care facilities. It has been found that in time of need for help, older people turn first to their spouses; in the absence of a spouse, they turn to their adult children, particularly to their daughters. In addition, family members play an active role in the care and provision of services for their older relatives. Friends and neighbors often play important roles in the provision of instrumental tasks as well. Therefore, effective linkages must be established between the care provided by informal support systems and the care provided by formal organizations and professionals for functionally dependent older people (Dobrof, 1992).

Contributors to Policy Failure in Care for Dependent Elders

Americans find it difficult to confront a physical handicap (Werner-Beland, 1980), dependency, and the inability of adults to contribute to society economically (Strauss, 1984). A policy of segregating those who have little chance for recovery has resulted. Few restrictions are placed on research and treatment dollars for efforts promising cure and full restoration of function, yet each innovation in long-term care is carefully scrutinized for cost effectiveness. A two-tiered system of care results: separate and unequal. In acute care for those with temporary dysfunction, money is no object. In chronic care, however, cost efficiency has long been the excuse for *not* spending money on compensation for disease. Although concerns about the high cost of medical care have been evident since the 1930s, the majority of health care dollars are spent in acute care settings. Tax reform legislation in 1982 brought the first meaningful reforms in financing of modern hospital care. Nonetheless, most Medicare dollars finance acute care rather than outpatient or preventive care. Acute care receives a more favorable reimbursement rate.

The sanctioned response to illness in American society is adoption of the sick role. There is little evidence of support for other models of living with illness, such as the impaired role described by Wu (1973). The sick role does not apply readily to the situation of the elderly, who are most likely to suffer from chronic disease. Benefits for chronic disease care based on the sick role model would quickly bankrupt any health insurance scheme. Medicare's answer has been to pay only for acute exacerbations of chronic illness. Focusing on acute care coverage has severely impeded the development of prevention programs for typical disabilities or chronic illnesses associated with old age.

Another contributor to problems associated with policy formulation for dependency in old age is the hierarchical power arrangement of health care professionals regarding impaired individuals (Rancho Owls, 1984). This relationship, based on an acute care model, emphasizes control of the professionals over the needs and treatment of dependent patients. This style of helping neither prepares the elderly client for self-care or

independence nor creates a comfortable environment for development of self-reliance among those with chronic dependencies. As a result, elderly persons and their families receive mixed messages about the degree to which they should turn to professionals for help and the extent to which they should attempt to manage matters on their own.

Finally, the interests of the medical-industrial complex favor a focus on acute, high-technology care rather than chronic care (Wohl, 1984; Madison, 1983). The high expense of technologically oriented care leaves little money to finance what Madison describes as "Cinderella services": those that lack the glitter and glamour of highly technological, rapidly health-restoring measures but that often result in greater benefit for greater numbers of people in the long run. Examples of these Cinderella services include educational services, organized prevention, home care, and care of the dependent. The dilemma posed by the nature of the American medical-industrial complex is described eloquently by Madison (1983, p. 1281):

He who writes the ticket determines the destination. When those in charge are addicted to technology, the services for sale, that people are told are essential, will be those that feed the addiction. Never mind how much healing results per dollar spent. The Cinderella services that are an essential part of COPC [community-oriented primary care] will inevitably be caught in the budget squeeze, not because they themselves are especially expensive, although they do cost; not because they are less effective, although they will never be credited with as many dramatic results; but simply because other more expensive destinations are more interesting to those who write the ticket, and getting there is budget busting.

Consequences of Policy Failure

Failure to set clear national policy for dependent older persons has led to a variety of problems. These include premature institutionalization, unclear expectations regarding the future of care for dependent older people, ambiguous rules and regulations for providers/consumers, focus on process rather than outcome in evaluating quality of services, fragmentation of services for older persons, and escalating cost of medical care (Callahan and Wallack, 1981).

Despite a national concern over cost containment in health services, care for dependent older persons is still offered in a highly inefficient manner. Numerous agencies, both public and private, are involved. Reimbursement structures are complex, overlapping, and institutionally biased. Services such as congregate housing have languished for lack of a stable funding base, despite the fact that they have demonstrated effectiveness in maintaining frail older persons in the community at a cost less than institutionalization.

The result of this lack of innovation in community-based service delivery to dependent older persons is an overreliance on institutional solutions for dependency. The assumption is that because institutions provide a relatively predictable amount and quality of dependent care at a moderate cost, they are preferable to community-based care. Institution-based care is also somewhat easier to supervise and monitor.

Impact on Nursing Practice

The current disarray of provisions for the needs of dependent older persons has considerable impact on the delivery of nursing care. Nurses play key roles in coordinating services and as advocates for the elderly seeking to obtain services appropriate to their level of functioning or disability.

The term *case management* comes from the social service literature but is gaining increasing acceptance in interdisciplinary human services circles (Koff, 1983; Beatrice, 1981). Although many professionals may serve in the case manager or care coordinator capacity, nurses are a logical choice. Nurses have generalist health preparation and broad assessment skills that include an emphasis on the patient's function, and they are already major providers of care in the community. As highly technological nursing care becomes commonplace in community-based care, it is essential that nurses not lose their perspective of the whole person and the need for well-organized, individualized systems of care.

Restrictions on reimbursement for services in the community become more prominent as the care needs of the elderly increase. There is a pernicious trend for professionals in health care to equate reimbursable services with needed services. For example, clinicians have been observed to conclude that if reimbursement is not available for provision of emotional support during a terminal illness, then the service is not truly needed by the client. Or if a client progresses less quickly than the norms established by a fiscal intermediary, the client is considered not a rehabilitation candidate and therefore no longer in need of physical or occupational therapy or restorative nursing care, regardless of whether maximal function has been obtained.

The inadequacies of reimbursement policies for defining professional services in care for the elderly have long been recognized (American Nurses' Association, 1975). The pressures for cost consciousness and cost containment will require renewed vigilance on the part of nurses to advocate articulately for needed services. Nurses are knowledgeable about the impact of services on the individual's response to illness. Such knowledge is useless if it is not communicated to those who control decisions regarding reimbursement for services.

Attempts to Resolve Policy Failure

Reform of the care system for dependent older persons has been characterized by incremental solutions. Only recently has there been serious examination of the assumptions that underlie the current nonsystem of care: the need for pluralism in health care; continuance of the national focus on acute, high-technology care; protection of proprietary interests in care; and the roles of the dependent older person, the family, and the federal government in providing care.

Projects to date have centered on two major strategies: changing the reimbursement structure and changing the service delivery structure. Some projects have focused on both strategies simultaneously. Most reform efforts have attempted to demonstrate both improved patient/client outcomes and reduced cost. Examples of innovations include waiver projects, channeling projects, prospective payment reimbursement systems, social HMOs, and congregate housing services.

Health care reform of the 1990s under the direction of Hillary Rodham Clinton was an attempt to deal with the complex problems of health care delivery to all citizens, including the dependent, chronically ill elderly. Health promotion, case management, primary care, and the prominent role of nurses as advanced practitioners are key concepts in future health care delivery.

ELDER NEGLECT AND ABUSE

Definition and Scope of the Problem

Elder abuse encompasses physical, psychological, financial, and social abuse or violation of an individual's rights (Benton and Marshall, 1991). Several key terms are used to define concepts related to elder abuse.

Abuse is defined as the willful infliction of

physical pain, injury, or debilitating mental anguish; unreasonable confinement; or the willful deprivation of services that are necessary to maintain physical and mental health. *Physical abuse* usually includes beatings, withholding personal or medical care, or failure to supervise an impaired person adequately enough to prevent injury. *Psychological abuse* consists of instilling fear through verbal assaults or demands to perform demeaning tasks, making threats, or isolating an older person. *Financial or material abuse* is characterized by the theft or mismanagement of money or personal belongings. *Social abuse* or violation of rights consists of being forced out of one's home or being denied the opportunity to exercise rights as an adult.

Neglect refers to a lack of services that are necessary for the physical and mental health of elderly persons living alone or not able to provide self-care. Neglect may be by self or another. According to Lachs and Fulmer (1993), neglect is more difficult to define than abuse because it is a more subtle form of mistreatment. The terms passive neglect and active neglect may help to clarify cases of neglect. *Passive neglect* describes the legitimate inability of the caregiver to perform caregiving activities, such as bathing, dressing, or changing an incontinent older person. *Active neglect* implies that a caregiver is intentionally withholding food or services to harm the elder.

Self-neglect, in which an older adult refuses medical care, services, or money, presents another form of neglect that is fraught with ethical problems. Elderly persons, unlike children, can choose their own lifestyle, and the right to self-determination is relinquished only when they are legally declared incapable or incompetent (Benton and Marshall, 1991).

Exploitation is the illegal or improper use of disabled adults or their resources for another's profit or advantage (Shiferaw et al., 1994).

Elder abuse is an international problem (Saveman et al., 1993; Saveman and Norberg, 1993; Jarde et al., 1992; Coyne et al., 1993; Roberts et al., 1993; McCreadie and Tinker, 1993; Kurrle et al., 1992; Homer and Gilleard, 1990; Leroux and Petrunik, 1990). In the United States, it has been estimated that 2.5 million older adults are abused or neglected yearly (Delunas, 1990). Abuse may occur among community-residing elderly or in institutional settings, such as domiciliary homes, nursing homes, or even hospitals. In reports from 21 states in 1991, it was found that persons most likely to abuse elders are family members who are direct caregivers;

the most frequent abusers are adult children (32.5 per cent), other relatives including grandchildren and siblings (19.2 per cent), and spouses (14.4 per cent). The incidence of abuse increases with advancing age (from 10.5 per cent for ages 65 to 69 to 23.1 per cent for age 85 and up), and older women are more than twice as likely to be abused as older men are (67.8 vs. 32 per cent) (Schick and Schick, 1994).

Elders who are the most likely victims of abuse are socially isolated women who retain some independence and on whom the abuser is dependent financially (Blomquist, 1993). Other risk factors for elder abuse are advanced age, a history of significant past generational conflict between the parent and child, alcohol abuse in either the caregiver or elder, stress, and a past history of abuse (Costa, 1993; Kurrle et al., 1992; Benton and Marshall, 1991). Elderly individuals who are most at risk for neglect are those with dependency needs related to confusion, immobility, and personal hygiene (Rounds, 1992).

Many incidences of elder abuse have gone unreported in the past. Now that all 50 states have enacted mandatory reporting laws and have instituted protective service programs, elder abuse has been increasingly recognized as a social problem. Unfortunately, both professionals and the public continue to underreport cases of abuse. Reasons cited include denial, reluctance to report abuse, and lack of awareness of abuse laws (Ehrlich and Anetzberger, 1991; Wolf and Pillemer, 1994; Benton and Marshall, 1991).

Theoretical Issues

Concept Clarification

The concept of elder abuse continues to be difficult to define and recognize. According to Lachs and Fulmer (1993), older adults who are abused and neglected may demonstrate signs and symptoms similar to the signs and symptoms of many common chronic medical conditions in elderly persons. In addition, many investigated reports of elder abuse have been determined to be unsubstantiated. In a study by Shiferaw and associates (1994), it was found that only 23 of 123 cases investigated were confirmed as elder abuse. Unconfirmed cases were more likely to occur in a nursing home or to involve elderly patients who were ill.

Ethical difficulties are also related to defining and describing elder abuse and neglect. These difficulties stem from differences among individuals and cultural groups in defining quality of life, survival needs, and well-being. For example, Moon and Williams (1993) found that there were significant group differences in perceptions of abuse among African-American, Caucasian-American, and Korean-American elderly women. Korean-American women were less likely to perceive a given situation as abusive, and all three groups would use formal and informal sources of help for abuse differently.

There are many gaps in the knowledge about elder abuse and neglect, and it is unlikely that there will be a definition of abuse that is accepted by everyone. Thus, nurses must continue to integrate their clinical experience and social skills to recognize the problem and provide appropriate intervention (Lachs and Fulmer, 1993; Weiler and Buckwalter, 1992). Nurses must also be aware of the values that underlie each definition of abuse and be prepared to use principles of ethical decision making as guides to intervention (see Chapter 3).

Contributors to Elder Neglect and Abuse

Several theories have been proposed to explain elder abuse and neglect: (1) social learning or transgenerational violence theory; (2) psychopathology of the abuser theory; (3) stressed caregiver theory; (4) dependency theory; and (5) isolation theory. According to the *social learning or transgenerational violence theory,* children who are abused tend to grow up to abuse their own children and then, in turn, abuse their elderly parents as well. The *psychopathology of the abuser theory* asserts that non-normal personality characteristics of the abuser result in abuse. The premise of the *stressed caregiver theory* is that stresses from caregiving or external stresses build up in the caregiver beyond some critical threshold. The *dependency theory* implies that functional frailty and medical illness lead to abuse. The *isolation theory* contends that a shrinking social network is a major risk factor for elder abuse and neglect (Lachs and Fulmer, 1993).

Family Violence

Family violence has been described as a learned behavior pattern that is transmitted to subsequent generations, and elders in such families are at high risk for receiving abuse (Strauss et al., 1981; O'Malley et al., 1983). Most cases of abuse involve family members, and many researchers have found high rates of elder abuse in families in which there have been long-standing conflicts. Characteristics of families in which elder abuse is most likely to occur are lack of family support, caregiver reluctance, overcrowding, isolation, marital conflict, and disharmony in shared responsibility. In some families, violence may be the norm, with multiple forms of abuse occurring simultaneously. Abusive behavior is often bidirectional (that is, both the elder and the caregiver behave abusively toward each other), and there is evidence that aggression by the care recipient toward the caregiver may precipitate a violent response (Saveman and Norberg, 1993; Kurrle et al., 1992; Benton and Marshall, 1991; Homer and Gilleard, 1990; Steinmetz, 1988; O'Malley et al., 1983).

Family dysfunction of many types is cited as a contributing factor to elder abuse or neglect. This ranges from dysfunctional interactional patterns, where dependence in the older person may be denied, to families who have "impaired caregivers" in their midst. Impaired caregivers are those who have particular personality traits or psychopathology that may lead to abuse, such as alcoholism, drug abuse, mental illness, or cognitive impairments that limit caregiving capability (Pillemer and Finkelhor, 1989; Homer and Gilleard, 1990). Other caregiver traits that increase the risk of abuse are caregiver inexperience, economic stress, being unengaged outside the home, blaming personality, unrealistic expectations, economic dependence on the elder, hypercritical personality, and poor self-esteem (Kosberg, 1988; Pillemer and Suitor, 1992).

According to Leroux and Petrunik (1990), elder abuse has emerged as a social problem that is a major new form of family violence. Unfortunately, elder abuse receives much less attention than other problems grouped under the family violence rubric.

Caregiver Stress

Caregiver stress is frequently mentioned as a causative factor in elder abuse. In a study of 119 dependent elders and their caregivers, it was found that caregivers who perceived caring as stressful and burdensome had higher levels of verbal, psychological, and physical abuse than those who did not (Steinmetz, 1988). In addition, a survey of victims in Canada revealed that nearly 50 per cent of married victims of verbal aggression described their spouses as being under a great deal of stress (Podnieks, 1990).

One factor that appears to play a part in caregiver stress is a relatively recent phenomenon—the "beanpole family" (Bengtson et al., 1990). This type of family structure is characterized by an increased number of generations living together with fewer members within each generation. The duration of family roles for husbands, wives, children, and caregivers lengthens, resulting in increased caregiver roles for older members of the family.

Stressful life events (external stress) experienced by the caregiver may also lead to elder abuse. Events that are not connected with the caregiving situation, such as the death of a friend, loss of a job, a move, pregnancy, or marital difficulties, may trigger inappropriate responses in which caregivers focus their anger on the dependent elder. Although not all studies support this hypothesis, several have found that abusive caregivers report more stressful life events than nonabusive caregivers do (Benton and Marshall, 1991).

Dependency

The caregiver role appears to become increasingly stressful as the older person becomes more frail and dependent. As the demands of the relationship grow for the caregiver and the rewards diminish, the exchange becomes perceived as unfair. Thus, caregivers who are locked into the caregiving role may become abusive (Pillemer and Suitor, 1992).

Studies of elder abuse and neglect confirm that victims are frequently physically and psychologically dependent (Saveman and Norberg, 1993; Coyne et al., 1993; Kurrle et al., 1992; Paveza et al., 1992; Rounds, 1992). However, dependency alone does not explain elder abuse. There are many dependent older persons who are not subject to abuse or neglect. It is more likely that physical dependency triggers an inappropriate caregiving response in some persons, resulting in neglect or abuse.

Consequences of Elder Neglect and Abuse

Health Status of Old People

Little research has been reported on the impact of elder abuse or neglect on the individual or family. Clearly, situations of neglect or physical abuse have deleterious effects on an individual's health status. Financial exploitation may limit the older person's ability to obtain necessities of daily life including health care. Finally, the consequences of emotional abuse are most difficult to quantify yet are likely to influence the older person's ability to participate in daily activities, rehabilitation, or other goals. The human tragedy of abuse of others is difficult to quantify but abhorrent to helping professionals.

Impact on Nursing Practice

The problem of elder neglect and abuse and speculations about its causes have important implications for nurses working with dependent elders and caregivers of all types. Because elders may suffer neglect or abuse at the hands of themselves, their peers, family members, paid helpers, and organizations designed to help them, nurses have an opportunity to affect the development and consequences of elder abuse and neglect in many ways. Specific opportunities presented by working with individuals, families, small groups, and complex organizations in a community are discussed in turn.

While working with elderly individuals, whether in the hospital, nursing home, clinic, or home setting, nurses should be alert for signs of abuse or neglect. Nurses frequently have intimate contact with older persons and may be able to observe firsthand the effects of abuse or neglect. Nurses may be the first helping professionals to identify abuse or neglect as a problem for the older client.

Nurses often monitor the patient's condition and family concerns in community settings. This is an excellent opportunity to identify family situations with high potential for abuse. Initial research points to families with a history of abusive behavior and family caregivers with multiple stressors as being at high risk for elder abuse. Once these families are identified, interventions designed to increase family coping resources or decrease family stressors may be instituted. Failing this, it may be important to help the older person identify an alternative source of care so that the abuse-prone situation is avoided entirely. Educational programs aimed at families who are caring for impaired elders may help reduce some of the frustration engendered by the misunderstanding of disease processes or the ignorance of management strategies.

At the community level, the gerontological nurse has a dual role with respect to elder neglect and abuse. Because elder abuse and neglect have only recently been identified as significant problems, nurses need to take leadership roles in raising the consciousness of community groups and institutions. Also, leadership in providing advocacy for older adults is often needed. Substandard staffing and funding of services designed to assist dependent elders are national problems. As nurses have more opportunity for input into

T A B L E   1 6 – 1
Common Indicators of Elder Abuse and Neglect

Abrasions	Injuries inconsistent with history
Lacerations	History of falls
Bruises	Untreated medical problems
Burns	Inappropriate clothing
Sprains	Poor hygiene
Fractures	Excessive drowsiness
Dislocations	Over/undermedication
Pressure sores	Malnutrition/dehydration

governmental and private-sector initiatives regarding standards for and funding of these services, there is potential for change of the institutionalized elder neglect and abuse that plagues American society.

Prevention and Resolution of Elder Neglect and Abuse

Process for Treatment

One process recommended for managing elder abuse and neglect involves five components: identification, access and assessment, intervention, follow-up, and prevention (O'Malley et al., 1983).

IDENTIFICATION. Identification of possible elder abuse/neglect victims involves, first, a high index of suspicion for the problem. Individuals at high risk include those who have considerable dependency but a limited informal support network, those whose primary caregivers express frustration or high levels of stress, those who come from families with a history of family violence, those who abuse alcohol or drugs, and those whose caregivers are substance abusers. Individuals with disorders that predictably have multiple disabilities, both physical and emotional, such as Parkinson's disease, Alzheimer's disease, and CVA, are thought to be at high risk as well (Delunas, 1990; Paveza et al., 1992; Hamel et al., 1990).

A detailed history and physical assessment are necessary to detect signs and symptoms of abuse (Table 16–1). A history may reveal inconsistencies in the handling of illnesses or trauma, such as an unusually long lapse between the reported onset of illness or trauma and the time when assistance is sought. Repeated visits to the hospital or clinic with unexplained or questionably explained injuries may indicate abuse. Frequent surgeries that may have been corrective for traumatic injury also arouse suspicion. A caregiver may insist on providing the medical history and offer implausible explanations for illnesses or injuries, often claiming that the older person is "acci-

dent prone." A family and social history should also be conducted to determine relationships and social interactions.

A physical assessment may provide clues to physical abuse, but it may be difficult to differentiate abuse from disease- or age-related physiological changes. However, any physical findings that do not fit the history of the injury should raise suspicion. The patient's general appearance and hygiene may indicate neglect, and an examination of the skin and other organs may reveal some of the most frequently found signs of abuse, including multiple bruising, burns, facial lacerations, absence of hair in patches, and fractures in various stages of healing. Mental status testing should be conducted to determine whether there is an underlying delirium or dementia and to determine competency, an issue that may be crucial in attempting to intervene (Roberts et al., 1993; Costa, 1993; Lachs and Fulmer, 1993; Benton and Marshall, 1991; Fulmer and Birkenhauser, 1992).

ACCESS AND ASSESSMENT. Access must be obtained before assessment can take place. Access may be a problem if the older person is in the home, because adults who are considered competent have the right to make their own personal care decisions. Access by police is permissible only if there is probable cause to suspect that a crime has been committed or if the older person has made a complaint. O'Malley and associates (1979) found that in 40 per cent of the cases, professionals were unable to obtain the access needed to assess and intervene. O'Malley and colleagues (1983) identify nursing personnel as key individuals in the process of gaining access. Keys to helping the older person and family accept help include a nonjudgmental style and negotiation and persuasion skills (Murdach, 1980).

Once access is obtained, assessment should focus on the following questions:

1. Is the person in immediate danger of bodily harm?
2. Is the person competent to make decisions regarding his or her care?
3. What are the degree and significance of the person's functional impairments?
4. What specific services might help to meet the unmet needs?
5. Who in the family is involved and to what extent?
6. Are the patient and family willing to accept intervention?

Assessment is best carried out in a multidisciplinary team context, for the issues involved are complex. Nurses have the assess-

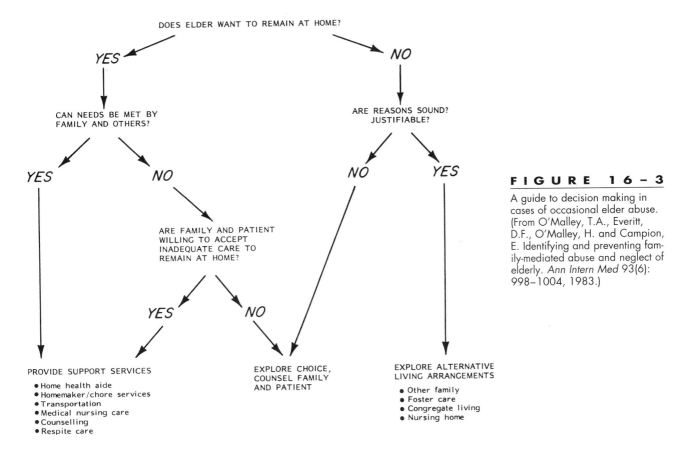

FIGURE 16-3

A guide to decision making in cases of occasional elder abuse. (From O'Malley, T.A., Everitt, D.F., O'Malley, H. and Campion, E. Identifying and preventing family-mediated abuse and neglect of elderly. *Ann Intern Med* 93(6): 998–1004, 1983.)

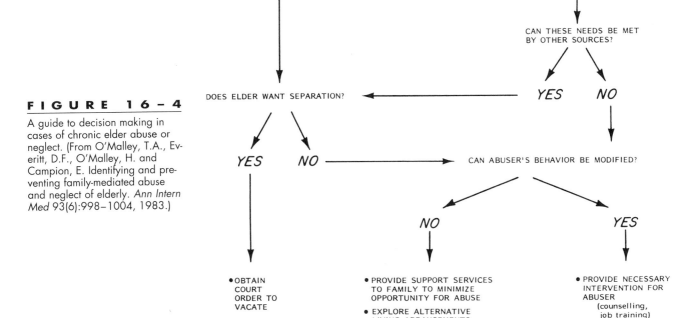

FIGURE 16-4

A guide to decision making in cases of chronic elder abuse or neglect. (From O'Malley, T.A., Everitt, D.F., O'Malley, H. and Campion, E. Identifying and preventing family-mediated abuse and neglect of elderly. *Ann Intern Med* 93(6):998–1004, 1983.)

T A B L E   1 6 – 2
Ideas for Reduction of Elder Abuse and Neglect

A classic prevention model, in which three levels of preventive efforts are defined, is a framework that suggests different strategies for reducing the prevalence of elder abuse. Each level of prevention is described, followed by a list of ideas for reduction of elder neglect and abuse at each level.

Primary Prevention

Efforts designed to foster well-being, such as the introduction of healthful lifestyle teaching in elementary school to promote activity and better nutrition.

Primary Prevention and Elder Abuse

1. Projects to interrupt cycles of family violence
2. Projects that increase family communication effectiveness
3. Projects that increase family understanding of the aging process
4. Projects that maximize nonfamily natural helping networks for dependent elders
5. Gray Panther, American Association of Retired Persons, National Council on the Aging efforts to enhance the image/status of the elderly

Secondary Prevention

Efforts directed toward early detection and treatment of disease before adverse effects have been felt. An example is hypertension and diabetes screening.

Secondary Prevention and Elder Abuse

1. Identifying elderly at risk for self-neglect or abuse
2. Identifying families at risk for elder abuse or neglect
3. Identifying communities at risk for elder abuse or neglect (migrant communities; communities that are over- or underpopulated with old people; certain ethnic groups, e.g., WASP women or blacks; mentally retarded elders; bag ladies; SRO occupants; nursing home chains with ageist corporate philosophies)
4. Monitoring of high-risk situations—advocacy groups, ombudsman programs
5. Counseling or therapy for those showing signs of neglect or abuse
6. Substance abuse programs

Tertiary Prevention

Efforts aimed at reducing morbidity from existing disorders, such as rehabilitation after cerebrovascular accidents or myocardial infarction.

Tertiary Prevention and Elder Abuse

1. Adult protective services programs—placement, guardianship
2. Family counseling
3. Maximizing support from sources other than the primary caregiver

---

ment skills to make initial judgments in each of these six areas.

INTERVENTION. Intervention is based on the findings of the assessment. The major goals of intervention are protection of the patient and prevention of further episodes of abuse or neglect. O'Malley and coworkers (1983) offer useful decision trees for use with those thought to be victims of abuse or neglect (Figs. 16–3 and 16–4). The intervention process should be augmented by considering guidelines for ethical decision making (see Chapter 3) when decisions, such as what are "sound and justifiable reasons" for wanting to remain at home, involve value judgments. The alternatives to staying in the current situation may not significantly improve the patient's situation, and the options for intervention are often limited.

FOLLOW-UP. There are few data reported on the impact of intervention on elder abuse over time. Careful follow-up is indicated in all situations of elder neglect or abuse, even if interventions are accepted, because the risk for further abuse remains high.

PREVENTION. Prevention efforts are most productive when they are targeted toward abuses early in a caregiving experience with elders and the community at large. Table 16–2 lists efforts that may help reduce the prevalence of elder neglect and abuse. To date, no research has been reported on this important area.

Evaluation of Treatment and Prevention Efforts

Unfortunately, the intervention efforts tried to date have yielded only marginally successful results. O'Malley and associates (1979) reported only a minority (45 per cent) of their cases resolved, and Block and Sinott (1979) concluded that the majority of their cases were not satisfactorily resolved (95.24 per cent). Part of the problem in evaluating the effectiveness of programs is the failure to adequately define criteria for success. Given the problems in defining elder neglect and abuse alone, agreement on criteria for success is likely to be difficult to achieve.

The interventions available for protection from and treatment of the abusive situation are limited. Many studies report institutional placement as the primary means of protecting abused or neglected clients. Given the problems with institutional care, this may be only a partial solution to the problem. Unfortunately, abuse of residents in nursing homes has been an ongoing concern. In an attempt to correct the problem, a model abuse prevention program was established for nursing assistants. Eight training modules were used to educate and sensitize nursing staff to abuse. The program was successful in reducing conflict with and abuse of residents (Pillemer and Hudson, 1993).

Several programs have been developed in the community, chiefly through the Area Agencies on Aging. They include an elder abuse task force, multidisciplinary teams, a senior advocacy volunteer program, a victim support group, and a master's level training unit in adult protective services. The outcomes of these programs appear positive; however, they are not quantified (Wolf and Pillemer, 1994; Foelker et al., 1990).

There is also the problem of gaining acceptance from the elderly individual or family to provide help. Rates of help refusal range from 58 (Boydston and McNair, 1981; O'Malley et al., 1979) to 77 per cent (Wolf et al., 1982). In addition, available services may not be appropriate to the family's or elderly person's needs. Agencies investigating abusive situations typically have no better funding mechanism than the ones currently implicated in fostering overburdened family caregivers.

Follow-up on abuse cases is another problem in successful intervention. This is particularly true with institution-based abuse or neglect cases; gaining access to investigate and multiple care providers may make follow-up difficult.

It is apparent from these early reports of treatment success that it is far preferable to prevent this problem than to treat it.

It is necessary to recognize elder abuse and neglect as a significant problem facing the aged and society today. The full extent of the problem is as yet unquantified, yet the specter of dependent old people living out their lives in fear, discomfort, or isolation is unacceptable to American society. Nurses have a clear function in early identification of those suffering from elder neglect and abuse. More important, because of the nursing profession's focus on promotion of development and health, nurses have an excellent opportunity for promoting client situations and professional and lay programs that help to prevent this tragic state from ever happening. The forces that foster the development of elder abuse and neglect are complex. This problem represents a stunning challenge to the nursing profession, calling for creativity and leadership.

WOMEN'S ISSUES IN AGING

Gerontological research has been criticized for considering the experience of the aging man to the exclusion of the experience of the aging woman. Beeson (1975) noted that the problems inherent in the majority of the research stem from two major sources: (1) the predominantly male frame of reference that identifies salient research topics (for example, retirement rather than menopause) and (2) the fact that the earliest longitudinal studies did not include women as subjects. Although this glaring omission has been rectified in subsequent studies, this early re-

search laid the groundwork for assumptions that underpin future research efforts. These assumptions have led to theoretically logical but empirically unfounded conclusions that aging is somehow smoother and less of a problem for women than for men. The "scholarly view" contradicts what is reported in the journalistic literature concerning the difficulties women encounter with aging.

Fortunately, the number of studies about aging women and their concerns is on the increase. For example, Heidrich and Ryff (1992) studied the problems women faced with aging. They found that the most frequent day-to-day concerns were evenly distributed among household management and activity limitations. The most frequent major concerns were their own health (35 per cent) and caring for others (29 per cent).

The woman's health literature has drawn attention to the adverse effects of assumptions based on research performed by and on men. It is suggested that a feminist perspective on the process of aging and its associated problems is necessary because aging affects women in unique ways. Specifically, the uniqueness of a woman's aging experience is due to the following factors:

- The majority of older persons are women.

- Women have a longer life expectancy than men.

- Women have more illnesses and functional limitations than men do.

- Women are the predominant caregivers of dependent older people (in both formal and informal caregiving systems).

- Through differential sex role socialization, older women have been less well prepared than their male counterparts to deal with certain aspects of late life, such as maintaining a household, paying bills, dealing with complex bureaucracies, and securing and maintaining adequate income.

Each of the issues identified has potential effects on older women as health care recipients.

Theoretical Issues

SEX ROLE SOCIALIZATION. Men and women receive different socialization into adult roles. Socialization has a powerful influence on expectations for achievement and maintenance of self-esteem. The traditional female role is currently devalued in our society. Women learn to undervalue themselves, leading to lower self-esteem, lower aspirations, and further devaluation.

DEMOGRAPHIC CONSIDERATIONS. Most women can expect to live longer than men. Along with this greater life expectancy are some negative aspects of increased longevity. Older women tend to have more illnesses, functional disabilities, caregiver demands, and economic problems. The greatest growth in the potential population in need of long-term care is for unmarried women aged 75 and older, with the largest increase projected for the population of women older than 85. The oldest-old—primarily women—most likely will be disadvantaged not only by increasing infirmity but also by outliving their close relatives who may provide supportive care (Johnson and Wolinsky, 1994; Arendell and Estes, 1991).

The fact that women represent a substantial majority of the elderly population is of note. It means that more women than men are unmarried. It means that age-segregated services and facilities will have disproportionately large numbers of women to serve, resulting in the slanting of activities and priorities of such facilities toward women's concerns and interests. Because women have a lesser social status in American society relative to men, such services and facilities may be devalued and underfunded.

Women as Caregivers of Dependent Elders

Women are the primary caregivers of dependent older family members (Dowler et al., 1992; Walker and Allen, 1991). This function has historical precedent and has remained almost exclusively in the domain of women's work, despite the change in work force participation by women in the past several decades. Caregiving traditionally has been an unpaid service to society, much like housekeeping and child rearing. Those without family to perform this function have had to turn to the marketplace for these services, at considerably higher monetary cost than if they received such help within the family.

Sexual Discrimination

The effects of a lifetime of sexual discrimination are difficult to measure. It is clear, however, that women are more likely to be impoverished, are less likely to be in the work force, and may have fewer social opportunities available because of a more narrow social world in earlier years. Elderly minority women have been at special risk for the consequences of sexual discrimination. Of the 18.6 million women older than 65, 11 per cent are minorities, most of whom are black. According to Dr. Mary Harper (Laurence, 1994), older minority women face "a quadruple jeopardy." Not only are they poor, but they must also deal with age, sex, and racial discrimination. One third of black women older than 55 work part-time and have no health insurance benefits. Many are unable to obtain mental health services and are less likely than white women to seek out other health care services. In addition, there is a dearth of research on elderly minority women, so that major gaps in knowledge exist. Of eight major national clinical trials, only one included minority women.

Economic Problems

Older women, particularly minority women, and most especially African-American women, have the highest rates of poverty in the United States (U.S. Department of Health and Human Services, 1991). Somers (1980) identified several factors contributing to poverty in older women:

1. *Sex discrimination* in employment results in sex discrimination in retirement.
2. Women are punished for *motherhood* by losing earning years.
3. *Early retirement* results in less income for the rest of one's life. Women frequently take early retirement because of few job opportunities and because men who do the hiring generally prefer younger women.
4. Women dependents may receive more if their husbands earn more than Social Security benefits on the same income combined and both received benefits based on their own work histories.
5. There is no credit for work in the home. This means that there is no coverage for disabled homemakers and that women who have worked have benefits only as "dependent." Older women with younger husbands must wait until the husband is of retirement age to receive benefits (Somers, 1980; O'Grady-LeShane, 1990).

Somers suggests that these difficulties for women in the Social Security system amount to institutionalized sexism.

Impact of the Feminist Movement

The effects of the women's movement on the status of elderly women have been mixed. In one way, the women's movement has helped to draw attention to discriminatory practices in the workplace, in health care, and in pension systems, resulting in reforms that have had an impact on the lives of older women. However, older women may experience lowered self-esteem if they measure their accomplishments without considering the changes in opportunities and expectations for women that have accompanied the women's movement. The current cohort of older women matured in a time when the opportunities open to women were considerably more restricted than today. The older woman who evaluates her life accomplishments by today's standards may be left with a negative self-image. Similarly, the older woman who was denied opportunity based on sex may actually grieve for the lost opportunity. The positive side of this situation is that some older women may choose this period in their lives to take advantage of opportunities that previously had been closed to them. The relative "normlessness" of old age allows considerable creativity in this period of life if physical and mental health permit.

Paucity of Research on the Aging of Women

In recent times, it has been noted that there are significant gaps in the research regarding older women. Large longitudinal and cross-sectional studies related to health and aging have systematically eliminated women; and studies related specifically to women, such as the response of women to their retirement, menopause, and other issues, have not been conducted (Szinovacz, 1983; Wenger, 1992; Gurwitz et al., 1992). Fortunately, the National Institutes of Health (NIH) have responded to concerns about this issue and are requiring all researchers to include women in their studies or provide an excellent rationale for exclusion. In addition, NIH announced a Women's Health Initiative in the early 1990s, which is the largest community-based clinical prevention and intervention trial ever conducted. The 10-year project will investigate the effect of diet and exercise, use of hormone replacement therapy, and smoking cessation on women's risk for disease as they age (Champlin, 1991). These initiatives are encouraging and will increase the amount of research carried out on the aging of women.

Impact of the Status of Women on Health

Several major influences on health and health care of older women can be inferred from the status of women in America. First, poverty negatively influences health and access to health care, and therefore the lower economic status of older women contributes to poorer health status. Second, the socialization of women in the early part of the 20th century has left many older women ill-prepared for the tasks of home maintenance, transportation, and financial management without a spouse. It is a testament to the adaptability of both women and older people that most women are able to cope with day-to-day living requirements in a complex bureaucratic world. Finally, the relative lack of research on women and the aging process means that there are even fewer norms for women in advanced age. This means that women remain at risk for receiving treatment based on scientific rumor or clinical fashion rather than on solid research. The erroneous but widely held notion that women are hypochondriacal is one example of how women are stereotyped rather than treated according to current research findings.

Nurses should be aware of the inadequacy of the gerontological research base with regard to women. They should be particularly alert to the effects of sexism in health care, because older women may find it more satisfactory to share concerns with a woman health care provider. Finally, nurses should be alert to the particular problems older women may encounter as a result of their socialization, increased longevity, and status in American society.

COMMON AGE-RELATED PSYCHOLOGICAL DISORDERS

Mental health problems in the elderly are significant in their frequency, impact on mental status, and influence on the course of physical illness in later life. It has been estimated that 20 to 25 per cent of people age 65 and older may exhibit signs and symptoms of significant mental illness at any given time. The problems are occurring in both community and institutional settings. For example, the number of people in nursing homes continues to rise, and although psychiatric admissions to state hospitals have declined in the past two decades, admissions to private psychiatric and general hospitals have increased.

Mental health services are notoriously underused by the elderly (Smyer et al., 1994; Cohen, 1990). Access to services has been hampered by the stereotypical views of care providers toward the elderly and their ability to be treated and by the suspicions with

TABLE 16 – 3
Medical Illnesses Associated with Depression

Metabolic disturbances	Pulmonary
Dehydration	Chronic obstructive lung disease
Azotemia, uremia	Malignant neoplasm
Acid-base disturbances	Gastrointestinal
Hypoxia	Malignant neoplasm (especially
Hyponatremia and hypernatremia	pancreatic)
Hypoglycemia and hyperglycemia	Irritable bowel
Hypocalcemia and hypercalcemia	Other (e.g., ulcer, diverticulosis)
Endocrine	Genitourinary
Hypothyroidism and	Urinary incontinence
hyperthyroidism	Musculoskeletal
Hyperparathyroidism	Degenerative arthritis
Diabetes mellitus	Osteoporosis with vertebral
Cushing's disease	compression or hip fracture
Addison's disease	Polymyalgia rheumatica
Infections	Paget's disease
Viral	Neurological
Pneumonia	Cerebrovascular disease
Encephalitis	Transient ischemic attacks
Bacterial	Strokes
Pneumonia	Dementia (all types)
Urinary tract infection	Intracranial mass
Meningitis	Primary or metastatic tumors
Endocarditis	Parkinson's disease
Other	Other
Tuberculosis	Anemia (of any cause)
Fungal meningitis	Vitamin deficiencies
Neurosyphilis	Hematological or other systemic
Cardiovascular	malignant neoplasm
Congestive heart failure	
Myocardial infarction	

From Kane, R.L., Ouslander, J.G. and Abrass, I.B. *Essentials of Clinical Geriatrics*, 3rd ed. New York: McGraw-Hill, 1994. Reproduced with permission of McGraw-Hill, Inc.

TABLE 16 – 4
Drugs That Cause Signs of Depression

Antihypertensives	Psychotropics	Steroids
Reserpine	Sedatives	Corticosteroids
Methyldopa	Barbiturates	Estrogens
Propranolol	Benzodiazepines	
Clonidine	Meprobamate	Analgesics
Hydralazine	Antipsychotics	Narcotic
Guanethidine	Chlorpromazine	Morphine
	Haloperidol (Haldol)	Codeine
Cardiovascular	Thiothixene	Meperidine
Preparations	Hypnotics	Pentazocine
Diuretics	Chloral hydrate	Propoxyphene
Digitalis	Benzodiazepines	Non-narcotic
Lidocaine	Antidepressants	Indomethacin
Procaine	Amitriptyline	
	Doxepin	Others
Antiparkinsonians		Cimetidine
Levodopa	Antimicrobials	Cancer
	Sulfonamides	chemotherapeutics
Hypoglycemics (oral)	Isoniazid	Alcohol

From Buckwalter, K.C. How to unmask depression. *Geriatr Nurs* July/August: 179–181, 1990.

which the older adults view the service providers. In a report conducted by Smyer and associates (1994), only one fifth of nursing home residents with a mental disorder received any mental health care services, even though more than 75 per cent of them lived in nursing homes that provided services.

The course of chronic mental illness in later life is characterized by exacerbations and remissions, closely resembling the course of chronic physical illness. When chronic mental disorders are exacerbated, they can be brought back under control, much like physical conditions; in many cases, the elderly are more responsive to treatment of mental illnesses (Cohen, 1990).

The most prevalent psychiatric disorders in later life are depressive syndromes and dementias (the dementias are discussed in Chapter 9). Other, less prevalent conditions include anxiety and somatoform disorders, schizophrenia and delusional disorders, and substance abuse. Many of these conditions are amenable to treatment with pharmacotherapy, psychotherapy, environmental manipulation, and family therapy (Finkel and Denson, 1990; Henderson, 1992; Schick and Schick, 1994; U.S. Department of Health and Human Services, 1991).

Depression

Depression, the most common psychiatric disorder in later life, has an estimated prevalence of approximately 15 per cent, with a range from 10 to 25 per cent. Late-life depression appears to be a result of a network of multiple internal and external causes. The disorder is characterized by sadness, low mood, pessimism about the future, self-criticism and self-blame, retardation or agitation, slow thinking, difficulty concentrating, and appetite and sleep disturbances (Blazer, 1993; Finkel and Denson, 1990).

The origins of depression in late life are related to biological factors, physical factors, psychological processes, and sociocultural influences (Muller-Spahn and Hock, 1994). *Biological* theories of late-life depression encompass genetic predisposition; changes in neuroanatomy, neurophysiology, and neuroendocrine regulation with aging; and disruption of biological rhythms. Genetic predisposition to depression appears to be more evident in early-onset depressive disorders than in disorders of later onset and is thought to have more of a role in bipolar depression than in unipolar depression. It is generally accepted that the more severe depressive disorders are strongly influenced by biological phenomena. Many of the psycho-biological changes that occur with aging are parallel to those that occur in depression, so that older people may be at greater risk for a depressive disorder with biological origins than are younger individuals (Blazer, 1993; Murphy, 1992).

Physical factors that may cause depression in older adults are specific diseases, chronic medical conditions, exposure to drugs, sensory deprivation (loss of vision or hearing), and loss of physical function (Buckwalter, 1990; Badger, 1993; Kane et al., 1994). Medical conditions most commonly associated with late-life depression (Table 16–3) are metabolic disturbances; disorders of the endocrine, cardiopulmonary, gastrointestinal, genitourinary, neurological, and musculoskeletal systems; and infections (Kane et al., 1994, pp. 124–125). Drugs that cause signs of depression (Table 16–4) include antihypertensives, cardiovascular preparations, psychotropics, steroids, and analgesics (Buckwalter, 1990, p. 180).

Psychological theories of depression in later life are based on the assumption that intrapsychic and psychosocial changes occur throughout life, and the inability to adapt to these challenges contributes to the symptoms, cause, and outcome of late-life depression. The psychological theories are closely related to Erikson's (1963) developmental stage of ego-integrity versus despair. The challenge of late life is to look back on one's life with acceptance and equanimity, derive wisdom from experiences, and look forward to the future. An older person who is not able to resolve the crises and challenges is likely to have depression and despair (Blazer, 1993).

Social factors, particularly increased social stressors and decreased social supports, are thought to contribute to late-life depression. Changes in self-image and identity as usual social roles are gradually taken away necessitate major adaptational tasks with advancing age. Many changes are viewed as losses, such as declines in physical vigor and stamina, decreased mental agility, decreased income and economic stability, and loss of loved ones. George (1991) identified three types of social environmental factors that may contribute to late-life depression: (1) life events (e.g., loss of a loved one), (2) chronic stress (e.g., challenges or threats to a person's well-being, such as financial deprivation), and (3) daily hassles (e.g., ordinary events such as household responsibilities or unpleasant interactions with neighbors). It has been found that chronic stress has a

TABLE 16–5
Symptoms and Signs of Depression in Late Life

SYMPTOMS	OBSERVABLE SIGNS
Emotional	**Appearance**
Dejected mood or sadness	Stooped posture
Decreased life satisfaction	Sad face
Loss of interest	Uncooperativeness
Impulse to cry	Social withdrawal
Irritability	Hostility
Emptiness	Suspiciousness
Fearfulness and anxiety	Confusion and clouding of consciousness
Negative feelings toward self	Diurnal variations of mood
Worry	Drooling (in severe cases)
Helplessness	Unkempt appearance (in severe cases)
Hopelessness	Occasional ulcerations of skin secondary to picking
Sense of failure	Crying or whining
Loneliness	Occasional ulcerations of cornea secondary to decreased blinking
Uselessness	Weight loss
	Bowel impaction
Cognitive	
Low self-esteem	**Psychomotor Retardation**
Pessimism	Slowed speech
Self-blame and criticism	Slowed movements
Rumination about problems	Gestures minimized
Suicidal thoughts	Shuffling slow gait
Delusions	Mutism (in severe cases)
Of uselessness	Cessation of mastication and swallowing (in severe cases)
Of unforgivable behavior	Decreased or inhibited blinking (in severe cases)
Nihilistic	
Somatic	**Psychomotor Agitation**
Hallucinations	Continued motor activity
Auditory	Wringing of hands
Visual	Picking at skin
Kinesthetic	Pacing
Doubt of values and beliefs	Restless sleep
Difficulty concentrating	Grasping others
Poor memory	
	Bizarre or Inappropriate Behavior
Physical	Suicidal gestures or attempts
Loss of appetite	Negativism, such as refusal to eat or drink and stiffness of the body
Fatigability	Outbursts of aggression
Sleep disturbance	Falling backward
Initial insomnia	
Terminal insomnia	
Frequent awakenings	
Constipation	
Loss of libido	
Pain	
Restlessness	
Volitional	
Loss of motivation or "paralysis of will"	
Suicidal impulses	
Desire to withdraw socially	

From Blazer, D.G. *Depression in Late Life,* 2nd ed. St. Louis: C.V. Mosby, 1993, p. 30.

stronger effect on the onset and outcome of depression than life events do, so that elders may be able to adapt better to specific changes in their lives but have more difficulty with ongoing sources of strain.

Symptoms of depression (Table 16–5) may be categorized into emotional, cognitive, physical, and volitional symptoms (Blazer,

TABLE 16-6
Presentations of Depression Unique to the Elderly

Cognitive	Psychomotor
Confusion	Apathy
Pseudodementia	Withdrawal
Memory impairment	
Inability to concentrate	Somatic
Low self-esteem	Pain
Fewer feelings of guilt	Fatigue
	Gastrointestinal problems
Emotional	
Anxiety	
Irritability	

1993, p. 30). Emotional symptoms are changes in the person's feelings in relation to the depression. The most common emotional symptom is sadness or dysphoria. Cognitive symptoms are related to thought processes, and the most common symptom is low self-esteem. Physical or endogenous symptoms are most often associated with depression in late life and are frequently the presenting symptoms in primary care settings (Zung et al., 1993). Sleep disturbances are among the most common complaints of depressed older adults; however, changes in sleep habits occur frequently with older age and may be related to other causes. Volitional symptoms are related to the impulse to strive. Older patients may regress or withdraw from activities that are too demanding.

The major categories of observable *signs* of late-life depression (Table 16–5) are appearance, psychomotor retardation or agitation, and bizarre or inappropriate behavior (Blazer, 1993, p. 30). Signs most characteristic of depression are sad expression, retardation or agitation, frequent crying, clinging, and other expressions of dependency and helplessness (Blazer, 1993).

Signs and symptoms of depression in the elderly may present differently from those in the younger population (Table 16–6). Chief among these differences are that older people may deny changes in mood or feelings of depression and instead may complain of somatic symptoms. In addition, elders may exhibit signs of confusion rather than depression (McCullough, 1991; Kane et al., 1994).

The course and outcome of late-life depression do not seem to be related to age of onset. Depressive disorders are chronic illnesses, and approximately one third of the patients recover with no remissions, one third recover from an episode and then re-lapse, and one third never recover or only partially recover (Blazer, 1993).

Major categories of depressive disorders in later life include major depression, minor depression and dysthymia, bipolar disorder, bereavement, and adjustment disorder with depressed mood.

MAJOR DEPRESSION. A major depression or unipolar depression is defined as a cluster of symptoms lasting at least 2 weeks consisting of five of the following symptoms: depressed mood, loss of interest or pleasure, significant weight loss or gain, insomnia or hypersomnia, psychomotor agitation or retardation, fatigue, feelings of worthlessness or guilt, diminished ability to think or concentrate, and recurrent thoughts of death or suicidal thoughts. At least one of the symptoms is either depressed mood or loss of interest or pleasure (American Psychiatric Association, 1994). Older people are more likely to exhibit loss of interest or pleasure than a depressed mood, weight loss rather than weight gain, insomnia rather than hypersomnia, and fatigue. They are less likely to have feelings of guilt and to report suicidal thoughts (Blazer, 1993).

Treatment for a major depression depends on the extent to which a person is suicidal or functionally impaired. Hospitalization and drug therapy are usually required for a person who is suicidal or severely functionally impaired; ambulatory care is required for those who are not suicidal and show mild-to-moderate functional impairment. Antidepressants, usually tricyclics, can be given for patients who do not respond to psychotherapy. Electroconvulsive therapy (ECT) may also be given for older persons with severe depression (Murphy, 1992; Finkel and Denson, 1990; Blazer, 1993).

DYSTHYMIA AND MINOR DEPRESSION. Minor depressions, including dysthymic disorders, are a chronic but less severe form of depression that appears to occur more frequently than major depression in late life. Minor depression is characterized by a depressed mood, marked loss of interest or pleasure in most activities, and other symptoms of depression. The symptoms are not of sufficient duration or severity to meet the criteria for a major depressive episode, and the periods of depression may be interspersed with months of normal mood.

Minor depressions seem to respond to drug therapy better than to psychosocial interventions. Therefore, people who are chronically and persistently depressed, even if they do not meet the criteria for major depression, should be treated with antidepressant medications. New medications such as fluoxetine (Prozac) appear to alleviate symptoms better than the traditional tricyclic antidepressants (Blazer, 1993; Kane et al., 1994).

BIPOLAR DISORDER. Older adults who suffer from bipolar disorders exhibit a manic episode after having had at least one depressive episode. An average of 10 years has lapsed between the depressive and the manic episodes, with depression appearing in mid-life and mania appearing in late life. Key characteristics of manic episodes are distinct periods of relatively persistent elevated or irritable mood, increased activity, restlessness, talkativeness, flight of ideas, inflated self-esteem, and distractibility. Studies are inconclusive regarding whether elderly persons have atypical presentations of mania (Blazer, 1993; Kane et al., 1994).

Medical treatment of older adults with a bipolar disorder includes antipsychotic medication (haloperidol or thioridazine) for acute agitated behaviors and lithium carbonate for prevention of recurrent symptoms of mania. If lithium carbonate cannot be tolerated because of existing cardiac or renal disease and the symptoms are not controlled by antipsychotic medications, ECT may be used as a therapeutic alternative. In addition, carbamazepine may be given if lithium therapy is ineffective. Hospitalization may be required during the acute onset of the illness. The prognosis is similar in the older and younger populations (Blazer, 1993).

BEREAVEMENT. Everyone suffers from loss as a part of living, and most people grieve appropriately, but some people suffer poor outcomes from grief or abnormal bereavement. Normal bereavement occurs within 2 to 3 months after the death of a loved one and is characterized by depression, guilt, preoccupation with thoughts of the deceased, and somatic complaints (tightness in the throat, shortness of breath, lassitude, loss of appetite). Symptoms of abnormal bereavement are delayed grief reaction, feelings of worthlessness, exhibition of symptoms similar to the last illness of the deceased, and altered social relationships. Risk factors for abnormal bereavement are situations in which the lost loved one was a spouse, the bereaved was dependent on the deceased, the deceased was overly dependent on the bereaved, or the bereaved had ambivalent feelings toward the deceased.

Treatment for abnormal bereavement in later life is primarily psychosocial, including promoting social interactions, maintaining independence, encouraging physical activity, and suggesting resources for dealing with administrative and legal problems. A cognitive behavioral approach to psychotherapy may be helpful, and patients are encouraged to discuss their feelings of bereavement and their relationship with the deceased. Medications are used sparingly, usually for promotion of sleep and appetite (Blazer, 1993).

ADJUSTMENT DISORDER WITH DEPRESSED MOOD. The chief characteristic of an adjustment disorder with a depressed mood is that the older person responds to an identifiable psychosocial or physical stressor. This is sometimes known as a "reactive depression" and is thought to occur frequently in later life as age-related losses accumulate. This type of depression usually appears within 3 months of the onset of the stressor and eventually disappears after the person adapts to the stressor or it ceases. Symptoms include a depressed mood, tearfulness, hopelessness, or other symptoms in excess of a normal response to a stressor.

Supportive measures, such as information and encouragement, physical and social activities, involvement with family and friends, and environmental alterations, as well as individual and group psychotherapy, are the treatments of choice for adjustment disorders. Drugs may be used for severe depression (Kane et al., 1994).

Assessment

An accurate psychiatric and medical history is the first step in assessment for late-life depression. A chronological life review can uncover past medical illnesses or previous episodes of depression that may have an influence on the present situation. Many physical illnesses, such as hypothyroidism, Cushing's disease, cancer, brain lesions, and malnutrition, may be accompanied by depressive features. Medications can also produce symptoms of depression, especially reserpine. These treatable diseases and medication problems should be either ruled out or treated before counseling or other forms of psychiatric treatment are begun.

Depressed older persons may have a number of physical complaints. They may deny all feelings, expressing discomfort and unhappiness only as they relate to the physical and concrete. Physical complaints commonly associated with depression include insomnia, anorexia, fatigue, shortness of breath, constipation, decreased sleeping or lethargy, increased appetite, decreased sexual drive, and restlessness.

A history of the presenting complaint

should be taken to determine the duration of symptoms and whether they have occurred in the past. Precipitating events should be identified; losses and changes, such as physical illness, widowhood, or retirement, should be noted. In addition, a determination must be made of the extent of the desire to commit suicide. Older people are often successful at suicide and may attempt a form of "passive suicide" by not eating or not taking medicine.

A mental status examination is useful for determining the confusion and disorientation that may accompany depression in older age. When a mental status examination is conducted, depressed older people may know the answers to questions but may respond by saying "I don't know." This may be due to lack of interest in answering or an inability to decide on an answer. Conversely, older persons with organic brain disease who are confused often make up answers rather than admit that they cannot remember.

Appearance and functional status should also be assessed. Depressed older persons may appear sad, burdened, unkempt, drab, tired, or underweight. They may be disinterested in caring for their personal appearance, dressing, keeping clean, or taking care of their immediate environment. Lack of interest and motivation in the daily effort of self-medication for chronic diseases such as diabetes, hypertension, and heart disease can be fatal. Lack of interest in personal hygiene activities may also increase the possibility of physical health problems. Depressed older persons may lose confidence in their ability to manage personal and financial affairs. They may literally feel that they cannot do anything, and even making out a grocery list and going to the store may seem to be insurmountable challenges.

Many instruments have been designed to assess depression in people of all ages, and most have been modified for use in the elderly. These tools are controversial because they do not detect the levels of depression in older people that clinicians seem to observe. Some of the scales are based on classic physical symptoms of depression, which may be normal concomitants of older age. Researchers are continuing to explore better and more exact ways to assess depression in the elderly.

Treatment

If the depression is severe enough that the older clients are losing weight, seem agi-

TABLE 16-7
Potential Side Effects of Tricyclic Antidepressants

Anticholinergic
Dry mouth
Blurred vision (impairment of lens accommodation)
Acute angle-closure glaucoma (unusual)
Constipation, fecal impaction, incontinence
Reflux esophagitis (diminished esophageal sphincter tone)
Urinary retention, overflow incontinence
Tachycardia
Psychosis ("anticholinergic crisis")

Cardiovascular
Postural hypotension
Decreased myocardial contractility
Prolonged cardiac conduction
Tachycardia
Exacerbation of angina or heart failure

Central Nervous System
Sedation
Cognitive impairment
Psychosis

From Kane, R.L., Ouslander, J.G. and Abrass, I.B. *Essentials of Clinical Geriatrics*, 3rd ed. New York: McGraw-Hill, 1994. Reproduced with permission of McGraw-Hill, Inc.

tated or retarded, feel suicidal, or have delusions or hallucinations, they almost certainly need to be medicated and, often, hospitalized. Drug therapy is effective in treating depression, and tricyclic antidepressants such as imipramine (Tofranil) and doxepin (Sinequan) are frequently used for older persons. Because older people are particularly sensitive to the effects of drugs, lower doses must be used (usually about one third of the usual adult dose). In addition, caregivers must be alert to signs of side effects that frequently occur, especially the anticholinergic symptoms associated with tricyclics, such as urinary retention, severe constipation, and orthostatic hypotension. Potential side effects of tricyclic antidepressants are listed in Table 16–7.

Many new drugs and treatments for depression have emerged during the past decade. New classes of tricyclic secondary amines, such as nortriptyline (Aventyl), protriptyline (Vivactil), and desipramine (Norpramin), have fewer side effects than the traditional tricyclics. Tetracyclics, trazodone, and fluoxetine are other drugs that have been successful in treating depression in late life.

Although it is not usually used until after a drug trial, ECT may be a treatment of choice for depressed older persons. The treatment is carried out in an inpatient setting and can be safer than long-term drug therapy. Major complications of ECT are not common but do include post-shock confusion and cardiac problems.

Whether medications, ECT, or hospitalization is used, some kind of talking therapy—either psychotherapy or supportive counseling—should be carried out. It must be kept in mind that depressed persons are sensitive to rejection and disapproval; therefore, formation of a therapeutic alliance is of utmost importance. Older depressed persons should be encouraged to replace lost objects by allowing other things and people to have meaning for them. However, this should not be done until grieving for the lost object has been completed. The supportive environment can also be increased and strengthened, using assistance from family and social supports. Group therapy or counseling can be helpful in strengthening support systems and helping older persons to work through their depression (Buckwalter, 1990).

Suicide

Suicide is a most unfortunate outcome of late-life depression. Suicide is a more frequent cause of death among the elderly than among any other age group, particularly among white men (U.S. Dept. of Health and Human Services, 1991) (Fig. 16–5). Suicide rates for African-American men older than 85 have tripled during the past 25 years (Blazer, 1991). The method used most frequently is firearms, usually handguns, and men are six times more likely to use a gun to commit suicide than are women. Of all suicide attempts, those involving firearms are most likely to result in death. Interestingly, individuals older than 65 are more likely than any other age group to commit suicide with firearms, even more so than adolescents and young adults (Kaplan et al., 1994).

Risks for suicide in older adults include age (75+), race (white), gender (male), living alone, comorbid physical and psychiatric illness, divorce, widowhood or bereavement, alcohol or drug problems, low income, and a history of suicide attempts (Blazer, 1993; Schmid et al., 1994; Kane et al., 1994) (Table 16–8). It has been estimated that depression is present in 60 to 80 per cent of older adults who commit suicide (Finkel, 1990).

Suicide can be masked as indirect self-destructive behavior. Examples of self-destructive behavior in the elderly are withdrawal from the social environment, disregard or abuse of health, and refusal to accept medical treatment. Some older patients have "a will to die," and they often die sooner than would be expected given their medical diagnoses. They may refuse to eat, not take medication, fail to follow specific orders, or smoke or drink alcohol against medical advice (Finkel, 1990).

Older adults may give clues to suicide, which may be classified as verbal, behavioral, situational, or syndromatic. Verbal clues may be direct, "I am going to kill myself," or indirect, "I just don't want to go on anymore." Behavioral clues indicate a history of suicide attempts. The majority of older people who attempt suicide kill themselves within 1 to 2 years after a suicide attempt. Other behavioral clues in later life that may indicate suicide ideation are changes in self-care; changes in social activities; and relationships that become hostile, angry, and argumentative. Indirect behavioral clues include making or altering a will, arranging for one's funeral, obtaining a weapon or means to commit suicide, and putting one's affairs in order.

Situational clues to suicide include death of a spouse, relative, or friend; development of a significant illness; a recent move to a new residence; and deterioration of relationships. A significant syndromatic clue is the presence of depression, especially with agitation or severe guilt. People who are recovering from depression are at particularly high risk for committing suicide because as the depressed mood lifts, the person has greater energy (Finkel, 1990).

Elders at risk for suicide should be asked

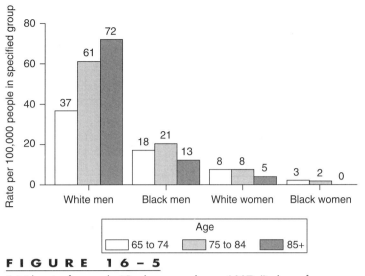

FIGURE 16 – 5

Suicide rates for people 65+, by age and race: 1987. (Redrawn from United States Department of Health and Human Services. *Aging America: Trends and Projections.* Washington, DC, 1991.)

TABLE 16-8
Factors Associated with Suicide in the Elderly

FACTOR	HIGH RISK	LOW RISK
Sex	Male	Female
Religion	Protestant	Catholic or Jewish
Race	White	Nonwhite
Marital status	Widowed or divorced	Married
Occupational background	Blue-collar, low-paying job	Professional or white-collar job
Current employment status	Retired or unemployed	Employed full- or part-time
Living environment	Urban Living alone Isolated Recent move	Rural Living with spouse or other relatives Living in close-knit neighborhood
Physical health	Poor health Terminal illness Pain and suffering	Good health
Mental health	Depression (current or previous) Alcoholism Low self-esteem Loneliness Feeling rejected, unloved	Happy and well adjusted Positive self-concept and outlook Sense of personal control over life
Personal background	Broken home Dependent personality History of poor interpersonal relationships Family history of mental illness Poor marital history Poor work record	Intact family of origin Independent, assertive, flexible personality History of close friendships No family history of mental illness No previous suicide attempts No history of suicide in family Good marital history Good work record

From Kane, R.L., Ouslander, J.G. and Abrass, I.B. *Essentials of Clinical Geriatrics,* 3rd ed. New York: McGraw-Hill, 1994. Reproduced with permission of McGraw-Hill, Inc.

directly whether they are contemplating suicide. Additional questions about the seriousness of the plan in relation to the availability of the means, details of time and place, and feasibility should be asked.

Interventions are geared toward reducing or eliminating the risk and then treating the underlying depression, if present. Removing the weapon or medications from the person at risk is the first step. Other people may be needed to monitor the potentially suicidal person. Individual and group psychotherapy, family therapy, pharmacotherapy, or ECT may be used to treat the depression. Liptzin (1991) has listed do's and don't's in

the treatment of elderly suicidal persons (Table 16–9).

Substance Abuse

Alcohol Abuse

According to the United States Department of Health and Human Services' National Institute on Alcohol Abuse and Alcoholism, alcoholism is a condition resulting from excessive ingestion of or idiosyncratic reaction to alcohol. Acute alcoholism is a state of acute intoxication with temporary and reversible mental and bodily effects; chronic alcoholism is the fact and consequence of habitual use. Problem drinkers are those who drink enough to cause problems for themselves and society.

The American Society of Addiction Medicine (1990) has proposed a definition of alcoholism that incorporates the disease concept and the multiple etiological factors suspected of contributing to the problem: "*Alcoholism* is a primary, chronic disease with psychosocial and environmental factors influencing its development and manifestations. The disease is often progressive and fatal. It is characterized by continuous or periodic impaired control over drinking, preoccupation with the drug alcohol, use of alcohol despite adverse consequences, and

TABLE 16-9
Do's and Don't's in Treatment of Elderly Suicidal Persons

Do
Arrange for a psychiatric evaluation
Hospitalize, even involuntarily, when there is a clear threat of suicide
Treat depression aggressively
Use neuroleptics or electroconvulsive therapy if delusions are present
Provide maintenance treatment
Treat associated alcohol or drug abuse
Treat associated personality disorder
Treat associated medical conditions
Monitor closely
Insist that firearms be removed
Try to increase social supports
Consult with colleagues
Thoroughly document assessment and treatment

Don't
Worry about offending the person by suggesting a psychiatric evaluation or admission
Undertreat the depression
Give prescriptions with amounts of medication that could be lethal in overdoses
Hesitate to use electroconvulsive therapy, even involuntarily with a court order

From Liptzin, B. The treatment of depression in older suicidal patients. *J Geriatr Psychiatry* 24:203–215, 1991.

distortions in thinking, most notably denial" (p. 3).

It is often difficult to detect alcoholism in older adults on the basis of standard definitions of the problem. Older adults may exhibit symptoms of alcoholism, such as memory loss and tremors, that mimic normal aging changes. Related health and financial problems that are indicators of alcoholism in a younger population frequently occur among the elderly. Employment problems do not emerge because most elders are retired. In addition, many older alcoholics drink in isolation, so the problem is often hidden (Marcus, 1993).

According to most surveys, at least 10 per cent of the population older than 65 has some form of drinking problem, and about half of these are alcohol dependent. Men are two to six times more likely to have documented alcohol problems than are women, especially young-old men. The incidence of problem drinking and heavy drinking declines sharply after age 70, and the proportion of abstainers increases with age. In a national cooperative Epidemiologic Catchment Area study conducted to determine prevalence of actual diagnoses of alcoholism according to DSM-III-R criteria, it was found that prevalence rates were higher for younger than for older adults and for men than for women. In addition, the remission rates rose consistently with increasing age (Robins et al., 1988; Miller, 1991).

It is thought that the apparent decline in heavy drinking with age is largely due to early morbidity and mortality associated with alcoholism. One difficulty in detecting the incidence of alcohol abuse in the elderly is the apparent lack of sampling among older drinkers in alcohol studies and the reluctance or inability of older adults to accurately report alcohol intake. Cross-sectional studies may not separate cohort effects from age effects, so that drinking habits may reflect the drinking-related social norms that prevailed in young adulthood rather than a decline with age (Bienenfeld, 1990; Atkinson et al., 1992).

There are two types of alcoholism in older age: (1) long-time alcoholism, i.e., those who have been lifelong alcoholics and have grown old; and (2) later-life alcoholism, i.e., those who become alcoholics in later life. About two thirds of elderly alcoholics belong to the first group (Beresford and Gordis, 1992). Controversy exists over what causes alcoholism, but major theories include genetic determination, a learned adaptation to psychological stress, and a reflection of various social conditions. Factors that

TABLE 16-10
Risk Factors for Alcohol Abuse in the Elderly

Demographic Factors
Male gender (alcohol, illicit substances)
Female gender (sedative-hypnotics)

Substance-Related Factors
Prior substance abuse
Family history (alcohol)

Increased Biological Sensitivity
Drug sensitivity
    Pharmacokinetic factors
    Pharmacodynamic factors
Medical illnesses associated with aging
    Cognitive loss
    Cardiovascular disease
    Metabolic disorders

Iatrogenic Factors
Prescription drug dependence
Drug-drug and alcohol-drug interactions
Caregiver overuse of *as needed* medication
Physician's advice or permission to use alcohol

Psychosocial Factors
Loss and other major life stress
Discretionary time, money
Social isolation
Family collusion

Psychiatric Factors
Depression
Dementia
Subjective symptoms of chronic illness

Cohort and Period Effects

From Atkinson, R.M., Ganzini, L. and Bernstein, M.J. Alcohol and substance-use disorders in the elderly. In Birren, J.E., Sloane, R.B. and Cohen, G.D. (eds.). *Handbook of Mental Health and Aging*, 2nd ed. San Diego: Academic Press, 1992, p. 520.

tend to promote alcohol abuse among the elderly are retirement, losses associated with the death of family and friends, poor health and discomfort, and loneliness. Risk factors for alcohol abuse in the elderly are listed in Table 16-10.

Alcohol seems to have unusual effects on older people, and they seem to be less tolerant of lower doses of alcohol. Not only are they more severely impaired after drinking, but they also recover more slowly. Alcoholism is especially detrimental to older people because (1) their blood levels of ethanol are higher than those in younger persons, and their brain neurons may be more sensitive to the drug; (2) ethanol can disturb their sleep and sexual performance; (3) their cognitive functions may be significantly impaired by ethanol; and (4) for older persons who take a variety of drugs, ethanol and drug interactions are particularly hazardous.

Moderate drinking (about 2 ounces per day) is thought to be healthful for older individuals; however, not all people can limit themselves to moderate drinking, and these people may have physical and mental problems from alcohol abuse. More alcohol drinking among older men accounts for higher rates of cirrhosis of the liver than is seen in women. Alcohol can cause permanent damage to cardiovascular functioning and the nervous system. Hypertension, cardiomyopathy with heart failure, irregularities in cardiac rhythm, and rapid heat loss because of vasodilation are problems associated with impaired cardiovascular functioning. A decrease in brain cells and enlargement of the ventricles can produce a loss of cognitive ability and, after prolonged alcohol abuse, dementia may develop (Thibault and Maly, 1993; Mathwig and D'Arcangelo, 1992).

Functional status can be seriously affected by alcoholism in the elderly, who are at risk for falls and other accidents, malnutrition, poor hygiene, and an inability to live alone. Transportation can be a problem, especially in relation to automobile driving. Family and social relationships are often affected, so that the older alcoholic may become increasingly isolated. Social isolation can produce sensory deficits and, along with the increased risk of mental confusion and dementia, can greatly increase the risk of institutionalization.

Alcohol withdrawal may occur within several hours after cessation of drinking in an alcohol-dependent older person. The major signs and symptoms are coarse tremors of the hands, tongue, or eyelids, along with nausea and vomiting; malaise; autonomic hyperactivity with rapid pulse, sweating, or increased blood pressure; anxiety, depression or irritability; and postural hypotension. Sleep is frequently fitful, with dreams that may merge into illusions or hallucinations. Withdrawal symptoms usually last 5 to 7 days, but the symptoms can last 2 to 3 weeks in the elderly.

Delirium tremens, now called alcohol withdrawal delirium, can begin 2 to 3 days after drinking cessation. In older people, alcohol withdrawal delirium can begin as late as the tenth day. Signs and symptoms include grand mal seizures, vivid and delirious hallucinations, and confusion. If treated, the delirium lasts about 2 or 3 days; if untreated, there may be a 15 per cent mortality rate.

Korsakoff's disease, which is related to thiamine deficiency, may develop after an episode of Wernicke's encephalopathy associated with acute and chronic alcoholism. Korsakoff's disease is an alcohol amnesia disorder with symptoms of confusion, memory deficits, staggering gait, eye movement problems, and other neurological signs. The disorder usually persists indefinitely (Solomon et al., 1993).

Drug Abuse

Older adults are at high risk for drug misuse and abuse. Drug *misuse* may be intentional or unintentional in the elderly and is defined as the underuse, overuse, or erratic

TABLE 16–11
Patterns of Drug Misuse in the Elderly

PATTERN OF USE	POSSIBLE CAUSE
Overuse	Deliberate: believe more will help
	Accidental: forgot that medication was already taken
Underuse	Forgetfulness
	Stretching the prescription for financial reasons
	No symptoms, therefore no drug needed
Erratic use	Both underuse and overuse apply

From Chenitz, W.C., Salisbury, S. and Stone, J.T. Drug misuse and abuse in the elderly. *Issues Ment Health Nurs* 11:1–16, 1990. Reproduced with permission of Taylor & Francis, Inc., Washington, D.C. All rights reserved.

use of a drug. *Abuse* is the use of a drug for other than the intended purpose and, in older adults, may constitute extreme cases of drug misuse. Drug misuse occurs when the risks of taking the medication as prescribed outweigh the benefits. Misuse may be in the form of overdosage, self-selection of medication, medication omission or duplication, automatic refills, medications taken on an as-needed basis, exchange of drugs with others, inappropriate prescriptions, and prescriptions by telephone. The possible causes for misuse are listed in Table 16–11 (Chenitz et al., 1990).

Illicit drug use ("street drugs" such as opiates and psychostimulants) is virtually nonexistent in the elderly population. However, prescription drug use is widespread, and older people are the largest consumers of legal drugs. Although people older than 65 represent 11 per cent of the population, they account for approximately 25 to 30 per cent of all prescription medications. In addition, the elderly are the largest users of sedative-hypnotic agents and benzodiazepines (Blazer, 1993; Miller, 1991; Chenitz et al., 1990; Montamat and Cusack, 1992). In a study of prescription drug abuse in community-residing elders, Jinks and Raschko (1990) found that the three most abused drugs were codeine, meprobamate, and flurazepam. Ninety-two per cent of the subjects were found to have a duration of prescription drug abuse in excess of 5 years.

Older adults have a high use of over-the-counter (OTC) medications, which tends to increase with age. Analgesics are the most popular OTC medications among community-residing elderly, whereas the use of psychoactive drugs is less common than the use of prescription medications with the same effects. Sleep medications contain antihistamines or anticholinergic agents, and many other combination drugs contain ingredients such as alcohol, caffeine, and antihistamines. All of these ingredients can produce side effects when used either alone or in combination with other prescription or nonprescription medications (Bienenfeld, 1990; Atkinson et al., 1992). Table 16–12 lists adverse effects of commonly used OTC medications.

Assessment

A thorough history is useful in detecting both alcohol and drug abuse. Older people may tend to hide their drinking habits and may be unaware of their overuse of medications. They may also think that drinking beer or wine rather than hard liquor does not produce alcohol-related problems, so these substances may not be mentioned in the history. Specific information must be gathered regarding types of liquor and drugs used. In addition, alcohol often interacts with drugs, so that their combined use can either potentiate or negate the action of many medications. A good history can help sort out these problems.

A physical examination and mental status examination can detect many signs and symptoms of drug and alcohol abuse. Tremors, alcohol on the breath, red palms, and an enlarged liver are physical signs suggestive of alcoholism; confusional states can indicate problems with either drug or alcohol abuse. Laboratory tests that are useful for detecting alcohol-related problems include blood sugar, liver function, electrolytes, serum magnesium (often low in chronic alcoholics), serum proteins, and folic acid. Sometimes an electroencephalogram or computed tomographic scan is done to detect diffuse brain damage or subdural hematoma from a fall (Blazer, 1993; Thibault and Maly, 1993; Atkinson et al., 1992).

A home visit can be most effective in detecting drug and alcohol abuse. All drugs and labels should be identified, including date of prescription and physician. A good detective can identify the various physicians who are used and the pattern of visits. Telltale signs of alcohol use can also be explored, albeit judiciously, because many alcoholics hide their liquor and become hostile if discovered.

Treatment

Because alcoholism is a complex psychosocial and physical problem, successful treatment is sometimes difficult. However, it has been found that treatment for older people

TABLE 16–12
Adverse Effects of Over-the-Counter Medications

AGENT	FOUND IN	ADVERSE EFFECTS
Salicylates	Analgesics and cold preparations	Acute: central nervous system stimulation, then depression; dizziness, hearing loss, tinnitus, nausea, and vomiting Chronic: dementia with psychosis, seizures, and hemiplegia
Antihistamines	Cold, allergy, and sleep preparations	Sedation Central anticholinergic syndrome: delirium; tachycardia; fever; and hot, dry, and flushed skin
Sympathomimetics (e.g., phenylpropanolamine)	Diet pills and cold and allergy preparations	Agitation, delirium, hallucinations, panic, insomnia, headache, tachycardia, and hypertension
Belladonna alkaloids (e.g., scopolamine)	Antidiarrheal, cold, and sleep preparations	Central anticholinergic syndrome (see antihistamines)
Phenacetin	Analgesics	Hemolysis, anemia, and renal papillary necrosis
Dextromethorphan	Cold preparations	Depression and seizures

From Bienenfeld, D. Substance abuse. In Bienenfeld, D. (ed.). *Verwoerdt's Clinical Geropsychiatry*, 3rd ed. Baltimore: Williams & Wilkins, 1990, p. 176. Copyright Williams & Wilkins, 1990.

is at least as successful as and often more successful than for younger people. The goal is always complete sobriety and abstinence. Treatment is carried out in several stages that involve attention to the patient's physical and psychological condition: (1) abstinence and medical detoxification, and treatment of milder withdrawal syndromes; (2) admission or acceptance of the concept that alcoholism is a disease; (3) compliance with treatment measures such as attendance in a 12-step program; (4) acceptance by persons that they are addicted to alcohol; and (5) surrender or maintenance of sobriety (Solomon et al., 1993).

For some older people, hospitalization or other institutional care is best for detoxification, because many of them are malnourished and have multiple medical problems. Treatment of withdrawal symptoms begins with administration of a depressant drug with properties similar to those of alcohol, then gradual withdrawal of the drug. Either short- or long-acting benzodiazepines are the drugs of choice. Older patients should also receive 100 mg of thiamine as well as multivitamins daily. Maintenance of hydration by means of either intravenous or oral intake is important, and fluid and electrolyte loss should be monitored (Miller, 1991). Good medical, nursing, and nutritional care should be carried out. Safety measures, especially when the older clients are experiencing seizures or delirium, should also be carried out.

Older people are less likely to receive specialized inpatient or outpatient treatment specifically directed toward their substance abuse. After detoxification has been completed, elders should be encouraged to participate in self-help groups such as Alcoholics Anonymous. Usually when they participate in formal programs such as these, they tend to be more responsive and more faithful in attendance. They should not be forced to join a group, however, especially one that is made up mostly of young people (Thibault and Maly, 1993; Blazer, 1993; Moos et al., 1993). One successful program for elderly substance abusers was established to provide an intervention that uses strategies employed by current treatment facilities combined with knowledge of and respect for normal aging changes. Called the Elders Health Program, the program is designed to offer education about chemical dependency and encourage change in substance use by elders that would ultimately lead to a healthier lifestyle. It was found that all older people have a network that can be employed or created to effect change, and older substance abusers are able to benefit from the intervention process (Lindblom et al., 1992).

Treatment for drug abuse can be as sophisticated as managing physical and psychological withdrawal symptoms or as simple as drug teaching and management. Old drugs and OTC medications should be destroyed, and various physicians should be advised of doctor-shopping and drug use behaviors. Families must be apprised of the risks involved in drug abuse and can be taught to help with drug administration and to look for signs of misuse.

Anxiety and Somatoform Disorders

Anxiety Disorders

Anxiety is a symptom and a category of disorders within DSM-IV. Anxiety as a symptom affects between 10 and 20 per cent of community-residing elderly. The DSM-IV category of primary anxiety disorders includes generalized anxiety disorder, panic disorder, phobias, and obsessive-compulsive disorder. The overall incidence of anxiety disorders in older age is relatively low, and they are more likely to appear in early life to midlife than later. However, one category, phobic disorders, frequently develops in

older adults, especially older women. Panic and obsessive-compulsive disorders are rare in older persons. People in whom an anxiety disorder develops in later life tend to have more feelings of loneliness, more actual physical illness, more difficulty caring for themselves, and fewer hobbies than those who have symptoms earlier (U'Ren, 1990; McCullough, 1992; Ruskin, 1990b); Abrams, 1991).

Anxiety

Anxiety as a symptom is defined as a subjective emotional state characterized by apprehension, fear, worry, and concern, accompanied by objective symptoms of autonomic nervous arousal such as sweating, heart palpitations, and discomfort in the pit of the stomach. It is often related to other psychiatric or physical conditions. Older people may worry about physical illness, crime, financial problems, institutionalization, dependency, senility, and loneliness. Much of their worry is related to feelings of vulnerability associated with the limitations of older age. Anxiety is frequently associated with depression and other psychiatric disorders. Studies of elders presenting with depression indicate that between 72 and 96 per cent had accompanying anxiety symptoms (Coplan and Gorman, 1990). Physical conditions associated with anxiety include cardiopulmonary problems such as coronary insufficiency, recurrent pulmonary emboli, and chronic pulmonary disease; endocrine disorders such as hypoglycemia and hyperthyroidism; and dementia, medications, nutritional deficiency, chronic pain, and carcinoma.

Treatment of anxiety symptoms depends on the cause. Benzodiazepines are usually the treatment of choice, but they must be used cautiously with older adults. Antidepressants are used when anxiety accompanies a depression. When stress or social problems have caused the anxiety, simply listening to the older person's problems may be therapeutic. Supportive therapy and relaxation techniques are also helpful (Bienenfeld, 1990; U'Ren, 1990; McCullough, 1992).

Anxiety States

Generalized anxiety disorder is characterized by excessive or unrealistic worry and anxiety that persists at least 6 months and is accompanied by motor tension, restlessness, autonomic hyperactivity, apprehension, irritability, vigilance, and difficulty sleeping. Treatment is the same as the treatment for anxiety as a symptom.

Panic disorder consists of discrete, brief (less than 30 minutes) episodes of recurrent, intense feelings of terror that occur spontaneously and are accompanied by physical symptoms such as chest pain, palpitations, choking, and fear of dying. Panic disorder is best treated with tricyclic antidepressants, monoamine oxidase (MAO) inhibitors, and benzodiazepines. However, tricyclic antidepressants are usually favored over the others because of the dietary restrictions with MAO inhibitors and the risk of dependence and withdrawal with benzodiazepines.

Phobias are persistent, irrational fears of specific objects or situations that lead to avoidance. Phobic disorders consist of three types: agoraphobia, social phobia, and simple phobia. Agoraphobia involves places that are perceived as possible entrapments when the person is either alone or in public places; social phobia involves the possibility of public humiliation or embarrassment; and simple phobia focuses on a simple object or situation. Panic attacks are often associated with agoraphobia. Older individuals are frequently socially isolated for a number of reasons, but it is important to assess for the possibility of some type of phobia as the cause. It is also important to assess whether fears such as going outside are justified (e.g., in high-crime areas). Management of phobias is multifaceted. The usual treatment involves behavior therapy with increasing exposure to the phobic stimulus. However, limitations in instrumental and physical ADLs that often accompany older age must be considered. An active approach must often be taken, such as arranging for transportation to social events. Antidepressants are usually the medications of choice for treatment of phobic disorders.

Obsessive-compulsive disorder is characterized either by obsessive and persistent ideas or thoughts or by compulsive, repetitive, seemingly purposeful behavior. The disorder rarely begins in older age; however, older individuals who experienced the disorder earlier in life may have a serious worsening of their condition in older age. Obsessive-compulsive states are often associated with depression, so treatment of symptoms is usually the treatment of clinical depression (McCullough, 1992; U'Ren, 1990; Bienenfeld, 1990).

Somatoform Disorders

Hypochondriasis is "the preoccupation with the fear of having, or the idea that one has, a serious disease based on the person's misinterpretation of bodily symptoms or bodily functions" (American Psychiatric As-

sociation, 1994, p. 445). It is characterized by the following traits:

1. The predominant disturbance is an unrealistic interpretation of physical signs or sensations that are abnormal and that lead to a preoccupation with the fear or belief of having a disease.
2. There must be an absence of physical disease that would account for the symptoms.
3. The belief must be persistent despite medical reassurance.
4. There is impairment in social, occupational, and recreational functioning.
5. The duration of the disturbance is at least 6 months (American Psychiatric Association, 1994).

The disease may appear for the first time during middle or older age and is equally common among men and women. About 10 per cent of older adults have exaggerated concern about their health. Hypochondriacal symptoms are particularly common among depressed people and those with actual medical diseases. Older people who had hypochondriasis early in life (chronic hypochondriacs) differ little from normal older adults, except they have more persistent physical complaints. Individuals with late-onset hypochondriasis more often have an actual physical illness and experience more loneliness and difficulty with self-care than normal older adults or chronic hypochondriacs do. There are several factors that may precipitate the onset of hypochondriasis at any age: (1) a stressful event that represents loss or threat, including an actual physical illness; (2) experiences earlier in life that taught the individual to use somatic symptoms as signals of distress; (3) experiences with pain or illness earlier in life; and (4) perception of the sick role as a means to obtain attention or support or to avoid demands and obligations (U'Ren, 1990).

Busse (1989) suggested four psychosocial and psychological causes that contribute to hypochondriasis in the elderly. First, symptoms may be used to explain a failure to meet personal or social expectations and to avoid or excuse recurrent failure. Second, older individuals may experience increased isolation and may respond to this isolation by withdrawing interest in those around and focusing that interest on themselves, especially the body and its functions. Third, the older adult may attempt to shift anxiety from specific psychological conflicts to a less threatening problem with a body function. Finally, older individuals may use hypochondriacal symptoms to punish themselves or to provide some type of atonement for unacceptable hostile feelings toward another person.

Secondary gains may be derived from hypochondriacal symptoms because the person may receive more attention from family and friends. In addition, the hypochondriacal person is able to assume the "sick role" and is able to avoid meeting social and other obligations (Blazer, 1990).

Hypochondriacs tend to doctor shop, and they may retain the services of a number of specialists. A major symptom of the condition is the endless discussion of every detail of every illness related to every organ system, a phenomenon often called the "organ recital." Although numerous drugs have usually been prescribed, they may have little effect in treating physical and emotional symptoms. Side effects are frequently noted, the drugs are discontinued, and new drugs are ordered (Gurian, 1991; Blazer, 1990; U'Ren, 1990; Barsky et al., 1991).

Assessment

Areas of assessment to be addressed include identification of the personal and situational factors that produce and maintain the symptomatic behaviors and assessment of the positive and negative consequences of the symptomatic behavior on day-to-day functioning.

A history of the client's symptoms is necessary to identify underlying causes and look for actual disease. In many cases, the symptoms can be linked to environmental changes, adaptation to stress, or losses. Sometimes the symptomatic responses can represent lifelong patterns of dealing with stressful situations. It is important to understand the factors that perpetuate hypochondriacal behavior and how these factors are related to achieving gains from the behavior, such as emotional gratification, support, or relief of depression. It is also important to assess the impact of the behavior on families, social supports, and members of the health care system.

Patterns of health care use should be identified, for the hypochondriacal older person may visit many physicians and health care professionals. Numerous drugs may have been prescribed, so that the older person is at risk for increasing the number of symptoms as a result of overmedication. It can be helpful to identify those health care providers who have developed a good relationship with the older client and those who have become "enemies" (Herman, 1984).

Treatment

It is generally thought that hypochondriasis is a prophylactic measure to ward off more incapacitating mental illness. According to Busse and Blazer (1980), health care providers should not directly confront older clients with their defensive systems; rather, a firm therapeutic alliance should be established that may eventually take on a psychotherapeutic cast. Clinicians should not attempt to convince clients that their symptoms or "illness" is not real, nor should they venture a diagnosis or prognosis of the condition. Instead, it should be emphasized that the individual does have a serious problem worthy of attention but that it does not appear dangerous or critical. Most hypochondriacs do not necessarily seek a cure, but they do seek understanding.

The focus of attention should be on the symptoms rather than on a causative disease. Attentive listening is imperative, and practical interventions should be offered to ease individual symptoms without any promise of marked success or total cure. This should demonstrate to the client that the problem is taken seriously while, at the same time, not reinforcing or encouraging the belief in an imaginary illness.

The client should establish a therapeutic relationship with a single care provider on a regular, ongoing basis. Visits should be frequent at the onset, then tapered off over time. The visits should take on a decidedly medical flavor, regardless of the discipline of the clinician. Trappings such as a medical office, white coat or uniform, and stethoscope can reassure the client that medical care is being provided. The focus should be on the discussion of symptoms initially, and exploration of feelings and emotions should not be forced. Casual inquiry into the client's living conditions, family, and relationships can gradually lead to a more indepth discussion of psychological issues later on.

Schizophrenia and Delusional Disorders

Schizophrenia

Approximately 1 per cent of the population suffers from schizophrenia. The condition usually develops in early life; however, a minority of people have schizophrenia after age 45. The disease is differentiated according to the age of onset: early-onset schizophrenia (EOS) and late-onset schizophrenia (LOS), formerly known as paraphrenia. More men than women suffer from EOS; more women than men suffer from LOS by a ratio of 2:1 to 10:1. It is not clear why more women than men have LOS, but some researchers think that estrogens might protect premenopausal women, or perhaps more women have schizophrenia late in life because they live longer.

The course of EOS is variable, but the results of several longitudinal studies have indicated that there appears to be a diminution of symptoms over time. One fairly common pattern is a decrease in positive symptoms such as delusions, hallucinations, and agitation, and an accentuation of negative symptoms such as blunt affect and social withdrawal. Predictors of a good outcome of the illness are good premorbid functioning, acute onset of illness, positive symptoms, and an undulating course. With the advent of new drugs to treat schizophrenia such as clozapine (Clozaril) and risperidone, there is hope for a positive outcome of the illness for greater numbers of people (Ruskin, 1990a).

Patients with EOS and LOS share similar symptoms, both positive (hallucinations, delusions, and disorganized thinking) and negative (social withdrawal, limited speech, and apparent inability to enjoy life). They also have similar deficits in verbal ability, attention, learning, abstraction, and motor skills. EOS and LOS have several differences. Most schizophrenics with onset after the age of 45 have paranoid symptoms (bizarre delusions and auditory hallucinations) and usually do not have thought disorder. Their personalities tend to remain basically unchanged from the premorbid state, although they are more likely to have premorbid schizoid and personality disorder. People with LOS are more likely to have married, held a job, and led a social life without serious problems than are people with EOS. They frequently remain clean and tidy and often are able to remain at home and carry out ADLs independently. Vision and hearing problems are more common among older schizophrenics, but they may be related more to age than to the disease state (Laitman and Davis, 1994; Jeste and Heaton, 1994; Ruskin, 1990a; Almeida et al., 1992).

Delusional Disorder

Delusional disorder, formerly known as paranoid disorder, usually begins in middle or late life. The average age of onset is 40 to 49 years in men and 60 to 69 years in women. Between 2 and 8 per cent of the

TABLE 16 – 13
Conditions in Which Paranoid Symptoms Occur in Elderly Persons

---

Organic Conditions
Delirium (any cause)
Dementia (any cause)
Auditory and visual impairment (any cause)
Stroke
Hypothyroidism and hypoparathyroidism
Head injury
Temporal lobe epilepsy
Multiple sclerosis
Vitamin B_{12} deficiency and pernicious anemia
Syphilis
Brain tumors

Drugs
Corticotropin (adrenocorticotropic hormone) and cortisone
Levodopa
Psychotropics (e.g., imipramine, benzhexol, monoamine oxidase inhibitors)
Phenytoin
Psychostimulants
Alcohol
Barbiturates
Bromides
Withdrawal from alcohol, minor tranquilizers, barbiturates, and hypnotics

Paranoid Symptoms Associated with Other Psychiatric Conditions
Mood disorders (depression, mania)
Paranoid personality disorders

Functional Paranoid States
Acute paranoid states secondary to any major procedure in hospital
Psychological stress (e.g., bereavement, loneliness, isolation)
Paraphrenia (late-onset schizophrenia)
Schizophrenics who have grown old
Monosymptomatic hypochondriacal delusions (e.g., parasitosis)

From U'Ren, R.C. Anxiety, paranoia, and personality disorders. *In* Cassell, C.K., Riesenberg, D.E., Sorenson, L.B. and Walsh, J.R. (eds.). *Geriatric Medicine,* 2nd ed. New York: Springer-Verlag, 1990, p. 495.

psychiatric population suffers from some type of paranoid symptom (Jeste et al., 1991; Ruskin, 1990a). Delusional disorder can be differentiated from paranoia, which is a symptom of a range of diseases and conditions including organic conditions, drug use, other psychiatric conditions, and functional paranoid states (Table 16–13).

Delusional disorder is characterized by nonbizarre delusions that are primarily persecutory in nature; however, other themes may emerge, such as erotomania, grandiosity, jealousy, somatic, or unspecified. The delusions involve situations that may occur in real life, such as the belief that others are conspiring against or harassing the person. Auditory and visual hallucinations are not prominent, and affective symptoms are rare. Paranoid patients are able to function well in their daily lives in all areas unrelated to the delusions. The disorder may cause family discord, especially if family members are part of the delusions (Ruskin, 1990a; U'Ren, 1990; Jeste et al., 1991; Moran and Thompson, 1990).

Assessment

Many older people who experience delusions or paranoia are never treated or hospitalized because they do not consider themselves ill. They are more likely to call the police, write to a government official, or be reported by their families or neighbors than they are to seek help on their own. Because they are brought to the health care provider by others, paranoid older people may be suspicious and hostile. It is best to be honest with them, letting them know that they are being examined to understand them and the reasons they were brought in, so that they may be helped in the best way possible.

A skillful history should be taken to determine not only the nature and scope of the problem but whether the suspicions are based in fact. A good rule of thumb for evaluating paranoid disorders is "Show me one truly paranoid person and I will show you ten who are truly persecuted" (Butler and Lewis, 1982). Because of their delusional systems, paranoid people see things differently, so the history should be obtained from both the client and some other informed individual. However, even paranoid people have enemies, and they may be within the family. If that is a possibility, it is helpful to talk to at least two family members or to some knowledgeable outside observer.

The content of the history should address the development and duration of the symptoms, the behavioral outcomes, and the effect of the behavior on daily life. Interruptions in sleeping and eating patterns, medicine taking, personal hygiene, bill paying, and relationships with the family should be noted. Peculiar behavior, such as calling the police for unfounded reasons, and violent behavior should also be noted.

A review of the past medical history, including physical illnesses, psychiatric conditions, and medications, provides important indicators for the development of paranoid ideation. A sudden onset of a paranoid delusion is suggestive of the possibility of delirium caused by physical illness or drugs. Symptoms of persecution are common in patients with dementia. Vision and hearing impairments have also been associated with paranoia. In addition, paranoid reactions may occur in relation to sensory deprivation, stress, immobility, apprehension, exhaustion, and unfamiliar surroundings.

An environmental assessment should be made, if possible, to identify real or imagined threats and safety hazards. Dangers should be identified, such as the possibility for physical violence and access to weapons. A home visit provides an excellent means of assessing the factors in the environment that may precipitate paranoid reactions (Whanger, 1984; U'Ren, 1990).

Treatment

Treatments usually prescribed for schizophrenia and delusional disorder include drugs, institutionalization, psychotherapy, and family therapy.

Neuroleptic therapy is effective for the treatment of EOS, LOS, and delusional disorder. The medication may not eliminate the paranoid beliefs entirely, but the intensity of the beliefs tends to diminish, along with the patient's likelihood of acting on them in a dangerous manner. Side effects vary with each drug and include postural hypotension, drowsiness, unsteadiness, and extrapyramidal disorders (U'Ren, 1990; Ruskin, 1990a).

Institutionalization can be effective for the treatment of acute cases of paranoia, especially if the client is extremely frightened, hostile, or suspicious in the environment. The use of drugs has alleviated much of the need for institutionalization, and outpatient treatment is preferable if possible. Psychotherapy can be effective by providing a supportive, nonthreatening environment in which paranoid clients can ventilate their fears and anxieties. Strategies for reducing perceived threats and stresses can be explored, and the client can be helped to "encapsulate" the delusional ideas so that they will be shared only with the therapist. Attempts should never be made to dissuade or confront paranoid persons with their delusions, for they will always turn to another delusion to explain their fears. An example is the 75-year-old woman who claimed to see her dead husband in a local nursing home while visiting a friend. She said that he was in a bed in the next room and was being mistreated. When the unsuspecting nurse took her into every room in the nursing home with no sign of the husband, the client said, "Well, they must have moved him to another nursing home."

Intervention for families is usually necessary because they are almost always involved in some way with the older delusional client. They may need supportive counseling because they may be the focus of the delusions or they may have reached their tolerance level. The family may need education concerning the disease, drug management, and how to approach a paranoid person. Because medication compliance is a problem with paranoid clients, families often must be responsible for administration. A home visit is useful to help the family maximize safety and minimize problems related to sensory deficits (Whanger, 1984).

Factors that predict a good outcome for LOS are immediate response to treatment, insight gained secondary to treatment, success in maintaining a longer period of drug treatment, marriage, younger age, and good premorbid relationships predicting cooperation during maintenance treatment. The outcome for older patients with delusional disorder is good in that most are discharged from hospitals back to the community, with fewer rehospitalizations than occur with schizophrenics. Patients with LOS and delusional disorder are equally able to function occupationally and socially despite their symptoms (Laitman and Davis, 1994; U'Ren, 1990).

PSYCHOSOCIAL ASSESSMENT OF THE ELDERLY

The purpose of psychosocial assessment is to characterize the client's functioning in a particular social environment. The principles that govern psychosocial assessment of the aged are the same as those for the conduct of any assessment of an older person. The clinician should consider pace, client fatigue, trust, validation of information with other sources, and the purposes for which the assessment is being made when selecting assessment techniques. In addition, knowledge of the most prevalent psychosocial problems encountered by older persons and their families, as well as knowledge of typical potential areas for growth, should guide the assessment.

It is difficult to compare psychosocial assessment data with normal standards for older people, mainly because the literature on aging presents conflicting findings regarding normal behavior. Norms are constantly changing for older people as more reach an advanced age and as ageist assumptions and practices of Western society are challenged. In addition, previously accepted norms for the elderly were based on cross-sectional rather than longitudinal stud-

ies; therefore, the findings may not apply to present and future cohorts of the aged.

Elements

Psychosocial assessment should include the individual, the family, and the community, with consideration for the cultural environment. Essential content in assessment of the *individual* includes

- Perception of current life situation
- Current roles and recent role changes
- Lifestyle
- Cultural background
- Location/residence
- Financial resources
- Mental status
- Goals and plans for the future

Essential content in the assessment of *family and significant others* includes

- Perception of the family or caregiver of the client's life situation and goals
- Family structure
- Family patterns of functioning
- Roles of client's significant others

Essential content in the assessment of the client's *community* includes

- Special resources in the current environment/community
- Special demands of the current environment/community

These elements of assessment are discussed in the context of three different types of assessment: screening, comprehensive assessment, and problem-specific assessment.

Screening

The purpose of screening is to identify potential client, family, or community attributes that may signify a need for either preventive action or treatment. Screening may be problem oriented, or it may identify potential for growth in some area of function. The emphasis on particular psychosocial screening techniques varies with the expectations of the health care setting, the perspective from which the nurse practices, and the purpose for the screening examination. In all health care settings, a wellness focus can be maintained, along with an illness perspective.

During the screening process, it is important to determine whether an individual has certain prevalent problems related to aging, such as depression, substance abuse, and elder abuse. Because the current population of elderly matured in an era when psychological problems were not openly discussed or acknowledged, it is sometimes difficult to detect whether they exist. However, simple screening maneuvers are useful, such as drug and alcohol histories; depression questionnaires; and observation of appearance, hygiene, and dress.

Psychological or social barriers may exist that interfere with achieving nursing care goals. These should be assessed during the screening process. These barriers may be economic, attitudinal, or cultural. Examples of economic barriers are insufficient funds with which to purchase medicines, equipment, food, or transportation to medical facilities; inability to pay for medical or nursing care; and lack of financial coverage for rehabilitation. Attitudinal barriers are related to health beliefs that interfere with prescribed medical or health care regimens, family issues that prevent rehabilitative measures because of the need to maintain dependence in the older member, or beliefs about services provided that may be viewed as "charity." Cultural barriers are related to religious, racial, or ethnic issues. Beliefs of older persons of particular racial or ethnic groups regarding the medical and health care system or its providers may lead to what appears to be "lack of compliance." Religious beliefs may also interfere with the carrying out of various medical and self-care regimens.

Mechanics of Screening and Assessment

At a screening level, the interview/assessment is necessarily superficial. In many cases, information may be gained through a social, conversational manner to put older clients at ease. An informal format is usually preferable to a structured interview, especially with older people who may be uncomfortable discussing psychological or social issues.

The interview should begin with open-ended questions and should focus on matters of primary importance to the client. This allows the client the opportunity to discuss issues of greatest concern and reinforces the impression that the nurse is truly concerned with the major problems. The following screening questions are particularly helpful in eliciting psychosocial data:

1. In a clinical setting with a high proportion of low-income elderly, ask whether *income* is sufficient to provide needed groceries, drugs, and medical supplies.

2. If the individual lives alone and volunteers no information about family or friends, determine whether the person has a close friend or family member who acts as a *confidant*. A confidant increases life satisfaction.

3. If the older person has obvious dependencies, note on the first encounter who is *assisting with care* and who else in the family or friendship network is available to provide assistance.

4. Identify any *major life changes* that have occurred within the past year and chart the dates of key life events, such as retirement, widowhood, death of close friends, and anniversaries.

5. By asking an older person to *describe a typical day*, it is possible to gain insight into role relationship patterns, self-concept, and demands of daily living.

6. Because many values and beliefs regarding health, illness, aging, and dying are culturally determined, it is beneficial to note the *racial and ethnic background* of an individual. Older persons are closer to their culture of origin than the young, and membership in a particular cultural group may influence health beliefs or self-care practices.

7. Finding out the *religious background* of an older person can assist in determining whether spiritual distress is being experienced. National survey data have shown that the current cohort of old people is more likely to be a part of organized religion than younger persons. Religious organizations may also provide an important source of informal support.

8. *Note recent losses,* because a high number of losses in a short amount of time can predispose to illness, including depression, in all ages.

9. Asking *what the client does for pleasure* is helpful in indicating whether depression is present. An inability to enjoy life is one of the cardinal symptoms of depression, and the individual who is unable to describe any pleasurable activity should be assessed further.

10. *Employment status* and *work history* should be assessed, including year of retirement, if applicable. This helps prevent inaccurate stereotyping of older people as universally retired and also identifies current roles that may be affected by an illness status.

After a screening, in-depth data gathering may be indicated. The nurse should judge the timing and depth of further assessment. Generally, primary care or continuing care nurses should prepare a comprehensive data base for their clients. Nurses in acute care settings will probably do so only if psychosocial problems affect the handling of an acute problem or result in discharge difficulties.

Comprehensive Psychosocial Assessment

The major areas to be addressed in a comprehensive psychosocial assessment are economic situation, role relationship patterns, sexuality, coping and stress tolerance, health perception, and value/belief patterns. The data may be gathered in a conversational style; sometimes structured questioning of the individual or a significant other may be necessary.

Economics

For any older individual in need of long-term care, economic assessment is essential. Most people who are retired are faced with diminished income and, at the same time, may encounter markedly increased expenditures for medical care. Long-term care services are costly and frequently not covered by insurance or Medicare. Failure to acknowledge economic realities impedes planning of resource allocation and may result in impoverishment without the client's goals being met.

For example, Mr. J. had always said that he would "sooner die than go to a nursing home." When he experienced inoperable lung cancer and became weak secondary to radiation therapy and the progress of his disease, his family assumed that home care would be prohibitively expensive. They arranged for admission to a skilled nursing home. He died 2 weeks later. Had his financial status been assessed, adequate financial resources to purchase 24-hour daily help for 9 months would have been found. Failure to assess his financial status thus resulted in Mr. J.'s not meeting an important goal despite adequate resources.

Role Relationship Patterns

Assessment of role relationship patterns provides information regarding self-concept and sources of social support. One method of determining the pattern of role relationships is to obtain detailed information about the day's activities. If the client is vague, this may indicate a paucity of social roles or lack of integration into the larger community. Vague responses may also indicate the presence of cognitive impairment or other mental disorders.

Sexuality

Several real or imaginary barriers may exist in assessment of the sexual patterns of older adults: generational barriers, myths about sexuality in old age, and taboos about discussion of sexual concerns. Nurses typically belong to a younger age cohort than their elderly clients, which may make discussion of sexual matters more difficult. In addition, when older persons matured, sexual mores were more restrictive and there was less explicit discussion of sexual matters. The myths that older persons are uninterested in sex, are unable to enjoy it, or are sexually inactive further complicate the issue, from both the nurse's and older person's standpoint. Not only is it believed that older people are asexual, there is also the belief that one does not discuss the issue.

Assessment of sexual patterns requires that the nurse project a nonjudgmental, matter-of-fact manner. Older clients should be asked whether they are sexually active or whether there have been recent changes in sexual patterns. If concerns about sexual function are expressed, an opportunity for further exploration is provided. In-depth assessment need not be pursued unless there is evidence of sexual dysfunction or the client is at risk for alterations in sexual function.

Coping and Stress Tolerance

Understanding an older individual's lifetime patterns of coping can greatly facilitate the planning of nursing care. It is important to know how major problems were handled in the past and how these techniques could be used to handle present and future problems. If the client has relied on family members or friends for support, are these individuals still living and in good health? How does the client typically cope with pain, uncertainty, or new situations? Does the client use alcohol or drugs to cope with stressful situations? How much does the client value religion as a means of coping with life's problems? The answers to these and similar questions affect the approach to client teaching and counseling and indicate areas of potential lifestyle modifications and growth.

Health Perception

In determining an older person's health perception, it is worthwhile to ask the following question: How do you rate your overall health—excellent, good, fair, or poor? Studies have shown that self-perception of health is significantly correlated with objective measures of health and longevity (Maddox, 1962). In addition, responses to this question may give the nurse important insight into the individual's self-concept, need for knowledge, and motivation for change. Many older individuals perceive their health as "good," despite long lists of chronic diseases; this may reflect excellent coping abilities or denial of illness.

Gordon (1982) advises asking individuals about practices they believe to be important in maintaining health, including folk remedies. They should also be asked about personal goals for health. This important step is often overlooked, resulting in frustration for clients and nurses alike. Older people do not necessarily have experience in deriving goals with their health care providers, so nurses should be prepared to explain the importance of the patient's involvement in the management and prevention of chronic disease.

Value/Belief Pattern

Maintaining certain beliefs and adhering to values may become more important as older people grow closer to death. Often, decisions about priorities in health care for dependent older people must be made; knowledge of the individual's values and beliefs is central to making these decisions in an ethical manner. Religious beliefs, concerns about dependency and control, and prolongation of life if severe functional impairment exists should be discussed with the older person and involved family members to plan thoughtfully for nursing and health care.

Problem-Specific Assessment

Assessment maneuvers for the various psychosocial problems are specified in each nursing diagnosis category included in Chapter 17.

SUMMARY

Psychosocial problems of the aged are varied in nature and often require interventions from members of different disciplines for successful resolution. Many of the social problems are not soluble without community or societal interventions. However, nurses should remain cognizant of the extent to which social problems influence the health status of older people.

The majority of people do not have psychiatric disorders in old age. However, the pervasiveness of social problems makes older people particularly vulnerable to the development of psychiatric disorders, and presentation is often atypical. The current cohort of old people is characterized as being less "psychologically minded" than today's younger adults. They are therefore less likely than younger adults to seek assistance for psychological problems. Nurses should have a higher index of suspicion for the presence of undetected psychological disorders and should be able to assess, refer, and intervene as indicated. Failure to do so may mean that older people suffer needless psychological pain or disability from undetected but treatable psychological disorders.

REFERENCES

Abrams, R. Anxiety and personality disorders. *In* Sadavoy, J., Lazarus, L.W. and Jarvik, L.F. (eds.). *Comprehensive Review of Geriatric Psychiatry*. Washington, D.C.: American Psychiatric Press, 1991.

Adelman, R.D., Fields, S.D. and Jutagir, R. Geriatric education. Part II: The effect of a well-elderly program on medical student attitudes toward geriatric patients. *J Am Geriatr Soc* 40(9):907–973, 1992.

Almeida, O.P., Howard, R., Forstl, H. and Levy, R. Should the diagnosis of late paraphrenia be abandoned? *Psychol Med* 22:11–14, 1992.

American Association of Retired Persons. *A Profile of Older Americans: 1992*. Washington, D.C.: AARP, 1993.

American Nurses' Association Committee on Skilled Nursing Care. *Nursing and Long-Term Care: Toward Quality Care for the Aging*. Kansas City, MO: American Nurses' Association, 1975. ANA Publication Code GE4-3m 4/75.

American Psychiatric Association. *Diagnostic and Statistical Manual of Mental Disorders—IV*. Washington, DC: American Psychiatric Association, 1994.

American Society of Addiction Medicine. Disease definition of alcoholism revised. *Addict Rev* 2(2):3, 1990.

Arendell, T. and Estes, C.L. Older women in the post-Reagan era. *Int J Health Serv* 21(1):59–73, 1991.

Atkinson, R.M., Ganzini, L. and Bernstein, M.J. Alcohol and substance-use disorders in the elderly. *In* Birren, J.E., Sloane R.B. and Cohen G.D. (eds.). *Handbook of Mental Health and Aging,* 2nd ed. San Diego: Academic Press, 1992, pp. 516–555.

Badger, T.A. Physical health impairment and depression among older adults. *Image* 25(4):325–330, 1993.

Barrow, G.M. and Smith, P.A. *Aging, Ageism, and Society*. St. Paul: West Publishing, 1979.

Barsky, A.J., Frank, C.B., Cleary, P.D. et al. The relation between hypochondriasis and age. *Am J Psychiatry* 148(7):923–928, 1991.

Bearon, L.B. No great expectations: The underpinnings of life satisfaction for older women. *Gerontologist* 29(6):772–778, 1989.

Beatrice, D.F. Case management: A policy option for long-term care. *In* Callahan, J.J., Jr. and Wallack, S.S. (eds.). *Reforming the Long-Term Care System*. Lexington, MA: Lexington Books, 1981.

Beeson, D. Women in studies of aging: A critique and a suggestion. *Soc Probl* 23:52–59, 1975.

Bell, J. In search of a discourse on aging: The elderly on television. *Gerontologist* 32(3):305–311, 1992.

Belling, B., Kenny, K. and Scholen, K. Home equity conversion. *Generations* 9(3):20–21, 1985.

Bengtson, V., Rosenthal, C. and Burton, L. Families and aging: Diversity and heterogeneity. *In* Binstock, R.H. and George, L.K. (eds.). *Handbook of Aging and the Social Sciences,* Vol. 3. San Diego: Academic Press, 1990, p. 263.

Bennett, C.L., Greenfield, S., Aronow, H. et al. Patterns of care related to men with prostate cancer. *Cancer* 67(10):2633–2641, 1991.

Benton, D. and Marshall, C. Elder abuse. *Clin Geriatr Med* 7(4):831–845, 1991.

Beresford, T.P. and Gordis, E. Alcoholism and the elderly patient. *In* Evans, J.G. and Williams, T.F. (eds.). *Oxford Textbook of Geriatric Medicine.* New York: Oxford University Press, 1992, pp. 639–646.

Bienenfeld, D. Substance abuse. *In* Bienenfeld, D. (ed.). *Verwoerdt's Clinical Geropsychiatry,* 3rd ed. Baltimore: Williams & Wilkins, 1990.

Binstock, R.H. The aged as scapegoat. *Gerontologist* 23(2):136–143, 1983.

Birren, J.E., Sloane, R.B. and Cohen, G.D. (eds.). *Handbook of Mental Health and Aging,* 2nd ed. San Diego: Academic Press, 1992.

Blazer, D. *Emotional Problems in Later Life.* New York: Springer Publishing Co., 1990.

Blazer, D. Suicide risk factors in the elderly: An epidemiological study. *J Geriatr Psychiatry* 24(2):175–190, 1991.

Blazer, D.G. *Depression in Late Life,* 2nd ed. St. Louis: C.V. Mosby, 1993.

Block, M. and Sinott, J. (eds.). *The Battered Elder Syndrome: An Exploratory Study.* College Park, MD: Center on Aging, University of Maryland, 1979.

Blomquist, K.B. Prevention: Older adults. *In* Knollmueller, R.N. (ed.). *Prevention Across the Life Span: Healthy People For the Twenty-First Century.* New York, American Nurses Publishing, 1993.

Boydston, L.S. and McNair, J.P. *Elder Abuse by Adult Care-takers: An Exploratory Study.* San Francisco: Select Committee on Aging—Physical and Financial Abuse of the Elderly. April 3, 1981. Publication 97–297, 1981.

Broad, J.B., Richmond, D.E. and Baskett, J.J. Dependency levels of people in aged care institutions in Auckland. *N Z Med J* 103(900):500–503, 1990.

Brown, D.S., Gardner, D.L., Perritt, L. and Kelly, D.G. Improvements in attitudes toward the elderly following traditional and geriatric mock clinics for physical therapy students. *Phys Ther* 72(4):251–257, 1992.

Buckwalter, K.C. How to unmask depression. *Geriatr Nurs* July/August: 179–181, 1990.

Burgess, J.W. A standardized mental status examination discriminating four major mental disorders. *Hosp Community Psychiatry* 43(9):937–939, 1992.

Busse, E.W. Somatoform and psychosocial disorders. *In* Busse, E.W. and Blazer, D.G. (eds.). *Geriatric Psychiatry.* Washington, D.C.: American Psychiatric Press, 1989, pp. 429–458.

Busse, E.W. and Blazer, D.G. Disorders related to biologic functioning. *In* Busse, E.W. and Blazer, D.G. (eds.). *Handbook of Geriatric Psychiatry.* New York: Van Nostrand Reinhold, 1980.

Butler, R. *Why Survive? Being Old in America.* New York: McGraw-Hill, 1975.

Butler, R.N. The poverty of living alone. *Geriatrics* 45(5), 1990.

Butler, R.N. Dispelling ageism: The cross-cutting intervention. *Generations* 17(2):75–78, 1993.

Butler, R. and Lewis, M. *Aging and Mental Health,* 3rd ed. St. Louis: C.V. Mosby, 1982.

Callahan, J.J., Jr. and Wallack, S.S. (eds.). *Reforming the Long-Term-Care System.* Lexington, MA: Lexington Books, 1981.

Cantor, M. Life space and social support. *In* Byerts, T.O. et al. (eds.). *Environmental Context of Aging.* New York: Garland STPM Press, 1979.

Carp, F. Housing and living environments of older people. *In* Binstock, R. and Shanas, E. (eds.). *The Handbook of Aging and the Social Sciences.* New York: Van Nostrand, 1976.

Carp, F.M. Lifestyle and location within the city. *In* Byerts, T.O. et al. (eds.). *Environmental Context of Aging.* New York: Garland STPM Press, 1979.

Cassel, C.K., Riesenberg, D.E., Sorensen, L.B. and Walsh, J.R. *Geriatric Medicine,* 2nd ed. New York: Springer-Verlag, 1990.

Champlin, L. Caring for older women: No more 'hand me down' medicine. *Geriatrics* 46(10):90–92, 1991.

Chenitz, W.C., Salisbury, S. and Stone, J.T. Drug misuse and abuse in the elderly. *Issues Ment Health Nurs* 11:1–16, 1990.

Clark, W.F., Pelham, A.O. and Clark, M.L. *Old and Poor: A Critical Assessment of the Low-Income Elderly.* Lexington, MA: Lexington Books, 1988.

Cohen, G. Lessons from longitudinal studies of mentally ill and mentally healthy elderly: A 17-year perspective. *In* Bergener, M. and Finkel, S.I. (eds.). *Clinical and Scientific Psychogeriatrics,* Vol. 1. New York: Springer Publishing, 1990.

Cohen, G.D. Journalistic elder abuse: It's time to get rid of fictions, get down to facts. *Gerontologist* 34(3):399–401, 1994.

Coplan, J.D. and Gorman, J.M. Treatment of anxiety disorder in patients with mood disorder. *J Clin Psychiatry* 51(10)(Suppl.):9–13, 1990.

Costa, A.J. Elder abuse. *Prim Care* 20(2):375–389, 1993.

Coyne, A.C., Reichman, W.E. and Berbig, L.J. The relationship between dementia and elder abuse. *Am J Psychiatry* 150(4):643–646, 1993.

Crowley, M. Living longer and better than expected. A wellness-based model keeps CCRC residents active, healthy, and out of nursing homes. *Health Prog* 73(10): 38–41, 1992.

Crystal, S. and Beck, P. A room of one's own: The SRO and the single elderly. *Gerontologist* 32(5):684–692, 1992.

Cullinane, P. Neighborhoods that make sense: Community allies for elders aging in place. *Generations* 16(2): 69–72, 1992.

Delunas, L.R. Prevention of elder abuse: Betty Neuman health care systems approach. *Clin Nurse Spec* 4(1):54–58, 1990.

Derby, S.E. Ageism in cancer care of the elderly. *Oncol Nurs Forum* 18(5):921–926, 1991.

Dobrof, R. Social support systems. *In* Calkins, E., Bord, A.B. and Katz, P.R. (eds.). *Practice of Geriatrics,* 2nd ed. Philadelphia: W.B. Saunders, 1992.

Dowler, J.M., Jordan-Simpson, D.A. and Adams, O. Gender inequalities in care-giving in Canada. *Health Rep* 4(2):125–136, 1992.

Ehrlich, P. and Anetzberger, G. Survey of state public health departments on procedures for reporting elder abuse. *Public Health Rep* 106(2):151–154, 1991.

Ensrud, K.E., Nevitt, M.C., Yunis, C. et al. Correlates of impaired function in older women. *J Am Geriatr Soc* 42(5):481–489, 1994.

Erikson, E. *Childhood and Society.* New York: W.W. Norton, 1963.

Falchikiov, N. Youthful ideas about old age: An analysis of children's drawings. *Int J Aging Hum Dev* 31(2): 79–99, 1990.

Ferraro, K.F. Self and older-person referents in evaluating life problems. *J Gerontol* 47:S105–S114, 1992.

Finkel, S.I. Suicide in later life. *In* Bergener, M. and Finkel, S.I. (eds.). *Clinical and Scientific Psychogeriatrics,* Vol. 1. New York: Springer Publishing, 1990.

Finkel, S.I. and Denson, M.W. Psychopathology in later life. *Compr Ther* 16(9):17–24, 1990.

Foelker, G.A., Jr., Holland, J., Marsh, M. and Simmons, B.A. A community response to elder abuse. *Gerontologist* 30(4):560–562, 1990.

Fogel, B.S. Psychological aspects of staying at home. *Generations* 16(2):15–19, 1992.

Forschner, B.E. A sense of community. Senior living communities must allow for mission, mutuality, and myth. *Health Prog* 73(5):34–37, 57, 1992.

Fulmer, T. and Birkenhauser, D. Elder mistreatment assessment as a part of everyday practice. *J Gerontol Nurs* March:42–45, 1992.

Galanos, A.N., Cohen, H.J. and Jackson, T.W. Medical education in geriatrics: The lasting impact of the aging game. *Educ Gerontol* 19:675–682, 1993.

Gamzon, M. Assisted living reigns. *Contemp Longterm Care* 16(6):30–32, 92, 94–95 passim, 1993.

George, L.K. *Social Factors and Depression in Late Life.* Paper prepared for the National Institute on Health Consensus Development Conference on the Diagnosis and Treatment of Depression in Late Life. November 4–6, 1991, Bethesda, MD.

Giles, H., Coupland, N., Coupland, J. et al. Intergenerational talk and communication with older people. *Int J Aging Hum Dev* 34(4):271–297, 1992.

Glasgow, N. Poverty among rural elders: Trends, context and directions for policy. *J Appl Gerontol* 12(3):302–319, 1993.

Gordon, M. *Nursing Diagnosis.* New York: McGraw-Hill, 1982.

Gornick, M., Greenberg, J.N., Eggers, P.W. and Dobson, A. Twenty years of Medicare and Medicaid: Covered populations, use of benefits, and program expenditures. *Health Care Financing Rev* (Suppl.):13–59, 1985.

Grembowski, D., Patrick, D., Diehr, P. et al. Self-efficacy and health behavior among older adults. *J Health Soc Behav* 34(2):89–104, 1993.

Gurian, B. Coping with hypochondriasis in older patients. *Geriatrics* 46(9):71–73, 1991.

Gurwitz, J.H., Col, N.F. and Avorn, J. The exclusion of the elderly and women from clinical trials in acute myocardial infarction. *JAMA* 268(11):1417–1422, 1992.

Hamel, M., Gold, D.P., Andres, D. et al. Predictors and consequences of aggressive behavior by community-based dementia patients. *Gerontologist* 30:206–211, 1990.

Heidrich, S.M. and Ryff, C.D. How elderly women cope: Concerns and strategies. *Public Health Nurs* 9(3):200–208, 1992.

Henderson, A.S. The epidemiology of mental disorders in elderly people. *In* Evans, J.G. and Williams, T.F. (eds.). *Oxford Textbook of Geriatric Medicine.* New York: Oxford University Press, 1992, pp. 617–620.

Henrichs, C., Roche, W. and Sirianni, C. *Working Time in Transition.* Philadelphia: Temple University Press, 1991.

Herman, S. Somatoform disorders. *In* Whanger, A.D. and Myers, A.C. (eds.). *Mental Health Assessment and Therapeutic Intervention with Older Adults.* Rockville, MD: Aspen Systems Corporation, 1984.

Hirshorn, B.A. and Hoyer, D.T. Private sector hiring and use of retirees: The firm's perspective. *Gerontologist* 34(1):50–58, 1994.

Homer, A.C. and Gilleard, C. Abuse of elderly people by their carers. *BMJ* 301(6765):1359–1362, 1990.

Howell, S. Home. *Generations* 9(3):58–60, 1985.

Hummer, M.L., Garstka, T.A., Shaner, J.L. and Strahm, S. Stereotypes of the elderly held by young, middle-aged and elderly adults. *J Gerontol* 49:P240–P249, 1994.

Jackson, J. *Minorities and Aging.* Belmont, CA: Wadsworth, 1980.

Janz, M. Clues to elder abuse. *Geriatr Nurs* Sept/Oct: 220–222, 1990.

Jarde, O., Marc, B., Dwyer, J. et al. Mistreatment of the aged in the home environment in northern France: A year survey (1990). *Med Law* 11(7–8):641–648, 1992.

Jeste, D.V. and Heaton, S. How does late-onset compare with early-onset schizophrenia? *Harv Ment Health Let* 10(8):8, 1994.

Jeste, D.V., Manley, M. and Harris, M.J. Psychoses. *In* Sadavoy, J., Lazarus, L.W. and Jarvik, L.F. (eds.). *Comprehensive Review of Geriatric Psychiatry.* Washington, D.C.: American Psychiatric Press, 1991.

Jinks, M.J. and Raschko, R.R. A profile of alcohol and prescription drug abuse in a high-risk community-based elderly population. *Ann Pharmacother* 24:971–975, 1990.

Johnson, R.J. and Wolinsky, F.D. Gender, race, and health: The structure of health status among older adults. *Gerontologist* 34(1):24–35, 1994.

Jones, P. Older patients are people first. *Health Visit* 66(6):214–215, 1993.

Kane, R.L., Ouslander, J.G. and Abrass, I.B. *Essentials of Clinical Geriatrics,* 3rd ed. New York: McGraw-Hill, 1994.

Kaplan, M.S., Adamek, M.E. and Johnson, S. Trends in firearm suicide among older American males: 1979–1988. *Gerontologist* 34(1):59–65, 1994.

Kearl, M.C. An inquiry into the positive personal and social effects of old age stereotypes among the elderly. *Int J Aging Hum Dev* 14(4):277–290, 1981–82.

Kendig, H. Comparative perspectives on housing, aging, and social structure. *In* Binstock, R.H. and George, L.K. (eds.). *Handbook of Aging and the Social Sciences.* San Diego: Academic Press, 1990.

Koff, T.H. *Case Management: A New Service for the Older Person.* Paper presented at the Twelfth Annual Symposium of the Western Division of the American Geriatric Society, October 28–29, 1983.

Kosberg, J.I. Preventing elder abuse: Identification of high risk factors prior to placement decisions. *Gerontologist* 28(1):43–50, 1988.

Kurrle, S.E., Sadler, P.M. and Cameron, I.D. Patterns of elder abuse. *Med J Aust* 157(10):673–676, 1992.

Kuypers, J.A. and Bengtson, V. Social breakdown and social competence. *Hum Dev* 16:181–201, 1973.

Lachs, M.S. and Fulmer, T. Recognizing elder abuse and neglect. *Clin Geriatr Med* 9(3):665–681, 1993.

Laitman, L.B. and Davis, K.L. Paraphrenias and other psychoses. *In* Hazzard, W.R., Bierman, E.L., Blass, J.P., et al. *Principles of Geriatric Medicine and Gerontology,* 3rd ed. New York: McGraw-Hill, 1994, pp. 1111–1117.

Laurence, L. Minority women in 'quadruple jeopardy.' Mary Harper quoted in *San Antonio Express News,* Images, June 26, 1994.

Lawton, M.P. How the elderly live. *In* Byerts, T.O. et al. (eds.). *Environmental Context of Aging.* New York: Garland STPM Press, 1979.

Lawton, M.P. Housing and living environments of older people. *In* Binstock, R. and Shanas, E. (eds.). *The Handbook of Aging and the Social Sciences,* 2nd ed. New York: Van Nostrand Reinhold, 1985, pp. 450–478.

Lawton, M.P. and Nahemow, L. Ecology and the aging process. *In* Eisdorfer, C. and Lawton, M.P. (eds.). *Psychology of Adult Development and Aging.* Washington, DC: American Psychological Association, 1973.

Learman, L.A., Avorn, J., Everitt, D.E. and Rosenthal, R. Pygmalion in the nursing home: The effect of caregiver expectations on patient outcomes. *J Am Geriatr Soc* 38(7):797–803, 1990.

Leroux, T.G. and Petrunik, M. The construction of elder abuse as a social problem: A Canadian perspective. *Int J Health Serv* 20(4):651–663, 1990.

Lindblom, L., Kostyk, D., Tabisz, E. et al. Chemical abuse: An intervention program for the elderly. *J Gerontol Nurs* April:6–14, 1992.

Liptzin, B. The treatment of depression in older suicidal patients. *J Geriatr Psychiatry* 24:203–215, 1991.

Lubomudrov, S. Congressional perceptions of the elderly: The use of stereotypes in the legislative process. *Gerontologist* 27:77–81, 1987.

MacDowell, N.M. and Clawson, K.R. Amenities that influence nursing home selection. *J Long Term Care Adm* 20(4):13–15, 1992.

Maddox, G.L. Some correlates of differences in self-assessments of health status among the elderly. *J Gerontology* 17:180–185, 1962.

Madison, D. The case for community-oriented primary care. *JAMA* 249(10):1279–1282, 1983.

Mandelblatt, J., Traxler, M., Lakin, P. et al. A nurse practitioner intervention to increase breast and cervical cancer screening for poor, elderly black women. The Harlem Study Team. *J Gen Intern Med* 8(4):173–178, 1993.

Manton, K.G., Corder, L.S. and Stallard, E. Estimates of changes in chronic disability and institutional incidence in the U.S. elderly population from the 1982, 1984, and 1989 National Long Term Care Survey. *J Gerontol* 48:S153–S166, 1993.

Marcus, M.T. Alcohol and other drug abuse in elders. *J ET Nurs* 20(3):106–110, 1993.

Mathwig, G. and D'Arcangelo, J.S. Module II.6: Drug misuse and dependence in the elderly. *In* Naegle, M.A. (ed.). *Substance Abuse Education in Nursing,* Vol. II. National League for Nursing, 1992, pp. 465–475. Publication 15–2463.

McCabe, B.W. Ego defensiveness and its relationship to attitudes of registered nurses toward older people. *Res Nurs Health* 12(2):85–91, 1989.

McCreadie, C. and Tinker, A. Review: Abuse of elderly people in the domestic setting: A UK perspective. *Age Ageing* 22(1):65–69, 1993.

McCullough, P.K. Geriatric depression: Atypical presentations, hidden meanings. *Geriatrics* 46(10):72–76, 1991.

McCullough, P.K. Evaluation and management of anxiety in the older adult. *Geriatrics* 47(4):35–44, 1992.

McDonald, D.D. and Bridge, R.G. Gender stereotyping and nursing care. *Res Nurs Health* 14(5):373–378, 1991.

McLaughlin, D.K. and Jensen, L.I. Poverty among older Americans: The plight of nonmetropolitan elders. *J Gerontol* 48:S544–S554, 1993.

McVey, L.J., Davis, D.E. and Cohen, J.J. The aging game: An approach to education in geriatrics. *JAMA* 262(1):1507–1509, 1989.

Meyer, D.R. and Bartolomei-Hill, S. The adequacy of supplemental security income benefits for aged individuals and couples. *Gerontologist* 34(2):161–172, 1994.

Mikelsons, M. and Turner, M. *Housing Conditions of the Elderly in the 1980s: A Date Book.* Washington, D.C.: Urban Institute, 1991.

Miller, N.S. Alcohol and drug dependence. *In* Sadavoy, J., Lazarus, L.W. and Jarvik, L.F. (eds.). *Comprehensive Review of Geriatric Psychiatry.* Washington, D.C.: American Psychiatric Press, 1991, pp. 387–401.

Montamat, S.C. and Cusack, B. Overcoming problems with polypharmacy and drug misuse in the elderly. *Clin Geriatr Med* 8(1):143–158, 1992.

Moon, A. and Williams, O. Perceptions of elder abuse and help-seeking patterns among African-American, Caucasian American, and Korean-American elderly women. *Gerontologist* 33(3):386–395, 1993.

Moos, R.H., Mertens, J.R. and Brennan, P.L. Patterns of diagnosis and treatment among late-middle-aged and older substance abuse patients. *J Stud Alcohol* 54:479–487, 1993.

Moran, M.G. and Thompson, T.L. Depression, suicide, and paranoia. *In* Schrier, R.W. (ed.). *Geriatric Medicine.* Philadelphia: W.B. Saunders, 1990.

Muller-Spahn, F. and Hock, C. Clinical presentation of depression in the elderly. *Gerontology* 40(Suppl. 1):10–14, 1994.

Murdach, A.D. Bargaining and persuasion with nonvoluntary clients. *Soc Work* Nov:458–461, 1980.

Murphy, E. Concepts of depression in old age. *In* Evans, J.G. and Williams, T.F. (eds.). *Oxford Textbook of Geriatric Medicine.* New York: Oxford University Press, 1992, pp. 620–634.

Mutschler, P.H. Where elders live. *Generations* 16(2):7–14, 1992.

Najman, J.M. Health and poverty: Past, present and prospects for the future. *Soc Sci Med* 36(2):157–166, 1993.

O'Gorman, H.J. False consciousness of kind: Pluralistic ignorance among the aged. *Res Aging* 2:105–128, 1980.

O'Grady-LeShane, R. Older women and poverty. *Soc Work* 35(5):422–424, 1990.

O'Malley, H.C., Segel, H.D. and Perez, R. *Elder Abuse in Massachusetts: A Survey of Professionals and Paraprofessionals.* Boston: Legal Research and Services for the Elderly, 1979.

O'Malley, T.A., Everitt, D.F., O'Malley, H. and Campion, E. Identifying and preventing family-mediated abuse and neglect of elderly. *Ann Intern Med* 93(6):998–1004, 1983.

O'Shea, E. and Blackwell J. The relationship between the cost of community care and the dependency of old people. *Soc Sci Med* 37(5):583–590, 1993.

Palmore, E.B. *Ageism: Negative and Positive.* New York: Springer, 1990.

Pastalan, L. Retirement communities. *Generations* 9(3):26–30, 1985.

Paul, M. A little help, a lot of independence. Retirement community advances the cause of aging with dignity. *Health Prog* 74(4):43–45, 1993.

Paveza, G.J., Cohen, D., Eisdorfer, C. et al. Severe family violence and Alzheimer's disease: Prevalence and risk factors. *Gerontologist* 32(4):493–497, 1992.

Phillips, L.R. Abuse and neglect of the frail elderly at home: An exploration of theoretical relationships. *J Adv Nurs* 8:379–392, 1983.

Pillemer, K.A. and Finkelhor, D. Causes of elder abuse: Caregiver stress versus problem relatives. *Am J Orthopsychiatry* 59:179–187, 1989.

Pillemer, K. and Hudson, B. A model abuse prevention program for nursing assistants. *Gerontologist* 33(1):128–131, 1993.

Pillemer, K. and Suitor, J.J. Violence and violent feelings: What causes them among family caregivers? *J Gerontol* 47(4):S165–S172, 1992.

Podnieks, E. *National Survey on Abuse of the Elderly in Canada, The Ryerson Study.* Toronto: Ryerson Polytechnical Institute, 1990.

Poole, G.G. and Gooding, B.A. Developing and implementing a community intergenerational program. *J Community Health Nurs* 10(2):77–85, 1993.

Pynoos, J. Option for mid-upper-income elders: Continuum of care retirement communities. *Generations* 9(3):26–33, 1985.

Rabushka, A. and Jacobs, B. *Old Folks at Home.* New York: Free Press, 1980.

Radecki, S., Kane, R., Solomon, D. et al. Do physicians spend less time with older patients? *J Am Geriatr Soc* 36:713–718, 1988.

Rancho Owls. Stop, look, listen. *Generations* 8(4):51–52, 1984.

Redfoot, D. and Gaberlavage, G. Housing for older Americans: Sustaining the dream. *Generations* 15:35–38, 1991.

Revenson, T.A. Compassionate stereotyping of elderly patients by physicians: Revising the social contact hypothesis. *Psychol Aging* 4(2):230–234, 1989.

Riley, M.W. and Riley, J.W., Jr. Age integration and the lives of older people. *Gerontologist* 34(1):110–115, 1994.

Roberts, L., Gwynedd, Y. and Nolan, B-M. Elder abuse: Raising the awareness of nurses working in A&E units. *Br J Nurs* 2(3):167–171, 1993.

Robins, L.N., Helzer, J.E., Przybeck, T.R. et al. Alcohol disorders in the community: A report from the Epidemiologic Catchment Area. *In* Barret, R.R. (ed.). *Alcoholism: Origins and Outcome.* New York: Raven Press, 1988, pp. 15–29.

Rounds, L. Elder abuse and neglect: A relationship to ·health characteristics. *J Am Acad Nurse Pract* 4(2):47–52, 1992.

Ruskin, P.E. Schizophrenia and delusional disorders. *In* Bienenfeld, D. (ed.). *Verwoerdt's Clinical Geropsychiatry,* 3rd ed. Baltimore: Williams & Wilkins, 1990a.

Ruskin, P.E. Anxiety and somatoform disorders. *In* Bienenfeld, D. (ed.). *Verwoerdt's Clinical Geropsychiatry,* 3rd ed. Baltimore: Williams & Wilkins, 1990b.

Ryan, E.B., Bourhis, R.Y. and Knops, U. Evaluative perceptions of patronizing speech addressed to elders. *Psychol Aging* 6(3):442–450, 1991.

Ryan, W. *Blaming the Victim.* New York: Vintage, 1971.

Saveman, B.I. and Norberg, A. Cases of elder abuse, intervention and hopes for the future, as reported by home service personnel. *Scand J Caring Sci* 7(1):21–28, 1993.

Saveman, B.I., Hallberg, I.R., Norberg, A. and Eriksson, S. Patterns of abuse of the elderly in their own homes as reported by district nurses. *Scand J Prim Health Care* 11(2):111–116, 1993.

Schick, F.L. and Schick, R. *Statistical Handbook on Aging Americans.* Phoenix, AZ: Orynx Press, 1994.

Schmid, A.H. The deficiency model: An exploration of current approaches to late-life disorders. *Psychiatry* 54(4):358–367, 1991.

Schmid, H., Manjee, K. and Shah, T. On the distinction of suicide ideation versus attempt in elderly psychiatric inpatients. *Gerontologist* 34(3):332–339, 1994.

Seccombe, K. and Ishii-Kuntz, M. Perceptions of problems associated with aging: Comparisons among four older age cohorts. *Gerontologist* 31(4):527–533, 1991.

Shenk, D. and Achenbaum, A. Changing perceptions of aging and the aged: Introduction. *Generations* 17(2):5–8, 1993.

Shiferaw, B., Mittelmark, M.B., Wofford, J.L. et al. The investigation and outcome of reported cases of elder abuse: The Forsyth County Aging Study. *Gerontologist* 34(1):123–125, 1994.

Skinner, J.H. Aging in place: The experience of African American and other minority elders. *Generations* 16(2):49–51, 1992.

Smyer, M.A., Shea, D.G. and Streit, A. The provision and use of mental health services in nursing homes: Results from the national medical expenditure survey. *Am J Public Health* 84(2):284–287, 1994.

Sofaer, S. and Abel, E. Older women's health and financial vulnerability: Implications of the Medicare benefit structure. *Women Health* 16(3–4):47–67, 1990.

Solomon, K. and Vickers, R. Attitudes of health workers toward old people. *J Am Geriatr Soc* 24:186–191, 1979.

Solomon, K., Manepalli, J., Ireland, G.A. and Mahon, G.M. Alcoholism and prescription drug abuse in the elderly: St. Louis University Grand Rounds. *J Am Geriatr Soc* 41(1):57–69, 1993.

Somers, T. Social Security: A woman's viewpoint. *In* Fuller, M.M. and Martin, C.A. (eds.). *The Older Woman: Lavender Rose or Gray Panther?* Springfield, IL: Charles C Thomas, 1980.

Staebler, R. Medicaid: Providing health care to (some of) America's poor. *Caring* 10(6):4–6, 8–10, 12–13, 1991.

Steinmetz, S.K. *Duty Bound: Elder Abuse and Family Care.* Newbury Park, CA: Sage Library of Social Research, 1988, Vol. 166:288.

Stern, R.S., Weissman, J.S. and Epstein, A.M. The emergency department as a pathway to admission for poor and high-cost patients. *JAMA* 266(16):2238–2243, 1991.

Stoller, E.P. and Stoller, M.A. The propensity to save among the elderly. *Gerontologist* 27(3):314–320, 1987.

Strauss, A. *Chronic Illness and the Quality of Life,* 2nd ed. St. Louis: C.V. Mosby, 1984.

Strauss, M., Gelles, R. and Steinmetz, S. *Behind Closed Doors.* New York: Anchor Press/Doubleday, 1981.

Szinovacz, M. *Women's Retirement: Policy Implications of Recent Research.* San Francisco: SAGE Publications, 1983.

Thibault, J.M. and Maly, R.C. Recognition and treatment of substance abuse in the elderly. *Prim Care* 20(1):155–165, 1993.

Thorslund, M. and Lundberg, O. Health and inequalities among the oldest old. *J Aging Health* 6(1):51–69, 1994.

Tobin, S.S. and Lieberman, M.A. *Last Home for the Aged.* San Francisco: Jossey-Bass, 1976.

U'Ren, R.C. Anxiety, paranoia, and personality disorders. *In* Cassel, C.K., Riesenberg, D.E., Sorenson, L.B. and Walsh, J.R. (eds.). *Geriatric Medicine,* 2nd ed. New York: Springer-Verlag, 1990.

U.S. Bureau of the Census. *Statistical Abstract of the United States: 1991,* 11th ed. Washington, D.C.: U.S. Government Printing Office, 1991.

U.S. Bureau of the Census and U.S. Department of Housing and Urban Development. *American Housing Survey of the United States in 1987.* Current Housing Reports, H–150–87, December 1989.

United States Department of Health and Human Services. *Aging America: Trends and Projections.* Washington, DC, 1991.

U.S. Senate. *Developments in Aging: 1992,* Vol. 1. Washington, D.C.: U.S. Government Printing Office, 1993.

Vetter, N.J., Lewis, P.A. and Llewellyn, L. Supporting elderly dependent people at home. *BMJ* 304:(6837):1290–1292, 1992.

Walker, A.J. and Allen, K.R. Relationships between caregiving daughters and their elderly mothers. *Gerontologist* 31(3):389–396, 1991.

Weiler, K. and Buckwalter, K.C. Abuse among rural mentally ill. *J Psychosoc Nurs Ment Health Serv* 30:32–36, 1992.

Weinberger, M., Saunders, A.F., Bearon, L.B. et al. Physician related barriers to breast cancer screening in older women [Special issue]. *J Gerontol* 47:111–117, 1992.

Wenger, N.K. Exclusion of the elderly and women from coronary trials. Is their quality of care compromised? *JAMA* 268(11):1460–1461, 1992.

Werner-Beland, J.A. Physical disability and grief resolution. *In* Werner-Beland, J.A. (ed.). *Grief Responses to Long-Term Illness and Disability: Manifestations and Nursing Interventions.* Reston, VA: Reston Publishing (Prentice-Hall), 1980.

Whall, A.L. The problem of missed psychiatric diagnoses in the elderly. *J Psychosoc Nurs Ment Health* 31(1):33–34, 1993.

Whanger, A.D. Paranoid and schizophrenic disorders. *In* Whanger, A.D. and Myers, A.C. (eds.). *Mental Health Assessment and Therapeutic Intervention with Older Adults.* Rockville, MD: Aspen Systems Corporation, 1984, pp. 89–123.

Wiener, J.M. and Illston, L.H. Health care reform in the 1990s: Where does long-term care fit in? *Gerontologist* 34(3):402–408, 1994.

Wilkin, D. Conceptual problems in dependency research. *Soc Sci Med* 24(10):867–873, 1987.

Wohl, S. *The Medical Industrial Complex.* New York: Harmony Press, 1984.

Wolf, R.S. and Pillemer, K. What's new in elder abuse programming? Four bright ideas. *Gerontologist* 34(1): 126–129, 1994.

Wolf, R.S., Strugnell, L.P. and Godkin, M.A. *Preliminary Findings from Three Model Projects on Elderly Abuse.* Worcester, MA: Center on Aging, University of Massachusetts Medical Center, 1982.

Wolfensberger, W. *The Principle of Normalization in Human Services.* Toronto: National Institute on Mental Retardation, 1972.

World Health Organization. *International Classification of Impairments, Disabilities and Handicaps: A Manual of Classification Relating to the Consequences of Diseases.* Geneva: World Health Organization, 1980.

Wu, R. *Behavior and Illness.* Englewood Cliffs, NJ: Prentice-Hall, 1973.

Zung, W.W., Broadhead, W.E. and Roth, M.E. Prevalence of depressive symptoms in primary care. *J Fam Pract* 37(4):337–344, 1993.

Zusman, J. Some explanations of the changing appearance of psychotic patients: Antecedents of the social breakdown syndrome concept. *Milbank Mem Fund* 44(Suppl.):363–396, 1966.

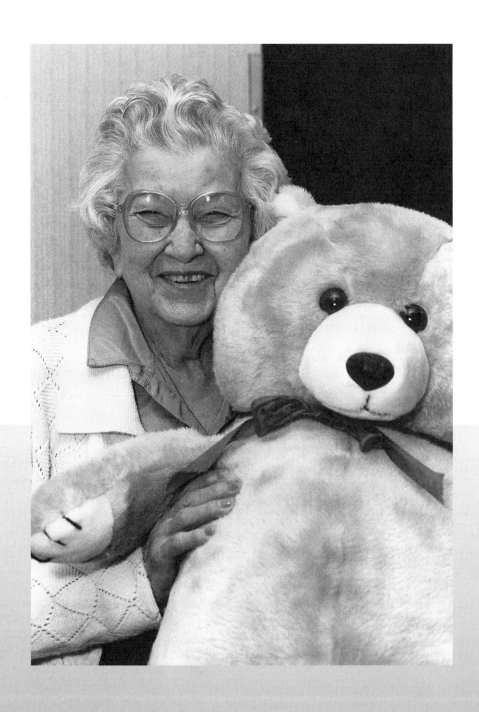

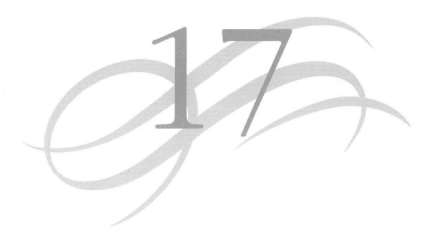

Nursing Diagnoses Related to Psychosocial Alterations

J. TAYLOR HARDEN *

* The opinions expressed in this chapter are those of the author and do not necessarily reflect those of the National Institutes of Health, the National Institute of Nursing Research, or the U.S. Department of Health and Human Services.

ANXIETY

INEFFECTIVE INDIVIDUAL COPING

ALTERATIONS IN FAMILY PROCESS AND INEFFECTIVE FAMILY COPING

DECISIONAL CONFLICT

FEAR

GRIEVING

HOPELESSNESS

KNOWLEDGE DEFICIT

RELOCATION STRESS SYNDROME

POWERLESSNESS

DISTURBANCES IN SELF-PERCEPTION: BODY IMAGE, SELF-ESTEEM, PERSONAL IDENTITY, AND ROLE PERFORMANCE

SOCIAL ISOLATION

SPIRITUAL DISTRESS

POTENTIAL FOR VIOLENCE

ANXIETY

Definition and Scope of Problem

Anxiety is variously defined as a feeling, a bodily reaction, a psychiatric symptom, and a psychiatric disorder. As a feeling, anxiety is characterized by a vague, uneasy sense of dread or apprehension that is related to a source that is either nonspecific or unknown to the individual. It is an endogenous feeling of helplessness and inadequacy. Anxiety-ridden people expect horrible things to happen and doubt their ability to cope with them. Further, anxiety is defined as a state of apprehension and worry, often associated with inability to cope with true or imaginary hardships. It is one of the three major mental disturbances; the other two are depression and stress. Almost all mental disorders are accompanied by anxiety symptoms (Wolman and Stricker, 1994). It is one of the most common psychiatric disorders in later life (Fernandez et al., 1995).

As a bodily reaction, anxiety is characterized by physiological responses such as palpitations, tachycardia, hyperventilation, respiratory distress, trembling, and dizziness.

Anxiety has been described as one of the most common responses to illness and diagnosis. The National Institute of Mental Health Epidemiological Catchment Area Survey (Reiger et al., 1988) revealed that anxiety disorders are the most common mental health problems, affecting 8.3 per cent of the population. These disorders outrank depression and substance abuse, yet only one of four patients ever receives treatment (Freeman and DiTomasso, 1994).

Anxiety is a universal human experience and is undoubtedly a common human emotion; however, it does not necessarily imply the presence of a clinically significant disorder. It may be an acute condition, with brief, unbearable levels of intensity known as "panic attacks," or it may be a chronic condition of physical and psychological tension.

The experience of anxiety in older persons, especially in its extreme forms such as panic attacks, can be extremely unpleasant when left untreated. Anxiety can interfere with functioning and can increase feelings of helplessness. It also may be self-perpetuating because it may lead the older individual to a position of exaggerated dependency on family members and support persons, who may in turn retreat from overwhelming responsibility. Physical health may be affected by physiological symptoms of anxiety, especially muscular tension and its associated fatigue, weakness, muscular pain, and sleep loss. These conditions may exacerbate the course of chronic diseases already present, and rapid deterioration of functional status may result (Abrams and Berkow, 1990). Finally, cognitive functioning may be impaired by high levels of anxiety, so that already-present losses in memory or calculation and problem-solving skills may be amplified.

In sum, a distinction is often made between transitory, situation-specific state anxiety, and the relatively stable characteristic trait anxiety. State anxiety refers to transitory, situation-specific anxiety, whereas trait anxiety refers to a relatively stable characteristic persisting across situations and over time (Spielberger, 1970). Further, there are many reasons to expect increased anxiety with advanced age. Nevertheless, research findings have been contrary to theoretical expectations. Trait anxiety appears unaffected by, or decreases slightly with, advanced age, whereas state anxiety is highly situation- and individual-specific. Further research is needed to address the relationship between multiple measures of anxiety and age (Schultz, 1987).

Contributing Factors

It is thought that anxiety may be related to the fear of separation or to the loss of essential sources of external support (Rank, 1929; Sullivan, 1953). Factors that contribute to anxiety can be summarized as follows (North America Nursing Diagnoses Association, 1994):

1. Unconscious conflict about essential values or goals of life
2. Threat to self-concept
3. Threat of death
4. Threat to or change in health status
5. Threat to or change in socioeconomic status
6. Threat to or change in role functioning
7. Threat to or change in environment
8. Threat to or change in interaction patterns
9. Situational or maturational crises
10. Interpersonal transmission or contagion
11. Unmet needs

Although feelings of anxiety may be experienced at any age, anxiety disorders usually begin in childhood, adolescence, or young adulthood; rarely is there a new onset in old age. However, anxiety states may become manifest for the first time in later life and may be linked to a significant, long-standing vulnerability to emotional stress (Turnbull, 1989; Devanand et al., 1994). Clinicians often note that in most cases of geriatric anxiety disorders the older person or family members indicate that the client has always had "bad nerves."

Assessment

Goals for assessment of the anxious client include determination of (1) the degree of anxiety the person is experiencing, (2) the events preceding the anxiety, and (3) what techniques help alleviate the anxiety. This information provides the foundation on which nursing care can proceed. However, two additional goals for assessment include differentiating anxiety disorders from other conditions in which anxiety is a factor, and determining the underlying cause of the anxiety.

Although the causes of anxiety in older persons differ little from those in young adults, two important differences in the development of anxiety in old people are pertinent. First, in older persons there are more likely to be multiple, concomitant factors contributing to the anxiety. Second, the early manifestations of anxiety may be masked by the presence of chronic disease. Many factors commonly found in an older person's life situation contribute to anxiety. Thus, the nurse should look closely for symptoms, especially in an encounter with a new client.

Specific items that should be included in this assessment are shown in Box 17–1.

The nurse should assess whether physical or mental diseases are present that could produce or potentiate symptoms of anxiety. Hyperthyroidism, carcinoma, cardiac failure, dementia, nutritional deficiency (folate, vitamin B_{12}), hypoglycemia, hypoxemia, cardiac arrhythmias, depression, paranoid states, and hypochondriasis may present in atypical fashion in some older people with symptoms of anxiety (McCullough, 1992). In addition, medications such as theophylline, anticholinergics, over-the-counter cough and cold preparations, caffeine, and psychoactive drugs may produce anxiety as a side effect or as a paradoxical reaction (Tueth, 1993).

A detailed psychosocial history may reveal life factors that may be exacerbating or maintaining the current level of anxiety. Recent bereavements, other significant losses, or changes in lifestyle should be noted particularly. The history should also include precipitating events and coping strategies used in stressful situations previously. Behavioral and physical assessments also yield valuable information about the individual's response to certain types of interventions and cues to anxiety levels. Assessment of a client's anxiety level is an ongoing process, so it is useful to keep an open mind and to carefully document signs indicating anxiety. Observations of behavior can also be made using data from the client and from family members. Hyperventilation, restlessness, pacing, inability to sit still in a chair, finger-tapping, irritability, sighing, and dizziness are all signs and symptoms associated with anxiety. Family members and older clients may be able to observe whether the behaviors are associated with particular life events or situations. The nurse also can observe whether the behaviors are associated with any segment of the discussion, such as particular problems or concerns.

Planning

Expected outcomes or objectives for nursing care of the older client with anxiety might include

---

BOX 17-1
Assessment Guide for Anxiety in Elderly People

History

Physical symptoms that may be stress-related such as chest pain, rapid pulse, palpitations, hyperventilation, sighing, nausea, constipation or diarrhea, anorexia or compulsive eating, sweating, itching, hives or rashes

Current worries, concerns, feelings (apprehensive, fearful, scared, regretful, worried, jittery)

Recent life changes

Coping methods normally used

Mood changes

Behavioral Assessment

Anxiety-related behaviors such as nail biting, sleep disturbance, finger tapping, foot swinging, distractability

Factors that worsen or improve anxiety-related behaviors

Client's insight into behaviors affecting feelings of anxiety

Physical Assessment

Presence or absence of physiological signs of anxiety

Objective

Sympathetic stimulation—cardiovascular excitation, superficial vasoconstriction, pupil dilation

Restlessness

Insomnia

Glancing about

Poor eye contact

Trembling or hand tremors

Extraneous movement (foot shuffling, hand/arm movements)

Facial tension

Voice quavering

Focus on "self"

Increased wariness

Increased perspiration

Physiological Manifestations

Increased blood pressure	Dry mouth
Rapid breath and pulse	Headaches
Muscular tension	Nausea
Pounding heart	Dizziness
Dilated pupils	Trembling
Perspiration	Cold, clammy hands
Gastric discomfort	

From North American Nursing Diagnosis Association. *Definitions and Classification 1995–1996.* Philadelphia: North American Nursing Diagnosis Association, 1994, pp. 86–87; and Nurseco. *Nursing Care Planning Guides in Long-Term Care.* Pacific Palisades, CA: 1984, p. 92.

---

1. Reducing the current level of anxiety (unless a mild anxiety is desired to facilitate learning or behavioral change)
2. Demonstrating effective coping skills
3. Preventing recurrence of extreme anxiety states
4. Learning early signs of anxiety and techniques for reducing anxiety. Teaching techniques might be directed to the older clients, family members, and other caregivers

It is particularly important to involve all caregivers in the plan of care because failure to do so can result in overstimulation of the anxious person through a diversity of approaches that are poorly tolerated by a severely anxious person.

Intervention

General Approaches

Four general approaches to the treatment of anxiety symptoms include environmental manipulation, medications, behavioral therapies, and psychotherapy (Eppley et al., 1989; Stetter et al., 1994).

The purpose of *environmental manipulation* is to alleviate the fears associated with the older person's feelings of dependency. Environmental manipulation can be applied to either the physical environment or the family and social support system. A more structured, safe, and protective physical environment and in some cases relocation to a group home or institutional setting may be required to alleviate symptoms of severe anxiety. Strengthening support systems can be accomplished by teaching family and friends about the older person's increasing dependency and fears of dependency characteristic of old age. Family members and significant others who understand the causes of anxiety are better prepared to offer structured support.

Antianxiety medications are used frequently for the elderly, and nurses have an important role in monitoring client responses. Drugs used to control anxiety can be classified into two major groups: the minor tranquilizers, such as the benzodiazepines and meprobamates, and the major tranquilizers, such as the phenothiazines and butyrophenones. Table 17–1 summarizes the major actions, uses, and side effects of and adverse reactions to the most commonly prescribed drugs in each category.

Minor tranquilizers, or anxiolytic drugs, are used for treating anxiety disorders because they act on the lower brain centers involved in the anxiety process. Benzodiaze-pines such as Librium (chlordiazepoxide) and Valium (diazepam) have been pre-scribed traditionally. However, they tend to accumulate in the body, resulting in unde-sirable side effects in older people such as unsteadiness or confusion. Drugs such as Ativan (lorazepam) and Serax (oxazepam) are used more frequently because they have shorter half-lives and are less likely to accu-mulate in the body and cause adverse ef-fects.

However, patients who take shorter-acting benzodiazepines are more likely to experience withdrawal symptoms if the drug is stopped abruptly than is the case with longer-acting benzodiazepines (Benson, 1990). Withdrawal symptoms have been re-ported with short-term use (4 to 8 weeks) and may include rebound anxiety, my-oclonus, fasciculations, delirium, psychosis, and seizures, among others. Tapering these drugs rather than abrupt discontinuation is therefore indicated to prevent acute with-drawal syndromes (Vanelle and Feline, 1994).

If the anxiety is severe, major tranquiliz-ers, such as Stelazine (trifluoperazine) or Mellaril (thioridazine), may be prescribed in small doses. If panic attacks or symptoms of depression are present, tricyclic antidepres-sants, including Tofranil (imipramine), Sine-quan (doxepin), and Asendin (amoxapine), may be helpful. Inderal (propranolol) has also been successful in treating panic attacks (Benson, 1990).

Several key problems with antianxiety medications merit discussion. First, medica-tions may lower the anxiety level to such an extent that clients lose any incentive to ex-plore the underlying problems and change their behaviors. Second, the drugs may be perceived by clients, families, or staff as a reasonable solution to the problem, since the anxiety is alleviated. Unfortunately, the drugs merely treat the symptom and not the underlying cause, so the root of the problem is not addressed. Third, antianxiety agents may produce serious side effects that may cause worse problems for the older person than the initial problem of anxiety (Todd, 1989). Finally, research on the effects of age-related changes in pharmacokinetics is inad-equate to predict reliably the responses of older persons to anxiolytic drugs.

Behavioral therapies may include systematic desensitization, progressive muscle relax-ation, hypnosis, biofeedback, massage, and exercise. Progressive relaxation and biofeed-back may be especially suitable for helping

TABLE 17–1
Drug Treatment of Anxiety in Elderly People

DRUG CATEGORY	ACTION	SIDE EFFECTS
Benzodiazepines Valium (diazepam) Librium (chlordiaze-poxide) Dalmane (flurazepam) Tranxene (chloraze-pate) *Xanax (alprazolam) *Serax (oxazepam) *Ativan (lorazepam)	Especially useful for so-matic symptoms of anxiety (e.g., head-ache, fatigue, and gastrointestinal dis-tress) (Blazer, 1990) Xanax thought to also have antidepressant properties	Drowsiness, ataxia, dys-arthria, coordination difficulties, and mental confusion (Blazer, 1990) Paradoxical reactions reported include agita-tion, insomnia, rage and hallucinations Habituation is a prob-lem, and withdrawal reactions are similar to those for barbiturate withdrawal
Propanediols Equanil, Miltown (me-probamate) Tybatran (tybamate)	Sedative and relaxant properties	Habituation and with-drawal problems greater than with ben-zodiazepines Risk of oversedation greater than with ben-zodiazepines
Diphenylmethanes Benadryl (diphenhydra-mine) Atarax, Vistaril (hydrox-yzine)	Sedative properties greater than anxiolytic properties	Anticholinergic side ef-fects predispose to an-ticholinergic delirium (Jenike, 1985)
Tricyclic Antidepressants Elavil (amitriptyline) Sinequan (doxepin) Tofranil (imipramine) Aventyl (nortriptyline) Prozac (fluoxetine) Zoloft (sertraline)	Anxiolytic properties in addition to antidepres-sant effects Offer the advantage of single drug if both anxiety and depres-sion are present	Anticholinergic and car-diotoxic side effects
Major Tranquilizers Mellaril (thioridazine) Stelazine (trifluopera-zine) Haldol (haloperidol) Wellbutrin (bupropion)	In low doses, have anti-anxiety effect Nonsedating; recom-mended for depressed cardiac patients	Extrapyramidal and an-ticholinergic side ef-fects can also cause hypotension
Other BuSpar (buspirone)		

* Preferred drug because of shorter half-life.

with panic attacks and generalized anxiety reactions (Eppley et al., 1989). Group train-ing in relaxation procedures has been found to be useful (Stetter et al., 1994) and may provide the social structure and support needed to alleviate dependency needs. Al-though the number of subjects in the study was small, massage therapy was shown to be of some benefit in decreasing anxiety in both psychiatric (Stetter et al., 1994) and cancer (Ferrell-Torry and Glick, 1993) patients. Guided imagery may be an enhancement to both muscle relaxation therapy and biofeedback. Exercise programs and assorted exercise therapies have been associated with decreases in both state and trait anxiety levels (Petruzzello et al., 1991).

Psychotherapy for anxiety should be based on a supportive relationship rather than on the development of insight. The older person should be reassured that the anxiety symptoms are emotionally related and are not signals of impending physical breakdown. Regular, frequent meetings help provide assurance that a caring, supportive person is available. The meetings may be gradually tapered off as the level of anxiety lowers. Therapy should aim at returning a sense of control over their own lives to clients (Stetter et al., 1994).

Short-Term and Long-Term Approaches to Anxiety Reduction

The specific techniques used to reduce anxiety are highly variable, because they depend not only on the individual's current level of function but also on coping strategies developed over a lifetime. It is important to capitalize on coping mechanisms and habit patterns that have been successful in the past. Use of familiar strategies may serve to heighten the client's sense of mastery over the situation, which itself contributes to anxiety reduction.

One way to elicit information about past coping strategies is through the "reminiscence interview." The nurse asks the patient to focus memories on past stressful situations in which he or she had "triumphed over obstacles" (Rybarczyk and Auerbach, 1990). This assessment strategy has been shown to be an effective intervention.

Short-term intervention goals are to reduce the current level of anxiety and to prevent further severe anxiety states. Useful techniques include the following:

1. Use consistent caregivers (i.e., do not change patient care assignments capriciously).
2. Use short, simple explanations for procedures.
3. Be predictable. Follow through on promises, especially regarding time.
4. Provide companionship in small, regular, frequent doses. During this time, gentle, firm touch may be useful rather than conversation. Spend quiet time with the client.

5. Consider the client's pace. It is likely to be slower than yours! A calm, unhurried manner is transmitted to the client.
6. Coach the client in deep breathing.

Long-term intervention goals are to prevent further severe anxiety states and to teach recognition of early signs of anxiety and techniques to reduce anxiety. Useful techniques include the following:

1. Explore with the client life events that contribute to anxiety.
2. Assess antecedents of anxiety with the client. The use of a diary may be helpful.
3. Document client responses to environmental stimuli, including drugs if they are used.
4. Document the effectiveness of interventions used in the short term.
5. Model or describe to caregivers behaviors that successfully reduce anxiety and praise their successes in reducing or preventing anxiety in the client.
6. Explore the need for referral for psychotherapy to deal with the anxiety problem on a long-term basis. Peer counseling programs are attracting increasing interest and respect as a viable treatment option for older persons who require supportive therapy (Tueth, 1993).

Interpersonal Techniques Keyed to Specific Contributing Factors

Interpersonal interventions are best when based on factors that contribute to the individual patient's anxiety. These interventions are powerful and have the advantage of no dangerous side effects of medication. An additional benefit is their potential for addressing the cause of the anxiety rather than simply alleviating the symptoms.

The effective use of interpersonal interventions requires careful assessment and communication with other care providers about strategies that effectively allay anxiety. Figure 17–1 is an algorithm that helps simplify the assessment of factors that contribute to anxiety. A variety of ways to elicit the data are needed to follow the algorithm, but the cornerstone is careful history taking and observation of patient responses. Differentiating one contributing factor from another may be accomplished only by trying several different interventions and noting the individual's response. Remember that several factors may be contributing to the anxiety simultaneously. The most common factors contributing to anxiety are discussed next,

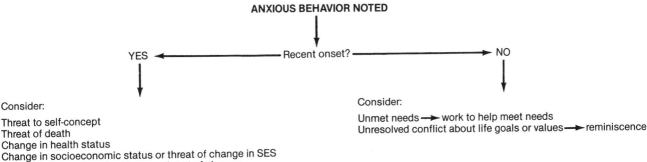

ANXIOUS BEHAVIOR NOTED

YES ← Recent onset? → NO

Consider:

Threat to self-concept
Threat of death
Change in health status
Change in socioeconomic status or threat of change in SES
Change in interactional patterns or threat of change
Change in environment or threat of change
Change in role functioning
Situational/maturational crisis
Interpersonal transmission

Consider:

Unmet needs → work to help meet needs
Unresolved conflict about life goals or values → reminiscence

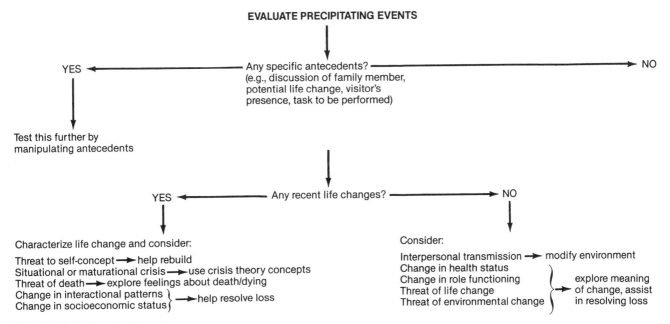

EVALUATE PRECIPITATING EVENTS

YES ← Any specific antecedents?
(e.g., discussion of family member,
potential life change, visitor's
presence, task to be performed) → NO

Test this further by
manipulating antecedents

YES ← Any recent life changes? → NO

Characterize life change and consider:

Threat to self-concept → help rebuild
Situational or maturational crisis → use crisis theory concepts
Threat of death → explore feelings about death/dying
Change in interactional patterns ⎫
Change in socioeconomic status ⎭ → help resolve loss

Consider:

Interpersonal transmission → modify environment
Change in health status
Change in role functioning ⎫ explore meaning
Threat of life change ⎬ → of change, assist
Threat of environmental change ⎭ in resolving loss

F I G U R E   1 7 – 1

Algorithm for assessing contributing factors to anxiety in the elderly.

and specific intervention techniques are described for each.

Unconscious Conflict About Essential Values or Goals

Conduct life review therapy to work through unresolved conflict. This may take place in a group or individually. Family members, interested volunteers, and paraprofessional workers can be taught the principles and techniques applicable to facilitating an individual's life review.

Threat to Self-Concept

- Explore client feelings about self at present and in the past.
- Assist clients to identify ways in which

they are important despite changes in roles.

- Help clients identify meaningful activities at which they can succeed.
- Teach new skills as indicated, or help the individual search for new meaning in previously learned skills.

Threat of Death

NONTERMINALLY ILL CLIENTS

- Clarify the prognosis for the individual's illness and explain available treatment options. Death anxiety in nonterminally ill people may serve as a motivator for improved control of chronic illness if properly managed. After a life-threatening exacerbation of a chronic disease such as diabetes mellitus, people who previously used denial as their main coping mechanism may become motivated to learn new techniques or to apply old techniques of disease management consistently. Likewise, individuals in the early recovery phase of a myocardial infarction may be motivated to learn about lifestyle modification to reduce their risk of a second infarction.

TERMINALLY ILL CLIENTS

- Nurses must explore their own feelings about dying and achieve some comfort in viewing dying as a part of living to avoid transmitting their anxieties to the patient.

- Give patients the opportunity to share feelings, fears, and concerns about the process of dying.

- Active listening techniques encourage patients to express concerns. Older people are more likely to talk about death and to express less fear, but there are few good predictors of persons who will experience death anxiety. Dying is a highly charged emotional issue to be worked through. Some patients prefer to talk with someone closer in chronological age or cultural background because they may be protective of younger people, including their health care providers, and will discuss matters such as dying or sexuality only with age peers.

- Monitor the patient's ability and willingness to discuss dying and initiate contact with other health team members such as the chaplain, social worker, or hospice team, as indicated by client wishes, stress level, and proximity of death. All members of the health care team should be knowledgeable about the importance of reflective listening for someone coping with death-related anxiety.

Change in Health Status

- Teach clients about current treatment options and prognoses of pertinent chronic diseases. Chronic diseases are now diagnosed earlier in the course of illness than was true earlier in the lives of most older people, and therefore some of the anxieties of older persons are based on outdated notions of the impact of disease. For example, a diagnosis of cancer no longer means an inevitably painful death. Advances in the treatment of chronic disease render old assumptions about the impact of certain diseases invalid. Many older persons fear prolonged dependency and disability more than death, and accurate information about current treatment options and their impact on function may allay anxieties based on misinformation.

Changes in health status usually result in changes in other role relationships, which represents a potential threat to self-concept. Assist individuals to acknowledge potential changes in roles, and then guide them in developing strategies to adapt to the upcoming changes.

- Assign a consistent provider of care for the individual. Information about diseases and their management is difficult to assimilate in one sitting. Discontinuities in care providers result in less efficient learning and increase the likelihood that the patient will be exposed to varying opinions and approaches to treatment of the disease.

Evaluation

The number and duration of extreme anxiety states are two critical outcome variables. These parameters can be monitored using a simple flow sheet (Fig. 17–2). In addition, observations of environmental factors that cause anxiety states should be identified and communicated to all persons involved in the care of an anxious client. If there is insufficient time to accomplish the goals and objectives of care, referral should be made to other care providers, such as home health nurses, psychotherapists, or staff in a nursing home, who can follow through with treatment for anxiety.

INEFFECTIVE INDIVIDUAL COPING

Definition and Scope of Problem

The ability to cope with stressful life circumstances is essential to living. Humans have an amazing ability to adapt to adverse physical and socioemotional conditions. There is a wide range of normal human coping responses. This range becomes larger rather than smaller with advanced age because there is increased diversity among individuals and lifestyles. It is therefore difficult to identify with consistency the characteristics of an older person who is ineffectively coping. Such judgments are necessarily related to the dominant culture influences, and therefore consensus about the effectiveness or appropriateness of a particu-

DATE/TIME	Anxiety State	Activities Since Last Assessment	Coping Strategies Used During Assessment Period (Client Perception)	Medications

FIGURE 17-2

Flow sheet for anxiety documentation.

lar coping response will never be achieved in all situations. However, within American culture there are certain standards against which the effectiveness of an individual's coping strategies can be measured.

Specific defining characteristics of the individual with ineffective coping include (NANDA, 1994)

1. Verbalization of inability to cope
2. Inability to meet role expectations
3. Inability to meet basic needs (neglect)
4. Inability to solve problems
5. Destructive behavior toward self or others
6. Alteration in societal participation
7. Inappropriate use of defense mechanisms
8. Change in usual communication patterns
9. Verbal manipulation
10. High illness rate
11. High rate of accidents

Ineffective coping is thus defined as a situation in which an individual displays behavior that shows that he or she is not able to solve problems or adapt to the basic de- mands for daily living. Requirements for daily living include needs for physical maintenance, emotional sustenance, interaction with others, and progress in achieving developmental milestones. Thus, ineffective coping is judged by the outcomes of the coping effort, rather then the choice of coping strategy. Denial and defensiveness can both be effective coping strategies at times. However, when the outcome results in inability to problem solve or adapt in a way to improve the individual situation, then the diagnoses of Ineffective Denial and Defensive Coping can be used. In ineffective denial, the reality of a situation is denied, and the denial impairs rather than supports. In defensive coping, the effect of a situation on the person is denied, and the ability to adapt function is decreased rather than increased (Carpenito, 1993).

The consequences of ineffective individual coping are wide-ranging. People who find it difficult to cope are more vulnerable to additional assaults (either physical, psychological, or social) and in the most extreme instances may die without intervention

(Miller, 1990). In less extreme circumstances, the individual may lead a more restricted life than necessary because of the inability to cope with new demands. The result is that the person expends more energy on meeting basic physical needs and less on other human needs such as the need to interact with others.

The individual who is coping ineffectively may be labeled deviant because no effective means for fulfilling a role in a socially acceptable manner has been found. "Behavior problem" patients are an excellent example of the deviance engendered by poor coping abilities. The individual with a behavioral problem seems to engage only in behavior that the staff or family finds offensive. Incontinence, screaming, inappropriate sexual expression, and wandering are just a few of the more common deviant types of behavior. Most of the reaction of staff or family toward the individual centers on the undesirable behaviors. There are frequent attempts to "modify" the behavior through negative reinforcement. Behavioral analysis of these individuals' daily life often shows that the person has no other role in relation to other people except as a deviant. It is difficult to extinguish such behavior if no other role is offered to take the place of the deviant role. This is an extreme but often overlooked form of ineffective coping. Professionals and lay persons often incorrectly view such behavior as an inevitable consequence of a dementing disorder, ignoring the fact that others with similar disorders do not have such serious behavior problems (Cox, 1991).

Contributing Factors

Coping is the result of the interaction between the demands made on an individual, the internal resources available to the individual for meeting those demands, and the resources available to the individual from the environment. Demands on the individual may be self-determined or they may originate from the physical or interpersonal environment. Coping resources or mechanisms refer to resources intrinsic to the individual, whereas social and environmental supports refer to resources that are external to the individual. Ability to cope with the demands of daily living requires integration of all these available resources. Ineffective coping is likely to occur when the demands on an individual increase to the point at which they overwhelm the resources of the individual or when the individual's resources diminish in the face of a constant level of demand. Both these situations may occur suddenly or gradually. Several theoretical perspectives inform the discussion of factors contributing to ineffective individual coping, including the self-care framework, person-environment interaction models, and stress and adaptation theory.

SELF-CARE FRAMEWORK. A stressor is any new demand that requires change in behavior patterns from the individual. Orem's concept of self-care demands is useful in illustrating the importance of this point for nurses (see Chapter 1) (Orem, 1985; Johnston, 1989). Recall that there are three types of self-care demands: universal, developmental, and health deviation. According to Orem, individuals meet their demands for self-care through both action from themselves (self-care agency) and assistance from others. Comparison of self-care demands with the self-care agency and the support system should yield valuable insights into the individual's ability to cope. Increased self-care demands and diminished self-care agency and support systems are stressors because any change in the nature of these three structures necessitates a change in behavior to meet the individual's self-care requirements.

PERSON-ENVIRONMENT INTERACTION MODELS. Ineffective coping may also occur when the individual is put into an environment that is so protective that it does not allow full utilization of her or his potential. This situation opposes the individual's innate drive to live to the fullest potential and, ironically, imposes a new type of demand on the individual (Kielhofner, 1985). The demand is to perform at a lower level than that suited to the individual's capabilities, requiring an alteration in self-perception. In institutional settings, individual initiative is often subdued because of routines or because of fear of incurring institutional liability if the individual becomes injured while attempting too demanding a task. For example, door alarms restrict access to all patients, even those who exercise appropriate judgment and who may desire to walk, spontaneously and unaccompanied, on the institution's grounds. Another, more subtle example of overprotectiveness is the individual recovering from a myocardial infarction who is sometimes kept from performing up to potential because of overanxious family.

The importance of the environment as an influence on the coping behavior of older persons cannot be overstated. Most older persons compensate for functional impairment by carefully structuring their environments. Interference with this structure, particularly if the older adult has little warning of the impending change, may be devastating. Seemingly trivial matters, such as chair placement, room lighting, or placement of possessions, may cause an individual who can normally function independently to become totally dependent on others for help.

An individual's environment may consist of several layers that influence behavior: objects, task demands, social groups, culture, space, and values. Each of these layers has its own dimensions that specifically influence the nature of the demands placed on the individual and the individual's level of arousal. The nurse who understands the contribution of these various environmental variables to the motivation, habit structure, and performance of older persons is in a powerful position to influence the environment to enhance the functional capacity of the client. Those who ignore such considerations will continually endure surprise at the unpredictability of their "best laid plans" to influence health outcomes and behavior of older clients successfully.

STRESS AND ADAPTATION THEORY.
The dynamics of ineffective coping are complex. An individual's ability to cope with a new demand or stressor is related to several characteristics of the stressor (Lazarus, 1993):

1. The nature of the stressor
2. The number of stressors occurring simultaneously
3. Duration of exposure to the stressor
4. Past experience with similar types of stressors

According to this framework, the person most at risk for ineffective coping is the individual who is exposed to multiple new demands that are threatening to the person's self-concept, likely to last for a long period of time, and have not been previously experienced. For example, a usually healthy movie star from a very healthy family who, in the middle of shooting a very important film, is faced with the prospect of disfiguring surgery or certain death is at high risk for ineffective coping. In contrast, if a retired gerontological nurse, who has accomplished the majority of her goals in life and has come to some acceptance of the inevitability of death, experiences a transient ischemic attack and undergoes a successful endarterectomy, she is at much smaller risk for ineffective coping.

A three-part classification for individuals at risk for ineffective individual coping is suggested:

1. Those undergoing *situational crises,* such as separation and loss, divorce, death, illness, natural disasters, and rapid social change,
2. Those undergoing *developmental crises,* such as marriage, the climacteric, or retirement, and
3. Those who have *personal vulnerabilities* in coping effectively, such as those with psychiatric disorders and those with limited environmental resources (Miller, 1990). Many older persons may fit into all three categories—for example, a 70-year-old individual who has recently lost a spouse and has just retired owing to increasing visual impairment secondary to diabetic retinopathy. Although not all older people suffer such dramatic losses simultaneously, it is far from uncommon (Garrett, 1987).

To reiterate, what makes older people cope ineffectively is not solely the nature of the stressor but the degree of risk or probability of having certain distressing experiences occur later rather than earlier in life. Many aging and older persons never experience a major loss of role, extended boredom, incapacitation, loss of autonomy, and other common sources of stress before they die (Birren and Schaie, 1990).

Unfortunately, older persons with few or undesirable adaptational skills are most vulnerable to ineffective coping and comprise the population most often seen by health care providers. This vulnerable group may cope ineffectively for several individual reasons. First, the demands of daily living often increase. The problems associated with adjustment to multiple new demands may overwhelm the individual's coping resources. Adjustments commonly demanded from vulnerable older persons include lifestyle changes imposed by chronic illness, adjustment to rapid societal change, and adaptation to forced role change with retirement, relocation, and death of close companions. Simultaneously, the vulnerable older person's support network, both physical and interpersonal, may be diminishing. The appropriateness of the physical environment may diminish with increasing frailty; the older person's sources of social support may become disabled or lost. Further, the support that is available may come from individuals who have unenlightened views of the aging process, producing more burden than support.

One important factor that serves to balance these contributors to ineffective coping in the vulnerable older individual is the likelihood of enhanced coping mechanisms. Older persons are survivors, which means that in most cases they have had considerable opportunity to master and refine coping mechanisms. Well-developed individual coping resources are a powerful means of maintaining homeokinesis in the face of diminishing support and increasing demand. Professional support and encouragement of time-tested coping mechanisms is important in promoting the well-being of older persons.

The possibility that we, as gerontological clinicians, might be able to influence coping, both preventively and therapeutically, to facilitate a better quality of life at any stage of development, including aging and old age, makes most attractive the investigation of coping in a microanalytic and process sense (McCrae, 1987).

Assessment

Ineffective coping can be understood as a rigid adherence to a defense mechanism that does not increase the individual's ability to deal with the new balance of demands and support. Potter and Perry (1993) suggest several parameters for nursing assessment of intensified stress states. These assessment parameters pertain to the assessment of individual coping, because display of high stress levels for a prolonged period of time is indicative of ineffective coping. The assessment should document

1. Accentuated use of one pattern of behavior
2. Alteration in the variety of activities usually undertaken
3. Behavior that is less organized, or organized at a lower level
4. Demonstration of greater sensitivity to the environment
5. Presence of behaviors reflecting alteration in usual physiological activity
6. Distortion of reality

The goals for assessment of the person suspected of ineffective individual coping are to establish the diagnosis, including the specific contributing factors, and to identify strategies that will bolster the individual's adaptation to the current situation. To accomplish this, the nurse should:

- Identify stressors that impinge on the individual at present

- Identify the client's perception of these stressors and their meaning
- Identify the client's previous experience with similar types of stressors
- Identify the individual's perception of his or her present coping ability
- Identify the individual's usual coping mechanisms
- Identify sources of support available to the client
- Determine significant other's perception of the client's coping ability at present
- Determine the client's anxiety level at present

Specific maneuvers that should be used include history taking, behavioral assessment, and physical assessment.

HISTORY. The history should include questions regarding recent changes in role relationships, health status, functional status, and living situation. Elicit the client's perception of the current stress level, coping adequacy, functional status, and adequacy of the support network. Determine the client's goals for the future and usual behavior patterns. Identify what medications are being taken. Have the older person describe coping strategies that have been successful in the past.

A reminiscence interview focused on past accomplishments can be used to accomplish this goal. Table 17–2 lists various theoretical perspectives of useful coping strategies. Familiarity with these approaches to coping may help the nurse listen more critically for themes and patterns in a patient's descriptions of stressful experiences.

BEHAVIORAL ASSESSMENT. The individual's response to the interview situation should be observed. Specifically, the individual's distractability, thought processes, match or mismatch between verbal and nonverbal behavior, and any distortion of reality should be noted. Responses to the heightened stress produced by an interview situation provide opportunity to observe coping mechanisms in action. For some clients the use of a diary to assess behaviors that may be interfering with effective coping may be helpful. Formal mental status testing is used to determine in an objective manner the cognitive resources available to the client. The individual who has severely impaired short-term memory requires different approaches to intervention than the individual with intact short-term memory. Similarly, validation of estimates of sensory-perceptual difficulties or abstract reasoning deficits is important, so that interventions may be tailored to the individual's strengths.

PHYSICAL ASSESSMENT. Measurement of pulse, respiration, and blood pressure provides objective information about the autonomic stress response of the individual. Additionally, observation for signs of neglect and functional impairment is the key in validating a presumptive diagnosis of ineffective coping. Presence of urine odor, unkempt appearance, and uncut toenails are suggestive of impaired coping ability. Quantify the demands of daily living for the individual by directly observing selected aspects of ADLs and IADLs (see Chapter 2).

If the client admits to having difficulty coping, or shows an inability to solve problems, then a diagnosis of ineffective individual coping is warranted. If two or more of the defining characteristics listed on p. 669 are present, then this diagnosis is justified.

Planning

Provision of immediate support for the areas of unmet need is the most important short-term goal. The central long-range goal is to establish a care system that will enable the individual to cope with life demands with a minimum of assistance. This usually involves a combination of helping the individual enhance coping skills and increasing the social and environmental support available to the client (Roy and Corliss, 1993; Spearman et al., 1993). Initially the client may require what the self-care model terms a wholly compensatory mode in which the nurse makes the majority of decisions, moving next through a partially compensatory care system, and finally achieving a supportive educative system, in which the older client has the primary decision-making role.

Interventions

Specific interventions depend to a great degree on the specific factors contributing to the coping difficulty and on the resources available for support in a given setting. Strategies for compensating for ineffective short-term coping include

1. Increasing the support available to the older person through use of formal agencies, such as home health agencies, social service agencies, clinics, and hospitals
2. Mobilizing informal support networks, such as church groups, extended family, vol-

TABLE 17-2
Selected Methods of Coping

SOURCE	COPING METHODS

Beckett (1991)	Moving against others
	   venting, demanding, resisting
	Moving toward others
	   accepting, seeking, focusing, choosing, giving
	Moving away from others
	   retreating

Folkman and Lazarus (1988)	Confrontive Distancing Self-controlling Seeking sound support Accepting responsibility Escape-avoidance Planful problem solving Positive reappraisal

Heidrick and Ruff (1992)	Direct action
	   get support
	Passive cognitive coping
	   ignore stress
	Positive cognitive coping
	   faith in others
	Emotional expression
	   cry

Jalowiec and Powers (1981)	Emotive
	   expressing emotions
	Evasive
	   evasive and avoidant activity
	Confrontive
	   constructive problem solving
	Fatalistic
	   pessimistic approach
	Optimistic
	   positive outlook
	Palliative
	   stress-reducing methods
	Self-reliant
	   self-initiated activities
	Supportive
	   supportive systems

Lazarus and Folkman (1984)	Emotion focused
	   strategies that regulate the emotional response to a problem
	Problem focused
	   strategies that manage or alter a problem

unteers to increase the support available to the older person
3. Institutionalization

Care should be offered in the least restrictive environment possible. Once the individual's immediate needs are addressed, the following specific factors contributing to the ineffective coping can be considered.

CLOUDED PERCEPTION OF LIFE EVENTS. Because of the frequency of atypical presentation of disease in the elderly, nurses should be alert for physiological imbalance as a contributor to ineffective coping. Any disorder that impairs tissue oxygenation or use of nutrients at the cellular level potentially affects the individual's perception of the external environment and problem-solving abilities, and thus may adversely affect the individual's ability to cope. The intervention of choice is correction of the physiological disturbance.

It is important to distinguish ineffective coping related to acute, reversible causes from that related to chronic impairments. Those with a chronic impairment in mentation that affects coping require some form of surrogate to provide ongoing support. Those with temporary and reversible coping difficulties require transient support but will later be able to resume former coping patterns.

REDUCED SOCIAL SUPPORT. Older persons often experience a gradual or sudden diminution of social supports as they age. Loss of a spouse, friendly neighbor, or confidant may result in the inability to maintain independent living. Assess the roles performed by the lost member of the support network in determining the appropriate intervention. Some losses can be compensated, particularly in the case of instrumental support services. Even in the case of loss of affective support contributing to ineffective coping, new, emotionally satisfying relationships can be formed although this requires an extended period of time. In the interim, the individual may require transient instrumental support to prevent deterioration of health status.

KNOWLEDGE DEFICIT. Information is a key coping resource. Some older persons may be at a disadvantage in acquiring new knowledge for several reasons, including slowed responses, memory impairment, sensory impairment, and ageism on the part of individuals in positions to share knowledge. There is every indication that older persons benefit from new knowledge if it is presented in a form that is perceptible and understandable and is paced appropriately (see Chapter 15). For a more detailed discussion of teaching methods available to enhance the knowledge of older persons, refer to the section on knowledge deficit in this chapter.

MASSIVE FUNCTIONAL DISABILITY. Although humans have an enormous capacity for adaptation, at some point the number or nature of the stressors in comparison to a person's coping resources and situational support becomes overwhelming. This may occur on a transient or chronic basis. For example, the individual who sustains bilateral cerebral infarctions with a total loss of function initially will be overwhelmed, even with excellent coping resources and social support. Although it is possible for such a person to adapt eventually, nursing action usually is required to compensate for overwhelmed psychological defenses. The key to intervention lies in maximizing the individual's remaining abilities, facilitating the grief process of the client and family, and helping the individual clarify on an ongoing basis both progress and prognosis. The patient's perception is most important because the patient and family often do not understand the powerful impact of skillful rehabilitation in helping individuals compensate for lost function. It is essential that patient and family be included in goal setting and prioritization.

ENVIRONMENTAL CHANGE. Nurses should have a high index of suspicion for environmental change as a factor that precipitates ineffective coping in the elderly because they are sensitive to such changes, those with sensory impairments or mobility impairments being particularly vulnerable. It is vital to determine the older person's functional level before the environmental change took place in order to ascertain whether the functional disability has been induced merely by a change in the environment. For example, older persons who have no difficulty maintaining continence at home may have extreme difficulty remaining continent in the hospital. This change in capacity may be inaccurately perceived by family or patient as an inevitable part of aging and a signal that the older person is losing the ability to cope independently. The true etiology of the functional impairment should be determined (in this case, for example, a new diuretic, lack of privacy, activity restriction, reduced mobility, or urinary tract infection), and both the causes and their treatment should be discussed with the patient and family. Failure to do so may well contribute to a downward spiral leading to increased dependency and reduced coping capacity. Sensitivity to the way in which changes in environmental conditions may precipitate ineffective coping greatly increases the range of the nurse's means of intervention.

Evaluation

Criteria for evaluation of nursing care for patients with ineffective coping should reflect expected outcomes of the desired health state of a patient and specify indicators addressing the extent of achievement of the patient goal. The critical outcome variable for the client with ineffective coping is developing an adequate response repertoire, evidenced by

1. Verbalizing or demonstrating cognitive knowledge learned, skills achieved, and new behaviors acquired; and

2. Using the new knowledge, behavior, and skill in daily life activities.

Additional outcomes might include meeting daily physical needs, realistic cognitive/perceptual domains, and a functional kin/social support network. Questions that might be relevant in evaluating the support network are: What is the nature of the social support available to the patient? Does the patient have a confidant? Has the patient identified a surrogate to act in his or her behalf should ineffective coping again be a problem? Have these support persons been included in plans for the patient's care? Will the patient receive support from any formal agencies? If the nature of this help is time limited, is there a mechanism to re-evaluate the need for support when these services are terminated?

ALTERATIONS IN FAMILY PROCESS AND INEFFECTIVE FAMILY COPING

Definition and Scope of Problem

The family is a unique social system with complex interactional patterns that function to support the attainment of needs for its members (Potter and Perry, 1993, p. 731). Most care of the elderly person is provided informally, within families or kin groups. It is not surprising, then, that understanding the impact of caregiving on caregivers has been and continues to be a major focus within gerontology and gerontological nursing (Kosloski and Montgomery, 1995; George, 1992). Family process is of interest to gerontological nurses because the family often is central to need attainment for older people. The structure, developmental level, and interactions within families vary, and these variations are important in determining the ability of a family to cope with the needs of its elderly members and societal demands.

With population aging, family networks (kin networks) take on new shapes. Multigenerational families are more common; family members have a growing number of relationships that bridge generational lines. Many grandparents are also great-grandparents, i.e., members of families with four generations or more.

Among individuals over age 65 years, more than half are married; nearly 80 per cent have living children; almost 80 per cent have at least one sibling; approximately 75 per cent are grandparents, and at least 40 per cent of the grandparents are also great-grandparents. Furthermore, the majority have other kin, such as cousins, nieces, and nephews. To this mix we also add divorced kin relationships without genetic links, and the questionable loyalties of the children of divorced or never-married parents (Hagestad, 1987; Himes, 1992). It is therefore necessary to be flexible in defining the family unit, paying particular attention to the perception of the older client. Failure to do so may result in the omission of crucial information about decision makers and support systems within the family.

Older people in the United States are well integrated into their family networks. The elderly are significant sources of assistance to the family unit when they are healthy. Most older people live with a spouse or alone, maintaining regular contact with children. Family members are frequently identified by older persons as confidants and they are also most likely to be named as the individuals to whom older persons would turn for assistance in time of need. Thus any loss of a family member represents a significant event in the older person's life. On the other hand, families are likely to experience more stress than ever before in caring for their elders because increases in life expectancy result in larger numbers of dependent older persons to support. Although the responses of the family to the aging of its members are complex, it is clear that a relationship exists between changes in family structures and processes and family coping.

Two major taxonomy patterns, choosing and relating, provide the context for describing five nursing diagnoses relevant to family functioning: Family coping—potential for growth; Ineffective disabling family coping; Ineffective compromised family coping; Altered family processes; and Caregiver role strain (NANDA, 1994). The first three diagnoses are grouped under the concept *choosing* and reflect, overtly or covertly, family choices from some theoretical and finite set of alternatives. Family coping—potential for growth is defined as effective managing of adaptive tasks by a family member involved with the client's health challenge, who now is exhibiting desire and readiness for enhanced health and growth in regard to self and in relation to the client. The second diagnosis, ineffective disabling family coping, is defined as behavior of a significant family or kin member who disables his or her own capacities and the client's capacities to address effectively tasks essential to either person's adaptation to the health challenge. Ineffective compromised family coping is defined as a usually supportive family providing insufficient, ineffective, or compromised support, comfort, assistance, or encouragement, which may be needed by the client to manage or master adaptive tasks related to the health challenge.

The two remaining family diagnoses are grouped under the broader taxonomy concept of *relating*. Altered family processes and caregiver role strain tend to represent relational problems and do not necessarily imply ineffective functioning. Altered family process is defined as the state in which a family that normally functions effectively experiences a dysfunction. Caregiver role strain or potential for caregiver role strain refers to the state in which a caregiver expresses felt difficulty in performing the family caregiver role.

NANDA definitions of these categories have been criticized by psychiatric nurse experts as unclear, although potentially of great use in practice. A major criterion of the standard definition of altered family process is that such alterations do not necessarily imply ineffective functioning (McFarland and Naschinski, 1987).

Family coping—potential for growth is the gold standard that gerontological health care providers seek for older clients and their family/kin networks. Unfortunately, what we see in clinical practice is mostly related to the remaining four diagnoses. While each diagnosis has a unique impact, the consequences common to all may include (1) a reduced support network available to the older person; (2) premature institutionalization; (3) psychiatric illness among family members, particularly depression; (4) abuse or neglect of elders; and (5) exacerbation of stress-related chronic diseases in client or caregivers.

Contributing Factors

Developmental Considerations

Alterations in family process may occur many times throughout the life cycle as a result of developmental events or as an unexpected situational occurrence. Structural changes within the family, such as marriage, birth, death, or divorce, changes in living arrangements, changes in health status or functional status, and role changes can also affect family process. The degree of impact that alterations in family process have on family coping is influenced by the following factors:

- The timing of the precipitating event—whether sudden or gradual, expected or unexpected
- The nature of the alteration, whether permanent or transient
- The degree to which the precipitating events affect individual family members' role relationships outside the family
- The family's previous experiences with alterations in process
- The strengths and weaknesses of the family prior to the precipitating event
- The physical and social environment in which the family is located

Structural changes in the family that may result from alterations in family process include older persons moving in with another relative, relatives moving in with older persons, or institutionalization of older persons. These changes have major ramifications for coping within the newly formed family units. New role relationships and interactional patterns must be formed, and individual needs for privacy, personal space, and affiliation must be considered. In addition, responsibilities for completion of day-to-day household tasks such as meal preparation and housekeeping must be negotiated.

It is difficult to predict which structural changes in households will result in increased coping effectiveness and which will be so stressful that they are worse than no change at all.

A variety of factors contribute to ineffective family coping when a dependent elder is a part of the family, including caregiver stress, impending death, lack of understanding of the aging process, and lack of knowledge about specific disease processes.

Caregiver Role Strain

The demands on caregivers of dependent elders are substantial. Caring for a chronically ill older person is emotionally demanding of both care recipient and caregiver. The course of the illness or multiple illnesses is often unpredictable. Unpleasant or inconvenient lifestyle modifications are often required. In addition, the problems associated with the illness usually result in death (barring a miraculous cure), which generates discouragement and ambivalence.

While caring for their older parents, children may have to take control over financial management, decision making, and physical care. Assuming major responsibility for a parent may involve significant ambivalence and loss for both parent and caregiver. Caregiver role strain, a situation that occurs when other roles and activities of the caregiver are subordinated to the demands of the caregiver role, may develop in children caring for chronically ill older parents. The development of role strain is gradual, as roles other than caregiver are relinquished owing to irreconcilable role conflict (Mui, 1992; Temple and Fawdry, 1992). Caregivers may also face considerable financial burden in supporting a dependent older person. Care for chronic disease is seldom adequately covered under insurance programs, including Medicare. Caregivers are often faced with the nonreimbursable needs of the elderly and must make the choice between paying for the needed services or watching a loved one do without.

Coping with these diverse sources of stress is difficult. Family members are the primary source of assistance for older adults with chronic impairments who continue to live outside of institutional settings (Stone et al., 1987). Caregiving can have pronounced negative effects on family members, although not all caregivers report these difficulties, and some positive effects have been described (Kinney and Stephens, 1989; Lawton et al., 1989; Lawton et al., 1992). Caregivers as well as care recipients may suffer.

Problems caregivers face have not only been conceptualized as strain but also as "burden," with the presumption that greater perceived burden leads to more likelihood of caregiver breakdown and possibly early departure from the caregiver role (Gallagher, 1987). Several negative effects have been reported in those caring for frail elders with varying diagnoses; these include constriction of social life, depression, conflict, and violence (Pillemer and Suitor, 1992).

Because of the essential role that families play in providing care to older persons, there is wide public policy interest in assisting family caregivers and an implicit reliance by public planners on their continued presence (Himes, 1992). Proposed changes in the health care system will probably create a greater reliance on families (Harvath et al., 1994). It is crucial that nurses practicing in a variety of settings be prepared to establish partnerships with family caregivers in order to attend to the long-term needs of older people.

Harvath and colleagues (1994) explored the concepts of local and cosmopolitan knowledge and described their use by gerontological nurses in conceptualizing partnerships with family caregivers to older people. Local knowledge is knowledge that is unique to the inhabitants of a culture—that is, the understanding and skills that the family brings to the caregiving situation. The term "cosmopolitan knowledge" refers to the knowledge and understanding that gerontological nurses bring to the caregiving situation. Four nursing interventions guided by the conceptualization of local and cosmopolitan knowledge were examined in research: (1) acknowledging and affirming the family's local knowledge when it is adequate; (2) developing or enhancing family caregivers' local knowledge when it is inadequate; (3) assisting family caregivers to apply their local knowledge in problem solving; and (4) blending local knowledge with cosmopolitan knowledge of gerontological nurses. The concepts of local knowledge and cosmopolitan knowledge are grounded in anthropological theory.

Pallet (1990) proposes a framework that may guide policy and effective intervention to maximize the caregiver's ability to provide care. The theoretical belief is posited that variables within four domains affect caregiver stress and well-being: (1) characteristics of the impaired relative; (2) characteristics of the caregiver; (3) characteristics of the relationship between the caregiver and recipient of care; and (4) the caregiver's social support resources (Fig. 17–3).

Clearly, several points can be made in summarizing caregiver concerns. First, gerontological nurses can make a significant contribution to this body of knowledge. Clearer conceptualization of the caregiving process is critical. Future studies need to differentiate between different types of family involvement in caregiving—e.g., hands on, paid caregivers, and shared households. Further, it may be appropriate to replace the concept of a caregiver with that of the network in order to study the family as a functioning unit (Barer and Johnson, 1990). Both the foregoing nursing perspectives can be useful in achieving these aims.

Impending Death

To work with dependent older persons is to confront the fact of death. There are many ambiguities in the handling of death and dying in the United States despite the work of Kubler-Ross (1969) and other thanatologists. Discussion of death is difficult, and the anxiety of losing a loved one increases

Characteristics of Cognitively Impaired Relative	Characteristics of Primary Family Caregiver	Characteristics of Dyadic Relationship	Social Support Resources of Primary Caregiver
Level of cognitive impairment	Age Gender	Type of relationship	Size of support network
Behavior problems Functional status	Marital status Health status	Quality of relationship prior to dementia	Type of informal supports available
			Type of formal supports available
Type and amount of care and supervision needed	Social roles Management ability	Quality of current relationship	Ease of contact with available supports
			Perceived supportiveness of social ties in network

F I G U R E   1 7 – 3

Variables within four domains that influence family caregiver stress and well-being in dementia. (From Pallett-Hehn, P.J. A conceptual framework for studying family caregiver burden in Alzheimer's-type dementia. *Image* 22(1):52–58, 1990.)

the difficulty. There is no universally accepted place to die or method by which the chronically ill aged can die. Each caregiver must confront these issues forthrightly with the older person or be forced on the mercy of the whims of the prevailing health care policy. For example, from the beginning of the twentieth century until just prior to the advent of the hospice movement in the United States, it had been almost "unmannerly" to die at home. Few supports were available to caregivers of the dying, and unless a person died at the hospital, doubts lingered that perhaps not everything appropriate had been done to support life.

Since high-quality in-home supportive care has become available (such as that provided by many hospice programs), dying at home has regained some acceptability. However, technology has changed the dying process. Decisions about when and whether to hospitalize, and when and to what extent resuscitative measures should be used are becoming increasingly complex. Changes in the financing of hospital care further complicate decision making for health care providers and family alike. These new ambiguities about an issue that is already fraught with emotional difficulties

produce a stressful situation for both old people and their caregivers. Their methods of coping depend on past coping mechanisms, family strengths, and role relationships.

Brass and Bowman (1990) examined two competing hypotheses about the relationship between care-related strain and the difficulty adjusting to the impaired relative's death. One hypothesis suggests that family members who perceive caregiving as stressful will experience some relief when their relative dies because caregiving responsibilities end.

An alternative hypothesis derived from several conceptualizations posits the opposite relationship, with greater care-related strain predictive of greater strain during the dying and bereavement process. Panel data from spouse and adult-child caregivers collected before and after death support the second hypothesis. Respondents who appraise caregiving as more difficult and those who report more negative caregiving consequences for the family assess bereavement as more difficult and report greater bereavement strain for the family. Consequently, alterations in family processes and ineffective family coping may surround and even remain problematic following the death of an older relative.

Lack of Understanding of the Aging Process

Another stressor for the families of older people is the general lack of knowledge and understanding of the aging process among the general public. Unfortunately, this ignorance extends to many members of the helping professions, making it difficult for older people and their families to gain access to up-to-date information about aging and its effects. Failure to understand the basic accompaniments of aging, such as slowed response time, sensory impairment, and the difference between benign senescent forgetfulness and senility can make life difficult. The family may come to believe that Grandfather is merely being uncooperative when the reality is that he cannot hear adequately to participate in the family's activities. A family that plans activities by taking into account slowed processing time and increased cautiousness in its older members may experience a far richer family gathering than if the activities are oriented only toward the children and younger adults.

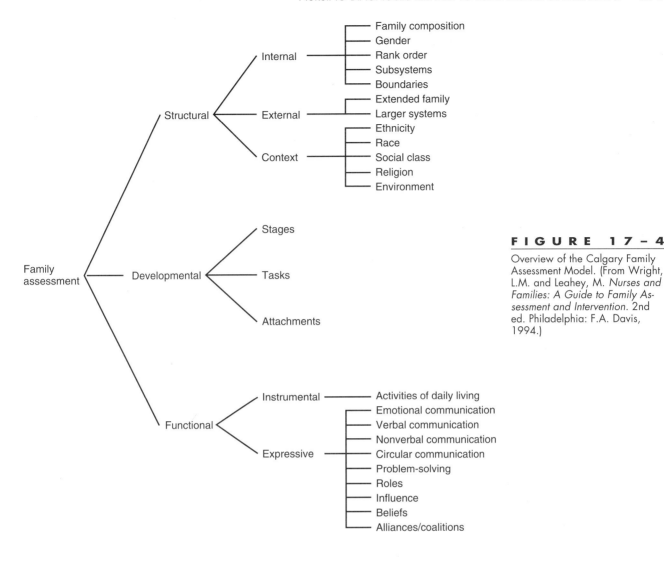

FIGURE 17 - 4

Overview of the Calgary Family Assessment Model. (From Wright, L.M. and Leahey, M. *Nurses and Families: A Guide to Family Assessment and Intervention.* 2nd ed. Philadelphia: F.A. Davis, 1994.)

Lack of Understanding of Specific Disease Processes

One of the most frustrating experiences for a caregiver is to work with someone who is "just not trying." Many of the diseases that cause functional impairment in older persons have fluctuating courses, leading to unpredictable functioning from day to day. Without proper counseling, families may assume that dysfunction is the result of laziness or poor motivation rather than neuronal dysfunction. Understanding and acceptance of the underlying causes of fluctuating function in chronic diseases results in more realistic expectations of the older person and a less stressful atmosphere for the entire family.

Assessment

The purposes of family assessment in working with elderly persons are (1) to de-

fine the nature of the support network available to the older person; (2) to identify demands on the older person; and (3) to identify sources of conflict within the family unit that impede its effective function.

Wright and Leahey (1994) have adapted the Calgary Family Assessment Model (Tomm and Saunders, 1983), dividing family assessment into three categories: structural assessment, developmental assessment, and functional assessment. All three aspects of the family should be assessed at each encounter because families are dynamic groups, and changes in one aspect of a family affect other aspects. These components of family assessment and their constituent elements are diagrammed in Figure 17–4.

Family Structure

GENOGRAM. The first step in family assessment is to define the structure of the everyday family unit and the extended family network. One efficient way to do this is to construct a genogram (Fig. 17–5). For older persons, three generations should be included at a minimum: (1) the older person's spouse, siblings, and cousins; (2) the offspring of the older person's generation; and (3) the grandchildren. If there are other significant family members (alive or dead), they are usually volunteered spontaneously by the informant. Additional information written into the genogram consists of the following: (1) names and ages of all family members; (2) exact dates of birth, marriage, separation, divorce, death, and other significant family life events; and (3) notations, with dates, about occupations, places of residence, illness and changes in life course (Visscher and Clore, 1992).

The next step is to identify key support persons who help in times of illness and who assist with instrumental activities of daily living. Information about the various roles that family members fulfill in regard to older members as well as the roles that older members fulfill in relation to the family should be defined. Older people may have work roles, child-raising responsibilities, or demands placed on them because of illness or other circumstances in the family.

THE FAMILY ECOMAP. The family ecomap (Dalton and Ranger, 1993) is another useful structural assessment tool (Wright and Leahey, 1994). It functions as a visual description of the relationships of family members outside the household, highlighting other strong attachments, competing roles, and the family's connectedness with the larger community. To construct an ecomap, the household or functional family is placed in the center of a circle, and relevant persons, agencies, or institutions are diagrammed outside the main circle. Specifics of the nature of the relationship between the individual in the family and the outside group are noted in the circle. Connections within the family are depicted by lines between the individual and the circle depicting the outside group, with symbols denoting strong bonds or conflicting bonds, as noted in the key to Figure 17–6.

FAMILY VALUES. The final piece of information related to family structure concerns family values. Values include religious beliefs and beliefs about how old people and sick people should be treated. Accurate information about belief systems may be difficult to elicit due to the influence of "social desirability." Social desirability is the tendency of individuals to tell professionals what

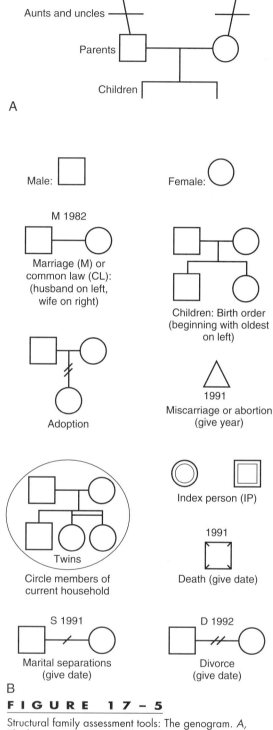

FIGURE 17–5

Structural family assessment tools: The genogram. *A,* Blank genogram; *B,* symbols used in genograms. (From Wright, L.M. and Leahey, M. *Nurses and Families: A Guide to Family Assessment and Intervention.* 2nd ed. Philadelphia: F.A. Davis, 1994.)

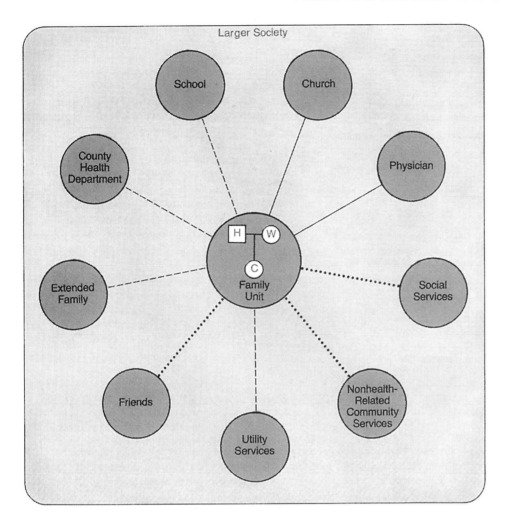

FIGURE 17–6

Structural family assessment tools: The family ecomap. Pictured here are but a few of the many external relationships that could be considered.

Key:

——— Strong, supportive, positive relationship

- - - - - Erratic, conflicted relationship, sometimes supportive and sometimes disruptive

· · · · · Negative, disruptive, or nonexistent relationship (From Betz, C.L., Hunsberger, M. and Wright, S. *Family-Centered Nursing Care of Children*. 2nd ed. Philadelphia: W.B. Saunders, 1994.)

---

they think the professional wants to hear rather than sharing the family's true beliefs. Therefore, a combination of careful observation and nonjudgmental communication techniques should be used in the data-gathering process. Suggesting that certain values may be held but are difficult to live up to may help family members share their beliefs more honestly.

Family Developmental Level

A number of family theorists advocate a life-stage or life-cycle approach to understanding family dynamics. Family development has been defined as

. . . the process of progressive structural differentiation and transformation over the family's history to the active acquisition and selective discarding of rules by incumbents of family positions as they seek to meet the changing functional requisites for survival and as they adapt to recurring life stresses as a family system (Hill and Mattessich, 1979).

Interpretations of family health based on rigid adherence to a model of family development should not be made because the universality of family life stages has not been established through cross-cultural research. A further difficulty with the use of developmental task models for study of aging families is that there is little consensus on what constitutes an appropriate set of roles for older people. Thus, family-stage models are somewhat confining and are inadequate to express the rich diversity of older families.

However, certain tasks do seem to prevail for families with aged members; these include (1) shifting from a focus on work roles to retirement and leisure roles, (2) maintaining the functioning of individuals and couples while adapting to aging-related changes, and (3) preparing for death and coping with the loss of spouse, siblings, and peers (Potter and Perry, 1993). Because difficulties in performing these tasks may create family conflict, assessing an older family in terms of its abilities to deal with these tasks has some merit.

Functional Assessment

Assessing the adequacy of the family's current ability to meet the material and affective needs of its members is done by observing the family in action.

MATERIAL NEEDS. Inferences about the family's ability to provide for the material needs of its members can be made by reviewing health status information about family members such as adequacy of nutritional status, financial status, presence of preventable problems associated with chronic disease, and need for assistance with basic needs.

AFFECTIVE NEEDS. Assessing the family's ability to meet the affective needs of its members requires the nurse to focus on the process of family communications, including verbal and nonverbal communication, ability to solve problems, the allocation of roles, the way in which control over family members is exercised, the expression of beliefs and values, the presence or absence of dysfunctional communication patterns, and the presence of alliances or coalitions among subgroups of the family. In-depth discussion of faulty communication processes is beyond the scope of this chapter. However, family therapy literature is replete with excellent discussions of assessment and treatment of dysfunctional communication patterns (see, for example, McCubbin et al., 1985; Olson et al., 1985; and Archbold and Stewart, 1991).

Conduct of Family Assessment

Assessment of family process should be conducted by direct observation of family interactions. Interview the family members about their estimation of the adequacy of family functioning and individual coping. Question the family about their goals, the quality and character of day-to-day life within the family unit, decision-making processes, and adequacy of resources to meet family needs. Note the degree to which the older person is involved in goal setting, decision making, and the activities of family life.

A comprehensive family assessment is time-consuming and requires some skill in interviewing techniques. Time can be saved by selecting certain aspects of the assessment for screening purposes and saving more in-depth assessment maneuvers for families that are at high risk for ineffective family coping. However, the importance of the family to the well-being of the older person, together with the relative stability of family relationships in advanced age, argues for gathering in-depth family assessment data as a baseline. If time is a major constraint, the minimum acceptable assessment should include identification of the everyday family, children, and key support persons. Interactions with family should be invited whenever appropriate, but the clients' agreement must be obtained, if possible. If clients are unwilling to grant consent to interact with family, then general questioning of clients regarding their perception of the adequacy of family supports is indicated.

Diagnostic Issues

Making a diagnosis of altered family process is not difficult as long as adequate baseline information is obtained. Any recent deviation from the usual patterns of decision making, communication, and need satisfaction is diagnostic. Whether the alteration in family process is indicative of ineffective family coping is a more difficult judgment to make.

Few widely accepted norms are available for assessing effective family coping in the geriatric population. The extreme case of ineffective family coping, elder abuse, is a subject of increasing research by nurses and others (see Chap. 16). The literature on caregiver burnout suggests certain criteria for identifying families with coping difficulties, including increased requests for assistance, increased alcohol and drug use, difficulty in maintaining employment because of care requirements of the older family member, lack of privacy in the home, and interference with parenting. Any of these defining characteristics or related factors may be indicative of ineffective family coping.

The diagnosis of a family with "potential for growth" can be even more difficult. Any family of an older person has a potential to adapt to changes inherent in the aging process; however, assessing the family's readiness to mature or change is imprecise at best. More research is needed to identify families with the greatest potential for change.

Planning

Regardless of the specific nursing diagnosis derived, planning should involve identifying the family unit that is to be the focus of nursing care. Ground rules then should be established regarding communication with other members of the family system. Measures should be taken to protect privacy of individuals, since some members of the family have conflicting goals. The family can be helped to establish specific goals for the family unit that are separate from the goals for individuals within the unit. For example, if the family goal is to have Grandmother live in her own house, regardless of her level of disability, then individual family members' goals may be subordinated to the collective goal. If, however, the predominant family goal is child raising within the nuclear family, without day-to-day participation from extended family members, then the support needs of the old person will have a lower priority.

Sometimes families have difficulty in establishing goals. In such situations, individual need satisfaction is likely to predominate, and goals that require collective action are probably unrealistic.

Intervention

The specific interventions indicated for a family with difficulty in coping or altered process depend on the factors contributing to the situation. Many of the factors that commonly contribute to problematic family situations are listed below, and interventions are discussed according to contributors. When working with families who have coping difficulties, the nurse has two general strategies at her disposal: counseling and referral to another professional for more indepth work.

Referral of the family for counseling or support services depends on the resources available in the community. Nurses should be knowledgeable about family counseling resources and be able to refer the family to a capable therapist, who can then aid in finding the appropriate community resources. The therapist may be another nurse, a social worker, or another professional with knowledge of community resources and family dynamics. Four factors dictate the extent of the nurse's continued involvement with the older person's family: (1) the skills of the nurse in counseling, (2) the time available for counseling, (3) the goals of the family, and (4) the skills and availability of other professionals in the community to accomplish these goals.

If the nurse must refer families to other resources often, it is important to obtain evaluative feedback from the families. A common mistake in referral is assuming that once the referral has been made, the nurse's responsibility ends. Although this view may be technically correct in the eyes of the agency, professional standards dictate that the nurse be aware of the adequacy of the referral network in the community to meet the needs of the client group. This is particularly important in working with the elderly because not all psychotherapists are trained or skilled in working with the problems that are of special concern to aged clients and their families. When deficiencies exist, the nurse should work to correct the service gaps.

Many experts advocate family counseling only with a co-therapist. The rationale is simple: Family systems are inevitably complex. In a co-therapy model it is possible for one therapist to attend to the process of the family, while the other therapist focuses on implementing interventions. Although it is not possible in all situations to work with a co-therapist, the complexity of family systems should be respected and appropriate assistance sought.

Alterations in Family Process

Interventions to assist families experiencing alterations in process are often within the skill level of the nurse. Anticipatory guidance, teaching about normal growth and development, teaching about disease process and its subsequent impact on role enactment, reflective listening, and support for group problem solving are all within the repertoire of generic nursing skills. A limiting factor for many nurses is lack of sufficient time to provide the necessary assistance as well as lack of knowledge of the varied responses to age-related changes within the family. It is important that nurses acquire this knowledge because deviations from normal family process can then be readily identified without misjudging families whose process may seem unusual, but in which need attainment for all members is achieved.

DEVELOPMENTAL EVENTS. Retirement, death, and changes in health status are three age-related events that alter family process.

Retirement. *Retirement* affects family process in several ways: (1) income is generally reduced, (2) the worker gives up the role of worker and has increased time in the household, and (3) there is generally less structure to the day than was the case during active employment. Reduction in income means that budgets may have to be planned more carefully, and sacrifices may have to be made. Whereas at one time unilateral budget decisions may have been the norm, with more restrictive financial circumstances, the spouse may become more active in decision making about money. Although the shift toward shared financial decision-making may be healthy, it may also be a source of additional friction in the marriage. Couples may need assistance in recognizing that the change in economic status with retirement is a nearly universal phenomenon and not the result of inadequate planning. Suggest methods of joint decision-making (if this is a new pattern for the couple) and assist them in practicing these methods with role play using examples less emotionally charged than money matters.

Role change accompanies retirement, usually affecting the spouse or other household members most acutely as the retiree explores new role options. Role relationships within the household undergo realignment. Men may assume more responsibility for household tasks, while women may have to relinquish some territory and privacy during the hours when the worker was away from the home. Anticipatory guidance in this situation can be extremely helpful. Although research on the effectiveness of preretirement planning or counseling sessions on the well-being of retirees is equivocal, this may be because the outcome measures have not focused on family functioning. There is considerable anecdotal evidence of the stressfulness of retirement for spouses, although the majority of families resolve this stressful period without external assistance.

The transition to retirement presents several challenges and some rewards for husbands, wives, and families (Vinick and Ekerdt, 1991). The term "retirement" signifies a set of economic and societal practices that manage the size of the labor force. It also designates a social status considered by some to be a historically new stage of the life course. Areas of nursing concern relate to health promotion and disease prevention during this time of transition. The maintenance of personal resources and health has a tremendous impact on the quality of the retirement experience. The effect of retirement on spouses' division of household tasks, including caregiving; subjective well-being of widows in retirement communities; and labor force participation rates are just a few of the areas in which nursing may have an impact on family coping (Hayward et al., 1994; Hong and Duff, 1994; Szinovacz and Harpster, 1994).

Death of a Family Member. Death results in irrevocable structural change within the family. Most people are familiar with situations in which an extended family network was maintained entirely by one strong family member. On the death of that person, many family customs and practices ended. On a more mundane level, the death of a family member may mean that a household is no longer able to function independently. A recently widowed spouse may require extensive skill training to function independently. Although such extreme situations exist, usually family or friends are available to buffer the immediate negative effects of the loss of a family member. However, for those who are unable or unwilling to learn new skills, loss of a family member can be devastating. For this reason it is important to identify family units that are particularly vulnerable to the adverse effects of alterations in family process and initiate plans to mitigate the effects of such changes if they should occur.

For example, S.J. is a 78-year-old woman with profound dementia and hypothyroidism. She lives with her husband, who is her primary caregiver. They have no children, and Mr. J.'s health is quite fragile. Should he predecease his wife, a crisis would occur because there would be no one readily available to provide S.J. with the care that she needs on an ongoing basis. Nursing intervention for this couple includes confronting the possibility that Mr. J. may predecease his wife and discussing available options for continuing care for her. A written plan for her continued care should be established, along with identification of a guardian authorized to implement the plan, to avoid such a predictable crisis.

Considerable debate continues regarding issues of advance directives, surrogate decision makers, and durable powers of attorney. For many years gerontological research was guided by the myth that old people were alienated from their families, that families did not care, and that children had abandoned their older relatives to institutions for care. This scenario is not completely true and lacks compelling empirical data. We know that families are a major source of help to older adults. As gerontological nurses we need more research and data on advance directives, on how and why family involvement in surrogate decision making goes awry, but also on how well it works, especially when elders are without adult children or other genetically linked relatives (High, 1991).

CHANGE IN HEALTH STATUS OF FAMILY MEMBER. Changes in health status of family members may precipitate changes in family process. Diseases that either cause functional disability or pose a serious threat to life are the common contributing factors in the aged family. When a family member cannot carry out some aspects of the role repertoire, another family member must carry the additional burden, or needs will go unfulfilled. Thus, a change in health status puts the family in double jeopardy: There is a change in family process because of the failure of role fulfillment and also because of the need to assume new role responsibilities.

Functional disability in the elderly is usually of a chronic and progressive nature. This means that ongoing arrangements for the altered capacity of the elder to fulfill certain roles must be made within the family unit. Cobe (1985) suggests that the central issue to be resolved between elders and their children is the provision of "appropriate independence" for the elders within the family unit. Brody (1985) contends that "parent care" has become a normative developmental event for adult children. She notes that care of the old-old has become a major new role for the young-old but questions its attractiveness compared to some of the other new roles being opened to young-old persons, such as creative pursuits, second careers, and volunteer activities. The stressful nature of parent care is underscored.

Teaching, guidance, and health promotion are of paramount importance. Family members will turn to professionals for guidance about the length of time impairment will be experienced, the nature of the impairment, and the factors that accentuate or reduce the impact of the impairment. The family will often need assistance in understanding the specific limitations imposed by the impairment. For example, expressive aphasia as a result of a CVA does not necessarily mean that the affected individual cannot comprehend what is being spoken. The family should understand that the patient may derive considerable benefit from continuing to function as a listener in family discussions, even if conversation is not possible. Preserving role function when possible is an impor-

tant goal when working with family members of those with recent changes in health status.

Identifying the full range of care options is an important intervention in families of older persons experiencing changes in health status. Although specific needs for care vary with the nature of the health impairment, the chronic nature of most impairments places great demands on family caregivers. Montgomery and Kosloski (1994) found that certain characteristics, stressors, and resources available to family caregivers were related to their attitudes toward institutionalization. Generally, those who experienced health problems related to caregiving responsibilities, feelings of being "tied down," and feelings of resentment, hopelessness, and guilt were more likely to consider institutionalization than those who did not experience these states.

Unfortunately, predicting outcomes of family caregiving and the likelihood of nursing home institutionalization is not a simple linear process. Montgomery and Kosloski's (1994) research using an event history framework indicates that the predictors of placement differ substantially for elders cared for by spouses from those cared for by adult children. There were differences not only in the conditions under which caregiving ends, but also apparent differences in when caregiving begins and how it is perceived by the caregiver. Some of the findings revealed that for elders cared for by spouses, women were more likely to be placed than men, and placement was more likely when the caregiver was not working.

Further, for both groups of caregivers, lower morale was associated with an increased probability of placement. As indicated in most research literature, the presence of Alzheimer's disease and a greater need for assistance with household activities of daily living predicted placement for both groups. Gerontological nurses must remember that the marital relationship is fundamentally different from the parent-child relationship in terms of implications related to changes in health status. Clearly, additional research is necessary to corroborate the findings from the Montgomery and Kosloski study, and to fill in gaps in our understanding of the implications of changes in health status and family coping.

RELOCATION. Geographic mobility is normal in American society. It is therefore important that families consider the impact of relocation on family process and plan means of preserving important functions despite relocation. A case in point is A.A., a

72-year-old retired home economist with chronic drug dependence problems who lives near her daughter and depends on her for assistance with household management. The daughter's husband takes a new job in a town 100 miles away. Without the regular support of the daughter in running the household, A.A. would probably forego regular meals and thus would not be able to meet all of her basic needs. Her family sought counseling about the options available to cope with the impending move without sacrificing need attainment for any of the family members. Reflective listening regarding the family's goals and resources and the individual family members' goals was important in helping this family. Additionally, information was provided about residential retirement communities in the state, which could substitute for some of the instrumental support provided by the daughter. Ultimately, the patient decided to cope with the relocation by moving to the same county as the daughter, at the same time selecting a residential retirement community as her new residence to decrease her vulnerability to future relocation of family members.

CHANGE IN HOUSEHOLD COMPOSITION. New household members may come from many sources. Recent attention has been focused on the "empty nest" that does not ever empty. Adult children may choose to move back to their parents' home because the children require or desire continued support. Although a myth persists in American culture that extended families are best, in reality, once separation from the nuclear family as an adult has taken place, sharing a household with family members of another generation may be problematic. Unresolved conflicts from childhood may resurface. The elders may be exploited if the adult children use a dependent parent's resources to further their own goals at the expense of the elder's well-being.

Another common source of change in household membership may occur in the case of a dependent older person. A "live-in" helper to assist the older person may be secured in the hope that this will prevent or forestall institutionalization. There is often a failure to recognize that this type of hired assistance inevitably becomes a part of the family unit and thus affects the family process. For some families this is a happy occurrence: There is a match between the older person's needs, the helper's skills, and congruence of values and interactional patterns. However, for others, this new addition be-

comes an ongoing nightmare. Differences in social class, time utilization, need for personal space and privacy, and interactional style may conspire to make life with the new family addition more stressful than it was before. Guidance pertaining to reasonable expectations for paid helpers and the complexities of adding a new household member may be the difference between a family who enters a new phase of its development and one that becomes severely stressed by the new situation.

INSTITUTIONALIZATION. The impact of institutionalization of a family member on the functioning of a family unit is highly variable. It depends on the characteristics of the institution and of the family. It also depends on the precipitating cause of the institutionalization. If the institutionalization was perceived to be an answer to an intolerable family situation by all members, then the effects of the move on family process may be more helpful than detrimental. More commonly, however, there is considerable ambivalence among family members regarding the change. This may result in unclear understanding of the role of the institution in providing for the patient's needs and the new roles of family members. Anticipatory guidance may be helpful in this regard, although more research is needed in this area.

Relocation of elderly individuals to an institution can, on occasion, enhance relations between the individual and members of the family. However, what remains less clear and less documented are the roles that families assume in the care of their family member in nursing facilities and the specific degree of family involvement in care. According to Schwartz and Vogel (1990), previous research studies have indicated substantial role ambiguity among nursing facility staff and relatives of residents. However, in their own research, considerable agreement was found among both groups. It is hypothesized that defining appropriate and workable roles for family would improve quality of care for residents in institutions.

Impaired Family Coping

OVERWHELMING NEEDS OF ONE FAMILY MEMBER. *Overwhelming* is a highly value-laden term. It is analogous to pain in that its experience contains a large subjective component. The perceptions of individual family members are extremely important.

Some families become dysfunctional because virtually all activities center on the attainment of needs for one member. An example of this is the multigenerational family that is committed to caring at home for an elder severely impaired by senile dementia of the Alzheimer's type. The patient requires constant attendance and assistance with all activities of daily living and has exhausted her own finances. The teen-aged granddaughter is not allowed to bring friends home because they might disturb the patient. The daughter and her husband have no private time together because the patient does not tolerate being left alone and sleeps less than anyone else in the household. When family life revolves around one member, other members' needs may go unmet. Respite services, if available, should be part of the plan of care. This intervention can allow time for the family to rest as well as provide noncrisis time for re-evaluation of family and caregiving goals.

Interventions should focus on helping the family unit to reassess and clarify their goals. Without the observations of others, the family decision makers may unwittingly overlook other important family goals. Sometimes "promises" have been made to an elder that may not be realistic to keep in altered family circumstances. This is a conclusion that some families may not be able to reach without professional assistance.

Support groups may be helpful to families with ineffective coping. Although it may be extremely difficult to get family members to attend a support group while they are in the midst of a crisis, the opportunity to hear the experiences of others who are coping with similar problems may offer fresh insights into the family situation (Glosser and Wexler, 1985). Some support groups offer services to individuals, so unwillingness to attend a group meeting is not always a barrier to this type of intervention.

INSUFFICIENT FINANCIAL RESOURCES. Care of the elderly can be an expensive enterprise. As noted elsewhere in this text, many care needs are not reimbursed by insurance companies, Medicare, or Medicaid. For example, dentures, a vital prosthesis for some, is not an expense that is covered by most third-party payers. Low- or moderate-income families must make difficult choices between individual and family goals. Is it more important for Grandmother to have her medicine or for the family to have a nutritious diet? Is it more important for one spouse to have physical therapy or for the roof to be repaired?

Two general strategies apply when finances are inadequate. The first is to ensure that the family is obtaining the maximum governmental benefits to which it is entitled. Although this may seem obvious, clinicians should remember that the intricacies of bureaucracies may seem overwhelming at first glance to overstressed families. Additionally, the older client and family may not be aware of the full range of income-related benefits available. Securing a trustworthy volunteer may make a tremendous difference in the family's ability to benefit from governmental services. The second strategy available to the nurse involves counseling to help the family clarify its goals and priorities. Communication patterns may be distorted in the family as a result of the increased demands on the family system. An "outsider" to the family is in an excellent position to observe such dysfunctional processes and either intervene directly or refer the family for therapy.

LACK OF UNDERSTANDING OF DISEASE PROCESSES. Misunderstandings regarding the nature, course, or treatment of a chronic illness may precipitate ineffective family coping. Fear that a disorder such as Alzheimer's disease is genetically determined may render a family member incapable of providing care. Lack of knowledge about the natural history of a disability may lead to unrealistic expectations on the part of the patient and subsequent resentment. This in turn may lead to abusiveness or neglect. Finally, lack of knowledge about the client's disabilities may lead to unrealistic expectations by the family unit. For example, failure to understand the progressive irremediable nature of some disorders may lead well-intentioned family members to take leaves of absence from jobs, simultaneously promising the client care until recovery has been achieved. This sets the stage for either broken trust or unexpected loss of income. Conversely, if the family perceives the client's problems to be more serious than is the case, jobs may be relinquished unnecessarily or inappropriate dependency fostered.

Prevention of knowledge deficits about chronic illness is the preferred mode of intervention. This is sometimes easier said than done. Merely conveying information does not ensure learning. Readiness to hear or to learn new information may not always coincide with the timing of patient or family teaching. Thus, it is useful when possible to build in opportunities for reinforcement of teaching about chronic illness, disabilities, and aging-related changes. Because families are dynamic systems, nurses should be alert for changes in family composition that may necessitate re-teaching of pertinent content.

IMPENDING LOSS OF FAMILY MEMBER. In a prolonged terminal illness, the impending loss of a family member may precipitate ineffective family coping. The family prepares for the patient to die, and the patient does not die on cue. A similar situation may occur in families anticipating major losses in the functioning capacity of the patient.

Anticipatory guidance serves a useful purpose for those near bereavement, but when terminally ill individuals are robbed of life roles, responsibilities, and opportunities in which they might participate, the family is not coping optimally. The key is to help the family re-assess the patient's current functioning level and aid the family in supporting that level.

DEATH OF FAMILY MEMBER. The same losses that may precipitate alterations in family processes may also trigger ineffective coping responses. Similar interventions are indicated. Clinicians should be alert to the need to promote the safety and security of elderly clients in situations in which family coping is clearly ineffective.

Evaluation

Evaluation of the effectiveness of nursing care with families is difficult for the same reasons that precise diagnosis is difficult: few norms exist. However, the criteria for evaluation of care are supported by the research that does exist.

1. Does the client belong to an identifiable family unit?
2. Does that family unit promote need attainment (physical and psychoemotional) for all members?
3. Does the family have clear understanding of the limitations and abilities of the client?
4. Does the family understand the full range of resources available to the older person?
5. Are the family goals and the older individual's goals compatible?

DECISIONAL CONFLICT

Definition and Scope of the Problem

Decisional conflict is the state of uncertainty about a course of action to be taken when choice among competing actions involves risk, loss, or challenge to personal life values (NANDA, 1994). The focus of the conflict should be specified when using this diagnosis and may include choices regarding health, family relationships, career, finances, or other life events.

For the individual's choice to be considered ethically and legally valid, three elements are required: voluntariness, mental capacity, and adequate information (Rozovsky, 1990).

The problem of decisional conflict is not implicated when decisional power transfers from the mentally incapacitated person to a proxy. Rather it refers to the mentally capable older person who needs a little help from family and kin networks to get by (Kapp, 1991). This discussion of decisional conflict will be presented in the context of health care decision-making, recognizing that the scope of this problem affects aspects of daily living and has profound biopsychosocial implications. One of the greatest concerns of older adults is that decisional conflict will be viewed as decisional incapacity, which would call into question the individual's mental competence.

Contributing Factors

Many factors can contribute to decisional conflict, particularly those that involve complex medical interventions of great risk. The conflictual nature of a situation may be compounded by the amount of information available to the elder, the ability of the person to process the information at the pace presented, and the degree to which the decision is viewed as voluntary. Problem situations include decisions about surgery, chemotherapy, enteral feedings (Krynski et al., 1994), marriage, divorce, institutionalization, retirement, and cessation of life-support systems. These examples are not exhaustive but reflect situations that may be problems (Carpenito, 1989).

Assessment

Assessing decisional capability and conflict is best completed in partnership with the client and family. Barring the presence of family, assessments might include a team of health professionals working with the elder client. The major areas to be addressed in a psychosocial assessment relative to decisional conflict include value/belief patterns, mental status, health perceptions, coping and stress patterns, role relationships, communication ability, and economic situation.

For each assessment parameter, some judgment about the cultural context in which the elder individual exists is also required. Few structured value/belief instruments exist, thus careful interview skill is required. Valid and reliable assessment tools can be used to determine the course of intervention, treatment, and outcomes (Harden, 1989). In assessing mental status, the gerontological nurse may find the Mini-Mental Status Questionnaire (Folstein and colleagues, 1975) useful in the initial assessment. The MMS Questionnaire is an 11-item form that provides a quantitative assessment of cognitive performance.

The major defining characteristics for decisional conflict include verbalized uncertainty about choices, verbalization of undesired consequences of alternative actions being considered, vacillation between alternative choices, and delayed decision making. These are the characteristics that the gerontological nurse should seek to discover during careful assessment.

Planning

The desired outcomes/goals for an older person experiencing decisional conflict include making an informed decision, stating advantages and disadvantages of the choices considered, and sharing fears and concerns about the choice made and responses of others. In developing a plan of action to address this problem, the gerontological nurse must consider individual, family, and community resources. Because of likely and recurring decisional conflict in later life, the nurse, in mutual cooperation with the client, should plan to increase the preparedness and confidence of the older adult in decision making regarding health care. From a health promotion perspective, the older adult might be encouraged to participate in empowerment and self-help groups. The plan might also include referral to the local library for additional information or instruction in the use of various telephone information services. The National Institute on Aging at the National Institutes of Health prints several information pamphlets under the topic of "Age Page." Each Age Page addresses a health concern of interest to older adults. The nurse might incorporate such a strategy into the plan of care. During clinic visits, the nurse could plan to inform and counsel the older adult and family members about decisions in conflict. Specific plans for interventions are discussed next.

Intervention

Interventions to increase preparedness for decision making and to resolve decisional conflicts should be based on scientific rationale. There is, however, a dearth of research in this area. For current purposes, the diagnosis of decisional conflict about initiation of enteral tube feeding will be the focus for discussion of intervention process (Carpenito, 1989; Ackley and Ladwig, 1993; Kim et al., 1993; Krynski et al., 1994). The goals remain as identified earlier. The nurse will

- Establish time for individual and family assessments.

- Explore with the older adult and family the stated health care goal and clarify alternatives and their possible consequences for accepting or rejecting enteral tube feeding.

- Realign unrealistic expectations; anticipating a negative consequence, such as death, when that likelihood is extremely low or anticipating a positive consequence when *that* likelihood is low—e.g., no diarrhea or additional weight loss— may increase decisional conflict.

- Identify with the client value tradeoffs implicit in making a choice for or against tube feeding: e.g., you will become weak—as your body becomes weaker from lack of food your mind becomes more confused; or, your body becomes stronger, you are able to go home from a hospital with a tube feeding, the tube feeding may be for a very short time.

- Supply the decision makers with appropriate and informative written materials.

- Identify printed materials, organizations, and persons that might be helpful in making a decision.

- Allow time for vacillation; decisions that have high negative consequences may be reversed.

- Be supportive of the family unit throughout the process, recognizing that a final decision may not be to everyone's satisfaction. If the family membership cannot be supportive, at least help them avoid destructive behaviors.

- Monitor previously resolved problems.

Evaluation

Evaluation of this problem should first focus on whether or not the outcomes/goals were achieved. Further evaluation will consider the quality and completeness of the assessment data and whether revisions and updates are planned. The nurse must also judge the extent to which the interventions were carried out as planned and how the process might be revised to better assist the client.

FEAR

Definition and Scope of Problem

Fear is a feeling of dread related to an identifiable source that the person validates. Fear is distinguished from anxiety by the fact that the patient can identify the source of the discomforting feeling. Although fear may be a realistic response to the client's self-appraisal of abilities or environmental circumstances, it may also be based on inadequate knowledge of the situation or on a lack of understanding of the full range of options that are open. For example, some people who fear placement in a nursing home may not have visited a nursing home for many years and are reacting to outdated information about conditions in nursing homes. Some patients who are fearful of falling are not aware of the potential effects of a structured program of rehabilitation to reduce the risk of falling and fall-related injury. Fears in elderly persons should therefore be identified and addressed forthrightly.

Contributing Factors

Any circumstance that threatens the individual's well-being, autonomy, preferred life style, or comfort is a potential source of fear. Most fears have some base in reality, but the older person's response to the reality may be immobilizing. Common fears expressed by older people include fear of falling, fear of dependency, fear of institutionalization, fear of crime, and fear of economic ruin.

Assessment

The key to assessment of fear is establishing a trusting relationship with the older person. Although some people are so consumed by fear that they will eagerly voice their concerns, other people may be more reluctant to share their fears because they do not want to appear childlike or silly. Nurses should therefore be alert for subtle signals that fear is an underlying problem. Cues pointing to undisclosed fears include excess dependency in activities of daily living, a reluctance to be discharged from an institutional environment, or frequent deferral to another family member or friend for decision making. Although these behaviors may also signal problems such as powerlessness, anxiety, or alteration in self-concept, fear should be considered a possible diagnosis.

Planning

One key planning issue is the identification of others who should be involved in resolving the patient's fear. Some fears can be treated within a counseling relationship between patient and nurse. Others require involvement of many persons. For example, fear of returning home following a hospitalization may be resolved by encouraging the patient to express the fear and then arranging for frequent home health visits immediately after discharge to monitor posthospital progress and reinforce teaching. This requires only a minimum of intervention by others. In contrast, fear of crime in a neighborhood may require facilitating an extensive network of volunteers, family, and police to allow the old person to venture outside the home.

Interventions

Interventions to reduce fear in older persons generally involve increasing the client's knowledge, competence, or awareness of the feared situation or object. Progressive relaxation and guided imagery are two stress reduction techniques that may be applicable to older persons experiencing fear (Zahourek, 1985; Rickard et al., 1994). Possible interventions for common sources of fear in older people are discussed below:

- Fear of pain: Use premedication, deep breathing, and systematic relaxation techniques and provide preparatory sensory information before painful procedures. Be with the older person during the procedure, if possible. Consider whether the patient is a candidate for self-management of pain medication and offer the option if feasible.

- Fear of nursing home placement: Encourage patient to express fantasies about nursing home life. Then enlist the assistance of family or friends to obtain first-hand information about local nursing homes regarding the feared attributes. If the fantasized fears are based in reality, try anticipatory problem solving to allow the patient opportunity to exert some control over the situation. Consider shopping for a nursing home that has the least number of feared characteristics.

- Fear of falling: Assess patient's previous fall patterns and risk factors for fall-related injury. Implement a plan to reduce risk for fall-related injury, and include the patient in establishing goals and evaluation criteria. Explore fears with patient more fully. Fears may be based on an experience in which situational elements were quite different—e.g., the patient's sister died after a fall, but the patient's risk of fall-related injury is not high. In institutional settings, if the problem is prevalent, consider establishing a self-help group including those who have successfully coped with the problem.

- Fear of crime: Contact local police department for information about neighborhood watch programs, other resources for frail, isolated individuals. Encourage client to express specific fears about crime and facilitate reality testing and problem solving.

- Fear of incontinence: Explore meanings and fears of incontinence with the individual. This may be the first opportunity offered to the client to discuss the human aspects of incontinence. Knowledge deficits about incontinence may be revealed, which in turn may suggest some strategies for intervention. For example, if a woman no longer goes to church because she fears the embarrassment associated with an episode of stress incontinence, then she could be counseled about the effectiveness of Kegel exercises and other behavioral therapies, as well as types and availability of pads for such an occasion.

Evaluation

Effectiveness of interventions for those with fears can be judged by two criteria:

1. Does the client identify the fear as resolved?
2. Have the signs of dysfunction or restricted activity associated with the fear(s) been alleviated?

There has been little nursing research to define realistic time schedules for resolution of fears. It is reasonable to assume that the more complex the intervention required, the more time will be required for resolution.

CASE EXAMPLE

A.N. was an 86-year-old woman admitted to the hospital because of a septic knee and uncompensated congestive heart failure. Prior to the hospitalization she was functionally independent in all domains and lived alone. She had not been hospitalized in the past 50 years. The knee inflammation caused her to have considerable pain on motion. As a result, she limited her mobility to such an extent that she performed no activities of daily living independently because she was afraid of inducing more pain. She became increasingly weak and developed a grade II sacral pressure sore.

To reverse this downward spiral of declining function secondary to fear of pain, the nurse began giving the patient regular doses of analgesia rather than administering pain medication only on an "as requested" basis. The nurse also instructed A.N. on the relationship between immobility and decreased strength and ability. Finally, the nurse stayed with the patient and assisted her in performing activities within her functional capacity, such as sitting on the bedside commode and bathing and grooming activities. Increased activity helped reduce the edema associated with the infection. The experience of increased activity without an increase in knee pain served to resolve the patient's fear of pain with increased activity.

GRIEVING

Definition and Scope of Problem

Grief is a natural human response to the loss or threatened loss of a loved object; it is a response that involves thoughts, feelings, and actions. Adaptation to losses is believed to occur gradually through a process of grief resolution. Two categories of grieving are currently recognized as nursing diagnosis categories: anticipatory grieving, or the response to a loss before it actually occurs, and dysfunctional grieving, a delayed or exaggerated response to a perceived, actual, or potential loss (NANDA, 1994).

As in many areas of daily living, a variety of terms are used to describe the processes associated with death and bereavement. In the literature we find bereavement, grief, grieving, and bereavement process. Many of the terms are overlapping or are used interchangeably. In this chapter, bereavement is defined as the action of having someone go permanently out of one's control, possession, or environment. The term as used will always pertain to the death of a person. Grief refers to the complex of feelings, cognitions, and behaviors of an individual in response to a loss. Grieving can be seen as experiencing sorrow, pain, distress, and sadness about a loss. Bereavement process will refer to the cognitive, affective, and behavioral changes in the bereaved individual after the loss (Cleiren, 1993).

It is generally believed that if the death can be anticipated, the period before the death will in some way influence adaptation after the death. Unfortunately, the extent to which stress as a response to anticipatory grief can be considered valuable for adaptation to the actual loss remains unclear.

Caserta and Lund (1992) compared the stress and coping levels of 108 older adults who recently lost their spouses with expectations of stress and coping reported by 85 matched nonbereaved controls. The bereaved reported moderately high stress levels over 2 years; however, their stress scores were lower and their coping scores were higher than those the nonbereaved anticipated their levels would be if their spouse died. The findings are consistent with evidence beginning to emerge in the bereavement literature demonstrating resiliency on the part of those who have suffered a loss; the ability to cope with loss is often underestimated. Further, for many older adults, death is not unanticipated. Consequently, some caution is warranted in the use of literature related to anticipatory grieving.

Aging is associated with many losses. Gerontological nurses should be knowledgeable about the grieving process and about means of facilitating resolution of losses. Unfortunately, there are serious limitations to the research based on grief as experienced by the elderly. First, most research on bereavement pertains to loss of a spouse. Many of the approaches to bereavement counseling are based on research done with younger subjects, and much of this research has serious methodological flaws (Cleiren, 1993). Second, not all losses associated with aging involve loss of an object outside the self. Many of the losses associated with aging involve losses of bodily function, structural change, or role. Grief associated with long-term illness or disability differs in important ways from grief associated with loss of a significant other. The distinctions include the magnitude of the loss and the continual confrontation of the loss (Cleiren, 1993).

When a loved one dies, there is hope of resolution of grief. That person is gone and one can learn to live without him. More important, he is not reappearing constantly to reactivate the feelings of loss. On the other hand, the loss of one's own functioning is always present. Although the feelings about this loss also diminish over time, events frequently occur that remind the person that he is less than perfect. Grief raises its ugly head each time the illness or disability becomes conspicuous or when it significantly interferes with hoped-for goal achievement (Warner-Beland, 1980, p. 4).

Despite the limitations of the literature on grief as applied to elderly people, individuals at high risk of dysfunctional grieving can be identified (Table 17–3), and coping strategies of the bereaved are well described.

Theoretical Issues

As indicated earlier, there is controversy about whether anticipatory grieving is helpful to those experiencing loss or a risk factor for adjustment problems following the loss. Part of the controversy stems from imprecise use of the term *anticipatory grieving*. Anticipatory grieving should be reserved for the actual response to the loss in advance, as distinguished from anticipatory guidance, which describes the help given by professionals in providing accurate information, support for expression of anticipatory anxiety, opportunity for continued interaction with the dying person, and structuring of opportunities for people to resolve "unfinished business" with the dying person (Clei-

TABLE 17–3
Risk Factors for Dysfunctional Grieving

TYPE OF DEATH
Sudden, unexpected, or untimely
Painful, horrifying, or mismanaged

CHARACTERISTICS OF RELATIONSHIP
Dependent or symbiotic
Ambivalent
Death of spouse

CHARACTERISTICS OF SURVIVOR
Grief-prone personality (clinging or pining behaviors)
Experience of anticipatory grief
Insecure, anxious, low self-esteem
Previous mental illness
Excessively angry
Excessively self-reproachful
Previous unresolved losses
Inability to express feelings (especially those with self-image that prohibits expressing feelings of grief)

SOCIAL CIRCUMSTANCES
Family absent or seen as unsupportive
Detached from traditional religious and cultural support systems
Low socioeconomic status
Other concurrent losses ("bereavement overload")

ren, 1993). The defining characteristics for anticipatory grieving are summarized by NANDA (1994):

1. Potential loss of significant object
2. Expression of distress at potential loss
3. Denial of potential loss
4. Guilt
5. Anger
6. Sorrow
7. Choked feelings
8. Changes in eating habits
9. Alterations in sleep patterns
10. Alterations in activity level
11. Altered libido
12. Altered communication patterns

Dysfunctional grief reactions may be absent, prolonged, delayed, or exaggerated responses to a loss (Ackley and Ladwig, 1993). When many symptoms of grief persist and remain intense for longer than 2 years or when the individual's functioning becomes significantly impaired or detrimental in relation to a loss, dysfunctional grieving may be diagnosed.

The process of grief resolution has been variously described, and Kubler-Ross's (1969) stages are familiar to most readers: denial, anger, bargaining, depression, acceptance. Although considerable disagreement exists regarding how people pass through these stages, most writers agree that most people experience these phases many times over during the process of adjusting to loss. Strong and often uncomfortable emotions accompany these phases, leading to strained relationships with others. Thus, unresolved grief should be understood as a potential barrier to rehabilitation and to establishment of new social networks.

Contributing Factors

The major contributing factor to anticipatory grieving is knowledge of an impending major loss, when the exact timing of the loss is uncertain. Also, caregivers and families of demented patients may experience intense grief reactions to the gradual loss of the patient's intellectual functioning and pre-illness personality. Thus, grief before the actual death of the person may be both anticipatory for loss of the person and actual for loss of the bodily function (Jones and Martinson, 1992).

The factors that contribute to dysfunctional grieving are not well understood in elderly people. However, three major factors appear to influence the bereavement process in the elderly: (1) support network, (2) presence of concurrent losses, and (3) individual

coping skills (Bateman et al., 1992; Curry and Stone, 1992; Watson, 1994). Individuals with more extensive support networks are more likely to make a successful adaptation to a loss (Lazarus, 1993). Those who experience multiple concurrent losses are thought to have more difficulty in adapting to the losses (Bateman et al., 1992). Individuals with well-developed coping skills, particularly the ability to solve problems rather than use defense mechanisms such as denial or projection, are more likely to resolve a loss successfully (Watson, 1994).

Parkes (1985) identifies four common patterns of dysfunctional grieving. The first pattern occurs when an individual has pre-existing tendencies toward psychiatric illness that are exacerbated by the loss. The second pattern, labeled the "unexpected grief syndrome," occurs when the loss is either unexpected or untimely, and denial is the major defense mechanism used. The individual typically manifests moderate-to-severe anxiety and experiences feelings of self-reproach and continued obligation to the lost person. A third pattern is the "ambivalent grief syndrome" in which in the early stages of bereavement the individual feels relief but later experiences anxiety, despair, and desire to make amends, with no satisfactory means of doing so. The bereaved person may become self-punitive. Finally, there is a chronic grief pattern, which is based on a relationship between the bereaved and the deceased characterized by dependency of one member on the other. The bereaved is left with feelings of helplessness even if he or she was the "stronger" of the two.

Assessment

Assessment for those experiencing anticipatory grief employs an approach similar to that used for individuals suffering from dysfunctional grieving. First, determine the individual's anxiety level and ability to process information. Next, specify the nature and extent of social support available to the older person. Attempt to elicit the meaning of the loss of the individual and previous experiences with similar losses. Finally, determine what specific functional impairment(s) the older person is experiencing, using data from the older person's perspective as well as that of family or friends.

Assessment of the person's anxiety level and level of cognition helps the nurse establish priorities and select interventions appropriate for the individual's cognitive and emotional level of function. If the individual's anxiety is extreme, this must be treated before the grief can be addressed.

Assessment of social support centers on determining the presence or absence of a confidant. Those without a confidant will require additional help in securing someone who will listen as they reflect on the loss. Some bereaved older persons may have difficulty in carrying out instrumental activities of daily living, and therefore require the presence of support people to assist with these needs. Determine the extent of the support network by asking the older person or the next of kin.

The meaning of the loss to the grieving individual is best determined by listening carefully to the individual's description of the loss and remaining alert throughout the encounter for references to the loss and its meaning. Explore allusions to changes in self-concept, self-esteem, role performance, habit patterns, and fears about the impact of the loss. Data should also be collected about the individual's previous experiences with losses generally and with the specific type of loss most recently experienced. The ability of the individual to grieve should be considered. Factors that potentially interfere with grieving include cognitive impairments, impaired verbal communication, and multiple concurrent stressors that do not leave any psychic energy for coping with the loss.

Functional impairments should be specified, using techniques described in Chapter 2. The older person may require assistance with self-care tasks until the grief problem is resolved. Functional status assessment also provides a valuable criterion against which to evaluate the effectiveness of interventions.

Planning

In those experiencing anticipatory grief, the primary goals are to facilitate the grieving process and to assist the bereaved person to focus on the here-and-now aspects of life. Anticipatory guidance, as described by Parkes (1985), is not precluded. However, promoting the individual's ability to function in the present is important because the dying individual needs support from family and friends, and "unfinished business" may remain. Resolution of such matters reduces feelings of ambivalence about the death, which in turn reduces the likelihood of dysfunctional grieving.

The primary goal for those who have already experienced a loss is to facilitate the grief process. This may involve the inclusion of other professionals and lay people in the therapeutic process. A secondary goal for those experiencing grief is to identify the ways in which the grieving process interferes with other goals or tasks of the older person, such as rehabilitation or strengthening of social networks.

Interventions

Although grief is not an illness, gerontological nurses and other health care professionals have important roles in caring for the bereaved. The sophistication of interventions and contributions of individual health professionals to the bereaved depends on the organizational setting in which the health professional works; the religious, psychosocial, and cultural characteristics of the bereaved; the individual characteristics, interest, competence, accessibility, and availability of the gerontological nurse; and the nature of the relationship with the bereaved. Although the exact nature of client interventions may vary, several professional tasks following bereavement are well documented (Osterweis et al., 1984; Lund and Caserta, 1992; Cleirin, 1993) and include

- Information and education, with sensitivity to what significant others want to know
- Emotional support
- Clinical recognition of dysfunctional grieving
- Management and appropriate referral to mental health resources
- Legitimization of the occurrence of death, so that the bereaved are assured that all appropriate measures were attempted

In planning specific interventions to assist clients and accomplish these professional tasks, the nurse will be prepared to

- Observe cause/contributing factors of potential loss.
- Monitor the stage of grief: e.g., anger, denial, bargaining, depression, acceptance.
- Use open, facilitative communications to aid emotional support and sharing.
- Use silence, touch with permission, or sit and make eye contact if appropriate to the situation.
- Review past experiences, role changes, coping skills, and strengths.
- Permit expressions of anger and fear free from judgment, but be cautious that all members of the bereaved party may not

feel the same and may be in conflict with some emotional states.

- Be honest in all responses; trust is usually enhanced and communication paths opened; do not give false reassurances.
- Identify and discuss problems of eating, activity, sexual desire, sleep, finances, and so on.
- Identify other social supports: friends, family, religious leaders, mental health support services, and self-help groups.
- Provide clear explanations of the cause of death that may prevent misconceptions and self-blame by the bereaved (NANDA, 1994; Ackley and Ladwig, 1993).

Other sources of intervention may involve mutual self-help group support, hospice, psychotherapy, and medication use. The gerontological nurse may be involved to some degree in each. The bereaved may avail themselves of one or more of these interventions sequentially or simultaneously. Self-help groups have been around since the 1800s and have grown till there are different groups targeted for just about every disease and major life stress known (Lund and Caserta, 1992). Generally, self-help groups consist of people voluntarily meeting together for treatment or to accomplish a specific purpose and resolve mutual needs. Lund and Caserta (1992) examined bereaved spouses' assessment of the effectiveness of mutual self-help groups in facilitating the adjustment process of recently bereaved older spouses. From a prior longitudinal study, the investigators had documented the somewhat unexpected discovery of a high degree of coping ability, resourcefulness, and resiliency among many of the bereaved spouses.

Research has focused on the bereaved persons' reasons for participating in the mutual self-help group support, the extent to which needs were met, and their perceptions of participation in and usefulness of the group meetings. Older bereaved spouses were positive about their participation in the group, regardless of the type of leadership or duration of the therapy (8 weeks versus 10 months). To receive emotional support was the most common need identified, and groups led by peer nonprofessionals were just as effective as those led by professionals. Further, the potential value of group support required attendance at more than just a few of the meetings.

Hospice, a recent form of health care delivery, has taken a prominent place in the health care industry. As defined by Flexner (1979), hospice is a "medically directed, nurse-coordinated program providing a continuum of home and inpatient care for the terminally ill client and family. It employs an interdisciplinary team acting under the direction of an autonomous hospice administrator." Nurses may refer clients to a hospice unit or simply educate the family and patient about the availability of such services. There are at least five predominant models of hospice: free-standing, hospital-affiliated, hospital-based, within a nursing facility, and the home care program. In planning interventions, the nurse might assist the client and family in deciding which type of hospice care would best meet needs (National Hospice Organization, 1993).

For individuals who feel overwhelmed by the pain and sad emotions attributable to grief or who are experiencing dysfunctional grief, psychotherapeutic intervention may be warranted. The gerontological nurse might refer clients to a psychiatric clinical nurse specialist for short-term crisis intervention or to other mental health professionals for longer treatments. Psychotherapeutic intervention should be offered to individuals, families, or groups of similarly bereaved persons.

Medications may be used alone or in combination with other interventions. The medications most often used to assist the bereaved are antianxiety agents, hypnotics, and antidepressants. The value of psychopharmacological agents for bereaved clients is unsubstantiated. Some researchers argue that the use of medications interferes with the "normal" process of grief and causes delays that may have detrimental consequences. As with all medications and issues of polypharmacy with older adults, the most stringent monitoring is necessary.

Evaluation

Evaluative criteria that suggest successful resolution of both anticipatory grieving and dysfunctional grieving include observations that the grieving individual

1. Performs activities of daily living and instrumental activities of daily living at functional baseline,
2. Has the ability to appropriately express feelings of anxiety and sadness,
3. Has developed new plans, habits, and relationships with others that acknowledge that life goes on despite the lost object,

4. Has the ability to approach life one day at a time.

HOPELESSNESS

Definition and Scope of Problem

Throughout the years, clinicians, scientists, philosophers, and theologians have been interested in the concepts of hopelessness and hope. Often it is easier to identify when hope is not present than to identify when and to what degree it is present. To more clearly understand the two concepts, a positive context is presented using the concept of hope, followed by a discussion of the negative concept, hopelessness. Hope has often been described as an elusive "soft" concept. It is used as a verb, noun, and adjective (Farran et al., 1995).

The concept of hope is also elusive because it can be expressed as a way of feeling (affectively), as a way of thinking (cognitively), and as a way of behaving (behaviorally). Hope can also function as both a state and a trait. As a state, it reflects the present feelings that a person has about a particular situation, it may fluctuate over time, and it can be influenced through growth or intervention. As a trait, hope functions as a more enduring attitude toward life, and is less subject to fluctuation in response to life's vagaries (Averill et al., 1990). Hope is defined as an essential experience of the human condition. It functions as a way of life, a way of thinking, behaving, and relating to oneself and the world. Hope is fluid in its expectations, and in the event that the desired object or outcome does not occur, hope can still be present (Farran et al., 1995).

In both clinical and research settings, the concept of hopelessness has not been considered elusive or "soft." Like hope, hopelessness expresses a way of feeling, thinking, or behaving. As a feeling, hopelessness is expressed as discouragement, despair, or a de-energizing force. Often, despair is used as a synonym for hopelessness and is frequently referenced in gerontological literature. Hopelessness may further be defined as a subjective state in which an individual sees limited or no alternatives or personal choices available and is unable to mobilize energy on one's own behalf (NANDA, 1994).

When people feel hopeless, there is a sense of entrapment, and thinking is often impaired, with little or no expectation for relief (Beck et al., 1990; Ferran et al., 1995). Hopelessness, defined, constitutes an essential human condition and is expressed as feelings of despair, dissatisfaction, and discouragement. As a thought process, little is expected, and behaviorally, few or no attempts to take action are evident (Farran et al., 1995).

During the latter stages of development, older adults face a variety of stressors that require adaptive responses. Erikson (1980) described eight stages of ego development from infancy to old age. Each stage represents a developmental task reflective of a choice of crises in the expanding ego. The final stage of adult development described by Erikson is ego-integrity versus despair or hopelessness. In later maturity, the older adult reviews life events to create a sense of uniqueness, accomplishment and life integration. Sometimes, the older adult may be confronted with unresolved goals and a sense of unfulfillment or dissatisfaction with the life course. In this scenario, the older adult is challenged to build on past strengths and use intergenerational interactions and resources to maintain a sense of accomplishment and ego-integrity versus a sense of despair and hopelessness (Harden, 1989; Thompson, 1992).

Hopelessness and helplessness often go hand in hand. Hopelessness has been identified as a major contributing factor to suicide among the aged. Researchers who have analyzed suicide notes of individuals of various ages have found that the elderly express a sense of hopelessness and psychological exhaustion in their notes and not the anger expressed by younger people (Harper, 1991). Hopelessness and helplessness also contribute to alcoholism, a significant factor in late life suicide.

Contributing Factors

Contributing factors or antecedents to hopelessness may be separated into three major categories—intrapersonal, interpersonal, and environmental/sociological. Intrapersonal factors are thought to arise from unmet childhood needs. Other theorists link hopelessness with personal experiences or attitudes and believe that hopelessness is learned. From this perspective, the individual is trapped in a sense of endlessness and confusion that leads to hopelessness and illness. The environmental/sociological perspective posits that hopelessness is determined by hopelessness in society or in one's class (Farran et al., 1995). Specific examples of contributing factors include chronic or terminal illness (pathophysiological factors), treatments that alter body image (treatment-related factors), inability to achieve goals that one values in life (environmental factors), and loss of trust in significant others, such as when a child loses trust in parents (intrapersonal/maturational factors) (Carpenito, 1989). As indicated above, hopelessness is associated with alcoholism, suicide, terminal illnesses, and a host of losses frequently encountered in later life.

Assessment

Every individual is entitled to careful assessment and prudent care regardless of age. Old age is not an antecedent of hopelessness. Thus, offering hope to older adults who feel despondent, abandoned, discouraged, and apathetic is a critical nursing function. Many health professionals support the idea that an individual's ability to hope and to believe in a higher power facilitates healing and a sense of well-being. Additionally, many clinicians have noted that people do not continue to live very long after losing hope. Further, a note of caution is rendered in an effort to raise the collective consciousness of health professionals to avoid stereotyping and ageism regarding hopelessness in older adults.

The nurse should assess the older adult for behaviors reflecting defining characteristics and related factors of the nursing diagnosis rather than specific medical or psychiatric conditions. The diagnosis of hopelessness is based on observations of behavior, thematic analysis of nurse patient interactions, and described indicators such as hypoactivation, general psychological discomfort, social isolation or withdrawal, and a sense of incompetence (McFarland and McFarlane, 1993).

The presence of the following defining characteristics indicates that the older adult may be experiencing hopelessness:

Major:

1. Passivity
2. Decreased verbalization
3. Decreased affect
4. Verbal cues (despondent content, "I can't," sighing)

Minor:

1. Lack of initiative
2. Decreased response to stimuli
3. Decreased affect
4. Turning away from the speaker
5. Closing eyes
6. Shrugging in response to the speaker

7. Decreased appetite
8. Increased/decreased sleep
9. Lack of involvement in care/passively allowing care

Related Factors:

1. Prolonged activity restriction creating isolation
2. Failing or deteriorating physiological condition
3. Long-term stress
4. Abandonment
5. Lost belief in transcendent values/God (NANDA, 1994)

Scientists recognize that assessment using reliable measurement tools provides a vital link between conceptualization and research. Two hopelessness scales may be useful to clinicians in further assessment and documentation of the diagnosis. Far fewer instruments have been developed to measure hopelessness than hope. Beck et al. (1974) constructed an instrument, entitled the Beck Hopelessness Scale (BHS), to measure negative future expectancies. It is a widely accepted instrument with 20 true/false items scored 0 or 1. It is designed to quantify hopelessness in psychopathological conditions. The BHS is the only instrument reported to give a reliable measurement of hopelessness in old, frail, multiply impaired nursing home residents (Herth, 1991).

The Geriatric Hopelessness Scale (GHS) was developed by Fry in the mid-1980s on the basis of the hopelessness themes derived from the contents of interviews with 60 subclinically depressed subjects who were asked to reminisce about stressful episodes in their life (Fry et al., 1989). The instrument was designed to assess hopelessness in nonpsychiatric older adults. The GHS is a 30-item scale with a score range of 0–30, with a higher score denoting greater hopelessness. This instrument has a reading level for 14 to 16 year olds. It should be noted that the average reading level among older adults is fifth grade level.

Planning

Lillis and Prophit (1991) suggest that nurses must become enablers of hope for the patient and family unit. Webster's defined the term "to enable" as to provide one with the means, opportunity, power, or authority to do something, as well as to make something possible or effective (Webster's, 1990). In planning interventions to assist the older adult during periods of hopelessness, the patient care goal should focus on uncovering and highlighting the older adult's multiple internal and external resources and the focus of his or her hope. The planning is highly individualized. Selected interventions to enable hope and prevent hopelessness need to be recorded in the health care record. Specified outcomes and evaluation methods must be delineated.

Interventions

Ersek (1992) proposes that a delicate interplay exists between dealing with the potential for hopelessness and keeping hope in place, and that this delicate interplay enables the individual to maintain hope while still acknowledging the potential for hopelessness. The nurse needs to create an atmosphere that fosters the expression and sharing of hopes, fears, questions, and expectations. Older adults may need to be reminded that both hope and hopelessness may coexist in a situation. For example, the older adult newly admitted to a nursing home may feel hopeless about the potential for independent living but may be hopeful about being in a safe, caring, and supportive environment. It is important for the integrity of the older adult to be protected even in the face of despair. A perspective that acknowledges hopelessness may be balanced by presenting options for thinking, feeling, and behaving.

Strategies for enhancing hope include providing physical and emotional comfort, encouraging the person to verbalize why and how hope is significant in his or her life. The nurse may assist the older adult to identify and express feelings to determine if there is a sense of entrapment. Sometimes the use of a diary (written or tape recorded) can facilitate the discovery process and relieve some of the emotional discomfort associated with hopelessness.

Some older adults feel abandoned and need to feel connected to someone or something. Nurses might attempt to create conditions that foster a caring relationship among peers, family members, professional caregivers, and pets. Use of community resources, including religious groups, may be helpful in restoring a sense of hope when few family members or significant others are available.

Because some older adults feel void of energy, the nurse may use energy-conserving and restoration actions. The nurse may initially plan to reduce unnecessary activities that expend energy. Playing uplifting music may be helpful to restore hopefulness. Progressive physical activity may also enhance energy and cognitive and emotional well-being. Mental imagery and relaxation may be utilized to promote positive thought processes and re-energize hopeless individuals (Farran et al., 1995).

Control and autonomy are significant factors in restoring hope. The older adult should be respected as a competent decision-maker and involved in obtaining information and making rational decisions.

Counseling by psychiatric nurses is available in most acute care settings. Unfortunately, community resources may be scant. The nurse should refer to psychiatric counseling older adults with suicidal ideation or threatening behaviors to self or others. Emergency services may be needed to help stabilize and restore some sense of hope for the older adult with dysphoria.

Evaluation

As indicated above, these clinical strategies must be documented and evaluated for effectiveness in sustaining hope and preventing hopelessness. Documentation is needed to determine which strategies work best with particular populations. Evaluation must also consider specific dose requirements. How much uplifting music is sufficient to lift a sense of hopelessness? What frequency of pet visitation offers the best prospect for health promotion and hopefulness? Future investigations also need to address wellness response to treatment and quality of life.

KNOWLEDGE DEFICIT

Definition and Scope of Problem

A knowledge deficit is characterized by a person's inability to express understanding of concepts pertaining to his/her specific disease, disorder, or developmental needs or an inability to perform selected psychomotor tasks related to a specific self-care activity. Knowledge deficit is very common. The older adult may have entered a new health condition, such as benign prostatic hyperplasia, may be undergoing newly prescribed treatments or taking a new medication, or may be beginning a new life transition, such as retirement. If one has not experienced these states before or learned about them from others in the family or culture, then knowledge deficit is probable.

Some cases of knowledge deficit are easily diagnosed—for example, persons with chronic diseases who cannot perform simple disease management tasks or those who ask for information. An individual with diabetes who cannot describe the importance of proper foot care or demonstrate systematic foot inspection has a knowledge deficit. The person with long-standing coronary artery disease who asks for an explanation of how exercise affects the disease process has a knowledge deficit. Individuals who are newly diagnosed with a disease have obvious knowledge deficits, and the challenge is to prioritize the deficits in a manner that is clinically relevant yet meaningful to the individual so the individual is not overloaded with information.

Knowledge deficits may also present in subtle ways. For instance, an older person who considers that the inability to sleep 8 hours per night without interruption signifies insomnia probably has a knowledge deficit regarding the effects of the aging process on sleep patterns. An individual who insists that failure to have a bowel movement once per day indicates a need for milk of magnesia that evening probably has a knowledge deficit. Defining characteristics for a knowledge deficit are present when a person

1. Verbalizes a problem in understanding a disease or health need or in performing a self-care task
2. Inaccurately follows instructions regarding health maintenance, promotion, or disease treatment
3. Performs inadequately on test of knowledge or performance ability
4. Behaves inappropriately or in an exaggerated manner—e.g., hostile, agitated, apathetic (NANDA, 1994).

Nurses should have a high index of suspicion for knowledge deficits in the elderly. Older persons are at risk for knowledge deficits for three reasons: (1) they are more likely to have chronic diseases, which require acquisition of new information for optimal management; (2) they are less likely to have received formalized health education and therefore have less understanding of how their body functions and the differences between normal aging and disease effects on body function; and (3) patient education materials and methods usually are not adapted to account for the sensory impairments and slowed pace of older persons, so they are less likely to receive adequate instruction originally.

Since 1982, 10 per cent of all AIDS cases reported to the Centers for Disease Control in Atlanta are people 50 years of age and older. Yet educational and prevention campaigns are rarely targeted to the older adult. As a result, knowledge deficit is common, and the older adult is at a disadvantage in effective health management or in helping younger family members to manage their therapeutic regimen. In a recent study that examined the differences in the knowledge and attitudes about AIDS among young and older adults, Rocket (1994) found two significant predictors of knowledge about AIDS: gender and whether an individual had a blood transfusion between 1977 and 1985. Further, the study provided evidence that programs and materials need to be developed and implemented differently for younger and older adults in order for education and prevention to reach older adults effectively. Some methods for adapting programs and teaching materials will be presented in the discussion of interventions.

Although knowledge deficit is usually a relatively simple diagnosis to make, it is important to remember that those with a knowledge deficit may be confused with individuals who have noncompliance, anxiety, or powerlessness. Distinguishing individuals with a knowledge deficit from those with other diagnoses is important because the goals and intervention strategies differ.

Contributing Factors

Factors that contribute to knowledge deficits in the aged include

- Lack of exposure to information:
  Sensory impairments (especially undiagnosed hearing loss)
  Educational aids not legible or comprehensible
  Assumption that old people cannot learn
- Inability to recall information:
  Disease processes such as dementing disorders
- Misinterpretation of information:
  Sensory impairment
  Anxiety
  Pace too rapid for older individual
  Educational level too high for individual
- Cognitive limitations:
  Diseases: for example, dementing disorders
  Lack of formal education
- Disinterest in learning about disease or developmental process:
  Acceptance of paternalistic model of

health care provision in which all control (and knowledge) remains with the health care professional

Overwhelmed by other demands of daily living

Unfamiliarity with traditional teaching techniques

Low self-esteem—disbelief that they *can* learn

- Unfamiliarity with information resources

- Outdated information

Contributing factors can also be grouped according to the following scheme: patient-related factors, environmental factors, and characteristics of the subject matter to be taught.

Patient-related factors include sensory impairment, cognitive impairment, polypharmacy, multiple diseases, multiple knowledge deficits, anxiety, altered pace, lack of desire or readiness to learn, and lower educational level. These factors influence the patient's ability to receive and process information and therefore determine in large part the complexity of the teaching task. For example, teaching about diabetes to a patient who has no other diseases or functional impairments and is taking no drugs is considerably easier than teaching the individual who has suffered a stroke and who takes other medications.

Environmental factors include both the objective characteristics of the learning environment and its interpersonal attributes. Objective attributes such as lighting intensity, background noise level, and access to teaching aids all vary according to where the teaching is being conducted—in the hospital, in the clinic, or at home. Interpersonal variables in the environment, such as privacy, attitudes of clinicians toward older people, attitudes toward patient education, time and space available for teaching, use of group versus individual instruction, and the quality and variety of instructional aids, will influence the learning of the older individual. These attributes of the environment can be manipulated to optimize learning for the individual. Often, however, the environment is designed for the convenience of the provider without considering its possible effects on the older person's learning.

Characteristics of the material to be taught may contribute to a knowledge deficit. Some information is easier to transmit than others. Teaching an individual about the need for potassium supplementation and good dietary sources of potassium is a relatively simple task. Teaching a family about the management of incontinence in a demented individual is considerably more complex. Environmental variables have some influence on the complexity of transmitting the necessary information. For example, the skill of the clinician in simplifying and segmenting material influences the complexity of the teaching task. The availability of teaching aids such as models, large-print handouts, and adaptive equipment also influences the complexity of the teaching/learning task.

Assessment

Assessment should define the nature of the knowledge deficit and identify the specific contributing factors. The client's baseline level of knowledge also should be documented, along with barriers to learning and individual strengths that will enhance the teaching/learning process. Nurses should be alert for cues suggesting the presence of a knowledge deficit, such as client verbalization, new diagnosis, or new prognosis of disease. Some clinical settings mandate specific assessment protocols for identifying knowledge deficits as a part of routine admissions procedures. Parameters for assessment of knowledge deficits are as follows:

- Baseline knowledge and skills already processed by client

- Interest in learning

- Barriers to learning:
  Sensory impairments
  Cognitive impairments
  Literacy problems

- Educational background

- Comprehension of written and verbal material

- Preferred learning style

- Support system available (e.g., family, community resources, friends)

Individuals who request further information about their diseases should receive a more in-depth assessment of their current knowledge of the problem, prior experience with the problem, and desire for more information. The client may have a true knowledge deficit or may simply be looking for affirmation that the information possessed is current and correct. Clients should have the opportunity to ask questions as a part of any nursing encounter. Permission to bring up a wide range of topics can be granted through such questions as: "I've asked you some questions today—do you have any that you'd like to ask me?" or "Do you have any questions about your health that you wish to discuss today?" Although the simple assessment techniques cited earlier are adequate for many situations, there are instances in which a more in-depth assessment is advisable.

In-depth assessments have been advocated by some workers for patients who have chronic diseases with complex management regimens. In general, assessment might center on several cognitive domains in an effort to isolate and better define the scope of the knowledge deficit. The domains include attention span, concentration, intelligence, judgment, learning ability, memory, orientation, perception, problem solving, psychomotor ability, reaction time, and social intactness (McDougall, 1990). Each domain may not be represented in a single assessment tool, but each is necessary to a complete and in-depth assessment of cognition as related to knowledge deficit. In in-depth assessment protocols, behavioral objectives are set, and documentation of patient knowledge is made on a flow sheet (Fig. 17–7). The nurse selects the aspects of the disease or care on which to focus attention during each patient encounter. It is thus possible to review progress in many dimensions of a knowledge deficit over a period of time. Assessment tools of this type are available for many chronic diseases, and the format lends itself to the development of individualized teaching plans for learning about developmental issues as well. One strength of the approach to assessment used in Figure 17–7 is that it emphasizes patient performance rather than a self-report of understanding. The importance of obtaining data in working with the aged cannot be overemphasized. Too often a self-report is used as the only source of information, which may be flawed.

The assessment approaches just outlined allow the nurse to determine whether a knowledge deficit exists and to specify the nature of the deficit. These techniques do not necessarily help the nurse define the etiology of the knowledge deficit. Gathering information about the client's previous opportunities to learn about the subject matter is therefore important. Individuals who have significant knowledge deficits about a longstanding problem despite previous learning opportunities require further assessment and a more individualized teaching plan than those who simply have never received any instruction.

Presence of sensory impairments, deficits in memory or problem-solving abilities, or anxiety should be assessed because these will influence the teaching/learning process.

Problems with literacy should also be identified. The majority of patient education materials are prepared at an educational level far above the abilities of the average patient (Potter and Perry, 1993). People with low literacy skills are not stupid, nor are they easy to identify by the prevailing stereotypes. People with low literacy skills are often stereotyped as poor, unkempt, inarticulate, and poorly educated. In fact, it is possible for people with low literacy levels to have average IQs, be verbally articulate, have completed high school, and be from virtually any socioeconomic stratum. The social stigma associated with illiteracy leads affected individuals to conceal their deficits. Therefore, the only way to identify people with low literacy accurately is by testing comprehension of teaching materials. Several techniques may be used, including the Cloze Test, the Listening Test, the Wide Range Achievement Test, and the Comprehension Restatement Test. These tests are described in Doake (1991).

The final areas of assessment are the individual's current level of knowledge about the subject, goals for learning new information, previous educational background, and preferred learning style. Trying to match an individual's learning style involves assessing the individual's primary mode of processing information—visual, kinesthetic, or auditory—and providing information in the mode preferred by the individual (Theis, 1991; Potter and Perry, 1993). Ask the clients which mode they prefer.

Knowledge of social factors such as family members who should be included in teaching, friends or family who have had a similar problem, and availability of other agencies or professionals in the community to participate in the teaching is also helpful in developing a teaching/learning plan for someone with a knowledge deficit.

Planning

In the planning phase, clarify the following matters: (1) the goals of the teaching, (2) who should participate in the sessions, (3) teaching methods and materials to be used, and (4) criteria for evaluation to be used.

Goals of the teaching plan should address the knowledge deficit, but the readiness of the learner and the abilities of the learner to acquire new information must be acknowledged. Sometimes nurses are expected to teach unrealistic amounts of information on a time schedule that bears little relation to the client's acceptance of the disease or developmental stage. Pressures from the pro-

THE NORTH CAROLINA MEMORIAL HOSPITAL
UNIVERSITY OF NORTH CAROLINA
Chapel Hill, N.C.
RECORD SHEET

Diabetic Education   Imprint

Name_____ Year	
Hospital Number _____ Month	
Others taught _____ Day	

PATHOPHYSIOLOGY
  Relates Basic Pathophysiology
    A. Cause
    B. Chronicity
    C. Complications

INSULIN OR ORAL AGENTS
  Names Drug (or Abbreviation) and Strength
  Names Dose
  States Times
  Selects Correct Insulin
  Selects Correct Syringe
  Draws up Correct Dose
  Displays Correct Drugs and Equipment from Home
  Relates Proper Storage
  Demonstrates Proper Disposal of Syringe
  Demonstrates Good Injection Technique
  States 4 Sites Used for Rotation
  Relates General Length of Action
  Patient Was Given Picture Pages for Insulin Injection

URINE TESTING
  Names or Describes Test
  States Times Correctly
  Displays Equipment from Home
  Relates Proper Storage
  Carries Out Procedure Accurately
  Records a Reading Correctly
  Displays Readable Record
  States Significance of Sugar
  Describes Double-Void Technique and Rationale
  Selects Correct Test

HYGIENE
  Verbalizes 3 Reasons for Foot Care
  Demonstrates Foot Examination and Foot Care
  Relates Proper Care of Skin and Mouth
  Picture Pages Have Been Given

HYPOGLYCEMIA
  Displays Identification
  States Realistic Early Symptoms
  States Proper Remedy
  Picture Pages Have Been Given

DIET INSTRUCTIONS
  Have been Given by Dietitian
  Relates Proper Times to Eat

◻ Initial teaching   ⊘ Done incorrectly; retaught   ⊠ Not applicable

◻ Done incorrectly   ■ Done correctly without teaching   ✳ See progress note

FIGURE 17–7

Flow sheet to document a patient's knowledge of a particular disease condition—in this case, diabetes. (Courtesy of North Carolina Memorial Hospital Endocrine Nursing Staff, University of North Carolina, Chapel Hill, North Carolina.)

spective payment systems under Medicare in hospitals and home health agencies emphasize rapid discharge. In the outpatient setting, there are often constraints that limit the time available for patient teaching. Thus, nurses should attend to realistic goal setting and prioritization of learning needs while remaining alert for other resources to assist with teaching the needed information and skills. When the knowledge deficit poses a serious risk to the patient and the usual time schedules for care do not allow for its adequate resolution, nurses must be prepared to advocate more time or more support for the older individual until the deficit is resolved.

Deciding who will participate in the teaching/learning process requires consideration of the older person's functional abilities, the support people regularly available to the old person, and the complexity of the information to be taught. For old people with little functional impairment, the teaching may be carried out on an individual basis, with little in the way of modification in methods used with younger adults. However, for older people with a memory or sensory impairment or those requiring complex teaching that must take place in a short amount of time, it is useful to involve a family member or close friend in the teaching. The possibility of reinforcement at home is enhanced and a mechanism for the older person to validate the new information or technique is established.

As with any age group, the methods used to teach the necessary information or skills depend to a large extent on the characteristics of the subject matter and the older person's abilities. When working with the aged, it is important to consider the problem of visual or hearing impairments. Therefore, if a group teaching method is considered optimal, scrupulous attention must be paid to environmental characteristics such as background noise, lighting intensity, glare, pace, and opportunity for individuals to ask questions. In individual or group learning situations, printed material should be evaluated for readability by those with moderate to severe visual impairments. Many older persons have had little formal education, and formal education for others was likely to have occurred some time ago. Therefore, these learners are most likely to benefit from strict adherence to the adult learning principles of building on experience and use of practical examples when presenting new information. Also, studies have shown that older persons learn as well as younger persons if the information is presented at a slower pace and in a larger number of sessions (see Chapter 15).

Individuals with literacy problems also require modification of teaching methods. A variety of approaches for the individual with low literacy skills is recommended. The use of specially designed audiotapes to enhance learning that include frequent opportunities for feedback, and the use of simplified drawings to compensate for comprehension difficulties may be helpful. If a task must be learned, the teacher should focus on the "how-to" aspects of the skill without concentrating on the principles of the technique.

Research exists about the kinds of techniques used to enhance and/or document learning in elderly people (Hultsch and Dixon, 1990; Kausler, 1991; Backman and Larsson, 1992). Backman and Larsson (1992) discuss the modifiability of deficits in episodic memory. In tasks involving cognitive support, such as cues, age differences tend to be reduced or eliminated. Suggested techniques to enhance recall include manipulating learning instructions to make sure older adults know what is expected, encoding cues in the text of content to be remembered—for example, "You need to remember this," visual distinctiveness, and item richness so the content has high recall appeal (Smith et al., 1990).

Interventions

Interventions to address a knowledge deficit should be based on the contributing factors identified during the assessment process. The full range of teaching strategies used with younger adults is available for use with older persons. Modifications in methods should be based on observed patient factors such as sensory impairment, cognitive impairment, or difficulty in coping. It is important not to overlook the possibility of using methods that have been developed with the younger populations in mind. There are excellent examples of the use of self-help and peer counseling in facilitating learning about age-related changes and chronic diseases (Siegler and Rudden, 1992).

Evaluation

Criteria for evaluation should be established in advance of the teaching to provide a benchmark for teacher and client alike. This helps prevent any discouragement engendered by not stating measurable goals. Each teaching session provides an opportunity for an evaluation of teaching/learning effectiveness. The high prevalence of literacy problems in adults suggests that modest goals should be set and should be evaluated at each session. Such goals also allow experience-based encouragement for the learner. Specific methods used for evaluation depend to a great extent on the learning objectives.

The principles and techniques of assessment apply equally well to evaluation. Use of flow sheets to document progress in resolving knowledge deficits promotes continuity of teaching in settings in which nurses share teaching responsibilities. Flow sheets also provide a tangible view of progress for the older person and the nurse, a source of positive reinforcement for behavior change.

RELOCATION STRESS SYNDROME

Definition and Scope of Problem

Relocation stress syndrome is defined as "physiological and/or psychosocial disturbance as a result of transfer from one environment to another" (NANDA, 1994). Although 1992 was the year that relocation stress syndrome was accepted as a nursing diagnosis, the phenomenon has been described in the literature for years under various conceptual labels, including transportation shock, transfer trauma, relocation trauma, and translocation syndrome. According to Coffman (1987), the term "relocation stress" has no distinct meaning apart from the term stress. In Selye's (1976) meaning, stress is a natural component of life and desirable in certain optimal amounts. Relocation stress therefore can be good, bad, or neutral depending on individual needs, environmental quality, and adaptational energy. A more recent term found in some literature is "relocation transition," which is thought to provide a naturalistic connotation (Engle, 1994).

Relocation refers to (1) moving from one's own residence to another (residential); (2) moving from one institution to another (interinstitutional); (3) moving from one's own room or unit to another within an institution (intra-institutional); or (4) moving from one's own residence to an institution or the reverse (residential/institutional) (Rosswurn, 1983). Defining characteristics of the syndrome, as specified by NANDA (1994) are

Major:
1. Change in environment or location

2. Anxiety
3. Apprehension
4. Increased confusion
5. Depression
6. Loneliness

Minor:
1. Verbalization of unwillingness to relocate
2. Sleep disturbance
3. Change in eating habits
4. Gastrointestinal disturbance
5. Increased verbalization of needs
6. Insecurity
7. Lack of trust
8. Restlessness
9. Sad affect
10. Unfavorable comparison of post-transfer with pretransfer staff
11. Verbalization of being concerned or upset about transfer
12. Vigilance
13. Weight change
14. Withdrawal

Contributing Factors

According to Coffman (1987) many factors have been implicated in positive and negative effects, but in complex and often opposing ways. Except for environmental quality, no single variable is consistent in predicting relocation outcomes. Rather, the challenge in predicting or assessing risk of relocation stress syndrome is to look to interaction effects. Some of the factors thought to interact and compound this syndrome include past, concurrent, and recent losses; losses involved with decision to move; feelings of powerlessness; lack of adequate support; little or no preparation for the impending move; moderate-to-high degree of environmental change; history and types of previous transfers; impaired psychosocial health status; and decreased physical health status.

Assessment

The ability to separate and define the relocation stress event correctly leads to prevention strategies and distress reduction. Since not all persons who relocate experience relocation stress syndrome, a principal focus of nursing assessment is detection of those older adults most at risk. Using an adaptation of the injury model of human-environment interaction (Haddon and Baker, 1981) for assessment of this stress syndrome might be helpful. The major components of the model include interactions among human factors, energy-adaptation sources/resources, and characteristics of the physical/psychosocial environment. Each of these components is considered at three points in time: prerelocation phase, relocation event phase, and postrelocation phase. Figure 17–8 depicts the model.

Prerelocation considers events and factors prior to the actual relocation event. It is not time limited. The relocation event phase refers to the week of relocation, the physical response, the intensity of energy, and the environmental situation. The postrelocation phase is not time-specific and refers to the body's response, energy expenditures, and resources after the move. The emphasis in this model is on the interaction of the components. Human factors include age, physical condition, cognition, fatigue level, and other personal characteristics in the data base. Energy-adaptation sources strengthen the individual and buffer distress. The sources may include information, prayer, religion, quiet reflection, or group mutual help. The environmental characteristics include, for example, the staff characteristics, power, governance, and support services. Family resources may be considered either an adaptation component or an environmental component.

Planning

Adaptation is the optimal goal for stress disorders. Adaptation is a matter of person-environment congruence involving not only particular individual and situational conditions but the totality of environmental stimulation in relation to the totality of individual capacities (Coffman, 1987). Given such a broad perspective, outcome goals related to

relocation stress syndrome might include maintenance of general well-being in the new environment, ability to meet and satisfy demands of daily living, ability to appraise benefits as well as perceived threats realistically, balanced energy conservation and expenditures, and the ability to share feelings about the transition from one location to another.

Interventions

Planning interventions for this diagnosis does not depend upon the client's level of cognition but arises from the gerontological nurse's knowledge of actual and potential risk associated with relocation, stress, and adaptation. With the relocation model (Figure 17–8) as a framework, prerelocation interventions might include dedicated time to share thoughts about the pending move, such as the actual location, people to be encountered, weather, governance, planned accommodations, plans for meeting the older client's needs, and identification of additional sources of aid and comfort. During the relocation phase, planned interventions may incorporate special arrangements for care during the packing stage, coordination of special care and equipment, plans for the client to help in the packing if energy permits, a formal or informal ritual for good-byes and to mark the event appropriately, and use of family and friends as additional energy resources and buffers for the transition.

Postrelocation interventions call for heightened awareness by family and professionals to potential changes in the client's physical well-being. Target human factors and energy sources for frequent reassess-

Phases	Human factors	Energy-adaption sources	Physical-psychosocial environment
Prerelocation			
Relocation event			
Postrelocation			

FIGURE 17 – 8
Relocation model.

ment. Help the client orient to the new environment; a map of the area and/or facility may be helpful to the client and family. Facilitate contact with friends in the old location, which may take the form of letter writing, phone calls, or visits. If appropriate, try to retain positive features of the old environment in the new environment. Allow for fluctuations in feelings. Some days will be happier than others.

Evaluation

Although evaluation is listed as the last action in this process, it is actually an integral part of each step in assessing and understanding relocation stress syndrome. The total stimulation of anticipating a move, moving, and environmental change can benefit those who are understimulated and exhaust those with lesser capacities. The evaluation is based on how well all factors have been balanced for the client and the resultant steady-state of the client's well-being.

POWERLESSNESS

Definition and Scope of Problem

The nursing diagnosis of powerlessness is defined as

"Perception that one's own action will not significantly affect an outcome; a perceived lack of control over a current situation or immediate happening" (NANDA, 1994).

Miller (1983) defines power as the ability to influence what happens to oneself. Seven power resources are identified:

- Physical strength and reserve
- Psychological stamina and support network
- Positive self-concept (self-esteem)
- Energy (force capable of doing work or being stored)
- Knowledge
- Motivation
- Belief system (hope)

Power and control are recognized by a number of gerontologically oriented health professionals as being integral elements inextricably linked with the psychology of aging and interwoven with aspects of personal and social identity and well-being of older adults (Fry et al., 1989). By the time individuals reach late adulthood, they may experience a decline in personal skills, capabilities,

and controls, and these perceptions of decline may contribute to older persons' beliefs that they possess little power to influence the environment (Seligman, 1975).

A compelling case for the adverse consequences of powerlessness can be made. According to an extensive body of research, powerlessness adversely affects learning and results in reduced tolerance for aversive stimuli, reduced task performance under adverse environmental conditions, depressive symptoms, increased stress levels, maladaptive coping responses, and even death (Fry et al., 1989). Figure 17–9 displays a model of the adverse effects of powerlessness.

Although the majority of the studies used to describe the phenomenon of powerlessness have not been conducted on elderly subjects, considerable research evidence points to the importance of power or control in the lives of older adults.

Nystrom and Segesten (1994) postulate that because feelings of identity and integrity are important for old people's efforts to maintain a healthy life, experiences of powerlessness ought to be prevented. Their research describes sources of powerlessness in nursing home life. Participant observations regarding lucid, elderly patients were undertaken in two Swedish nursing home wards. The observations focused on interactions on the wards and observed patient reactions and structural/functional conditions of life. The constant comparative method of analysis was used to search for events or conditions that result in reactions signifying positive or negative experiences. Tender, loving care and strong cohesion and affection between patients and personnel were typical observations, yet patients complained of imprisonment, powerlessness, and hopelessness.

The research observation data are categorized as reflective of power (legitimate, reward, expert, informational, or reference), self-confidence and respect, or socialization. Additionally, the authors identify existential sources of powerlessness, for example, death, guilt, and suffering. Most of the subjects were female, widows, and homemakers with brief formal education. Reference to experiences of powerlessness was a recurrent theme in interview data.

In this study, the experiences of powerlessness stemmed from existential experiences of death and suffering, deteriorating somatic and mental functions with increased physical dependency and submission, lack of reciprocity, and feelings of inferiority, as well as feelings of despair from lack of au-

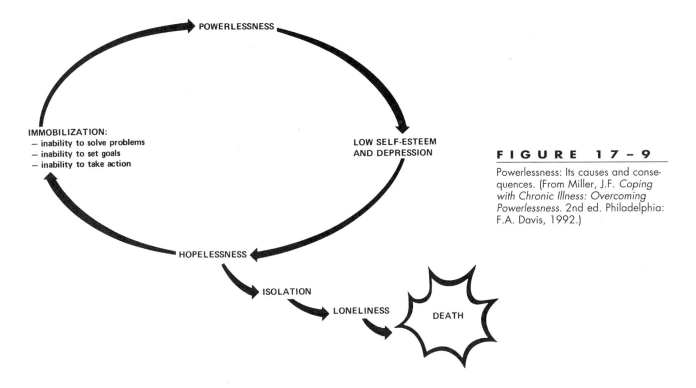

FIGURE 17 – 9

Powerlessness: Its causes and consequences. (From Miller, J.F. *Coping with Chronic Illness: Overcoming Powerlessness.* 2nd ed. Philadelphia: F.A. Davis, 1992.)

tonomy. The authors suggest organizational, interactional, and personal empowerment measures to address the problem of powerlessness.

According to White and Roberts (1993), everyone wants to maintain control over events in their life. The need for personal control does not end when a person is hospitalized; instead, the patient's need for personal control usually intensifies in critical and acute care situations. The nursing diagnosis of powerlessness is common for most critical care patients, and especially so for the patient experiencing respiratory difficulties. These investigators describe a model of powerlessness that suggests strategies for increasing the patient's control over his or her situation.

High morale among elderly nursing home residents has been associated with higher degrees of perceived choice in entering the institution (Fuller, 1978) and with internal locus of control (Chang, 1978). The external locus of control has been correlated with depression (Hanes and Wild, 1977). The desired amount of control correlates with health status and knowledge of services in community old people; in institutional settings, it is positively correlated with life satisfaction, self-concept, and tranquility (Ziegler and Reid, 1979). Boettcher (1985) contends that old people are vulnerable to

powerlessness because of diminished social opportunities and because of the greater likelihood of physical dependence with advanced age.

Nurses should be alert for signs of powerlessness and should consider this along with the more familiar diagnostic labels with similar defining characteristics. Relational diagnoses include noncompliance, anxiety, fear, knowledge deficit, self-care deficit, and altered self-concept. Defining characteristics are listed by NANDA (1994):

1. Severe
   a. Verbal expressions of having no control or influence over situation
   b. Verbal expressions of having no control or influence over outcome
   c. Verbal expressions of having no control over self-care
   d. Depression over physical deterioration that occurs despite patient compliance with regimens
   e. Apathy
2. Moderate
   a. Nonparticipation in care or decision making when opportunities are provided
   b. Expressions of dissatisfaction and frustration over inability to perform previous tasks or activities

c. Failure to monitor progress
d. Expression of doubt regarding role performance
e. Reluctance to express true feelings
f. Fearing alienation from caregivers
g. Passivity
h. Inability to seek information regarding care
i. Dependence on others that may result in irritability, resentment, anger, and guilt
j. Does not defend self-care practices when challenged
3. Low
a. Expressions of uncertainty about fluctuating energy levels
b. Passivity

Contributing Factors

Three categories of contributing factors for powerlessness can be defined: personality factors, characteristics of disease states, and environmental factors. Generally, no single factor is responsible—the condition results from the interaction of many factors.

Locus of control is the individual's viewpoint about why events happen as they do. Those people who believe that life events are primarily the result of chance, fate, or luck are said to have an external locus of control, whereas those who view their own behavior as responsible for much of what happens are said to have an internal locus of control. Locus of control is a fairly stable personality trait, and it is therefore distinguished from powerlessness, which is situation specific. Knowledge of the patient's locus of control tendencies allows the nurse to anticipate the level of independence the patient will seek, to understand the importance of mastering control-related information for those with an internal locus of control, and to anticipate the anxiety induced by powerless situations. Those with internal control tendencies are likely to experience more anxiety in powerless situations. Locus of control tendency affects coping strategies, those with internal control using approach and direct confrontation methods more frequently, and those with external control using withdrawal, hostility, and aggression (Anderson et al., 1994).

The complexity of self-care regimens varies by disease state. Management of some diseases places more demands and restrictions on the individual's time and lifestyle than others. For example, individuals with chronic renal failure who are dialysis dependent have many more limitations on diet and activity than those who have been recently diagnosed as hypertensive. The greater the amount of control demanded by a therapeutic regimen or disability, the less control individuals are likely to perceive over their own lives.

The environment of the individual contains factors that can promote powerlessness. The rigidity or flexibility of an institution's or household's routines has a tremendous influence on the individual's feelings of control. For example, does the institution allow patients to take baths when they desire, or are baths available only on a predetermined schedule? Are visiting hours unrestricted, or are the times when patients may see family and friends strictly limited? Although routines may have therapeutic benefits or may be essential to the efficient running of an institution or household, they are a potential contributor to feelings of powerlessness.

Another environmental factor to be considered in the etiology of powerlessness is interpersonal relationships. Institutional policy combined with reduced mobility may result in severe restrictions on the freedom of older persons to choose their associates. This basic human right is sometimes abridged in the name of therapeutic benefit or is simply neglected because the older person is depersonalized. The character of the interpersonal relationships in which the older person engages is also important. Interactions that are primarily of a professional rather than a friendly nature represent a discontinuity in lifestyle for most that is not welcome. A preponderance of interactions with caregivers rather than peers may convey the message that the old person is frail, dependent, and not very competent. Such interactions are likely to lead to feelings of powerlessness.

Poverty is another factor that may be associated with powerlessness. Some people learn to adapt to having a small amount of money. Others have great difficulty. The special problems of the elderly related to poverty are described in Chapter 16. It is noteworthy, however, that in Western society, money can sometimes buy influence and therefore power. Certainly, the ability to procure certain services in health care depends on adequate finances.

Assessment

Identification of those with powerlessness requires some skill in collecting information from nonverbal cues and inference. Before focusing on patient cues, nurses should periodically examine their own professional practice habits for evidence of unconscious reinforcement of dependency and for failure to allow sufficient opportunity for clients to participate in decisions about care. Without this self-assessment, natural patient responses to the nurse's direction may be misinterpreted as a more general pattern of powerlessness (Hendricks and Leedham, 1989).

Nurses should be alert throughout each encounter with an older person for cues of powerlessness, including excessive dependency, unexplained outbursts of anger, and apathy toward therapeutic decisions or outcomes. Repeated identification of any of these cues, plus any direct expressions of feeling out of control, justifies the diagnosis.

Miller (1983) has developed a behavioral assessment tool for powerlessness that helps systematize patient assessment (Fig. 17–10). Although the tool has not been rigorously evaluated, it is a promising beginning for a difficult diagnosis.

The next step in assessment is determining the relevant factors that contribute to the client's powerlessness, which requires skill at pulling together diverse bits of information. Examine the environment for attributes that contribute to powerlessness, such as household or institutional routines. Consider the impact of various disease management regimens on the patient's lifestyle. Gather detailed information about the client's other roles. Is there a consistent pattern of dependency on others in family and friend relationships? What freedom of choice exists

	Patient Behaviors	Nurse Rating of Behaviors			
		1 Never	2 Occasionally	3 Frequently	4 Always
VERBAL RESPONSE	Verbal expressions of lack of control over what is happening.				
	Verbal expressions of doubt that self-care measures can affect outcome.				
	Verbal expressions of giving up.				
	Verbal expressions of fatalism.				
EMOTIONAL RESPONSE	Withdrawal.				
	Pessimism.				
	Undifferentiated anger.				
	Diminished patient-initiated interaction.				
	Submissiveness.				
PARTICIPATION IN ACTIVITIES OF DAILY LIVING	Nonparticipation in daily personal hygiene.				
	Noninterest in treatments.				
	Refusal to take food or fluids.				
	Inability to set goals.				
	Lack of decision making when opportunities are provided.				
	Dependency on others for activities of daily living.				
INVOLVEMENT IN LEARNING ABOUT CARE RESPONSIBILITIES	Lack of questioning concerning illness.				
	Low level of knowledge of illness after being given information.				
	Lack of knowledge related to treatment.				
	Lack of motivation to learn.				

FIGURE 17–10

Tool for assessing powerlessness in the elderly. (From Miller, J.F. *Coping with Chronic Illness: Overcoming Powerlessness*. 2nd ed. Philadelphia: F.A. Davis, 1992.)

in other aspects of this individual's life? Are finances so limited that there is little choice in leisure activities or food? These determinations provide important clues to interventions.

Planning

Successful intervention with an individual who experiences powerlessness requires a team effort. The team membership may be client and nurse, or it may span a much larger group, including family, staff members in a clinic, several community agencies, or staff in an institution such as a hospital or nursing home. Planning is important because powerlessness is predominantly a socially constructed experience. Its resolution, therefore, depends to a large extent on social solutions. Additionally, poor control of physical health problems further saps the older person's compensatory reserves, making successful intervention more difficult (Fry et al., 1989).

If the team is composed of a client and a nurse only, an explicit contract with the client may be useful. A contract specifying nurse and client responsibilities and privileges immediately restructures the nurse-client relationship on a more egalitarian basis, returning some power to the individual. If the client refuses to contract or is unable to do so because of physical or emotional impairment, develop a written plan of approach with other team members to enhance consistency.

Interventions

Five general categories of interventions for patients with powerlessness can be identified (Fry et al., 1989; Ackley and Ladwig, 1993).

- Modifying the environment
- Helping the patient set realistic goals and expectations
- Increasing the patient's knowledge
- Sensitizing the health-team members and significant others to the imposed powerlessness
- Encouraging verbalization of feelings

Examples of interventions keyed to similar categories can be summarized as follows:

1. Modify the environment
   Help patient take control over routines

Help patient take control over interpersonal relationships
Modify nature of staff interactions: establish clear ground rules, practice to achieve desired effects
Examples: encourage patient to make choices and to refuse to engage in dependency-promoting behaviors

Kari and Michels (1991) argue that as long as either a medical model or a therapeutic model defines the structure for organizational governance in an institution that provides care for the elderly, powerlessness is inevitable. They propose a community model that gives residents true power in the organizational operations.

2. Modify patient
   Contract for goal-directed behavior change:
   a. Increase comfort with risk taking
   b. Increase assertiveness
   c. Increase knowledge of disease process
   d. Actively listen to client's expressions of frustration about current situation
3. Modify disease regimen
   Make changes based on mutually acceptable compromises between goals of therapy and lifestyle issues

Self-esteem and spiritual well-being are two important power resources, and therefore any impairment in either of these domains will enhance feelings of powerlessness experienced by the client. Thus, nurses should be alert for signs of decreased self-esteem and spiritual distress. Assessment and intervention for these diagnoses are discussed elsewhere in this chapter.

Evaluation

Patient responses indicating successful resolution of powerlessness include (1) verbalizing feelings of increased control over the situation, and (2) making more active choices about life situation or care regimen.

Powerlessness is not a state of being that develops quickly; therefore, it is unrealistic to expect that reversing the factors contributing to powerlessness will be simple. However, focusing on the day-by-day activities of the patient's world and setting day-by-day goals for increasing frequency of choice provides ample opportunity to measure progress toward enhancing the individual's control.

DISTURBANCES IN SELF-PERCEPTION: BODY IMAGE, SELF-ESTEEM, PERSONAL IDENTITY, AND ROLE PERFORMANCE

Definition and Scope of Problem

Disturbances in self-perception are conceptualized as disruptions in the way one perceives body image, personal identity, or role performance (Kerr et al., 1991) and fits the human patterns of relating and perceiving. NANDA (1994) classifies altered role performance with relating patterns and other social function diagnoses. This classification will be considered here because it is defined as disruption in the way one *perceives* role performance. Both the aging process and diseases influence self-perceptions by affecting the individual's body image, the roles available to an older person, role performance, and expectations of self. Self-esteem, the comparison of the individual's idealized self to self-concept, is also likely to be affected. NANDA (1994) defines a disturbance in self-esteem as a negative self-evaluation/feelings about self or self-capabilities, which may be directly or indirectly expressed. It may be situational or chronic. The paucity of normative standards for accomplishment and behavior for those of advanced age adds to problems with self-esteem because youthful models may be the only reference when evaluating self-performance. Disturbance in self-concept is therefore a diagnostic category with particular relevance for older persons. Defining characteristics for each subcategory of disturbance in self-perception are identified as follows (NANDA, 1994):

I. Body image disturbance
  A. Verbal response to actual or perceived change in structure or function*
or
  B. Nonverbal response to actual or perceived change in structure or function*

The following clinical cues may be used to validate the presence of one of the critical defining characteristics cited above:

  1. *Objective*
    a. Missing body part
    b. Actual change in structure or function
    c. Not looking at body part
    d. Not touching body part
    e. Hiding or overexposing body part (intentional or unintentional)
    f. Trauma to nonfunctioning part
    g. Change in social involvement
    h. Change in ability to estimate spatial relationship of body to environment
  2. *Subjective*
    a. Verbalization of
      (1) Change in lifestyle
      (2) Fear of rejection or of reaction by others
      (3) Focus on past strength, function, or appearance
      (4) Negative feelings about body
      (5) Feelings of helplessness, hopelessness, or powerlessness
    b. Preoccupation with change or loss
    c. Emphasis on remaining strengths, heightened achievement
    d. Extension of body boundary to incorporate environmental objects
    e. Personalization of part or loss by name
    f. Depersonalization of part or loss by impersonal pronouns
    g. Refusal to verify actual change
II. Self-esteem disturbance
  Self-negating verbalization
  Expressions of shame or guilt
  Evaluates self as unable to deal with events
  Rationalizes away or rejects positive feedback and exaggerates negative feedback about self
  Hesitant to try new things or situations
  Denies problems obvious to others
  Projects blame or responsibility for problems
  Rationalizes personal failures
  Hypersensitive to slight or criticism
  Grandiose
  A. Chronic low self-esteem
    1. *Major*
      Self-negative verbalization
      Expressions of shame or guilt
      Evaluates self as unable to deal with events
      Rationalizes away or rejects positive feedback and exaggerates negative feedback about self
      Hesitant to try new things or situations

---

*Denotes critical defining characteristic.

2. *Minor*

Frequent lack of success in work or other life events

Overly conforming, dependent on other opinions

Lack of eye contact

Nonassertive/passive

Indecisive

Excessively seeks reassurance

B. Situational low self-esteem

1. *Major*

Episodic occurrence of negative self-appraisal in response to life events in a person with a previous positive self-evaluation

Verbalization of negative feelings about the self (helplessness, uselessness)

2. *Minor*

Self-negating verbalizations

Expressions of shame or guilt

Evaluates self as unable to handle situations or events

Difficulty in making decisions

III. Role performance disturbance

Change in self-perception of role

Denial of role

Lack of knowledge of role

Change in others' perception of role

Change in usual patterns or responsibility

Conflict in roles

Change in physical capacity to resume role

IV. Personal identity disturbance (currently under development by NANDA)

Theoretical Issues

Relationships Among Concepts

Body image, personal identity, role performance, and self-esteem are overlapping and interrelated concepts. Each of these concepts is related to personality structure and earlier life development. Understanding the relationships among them facilitates discussion of the various factors contributing to a disturbance of self-perception. Self-perception is a significant contributor to mental and psychosocial health.

Current literature presents a number of inconsistencies in terms, definitions, and assumptions about self-perception, self-concept, and self-esteem. The notion of self-perception is abstract. Part of the self-perception is an appraisal of the body's capability of effectively coping with the environment and demands of daily living in that environment. Physical functioning, for exam-

ple, the ability to prepare a meal, as well as others' judgments of physical appearance and function are included. Further, individuals tend to develop self-appraisals within the context of role relationships and performance. The older adult's self-perception may be a reflection of independence in activities of daily living and the ability to work outside the home well into the seventh decade of life. Research supports the notion that role performance, for example, grandparenting, is essential to the continued development of self-perception. Self-perception is an internal psychodynamic process.

Older adults whose investment in self is healthy and whose body image is realistic may experience diminished self-esteem as a result of physical and mental decline. Decline in physical ability, restrictions in social roles and economic resources, and diminished physical attractiveness can attack the essential sense of self and undermine self-esteem and one's self-perception (Birren et al., 1992). Relationships between the concepts are depicted in Figure 17–11. The contributing factors for each category are described separately for purposes of clarity.

Contributing Factors

Body Image

Body image is based on past body experiences and current neuronal information, organized primarily in the parietotemporal areas of the cerebral cortex. It includes the

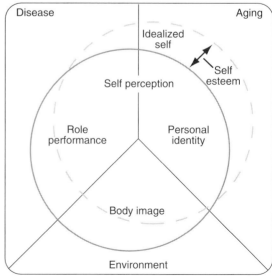

F I G U R E   1 7 – 1 1

Factors influencing self-concept in the elderly.

values and fantasies that individuals hold about their bodies (Ebersole and Hess, 1994). Body image is influenced by structural changes in the body, the ability of the body to process sensory inputs, and environmental factors such as opportunities for viewing the self through either interpersonal relationships or props such as pictures or mirrors. Integration of changes in body structure or function involve a complex process whereby the individual must relinquish the previously developed body image intrapsychically, resulting in anxiety and grief as a new body image is assumed. Disturbances in body image may therefore be linked to unsuccessful resolution of the bereavement associated with changes in body function or appearance. The two major categories of contributors to disruption in body image are age-related physical changes and the effects of disease.

AGE-RELATED CHANGES. Changes that commonly produce disruptions in body image include graying of hair, redistribution of body fat, wrinkling of skin, and changes in neuromuscular performance. Most individuals have little difficulty assimilating these changes in appearance; however, anecdotes of older individuals who feel youthful and "don't recognize that old lady in the mirror" are commonplace. Reduced efficiency of movement is more troublesome for older people because it may lead to dependency on others or fears of dependency, resulting in a diminished sense of competence.

DISEASE EFFECTS. Disease effects on body image are further categorized into *effects of the disease* itself, and *effects of treatment* for the disease. Hemiplegia, a consequence of cerebral infarction, results in a disturbed body image. In hemiplegia, the combination of altered sensory inputs, disturbed neural pathways, central nervous system integration of sensory stimuli, loss of functional abilities, and altered role performance results in severe alterations in body image and self-concept. Other diseases have effects resulting in less profound but significant changes in body image, such as autonomic neuropathy in diabetes or tumor growth in cancer. The degree of disturbance may be related to the degree to which the body change disrupts the individual's sense of continuity of self over time, an important aspect of self-concept in the elderly.

All forms of medical therapy potentially influence body image. Significant problems with body image result from traumatic surgery, such as that required for malignancies or vascular disease. Amputation of body parts, prostatectomy in men, and creation of ostomies produce major disturbances in body image that require gradual resolution. Radiation therapy may result in a disturbance in body image by destroying functional tissues. Pharmacologic agents may also disturb body image by altering the rates of body system functions or the responsiveness of end organs. For example, many antihypertensive drugs interfere with sexual responsiveness to the point of impotence. Drugs with anticholinergic properties produce unpleasant sensations such as dry mouth and constipation that affect body image.

Consequences of disturbance in body image are wide-ranging, and include self-neglect, preoccupation with weight control and achieving a "youthful" appearance, social isolation, and failure to learn to cope with a chronic disease because of inability to acknowledge the changes in body structure or function. Body image changes may also lead to alterations in role performance, disturbances in personal identity, and reduced self-esteem.

Role Performance

Role performance is the repetitive performance of tasks within a social group. Disturbance in role performance is present when a role change is perceived as unacceptable by the individual (Doenges and Moorhouse, 1985). Unacceptable role changes are grouped into the following categories: (1) inadequate role fulfillment, (2) undesired role loss, and (3) role overload.

Body image influences role performance. Individuals who perceive their bodies to be incomplete, too clumsy, or too slow either shy away from roles that they fear will require too much challenge for their bodies or perform badly in the role because of unrealistic perceptions of their bodies. Other physical changes influence role performance. For example, mobility problems reduce the efficiency of performing tasks. In some roles, decreased efficiency or competence is not important. For example, reduced efficiency in sewing clothes does not endanger health or safety. However, in time, an individual with decreased physical competence either relinquishes some roles or adjusts, along with family and friends, to a new level of task performance. If neither role loss nor adjustment takes place, then disturbance in role performance is the result. In the sewing example, the older person may cease to enjoy sewing or may experience hurt feelings when the family obtains their clothes elsewhere. Body image disturbance, decreased self-esteem, social factors, and role overload are four key contributors to disturbance in role performance.

Social factors that contribute to disturbance in role performance include inadequate socialization to new roles, rigid role expectations, and loss of continuity in role. Expectations for role performance come from within the individual and from environmental sources such as other social group members or physical attributes of the environment, such as accessibility of transportation or accessibility of toilets.

For example, the older individual who is admitted to a nursing home is at high risk for role disturbance for two reasons. (1) The old person has little experience in the role of nursing home resident, and (2) most institutions define fairly narrow ranges of acceptable behavior, expecting new residents to follow institutional routines and allowing few opportunities to continue preadmission roles.

Role overload, in which the individual is introduced to too many new roles simultaneously or has limited resources for enacting roles, is a fourth factor contributing to role disturbance. For example, an elderly man with marginal health status who suddenly finds himself thrust into the role of caregiver for his wife who has just had a stroke has many new roles to assume simultaneously. Unless the husband is extremely resourceful, role disturbance is likely to result.

Psychological factors and attributes of the social environment are determinants of role opportunities for the aged. For example, the societal expectation that old people perform less competently than younger people limits role opportunity and may result in rolelessness. In contrast, role overload may occur because of social circumstances, such as a spouse's need for caregiving or a financial requirement for late life employment despite an active leisure life.

The interplay between role performance and health status should be remembered. Ill health reduces the amount of time and energy available to initiate new activities or to maintain old roles in the accustomed manner. Evaluation of role performance is based on others' reflected appraisals of task performances. Limited opportunity to interact with others may result in a distorted view of role performance. Consequences of disturbance in role performance include feelings of inadequacy and lowered self-esteem and declines in health status.

Personal Identity

Personal identity results from a synthesis of information from role-performance experiences and body image. Words often used to describe an individual's identity include competent, independent, cheerful, sexy, creative, reliable. Changes in performance level or variety of roles, and changes in body image, may combine to cause a person to lose confidence in abilities that are present, resulting in a vicious cycle of ever-increasing dependency (see social breakdown model in Chapter 1, Fig. 1–7). Other consequences of disturbances in personal identity include anxiety, ranging from mild to extreme, and reduced self-esteem.

Self-Esteem

Self-esteem is a positive regard for oneself and may be expressed as a sense of competency, security, worthiness, and feelings of being loved (Skipwith, 1991). Disturbances in self-esteem stem from the individual's perception of negative appraisals from significant others or from a negative self-appraisal resulting from a significant difference between the "ideal" and the "real" self. Negative appraisals may be related to negative statements from significant others or to role changes. Those who view themselves as workers may experience difficulty when the work role is lost through retirement (Skipwith, 1991). Illness situations have a high likelihood of disturbing self-esteem because these situations may result in disfigurement, reduced role competence, and increased dependency, none of which is highly valued in Western society. The same may be said of age-related changes, which cause negatively valued changes in appearance and may affect role performance and independence negatively.

The second major category of contributors to decreased self-esteem is unrealistic expectations of self. Denial of the effects of decremental changes or poor judgment as a result of cognitive impairment results in situations in which the older person is prone to failure. Negative societal attitudes toward the elderly predispose them to reduced self-esteem by influencing the development of the idealized self. If an "old" appearance or behavior is valued negatively by society as a whole, the older adult is likely to have internalized these values. Also, stereotypical attitudes toward older adults may result in premature judgments that have nothing to do with actual performance. The older adult never has a "fair chance" to perform and therefore must perform exceptionally well in order to obtain a positive appraisal from the person who is stereotyping. In an initial clinical study designed to investigate the validity of the defining characteristics of self-esteem disturbance and test the assumptions of the three-component model derived from concept analysis, Norris and Kunes-Connell (1987) found that none of the defining characteristics as measured in this study reached the desired level of validity (.80), and only three of the characteristics achieved a minimal level of validity (.50). Additional empirical work is needed to validate the defining characteristics of self-esteem given the clinical association with such diverse conditions as substance abuse, psychological dysfunctions, psychiatric disturbances, and chronic physical illness.

Assessment

Systematic assessment of self-concept/self-perception disturbances requires gathering information in the following areas:

- Structural integrity of the body
- Integrity of neuroprocessing apparatus
- Predominant values regarding appearance and the importance of work and leisure, dependence and independence
- Self-expressed impact of existing changes or abnormal structural processes on the individual
- Observation of behaviors that are cues to inadequate coping with aging or disease-related changes, including (1) general physical appearance: well-kept vs. disheveled, (2) posture: erect and open vs. hunched over or withdrawn, (3) eye contact, (4) congruence between body language and speech content, (5) range of emotionality, and (6) range of role-relationships described.

If disturbed self-perception is suspected, more in-depth assessment regarding prior lifestyle and extent of support network is indicated to delineate the specific contributing factors and provide the basis for design of appropriate interventions.

Planning

Preventive approaches to disturbances in self-perception are worth consideration because nurses have numerous opportunities to implement or foster the development of effective prevention strategies. Nurses are involved in many of the situations that pre-cipitate self-perception disturbance in the aged. Disease-related changes, such as sequelae from an acute or chronic disease process and treatment, are key offenders. A primary goal of nurses who work with individuals who are faced with disease-related assaults should be to help the individual compensate for losses and make sense of those losses. Nurses are intimately involved in assisting with self-care activities, and in this capacity they may facilitate reintegration of self-image. The powerful influence of the nurse's attitudes and approaches to dependency, functional change, and lost or altered body parts on the older person's development cannot be overstated. The nurse can support older people's self-esteem by praising them, recognizing their contributions, and helping them identify situations in which they can be successful (Skipwith, 1991).

Nurses are in a prime position to offer anticipatory guidance to those adopting new roles, as when, for instance, a family member must assume caregiving responsibilities for an older person. Nurses in occupational health settings can promote the development of preretirement counseling programs to allow socialization for the retiree. Nurses have also taken active roles in developing support groups for those who must cope with chronic illness, facilitating adoption of the impaired role rather than maladaptive continuation in a sick role.

Intervention

Many interventions have been successfully applied to the problem of disturbances in self-concept and self-perception. Individual counseling, group approaches, network interventions, exercise, and environmental modification all have a place in the nurse's armamentarium.

Individual Counseling

Individual counseling is aimed at helping the individual resolve losses by facilitating the grief process. This intervention is particularly useful for those who are experiencing disturbances in role performance, personal identity, and body image (Norris, 1992). For those with disturbances in self-esteem, the focus of individual therapy is helping the individual identify strengths and lower unrealistic expectations (Fig. 17–12). Reminiscing is particularly useful in achieving both objectives (Burnside, 1994). Individual counseling need not take place only in an office

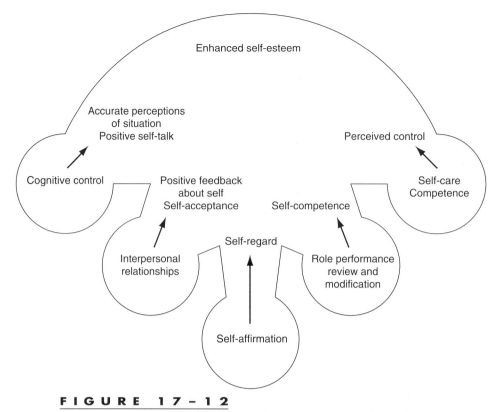

FIGURE 17-12

Interventions for altered self-esteem. (From Miller, J.F. *Coping with Chronic Illness: Overcoming Power-lessness.* 2nd ed. Philadelphia: F.A. Davis, 1992.)

setting or with an explicitly formulated contract for counseling. Nurses have numerous opportunities at the bedside or chairside to provide the active listening, guided reminiscence, gentle confrontation, and support needed by an older person who is grieving or working to reduce unrealistic expectations of self.

Exercise

Exercise addresses several aspects of disturbance in self-perception and image simultaneously. Development of increased strength, endurance, or coordination in selected tasks enhances the individual's competence, which in turn favorably influences self-esteem and increases the person's ability to assume new roles. A greater variety of role opportunities may thus become available. Personal identity is enhanced by the successful fulfillment of roles.

Setting realistic goals for the exercise program is important because an overly ambitious program will only serve to reinforce feelings of inadequacy. (See Chapter 14 for a detailed discussion of exercise programming.) However, carefully individualized exercise programs are associated with enhanced self-image, self-perception, and self-esteem, as well as other physiological benefits (Buchner et al., 1993; Mulrow et al., 1993).

Network Interventions

The purpose of network interventions is to increase the role opportunities available to older persons, thus affecting personal identity, self-esteem, and role performance. Ehrlich (1979) reports that the development of mutual support networks in residential neighborhoods provides older persons with meaningful work and social and service roles and enhances both the level of informal support in the community and individual morale.

Network interventions are applicable to both community and institutional care settings. They are a form of primary prevention for self-concept disturbance but can also be used therapeutically in communities where there is a high prevalence of self-concept disturbance, for example, in nursing home or age-segregated communities.

Group approaches to self-concept disturbance have the following advantages: efficient use of the nurse's or therapist's time, increased social contact for group members, enhanced feeling of universality of human responses to age-related changes, and exposure to new models for resolving problems (Frey et al., 1992). Lappe (1987) contends that groups are the preferred mode for conducting reminiscence therapy.

Educational interventions to increase the older person's understanding of developmental processes and change as a means of enhancing ego integrity in the elderly are encouraged (Foxall, 1991). A closed group model combining didactic and discussion methods is proposed. A preventively oriented educational group that prepares people for retirement is described by Ebersole and Hess (1994). The group focuses on preparation for postretirement roles with the goals of helping the older person clarify values and enhancing mastery of new roles.

Exercise groups are used successfully in all settings of care for the elderly. Participants should be allowed to follow their own pace. Music can be a useful adjunct. Individual participants may require extra attention from the group leader to maintain participation or to receive accurate directions about exercises.

Reminiscence groups are another form of intervention for self-concept disturbance (Stevens-Ratchford, 1993). In addition to the general advantages of group treatment, reminiscence groups have the added advantage of providing the experiences of many people to stimulate reminiscence, increasing the possibility of empathic responses by group members of a similar life station and birth cohort. Points to consider in organizing these groups are:

A. Minimum skill requirements for a reminiscence therapist*
   1. Someone who can serve as an active listener, helping the individual summarize the reflections stimulated
   2. Someone knowledgeable about techniques that stimulate reminiscence
B. Therapist's attitudes*
   1. Empathy for the older person's frame of reference
   2. Tolerance for defensive distortion of memories
   3. Positive concern for the patient's emotional struggle and progress in that struggle
   4. Sense of professional purpose and the ability to persevere

C. Considerations in group reminiscence therapy†
   1. Keep group size small, no more than five or six people, with men and women participants
   2. The group should meet at the same time and place on a regular basis
   3. Groups may be short-term or long-term
   4. Props, such as food, pictures, or objects, are excellent stimuli for discussion and reminiscence
   5. Relaxation exercises at the beginning of the group meeting stimulate awareness and facilitate discussion

Nurses who establish reminiscing groups should review an authoritative reference on group process and therapy with the aged, such as Burnside (1983).

Environmental Modification

Environmental modification encompasses a variety of interventions and has the greatest potential for impact on the individual's self-concept. Simplification of the environment to enhance the individual's abilities for self-care will enhance self-esteem (Orth, 1991). Making optimum use of the attitudes and nonverbal behaviors of helpers in the old person's environment is a powerful intervention. The attitude that old people are just like children makes it difficult for the older person to maintain a positive adult self-image continuous with earlier development. Nurses must educate caregivers about the importance of treating the elderly as adults to prevent deterioration of the older person's self-image as an adult.

Touch from caregivers is positively associated with self-esteem, warmth, and recognizing the wholeness of the individual (Osgood and Brant, 1991). In one study of hospitalized patients, the elderly were the age group least likely to be touched (Barnett, 1972). However, the nature of the touch and the social background of the elderly individual influence perception of touch as comforting or uncomfortable (Potter and Perry, 1993). Nurses are in a key position to influence the use of touch with older persons because lay and paraprofessional caregivers often look to professionals for guidance. Modelling therapeutic use of touch and teaching this to

---

*From Butler, 1960, 1968; quoted in Blum and Tross, 1980.

† From Ebersole, 1984

caregivers modifies the interpersonal environment of the older person in a manner that should promote increased self-esteem.

Another environmental intervention is encouraging the elderly to retain personal possessions, particularly in institutional settings. The positive effects of nursing home residents owning personal possessions have been documented by research (Holzapfel, 1982; 1992). Individuals have an emotional investment in possessions, and this contributes to the maintenance of self-identity (Rubenstein, 1989). Possessions can also be helpful in facilitating reminiscence.

Respecting personal space, territory, and promoting privacy are environmental interventions that prevent disturbances in self-concept. Territory is the area that an individual lays claim to, whereas personal space is an invisible boundary around the individual that varies with mood and circumstance (Potter and Perry, 1993). Size of personal space is believed to increase with lowered self-esteem (Rubenstein, 1989). In hospital and nursing home settings, needs for space are difficult to meet and are often belittled or ignored. The older person's insistence on fixed seating arrangements in the dining room is an attempt to establish and protect a territory—a very normal human response. The distress of nursing home residents at other residents rummaging through their drawers is understandable as a response to violated territory. It is important for staff to make every attempt not to violate territory and personal space. It is risky for a patient to become upset with staff members, yet the insult to self-concept is just as real. A reasonable alternative is to request permission before entering established territory or personal space.

Evaluation

Disturbances in self-concept are manifested by subtle behavioral cues. Therefore, descriptions of target behaviors are necessary for accurate monitoring of progress toward resolving a self-care disturbance. Self-care behaviors, eye contact, posture, statements about self, and extent of role repertoire are all measurable behaviors that may be used when evaluating the effectiveness of nursing care for those with self-concept disturbances.

SOCIAL ISOLATION

Definition and Scope of Problem

The observation that many elderly people are relatively isolated and socially inactive requires little documentation. Many elderly persons experience widowhood and diminished contact with their children. For most men, and for an increasing number of women, the loss of the job role at retirement brings with it the loss of many important social contacts that may never be satisfactorily replaced. The death of peers progressively constricts the range of friendships, at a time when some elders have fewer opportunities to make new friends (Engels, 1991). Loneliness and social isolation are two separate but related problems affecting older persons. Many overlapping definitions for these conditions are in use. NANDA (1994) defines social isolation as a

condition of aloneness experienced by the individual and perceived as imposed by others and as a negative or threatened state.

This is a considerably more restrictive definition than some used by researchers in social gerontology. Bennett (1980, p. 15) offers the following definition for social isolation:

. . . the absence of specific role relationships which are generally activated and sustained through direct personal face to face interaction.

In contrast, loneliness is defined as a subjective feeling of insufficient human contact, regardless of the frequency with which others are seen (Bennett, 1980). Separating these two concepts is useful in gerontological nursing because of the importance of respecting individual lifestyles. Although social isolation is a risk factor for loneliness and institutionalization, there are many examples of individuals who adopt an isolated lifestyle without experiencing loneliness. A second advantage to separating social isolation and loneliness is that it is possible to take advantage of the research into these problems as they are classically defined. Because social isolation, apart from consideration of feelings of loneliness, is associated with many negative outcomes for older persons, the concept of social isolation as defined by Bennett has clinical utility for nurses. Holmen and colleagues (1993) place the prevalence of loneliness among the elderly as high as 35 per cent. Other researchers indicate that findings on the frequency of loneliness among the older population are inconsistent, although there is clear general consensus on the negative impact of loneliness on later life (Dugan and Kivett, 1994).

Social isolation stems from a disruption in linkages to a supportive network and may prompt feelings of vulnerability, marginality, tension, and boredom (Weiss, 1989). Social isolation may have far-reaching consequences in the elderly. First, it may be a precursor to development of loneliness. Second, the frail older person's ability to remain in the community may be diminished because of a lack of family or friends to assist with personal care or instrumental activities of daily living. Third, social isolation may result in an alteration in self-concept. For example, the schoolteacher who was surrounded by students and other faculty may find on retirement that the lack of social outlets causes her to question her continued worth to society. Fourth, social isolation may result in further alterations in role relationships. The schoolteacher in the example just cited enacted a variety of roles, including confidant, teacher, counselor, and friend. In a socially isolated environment there is limited opportunity to conduct such role relationships because of insufficient "others."

Fifth, social isolation may result in alterations in family process. If the aged individual's social circle shrinks, she or he may increasingly turn to family members for assistance and for satisfaction of role-enactment. This may result in disequilibrium in the family unit. For example, the retirement of the parish minister may precipitate such a change. The pastor, long used to luncheon engagements as a means of transacting parish business, suddenly finds himself without luncheon partners. He has expected that his wife will be only too happy to join him for lunch, failing to take into account her routines of visiting or lunching with friends.

Finally, social isolation may result in deterioration of social skills (Bennett, 1980). Diminished opportunity to interact with others was found to be related to adjustment difficulties in other social situations, such as nursing homes or senior centers. Patterns of social isolation or a lack of social connectedness may be predictive of the older person's development of mental disorder (Engels, 1991).

Contributing Factors

Physical Impairment

Physical impairment alone is unlikely to cause social isolation unless it is severe. Obviously, individuals who cannot leave their beds because of severe functional impairments are at high risk for social isolation regardless of other factors. Hearing and visual losses are two examples of socially isolating physical impairments common among the elderly. Insecurity about navigating in unfamiliar environments leads many to remain at home rather than risk injury or embarrassment in unfamiliar surroundings. More commonly, however, physical impairment is only one predisposing factor that interacts with others to produce someone who is socially isolated or lonely.

American society as a whole has done a poor job of making the activities of mainstream life accessible to those with physical handicaps. Although work and recreational settings are increasingly being freed from barriers to wheelchairs and crutches through the use of ramps and modified toilet facilities, many areas remain problematic. Use of public transportation for those with physical handicaps remains difficult. These barriers, coupled with the older person's generally slowed response time and the sensory losses that often accompany advanced age, make travel outside the home a taxing endeavor. A new physical impairment in a person with other factors predisposing to social isolation may be the problem that tips the balance toward social isolation.

Diminished Social Status

Diminished social status is a problem that faces most older persons. This may result in a reluctance to seek out new acquaintances because the social opportunities that exist may not yield the desired contacts. For example, many older persons spurn the chance to go to meetings of a senior citizens' club or group even if the activity is one previously enjoyed because that person does not want to be around "all those old people." In the same breath, the same person may complain about the noisy children in the neighborhood. This negative view of one's age peers because society has a negative image of the elderly may be a significant contributor to social isolation in the elderly, particularly among those who relocate late in life.

Diminished Economic Resources

Just as physical impairment may limit social opportunities, so may economic constraints. Persons with sufficient income may join recreational clubs, travel, and entertain. Those whose income meets only basic needs have fewer social outlets. This is not to say that social outlets do not exist for those of limited income. Poor people, however, are at particular disadvantage if they do not have family, church, or neighborhood ties.

Relocation

Relocation may be one of the greatest contributors to social isolation and loneliness. It is simply not possible to replicate the social network and feelings of closeness developed over a lifetime in a few months. However, some people relocate as a result of diminished social contact (through death, disability, or relocation of friends). Sometimes such a move may result in a remedy for social isolation, with the result that the older person is less lonely.

Loss of Peer Contact

Death or disability of friends may limit the number of peers available. For example, it is not uncommon to hear widows complain that they seldom see some old friends because their social contacts typically centered on "couple"-type activities. Also, if the friend who was formerly the usual luncheon companion is suddenly no longer able to go out to eat independently, this may result in a constriction of social activity and interaction for the otherwise healthy partner.

Lifestyle

Lifelong socializers and joiners are at far less risk for social isolation than those who have been loners or isolates all their lives.

Psychological Factors

Individuals with personality disorders or chronic mental impairments may be at greater risk for social isolation than those without such impairments (Harper, 1991). High rates of psychological impairment in the elderly are typically associated with depression. Depressive illness may present as loss of interest in social roles, isolation, and loss of appetite with attendant loss of socialization.

Fear of Criminal Victimization

Although it has been shown that the prevalence of violent crime is not greater among elderly people, the disproportionate impact of victimization on their economic and physical well-being may help explain the widespread fear of crime. Such fear may reduce social integration.

Loneliness

Determinants of loneliness vary widely, but most researchers include major losses as a prime contributor (Harper, 1991; Ebersole and Hess, 1994). Loss of a spouse, decreased vision, low self-assessment of health, transportation problems, frequent use of telephones, being female, and low participation in formally organized social activities may help distinguish people who are characterized as often lonely from those who might be labeled almost never lonely (Haight,

1991; Engels, 1991). Austin (1989) reviewed the literature on loneliness among elderly persons and identified personality characteristics that increase or decrease the risk of loneliness. Poor social skills, a negative affect, self-centeredness, and the inability to enjoy activities while alone may predispose to loneliness. Openness, receptivity, and creative use of alone time may buffer against loneliness. Loneliness is an internal process.

Assessment

Bennett (1980) has developed a set of scales to measure social isolation in the elderly, which also could be adapted for clinical use. The first measure is the Past Month Isolation (PMI) Index (Table 17–4). It rates the older person's current role contacts with five groups: organizations, children, siblings, friends, and other relatives. It provides a measure of the older person's current social connectedness. The second is the Adulthood Isolation Index (Table 17–5). It rates the older person's life pattern of role contacts with the same five groups used in the PMI but additionally includes contacts with parents, spouse, and job. The measures of these three units provide important information on the older person's life patterns of socialization. The PMI was constructed with possible scores ranging from 0 to 10, and the Adulthood Isolation Index has possible scores ranging from 0 to 32. In using the scales, individuals are to be compared to each other on the dimension of social isolation. Thus, individuals are designated as isolates (low scores) and nonisolates (high scores), bearing in mind that these terms and numbers are used as relative ones within a comparatively isolated population. These measures have proved useful in studies of community elderly but are less reliable in studies of hospitalized mental patients (Bennett, 1980). Four patterns of social interaction have been identified:

- Older people who have been integrated throughout their lifetimes
- "The early isolate"—someone who was isolated as an adult but is relatively active in old age
- "The recent isolate"—someone who was active in early adulthood but is not in old age
- "The lifelong isolate"—a person whose lifestyle is one of isolation

Loneliness is somewhat easier to assess. Simply asking individuals how often they experience loneliness is likely to produce a lengthy unburdening from those who are lonely and a shorter, more direct response from those with a limited or nonexistent problem with loneliness.

Planning

Selecting interventions for socially isolated or lonely people depends on the location of the individual and the pattern of isolation identified. In community settings, coordination with other agencies or family members or friends is often necessary to set up the desired interventions or circumstances needed for goal achievement. In institutional settings, facilitating adaptation to the institutional environment may be a key issue in resolving social isolation. There is enhanced opportunity for behavioral interventions, but communication with other team members is essential for success.

Categorizing the pattern of isolation facilitates selection of interventions. Intervention with individuals who are lifelong isolates must be approached with great care. It is inappropriate for nurses to impose their own values regarding social interaction on individuals who believe that their patterns are functional. However, as life circumstances change, isolated individuals may choose to increase their connectedness with others and may need assistance developing basic social skills to do so. Nurses should remain alert for cues from lifelong isolates that they desire help in changing their isolated situation. In continuing-care settings such as outpatient clinics, nursing homes, or home health agencies, nurses can use the periodic health assessment as an opportunity to comment on the individual's isolation, providing an invitation to the older person to discuss whether the isolation is bothersome.

Recent isolates require interventions addressed to the factors that precipitated their isolation. These individuals have developed social interaction skills previously but may need help strengthening those skills or assistance in coping with a particularly isolating experience or set of circumstances, such as widowhood or physical disability.

Interventions

Studies show that social isolation in elderly people responds to a wide range of interventions, including behavior modification techniques (Ebersole and Hess, 1990), health education approaches (Potter and Perry, 1993), group therapeutic activities (Miller, 1990), mutual help groups (Ebersole and Hess, 1990), multipurpose senior centers, adult day centers, and activation of ex-

T A B L E   1 7 – 4

Assessment of Social Isolation in Elderly People: Past Month Isolation Index

CATEGORY	NUMBER OF ROLE CONTACTS	SCORE
Organization	A. Individual did not report membership in any organization such as church, social club, or political club during the past month.	0
	B. Individual reported membership in one organization during the past month.	1
	C. Individual reported membership in two or more organizations in the past month.	2
Children	A. Individual did not report any contact with children during the past month.	0
	B. Individual reported contact with one child during the past month.	1
	C. Individual reported contact with two or more children during the past month.	2
Siblings	A. Individual did not report any contact with siblings during the past month.	0
	B. Individual reported contact with one sibling during the past month.	1
	C. Individual reported contact with two or more siblings during the past month.	2
Friends	A. Individual did not report any contact with friends during the past month.	0
	B. Individual reported contact with one friend during the past month.	1
	C. Individual reported contact with two or more friends during the past month.	2
Relatives	A. Individual did not report any contact with relatives other than children or siblings during the past month.	0
	B. Individual reported contact with one such relative during the past month.	1
	C. Individual reported contact with two or more such relatives during the past month.	2

From Bennett, R. *Aging, Isolation, and Resocialization.* New York: Van Nostrand Reinhold, 1980.

isting support networks such as religious groups. Successful implementation of these interventions depends on sensitive matching of available programs to the needs of the individual. A description of attributes characterizing successful interventions follows.

Behavior Modification

Behavioral modification is most commonly conducted in institutional settings, although with the proper linkages, these techniques may be applied to old people living in the community. Hallmarks of successful interventions include analysis of the antecedents and consequences of the behavior to be changed, specification of a realistic, measurable goal, development of an appropriate reward system, and support people who understand that neutral behavior rather than negative reinforcement is the necessary response to the undesirable behavior. The importance of consistency in approach cannot be overstated when using behavioral inter-

TABLE 17-5

Assessment of Social Isolation in Elderly People: Adulthood Isolation Index

CATEGORY	NUMBER OF ROLE CONTACTS	SCORE
Organization	A. Individual did not report membership in any organization during adulthood.	0
	B. Individual reported membership in one organization.	1
	C. Individual reported membership in two organizations.	2
	D. Individual reported membership in three organizations.	3
	E. Individual reported membership in four or more organizations.	4
Children	A. Individual did not report direct contact with any children at all or with children beyond their infancy.	0
	B. Individual reported direct contact with one child.	1
	C. Individual reported direct contact with two children.	2
	D. Individual reported direct contact with three children.	3
	E. Individual reported direct contact with four or more children.	4
Siblings	A. Individual did not report direct contact with any siblings at all or with siblings beyond their infancy.	0
	B. Individual reported direct contact with one sibling.	1
	C. Individual reported direct contact with two siblings.	2
	D. Individual reported direct contact with three siblings.	3
	E. Individual reported direct contact with four or more siblings.	4
Relatives	A. Individual did not report direct contact with any relatives in adulthood.	0
	B. Individual reported direct contact with one relative.	1
	C. Individual reported direct contact with two relatives.	2
	D. Individual reported direct contact with three relatives.	3
	E. Individual reported direct contact with four or more relatives.	4
Friends	A. Individual did not report any friends in adulthood.	0
	B. Individual reported direct contact with one friend.	1
	C. Individual reported direct contact with two friends.	2
	D. Individual reported direct contact with three friends.	3
	E. Individual reported direct contact with four or more friends.	4
Mother	A. The individual reported he maintained no contact with his mother during adulthood.	0
	B. Individual reported that he either maintained some contact with his mother over a period of 15 years, or that he saw her frequently for a period of less than 15 years.	1
	C. The individual reported that he maintained frequent contact with his mother; i.e., he saw her at least once a month, for a minimum of 15 years in adulthood.	2
Father	A. The individual reported that he maintained no contact with his father during adulthood.	0
	B. Individual reported that he either maintained some contact with his father over a period of 15 years, or that he saw him frequently for a period of less than 15 years.	1
	C. The individual reported that he maintained frequent contact with his father; i.e., he saw him at least once a month, for a minimum of 15 years in adulthood.	2
Spouse	A. Never married.	0
	B. Married less than 15 years.	2
	C. Daily contact with spouse for a period of at least 15 years.	4
Job	A. Individual never worked in adulthood.	0
	B. Individual held any job.	1
	C. Individual worked at least 10 years.	2
	D. Individual held several types of jobs and worked during his entire adult life.	3
	E. Individual maintained one job or worked in the same field during most of his adult life.	4

From Bennett, R. *Aging, Isolation, and Resocialization.* New York: Van Nostrand Reinhold, 1980.

ventions. In institutional settings consistency can be extremely difficult to achieve unless the number of staff involved in the intervention is small or the staff group is highly motivated. However, MacDonald (1978) demonstrated the efficacy of a simple behavioral intervention to combat chronic social isolation in a nursing home that did not require intensive staff training or extensive communications with other staff members. The intervention consisted of the investigator initiating conversation during a meal and providing social reinforcement for appropriate conversation. All the hallmarks of successful behavioral intervention are exemplified by this study, and the author concludes that there are many opportunities in institutional settings to use staff attention and expectations to reduce social isolation.

Family and friends may be motivated to learn techniques of behavior modification to assist an older person. For example, one family member requested nursing consultation because Grandmother seldom left the house but complained about being lonely. The intervention was a change in the family visiting pattern from the extended family unit running all the errands for Grandmother to inviting Grandmother to assist with the shopping, concluding the errand trip with a brief visit with the great-grandchildren. This provided an appropriate reinforcement (seeing the great-grandchildren more often) with a regular outing that included interactions with people outside the family network.

Mutual Aid Groups

Mutual aid groups are useful for individuals with socially acceptable, easy to label conditions that are associated with isolation. Examples include "Widow-to-Widow" groups, "I Can Cope" or "Reach to Recovery" support groups for cancer patients, and groups for the vision-impaired or hearing-impaired. Such groups have been established for nearly every chronic disease, but their presence in a specific community is far from assured. Nurses should include as part of their community assessment an inventory of the mutual aid groups available and determine the ease of entry and extent of support available for members. For many, support groups provide ideal assistance in coping with role changes associated with chronic disease or bereavement as well as a useful social outlet. However, depending on the skill of the group leaders, individuals who have multiple impairments or limited social skills may have difficulty taking full advantage of these groups.

Therapeutic Groups

Structured activity programs, exercise classes, and health education groups provide a useful means of combining socialization with other therapeutic objectives. Ebersole and Hess (1994) describe impressive social and physiological benefits from structured activities. Reminiscence groups provide a forum for enactment of the socially expected role behavior of older adults, especially as related to the role of oral historian. In addition to convening a group of older persons, therapeutic groups often enhance the older person's confidence in living with a problem that is a self-perceived barrier to social interaction. For example, the increased endurance and flexibility developed in an exercise class may influence the older person's willingness to go on outings with the church or with family. The greatest obstacle to success in using a therapeutic group intervention may be convincing the older person to attend the first meeting. Resistance to attending a group may stem from low self-esteem, caution about trying new activities, or more mundane difficulties such as inconvenient meeting times or problems arranging transportation.

Group approaches are also appropriate for institutional populations, although modifications for the relative frailty of the participants are often indicated. Burnside (1983) offers excellent suggestions for group work with older persons. Groups are least often used in hospital settings but can be used effectively if the special constraints on group work in the hospital setting such as time, scheduling, and space are acknowledged (Dobson and Culhane, 1991). Maintaining social activity may help to counter hospital-acquired confusion by preserving the usual patterns of adult social interaction that are disrupted by the hospital environment. A clinical nurse specialist in one private acute care hospital developed an early morning group for elderly patients who had sleep difficulties as an alternative to sleep medications or restraint.

Multipurpose Senior Centers

Senior centers are important community resources in combating social isolation in elderly people. Designed to be a focal point for aging services, these centers all include a gathering place for older persons and, depending on funding and the sophistication of the staff, may also include a wide variety of recreational and social activities, including meals, travel, educational offerings, and exercise groups, as well as opportunities for health assessment, health counseling, and health services. The target population is the older person living independently in the community. Education of old people or family about the resources at a senior center is a useful intervention to prevent social isolation.

Adult Day Care

Adult day care programs serve individuals operating at a lower functional level than those attending a senior center. Models of adult day care range from a social model of care, which stresses socialization and purposeful activity, to a medical model, which emphasizes provision of therapies to promote recovery from disease. Many mixed models are in existence. They all share some form of structured activity program throughout the day and usually provide individualized, goal-oriented care planning for participants (Fulmer and Edelman, 1991). There are no universally accepted standards for day care programs, and few states require licensure. The advantage of a day program to reduce social isolation in the elderly is that it is a much more intensive program than that found in individual group or behavioral approaches.

Evaluation

Criteria for evaluation of nursing care for the socially isolated include the following:

1. Contributors to isolation are identified.
2. Interventions to address contributors are implemented.
3. Patient has increased number of social contacts per week.
4. Patient expresses increased confidence in social skills.
5. Patient expresses increased self-worth.

SPIRITUAL DISTRESS

Definition and Scope of Problem

Spiritual well-being is "the affirmation of life in a relationship with God, self, community and environment which nurtures and celebrates wholeness." It is explicitly included in the World Health Organization's definition of health, and spirituality is consistently identified as an important aspect of the health of older persons (Brock, 1991; Di, 1991; Cole, 1992; Stepnick and Perry, 1992). Moberg (1990) has defined spirituality as the totality of people's inner resources, the ultimate concerns around which all other values are focused, the central philosophy of life that guides conduct, and the meaning-giving center of human life that influences all individual and social behavior.

Spiritual distress is defined by NANDA (1994) as "disruption in the life principle which pervades a person's entire being and which integrates and transcends one's biological and psychosocial nature." As with most emerging topics within such fields as nursing and social gerontology, published research has been largely descriptive and focused primarily on white males (Levin et al., 1994). As a result, there has been little attention to religiosity in older adult women and members of ethnic minority populations, save the programmatic work of Taylor and Chatters on African Americans (1991) and of Levin and Markides (1986) on Mexican Americans. Given this state of science, the seminal work of Moberg (1953), more than 40 years ago, will continue to be the common point of discourse. In 1971, the White House Conference on Aging defined spiritual concerns as the human need to deal with sociocultural deprivations, anxieties and fears, death and dying, personality integration, self-image, personal dignity, social alienation, and philosophy of life (Moberg, 1984).

Theoretical Issues

Spirituality is sometimes equated with religiosity, but these two concepts are distinct. Religiosity refers to outward signs of spiritual belief, whereas spirituality is a much broader concept that does not always include religious aspects (Vaillot, 1970). Religion has been cited by some researchers as an important aspect of the older person's life and has been associated with psychological well-being (Markides, 1983). The importance of religion to older persons has been described as a need for affirmation in facing death and coming to terms with life as a whole. Additionally, religious activities and faith provide support to the elderly (Jackson et al., 1990).

Participation in religious communities provides members with a framework for deriving meaning from their life experiences and with structured opportunities to interact with others who are alike with respect to values, beliefs, and attitudes (Levin et al., 1994).

Contributing Factors

Factors that are believed to contribute to spiritual distress include the following:

- Heightened awareness of aging
- Separation from religious or cultural ties
- Challenged belief and value system, such as that occurring from intense suffering or due to the moral or ethical implications of therapy
- Disfigurement
- Disability
- Chronic pain
- Unresolved feelings about death
- Anger toward God (Carpenito, 1989; Ackley and Ladwig, 1993)

These life experiences are believed to stimulate questioning of lifestyle, meaning of existence, and meaning of suffering.

Assessment

Spirituality is highly personal and must be approached in a nonobtrusive and sensitive manner. Spiritual needs change during different phases of illness and life transition, so nurses must be aware of these changes and responsive to these concerns. Forbes (1994) utilized the Spiritual Well-Being (SWB) scale in pilot work to examine the concept of spirituality and the relationship between the caregiver's and care recipient's concept of spirituality, in order to identify its influence on emotional well-being and coping ability. This 20-item Likert scale measures the individual's relationship with God and satisfaction with life (Paloutzian and Ellison, 1982). Using tested outcome measures as assessment tools may assist the nurse in this complex area.

In addition, Forbes (1994) developed a 10-question structured interview guide as a companion to the SWB scale. Selected sample questions include

- To whom do you turn when you need help? God/Family and friends

- Has being sick or caring for someone sick made any difference in your feelings toward God? Toward yourself? Yes/No

- Does your faith help you make decisions? Yes/No

- How often do you pray privately? Prayed _____.

- When do you feel closest to God? When things are going well/When I am praying to God/I am not sure there is a God

Nurses should also be alert for signs and cues that suggest spiritual distress. Nonverbal cues such as crying, use of religious symbols, use of silence, and facial expressions should all be considered. Remember that many of the cues that are used to make the diagnosis of various psychoemotional disorders such as anxiety or grieving may also indicate spiritual distress. It is therefore important to be aware of the factors in the client's life situation that may predispose to spiritual distress, as noted earlier.

Defining characteristics of spiritual distress (NANDA, 1994) are

- Expresses concern with meaning of life and death or belief systems (this is the critical defining factor)

- Anger toward God

- Questions meaning of suffering

- Verbalizes inner conflict about beliefs

- Verbalizes concern about relationship with deity

- Questions meaning of own existence

- Unable to participate in usual religious practices

- Seeks spiritual assistance

- Questions moral or ethical implications of therapeutic regimen

- Gallows humor

- Displacement of anger toward religious representatives

- Description of nightmares or sleep disturbances

- Alteration in behavior or mood evidenced by anger, crying, withdrawal, preoccupation, anxiety, hostility, apathy

Planning

Readiness to deal with spiritual aspects of care for older persons is a key issue in planning. Unless the nurse regards the spiritual needs of the patient on a par with other needs for care, cues and signs of spiritual distress may be overlooked. Nurses must be particularly alert for cues that may indicate spiritual distress because the nurse's own conflicts regarding spiritual issues may interfere with correct diagnosis. Further, spiritual distress is not always manifested in religious language. Finding spiritual meaning in life is a uniquely individual task and does not come quickly or necessarily through the efforts of another. Plans may be apparent, transparent, or totally obscure (Ebersole and Hess, 1994).

Another important planning task is to identify possible resource people to assist those with spiritual distress. Some nurses and other health care providers are more comfortable than others in assisting those with spiritual distress. Although nurses clearly have great opportunities to assist people with spiritual needs, not all nurses have strong spiritual beliefs, and it may therefore be difficult for them to assist those with spiritual distress (Ebersole and Hess, 1994). However, it should not be assumed that only chaplains, pastors, or rabbis have the expertise to help patients with spiritual distress because many nurses are able to intervene successfully with those experiencing this problem (Stepnick and Perry, 1992; Forbes, 1994).

Planning and Interventions

No protocols are available for assisting individuals with spiritual distress. Several guidelines consistently appear in the nursing literature. These include

- The importance of awareness of spiritual issues in care

- Being available to listen to the individual's concerns

- A willingness to be nondirective, open-minded, and nonjudgmental and to allow individuals to create their own frameworks for understanding their spiritual dilemmas

Referral to clergy may be appropriate, but nurses should not overlook or underestimate the importance of their own proximity and trust relationships in intervening with those experiencing spiritual distress. Two case examples follow that show the importance of skillful nursing intervention for those with spiritual distress.

Evaluation

Criteria for evaluation of nursing care for older persons with spiritual distress include

1. Individual attaches meaning to suffering or current life experience.
2. Individual no longer experiences loneliness.
3. Individual has reduced physical pain.

CASE EXAMPLES

C.L. was a 74-year-old retired Protestant clergyman, admitted to the nursing home for terminal care with inoperable lung cancer. He had just finished a course of palliative radiation therapy, and his pain was controlled with Tylenol #3. Prior to his diagnosis, he had been the primary caregiver for his wife, who had multiple chronic illnesses. His wife was now also a patient in the nursing home. The L's had many supportive friends in the area, who visited regularly. Additionally, his only son and his family lived in the community and visited. Mr. L. experienced terrible nightmares and daytime weakness following his admission. He demanded large amounts of nursing staff time for seemingly minor needs, such as ice water several times per shift and being with him when he was frightened. He gradually reached the point where he was frightened to sleep at night because of bad dreams and thus sought support from the night nurse. Rather than interpreting this as a nuisance or turning to sleep medication, the nurse used Mr. L.'s "insomnia" as an opportunity to give him much-needed time with an active listener. They developed a regular time for meeting, which typically lasted about 45 minutes and generally included a nourishing snack. Sometimes Mrs. L. joined them. Mr. L. was then able to sleep during the daytime. Through this outlet, coupled with regular visits from the local pastor, Mr. L. was able to resolve his extreme anxiety about

death. It was significant that this individual had spent many years of his own ministry working with terminally ill people, yet experienced significant distress when his own mortality had to be confronted. It is likely that without the thoughtful intervention of the night nurse Mr. L. would have experienced a much more painful, anxiety-ridden dying process because his needs for counseling exceeded the resources of the parish clergyperson.

L.T. is a 7-year resident of an intermediate care facility. Her major problems included rheumatoid arthritis, spinal stenosis, immobility, congestive heart failure, chronic pain, stress incontinence, and dependent edema. Trials on several different antidepressants have been ineffective relieving her symptoms. Ms. T. is an excellent example of an individual with unresolved spiritual distress. She complains of hurting all over and is unable to localize pain despite the use of myriad assessment techniques. She describes her existence as a "test" handed to her by the Lord, and sometimes she simply doesn't know if she can go on living this way. She exists in a recliner wheelchair, getting up each morning at 6:30 A.M. and returning to bed at 9:30 P.M. She refuses to go to bed in the afternoon because "I'm afraid. When I go back to bed, I don't have anything to think about except myself." She describes her existence as miserable, but she "just tries to do what the doctors tell me to."

With encouragement, she is able to function at a much higher level, bearing the majority of her weight in transfer. She expresses the idea that she has found some meaning in her suffering, yet this does little to relieve it.

POTENTIAL FOR VIOLENCE

Definition and Scope of Problem

Violence, either self-directed or directed toward others, is not widely discussed in the geriatric literature. The paucity of information on violence in the aged probably results both from the tendency to idealize older people as incapable of violence and from the reduced prevalence of violence directed toward others in the older age group. Diminished physical capacity leads to diminished impact of violent behavior. However, we do know that violent outbursts in non-psychiatric residents tend to catch staff members off guard (Burnside, 1980; Burnside, 1984); as a result, restraints are used, even though these may further intensify aggression (Cox, 1991).

The question of what constitutes violent behavior is not always simple. As in many areas of daily living and health care, a variety of terms are used to describe the behaviors associated with violence. In the literature we find terms such as anger and hostility (Cox, 1991), aggression, agitation (Birkett, 1991), and problem behaviors (Evans, 1991). Most of what is known about violence among elderly adults is documented in literature from nursing home environments.

The slightest question of violence by staff against patients or residents is rigorously investigated by state authorities, whereas violence by patients or residents is governmentally ignored. Paranoia can be associated with sustained and dangerous behavior. In board and care facilities, there is a mixture of all types of mental illness, alcoholism, and drug addiction. Consequently, the potential for violence is high and may include rape and homicide.

Within nursing facilities, the most likely drugs associated with violence are the benzodiazepines. In small doses, these drugs may cause a drunken belligerence (Birkett, 1991). Among mental illnesses, dementia is the most likely to be associated with violence. However, these acts of violence are usually limited by the person's age, weakness, and physical incapacity.

Over 60 per cent of nursing home residents suffer from cognitive or psychiatric impairments that may contribute to management and violence problems. Violent acts may include such diverse behaviors as scratching, spitting, combativeness, ramming gerichairs, grabbing and mauling passersby, wandering into others' rooms or beds, and rape. Prior to the AIDS epidemic, spitting was regarded as a nonviolent act of aggression. This perspective is changing.

Suicide, the most extreme form of self-directed violence, is one of the ten leading causes of death for elderly people in the United States. The rate of suicide in men climbs steadily with advancing age. Compared with younger individuals, elderly people less frequently communicate their suicidal intent openly, use more violent and lethal means, and less often attempt suicide as a means of gaining attention (Osgood and Brant, 1991).

Defining characteristics of violent behavior differ for self-directed violence and other-directed violence. Violence directed toward others is characterized by

- Verbal attacks on others, including cursing and swearing
- Threats of physical attack on another
- Physical attacks on other family members, patients, or staff members, including biting, scratching, hitting or tripping, and fighting

Self-directed violence can be characterized by self-neglect or by signs of overt self-injurious behavior such as

- Refusal to perform self-care activities despite cognitive and physical ability to do so
- Presence of objective signs of tissue trauma, such as cigarette burns, lacerations, and bruises
- Refusal to eat
- Refusal to take medications

Contributing Factors

The literature on aggression is divided into two major theories: one that considers aggression an internally generated drive that motivates behavior, and one that considers aggression the result of frustrated goal attainment (Fox, 1991). Those who view aggression as an innate drive consider hostility the result of inadequate socialization. Violent behavior thus results from failure to learn nonviolent means of defending self or territory, resulting in a life-long pattern of hostile behavior. Viewing aggression as a response to frustration focuses attention on environmental factors and life events. Violence is attributed to lack of control over life or the environment or as a response to overwhelming stress. The two schools of thought are not mutually exclusive. Violence in the elderly is probably due to a combination of factors, both intrinsic and environmental. Consideration of violence in the elderly must also account for the contribution of brain damage to violent behavior. Brain damage may result in loss of inhibitory centers that control aggression, or it may be a source of frustration for the individual, also precipitating violent behavior. Lanza (1983) has synthesized a theoretical model of aggression that includes both viewpoints (Fig. 17–13).

Factors associated with violence directed toward others in the general psychiatric

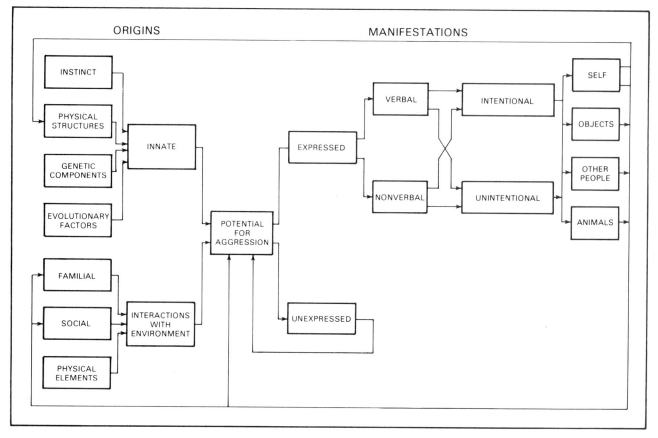

FIGURE 17-13

A model of causation of aggression. (From Lanza, M.L. Origins of aggression. *J Psychosoc Mental Health Nurs* 21(6):11-16, 1983.)

population include a history of violent behavior and a diagnosis of psychosis, intoxication, or confusion. Self-directed violence is associated with depression, low self-esteem, and altered body image.

Violence may occur in individuals who have exhausted their repertoire of coping responses. Two general types emerge: those with limited coping resources, such as those with aphasia, delirium, or dementia; and those living in environments totally alien to their lifestyle, in which the individual's coping resources are simply overwhelmed by the extreme nature of the environment. For example, those accustomed to considerable autonomy and flexibility in lifestyle may find the confinements of physical limitations and institutional policy unbearable. The inability to decide when or how the most basic activities of daily living will be achieved is difficult at best for most people. For those who place high value on privacy and self-determination, such environmental constraints may stress an individual into violent behavior.

Suicide

In the case of suicide, cultural factors influence the violent behavior. In some premodernized cultures suicide is considered an honorable response to certain life circumstances, including advanced age, whereas in postindustrial cultures it is considered immoral or insane (Bromberg and Cassell, 1983). A more recent but related phenomenon is the assisted suicide of older adults who freely choose to terminate their lives through drugs. Major ethical controversy has emanated from this type of act.

Bereavement is considered an important contributor to suicidal behavior in the elderly. Two formulations are possible: (1) bereavement is a stressor that overwhelms the coping resources of the old person, resulting in self-injurious behavior, or (2) bereavement is a major threat to the individual's self, and the response is heightened aggressiveness in the form of extreme self-directed violence.

Assessment

Violence Toward Others

Assessment of the potentially violent and self-injurious person includes an inventory of coping resources and deficits. Sensory impairments should be noted, along with testing of cognitive abilities, including problem solving and judgment. The assessment should include inquiry into use of violence in the past as a means of solving problems. Recent losses and changes in the support network or living situation should be determined, along with the meaning of the change for the individual. Finally, recent changes in health and functional status should be determined because they may represent frustrations leading to aggressive behavior. Body image disturbance, resulting from stroke, amputation, or other sensory impairment, should also be assessed.

Adequacy of the individual's coping resources must be evaluated within the context of environmental demand. Does the environment allow freedom of movement for the individual? Is there respect for personal space and territory? Some theorists interpret aggressive behavior as a response to protect territory, which is difficult for older persons to claim in institutional environments or in another person's home. Are there resources within the environment to help the older person cope with recent losses in function or health status?

Although environmental and personal contributors to violent behavior are linked, identification of the major contributor aids in the development of interventions. For example, if the key contributor to violent behavior is loss of control over the immediate environment, attempts to further restrict the individual's choices by setting limits will only exacerbate the problem. If the problem is primarily one of inability to handle too many stimuli or too many choices, the intervention of choice is *not* giving the individual more choices, but simplifying the environment.

Suicide

Prediction of violence is more art than science. The one criterion generally accepted as predictive of violence is the history of previous violence. For suicidal elders this caveat must be interpreted with caution. A suicide gesture in an older person must be taken quite seriously because old people tend to make fewer gestures and to be more "successful" in their attempts than younger people (Osgood and Brant, 1991). However, this means that clinicians cannot wait for a suicide attempt before diagnosing a potential for self-directed violence: suicide in the elderly. Increasing attention is being paid to assessment of more subtle signs of hostility as useful predictors of violence (Yeasavage, 1983). The following factors have been associated with increased suicide risk and therefore should be included in the assessment of suicide potential: social isolation, presence of negative expectations (hopelessness), prior suicide attempts, depression, spousal loss, and family history of suicide (Osgood and Brant, 1991). In the elderly, unresolved bereavement should be added as a risk factor. Directly inquiring about suicidal ideation is indicated in depressed older clients as it is for younger adults.

Planning

Setting consistent limits on the violent behavior is a key planning issue when one is faced with a client with a potential for either self- or other-directed violence. For dependent elders, this involves achieving consensus among the caregivers about what behaviors will and will not be tolerated. It is also important to attempt to identify behaviors or signs for each individual that are predictive of violent episodes. Examples of predictors of violence toward others include increased agitation, increased confusion, and changes in routines. Sample predictors of increased likelihood of self-inflicted violence for some individuals include increased alcohol intake and decreased frequency of social interaction. If an episode of violence can be predicted, interventions may be applied that will avert an episode of violence.

Elder suicidal clients are encountered in many diverse settings. The gerontological nurse's professional responsibility is to intervene and if possible prevent precipitous acts of self-violence. However, this must be balanced with some regard for personal determination. For some elders, their final statement of dignity will be in the control of their death (Ebersole and Hess, 1994). In some instances, interventions with depressed elders may be applied to suicidal elders.

Interventions

Interventions with the potentially violent older person can be grouped into three categories:

- Environmental modifications
- Behavior modification
- Pharmacological interventions

Environmental Modifications

Environmental modifications are typically the most restrictive and are usually only short-term measures. This category includes hospitalization, seclusion, the use of restraints, and removal of potentially injurious agents from the patient. Environmental interventions are indicated for those at high risk of violence or suicide. For those with lower degrees of risk of suicide, the use of a psychiatric day hospital program for suicidal patients is a reasonable option. Busteed and Johnstone (1983) critically review the recommendations for suicide precautions in inpatient settings and note that the environmental control inherent in suicide precautions runs counter to many of the goals of psychotherapy, such as increasing patient control of behavior and reducing anxiety. Other environmental modifications used for violent patients include seclusion and restraint. The last two interventions, while sometimes necessary to prevent serious injury, address only the symptom and therefore should be used in conjunction with other interventions more likely to address the underlying etiology. Environmental interventions are insufficient if used alone; therefore, behavioral techniques should always be incorporated into a violence prevention program.

Behavior Modification

Behavioral interventions depend on the nature of the violent behavior. For those at risk of self-injurious behavior, contracting with the patient not to engage in the behavior for a specified period of time is considered effective in some cases. Additional strategies for intervention center on addressing the underlying contributors to the self-injurious behavior such as low self-esteem, depression, or ineffective individual coping. Haley (1983) advocates a self-management behavioral approach for those involved in violent behavior directed toward others. He describes a case example in which a self-management technique was used with a nursing home resident who had frequent angry outbursts directed at other residents and staff. The self-management technique included assertiveness training combined with progressive relaxation to help the resident cope with particularly stressful circumstances. Episodes of aggressive behavior were reduced by over one half, and the resident's antipsychotic medicine was reduced to an infrequent PRN dosage. The advantage of a self-management approach is that the emphasis is on increasing the individual's coping skills generally rather than focusing more narrowly on symptom extinction.

Pharmacological Interventions

Psychotropic drugs such as the major tranquilizers and the benzodiazepines are the main pharmacologic agents used in the treatment of violence in people of all ages. Their use with the elderly is associated with a variety of adverse side effects, including sedation, extrapyramidal side effects resulting in a parkinsonian syndrome, and anticholinergic side effects such as dry mouth, constipation, and orthostatic hypotension (Jenike, 1985a). The choice of drug and dose are highly individual matters. More recently, there have been reports of the effectiveness of propranolol (Inderal) in the treatment of aggressive behavior in demented elderly individuals (Jenike, 1985a), without any concomitant effect on memory, cognition, or confusion. Symptoms in these individuals were not controlled on neuroleptic agents.

The mechanism of propranolol's effect on violent or aggressive behavior is not known at present, although two hypotheses are currently advanced. Propranolol may act peripherally to diminish the body's responses to frustration, rage, and fear. The second hypothesis is that propranolol acts directly at the central level to interfere with the disinhibition of rage responses caused by the central nervous system lesions of the patient.

It should be emphasized that propranolol is not currently recommended by the FDA for use in treatment of behavioral disorders, although its use for behavioral disturbance related to organic brain pathology has been reported over 15 years. According to Jenike (1985b), this does not make such therapy illegal, but the therapy remains in the category of innovations in practice. Therapeutic effects are typically not noted for 10 days to 3 weeks on doses ranging from 60 to 320 mg per day.

Evaluation

Criteria for evaluation of violent behavior are not difficult to establish. The ultimate goal is to prevent injury without unduly restricting the client. Effectiveness of interventions can be measured by the number of violent or self-injurious episodes per unit of time and by the amount of medication or physical restraint required to achieve the pre-established goal.

REFERENCES

Abrams, W. and Berkow, R. *The Merck Manual of Geriatrics*. Rahway, N.J.: Merck and Company, Inc, 1990, pp. 1006–1009.

Ackley, B. and Ladwig, G. *Nursing Diagnosis Handbook: A Guide to Planning Care*. St. Louis: C. V. Mosby, 1993.

Anderson, C., Miller, R., Riger, A. et al. Behavioral and characterological attributional styles as predictors of depression and loneliness: Review, refinement, and test. *J Personal Sociol Psychol* 66(3):549–558, 1994.

Archbold, P. and Stewart, B. The PREP project: Development of interventions to be used by home health nurses with older people and their family caregivers. *Gerontologist* 31(11):281, 1991.

Austin, A. Becoming immune to loneliness: Helping the elderly fill a void. *J Gerontol Nurs* 15(9):25–28, 1989.

Averill, J., Catlin, G. and Chon, K. *Rules of Hope*. New York: Springer-Verlag, 1990.

Backman, L. and Larsson, M. Recall of organizable words and objects in adulthood: Influences of instructions, retention interval, and retrieval cues. *J Gerontol Psychol Sci* 47(4):273–278, 1992.

Barer, B. and Johnson, A. A critique of the caregiving literature. *Gerontologist* 30(1):26–29, 1990.

Barnett, K. A survey of the current utilization of touch by health team personnel with hospitalized patients. *Intl J Nurs Sci* 9:195–209, 1972.

Bateman, A., Broderick, D., Gleason, L. et al. Dysfunctional grieving. *J Psychosoc Nurs Mental Health Serv* 30(12):5–9, 1992.

Beck, A., Brown, G., Berchick, R. et al. Relationships between hopelessness and ultimate suicide: A replication with psychiatric outpatients. *Am J Psychiatry* 147(2):190–195, 1990.

Beck, A., Weissman, A., Lester, D. and Trexler, L. The measurement of pessimism: The Hopelessness Scale. *J Consult Clin Psychol* 42(6):861–865, 1974.

Beckett, N. Clinical nurses' characterizations of patient coping problems. *Nurs Diagn* 2(2):72–78, 1991.

Bennett, R. (ed.). *Aging, Isolation and Resocialization*. New York: Van Nostrand Reinhold, 1980.

Benson, D. *Nursing Meds*. Norwalk, CT: Appleton & Lange, 1990.

Birkett, D. *Psychiatry in the Nursing Home: Assessment, Evaluation and Intervention*. New York: Haworth Press, 1991.

Birren, J. and Schaie, K. *Handbook of the Psychology of Aging*. 3rd ed. San Diego: Academic Press, 1990.

Birren, J., Sloane, R. and Cohen G. (eds.). *Handbook of Mental Health and Aging*. 2nd ed. San Diego: Academic Press, 1992.

Blazer, D. Anxiety disorders. *In* Abrams, W. and Berkow, R. *The Merck Manual of Geriatrics*. Rahway, NJ: Merck and Company, Inc, 1990, pp. 1007–1009.

Blum, J.E. and Tross, S. Psychodynamic treatment of the elderly: A review of issues in theory and practice. *In* Eisdorfer, C. (ed.). *Annu Rev Gerontol Geriatr* 1:204–234, 1980.

Boettcher, E.G. Linking the aged to support systems. *J Gerontol Nurs* 11(3):27–33, 1985.

Brass, D. and Bowman, K. The transition from care-giving to bereavement: The relationship of caregiving strain and adjustment to death. *Gerontologist* 30(1):35–42, 1990.

Brock, A. Economics of aging. *In* Baines, E. (ed.). *Perspectives in Gerontological Nursing*. Newbury Park, CA: Sage Publications, 1991, pp. 170–184.

Brody, E. Parent care as a normative family stress. *Gerontologist* 25:19–29, 1985.

Bromberg, S. and Cassel, C.K. Suicide in the elderly: The limits of paternalism. *J Am Geriatr Soc* 31(11):698–703, 1983.

Buchner, D., Cress, M., Wagner, E. et al. The Seattle FICSIOT/Moveit Study: The effect of exercise on gait and balance in older adults. *J Am Geriatr Soc* 41:321–325, 1993.

Burnside, I. (ed.). *Psychosocial Nursing Care of the Aged*. New York: McGraw-Hill, 1980.

Burnside, I. *Working with the Elderly: Group Processes and Techniques*. 2nd ed. North Scituate, MA: Duxbury Press, 1983.

Burnside, I. *Working with the Elderly: Group Process and Techniques*. (2nd Ed.). Monterey, CA: Wadsworth Health Science, 1984.

Burnside I. Reminiscence: Program abstracts. *Gerontologist* (Spec. Issue)34:51, 1994.

Busteed, E.L. and Johnstone, C. The development of suicide precautions for an inpatient psychiatric unit. *J Psychiatr Nurs Ment Health Serv* 21(5):15–19, 1983.

Butler, R.N. Intensive psychotherapy for the hospitalized patient. *Geriatrics* 15:653–664, 1960.

Butler, R.N. Toward a psychiatry of the life-cycle: Implications of socio-psychologic studies of the aging process for the psychotherapeutic situation. *Psychiatr Res Rep* 23:233–248, 1968.

Carpenito, L. *Handbook of Nursing Diagnosis 1989–90*. Philadelphia: J. B. Lippincott, 1989.

Carpenito, L. *Nursing Diagnosis: Application to Clinical Practice*. 5th ed. Philadelphia: J.B. Lippincott, 1993.

Caserta, M. and Lund, D. Bereavement stress and coping among older adults: Expectations versus the actual experience. *Omega* 25(1):33–45, 1992.

Cleiren, M. *Bereavement and Adaptation: A Comparative Study of the Aftermath of Death*. Washington, D.C.: Hemisphere Publishing Corporation, 1993.

Cobe, G.M. The family of the aged: Issues in treatment. *Psychiatr Ann* 15:343–347, 1985.

Coffman, T. Relocation and survival of institutionalized aged: a re-examination of the evidence. *Gerontologist* 21:483–500, 1981.

Coffman, T. Relocation/relocation stress. *In* Maddox, G. et al. (eds.). *The Encyclopedia of Aging*. New York: Springer Publishing Company, 1987, pp. 563–564.

Cole, T. The aging spirit: agism and the journey of life in America. *Aging Today* 13(4):17, 1992.

Connidis, I.A. and Davies, L. Confidants and companions: Choices in later life. *J Gerontol Soc Sci* 47(3):S115–122, 1992.

Cox, C. Anger and hostility in the nursing home. *In* Harper, M. (ed.). *Management and Care of the Elderly: Psychosocial Perspectives*. Newbury Park, CA: Sage Publications, 1991, pp. 104–114.

Curry, L. and Stone, J. Moving on: Recovering from the death of a spouse. *Clin Nurse Special* 6(4):180–190, 1992.

Dalton, C. and Ranger, C. Integration of a nursing model into a local community service center. *Can Nurse* 89(3):37–40, 1993.

Devanand, D., Nobler, M., Singer, T. et al. Is dysthymia a different disorder in the elderly? *Am J Psychiatry* 151(11):1592–1599, 1994.

Di, M. Rx for spiritual distress. *RN* 54(3):22–24, 1991.

Doake, D. *Literacy Learning: A Revolution in Progress*. Bothell, WA: The Wright Group, 1991.

Dobson, H. and Culhane, M. Groupwork. *In* Jacoby, R. and Oppenheomer, C. *Psychiatry in the Elderly.* Oxford, United Kingdom: Oxford University Press, 1991.

Doenges, M.E. and Moorhouse, M.F. *Nurse's Pocket Guide: Nursing Diagnoses with Interventions.* Philadelphia: F.A. Davis, 1985.

Dugan, E. and Kivett, V. The importance of emotional and social isolation to loneliness among very old rural adults. *Gerontologist* 34(3):340–346, 1994.

Ebersole, P.P. Establishing reminiscing groups. *In* Burnside, I. (ed.). *Working with the Elderly: Group Process and Techniques.* 2nd ed. North Scituate, MA: Duxbury Press, 1984, pp. 236–254.

Ebersole, P. and Hess, P. *Toward Healthy Aging.* St. Louis: C. V. Mosby, 1994.

Ehrlich, P. *Mutual Help for Community Elderly: Mutual Help Model.* Carbondale, IL: Southern Illinois University, 1979.

Engels, M. The promotion of positive social interaction through social skills training. *In* Wisocki, P. (ed.). *Handbook of Clinical Behavior Therapy with the Elderly Client.* New York: Plenum Press, 1991, pp. 185–202.

Engle, V. Personal communique: Relocation stress. Grant funded by the National Institute for Nursing Research, Bethesda, MD, 1994.

Eppley, K., Abrams, A. and Shear J. Differential effects of relaxation techniques on trait anxiety: A meta-analysis. *J Clin Psychol* 45(6):957–974, 1989.

Erikson, E. *Identity and Life Cycle.* New York: Norton, 1980.

Ersek, M. The process of maintaining hope in adults undergoing bone marrow transplantation for leukemia. *Oncology Nursing Forum* 19(6):883–889, 1992.

Evans, L. Nursing care and management of behavioral problems in the elderly. *In* Harper, M. (ed.). *Management and Care of the Elderly: Psychosocial Perspectives.* Newbury Park, CA: Sage Publications, 1991, pp. 191–206.

Farran, C., Herth, K. and Popovich, J. *Hope and Hopelessness: Critical Clinical Constructs.* Thousand Oaks, CA: Sage Publications, 1995.

Fernandez, F., Levy, J., Lachar, B. and Small, G. The management of depression and anxiety in the elderly. *J Clin Psychiatry* 56(2):20–29, 1995.

Ferrell-Torry, A. and Glick, O. The use of therapeutic massage as a nursing intervention to modify anxiety and the perception of cancer pain. *Cancer Nursing* 16(2):93–101, 1993.

Flexner, J. The hospice movement in North America— Is it coming of age? *South Med J* 72:248–250, 1979.

Folkman, S. and Lazarus, R. *Manual for the Ways of Coping Questionnaire.* Palo Alto, CA: Consulting Psychologist Press, 1988.

Folstein, M., Folstein, S. and McHugh, P. Mini-mental state: A practical method for grading the cognitive state of patients for clinicians. *Psychiatr Res* 12:189–198, 1975.

Forbes, E. Spirituality, aging, and the community-dwelling caregiver and care recipient. *Geriatr Nurs* 15(6): 297–301, 1994.

Foxall, M. Health education of the older client. *In* Baines, E. (ed.). *Perspectives in Gerontological Nursing.* Newbury Park, CA: Sage Publications, 1991, pp. 107–125.

Freeman, C. and DiTomasso, A. Treatment Issues. *In* Wolman, G. and Stricker, G. (eds.). *Anxiety and Related Disorders: A Handbook.* New York: John Wiley & Sons, 1994.

Frey, D., Kelbley, T., Durham, L. and James, J. Enhancing the self-esteem of selected male nursing home residents. *Gerontologist* 32(4):552–557, 1992.

Fry, P., Slivinske, L. and Fitch, V. Power, control and well-being of the elderly: A critical reconstruction. *In* Fry, P. *Psychological Perspectives of Helplessness and Control in the Elderly.* New York: Elsevier Press, 1989, pp. 319–338.

Fuller, S. Inhibiting helplessness in elderly people. *J Gerontol Nurs* 4:18, 1978.

Fulmer, T. and Edelman, C. Adult day care. *In* Harper, M. (ed.). *Management and Care of the Elderly: Psychosocial Perspectives.* Newbury Park, CA: Sage Publications, 1991, pp. 269–292.

Gallagher, D. Caregivers of chronically ill elders. *In* Maddox, G. et al. (eds.). *The Encyclopedia of Aging.* New York: Springer Publishing Company, 1987, pp. 89–91.

Garrett, J. Multiple losses in older adults. *J Gerontol Nurs* 13(8):8–12, 1987.

George, L. Community and home care for mentally ill older adults. *In* Birren, J., Sloan, R. and Cohen, G. (eds.). *Handbook of Mental Health and Aging.* San Diego: Academic Press, 1992.

Glosser, G. and Wexler, D. Participant's evaluation of education/support groups for families of patients with Alzheimer's disease and other dementias. *Gerontologist* 25:232–236, 1985.

Haddon, W. and Baker, S. Injury control. *In* Clark, D. and MacMahon, B. (eds.). *Preventive Medicine.* 2nd ed. Boston: Little, Brown, 1981.

Hagestad, G. Family. *In* Maddox, G. et al. (eds.). *The Encyclopedia of Aging.* New York: Springer Publishing Company, 1987, pp. 247–249.

Haight, B. Psychological illness in aging. *In* Baines, E. (ed.). *Perspectives in Gerontological Nursing.* Newbury Park, CA: Sage Publications, Inc., 1991.

Hanes, C. and Wild, B. Locus of control and depression among noninstitutionalized elderly persons. *Psychol Rep* 41:581, 1977.

Harden, J. T. Psychosocial care. *In* Burggraf, V. and Stanley, M. (eds.). *Nursing the Elderly: A Care Plan Approach.* Philadelphia: J.B. Lippincott, 1989, pp. 369–393.

Harper, M. (ed.) (1991). *Management and Care of the Elderly: Psychosocial Perspectives.* Newbury Park, CA: Sage Publications, Inc., 1991.

Harvath, T., Archbold, P., Stewart, B. et al. Local and cosmopolitan knowledge: Establishing partnerships with family caregivers in caring for older persons. *J Gerontol Nurs* 20(2):29–35, 1994.

Hayward, M., Crimmins, E. and Wray, L. The relationship between retirement life cycles and older men's labor force participation rates. *J Gerontol Soc Sci* 49(5): S219–230, 1994.

Heidrich, S. and Ruff, C. How elderly women cope: Concerns and strategies. *Public Health Nurs* 9(3):200–208, 1992.

Hendricks, J. and Leedham, C. Creating psychological and societal dependency in old age. *In* Fry, P. *Psychological Perspectives of Helplessness and Control in the Elderly.* New York: Elsevier Press, 1989, pp. 369–394.

Herth, K. Development and refinement of an instrument to measure hope. *Scholarly Inquiry for Nursing Practice* 5(1):39–51, 1991.

High, D. A new myth about families of older people? *Gerontologist* 31(5):611–618, 1991.

Hill, R. and Mattessich, P. Family development theory and lifespan development. *In* Baltes, P. and Brown, R. (eds.). *Lifespan Development and Behavior.* Vol. 2. New York: Academic Press, 1979, pp. 161–204.

Himes, C. Future caregivers: Projected family structures of older persons. *J Gerontol* 47(1):S517–526, 1992.

Holmen, K., Ericsson, K., Anderson, L. and Winblad, B. ADL capacity and loneliness among elderly persons with cognitive impairment. *Scand J Primary Health Care* March 11(1):56–60, 1993.

Holzapfel, S.K. The importance of personal possessions in the lives of the institutionalized elderly. *J Gerontol Nurs* 8(3):156–158, 1982.

Holzapfel, S., Schoch, C., Dodman, J. and Grant, M. Responses of nursing home residents to instrainstitutional relocation. *Geriatr Nurs* 13(4):192–195, 1992.

Hong, L. and Duff, R. Widows in retirement communities: The social context of subjective well-being. *Gerontologist* 34(3):347–352, 1994.

Hultsch, D. and Dixon, R. Learning and memory in aging. *In* Birren, J. and Schaie, K. (eds.). *Handbook of the Psychology of Aging.* San Diego: Academic Press, 1990, pp. 258–274.

Jackson, J., Antonucci, T. and Gibson, R. Cultural, racial, and ethnic minority influences on aging. *In* Birren, J. and Schaie, K. (eds.). *Handbook of the Psychology of Aging.* San Diego: Academic Press, 1990.

Jalowiec, A., Murphy, S. and Powers, M. Psychometric assessment of the Jalowiec Coping Scale. *Nurs Res* 33: 157–161, 1984.

Jalowiec, A. and Powers, M. Stress and coping in hypertensive and emergency room patients. *Nurs Res* 30: 10–15, 1981.

Jenike, M.A. Treating the violent elderly patient with propranolol. *Geriatrics* 38:29–30, 1983.

Jenike, M. *Handbook of Geriatric Psychopharmacology.* Littleton, MA: PSG Publishing, 1985a.

Jenike, M.A. Propranolol as treatment for aggressive behavior in elderly brain-damaged patients. *Clin Gerontol* 3(3):36–39, 1985b.

Johnston, R. Orem's self-care model for nursing. *In* Fitzpatrick, J. and Whall, A. (eds.) *Conceptual Models of Nursing.* 2nd ed. Norwalk, CT: Appleton & Lange, 1989.

Jones, P. and Martinson, I. The experience of bereavement in caregivers of family members with Alzheimer's disease. *Image* 24(3):172–176, 1992.

Kapp, M. Health care decision making by the elderly: I get by with a little help from my family. *Gerontologist* 31(5):619–623, 1991.

Kari, N. and Michels, P. The Lazarus Project: The politics of empowerment. *Am J Occup Ther* 45(8):719–725, 1991.

Kausler, D. *Experimental Psychology, Cognition, and Human Aging.* 2nd ed. New York: Springer-Verlag, 1991.

Kerr, M., Hoskins, L., Fitzpatrick, J. et al. From taxonomy I to taxonomy II. *Nurs Diagn* 2(3):131–136, 1991.

Kielhofner, G. The human being in an open system. *In* Kielhofner, G. (ed.). *A Model of Human Occupation: Theory and Application.* Baltimore: Williams & Wilkins, 1985.

Kim, M., McFarland, G. and McLane, A. *Pocket Guide to Nursing Diagnoses.* St. Louis: C.V. Mosby, 1993.

Kinney, J. and Stephens, M. Hassles and uplifts of giving care to a family member with dementia. *Psychol Aging* 4:402–408, 1989.

Kosidlak, J.G. Self-help for senior citizens. *J Gerontol Nurs* 6(11):663–668, 1980.

Kosloski, K. and Montgomery, R. The impact of respite use on nursing home placement. *The Gerontologist* 35(1):67–73, 1995.

Krynski, M., Tymchuk, A. and Ouslander, J. How informed can consent be? New light on comprehension among elderly people making decisions about enteral tube feeding. *Gerontologist* 34(1):36–43, 1994.

Kubler-Ross, E. *On Death and Dying.* New York: Macmillan, 1969.

Lanza M.L. Origins of aggression. *J Psychsoc Ment Health Nurs* 21(6):11–16, 1983.

Lappe, J.M. Reminiscing: The life review therapy. *J Gerontol Nurs* 13(4):12–16, 1987.

Lawton, M., Powell, J., Brody, E. and Saperstein, A. A controlled study of respite service for caregivers of Alzheimer's patients. *Gerontologist* 29:8–15, 1989.

Lawton, M., Powell, J., Rajagopal, D. et al. The dynamics of caregiving for a demented elder among black

and white families. *J Gerontol Soc Sci* 47(4):S156–164, 1992.

Lazarus, R. Coping theory and research: Past, present and future. *Psychosom Med* 55(3):234–247, 1993.

Lazarus, R. and Folkman, S. *Stress, Appraisal and Coping.* New York: Springer Publishing Company, 1984.

Levin, J. and Markides, K. Religious attendance and subjective health. *J Sci Study Relig* 25:31–40, 1986.

Levin, J., Taylor, J. and Chatters, L. Race and gender differences in religiosity among older adults: Findings from four national surveys. *J Gerontol Soc Sci* 49(3): S137–S145, 1994.

Lillis, P. and Prophit, P. Keeping hope alive. *Nursing 1991,* pp. 65–66, 1991.

MacDonald, M.L. Environmental programming for the socially isolated aging. *Gerontologist* 18(4):350–354, 1978.

Markides, K.S. Aging, religiosity and adjustment. *J Gerontol* 38(5):621–625, 1983.

Markides, K. Religion. In Maddox, G. (ed.). *The Encyclopedia of Aging.* New York: Springer, 1987.

McCrae, R.R. Stress and stressors. *In* Maddox, G.L. (ed.). *The Encyclopedia of Aging.* New York: Springer Publishing Company, 1987, pp. 649–650.

McCubbin, H., Larsen, A. and Olson, D. Family crisis oriented personal evaluation scales (F-COPES). *In* Olson, D. H. (ed.). *Family Inventories.* St. Paul: University of Minnesota Press, 1985.

McCullough, P. Evaluation and management of anxiety in the older adult. *Geriatrics* 47(4):35–38, 1992.

McDougall, G. A review of screening instruments for assessing cognition and mental status in older adults. *Nurse Practit* 15:11, 1990.

McFarland, G. and McFarlane, E. *Nursing Diagnosis and Intervention.* 2nd ed. St. Louis: C.V. Mosby, 1993.

McFarland, G.K. and Naschinski, C.E. Validation of nursing diagnoses labels for psychiatric mental health nursing practice. *In* McLane, A.M. (ed.). *Classification of Nursing Diagnoses.* Proceedings of the Seventh Conference. St. Louis: C.V. Mosby, 1987, pp. 174–181.

McLane, A. (ed.). *Classification of Nursing Diagnoses: Proceedings of the Seventh National Conference.* St. Louis: C.V. Mosby, 1987.

Miller C. *Nursing Care of Older Adults.* Glenview, IL: Scott, Foresman/Little, Brown Higher Education, 1990.

Miller, J. *Powerlessness: Coping with Chronic Illness.* Philadelphia: F.A. Davis, 1983.

Miller, J. and Oertel, C.B. Powerlessness in the elderly: Preventing hopelessness. *In* Miller, J. ed.: *Chronic Illness: Overcoming Powerlessness.* Philadelphia: F.A. Davis, 1983, pp. 109–132.

Moberg, D. Church membership and personal adjustment in old age. *J Gerontol* 8:207–211, 1953.

Moberg, D.O. Religion and the aging family. *Family Coordinator* 21:47–60, 1972.

Moberg, D. *The Church as a Social Institution.* Grand Rapids, MI: Baker Book House, 1984.

Moberg, D. Religion and aging. *In* Ferraro, K. (ed.). *Gerontology: Perspective and Issues.* New York: Springer Publishing Company, 1990.

Montgomery, R. and Kosloski, K. A longitudinal analysis of nursing home placement for dependent elders cared for by spouses vs. adult children. *J Gerontol Soc Sci* 49(2):S62–74, 1994.

Mui, A. Caregiver strain among black and white daughter caregivers: A role theory perspective. *Gerontologist* 32(2):203–212, 1992.

Mulrow, C., Gerety, M., Kanten, D. et al. Effects of physical therapy on functional status of nursing home residents. *J Am Geriatr Soc* 41:326–328, 1993.

National Hospice Organization: Standards of a Hospice Program. Arlington, VA: National Hospice Organization, 1993.

Norris, J. Nursing interventions for self-esteem disturbances. *Nurs Diagn* 3(2):48–53, 1992.

Norris, J. and Kunes-Connell, M. Self esteem disturbance: A clinical validation study. *In* McLane, A. (ed.). *Classification of Nursing Diagnoses.* St. Louis, C.V. Mosby, 1987.

Norris, J. and Kunes-Connell, M. A multimodal approach to validation and refinement of an existing nursing diagnosis. *Arch Psychiatr Nurs* 2(2):103–109, 1988.

North American Nursing Diagnosis Association. *NANDA Nursing Diagnoses; Definitions and Classification 1995–1996.* Philadelphia: North American Nursing Diagnosis Association, 1994.

Nystrom, A. and Segesten, K. On sources of powerlessness in nursing home life. *J Adv Nurs* 19(1):124–133, 1994.

Olson, D., Fournier, D. and Druckman, J. ENRICH Family Communication Scale. *In* Olson, D. H. (ed.). *Family Inventories.* St. Paul: University of Minnesota Press, 1985.

Orem, D. *Nursing: Concepts of Practice.* 3rd ed. New York: McGraw-Hill, 1985.

Orth, R. Restorative dining promotes independence, self-esteem. *Provider,* Dec. 1991, p. 33.

Osgood, N. and Brant, B. Suicide among the elderly in institutional and community settings. *In* Harper, M. (ed.). *Management and Care of the Elderly: Psychosocial Perspectives.* Newbury Park, CA: Sage Publications, 1991, p. 218–224.

Osterweis, M., Solomon, F. and Green, M. *Bereavement: Reactions, Consequences, and Care.* Washington, D.C.: National Academy Press, 1984.

Pallet, P. A conceptual framework for studying family caregiver burden in Alzheimer's type dementia. *Image* 22(1):52–58, 1990.

Paloutzian, R. and Ellison, C. Loneliness, spiritual well-being, and the quality of life. *In* Peplau, A. and Perlman, D. (eds.). *Loneliness: A Source Book of Current Theory, Research, and Therapy.* New York: John Wiley and Sons, 1982.

Parkes, C.M. Bereavement. *Br J Psychiatry* 146:11–17, 1985.

Petruzzello, S., Landers, D., Hatfield, B. et al. Meta-analysis on the anxiety-reducing effects of acute and chronic exercise. *Sports Med* 11(3):143–182, 1991.

Pillemer, K. and Suitor, J. Violence and violent feelings: What causes them among family caregivers? *J Gerontol Soc Sci* 47(4):S165–172, 1992.

Potter, P. and Perry, A. *Fundamentals of Nursing: Concepts, Process, and Practice.* St. Louis: Mosby–Year Book, 1993.

Rank, O. *The Trauma of Birth.* New York: Harcourt Brace, 1929.

Regier, D., Boyd J., Burke J., Jr. et al. One-month prevalence of mental disorders in the U.S. *Arch. Gen. Psychiatry* 45:977–986, 1988.

Rickard, H., Scoggin, F. and Keith, S. One-year follow-up of relaxation training for elders with subjective anxiety. *Gerontologist* 34(1):121–122, 1994.

Rocket, C. Acquired immunodeficiency syndrome and the older adult: Program abstracts. *Gerontologist* (Spec. Issue)34:51, 1994.

Rosswurn, M. Relocation and the elderly. *J Gerontol Nurs* 9:632–637, 1983.

Roy, S. and Corliss, C. The Roy Adaptation Model: Theoretical update and knowledge for practice. *NLN Publication* Aug 15-2548:215–229, 1993.

Rozovsky, F. *Consent to Treat: A Practical Guide.* 2nd ed. Boston: Little, Brown, 1990.

Rubenstein, R. The home environments of older people: A description of the psychosocial processes linking person to place. *J Gerontol* 44(2):545–553, 1989.

Rybarczyk, B. and Auerbach, S. Reminiscence interviews as stress management interventions for older patients undergoing surgery. *Gerontologist* 30(4):522–528, 1990.

Schultz, N. Anxiety. *In* Maddox, G. et al. (eds.). *The Encyclopedia of Aging.* New York: Springer Publishing Company, 1987, pp. 563–564.

Schwartz, A. and Vogel, M. Nursing home staff and residents' families' role expectations. *Gerontologist* 30(1):49–53, 1990.

Seligman, M. *Helplessness: On Depression, Development, and Death.* San Francisco: Freeman and Company, 1975.

Selye, H. *The Stress of Life.* 2nd ed. New York: McGraw-Hill, 1976.

Siegler, E. and Rudden, A. Patient education: Resources to recommend to elders and their families. *Geriatrics* 47(4):73–78, 1992.

Skipwith, D. Nursing care in acute and long-term care settings. *In* Harper, M. (ed.). *Management and Care of the Elderly: Psychosocial Perspectives.* Newbury Park, CA: Sage Publications, 1991, pp. 218–224.

Smith, A., Park, D., Cherry, K. and Berkovsky, K. Age differences in memory for concrete and abstract pictures. *J Gerontol Psychol Sci* 45:P205–P209, 1990.

Spearman, S., Duldt, B. and Brown, S. Research testing theory: A selective review of Orem's self-care theory. *J Adv Nurs* 18(10):1626–1631, 1993.

Spielberger, C., Gorsuch, R. and Lushene, R. *State-Trait Anxiety Inventory.* Palo Alto, CA: Consulting Psychologists Press, 1970.

Stepnick, A. and Perry, T. Preventing spiritual distress in the dying client. *J Psychosoc Nurs Mental Health Serv* 30(1):17–24, 1992.

Stetter, F., Walter, G., Zimmermann, A. et al. Ambulatory short-term therapy of anxiety patients with autogenic training and hypnosis. *Psychother Psychosom Med Psychol* 44(7):226–234, 1994.

Stevens-Ratchford, R. The effect of life review activities on depression and self-esteem in older adults. *Am J Occup Ther* 47(5):413–420, 1993.

Stone, R., Cafferata, M. and Sangl, J. Caregivers of the frail elderly: A national profile. *Gerontologist* 27:616–626, 1987.

Sullivan, H.S. *The Interpersonal Theory of Psychiatry.* New York: Norton, 1953.

Szinovacz, M. and Harpster, P. Couple's employment/retirement status and the division of household tasks. *J Gerontol Soc Sci* 49(3):S125–136, 1994.

Taylor, J. and Chatters, L. Nonorganizational religious participation among elderly Black adults. *J Gerontol Soc Sci* 46(3):S103–S111, 1991.

Temple, A. and Fawdry, K. King's theory of goal attainment: Resolving filial caregiver role strain. *J Gerontol Nurs* 18(3):11–15, 1992.

Theis, S. Using previous knowledge to teach elderly clients. *J Gerontol Nurs* 17(8):34–38, 1991.

Thompson, P. I don't feel old. *Ageing and Society* 12:23–48, 1992.

Todd, B. Disabling anxiety. *Geriatr Nurs* May-June, 1989, pp. 152–156.

Tomm, K. and Saunders, G. Family assessment in a problem-oriented record. *In* Hansen, J.C. and Keeney, B.F. (eds.). *Diagnosis and Assessment in Family Therapy.* Rockville, MD: Aspen Systems Corporation, 1983, pp. 101–122.

Tueth, M. Anxiety in the older patient: Differential diagnosis and treatment. *Geriatrics* 48(2):51–54, 1993.

Turnbull, J. Anxiety and physical illness in the elderly. *J Clin Psychiatry* 50(Suppl.):40–45, 1989.

Vaillot, M.C. Living and dying. Part 1: Hope, the restoration of being. *Am J Nurs* 70:268–273, 1970.

Vanelle, J. and Feline, A. Drug discontinuation in depression. *Encephale* (Spec. No. 1):223–229, 1994.

Vinick, B. and Ekerdt. The transition to retirement: Responses of husbands and wives. *In* Hess B. and Markson, E. (eds.). *Growing Old in America.* 4th ed. New Brunswick, NJ: Transaction Books, 1991.

Visscher, E. and Clore, E. The genogram: A strategy for assessment. *J Pediatr Health Care* 6(6):361–367, 1992.

Watson, M. Bereavement in the elderly. *AORN J* 59(5): 1079–1080, 1083–1084, 1994.

Webster's Ninth New Collegiate Dictionary. Springfield, MA: Merriam-Webster, Inc., 1990.

Weiss, R. Reflections on the present state of loneliness research. *In* Hojat, M. and Crandall, R. (eds.). *Loneliness: Theory, Research and Applications.* Newbury Park, CA: Sage Publications, 1989, pp. 1–16.

Werner-Beland, J.A. (ed.). *Grief Responses to Long-Term Illness and Disability.* Reston, VA: Reston Publishing Company (Prentice-Hall), 1980.

Wolman, G. and Stricker, G. *Anxiety and Related Disorders: A Handbook.* New York: John Wiley & Sons, 1994.

White, B. and Roberts, S. Powerlessness and the pulmonary alveolar edema patient. *Dimensions Crit Care Nurs* 12(3):127–137, 1993.

White, N., Richter, J. and Fry, C. Coping, social support and adaptation to chronic illness. *West J Nurs Res* 14(2):211–224, 1992.

Wright, L.M. and Leahey, L.M. *Nurses and Families: A Guide to Family Assessment and Intervention.* 2nd ed. Philadelphia: F.A. Davis, 1994.

Yeasavage, J.A. Relationships between measures of direct and indirect hostility and self-destructive behavior by hospitalized schizophrenics. *Br J Psychiatry* 143:173–176, 1983.

Zahourek, R.P. (ed.). *Clinical Hypnosis and Therapeutic Suggestion in Nursing.* New York: Grune & Stratton, 1985.

Ziegler, M. and Reid, D. Correlates of locus of desired control in two samples of elderly persons: Community residents and hospitalized elderly patients. *J Consult Clin Psychol* 47:977, 1979.

The
Clinical
Sciences

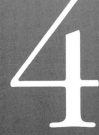

4

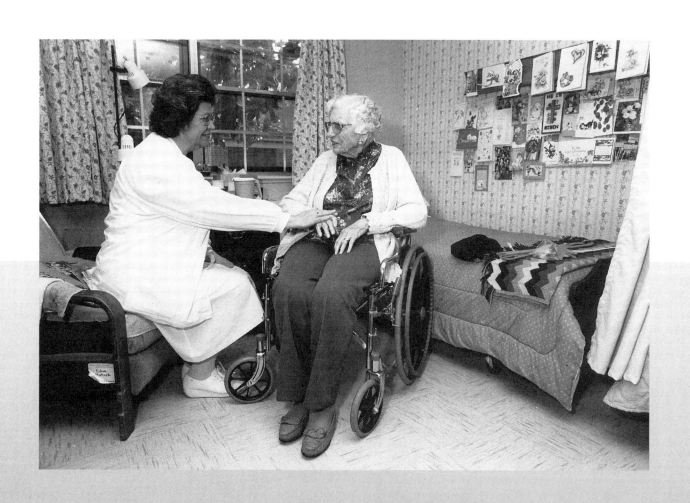

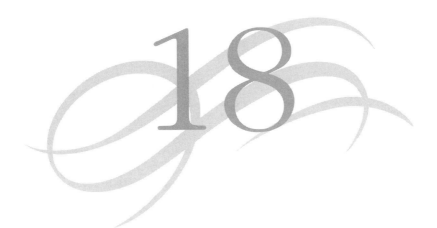

Pharmacological Considerations

ELEANOR S. McCONNELL
ADRIANNE DILL LINTON
JOSEPH T. HANLON

OBJECTIVES

Discuss sociocultural factors that affect drug responses in elderly clients and describe their impact on nursing care.

❖

List and describe age-related changes in pharmacokinetics and pharmacodynamics.

❖

Analyze the common adverse drug reactions in older persons, including confusion, falls, incontinence, and immobility.

❖

Conduct a drug assessment with an older client.

❖

Develop a plan of care and demonstrate interventions for administration of medications for an older client.

Drugs are potent therapeutic agents with the potential to cause great harm in elderly people as well as alleviate symptoms and cure disease. Nurses have tremendous opportunities through assessment, monitoring, teaching, and evaluation to intervene so that maximum benefit and minimal harm come to the older client undergoing drug therapy.

An understanding of the psychological and social influences on drug utilization, age-related changes in pharmacokinetics and pharmacodynamics, and the potential for drug-related health problems such as adverse drug reactions and drug withdrawal syndromes should guide nurses' approaches to care of the elderly patient receiving pharmaceutical agents.

SOCIOCULTURAL INFLUENCES ON DRUG RESPONSES OF OLDER PERSONS

Sociocultural factors and the health status of the older person contribute to altered drug responses.

Sociocultural Factors

Individual Values

The older person's response to drugs is influenced by the individual's value system. Today's older population has witnessed first hand the transformation of medical care through the miracles of modern pharmacotherapy, including the development of such effective drugs as antibiotics, insulin, antihypertensive agents, and psychotropic medications. It is not surprising that many of these individuals expect to receive "a pill for every ill." Unfortunately, health care practitioners sometimes support this belief by substituting medications for time in dealing with a patient's problems. Although this practice may lead to greater problems for the patient later on, it is nonetheless widespread. According to National Center for Health Sciences statistics, internists and general practitioners are more likely to spend less time with their elderly patients than with their younger patients and are more likely to prescribe medication for elderly patients than for younger patients. Nurses sometimes seek sedation for patients rather than taking the time to understand the underlying cause of the agitation or behavior problem.

Health Care System Influences on Drug Utilization

Many aspects of the health care system reinforce the tendency to use drugs as the first line of therapy for diseases, which can lead to suboptimal utilization of drugs. How drugs are marketed, emphasis on technological rather than human solutions to the problems associated with chronic disease, and ageism all affect drug utilization in the aged.

DRUG MARKETING. Drugs are developed in a market-oriented environment. Kessler (1991) reports estimates that drug companies spend 5 billion dollars annually on marketing and advertising. Profit is an important incentive in drug marketing. Regardless of the health care setting, drugs are featured prominently. In clinics, nursing homes, and hospitals, drug advertising is subtle but ever present. Basic tools like rulers, tape measures, pens, and note pads are emblazoned with names of drugs. In the home, television, radio, and print media all contain over-the-counter drug advertisements of various descriptions. Many of the drugs advertised are designed to treat ailments common in older persons, such as constipation, pain, and insomnia. Laxatives, analgesics, sleep aids, and cold preparations are often taken without the knowledge of the individual's health care provider, and they are not benign agents. Significant problems for older persons may develop due to interactions with other drugs and age-related physiological changes that predispose to adverse drug reactions.

The multiple names given to the same drug produced by different companies add to the dilemma. A classic example of the harm this may cause is the individual who comes to the clinic complaining of "ringing ears." Her drug history reveals that she takes Bufferin, Anacin, B.C. powders, and Pepto-Bismol for indigestion. The individual has unwittingly become the victim of salicylate intoxication, without ever having taken an "aspirin."

For professionals, drug advertising is even more pervasive. Few professional journals could exist without pharmaceutical advertising. Many professional meetings and continuing education offerings are in part (or in whole) underwritten by the pharmaceutical industry. Although no coercion is involved, the degree of oversimplification expressed in some drug advertisements borders on the unethical. For example, one laxative advertisement chides the professionals for "complicating a simple problem." The solution suggested is a saline cathartic, which has the potential for inducing fluid and electrolyte imbalance, not to mention laxative dependency, in older persons.

TECHNOLOGICAL VERSUS HUMAN RESPONSES TO CHRONIC DISEASE. American society values technological solutions to problems over more mundane remedies that may involve greater expenditures of time. Note the proliferation of weight reduction plans to which people willingly subscribe that remove any recognizable foodstuff from the plan. Similarly, prescriptions for lifestyle change, counselling, or exercise regimens are seldom as well received as plans for elaborate diagnostic studies or prescriptions. Indeed, some patients feel slighted if they leave the physician's or nurse practitioner's office *without* a prescription.

AGEISM. Ageism on the part of health care providers may also contribute to the overprescription of drugs to the elderly. This concern is not new. In 1980, Besdine noted that older persons "often bear the brunt of reflexive prescribing for uninvestigated symptoms." He noted that the average older American filled 13 prescriptions per year and took three times the number of drugs as the average younger American. More recent studies continue to reflect a high rate of prescribing for the elderly.

Impact on Care of the Elderly

Old people are more likely to receive a prescription from an outpatient visit to a physician than any other age group, yet the

TABLE 18 – 1
Drugs Most Commonly Prescribed for Elderly People

Cardiovascular drugs, including diuretics
Analgesics
Gastrointestinal agents
Nutritional supplements
Endocrine/metabolic drugs

length of an office visit with older people is *less* than that of any other age group. The result is less time spent in patient education about drugs in a population that requires more time to learn new information.

In the United States, where only 12 per cent of the population is over age 65 years, older people are reported to consume 30 to 32 per cent of all prescription drugs and to take two to three times as many drugs as younger people (Bressler and Katz, 1993; Baum et al., 1988; Michocki et al., 1993). The categories of drugs most commonly prescribed for the elderly are listed in Table 18–1. Bressler and Katz (1993) also found that 40 per cent of physician office visits by older people resulted in at least two prescriptions. Delafuente and colleagues (1992) caution that the interpretation of statistics on prescription drug use may be clouded by mixing data from subjects without regard to health status. Among a probability-based sample of over 2000 community-dwelling older adults, Hanlon and colleagues (1992) found a mean prescription drug rate of 2.23 per person and over-the-counter use of 1.31 drugs per person. A study of 2800 community-dwelling elderly Australians revealed that 18 per cent of the women and 25 per cent of the men were taking three or more prescription drugs. Also, 29 per cent of the men and 44 per cent of the women in that study took two or more nonprescription drugs (Simons et al., 1992).

Few studies report the number of medicines used in hospitalized older adults; however, several investigators have reported the average number of medicines used as between four to five per day. More importantly, as many as 75 per cent of older patients have one or more medicines discontinued and new ones started during a hospital stay.

The widespread use of drugs in the elderly along with their enhanced vulnerability to the adverse effects of drug treatment provides a strong rationale for gerontological nurses to study drug utilization patterns, drug handling, and potential for adverse effects in the elderly. Such knowledge should enhance the gerontological nurse's ability to help prevent adverse drug reactions, or assist in their early identification. Moreover, nurses can play an important role in optimizing drug therapy.

AGE-RELATED CHANGES IN DRUG PHARMACOKINETICS AND PHARMACODYNAMICS

An understanding of drug pharmacokinetics and pharmacodynamics is necessary to obtain the desired therapeutic efficacy and avoid drug-related problems. This is particularly important to consider for elderly patients since it is often difficult to discriminate whether observed changes are due to age alone or to chronic diseases that elderly people are more likely to have.

Altered Pharmacokinetics

Pharmacokinetics can be defined as the study of drug absorption, distribution, metabolism, and elimination. The following summarizes what is known about *how aging affects* each of the four major components of pharmacokinetics (Dawling and Crome, 1989; Montamat et al., 1989; Bennett, 1990; Woodhouse and Wynne, 1992).

Absorption

Although a number of age-related changes in gastrointestinal physiology, such as increased gastric pH and decreased gastric emptying, could potentially affect the absorption of medications, they appear to have little influence since most medications are absorbed via passive diffusion (Dawling and Crome, 1989; Montamat et al., 1989). However, the bioavailability of drugs such as propranolol and morphine that undergo extensive first-pass metabolism appears to be increased, leading to higher plasma concentrations. The absorption of certain nutrients such as calcium that require active transport and an acidic pH may be reduced in elderly people as well.

Distribution

The distribution of medications in the body depends on factors such as blood flow, plasma protein binding, and body composition. The relative decrease in body water and lean body weight with an accompanying increase in fat body weight that is seen with aging can alter drug distribution. The volume of distribution, defined as the apparent volume into which a drug distributes in

the body at equilibrium (Rowland and Tozer, 1995), of water-soluble drugs such as ethanol is decreased. Lipophilic drugs such as diazepam exhibit an increased volume of distribution. Changes in the volume of distribution of medications can have a direct impact on the half-life of medications and the amount of medication needed as a loading dose.

The two major plasma proteins that medications can bind to are albumin and alpha-1-acid glycoprotein. There is conflicting evidence as to whether the slight decrease in serum albumin is due to age alone or due to chronic diseases. For acidic drugs such as naproxen, phenytoin, tolbutamide, and warfarin, decreased serum albumin may lead to an increased free fraction of the drug. There is some evidence that alpha-1-acid glycoprotein levels increase with age as well as with certain conditions such as rheumatoid arthritis, myocardial infarction, and certain malignancies. This may lead to a decreased free fraction of basic medications such as lidocaine, propranolol, quinidine, and imipramine. While the clinical effects of these potential changes may be unclear, they are important to consider when interpreting serum drug levels since generally only total concentrations (i.e., free and bound drug) are reported.

A good example of a drug that is affected by hypoalbuminemia is phenytoin. If an individual has decreased serum albumin, the patient's total concentration is likely to be reduced, yet the free fraction of phenytoin (and hence, the pharmacological effect) is increased because of decreased binding, since unbound drug is responsible for pharmacological effects.

Metabolism

The liver is the major organ responsible for drug metabolism. Hepatic metabolism can be divided into either phase I, or preparative reactions, which include oxidation and reductive and hydrolytic biotransformations, or phase II, conjugative reactions, which include glucuronidation, sulfation, and acetylation biotransformations. Previously, it was thought that elderly people may have decreased enzymatic activity, but recently changes in metabolism have been attributed to reduced liver volume and thus a reduced amount of enzymes (Woodhouse and Wynne, 1992). The clearance of antipyrine, a marker of oxidative metabolism, decreases with increasing age. This decrease is more marked in men than women and may be selective for *N*-demethylation oxidative pathways. Decreased metabolism and clearance with associated increased half-life has been reported for medications such as diazepam, piroxicam, theophylline, and quinidine. Medications such as oxazepam that undergo phase II glucuronidation appear not to be as affected by age. Age-related decreases in liver blood flow can also significantly decrease the metabolism of high-hepatic-extraction ratio drugs, such as imipramine, lidocaine, and propranolol. Moreover, a number of confounding factors, including frailty, smoking, diet, and drug interactions, can significantly affect hepatic metabolism. For example, theophylline metabolism is increased by smoking and phenytoin, whereas cimetidine decreases theophylline metabolism (Vestal et al., 1993).

Elimination

Renal excretion is the primary route of elimination for many drugs. Age-related reductions in renal blood flow and glomerular filtration can significantly impair the excretion of water-soluble drugs. It should be noted, however, that as many as a third of "normal" elderly subjects in one study had no decrease in renal function as measured by creatinine clearance (Bennett, 1990). The estimation of creatinine clearance by using equations, although not entirely accurate in all patients, can serve as a useful screening approximation. One of the most commonly used equations, created by Cockcroft and Gault (1976), is

Creatinine clearance
(Men)

$$= \frac{(140 - age)\ (lean\ body\ weight\ in\ kg)}{(72)\ (serum\ creatinine)}$$

For women the result is multiplied by 0.85.

The doses of medications that are primarily renally excreted, such as acetazolamide, amantadine, aminoglycosides, atenolol, cimetidine, digoxin, lithium, and vancomycin, generally should be reduced to compensate for their decreased clearance. It is important to note that some hepatically metabolized medications can yield active metabolites that are primarily excreted renally and need to be taken into account when designing dosage regimens. For example, a procainamide metabolite is N-acetylprocainamide, meperidine yields normeperidine, and morphine sulfate yields morphine-6-glucuronide.

Altered Pharmacodynamics

Drug pharmacodynamics, defined in the broadest sense, is the effect that medications have on the body. A narrower definition is the pharmacological effect that results from a drug interacting with receptors at the site of action. There is some evidence in elderly people of enhanced drug response, or "sensitivity." This may be due to changes in receptor numbers or affinity, or to postreceptor alterations or age-related impairment of homeostatic mechanisms (Swift, 1990).

One of the best-studied therapeutic drug classes are the benzodiazepines. Evidence from epidemiological and experimental studies suggests that, independent of pharmacokinetic alterations, elderly people are more sensitive to the central nervous system effects of benzodiazepines (Roberts and Turner, 1988; Swift, 1990). This may contribute to an increased risk of falls, hip fractures, incontinence, and cognitive impairment in older persons. There is also evidence that elderly people have a greater analgesic response to narcotics when compared with their younger counterparts (Roberts and Turner, 1988; Swift, 1990). Older people may have enhanced response to anticoagulants, such as warfarin, and heparin and thrombolytic agents (Roberts and Turner, 1988; Swift, 1990). Knowledge of these and other medications that demonstrate enhanced pharmacodynamic sensitivity can allow clinicians and patients to use these drugs safely by making the appropriate adjustments in dosage.

There is also evidence that certain drugs, including beta-blockers and beta-agonists, exhibit decreased pharmacodynamic sensitivity. Another example of altered response in elderly people is the absence of reflex tachycardia, which is commonly seen with vasodilators in younger people. It is possible that this is due to dampened baroreceptor response.

It is important to consider that some drugs simultaneously demonstrate both enhanced and decreased sensitivity. For example, with calcium channel blockers, enhanced sensitivity is demonstrated by greater reduction in blood pressure, and decreased sensitivity is demonstrated by reduced AV node blockade. Because drugs can also simultaneously show alterations in drug pharmacokinetics, it is prudent for the clinician not to consider alterations in isolation.

DRUG-RELATED PROBLEMS: ADVERSE DRUG REACTIONS

Although drug therapy can be beneficial for elderly people, the potential for drug-related problems also exists. These problems

T A B L E   1 8 – 2
Common Medications That Cause Adverse Drug Reactions in Elderly People

POPULATION	COMMON DRUGS OR DRUG CLASSES IN DECREASING RANK ORDER
U.S. population	Antidepressants, antilipemics, antineoplastics, gastrointestinal, hypotensives
Community dwelling	Aspirin, ibuprofen, digoxin, propranolol, prednisone
Community dwelling to hospital	Beta blockers, corticosteroids, digoxin, thiazide diuretics, nonsteroidal anti-inflammatory drugs
Hospital	Furosemide, nifedipine, nitroglycerin, ampicillin, captopril
Nursing home	Cardiac, central nervous system, analgesics, gastrointestinal

Modified from Hanlon, J.T., Schmader, K. and Lewis, I. Adverse drug reactions. *In* Delafuente, J.C. and Stewart, R.B. (eds.). *Therapeutics in the Elderly.* 2nd ed. Cincinnati: Whitney Books, 1995, p. 215.

include adverse drug reactions (ADRs) and triggering or exacerbation of common geriatric syndromes such as cognitive impairment, falls, dysmobility, and incontinence. The epidemiology of ADRs follows, along with a discussion of predisposing factors.

Epidemiology

A well-accepted definition of ADRs is "any response to a drug that is noxious and unintended and that occurs in doses in man for prophylaxis, diagnosis, or therapy, excluding failure to accomplish the intended purpose" (Karch and Lasagna, 1975). ADRs can be further classified as either type A or type B reactions (Rawlins, 1981). Type A, or "augmented" reactions, the most common type, are predictable, dose-dependent and an exaggeration of the expected pharmacological effect of a drug. Type B, or "bizarre," reactions are idiosyncratic or due to allergic reactions, are not predictable, and are associated with low morbidity but high mortality.

Several investigators have reviewed the epidemiology of ADRs (Jue, 1984; Editorial in *Lancet*, 1988; Nolan and O'Malley, 1988; Stewart, 1988; Manasse, 1989; Brawn and Castleden, 1990; Denham, 1990). An overview of reports of ADRs in various settings of care follows.

Hospitalization is a serious consequence of drug therapy. The prevalence of ADRs leading to hospitalization in studies of ambulatory elderly people ranges from 3 to 16.8 per cent (Hanlon et al., 1993). Few investigations of ADRs in older adults in outpatient settings have been reported. The prevalence rates found in existing studies vary considerably (2.5 to 50.6 per cent) owing to different methods of ascertainment and different-

ences in study design. A study by Koronkowski and colleagues (1993) examined the prevalence of adverse drug events (ADEs) in a group of 167 ambulatory elderly people who were taking five or more medications. Thirty-five per cent of these subjects reported an ADR in the previous year. Studies of ADRs in the nursing home setting have revealed a prevalence of from 9.5 to 50.2 per cent (Hanlon et al., 1993). In contrast, many studies have been published on the prevalence of ADRs in hospitalized elderly people, in which the prevalence varies widely, ranging from 1.5 to 44 per cent (Nolan and O'Malley, 1988). Collectively, the studies document that ADRs are a common phenomenon in elderly people regardless of the setting of care. Table 18–2 presents the most common drugs found to cause ADRs in elderly people. These drugs are also among the most commonly prescribed for them.

Risk Factors

A number of factors may predispose elderly people to ADRs: the presence of multiple diseases, poor health status, and polypharmacy or multiple medications (Grymonpre, et al., 1988; Col et al., 1990; Carbonin et al., 1991; Chrischilles et al., 1992; Gerety et al., 1993). The association with polypharmacy is an important finding because multiple medication use is potentially modifiable, unlike some other risk factors. Whether age and gender are associated with ADRs is controversial. Older studies demonstrated that elderly groups were more likely to have higher rates of ADRs; however, they did not control for other known risk factors, such as number of medications, comorbidity, and disease severity. Recent studies with these controls have not found an association between age and ADRs (Grymonpre et al., 1988; Carbonin et al., 1991; Chrischilles et al., 1992; Gerety et al., 1993). It has been reported that women may be more susceptible to ADRs, but newer studies controlling for known risk factors have failed to find a gender association (Grymonpre et al., 1988; Col et al., 1990; Carbonin et al., 1991; Chrischilles et al., 1992; Gerety et al., 1993). Other factors that are suspected of being associated with ADRs include previous history of an ADR, age-related alterations in pharmacokinetics and pharmacodynamics, fragmented medical care, inappropriate prescribing, drug interactions, and medication dispensing and administration errors. The three latter subjects deserve further discussion.

Prescribing Errors

Prescribing errors involve incorrect drug selection, dose, dosage form, quantity, route, concentration, rate of administration, and instructions for use (American Hospital Formulary Service, 1994). A study of drug-prescribing appropriateness for older adults in the ambulatory care setting by Lipton and colleagues (1992) showed that 22 per cent of the subjects had a serious prescription medication problem, either improper schedule, inadequate dosage, potential drug interaction, therapeutic duplication, no indication for use, or allergy present. In a study of medication appropriateness in 208 ambulatory elderly patients with polypharmacy, 74 per cent of the prescribed drugs had one or more inappropriate ratings (Hanlon, Schmader, et al., 1992). The researchers concluded that medication prescribing was generally appropriate but improvement was needed in selecting less expensive drugs and in providing more exact and practical directions to patients.

Inappropriate prescribing has also been documented in the nursing home setting. A study by Beers and colleagues (1992) conducted in 12 nursing homes in the Los Angeles area showed that 7 per cent of all prescriptions were inappropriate; 40 per cent of residents received at least one inappropriate drug, with 10 per cent of residents receiving two or more inappropriate prescriptions. The size of the nursing home was positively associated with an increased number of inappropriate prescriptions. Inappropriate prescription of specific classes of medications, such as H_2 antagonists (Gurwitz et al., 1992) and antipsychotic drugs (Ray et al., 1980; Svarstad and Mount, 1991), in nursing home patients is common. The magnitude of the risk of adverse drug reactions or negative consequences of inappropriate prescribing is unclear. Bero and colleagues (1991), in their study of 48 drug-related readmissions of elderly people, concluded that 35 per cent of the drug-related hospital readmissions could be attributed to inappropriate prescribing, such as drugs that were contraindicated, allergy, inappropriate choice, overdose, and underdose. In contrast, they found that only 0.4 per cent of the readmissions could be attributed to drug interactions. Lindley and associates (1992), who studied the appropriateness of medications in an elderly population, related inappropriate prescriptions to 50 per cent of the hospital admissions that were associated with adverse drug reactions. Inappropriate prescriptions included those that could result in drug interactions, contraindicated drugs, and unnecessary drugs. However, neither the work of Bero and colleagues (1991) nor Lindley and associates (1992) identified inappropriate prescribing as an independent risk factor for adverse outcomes.

Drug Interactions

Drug interactions are one type of inappropriate prescribing that may lead to ADRs. Drug interactions can be defined as the effect that the administration of one medication has on another drug. Drug interactions can also be considered in a broader sense as involving medications that can affect and be affected by patients' diseases, nutrition, and biochemical status.

Studies of drug interactions in the elderly, although limited, have reported potential drug-drug interactions involving 6 to 42 per cent of all patients and 2 to 17 per cent of all prescriptions (Lamy, 1986). In a study of drug prescriptions generated during emergency room visits, Beers and colleagues (1990) found that 18 per cent of elderly patients received prescriptions that could interact with other drugs that they were already taking. Only 4 per cent of younger patients received potentially interacting prescriptions.

Not all potential drug-drug interactions are clinically significant. In their study of geriatric drug prescribing for ambulatory elderly people, Lipton and colleagues (1992) found potential drug interactions for 113 of 236 (48 per cent) of the subjects. However, an expert panel classified only 2 per cent of those interactions as potentially serious. A larger study found only 88 clinically significant drug-drug interactions for 2800 elderly community-dwelling subjects. However, it is interesting to note that Schmader and colleagues (1994) found zero instances of drug-drug interactions resulting in adverse clinical outcomes in 208 outpatients with polypharmacy.

Although potential drug interactions may be common, they rarely result in clinically significant adverse events. That is not to say, however, that health care professionals should not be vigilant about this issue, as older people are more vulnerable to serious consequences if a clinically significant interaction were to occur.

Medication Errors

Medication errors can be defined as drug misadventures that involve the prescribing, dispensing, or administration of medications. Although this problem has been most extensively considered for patients in institutional settings, it is pertinent to elderly people in all settings of care. The possibility of medication errors should be considered when evaluating the effects of drug regimens in elderly people.

Noncompliance

Adverse drug reactions may occur as a result of noncompliance. Failure to adhere to prescribed regimens, intentionally or unintentionally, is thought to be common among older patients (Stewart and Caranosos, 1989). However, there is no consistent evidence from the literature that age per se increases the risk of medication noncompliance. Noncompliance tends to be associated with underuse rather than overuse of medicines. In fact, overuse of drugs seems to be less common in elderly than in younger people. Darnell and associates (1986) studied medication use by ambulatory community-dwelling elders; they found drug overuse in only 7.5 per cent of the subjects.

In some cases, underuse of drugs may prevent adverse reactions. Problems may occur, however, if the patient is hospitalized and administered the drug dose that the physician believed was being taken at home. For example, a patient who has been noncompliant with antihypertensive medicines at home may become hypotensive and sustain a fall-related injury if given three-drug therapy for hypertension control when only one medicine is needed.

The concept of noncompliance has limited usefulness unless it is considered as a symptom of an underlying problem to be discovered and addressed rather than as a label to apply to a patient. The failure of the term to give meaningful guidance to care is highlighted by use of the term "intelligent noncompliance," which distinguishes failure to comply with medication regimens that have clear objective benefits from noncompliance with regimens that serve little apparent purpose or that are actually harmful. Some people prefer the term "nonadherence" as being less value-laden. A more complete discussion of this problem is in Chapter 21.

After discussing the magnitude and key risk factors of ADRs in elderly people, it is important to consider the most common medications reported to cause them in older people. Refer to Table 18–2 for the most common drugs implicated in ADRs across settings of care, which are also the most commonly prescribed classes of drugs in the aged. In particular, nurses should be vigilant about the potential for serious adverse reactions caused by drugs with a narrow therapeutic index, such as digitalis, lithium, anticoagulants, theophylline, anticonvulsants, antiarrhythmics, and aminoglycoside antibiotics. Although the range of ADRs is enormous, it is particularly important to recognize that certain common geriatric syndromes may be triggered or exacerbated by ADRs. These syndromes include cognitive impairment, falls, dysmobility, and incontinence, discussed next.

Drug-Related Pathology

Cognitive Impairment

Alterations in thought processes are a common adverse side effect of medication use in the elderly. Unfortunately, changes in mentation often go undiagnosed because of the erroneous belief that mental impairment is normal in older persons. Symptom reporting by older people themselves and their families is affected by this belief, and many health care professionals do not carefully consider drugs as the source of cognitive impairment.

The high incidence of cognitive impairment as a drug side effect is linked to several age-related factors, including diminished functional reserve of the central nervous system, altered sensitivity of the brain to some drug effects, altered drug pharmacokinetics associated with changes in the perfusion of the brain and cardiac tissues, and increased prescription of drugs in the elderly (Feely and Coakley, 1990; Lipowski, 1994; Jarvik et al., 1994). The drugs most commonly associated with altered mental function are listed in Table 18–3 (Bliwise et al., 1992; Lipowski, 1994; Bowen and Larson, 1993; American Psychiatric Association, 1994; Jarvik et al., 1994; Kane et al., 1994; Lipowski, 1994). Delirium is sometimes a presenting feature of drug intoxication. The *Diagnostic and Statistical Manual of Mental Disorders* (APA, 1994) classifies disturbances in consciousness and changes in cognition that are associated with medication side effects, as well as substance intoxication or withdrawal, as substance-induced delirium.

Although many patients cannot function without some of these agents, thoughtful drug choice and dosage in light of the age-related changes in pharmacokinetics and pharmacodynamics can alleviate drug-induced mental alterations in many cases. For example, a patient taking methyldopa for hypertension and showing signs suggestive of thinking and memory problems may be helped by a change to an alternative agent that is less likely to have adverse CNS side effects, such as a diuretic, calcium channel blocker, or angiotensin-converting enzyme (ACE) inhibitor.

The high incidence of mental confusion associated with adverse medication effects points to the need for baseline mental status testing in older persons before new regimens are instituted. Failure to do so results in an inadequate data base with which to evaluate possible drug side effects. Many simple, valid screening tests are available (see Chapters 2 and 10 for further detail).

When mental alterations due to drug side effects are suspected, nurses should specify the domains of function that are impaired and communicate those findings to the prescriber. Data including nature of the symptom, duration of symptom relative to starting the new medication, severity of the symptom, and aggravating factors are most important. Having information regarding suitable alternative treatments in hand before discussing the case with the prescriber makes the consultation process more efficient. Examples of alternative treatments include (1) use of different drugs with lower potential for adverse side effects, (2) dosage reductions to produce the same therapeutic effect but with fewer adverse side effects, and (3) use of nonpharmacological interventions, such as environmental modification or relaxation techniques.

For example, sometimes depressed patients have sleep difficulties, and hypnotic medications are prescribed. If the patient is subsequently placed on an antidepressant, the hypnotic may no longer be required, as many antidepressants have sedative effects. Failure to discontinue the hypnotic before beginning the antidepressant may result in depressed mental function. Tapering and discontinuation of the hypnotic when the antidepressant is started should prevent the unwanted side effect.

Careful choice of the drug may make the difference between an effective therapy and one that exacerbates the problem for which it was initially prescribed. It is possible for an "atropine-like psychosis" to be induced in patients if multiple drugs with anticholinergic properties are used simultaneously (Ahronheim, 1992). Since antipsychotic agents have varying degrees of anticholinergic properties, choice of drug will affect the degree of side effects.

T A B L E 1 8 – 3
Common Medications Causing Delirium in the Aged

DISORDER	MEDICATION TYPE	COMMON EXAMPLES
Cardiovascular	Antiarrhythmics	Procainamide, propranolol, quinidine, lidocaine
	Antihypertensives	Clonidine, methyldopa, reserpine
	Cardiac glycosides	Digitalis
Gastrointestinal	Antidiarrheals	Atropine, belladonna, homatropine, hyoscyamine, methantheline
	Antinauseants	Phenothiazines
	Antispasmodics	Phenothiazines, scopolamine
	Antiulcer agents	Propantheline, cimetidine, ranitidine, metaclopramide
Musculoskeletal	Anti-inflammatory agents	Corticosteroids, indomethacin, phenylbutazone, salicylates
	Muscle relaxants	Carisoprodol, diazepam
Neurological-psychiatric	Anticonvulsants	Barbiturates, phenytoin
	Antiparkinsonian agents	Amantadine, benztropine, bromocriptine, levodopa, trihexyphenidyl, selegiline
	Hypnotics and sedatives	Barbiturates, bromides, chloral hydrate, glutethimide, hydroxyzine
	Psychotropics	Benzodiazepines, lithium salts, neuroleptics, antidepressants
Respiratory/allergic	Antihistamines	Brompheniramine, chlorpheniramine, cyproheptadine, diphenhydramine, tripelennamine
	Bronchodilators	Theophylline
Miscellaneous	Analgesics	Narcotics
	Antidiabetic agents	Insulin, oral hypoglycemics
	Antineoplastic agents	Methotrexate, mitomycin, procarbazine
	Anti-infectives	Acyclovir, amphotericin B, cotrimoxazole, isoniazid, ketoconazole, rifampin

Falls

Falls are an important source of both morbidity and mortality among elderly people. Although falls are commonly attributed to medication use, Campbell (1991) contends that it is difficult to establish a cause and effect relationship. Tinetti (1994) acknowledges some contradictions among studies but reports adequate evidence that sedatives and antidepressants increase the risk of falls, particularly when longer-acting drugs are used. The risk of falls also rises with the number of drugs the person is taking (Sattin and McNevitt, 1992; Grissot and Kaplan, 1994; Tinetti, 1994; Tinetti et al., 1994). In addition to sedatives and antidepressants, classifications of drugs that have been implicated in falls are diuretics, antihypertensives, antipsychotics, hypoglycemics, psychotropics, analgesics, antiparkinsonian agents, antiarrhythmics, and alcohol (Campbell, 1991;

TABLE 18–4
Drugs Associated with Syncope, Falls, and Hip Fractures

DRUG CLASS	TYPE
Analgesics	Narcotic analgesics Nonsteroidal anti-inflammatory drugs
Cardiovascular agents	Alpha-antagonists Angiotensin-converting enzyme inhibitors Antiarrhythmics Beta blockers Calcium channel blockers Diuretics* Nitrates Vasodilators
Central nervous system drugs	Anticonvulsants Antidepressants Antiparkinsonian agents Antipsychotics Benzodiazepines Other sedatives/hypnotics
Endocrine-metabolic agents	Insulin Oral hypoglycemics

* Thiazide diuretics may be protective against hip fractures.
From Hanlon, J.T., Schmader, K.E. and Lewis, I.K. Adverse drug reactions. *In* Delafuente, J.C. and Stewart, R.B. (eds.). *Therapeutics in the Elderly.* 2nd ed. Cincinnati: Whitney Books, 1995, pp. 212–226.

Cwikel, 1992; Sattin and McNevitt, 1992; Grissot and Kaplan, 1994; Kane et al., 1994). Glynn and coworkers (1991) also found a positive relationship between falls and the use of nonmiotic topical eye medications in glaucoma patients. Table 18–4 summarizes drugs commonly associated with syncope, falls, and hip fractures.

A number of etiological mechanisms have been postulated to explain the relationship between drug use and falls. They include impaired postural control, impaired balance and reaction time, hypotension, diminished perceptual ability, impaired judgment, and memory impairment.

Drugs that interfere with postural control by acting on the autonomic nervous system include beta-blockers, antidepressants, and antipsychotics. Postural hypotension may occur with antihypertensives, nitrates, tricyclic antidepressants, and antipsychotics (Kane et al., 1994). Hypoglycemics can cause acute hypoglycemia with weakness, confusion, and impaired consciousness. Volume depletion caused by diuretics may also interfere with postural control. Dizziness and syncope are important causes of falls in elderly people. Dizziness is an adverse effect of phenytoin, lithium, and the benzodiaze-pines. Syncope can be associated with arrhythmias and with hypotension caused by vasodilators, antihypertensives, antidepressants, neuroleptics, diuretics, and dopaminergics (Jonsson and Lipsitz, 1994). Ototoxic drugs such as diuretics, salicylates, and some antibiotics may produce disturbances in balance. Digitalis, quinidine, and tricyclic antidepressants can cause arrhythmias with a resulting decrease in cardiac output and cerebral perfusion. The phenothiazines and diltiazem may cause drug-induced parkinsonism, with impaired motor function and muscle rigidity (Campbell, 1991).

Diminished mental acuity may result in diminished perception of obstacles to ambulation. Impaired judgment may cause older people to overestimate their abilities, resulting in falls when the environment is too challenging for their capabilities. Sedative medications may reduce the older person's ability to remember to use assistive devices, resulting in diminished competence and falls. Any drug that produces sedation may cause excessive drowsiness and contribute to falls. Grissot and Kaplan (1994) reported an increased incidence of hip fractures in people on hypnotics, anxiolytics, antidepressants, and antipsychotics.

The addition of a new medication to the older person's therapeutic regimen should trigger an assessment of the individual's likelihood of sustaining serious injury in a fall. If the risk is considered to be substantial, the need for the new drug should be closely scrutinized.

If the drug is essential, appropriate supportive measures should be taken to reduce the possibility of injury and enhance the access of the older person to postfall assistance, including having someone assess the home environment for specific hazards. Additionally, the patient should be instructed in measures that may reduce the likelihood of falls. These must be tailored to the individual but include environmental modification as well as instructions regarding gradual postural changes. For more detail on prevention of fall-related injury, see Chapter 21.

Incontinence

Another functional problem associated with drug side effects in elderly people is incontinence, both urinary and fecal. Incontinence related to drug therapy can be due to either therapeutic actions such as smooth muscle relaxation or to adverse effects such

TABLE 18–5
Medications That Can Affect Urinary Continence

DRUG OR THERAPEUTIC CLASS	MECHANISM
CNS sedatives	Affect sensory input
Diuretics Lithium	Cause polyuria
Anticholinergics Beta-agonists Prostaglandin inhibitors (NSAIDs) Calcium channel blockers Bromocriptine Tricyclic antidepressants Muscle relaxants	Decrease bladder contractility
Beta blockers Cholinergics	Increase bladder contractility
Alpha-adrenergic antagonists Muscle relaxants Neuroleptics Metoclopramide	Decrease outlet resistance
Narcotic analgesics Alpha-adrenergic agonists Estrogens	Increase outlet resistance

Data compiled from Shimp, L.A., Wells, T.J., Brink, C.A. et al. Relationship between drug use and urinary incontinence in elderly women. *Drug Intel Clin Pharm* 22:786–787, 1988; Wein, A.J. Pharmacologic treatment of incontinence. *J Am Geriatr Soc* 38: 317–325, 1990; and Gormley, E.A., Griffiths, D.J., McCracken, P.N. and Harrison, G.M. Polypharmacy and its effect on urinary incontinence in a geriatric population. *Br J Urology* 71:265–269, 1993.

as sedation, confusion, and motor impairment.

Some drugs affect the function of the organ systems responsible for excretion. For example, drugs that have anticholinergic properties may cause incomplete bladder emptying through inhibition of the detrusor muscle, predisposing to infection and possibly overflow incontinence. Common offending agents include antihistamines, antidepressants, antipsychotics, disopyramide, antispasmodics such as oxybutynin and flavoxate, and antiparkinson agents (Urinary Incontinence Guideline Panel, 1992). Other agents that inhibit detrusor muscle contractility include calcium channel blockers, beta-agonists, and nonsteroidal anti-inflammatory drugs (NSAIDs). Drugs like neuroleptics and alpha-adrenergic blockers can relax the internal sphincter and interfere with the patient's ability to inhibit bladder emptying (Romanowski et al., 1988). Alpha-adrenergic agonists (i.e., decongestants, narcotics, and estrogen) impede bladder emptying by increasing sphincter tone (Urinary Incontinence Guideline Panel, 1992). For a review of drug effects on the detrusor and urethral sphincters, see Table 18–5.

Anticholinergics and calcium channel blockers reduce peristalsis, setting up a cascade of events that may lead to fecal incontinence (Ouslander, 1994). Reduced peristalsis

TABLE 18–6
Comparison of Selected Effects of Neuroleptic Agents

DRUG (Brand Name)	RELATIVE POTENCY (mg)	EXTRA-PYRAMIDAL SIDE EFFECTS	SEDATION	ANTI-CHOLINERGIC EFFECT	ORTHOSTATIC HYPOTENSION
Aliphatic phenothiazine Chlorpromazine (Thorazine)	100	++	++	++	+++IM ++PO
Piperidine phenothiazine Thioridazine (Mellaril)	100	+	+++	+++	++
Piperazine phenothiazines Trifluoperazine (Stelazine)	5	+++	+	+ to ++	+
Fluphenazine* (Prolixin)	2	+++	+	+ to ++	+
Thioxanthenes Thiothixene (Navane)	2	++ to +++	+ to ++	+ to ++	++
Butyrophenone Haloperidol (Haldol)	2	+++	+	+	+
Dibenzoxazepine Loxapine (Loxitane)	10	++ to +++	+ to ++	+ to ++	+
Dihydroindolone Molindone (Moban)	10	++	+ to ++	+ to ++	+

*Facts and Comparisons, 1994.
From American Hospital Formulary Service. *Drug Information*. Bethesda, MD: American Society of Hospital Pharmacists (ASHP), 1994.

permits excessive water reabsorption in the colon, producing hardened feces that are more likely to become impacted. Continuous stooling around the impaction results, producing fecal incontinence.

Drugs that diminish mental acuity may interfere with the perception of the need to void or defecate and may prevent an appropriate response. The abilities needed to sense the urge to urinate or defecate, find the toilet, and undress and redress involve complex mental functions. Impairment in sensation, alertness, judgment, memory, or problem solving as a result of a drug side effect may precipitate incontinence. Drugs that may contribute to decreased mental acuity include long-acting benzodiazepines, sedatives-hypnotics, alcohol, and others listed in the previous section of this chapter.

Mobility is a critical factor in maintaining continence. Older persons are predisposed to mobility problems because of age-related chronic illness such as arthritis, stroke, Parkinson's disease, and dementing disorders. With decreased mobility, the time needed to respond to the urge to urinate or defecate is increased. An important mechanism for drug-induced incontinence is that the speed required to respond to the urge to urinate or defecate exceeds the individual's capacity to respond because of a drug effect. Drugs that increase the frequency of excretion or the amount of excrement may precipitate incontinence in elderly people who are unable to reach the toilet quickly enough. Such drugs may include diuretics, Kayexalate (potassium binding/exchange resin), laxatives, and antibiotics that cause diarrhea. Also, antipsychotic and antiparkinsonian drugs can indirectly affect continence by causing sedation, rigidity, and immobility. Table 18–6 contains a summary of the side effect profiles of many commonly used antipsychotic agents. Information on side effect profiles can be used to guide selection of a drug that has the least likelihood of adversely affecting mobility.

NURSING PROCESS AND PHARMACOLOGICAL INTERVENTIONS

Nurses often are responsible for administering medications and always are responsible for assessing individual responses to drugs. It is important to establish consciously a system for monitoring patient response to medications. Nurses should be knowledgeable about the conditions for drug administration that promote the desired effect. This knowledge is used by the nurse as drugs are administered but should also be taught to patients and family members if they are responsible for drug administration.

Assessment

Assessment of the older person requiring medications should include (1) the amount, type, frequency, and purpose of medications taken; (2) the individual's ability to take drugs independently; (3) the potential for drug interactions and adverse drug reactions; (4) a baseline from which to evaluate effectiveness of therapeutic regimen; and (5) whether any drugs can be discontinued or decreased in dose.

Drug Inventory

The drug inventory should include prescription medications as well as over-the-counter and social drugs (alcohol, caffeine, tobacco). Failure to perform an adequate drug assessment may result in inaccurate diagnosis of patient problems. For example, laxatives may have dangerous side effects, such as fluid and electrolyte disturbances, cathartic colon, and fat-soluble vitamin deficiency. It is important to consider the use or misuse of laxatives when addressing a variety of problems in elderly people, including diarrhea, constipation, dehydration, electrolyte imbalance, and vitamin deficiency. Finally, social drugs may interact with other drugs by affecting biotransformation or, in the case of alcohol, potentiating the effects of sedative medications.

Patient Perception of Purpose of Drug Therapy

Determining the elderly person's perception of the purpose of the medication is a key aspect of the drug assessment. People sometimes use medications for purposes that differ from the ones intended by the prescriber (Semla et al., 1991). Misconceptions about the purpose of a drug may lead to tragic results. Consider the following case. An elderly woman was found to be taking fluphenazine (Prolixin) to relieve "heartburn." She had borrowed the medicine from a friend and then talked her physician into prescribing this for her. A careful history of symptoms showed that she received little benefit from the fluphenazine, yet she was exposed to potentially irreversible adverse effects of parkinsonism and tardive dyskinesia. When the potential for adverse effects of the drug was explained to her, the patient willingly gave up the medicine.

Ability to Administer Medications Safely

Not all patients are able to self-administer their drugs accurately or independently. Factors affecting self-administration include vision, reading ability, memory, reasoning ability, judgment, motivation, and fine motor coordination. The complexity of the medication administration dictates that nurses should ask elderly people what approaches they have tried to help them take their medications accurately. Have the older person demonstrate key elements of medication taking, including opening pill bottles and reading the bottle labels so that impediments to accurate drug taking may be assessed. When serious visual, motor, or memory deficits exist, assistive devices may resolve the problem. When motivation, judgment, or reasoning is the problem, ongoing help from family or friends may be necessary to ensure adequate therapy.

Baseline Measures

Baseline measures of functions expected to be affected by medications should be taken as part of the medication assessment. In addition to assessing whether the desired therapeutic end-point has been achieved, standardized approaches to detecting common adverse side effects should be developed. For example, pulse rate is commonly used to monitor the effectiveness of digitalis preparations. However, a history of nausea or a mental status assessment is seldom elicited before the patient starts to take digitalis preparations. The latter two evaluations are important, for nausea and mental status impairment are two signs of digitalis toxicity often seen in elderly people. If the individual has chronic problems with nausea, digitalis toxicity may be incorrectly inferred. Conversely, if the patient's mental status is not carefully evaluated prior to the initiation of the drug, subtle changes may not be noted or may be attributed to dementia.

Problems encountered by those taking drugs with anticholinergic properties also highlight the need for accurate baseline assessment. Once again, mental status assessment is important as anticholinergics may precipitate delirium or diminished cognition (Tune et al., 1992).

Planning

The key aspects of planning pharmacological interventions in elderly people include (1) setting up systems for prevention and early identification of adverse drug effects, (2) anticipating the occurrence of new nursing diagnoses, and (3) selecting an individual to be responsible for monitoring the patient's day-to-day responses to the medication regimen. Drug therapy in elderly people is often complicated by psychosocial factors such as cognitive impairment, affective disorders, multiple prescribers, multiple daily dosage regimens, and poverty, necessitating further individualization of implementation and monitoring.

Prevention and Early Identification of Adverse Drug Reactions

The potential for drug interactions and adverse drug reactions in elderly people is great. Many are predictable, making it possible to assess the impact of drug therapy systematically on the function and comfort of the older person. Knowledge of common adverse drug reactions and interactions allows nurses to develop plans for early identification of unwanted drug effects. Every patient should have a periodic, systematic assessment to detect untoward drug effects.

Anticipating New Nursing Diagnoses

Many nursing diagnoses are linked to the effects of pharmacotherapy. Table 18–7 summarizes frequently occurring nursing diagnoses, with common etiologies and suggestions for treatment. The list is not intended to be exhaustive, but it should serve as a quick summary of the more common drug-related problems. In-depth material about these diagnoses and their treatments is contained in Chapters 14, 17, and 21. Predicting common nursing diagnoses associated with drug therapy requires some skill and experience in working with the aged. The paucity of research on specific diagnostic categories impedes prediction. However inexact the science at present, the expert gerontological nurse should strive to gain facility with predicting adverse functional effects of drugs, for there is great potential for precluding functional dependency through prevention or early identification of problems associated with drug therapy.

Supervising Drug Regimens

Every drug regimen requires someone to supervise its implementation on a day-to-

T A B L E   1 8 – 7
Common Nursing Diagnoses Associated with Pharmacotherapy in the Aged

CATEGORY	COMMON ETIOLOGIES	POSSIBLE TREATMENTS
Body image disturbance	Weight gain secondary to tricyclic antidepressant use	Assess motivation to modify diet Teach methods of weight reduction Refer to support group for weight reduction Be alert for noncompliance; instruct about the dangers of sudden withdrawal of antidepressants
High risk for fluid volume deficit	Iatrogenic effect of diuretic therapy Diarrhea or vomiting secondary to drug side effect	Monitor hydration status, including intake and output Hold diuretic if dehydrated and consult with prescriber Obtain order for antiemetic or antidiarrheal if drug will only be taken for short term. If long-term drug therapy indicated, consider changing to another drug
Altered thought processes	Anticholinergic delirium secondary to polypharmacy with anticholinergic agents Sedative effects of medication Depression secondary to drug effect (e.g., adrenergic drugs such as propranolol, reserpine, and methyldopa)	Consider reduced dosage Consider alternative drug Instruct caregivers regarding limitations and assistance needed to prevent injury Monitor emotional status
Constipation	Anticholinergic effects of medications Mobility-reducing effects of medications Dehydration secondary to overly aggressive diuresis	Consider alternative medication or reduced dosage; consider use of laxatives Institute exercise regimen to enhance mobility, especially around trunk and abdominal muscles Increase fluid intake, unless contraindicated because of cardiac or renal problems
Diarrhea	Reduced gastrointestinal flora secondary to broad-spectrum antibiotic use Cholinergic stimulation secondary to medication side effect	Try replacing flora through dietary means such as yogurt or buttermilk or with pharmacy-supplied agents such as Lactinex granules If medication needed on ongoing basis, consider use of bulk formers while restricting fluid intake to provide bulkier stool Use antidiarrheal medications if drug is to be used for the short term to prevent excessive fluid loss and promote comfort
Impaired physical mobility	Extrapyramidal side effects of neuroleptic drugs Sedative effects of drugs or adverse effects on balance	Consider reduced dosage Consider alternative drug Instruct caregivers regarding limitations and assistance needed to prevent injury
Functional urinary incontinence	Decreased time to respond secondary to diuretic use Sedative effects of medications Pharmacological effects on micturition	Evaluate need for diuretic therapy. Schedule diuretics in A.M. Is patient now motivated to try sodium restriction to eliminate need for diuretic and hence incontinence? Evaluate need for medication. Is therapeutic benefit worth induction of incontinence? Consider alternative medications that may be less sedating Institute toileting schedule Consider alternative medication Institute toileting schedule
Urinary retention	Secondary to anticholinergic effects of medication	Consider alternative medication Consider altered dose If on other anticholinergics, could some of those be discontinued or changed to medication with fewer anticholinergic side effects?
High risk for injury	Orthostatic hypotension Dizziness	If possible, give medication at bedtime, because peak effect will be felt shortly after dosage Teach patient to get up slowly, especially from reclining position, to use assistive devices, such as furniture or walker, and to re-equilibrate before moving Consider another drug with less propensity to cause orthostatic hypotension Consider reducing dosage to see if therapeutic effect can be obtained without dizziness Consider different drug Instruct family or paid caregivers of temporary hazard due to drug therapy and instruct them on ways to provide assistance with ambulation and transfer appropriate to the patient's functional capacity

TABLE 18 – 7
Common Nursing Diagnoses Associated with Pharmacotherapy in the Aged *Continued*

CATEGORY	COMMON ETIOLOGIES	POSSIBLE TREATMENTS
	Visual disturbances	Consider reducing dose to see if therapeutic effect can be obtained without side effect Consider different drug Instruct family or paid caregivers of temporary hazard due to drug therapy and instruct them on ways to assist with ambulation and transfer appropriate to the patient's functional capacity
	Impaired judgment	Consider reduced dosage Consider alternative drug Instruct caregivers regarding limitations and assistance needed to prevent injury
	Disturbance in balance or postural control	Consider reduced dosage Consider alternative drug Instruct caregivers regarding limitations and assistance needed to prevent injury
	Sedation	Consider reduced dosage Consider alternative drug Instruct caregivers regarding limitations and assistance needed to prevent injury
Noncompliance	Too many medications	Review medications for possibility of discontinuing some, e.g., dietary potassium supplements, tranquilizers, antihypertensives
	Noxious side effects	Consider alternative agent within the same class of drug or a different type of drug to accomplish the desired effect, e.g., antihypertensives, antidepressants, NSAIDs Consider nonpharmacological interventions: relaxation exercises, psychotherapy, massage
	Complex or frequent dosing regimen	For drugs with long half-lives, consider fewer doses per day (e.g., many psychotropic medications, Dilantin) Can drug dosage be reduced to maintenance schedule, allowing for less frequent dosing? Consider changing to similar drug that allows for less frequent dosage Use drug calendar or prepoured medications to simplify task of preparing medications
	Insufficient funds	Consider less expensive drugs that accomplish same therapeutic objective Consider nonpharmacological interventions If therapy is short term, consider drug samples
	Insufficient understanding of medications	Explain time is needed to see full therapeutic effect. Explain purpose, time it will require to take effect, importance of dosage schedule, common side effects Consider linking patient with another individual with similar problems but with successful drug therapy
Altered nutrition: less than body requirements	Anorexia secondary to gastrointestinal side effects of drug	Consider administering medications with meals, to decrease gastric irritation, unless contraindicated because of drug-food interaction Evaluate for possibility of toxic drug reaction, e.g., digitalis Monitor severity of nutritional alteration by assessing weight changes, actual food intake, and frequency and amount of vomiting, diarrhea Consider alternative medication If medication is short term, teach patient/family about temporary nature of symptoms If patient has borderline adequate nutritional status, consider supplementation between meals
	Hypo- or hyperglycemia	Monitor serum blood glucose levels on periodic basis and increase frequency of monitoring during initiation and with dose increases
Altered oral mucous membranes	Side effects of anticholinergic medications	Consider reduction in dosage or change in medication Use oral lubricant Teach regarding use of sugarless candy to relieve symptoms of dry mouth

Table continued on following page

T A B L E   1 8 – 7
Common Nursing Diagnoses Associated with Pharmacotherapy in the Aged *Continued*

CATEGORY	COMMON ETIOLOGIES	POSSIBLE TREATMENTS
	Dehydration	Evaluate continued need for diuretic if taking one Monitor hydration status Encourage fluid intake unless contraindicated by cardiac or renal status Pay scrupulous attention to mouth care in dependent patients until dehydration resolved
Sensory/perceptual alterations: visual, auditory, sensory	Neurotoxic side effects of drugs	Teach about risk of side effect and encourage patient to notify when changes occur Monitor for changes in sensory perception If symptoms develop, consider using different drug Teach patient compensatory responses to alteration, e.g., peripheral neuropathy, to examine feet daily for ulceration

day basis. In most cases older people themselves are quite capable of carrying out this function independently. Requirements for being an effective supervisor of a drug regimen include (1) intact memory, (2) ability to comprehend instructions about dosage, timing, and toxic effects, (3) ability to recognize adverse effects and take appropriate action, (4) ability to select the proper dosage from a stock supply, and (5) ability to procure the drugs.

Nurses caring for individuals who lack any of these abilities must consider alternative arrangements to ensure that the regimen is followed as prescribed. The incidence of memory and cognitive disturbances increases with age. The use of drug calendars or other memory aids such as pill boxes may suffice for those who simply have memory deficits. For those with more global impairments, support personnel may be necessary, such as family or paid helpers. Prescribers need to be aware of the arrangements for supervising the drug regimen so that the scheduling of doses is consistent with the aids or support available and changes in drug regimens are communicated in a meaningful way to the drug regimen supervisor. Whenever possible, prescribers should strive to use once or twice per day dosage schedules.

Financial Issues

Economics influence drug taking in the elderly, because many older people live on fixed incomes and take increasingly higher numbers of drugs with advancing age. Yet their primary insurance program, Medicare, does not pay for outpatient medications.

Most people economize on medications before more basic necessities, such as food or shelter. Thus, consideration of the price of a medication and its impact on the old person's budget should be a routine part of the prescription planning process. Increased cost consciousness throughout the health care industry may stimulate economically sound prescribing practices, but at present such behavior is far from reflexive (Glickman et al., 1994). Table 18–8 compares the costs of various commonly prescribed drugs. It is worthwhile noting that the Average Wholesale Price (A.W.P.) is the price a pharmacy can expect to pay a wholesaler for the drug. It is not possible to predict an individual prescription price from this figure; however, the A.W.P. is useful when contrasting the relative cost of various therapeutic agents within the same class. Similar information is available in sources such as *Medical Letter* and *Facts and Comparisons.*

Several general strategies for containing the costs of drug therapy are worthy of consideration. First, encourage patients to request the use of generic brand drugs when there is no evidence that a particular brand of drug affects bioavailability. Second, for patients who are on stable doses of medicines for chronic illnesses, encourage the prescriber to order larger quantities for each refill, such as a 90-day supply instead of a 1-month supply. This saves the patient the cost of the filling fee for 2 months. Third, avoid the use of newer agents, unless the therapeutic advantages are clear. Fourth, encourage the patient to request a review of medicines with their prescriber every 6 months, so that obsolete prescriptions can be discontinued. Finally, encourage patients to

TABLE 18-8
Cost Comparisons of Selected Drugs Commonly Prescribed for Elderly People

DRUG	REGIMEN	A.W.P.*
Analgesics		
Acetaminophen	975 mg po qid	3.60
Salsalate	500 mg po bid	10.54
Ibuprofen	400 mg po tid	6.70
Naproxen	375 mg po bid	50.19
Daypro	1200 mg po qd	72.20
Calcium Channel Blockers		
Norvasc	2.5 mg po qd	35.36
Nifedipine	10 mg po tid	30.51
Procardia XL	30 mg po qd	38.21
Cardizem CD	120 mg po qd	29.78
Diltiazem	30 mg po qid	42.48
ACE Inhibitors		
Capoten	12.5 mg po tid	57.45
Prinivil	5 mg po qd	22.68
Vasotec	5 mg po qd	27.36
Treatment for Peptic Ulcer Disease		
Prilosec	20 mg po qd	113.44
Cimetidine	400 mg po bid	79.43
Zantac	150 mg po bid	99.20
Carafate	1 gram po qid	84.17

* A.W.P., Average wholesale price for 1 month's supply for regimen indicated.
Data from *Drug Topics: Red Book*. Montvale, NJ: Medical Economics Data, 1995.

review their drug regimens with a clinical pharmacist if one is not already a regular member of the team. The pharmacist may be able to suggest methods of simplifying the drug regimen or be able to propose less costly alternatives to the patient and prescriber.

Using mail order pharmacies as the primary approach to cost containment may prove a false economy. Although costs of individual prescriptions may be somewhat less because of the high-volume business, the patient loses access to a personal relationship with a clinical pharmacist who can provide medication counseling on such important matters as the rationale for the drug, administration considerations, and common side effects that are key in optimizing drug therapy. Moreover, when using a mail order pharmacy, reordering of medicines must be planned carefully and adjustments in dosage or short-term medication use may not be accommodated easily.

Multiple Prescribers

Many older people must contend with multiple prescribers because of the effect of multiple chronic diseases and specialization in medical care. Undiagnosed and preventable drug interactions are one risk of having multiple prescribers. Nurses in ambulatory care and home health settings especially should be alert to the possibility of multiple prescribers and be prepared to intervene when possible therapeutic duplication or drug interactions are identified. When obtaining a drug inventory from an older person, ask about the various health care providers seen regularly who may prescribe drugs, including dentists and podiatrists. Consider teaching the older person to develop and use a medication list that can be brought to all providers of care.

Intervention

Nursing interventions in drug therapy can be divided into the following categories: (1) administering medication, (2) monitoring responses to therapy including identifying adverse drug reactions and titrating dosage, (3) teaching about medications, and (4) collaborating with prescribers regarding alternative forms of treatment.

Medication Administration

Nurses are experts in medication administration techniques. They can teach patients and families about ways to promote comfort and drug effectiveness as well as prevent or ameliorate side effects. Maximizing the effectiveness of drug therapy requires a knowledge of drug absorption and metabolism and an understanding of the nonpharmacological factors that potentiate or inhibit drug effects. For example, knowing that absorption of tetracycline is diminished by calcium leads the nurse to administer this drug between meals or snacks. Likewise, knowing that ethanol potentiates the sedative effects of benzodiazepines and antihistamines leads the nurse to a variety of possible interventions, including instructing the patient to abstain from alcohol while using benzodiazepines or antihistamines, suggesting a lower dose of these drugs for patients who habitually drink alcohol, and administering alcohol-containing elixirs at another time of day.

Deep breathing and relaxation techniques are examples of interventions that may be used to hasten the relief associated with some drug interventions. Their use may also result in lowering the doses required for symptom relief. Administering regular doses of analgesics and tranquilizers rather than waiting until the patient requests a dose may result in decreased dosage requirements. Techniques that promote relaxation may also diminish the discomfort associated with invasive administration methods such as injections, venipuncture, and rectal administration.

Taking medications may be complicated by physiological disturbances common to older people, including dysphagia, tremor, constipation, decreased muscle mass, and poor tissue perfusion. Nurses should be alert for these problems and knowledgeable about their impact and successful remedies. For example, difficulty in swallowing pills may be the result of decreased esophageal motility, poor positioning, anxiety, or a combination of these. Use of liquid medications rather than pills may alleviate swallowing problems. However, if positioning is incorrect, both pills and liquids will present problems. Figure 18–1 illustrates common positioning errors and proper positioning for swallowing. Hyperextension of the neck puts the individual at much greater risk for aspiration and makes swallowing of any substance more difficult. Demented individuals with swallowing difficulty may not tell a caregiver about their problem but may spit out the pill instead. Suspect swallowing difficulties in demented individuals who do not obtain the expected therapeutic effect from a drug despite presumably adequate dosage, and attempt a trial of a liquid form of the drug before changing to a new agent or assuming that the patient is refractory to therapy.

When a patient has difficulty in swallowing or has a feeding tube, the nurse must make a decision about whether or not it is acceptable to crush a tablet or open a capsule and dissolve its contents. While charts listing medicines that should not be crushed or opened are available, it is possible to make this decision by considering several characteristics of the tablet or capsule. Tablets or capsules often are prepared with special coatings to delay the release of the medication in the gut. This is generally done either to promote absorption, as in the case of omeprazole; to protect the gastric lining from irritation, as in the case of bisacodyl tablets or enteric-coated aspirin; or to prolong the release of the active medication to allow less frequent dosing intervals, as in the case of sustained-release theophylline. Many classes of drugs have at least one medication available as a liquid. Lists of medicines that should not be crushed and alternative preparations are available through the journal *Hospital Pharmacy* (Mitchell, 1992). Additional sources of this information include compilations often available through pharmacy organizations or pharmaceutical manufacturers.

Monitoring Responses to Therapy

As noted earlier, nurses are often the main caregivers responsible for noting patient responses to drug therapy. As such, it is imperative that they be knowledgeable about common adverse drug reactions. Nurses are also in an excellent position to use their knowledge of patient behaviors, drug effects, and other factors affecting the symptom under treatment to titrate dosage of medication to obtain maximum effectiveness with minimum adverse side effects.

Patient Education

National survey data show that older persons receive very little information about the drugs they take from physicians or pharmacists (National Association of Boards of Pharmacy, 1994). Because of the subtlety of disease presentation in the aged, it is particularly important that someone in the older person's immediate environment is knowledgeable about drug effects and toxicity. Furthermore, practicing physicians, pharmacists, and other nurses may not be knowledgeable about the increased susceptibility of older persons to adverse drug reactions or the altered pharmacokinetics seen in the aged. Nurses, therefore, should focus particular attention on teaching older persons and their caregivers about drugs and be prepared to educate other health professionals about altered responsiveness to drugs in the aged.

Collaboration with Prescribers on Alternative Forms of Therapy

A key function of nurses is to raise awareness regarding the feasibility of other forms of chronic disease treatment or symptom relief. Many chronic diseases can be managed with a multipronged approach to care that includes dietary management, psychosocial care, and activity or mobility modifications in addition to pharmacotherapy. Constipation can often be alleviated without the use of medications in this manner (see Chapter 14). Other clinical problems of older people, such as peripheral edema and chronic pain, often benefit from nonpharmacological inter-

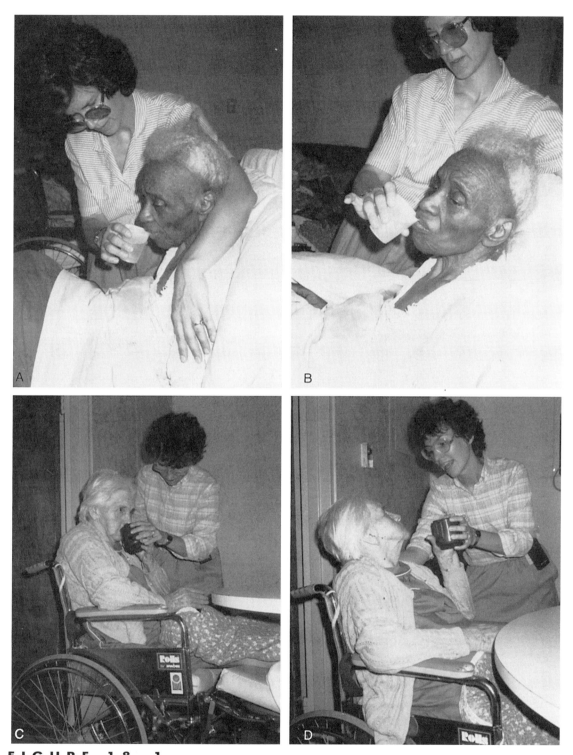

FIGURE 18-1

A, Correct position for medication administration to a reclining patient to prevent aspiration: head forward, neck slightly flexed. *B,* Incorrect position: head back, neck hyperextended. The patient is at high risk for difficulty in swallowing and aspiration. *C,* Correct medication position for a seated patient. *D,* Incorrect position.

ventions, but without a clinician to advocate their use, pharmacotherapy is often the only treatment utilized. Important nursing functions include encouraging the participation of other health care providers, sharing observations of patients' responses to alternative forms of therapy, and obtaining modifications in drug therapy as appropriate.

Evaluation

Individuals receiving drug therapy require ongoing evaluation of the impact of the drug regimen on their self-care abilities. Although the responsibility for evaluation of the efficacy of medications ultimately lies with the prescriber, nurses function in a collaborative role with prescribers, pharmacists, and other health care providers to evaluate patients' responses to medications and facilitate adaptation to side effects. In many settings nurses are responsible for titrating dosage within pre-established parameters according to patient response. The diverse responsibilities of nurses in drug therapy and the overlapping roles among health care professionals necessitate a clear plan for timing of interventions and evaluation.

Many models of evaluation of drug therapy are available. A sample appears here

---

BOX 18-1
Medication Appropriateness Index*

To assess the appropriateness of the drug, please answer the following questions and circle the applicable score:

1. Is there an indication for the drug? Comments:	1 _____ Indicated	2 _____	3 _____ Not Indicated	9 DK†
2. Is the medication effective for the condition? Comments:	1 _____ Effective	2 _____	3 _____ Ineffective	9 DK
3. Is the dosage correct? Comments:	1 _____ Correct	2 _____	3 _____ Incorrect	9 DK
4. Are the directions correct? Comments:	1 _____ Correct	2 _____	3 _____ Incorrect	9 DK
5. Are the directions practical? Comments:	1 _____ Practical	2 _____	3 _____ Impractical	9 DK
6. Are there clinically significant drug-drug interactions? Comments:	1 _____ Insignificant	2 _____	3 _____ Significant	9 DK
7. Are there clinically significant drug-disease/condition interactions? Comments:	1 _____ Insignificant	2 _____	3 _____ Significant	9 DK
8. Is there unnecessary duplication with other drug(s)? Comments:	1 _____ Necessary	2 _____	3 _____ Unnecessary	9 DK
9. Is the duration of therapy acceptable? Comments:	1 _____ Acceptable	2 _____	3 _____ Unacceptable	9 DK
10. Is this drug the least expensive alternative compared with others of equal utility? Comments:	1 _____ Least expensive	2 _____	3 _____ Most expensive	9 DK

*Complete instructions for use are available upon written request from Joseph T. Hanlon, MS PharmD, Duke University Center for the Study of Aging and Human Development, Box 3003, Duke University Medical Center, Durham, NC 27710.
† Don't know.
From Schmader, K.E., Hanlon, J.T., Weinberger, M. et al. Appropriateness of medication prescribing in ambulatory elderly patients. J Am Geriatr Soc 42:1241–1247, 1994.

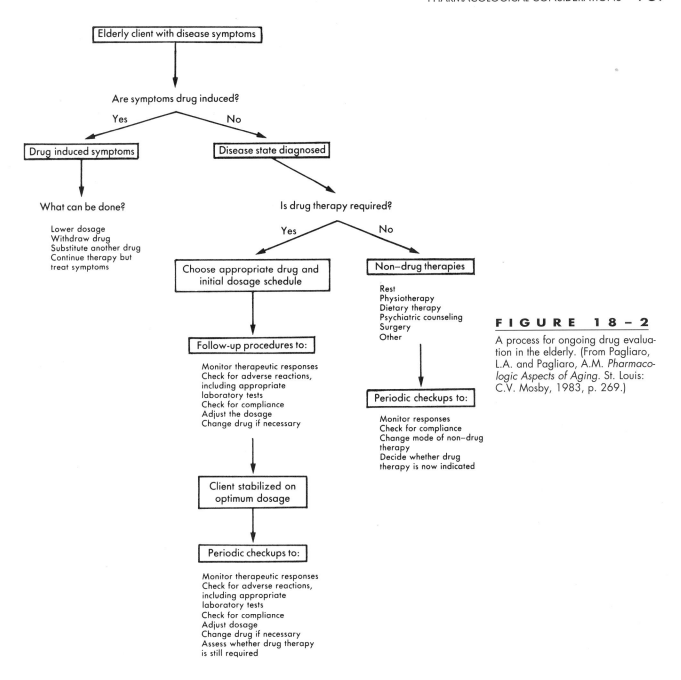

FIGURE 18–2

A process for ongoing drug evaluation in the elderly. (From Pagliaro, L.A. and Pagliaro, A.M. *Pharmacologic Aspects of Aging*. St. Louis: C.V. Mosby, 1983, p. 269.)

(Box 18–1). It can be followed before initiating drug therapy or whenever a patient's drug regimen is reviewed. Pagliaro and Pagliaro (1983, p. 269) offer a helpful algorithm for evaluating drug therapy (Fig. 18–2). Both models should be viewed as part of an ongoing process of assessment, planning, and intervention as well as evaluation.

Timing of the evaluation should be based on the nature of the individual patient's problems and therapy. Some conditions require daily or more frequent monitoring,

e.g., unstable diabetes, initiation of anticoagulant therapy, or titration of psychotropic medications for an acute behavioral disturbance. Other conditions require less frequent monitoring for several reasons, e.g., more stable disorders, less serious adverse drug effects, or adverse effects seen only with long-term therapy.

An often overlooked aspect of drug evaluation is assessment of whether the drug is still necessary. The patient is functioning at baseline, not complaining about drug therapy, and, as the saying goes, "If it ain't broke . . . don't fix it!" However, because older persons may be more likely to experience adverse drug reactions and because adverse drug reactions increase with the number of drugs taken, opportunities to stop medications should not be overlooked. In the past the use of "drug holidays" (a day during which most or all of a patient's drugs are withheld) was advocated. However, current knowledge suggests that drug holidays are not helpful and may be harmful. A more reasonable approach is a supervised withdrawal of certain medications, particularly if the indication for the medication is not clear or if the side effects are no longer tolerated.

Most medications can be discontinued abruptly without adverse complications. However, certain medications are associated with withdrawal syndromes, or exacerbation of underlying disease. Safe withdrawal of a drug requires understanding of the risks of withdrawal syndromes. A withdrawal syndrome is a clinically significant set of symptoms that occurs when a drug is discontinued. The syndrome may reflect recurrent symptoms that had been experienced before. For example, abrupt withdrawal of an antihypertensive may precipitate possibly severe rebound hypertension. Withdrawal from corticosteroids can result in weakness and nausea unrelated to the condition for which it had been prescribed. One other consequence of drug withdrawal is exacerbation of the condition that had been treated with the drug.

Medications commonly used by elderly people that are associated with withdrawal syndromes or exacerbations include alpha-antagonist antihypertensives, antianginals, anticonvulsants, antiparkinsonians, antipsychotics, muscle relaxants, benzodiazepines, beta-adrenergic blockers, corticosteroids, narcotic analgesics, sedatives-hypnotics, and tricyclic antidepressants (Hodding et al., 1980; Owens et al., 1989).

Case reports of withdrawal reactions are common, but few studies have addressed the phenomenon of withdrawal syndromes in a systematic manner. One study of adverse events related to drugs and drug withdrawal in nursing home residents reported 201 adverse drug withdrawal reactions in 95 residents, with an incidence of 0.44 per patient month (Gerety et al., 1993). In the study period, however, the investigators determined that the adverse drug withdrawal reactions were less common and less severe than other adverse drug reactions. Further study is needed to confirm the generalizability of these findings, as the investigators in this particular study were especially vigilant and skillful in their discontinuation of the drugs (Hanlon et al., 1993).

Slow, careful withdrawal from a medication can decrease or eliminate the risk of adverse effects. The lack of specific guidelines on withdrawal of most drugs requires the practitioner to devise a withdrawal schedule based on the pharmacokinetics of the drug. In a study of 124 elderly outpatients, in which 238 medications were stopped, 62 drugs resulted in 72 adverse drug withdrawal effects in 38 patients. The investigators concluded that the majority of medications can be discontinued without the occurrence of an adverse drug withdrawal event (Graves et al., 1995).

SUMMARY

Nurses play a significant role in monitoring and modifying drug regimens in the elderly. Given the high rate of adverse drug reactions in the elderly and the serious implications of these reactions for the functional status of older people, this is a responsibility that nurses should take very seriously. To intervene successfully, knowledge about altered drug handling resulting from the aging process and a chronic disease should be understood. Additionally, the particular hardships faced by older persons with functional limitations if an adverse drug reaction occurs must be recognized. With this knowledge in hand, nurses can be powerful resources for preventing disability related to adverse drug effects.

REFERENCES

Ahronheim, J.C. *Handbook of Prescribing Medications for Geriatric Patients.* Boston: Little, Brown, 1992.

American Hospital Formulary Service. *Drug Information.* Bethesda, MD: American Society of Hospital Pharmacists, 1994.

American Nurses' Association adopts position on polypharmacy. *Am J Hosp Pharm* 48:862, 1991.

American Psychiatric Association. *Diagnostic and Statistical Manual of Mental Disorders.* 4th ed. Washington, D.C.: 1994.

Baum, C., Kennedy, D.L., Knapp, D.E. et al. *Drug Utilization in the U.S.: 1986.* Springfield, VA: Center for Drug Evaluation and Research, Office of Epidemiology and Biostatistics, U.S. Food and Drug Administration, 1987.

Baum, C., Kennedy, D.L., Knapp, D.E. et al. Prescription drug use in 1984 and changes over time. *Med Care* 26:105–114, 1988.

Beers, M.H., Ouslander, J.G., Fingold, S.F. et al. Inappropriate medication prescribing in skilled nursing facilities. *Ann Intern Med* 117:684–689, 1992.

Beers, M.H., Storrie, M. and Lee, G. Potential adverse drug interactions in the emergency room. *Ann Intern Med* 112:61–64, 1990.

Bennett, W.M. Geriatric pharmacokinetics and the kidney. *Am J Kidney Dis* 16:283–288, 1990.

Bero, L.A., Lipton, H.I. and Bird, J.A. Characterization of geriatric drug-related hospital readmissions. *Med Care* 29:989–1003, 1991.

Besdine, R. Geriatric medicine: An overview. *In* Eisdorfer, C. (ed.). *Annual Review of Geriatrics and Gerontology.* Vol. 1. New York: Springer, 1980.

Bliwise, D.L., Pascualy, R.A. and Dement, W.C. Sleep disorders. *In* Evans, J.G. and Williams, T.F. (eds.). *Oxford Textbook of Geriatric Medicine.* Oxford: Oxford University Press, 1992, pp. 507–521.

Bowen, J.D. and Larson, E.B. Drug-induced cognitive impairment: Defining the problem and finding solutions. *Drugs Aging* 3(4):349–357, 1993.

Brawn, L.A. and Castleden, C.M. Adverse drug reactions: An overview of special considerations in the management of the elderly patient. *Drug Safety* 5:421–435, 1990.

Bressler, R. Adverse drug reactions. *In* Bressler, R. and Katz, M.D. (eds.). *Geriatric Pharmacology.* New York: McGraw-Hill, 1993, pp. 41–62.

Calkins, E., Ford, A.B. and Katz, P.R. *Practice of Geriatrics.* 2nd ed. Philadelphia: W.B. Saunders, 1992.

Campbell, A.J. Drug treatment as a cause of falls in old age. *Drugs Aging* 1(4):289–304, 1991.

Carbonin, P., Pahor, M., Bernabei, R. and Sgadari, A. Is age an independent risk factor for adverse drug reactions in hospitalized medical patients? *J Am Geriatr Soc* 39:1093–1099, 1991.

Chrischilles, E.A., Segar, E.T. and Wallace, R.B. Self-reported adverse drug reactions and related resource use: A study of community-dwelling persons 65 years of age and older. *Ann Intern Med* 117:634–640, 1992.

Cockcroft, D.W. and Gault, M.H. Prediction of creatinine clearance from serum creatinine. *Nephron* 16:31, 1976.

Col, N., Fanale, J.E. and Kronholm, P. The role of medication noncompliance and adverse drug reactions in hospitalizations in the elderly. *Ann Intern Med* 150:841–845, 1990.

Cwikel, J. Falls among elderly people living at home: Medical and social factors in a national sample. *Israel J Med Sci* 28:446–453, 1992.

Darnell, J.C., Murray, M.D., Martz, B.L. and Weinberger, M. Medication use by ambulatory elderly: An in-home survey. *J Am Geriatr Soc* 34:1–4, 1986.

Dawling, S. and Crome, P. Clinical pharmacokinetic considerations in the elderly: An update. *Clin Pharmacokinet* 17:236–263, 1989.

Delafuente, J.C., Meuleman, J.R., Conlin, M. et al. Drug use among functionally active, aged, ambulatory people. *Ann Pharmacother* 26:179–210, 1992.

Denham, M.J. Adverse drug reactions. *Br Med Bull* 46:53–62, 1990.

Drugs that cause psychiatric symptoms. *Med Lett* 35(901):65–70, 1993.

Editorial. Need we poison the elderly so often? *Lancet* 2:20–22, 1988.

Facts and Comparisons (1994).

Feely, J. and Coakley, D. Altered pharmacodynamics in the elderly. *Clin Geriatr Med* 6(2):269–283, 1990.

Frankhauser, M.P. Anxiolytic drugs and sedative-hypnotic agents. *In* Bressler, R. and Katz, M.D. (eds.). *Geriatric Pharmacology.* New York: McGraw-Hill, 1993, pp. 165–206.

Gerety, M., Cornell, J.E., Plichta, D. and Eimer, M. Adverse events related to drugs and drug withdrawal in nursing home residents. *J Am Geriatr Soc* 41:1326–1332, 1993.

Gibian, T. Rational drug therapy in the elderly or how not to poison your elderly patients. *Aust Family Phys* 21(2):1755–1760, 1992.

Glickman, L., Bruce, E.A., Caro, F.G. and Avorn, J. Physicians' knowledge of drug costs for the elderly. *J Am Geriatr Soc* 42:992–996, 1994.

Glynn, R.J., Seddon, J.M., Krug, J.H. et al. Falls in elderly patients with glaucoma. *Arch Ophthalmol* 109:205–210, 1991.

Graveley, E.A. and Oseasohn, C.S. Multiple drug regimens: Medication compliance among veterans 65 years and older. *Res Nurs Health* 14:51–58, 1991.

Graves, T., Hanlon, J.T., Schmader, K.E. et al. Adverse events after discontinuing medications in elderly outpatients. *J Am Geriatr Soc* 45:SA:5, 1995.

Grissot, J.A. and Kaplan, F. Hip fractures. *In* Hazzard, W.R., Bierman, E.L., Blass, J.P. et al. (eds.). *Principles of Geriatric Medicine and Gerontology.* 3rd ed. New York: McGraw-Hill, 1994, pp. 1321–1327.

Grymonpre, R.E., Mitenko, P.A., Sitar, D.S. et al. Drug-associated hospital admissions in older medical patients. *J Am Geriatr Soc* 36:1092–1098, 1988.

Gurian, B.S., Baker, E.H., Jacobson, S. et al. Informed consent for neuroleptics with elderly patients in two settings. *J Am Geriatr Soc* 38:37–44, 1990.

Gurwitz, J.H. and Avorn, J. The ambiguous relation between aging and adverse drug reactions. *Ann Intern Med* 114:956–966, 1991.

Gurwitz, J.H., Noonan, J.P. and Soumerai, S.B. Reducing the use of H_2 receptor antagonists in the long-term care setting. *J Am Geriatr Soc* 40:359–364, 1992.

Hale, W.E., May, F.E., Marks, R.G. and Stewart, R.B. Drug-drug and drug-disease interactions in the elderly: A report from the Dunedin program. *J Geriatr Drug Ther* 3:67–86, 1989.

Hanlon, J.T., Fillenbaum, G.G., Burchett, B. et al. Drug-use patterns among black and nonblack community-dwelling elderly. *Ann Pharmacother* 26:679–685, 1992.

Hanlon, J.T., Schmader, K.S., Samsa, G. et al. Medication appropriateness in ambulatory elderly (abstract). *J Am Geriatr Soc* 40:SA69, 1992.

Hanlon, J.T., Schmader, K.E. and Lewis, I.K. Adverse drug reactions. *In* Delafuente, J.C. and Stewart, R.B. (eds.). *Therapeutics in the Elderly.* 2nd ed. Cincinnati: Whitney Books, 1993, pp. 212–226.

Herrier, R.N. and Boyce, R.W. Compliance with prescribed drug regimens. *In* Bressler, R. and Katz, M.D. (eds.). *Geriatric Pharmacology.* New York: McGraw-Hill, 1993, pp. 63–78.

Hodding, G.C., Jann, M. and Ackerman, I.P. Drug withdrawal syndromes. *West J Med* 133:383–391, 1980.

Isaac, L.M., Tamblyn, R.M. and the McGill-Calgary Drug Research Team. Compliance and cognitive function: A methodological approach to measuring unintentional errors in medication compliance in the elderly. *Gerontologist* 33(6):772–778, 1993.

Jarvik, L.F., Lavretsky, E.P. and Neshkes, R.E. Dementia and delirium in old age. *In* Brocklehurst, J.C., Tallis, R.C. and Fillit, H.M. (eds.). *Textbook of Geriatric Medicine and Gerontology.* 4th ed. Edinburgh: Churchill Livingstone, 1994, pp. 326–348.

Jones-Grizzle, A.J. and Draugalis, J.R. Demographics. *In* Bressler, R. and Katz, M.D. (eds.). *Geriatric Pharmacology.* New York: McGraw-Hill, 1993, pp. 1–8.

Jonsson, P.V. and Lipsitz, L.A. Dizziness and syncope. *In* Hazzard, W.R., Bierman, E.L., Blass, J.P. et al. (eds.). *Principles of Geriatric Medicine and Gerontology.* 3rd ed. New York: McGraw-Hill, 1994, pp. 1165–1181.

Jue, S. Adverse drug reaction in the elderly. *In* Vestal, R.E. (ed.). *Drug Treatment in the Elderly.* Sydney: ADIS, 1984.

Kane, R.L., Ouslander, J.G. and Abrass, I.B. *Essentials of Geriatric Medicine*. 3rd ed. New York: McGraw-Hill, 1994.

Karch, F.E. and Lasagna, L. Adverse drug reactions: A critical review. *JAMA* 234:1236–1241, 1975.

Kessler, D.A. The FDA and drug marketing expenditures (letter). *JAMA* 265(12):1528, 1991.

Koronkowski, M.J., Hanlon, J.T., Schmader, K.E. et al. Adverse drug events in high-risk elderly outpatients. *J Am Geriatr Soc* 41:SA7, 1993.

Lamy, P. Drug interactions. *J Gerontol Nurs* 12(2):36–37, 1986.

Lindley, C.M., Tully, M.P., Paramsothy, V. and Tallis, R.C. Inappropriate medication is a major cause of adverse drug reactions in elderly patients. *Age and Ageing* 21(4):294–300, 1992.

Lipowski, Z.J. Update on delirium. *Psychiatr Clin North Am* 15(2):335–346, 1994.

Lipton, H.L., Bero, L.A., Bird, J.A. and McPhee, S.J. The impact of clinical pharmacists' consultations on physicians' geriatric drug prescribing. *Med Care* 30:646–658, 1992.

Lipton, H.L. and Bird, J.A. The impact of clinical pharmacists' consultations on geriatric patients' compliance and medical care use: A randomized controlled trial. *Gerontologist* 34(3):307–315, 1994.

Manasse, H.R. Medication use in an imperfect world: Drug misadventures as an issue in public policy; Part I. *Am J Hosp Pharm* 46:929–944, 1989.

McInnes, G.T. and Brodie, M.J. Drug interactions that matter. A critical reappraisal. *Drugs* 36(1):83–110, 1988.

Meyer, R.R. and Reidenberg, M.M. Clinical pharmacology and aging. *In* Evans, J.G. and Williams, T.F. (eds.). *Oxford Textbook of Geriatric Medicine*. Oxford: Oxford University Press, 1994, pp. 107–116.

Michocki, R.J., Lamy, P.P., Hooper, F.J. and Richardson, J.P. Drug prescribing for the elderly. *Arch Family Med* 2:441–444, 1993.

Mitchell, J.F. Oral dosage forms that should not be crushed: 1992 revision. *Hosp Pharm* 27:609–612, 695–699, 1992.

Montamat, S.C., Cusack, B.J. and Vestal, R.E. Management of drug therapy in the elderly. *N Engl J Med* 321:303–309, 1989.

National Association of Boards of Pharmacy (NABP). Patient Counselling Survey. Report abstracted in "News: Only 4 of 10 patients report receiving pharmacist counseling on outpatient prescriptions." *Am J Hosp Pharm* 51:3020, 1994.

Nolan, L. and O'Malley, K. Prescribing for the elderly. Part I: Sensitivity of the elderly to adverse drug reactions. *J Am Geriatr Soc* 36:142–149, 1988.

Ostrum, F.E., Hammarlund, E.R., Christensen, D.B. et al. Medication usage in an elderly population. *Med Care* 23:157–164, 1985.

Ouslander, J.G. Incontinence. *In* Hazzard, W.R., Bierman, E.L., Blass, J.P. et al. (eds.). *Principles of Geriatric Medicine and Gerontology*. 3rd ed. New York: McGraw-Hill, 1994, pp. 1229–1249.

Owens, N.J., Silliman, R.A. and Fretwell, M.D. The relationship between comprehensive functional assessment and optimal pharmacotherapy in the older patient. *DICP Ann Pharmacother* 23:847–854, 1989.

Pagliaro, L.A. and Pagliaro, A.M. (eds.). *Pharmacologic Aspects of Aging*. St. Louis: C.V. Mosby, 1983.

Rawlins, M.D. Adverse reactions to drugs. *Br Med J* 282:974–976, 1981.

Ray, W.A., Federspeil, C.F. and Schaffner, W.A. A study of antipsychotic drug use in nursing homes: Epidemiologic evidence suggesting misuse. *Am J Public Health* 70:485–491, 1980.

Roberts, J. and Turner, N. Pharmacodynamic basis for altered drug action in the elderly. *Clin Geriatr Med* 4:127–148, 1988.

Rollins, C.J. and Thomson, C. Nutrition. *In* Bressler, R. and Katz, M.D. (eds.). *Geriatric Pharmacology*. New York: McGraw-Hill, 1993, pp. 9–39.

Romanowski, G.L., Shimp, L.A., Balsom, A.B. and Cahn, M.I. Urinary incontinence in the elderly: Etiology and treatment. *Drug Intell Clin Pharm* 22:525–533, 1988.

Rowland, M. and Tozer, T.N. *Clinical Pharmacokinetics: Concepts and Applications*. 3rd ed. Baltimore: Williams & Wilkins, 1995.

Rumble, R. and Morgan, K. Hypnotics, sleep, and mortality in elderly people. *J Am Geriatr Soc* 40:787–791, 1992.

Sattin, R.W. and McNevitt, J. Epidemiology and environmental aspects. *In* Evans, J.G. and Williams, T.F. (eds.). *Oxford Textbook of Geriatric Medicine*. Oxford: Oxford University Press, 1992, pp. 81–87.

Schenker, S. and Bay, M. Drug disposition and hepatotoxicity in the elderly [review]. *J Clin Gastroenterol* 18(3):232–237, 1994.

Schmader, K.E., Hanlon, J.T., Weinberger, M. et al. Appropriateness of medication prescribing in ambulatory elderly patients. *J Am Geriatr Soc* 42:1241–1247, 1994.

Schneider, J.K., Mion, L.C. and Frengley, J.D. Adverse drug reactions in an elderly outpatient population. *Am J Hosp Pharm* 49:90–96, 1992.

Semla, T.P., Lemke, J.H., Helling, D.K. et al. Perceived purpose of prescription drugs: The Iowa 65+ Rural Health Study. *Drug Intel Clin Pharm* 25(4):10–13, 1991.

Shorr, R.I., Griffin, M.R., Daugherty, J.R. and Ray, W.A. Opioid analgesics and the risk of hip fractures in the elderly: Codeine and propoxyphene. *J Gerontol* 46:M111–M115, 1992.

Simons, L.A., Tett, S., Simons, J. et al. Multiple medication use in the elderly. Use of prescription and nonprescription drugs in an Australian community setting. *Med J Aust* 157(4):242–246, 1992.

Sloan, R.W. Principles of drug therapy in geriatric patients [review]. *Am Family Phys* 45(6):2709–2718, 1992.

Stewart, R.B. Adverse drug reactions. *In* Delafuente, J.C. and Stewart, R.B. (eds.). *Therapeutics in the Elderly*. Baltimore: Williams & Wilkins, 1988, pp. 121–131.

Stewart, R.B. Drug use in the elderly. *In* Delafuente, J.C. and Stewart, R.B. (eds.). *Therapeutics in the Elderly*. 2nd ed. Cincinnati: Whitney Books, 1995.

Stewart, R.B. and Caranasos, G.J. Medication compliance in the elderly. *Med Clin North Am* 73:1551–1560, 1989.

Svarstad, B.L. and Mount, J.K. Nursing home resources and tranquilizer use among the institutionalized elderly. *J Am Geriatr Soc* 39:869–875, 1991.

Swift, C.G. Pharmacodynamics: Changes in homeostatic mechanisms, receptor and target organ sensitivity in the elderly [review]. *Br Med Bull* 46(1):36–52, 1990.

Tinetti, M.E. Falls. *In* Hazzard, W.R., Bierman, E.L., Blass, J.P. et al. (eds.). *Principles of Geriatric Medicine and Gerontology*. 3rd ed. New York: McGraw-Hill, 1994, pp. 1313–1320.

Tinetti, M.E., Baker, D.I., McAvay, G. et al. A multifactorial intervention to reduce the risk of falling among elderly people living in the community. *N Engl J Med* 331(13):872–873, 1994.

Tune, L., Carr, S., Hoag, E. and Cooper, T. Anticholinergic effects of drugs commonly prescribed for the elderly: Potential means for assessing risk of delirium. *Am J Psychiatry* 149:1393–1394, 1992.

Urinary Incontinence Guideline Panel. *Urinary Inconti-*

nence in Adults: Clinical Practice Guideline. AHCPR Pub. No. 92-0038. Rockville, MD: Agency for Health Care Policy and Research, Public Health Service, U.S. Department of Health and Human Services, March 1992.

Vaughn, K., Yung, B.C., Rice, R. and Stoner, M.H. A retrospective study of patient falls in a psychiatric hospital. *J Psychosoc Nurs Mental Health Serv* 31(9):37–42, 1993.

Vestal, R.E., Cusak, B., Crowley, J.J. and Loi, C.M. Aging and the response to inhibition and induction of theophylline metabolism. *Exp Gerontol* 28:421–433, 1993.

Williams, L. and Lowenthal, D.T. Drug therapy in the elderly. *South Med J* 85(2):127–131, 1992.

Woodhouse, K. and Wynne, H.A. Age-related changes in hepatic function. *Drugs Aging* 2:243–255, 1992.

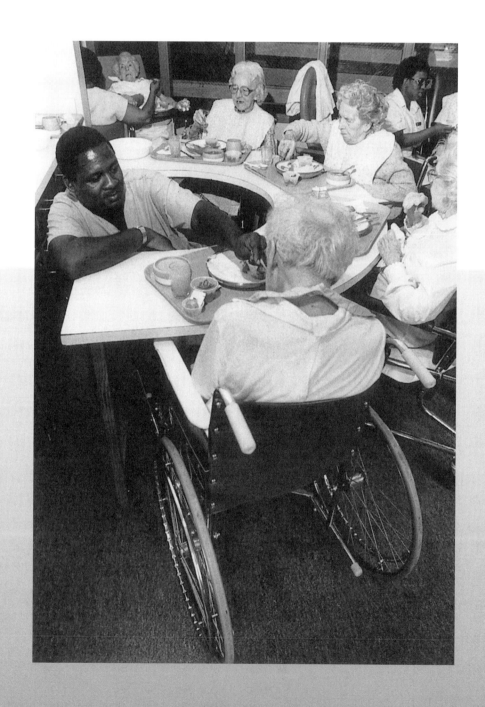

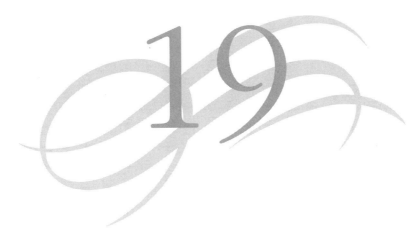

Nutritional Considerations

MARGARET L. BELL

Nutrition is fundamental to health promotion and maintenance. A good nutritional status helps prevent the development and progress of diseases and disabilities in later life as well as promoting successful medical treatment outcomes, thereby significantly contributing to the quality of life. Factors affecting nutritional status are multidimensional and interrelated at any age. For older adults, age-related changes in body composition and function, lifestyle, medication use, and the prevalence of chronic disease challenge maintenance of good nutrition. Lifetime eating habits and heredity, as well as psychosocial factors such as income, social interactions, and access to transportation, all can affect the client's nutritional status. Measures to promote good nutrition must specifically address the needs and problems of older adults in order to be effective.

This chapter provides an overview of the physiological and psychosocial factors affecting nutritional status in later life, assessment guidelines specific to older adults, and relevant measures for managing problems of under- and overnutrition.

AGE-RELATED FACTORS AFFECTING NUTRITIONAL STATUS

Physiological Factors

Sensory Changes

A progressive decline in sensory acuity occurs with aging (see Chapter 13). Comparisons between young and older adults suggest that the sense of smell declines more than the sense of taste (Murphy, 1993). Research shows that perceived loss of taste and smell are reasons for diminished enjoyment in eating, which in turn is associated with poor dietary intake (Horwath, 1991). Food seasonings can help compensate for this loss. Schiffman and Warwick (1993) found that flavor enhancement of food for elderly people resulted in increased food intake, increased bilateral hand grip strength, and improved immune status. The six flavors used in this study were primarily odors and contained no salt, monosodium glutamate, or sweeteners.

Reduced visual acuity makes reading fine print on food labels difficult. If an older adult cannot see adequately, food preparation also may become difficult and even hazardous. Hearing loss interferes with participation in conversation, possibly creating embarrassment or frustration, resulting in social isolation and increased risk of inadequate dietary intake.

Gastrointestinal Changes

Gastrointestinal changes with aging (see Chapter 10) may affect nutritional status negatively. Diminished saliva secretion decreases ability to chew and swallow food, which may be compounded by the use of medications that cause dry mouth. Decline of the opioid feeding system and increased satiety action of cholecystokinin may account for anorexia and hypophagia in advanced age (Morley and Silver, 1988; Morley, 1990). Abdominal distention and lack of appetite may result from delayed gastric emptying.

The prevalence of gastric atrophy and atrophic gastritis increases with age, so that secretion of intrinsic factor, hydrochloric acid, and pepsin is impaired (Bowman et al., 1991). Lack of gastric secretions may result in malabsorption of vitamin B_{12}, folate, and nonheme iron and increase the risk of bacterial overgrowth in the small intestine (Rudman and Cohan, 1992).

Metabolic Changes

Decreased metabolic rate and physical activity in old age result in reduced caloric need. When calories are reduced, less food is eaten, which may have a negative impact on the intake of other essential nutrients. Food must be chosen carefully to ensure an adequate intake of protein, vitamins, and minerals. Emphasis should be placed on choosing nutrient-dense foods (fish, poultry, dairy products, vegetables, fruits) rather than nutrient-empty foods (candy, rich desserts, alcohol) (Rudman and Cohan, 1992).

Impact of Health Problems

CHRONIC DISEASES. The nutritional status of the elderly may be affected by chronic diseases such as diabetes mellitus, atherosclerosis, and arthritis. Nutritional problems occur because of dietary restrictions, the inability or reduced desire to obtain and consume appropriate food, or the inability to utilize ingested food properly. In addition, many chronic diseases require drug therapy that may affect nutrient intake or absorption.

In most circumstances therapeutic diets should be liberalized for older adults who have chronic diseases that are treated with diet modification (Chernoff, 1991). Restrictive diets frequently are not palatable and differ markedly from long-standing eating habits.

The dependent older adult who finds eating less enjoyable because of dietary restrictions will likely consume less food. An adequate intake of essential nutrients is necessary to maintain maximum functional ability and to prevent complications that occur with immobility.

Opheim and Wesselman (1990) evaluated the effect of using a liberalized diet in six long-term care centers. Residents with adult-onset diabetes mellitus were served a regular diet with limited concentrated sweets and no sugar packet, and residents on low sodium diets were served a regular diet with no salt packet or table salt. No significant changes in edema, blood pressure, or weight resulted from returning to a regular diet, and residents were more satisfied with the variety of food choices.

When the independent older adult finds recommended dietary changes too restrictive, noncompliance may result, negating any benefit that may be realized from diet modification. In a survey of 3021 noninstitutionalized rural adults, 65 to 106 years of age, nearly 45 per cent reported following a special diet. The compliance rate was low for this group of independent older adults and was attributed to the difficulty in changing established dietary habits without adequate dietary counseling (Lee et al., 1993).

PHARMACOTHERAPY. Drugs can affect nutritional status by altering food intake and/or the absorption, metabolism, and excretion of nutrients (Table 19–1). Drug-nutrient interactions can also alter drug efficacy (see Chapter 18). Factors that increase the risk of adverse drug-nutrient interactions include

(1) inadequate or marginal nutrient intake;
(2) increased nutritional needs due to catabolic illness;
(3) impaired ability to absorb, metabolize, or excrete drugs and nutrients;
(4) long-term drug therapy; and
(5) multiple drug use (Ausman and Russell, 1994; Dudek, 1993; Robinson et al., 1993; Roe, 1986).

FLUID IMBALANCE. Water is an essential component of body tissues and the metabolic and excretory processes necessary to sustain life. Total body water decreases significantly with age due to reduced lean body mass and increased body fat (Fig. 19–1). The older adult needs 30 ml per kg of body weight (Ausman and Russell, 1994) or 6 to 8 glasses of water daily, enough to produce about 1.5 liters of urine (Lutz and Przytulski, 1994).

Dehydration is a frequent problem in older age and a common cause of acute confusion (Lipschitz, 1992). Decreased fluid intake and decreased ability to concentrate urine are contributory factors (Silver, 1990). Inadequate fluid intake may result from immobility, cognitive impairment, an inappropriate attempt to control urinary incontinence, and diminished thirst drive. Thirst deficit may be due to an age-related insensitivity of the hypothalamus; however, the reason for thirst deficit in the elderly is not yet clear (Phillips et al., 1984; Rolls, 1989).

DENTAL AND PERIODONTAL DISEASE. Poor dentition results from the loss of teeth due to periodontal disease or chronic poor hygiene. Although national surveys show a general trend toward a decrease in edentulism among elderly people (Dolan et al., 1990), it is estimated that 40 per cent of Americans by age 65 years have lost all their teeth, and 20 per cent have lost more than half their teeth (Martin, 1991). Edentulous people may have difficulty consuming a normal diet; however, many clinicians have observed edentulous people who can eat anything. When chewing becomes difficult or impossible, soft foods, many of which are high in fat and low in noncaloric nutrients, may be chosen. Foods high in fiber often are avoided. Even for people with optimally fitted dentures, the palatability of food may decrease, predisposing to dietary insufficiency. Dental problems may be a cause of current dietary problems or may reflect previous episodes of malnutrition.

CANCER. Rapid and substantial weight loss is often the first sign of an occult malignancy. Individuals undergoing treatment for cancer are therefore likely to have marginal or depleted nutritional reserves. Cancer treatments such as chemotherapy and radiation therapy are frequently associated with anorexia and weight loss. Malnutrition results when food intake does not meet the body's increased need for calories and other nutrients. People undergoing therapy may complain of nausea, changes in taste and smell, and feelings of fullness early in a meal. Foods not tolerated are often reported as tasting sour, bitter, salty, or spoiled. Treatment-induced stomatitis also increases the risk of inadequate intake. A systematic regimen of oral hygiene care has been shown to reduce the incidence and severity of stomatitis associated with chemotherapy and radiation therapy (Graham et al., 1993; Kenny, 1990). Other measures to provide nutritional support often are necessary, ranging from creative menu planning to nutritional supplementation.

DEMENTIA. The most common forms of dementia are primary neurodegenerative or Alzheimer's disease and vascular or multi-infarct dementia. The loss of functional capacity characteristic of dementia causes difficulty in obtaining, preparing, and eating food. Alterations in food intake may range from overeating, resulting in excessive

T A B L E   1 9 – 1
Influence of Some Drugs on Nutritional Status

DRUG	EFFECT ON NUTRITIONAL STATUS
Antacid	
Magnesium hydroxide and aluminum hydroxide	Decreased absorption of folacin, B_{12}, calcium, phosphate, and iron
Antiarrhythmic	
Digoxin	Anorexia; marked nausea with high doses
Antibiotic	
Gentamicin	Decreased appetite; increased urinary excretion of potassium, magnesium
Tetracycline	Decreased absorption of calcium with long-term therapy
Neomycin	Decreased absorption of folacin, B_{12}, fat-soluble vitamins, calcium, iron, sodium, potassium, lactose, sucrose, nitrogen, fat
Anticonvulsant	
Phenytoin	Decreased absorption of folate, calcium
Phenobarbital	Decreased absorption of calcium
Diphenylhydantoin	Decreased absorption of calcium
Primidone	Decreased absorption of calcium
Antidepressant, tricylic	
Amitriptyline	Increased appetite
Antihistamine	
Cyproheptadine	Increased appetite
Antihypertensive	
Hydralazine	Increased excretion of B_6
Methyldopa	Decreased absorption of B_{12}
Nitroprusside	Decreased absorption of B_{12}
Anti-inflammatory	
Colchicine	Decreased absorption of folacin, B_{12}, carotene, calcium, sodium, potassium, lactose, fat
Sulfasalazine	Decreased absorption of folacin, iron
Aspirin	Increased urinary excretion of ascorbic acid; iron deficiency due to gastrointestinal blood loss
Indomethacin	Increased urinary excretion of ascorbic acid; iron deficiency due to gastrointestinal blood loss
Penicillamine	Anorexia due to impaired taste acuity secondary to chelation of zinc, copper; inhibited B_6 metabolism

TABLE 19 - 1

Influence of Some Drugs on Nutritional Status *Continued*

DRUG	EFFECT ON NUTRITIONAL STATUS
Antilipemic	
Cholestyramine	Decreased absorption of folacin, B_{12}, fat-soluble vitamins, calcium, iron, fat
Antineoplastic	
Methotrexate	Anorexia
Mithramycin	Anorexia
Carmustine	Anorexia
Antitubercular	
Isoniazid	Decreased absorption of B_6
Para-aminosalicylic acid	Decreased absorption of folacin, B_{12}, fat
Cycloserine	B_6 antagonist
Corticosteroid	
Prednisone	Increased urinary excretion of ascorbic acid; decreased absorption of calcium with long-term therapy
Diuretic	
Thiazides	Increased urinary excretion of potassium, magnesium
Furosemide	Increased urinary excretion of potassium, magnesium, calcium
Ethacrynic acid	Increased urinary excretion of potassium, magnesium, zinc
H_2-Receptor Antagonist	
Cimetidine	Decreased absorption of B_{12}, calcium, iron
Laxative	
Phenolphthalein	Decreased absorption of vitamin D, calcium, potassium, fat
Bisacodyl	Decreased absorption of vitamin D, calcium, potassium, fat
Senna	Decreased absorption of vitamin D, calcium, potassium, fat
Mineral oil	Decreased absorption of fat-soluble vitamins
Tranquilizer	
Lithium carbonate	Increased appetite
Benzodiazepines	Increased appetite
Phenothiazines	Increased appetite
Sedative	
Glutethimide	Decreased absorption of calcium
Slow-Release Potassium Replenishers	Decreased absorption of folacin, B_{12}

Data from Roe, D.A. Drug-nutrient interactions in the elderly. *Geriatrics* 41(3):57–74, 1986; Roe, D.A. *Diet and Drug Interactions.* New York: Van Nostrand Reinhold, 1989, pp. 83–96; Garrison, R.H. and Somer, E.S. *The Nutrition Desk Reference.* 2nd ed. New Canaan, CT: Kents Publishing, Inc., 1990, pp. 273–282; Weinsier, R.L. and Morgan, S.L. *Fundamentals of Clinical Nutrition.* St. Louis: C.V. Mosby, 1993, pp. 187–188; and Lutz, C.A. and Przytulski, K.R. *Nutrition and Diet Therapy.* Philadelphia: F.A. Davis, 1994, pp. 404–415.

weight gain, to anorexia, resulting in significant weight loss (Dwyer et al., 1993; Hall, 1994). Other threats to nutritional status during the ambulatory phase of dementia include decreased attention span, not perceiving food as food, constant pacing, agitation, motor apraxia, fatigue, and extreme slowness (Hall, 1994). Supervised eating with verbal prompting, nonverbal prompting, or physical guiding; small, frequent meals with few choices; a nondistracting eating environment; use of modified eating utensils; and supplemental formulas are relevant support measures (Hall, 1994). During the nonambulatory phase of dementia, optimal intake is associated with skillful feeding, appropriate food consistency, adequate feeding time, and capitalizing on the midday meal when cognitive abilities tend to peak (Suski and Nielsen, 1989).

Psychosocial Factors

Some older adults have an inadequate retirement income. Poor dietary intake is associated with low income (White, 1991). Limited access to food and food choices plus inadequate facilities for food storage and preparation have a significant impact on both the quantity and quality of food intake.

Lack of transportation, loss of functional ability, immobility, limited income, and living alone may lead to social isolation. Older adults living alone may be deprived of stim-

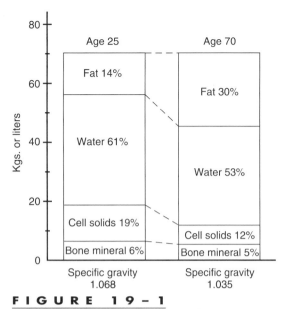

FIGURE 19-1

Changes in total body water with age. (Redrawn from Albanese, A.A. *Nutrition for the Elderly.* New York: A.R. Liss, 1980, p. 29.)

ulating interaction with others and thus lack incentive to cook and eat meals.

Depression frequently accompanies a sense of loss experienced with the death of a spouse or friends, retirement, changes in body appearance, impaired vision, and poor physical fitness. Lack of interest in eating and anorexia, common symptoms of depression, result in limited food intake. Opportunities for social interaction and a lifestyle of varied social and physical activities have a positive impact on morale, life satisfaction, and food intake (Horwath, 1991; Walker and Beauchene, 1991).

NUTRIENT AND DIETARY GUIDELINES

Recommended Dietary Allowances

Recommended Dietary Allowances (RDAs) are the intake levels of essential nutrients considered by the Food and Nutrition Board of the National Research Council–National Academy of Sciences as adequate to meet the known nutrient needs of practically all healthy people in the United States. These recommendations are for the average amounts of nutrients to be consumed daily from a normal diet consisting of a variety of foods that provide adequate energy. Although intended for group application, RDAs can be appropriately used to estimate the risk of deficiency for individuals. RDAs

do not cover special needs associated with chronic diseases, drug therapies, metabolic disorders, or other medical conditions.

Table 19–2 shows the RDAs for adults aged 51 years and older. The recommended energy intake is 30 kcal per kg of body weight per day for persons engaged in light-to-moderate activity. The recommended protein intake is 0.8 gm per kg of body weight per day. The iron RDA for older women is the same as that for men, owing to cessation of menstruation. When compared with younger adults, the RDAs for thiamin, riboflavin, and niacin are lower because of decreased energy requirements of older adults attributable to reduced basal metabolism and physical activity. There are no RDAs for dietary carbohydrate and fat. However, the U.S. Department of Agriculture recommends that 55 to 60 per cent of daily caloric intake be from carbohydrates, while total fat should be 30 per cent or less and saturated fat less than 10 per cent of daily caloric intake.

The RDAs are revised periodically to incorporate advances in scientific knowledge. Recent studies indicate that the 1989 RDAs for riboflavin, vitamin B_6, vitamin D, and vitamin B_{12} may be too low, and too high for vitamin A for the elderly population (Russell and Suter, 1993). Nutritional and dietary knowledge of the older adult is rapidly expanding, so it is likely that the next revision of the RDAs will have age categories with recommended nutrient levels for adults 50 to 70 years and over 70 years.

Dietary Guidelines and Food Guide Pyramid

The 1990 Dietary Guidelines for Americans (Table 19–3), issued jointly by the U.S. Department of Agriculture and the U.S. Department of Health and Human Services, provides guidance on food choices to promote and maintain good health. These guidelines represent current federal policy on nutrition.

In 1992, a Food Guide Pyramid (Fig. 19–2) was issued by the U.S. Department of Agriculture, replacing prior illustrations of four food groups. This graphic pyramid depicts six food groups based on recommendations set forth in the Dietary Guidelines, emphasizing the concepts of proportion, variety, and moderation. The pyramid is being promoted in nutrition programs for elderly people and through food labels and advertisements. It is an easy-to-use guide for teaching and evaluating dietary intake.

TABLE 19-2

Food and Nutrition Board, National Academy of Sciences–National Research Council Recommended Dietary Allowances,[a] Revised 1989

Designed for the maintenance of good nutrition of practically all healthy people in the United States

CATEGORY	AGE (years) OR CONDITION	WEIGHT[b] (kg)	(lb)	HEIGHT[b] (cm)	(in)	PROTEIN (g)	FAT-SOLUBLE VITAMINS Vitamin A (μg RE)[c]	Vitamin D (μg)[d]	Vitamin E (mg α-TE)[e]	Vitamin K (μg)	WATER-SOLUBLE VITAMINS Vitamin C (mg)	Thiamin (mg)	Riboflavin (mg)	Niacin (mg NE)[f]	Vitamin B6 (mg)	Folate (μg)	Vitamin B12 (μg)	MINERALS Calcium (mg)	Phosphorus (mg)	Magnesium (mg)	Iron (mg)	Zinc (mg)	Iodine (μg)	Selenium (μg)
Infants	0.0–0.5	6	13	60	24	13	375	7.5	3	5	30	0.3	0.4	5	0.3	25	0.3	400	300	40	6	5	40	10
	0.5–1.0	9	20	71	28	14	375	10	4	10	35	0.4	0.5	6	0.6	35	0.5	600	500	60	10	5	50	15
Children	1–3	13	29	90	35	16	400	10	6	15	40	0.7	0.8	9	1.0	50	0.7	800	800	80	10	10	70	20
	4–6	20	44	112	44	24	500	10	7	20	45	0.9	1.1	12	1.1	75	1.0	800	800	120	10	10	90	20
	7–10	28	62	132	52	28	700	10	7	30	45	1.0	1.2	13	1.4	100	1.4	800	800	170	10	10	120	30
Males	11–14	45	99	157	62	45	1,000	10	10	45	50	1.3	1.5	17	1.7	150	2.0	1,200	1,200	270	12	15	150	40
	15–18	66	145	176	69	59	1,000	10	10	65	60	1.5	1.8	20	2.0	200	2.0	1,200	1,200	400	12	15	150	50
	19–24	72	160	177	70	58	1,000	10	10	70	60	1.5	1.7	19	2.0	200	2.0	1,200	1,200	350	10	15	150	70
	25–50	79	174	176	70	63	1,000	5	10	80	60	1.5	1.7	19	2.0	200	2.0	800	800	350	10	15	150	70
	51+	77	170	173	68	63	1,000	5	10	80	60	1.2	1.4	15	2.0	200	2.0	800	800	350	10	15	150	70
Females	11–14	46	101	157	62	46	800	10	8	45	50	1.1	1.3	15	1.4	150	2.0	1,200	1,200	280	15	12	150	45
	15–18	55	120	163	64	44	800	10	8	55	60	1.1	1.3	15	1.5	180	2.0	1,200	1,200	300	15	12	150	50
	19–24	58	128	164	65	46	800	10	8	60	60	1.1	1.3	15	1.6	180	2.0	1,200	1,200	280	15	12	150	55
	25–50	63	138	163	64	50	800	5	8	65	60	1.1	1.3	15	1.6	180	2.0	800	800	280	15	12	150	55
	51+	65	143	160	63	50	800	5	8	65	60	1.0	1.2	13	1.6	180	2.0	800	800	280	10	12	150	55
Pregnant						60	800	10	10	65	70	1.5	1.6	17	2.2	400	2.2	1,200	1,200	320	30	15	175	65
Lactating	1st 6 months					65	1,300	10	12	65	95	1.6	1.8	20	2.1	280	2.6	1,200	1,200	355	15	19	200	75
	2nd 6 months					62	1,200	10	11	65	90	1.6	1.7	20	2.1	260	2.6	1,200	1,200	340	15	16	200	75

[a] The allowances, expressed as average daily intakes over time, are intended to provide for individual variations among most normal persons as they live in the United States under usual environmental stresses. Diets should be based on a variety of common foods in order to provide other nutrients for which human requirements have been less well defined. See text for detailed discussion of allowances and of nutrients not tabulated.

[b] Weights and heights of Reference Adults are actual medians for the U.S. population of the designated age, as reported by NHANES II. The median weights and heights of those under 19 years of age were taken from Hamill, P.V.V. et al. Physical growth: National Center for Health Statistics. *Am J Clin Nutr* 32:607–629, 1979. The use of these figures does not imply that the height-to-weight ratios are ideal.

[c] Retinol equivalents. 1 retinol equivalent = 1 μg retinol or 6 μg β-carotene. See text for calculation of vitamin A activity of diets as retinol equivalents.

[d] As cholecalciferol. 10 μg cholecalciferol = 400 IU of vitamin D.

[e] α-Tocopherol equivalents. 1 mg d-α-tocopherol = 1 α-TE. See text for variation in allowances and calculation of vitamin E activity of the diet as α-tocopherol equivalents.

[f] 1 NE (niacin equivalent) is equal to 1 mg of niacin or 60 mg of dietary tryptophan.

From Food and Nutrition Board. *Recommended Dietary Allowances.* 10th ed. Washington D.C.: National Academy of Sciences–National Research Council, 1989.

TABLE 19 – 3
Dietary Guidelines for Americans

- Eat a variety of foods
- Maintain healthy weight
- Choose a diet low in fat, saturated fat, and cholesterol
- Choose a diet with plenty of vegetables, fruits, and grain products
- Use sugars only in moderation
- Use salt and sodium only in moderation
- If you drink alcoholic beverages, do so in moderation

From U.S. Department of Agriculture and U.S. Department of Health and Human Services. *Nutrition and Your Health: Dietary Guidelines for Americans.* 3rd ed., 1990; Home and Garden Bulletin No. 232.

NUTRITIONAL ASSESSMENT

Nutritional assessment is the evaluation of dietary and other nutrition-related indicators to determine the need for intervention. Assessment includes a nutritional history, anthropometric measurement, physical examination, and laboratory analysis.

Nutritional History

Dietary intake is an essential component of a nutritional history. Methods for obtaining dietary intake include 24-hour recall, food frequency questionnaires, food records, and observation of food intake. The 24-hour recall method requires remembering food consumption from the previous day, whereas a food frequency questionnaire requires remembering the number of times per day, week, or month that particular foods are eaten. The 24-hour recall and food fre-

quency methods are sometimes used together to gather more complete information about intake. The food record or diary involves recording all intake for at least 3 days, to include 2 weekdays and 1 weekend day, which is then calculated to provide an average daily intake. The method of observation of food intake is time consuming and most easily used in an institutional setting. It involves unobtrusive observation and recording of actual intake and enables identification of factors affecting intake, such as mealtime social milieu and inappropriate feeding or assistive techniques used by caregivers. Dietary intake is evaluated by food group (Dietary Guidelines and Food Guide Pyramid) and/or nutrient composition (RDAs). Computer software programs are available to enable rapid calculation of nutrients.

A nutritional history should also include the following information:

- adequacy of income to purchase food
- educational level
- religious and cultural dietary practices
- food shopping accessibility
- adequacy of food preparation facilities
- physical activity
- functional ability
- food allergies and intolerances
- intentional or unintentional recent weight changes
- problems with chewing and swallowing
- gastrointestinal problems such as ano-

FIGURE 19 – 2

Food Guide Pyramid. (From U.S. Department of Agriculture and U.S. Department of Health and Human Services, Washington, D.C.)

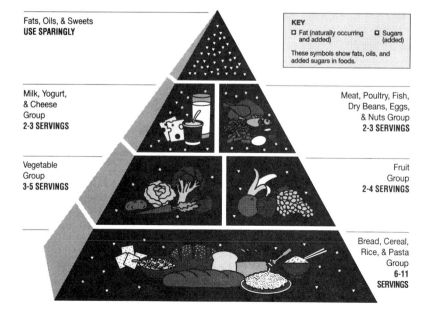

rexia, heartburn, indigestion, nausea, vomiting, bloating, flatulence, diarrhea, and constipation

- medical and psychiatric conditions
- over-the-counter and prescription medication use

Anthropometric Measurement

Anthropometric measurement includes height, weight, skinfold thickness, and circumferences. These measurements provide estimates of body fat and muscle mass for determining nutritional status when compared with available standards. The usefulness of these values depends upon accurate measurement technique. The *Anthropometric Standardization Reference Manual* (Lohman et al., 1988) provides detailed descriptions of standard techniques.

Height and Weight

Height should be measured with the person standing erect against a wall without shoes. Since arm span approximates height at maturity and changes little with aging, it has been used as an alternative method to estimate true height. Measurement is taken from fingertip to fingertip, with the measuring tape passing over the clavicles. Arm span is not recommended for the nonambulatory person because it is difficult to obtain a reliable measurement. Knee height can be used to estimate true height for the nonambulatory older adult, or when standing erect is not possible due to spinal curvature deformity (Chumlea, 1991). A sliding broad-blade caliper is used to measure the distance from the heel to 2 inches above the patella with the knee flexed. Knee height in the adult does not change with age and is more highly correlated with stature than total arm length or other length measurements. Estimation of height is made easily by using a nomogram (Chumlea et al., 1985). Knee height can also be used to estimate body weight (Chumlea, 1991).

Whenever possible a beam balance scale should be used to measure weight. The person should be weighed in light clothing without shoes. A bed scale should be used for persons who are nonambulatory. Weight provides an estimate of body energy stores. Well-validated, age-appropriate weight norms for older adults have not yet been established. One acceptable reference standard for determining desirable weight, based on available data, is presented in Table 19–4. Another method for determining

TABLE 19 – 4

Age- and Gender-Specific Reference Values for Weight in Kilograms (Pounds)

AGE (YEARS)	PERCENTILE		
	5th	50th	95th
Men			
65	62.6(138.0)	79.5(175.0)	102.0(224.9)
70	59.7(131.6)	76.5(168.7)	99.1(218.5)
75	56.8(125.2)	73.6(162.3)	96.3(212.3)
80	53.9(118.8)	70.7(155.9)	93.4(205.9)
85	51.0(112.4)	67.8(149.5)	90.5(199.5)
90	48.1(106.0)	64.9(143.1)	87.6(193.1)
Women			
65	51.2(112.9)	66.8(147.3)	87.1(192.0)
70	49.0(108.0)	64.6(142.4)	84.9(187.2)
75	46.8(103.2)	62.4(137.6)	82.8(182.5)
80	44.7 (98.5)	60.2(132.7)	80.6(177.7)
85	42.5 (93.7)	58.0(127.9)	78.4(172.8)
90	40.3 (88.8)	55.9(123.2)	76.2(168.0)

From Chumlea, W.C., Roche, A.F. and Mukherjee, D. *Nutritional Assessment of the Elderly through Anthropometry.* Used with permission of Ross Products Division, Abbott Laboratories, Columbus, Ohio.

appropriateness of weight is body mass index (BMI) or Quetelet index (weight in kilograms divided by the square of height in meters). The desirable BMI is 24 to 29 for persons over age 65 years (Committee on Diet and Health, 1989). Figure 19–3 shows a nomogram for estimating BMI.

Skinfold Thickness

Triceps and subscapular skinfold thicknesses provide measures of subcutaneous fat on the arm and trunk that significantly correlate with total body fat, indicating energy or caloric reserves. Subscapular skinfold thickness is measured 1 cm below the inferior angle of the scapula. Triceps skinfold (TSF) thickness is measured with calipers at midpoint between the olecranon and acromion processes on the posterior aspect of the arm. Percentile norms for TSF are presented in Table 19–5.

Circumference Measurements

Calf circumference measurement is recommended to monitor muscle loss from reduced physical activity. Measurement is done at the largest circumference of the calf with an inelastic tape measure.

Midarm circumference is measured halfway between the olecranon and acromion processes using an insertion tape. Midarm circumference and triceps fold thickness are used to calculate midarm muscle circumfer-

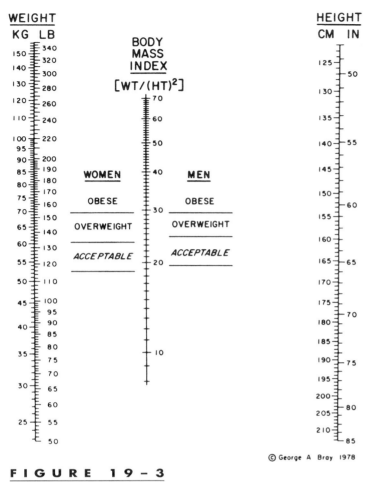

FIGURE 19-3

Nomograph for estimating body mass index. (From Shils, M.E., Olson, J.A. and Shike, M. (eds.). *Modern Nutrition in Health and Disease.* 8th ed. Philadelphia: Lea & Febiger, 1994; redrawn from Thomas, E., McKay, D.A. and Cutlin, M.B. Nomograph for body mass index [kg/m²]. *Am J Clin Nutr* 29:302-304, 1976. © American Society for Clinical Nutrition.)

ence (MAMC) and midarm muscle area (MAMA).* Both MAMC and MAMA are estimates of the amount of body muscle, an indication of muscle protein reserve. Visceral protein status is estimated by serum albumin and transferrin levels. Figure 19-4 shows a nomogram for rapid calculation of MAMC and MAMA; percentile norms are presented in Table 19-5.

The waist/hip or abdominal/gluteal ratio is an index for body fat distribution. To determine this ratio, waist measurement (smallest circumference below the ribs and above the umbilicus) is divided by hip measurement (largest circumference at the posterior extension of the buttocks). A waist/hip ratio of 0.8 or greater in women and 1.0 or greater in men indicates excess abdominal fat, which is a risk factor for hypertension,

cardiovascular disease, gallbladder disease, and noninsulin-dependent diabetes mellitus (Mahan and Arlin, 1992).

Physical Examination

Physical examination is important in the detection of nutritional deficiencies or excesses. Special attention should be given to the skin, oral cavity, eyes, abdomen, muscle tone and strength, and neurological integrity (Table 19-6). Physical signs and symptoms require confirmation with a dietary history and laboratory analysis.

Laboratory Analysis

Biochemical and hematological indices are more sensitive indicators of nutritional deficiency than are manifest physical signs and symptoms (Roe, 1983). Hemoglobin, hematocrit, complete blood count with differential, serum albumin, total protein, serum glucose, urinalysis, and stool guaiac for occult blood have been recommended as a minimum evaluation (Drugay, 1986). The normal values of common biochemical indices of nutritional status are summarized in Table 19-7.

NURSING DIAGNOSES/ NUTRITIONAL PROBLEMS

Three nursing diagnoses addressing nutritional problems are Altered Nutrition: More Than Body Requirements; Altered Nutrition: Less Than Body Requirements; and Impaired Swallowing. The diagnoses Health Seeking Behaviors and Knowledge Deficit are useful to focus attention on nutrition education and screening for the older adult. Other relevant nursing diagnoses, such as Fluid Volume Deficit or Excess and Altered Oral Mucous Membranes, are presented in Chapter 14.

Altered Nutrition: More Than Body Requirements/Obesity

Definition and Scope

Obesity refers to excess body fat and is generally defined as a body mass index above 30, or as a weight 20 per cent or more than ideal or desirable (Bray and Gray, 1988a; Rudman & Cohan, 1992). Overweight is defined as a weight 10 per cent more than ideal or desirable. Although weight for height is the most frequently used criterion to define obesity in elderly people, skinfold thickness and abdominal/gluteal ratio pro-

---

* MAMC (cm) = arm circumference (cm) − ($\pi \times$ triceps skinfold thickness in mm). MAMA = MAMC² ÷ 4π.

T A B L E   1 9 – 5

Percentile Norms for Upper Arm Anthropometric Measurements, CASE*

SEX AND AGE (YEAR) GROUP	NO. IN SAMPLE	MEAN	PERCENTILE						
			5th	10th	25th	50th	75th	90th	95th
Triceps Skinfold Thickness			**mm**						
Women									
60–89	496	25.2	12.5	14.4	18.5	24.0	30.8	38.1	43.6
60–69	146	27.2 ± 10.2†	13.0	14.7	20.7	26.2	33.0	40.3	47.2
70–79	239	25.1 ± 9.3	13.0	15.0	18.0	23.7	31.0	38.3	41.5
80–89	111	23.3 ± 9.7	10.9	12.9	16.7	21.8	27.5	34.6	43.4
Men									
60–89	250	22.5	5.7	7.6	11.5	20.4	31.8	42.1	45.8
60–69	86	21.9 ± 13.6	4.9	6.9	10.8	18.0	31.9	45.1	49.3
70–79	115	23.5 ± 13.3	6.3	7.9	12.0	22.0	32.7	41.8	45.4
80–89	49	21.6 ± 11.0	5.8	8.0	11.5	21.0	29.6	37.5	40.5
Mid-Upper-Arm Circumference			**cm**						
Women									
60–89	496	30.0	23.3	25.1	27.0	29.7	32.7	35.9	38.1
60–69	146	31.1 ± 4.8	23.5	25.6	27.7	30.6	33.7	37.5	39.9
70–79	239	30.0 ± 4.1	23.5	25.5	27.1	29.5	32.5	35.5	37.8
80–89	111	28.8 ± 4.6	22.5	23.5	26.0	28.8	31.6	34.5	36.4
Men									
60–89	250	30.4	24.9	26.6	28.7	30.4	32.2	34.6	36.3
60–69	86	30.5 ± 3.0	25.1	27.3	29.0	30.5	32.4	34.2	35.7
70–79	115	30.7 ± 3.1	25.3	26.8	29.0	30.7	32.4	34.6	36.6
80–89	49	29.6 ± 3.5	23.4	24.9	27.6	29.6	31.5	35.3	36.5
Mid-Upper-Arm Muscle Circumference			**cm**						
Women									
60–89	496	22.0	16.7	17.7	19.8	21.9	24.3	26.9	28.3
60–69	146	22.6 ± 3.6	17.8	18.4	20.2	22.3	24.6	27.5	29.2
70–79	239	22.1 ± 3.5	16.7	17.8	19.8	21.9	24.2	26.7	28.2
80–89	111	21.4 ± 4.1	15.2	16.7	19.1	21.3	24.2	26.7	27.5
Men									
60–89	250	23.3	16.6	18.1	20.5	23.4	26.2	28.4	29.7
60–69	86	23.7 ± 4.4	16.1	18.0	20.5	23.7	26.7	28.9	31.7
70–79	115	23.3 ± 4.1	17.0	18.2	20.4	23.4	26.3	28.4	28.7
80–89	49	22.8 ± 3.3	16.6	18.2	20.7	22.8	24.9	27.3	28.6
Mid-Upper-Arm Muscle Area			**cm²**						
Women									
60–89	496	39.9	22.2	25.0	31.1	38.0	47.1	57.7	63.8
60–69	146	41.6 ± 13.5	25.1	27.0	32.6	39.6	48.3	60.3	67.6
70–79	239	39.8 ± 12.7	22.1	25.1	31.2	38.0	46.7	56.6	63.2
80–89	111	37.9 ± 13.3	18.4	22.3	29.0	36.1	46.5	56.8	60.2
Men									
60–89	250	44.6	22.0	26.2	33.5	43.6	54.4	64.1	70.4
60–69	86	46.0 ± 16.5	20.7	25.8	33.4	44.8	56.8	66.7	79.7
70–79	115	44.6 ± 14.6	23.0	26.4	33.3	43.7	54.8	64.3	65.7
80–89	49	42.3 ± 11.8	21.9	26.5	34.2	41.5	49.4	59.1	64.9

* The Cincinnati Anthropometric Survey for the Elderly.

† Mean ± standard deviation.

Modified from Falciglia, G., O'Connor, J.O. and Gedling, E. Upper arm anthropometric norms in elderly white subjects. *J Am Diet Assoc* 88(5):569–574, 1988. Copyright The American Diatetic Association. Reprinted by permission from Journal of the American Diatetic Association.

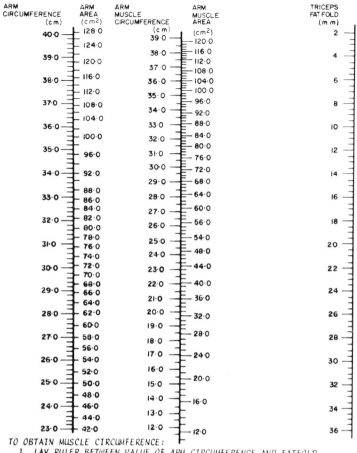

ARM CIRCUMFERENCE (cm)	ARM AREA (cm²)	ARM MUSCLE CIRCUMFERENCE (cm)	ARM MUSCLE AREA (cm²)	TRICEPS FATFOLD (mm)

TO OBTAIN MUSCLE CIRCUMFERENCE:
1. LAY RULER BETWEEN VALUE OF ARM CIRCUMFERENCE AND FATFOLD
2. READ OFF MUSCLE CIRCUMFERENCE ON MIDDLE LINE

TO OBTAIN TISSUE AREAS:
1. THE ARM AREA AND MUSCLE AREA ARE ALONGSIDE THEIR RESPECTIVE CIRCUMFERENCES
2. FAT AREA = ARM AREA-MUSCLE AREA

FIGURE 19-4

Arm anthropometry nomogram for adults. (From Gurney, J.M. and Jelliffe, D.B. Arm anthropometry in nutritional assessment: Nomogram for rapid calculation of muscle circumference and cross-sectional muscle and fat area. *Am J Clin Nutr* 26:912–915, 1973. © American Society for Clinical Nutrition.)

vide additional information for defining the degree of obesity.

Recent surveys show that Americans are more likely to be overweight than underweight at retirement age and obesity to be more prevalent among persons of lower economic status (Bray and Gray, 1988a; Pi-Sunyer, 1994). It is estimated that approximately 20 per cent of adults over 65 years of age are significantly overweight (Lipschitz, 1992). Health risks associated with excess weight include hypertension, hyperlipidemia, coronary artery disease, noninsulindependent diabetes mellitus, gallbladder disease (cholecystitis, cholelithiasis), osteoarthritis, and cancer (Weinsier and Morgan, 1993).

Etiology

Obesity results when caloric intake is greater than energy expenditure. Factors contributing to obesity in elderly people include inactivity, reduced metabolic rate, a lifelong pattern of obesity, limited social contacts, poor dentition, reduced mobility, and appetite-stimulating medications. Other causes, such as endocrine and hypothalamic disorders, rarely account for obesity in the older adult (Rudman and Cohan, 1992; Weinsier and Morgan, 1993).

Management

Weight reduction is achieved by reducing calorie intake, increasing energy expenditure through exercise, and behavior modification.

A well-balanced, reduced-calorie diet designed to promote a weight loss of 1 to 2 pounds per week is recommended for the overweight or obese older adult. The goal is weight reduction while conserving lean body mass. A daily intake 500 to 1000 calories less than energy requirements will promote a safe loss of 1 to 2 pounds per week. The Food Guide Pyramid (see Fig. 19–2) can be used to simplify diet instructions and meal planning. A diet consisting of the lowest number of servings on this guide and emphasizing low-fat foods will provide about 1600 calories a day.

Combined with diet, moderate exercise involving gross movement of large muscles promotes weight loss and conserves lean body mass. Exercise also improves muscle tone, cardiovascular condition, and body image. To sustain motivation, an exercise regimen needs to be compatible with the older adult's lifestyle. A person should exercise at least 30 minutes, three times a week; daily exercise will maximize weight loss.

Behavior modification promotes immediate weight loss and is necessary for longterm weight control. The essential elements of behavior modification are self-monitoring, stimulus control, and self-reward (Bray and Gray, 1988b). Self-monitoring involves writing down what foods are eaten, how much is eaten, where food is eaten, and the emotional circumstances at the time of consumption. This information is then used to identify cues that lead to overeating and behavior that needs changing. Stimulus control focuses on using techniques to control eating. Examples of control techniques are eating more slowly, taking smaller bites, not skipping meals, and eating only at pre-scribed times. Self-reward provides positive reinforcement to encourage change. Rewards should be established in advance and self-determined.

At the beginning of counseling, the older adult should be assisted in establishing personal weight goals and identifying the support needed to achieve those goals. Evaluation of weight loss should not occur too frequently, as day-to-day fluctuations in weight may be discouraging. An evaluation form completed by the older adult provides a concrete record of goal achievement.

Altered Nutrition: Less Than Body Requirements/Protein-Calorie Undernutrition

Definition and Scope

Inadequate intake of protein and calories to meet metabolic requirements results in a progressive loss of lean body mass and body fat. Major indicators of protein-calorie undernutrition (PCU) include

(1) loss of 5 per cent or more of body weight in one month (10 per cent or more in 6 months) or a weight 20 per cent below ideal or desirable body weight for height;
(2) midarm circumference and skinfold thickness less than the 10th percentile (see Table 9–5);
(3) serum albumin less than 3.5 gm/dl; and
(4) serum cholesterol less than 160 mg/dl (Ham, 1992; Silver, 1993).

Other objective measures include reduced serum hemoglobin, transferrin level, total lymphocyte count (less than 1500/mm^3), and cell-mediated immunity (Sullivan et al., 1990; Grant, 1992; Silver, 1993). Vitamin and mineral deficiencies may also be present with PCU and are confirmed through physical examination and laboratory analysis.

The exact prevalence of PCU among older adults is not known. Population surveys have indicated that 15 per cent of older adults experience PCU, whereas the incidence of PCU has been reported to range from 17 to 65 per cent in acute care settings and 30 to 85 per cent in long-term care facilities (Rudman and Feller, 1989; Fischer and Johnson, 1990; Powers and Folk, 1992; Sullivan, 1992; Keller, 1993).

PCU increases the risk of infection (Sullivan et al., 1990), delays wound healing and increases the risk of pressure sores (Welch et

TABLE 19–6
Symptoms of Nutritional Deficiency

Calories	Weakness, physical inactivity, weight loss, bradycardia, delayed wound healing
Protein	Dyspigmented, sparse, easily plucked hair; atrophic lingual papillae; parotid enlargement; muscle wasting; flaky dermatitis; edema; hepatomegaly; poor wound healing
Linoleic acid	Xerosis, desquamation, thickening of skin, hair loss, delayed wound healing
Vitamin A	Night blindness, xerophthalmia, keratomalacia, Bitot's spots, hypogeusia, hyposmia, skin xerosis, follicular hyperkeratosis, scaling
Vitamin D	Osteomalacia, tetany
Vitamin E	Anemia
Vitamin K	Bleeding tendency, purpura
Vitamin C	Spongy, bleeding gums if not edentulous; petechiae; ecchymoses; perifollicular hemorrhage; follicular hyperkeratosis; poor wound healing
Thiamin	Ophthalmoplegia; peripheral neuropathy: muscle weakness, paresthesias, ataxia, hyporeflexia, decreased vibratory/fine tactile/position sense; cardiomegaly; tachycardia; congestive heart failure; edema; mental changes: confabulation, disorientation
Riboflavin	Nasolabial seborrhea, angular stomatitis, cheilosis, magenta tongue, glossitis, atrophic lingual papillae, scrotal/vulvar dermatosis
Niacin	Nasolabial seborrhea, angular stomatitis, cheilosis, glossitis, atrophic lingual papillae, tongue fissuring, pellagrous dermatosis, malaise, headache, nausea, diarrhea, mental confusion
Pyridoxine	Nasolabial seborrhea, angular stomatitis, cheilosis, glossitis, peripheral neuropathy, irritability, muscular twitching, convulsions, microcytic anemia, depression
Folacin	Glossitis, stomatitis, pallor, anemia, diarrhea, depression
Vitamin B$_{12}$	Anorexia, atrophic lingual papillae, glossitis, optic neuritis, pallor, peripheral neuropathy, mental changes, diarrhea
Calcium	Osteomalacia, tetany, convulsions
Phosphorus	Osteomalacia, weakness, ophthalmoplegia, heart failure
Magnesium	Weakness, tremor, tetany, seizures, cardiac arrhythmias

Table continued on following page

TABLE 19-6
Symptoms of Nutritional Deficiency *Continued*

| Iron | Pallor, weakness, fatigability, angular stomatitis, atrophic lingual papillae, koilonychia, impaired wound healing |
| Zinc | Hypogeusia, hyposmia, photophobia, psoriasiform rash, eczematous scaling, poor wound healing |

Data from Mitchell, C.O. and Chernoff, R. Nutritional assessment of the elderly. *In* Chernoff, R. (ed.). *Geriatric Nutrition*. Gaithersburg, MD: Aspen Publishers, 1991, pp. 365–366; Grant, J.P. *Handbook of Total Parenteral Nutrition*. 2nd ed. Philadelphia: W.B. Saunders, 1992, p. 18; Mahan, L.K. and Arlin, M. *Krause's Food, Nutrition, and Diet Therapy*. Philadelphia: W.B. Saunders, 1992, p. 304; Rudman, D. and Cohan, M.E. Nutrition in the elderly. *In* Calkins, E., Ford, A.B. and Katz, P.R. *Practice of Geriatrics*. 2nd ed. Philadelphia: W.B. Saunders, 1992, pp. 20–21; and Weinsier, R.L. and Morgan, S.L. *Fundamentals of Clinical Nutrition*. St. Louis: C.V. Mosby, 1993, pp. 136–137.

al., 1991), prolongs hospital stay (Shaw-Stiffel et al., 1993), is a significant factor for hospital readmission within 3 months of discharge (Sullivan, 1992), and shortens life expectancy (Campillo et al., 1992).

Etiology

Usually more than one factor contributes to PCU in older adults. Age-related physical changes may alter food intake and the ability to utilize and metabolize essential nutrients. Social factors such as poverty, isolation, and lack of knowledge about nutritional requirements and appropriate food selection contribute to inadequate intake. Acute and chronic diseases may cause anorexia, increase energy utilization, cause nitrogen loss, alter vitamin and mineral metabolism, and/or alter ability to self-feed. Medical treatments such as surgery and chemotherapy may alter intake while simultaneously increasing metabolic demands. Drug-nutrient interactions and anorexia associated with medications may also contribute to undernutrition. Anticipatory guidance and early intervention to reduce risk can prevent many causes of PCU.

Management

Adequate assessment of the older adult is necessary to identify risk and causative factors as well as the degree of PCU. Intervention must address specific contributory and causative factors. Nutritional support will vary depending on the older adult's medical condition and degree of PCU. Interventions to improve access to food and increase oral intake include provision of congregate and home delivery meals, measures to promote self-feeding, and use of appropriate feeding techniques. When oral intake is insufficient in spite of conservative measures and supplementation, enteral and parenteral nutrition are alternative means for feeding.

CONGREGATE AND HOME-DELIVERED MEALS. Two types of resources in the community that address the problem of undernutrition are congregate nutrition programs and home-delivered meals. Most congregate nutrition programs have been developed for socially isolated older adults whose nutritional problems are related more to access and social stimulation than to mechanical eating difficulties. For older adults lacking the ability to go to a nutrition site, many communities also have home-delivered meal programs that provide at least one hot meal per day, which is equivalent to one third of the daily nutrient requirements for older adults.

PROMOTING SELF-FEEDING. The institutional long-term care environment may contribute to reduced self-feeding behavior in the aged (Rogers and Snow, 1982; Bonnel, 1993; Osborn & Marshall, 1993). Therefore, measures to enhance the self-feeding capacities of nursing home patients are advocated. These measures include:

TABLE 19-7
Reference Values for Biochemical Assessment of Adults

Hematocrit	
Male	40%–54%
Female	36%–46%
Hemoglobin	
Male	13.5–17 g/dl
Female	12–15 g/dl
Total lymphocytes	1700–3500 μl (mm^3)
	25%–35%
Serum albumin	3.5–5 g/dl
Serum total protein	6.0–8.0 g/dl
Serum transferrin	200–430 mg/dl
Transferrin saturation	
Male	30%–50%
Female	20%–35%
Serum ascorbic acid	0.2–2.0 mg/dl
Serum iron	50–150 μg/dl
Vitamin A	30–95 μg/dl
Serum carotene	60–200 μg/dl
Serum vitamin B_1	10–60 ng/ml
Plasma vitamin B_6	5–30 ng/ml
Serum vitamin B_{12}	200–900 pg/ml
Serum folate	200–700 ng/ml (RBC)
Serum vitamin E	5–20 μg/ml

From: Kee, J.L. *Laboratory & Diagnostic Tests with Nursing Implications*. 4th ed. Norwalk, CT: Appleton & Lange, 1995.

(1) attention to making the social environment of a meal more homelike through the use of small groups, removal of trays, and use of tablecloths and centerpieces;

(2) individualized adaptive equipment to promote self-feeding, such as plate guards, built-up utensil handles, universal cuffs, and proper set-up of plates; and

(3) staff training to emphasize techniques that promote self-feeding, such as proper positioning, the use of finger food, enhancing social exchange during the meal, and avoiding feeding the patient unless absolutely necessary to ensure adequate nutritional intake.

The older adult is more likely to have a positive attitude toward food and mealtime when self-feeding is fostered, thereby reducing the risk of inadequate intake and nutritional deficiency.

The principles of maintaining or restoring self-feeding ability apply to homebound older adults as well. Home health agencies provide assistance by teaching caregivers how to compensate for disabilities and create a conducive eating environment.

FEEDING TECHNIQUES. For older adults who lack the capacity to feed themselves, it is important to make intrusive feeding as risk-free and pleasant as possible. Relinquishing the self-care task of eating may have devastating psychological consequences. Failure to pay meticulous attention to position, pace of feeding, food preferences, and nonverbal communication during feeding is likely to result in the person's refusal to eat. Two studies have demonstrated increased protein and caloric intake with the use of touch and verbal cueing during feeding of both the cognitively impaired and the unimpaired older adult (Eaton et al., 1986; Lange-Alberts and Shott, 1994).

Careful attention must be paid to *positioning* the older adult who is sufficiently dependent to require feeding. The proper position is with the person sitting up, feet supported, head down, and chin tucked in (Welnetz, 1983). Inattention to positioning promotes fatigue, increased difficulty with feeding, and aspiration. Nurses and other caregivers need to ensure proper positioning and be knowledgeable about the risks associated with improper positioning.

Some older adults with sensory impairment are unable to determine when food is left in their mouth following a meal. They should be instructed to sweep the inside of their mouth with their tongue and then either swallow any remaining food or spit it into a napkin. *Mouth inspection* should be done at the end of each meal for older adults who pocket food or are unable to determine when food is left in their mouth. The caregiver should remove the food using a gloved finger, if the older adult is unable to perform the tongue sweeping maneuver successfully, to prevent aspiration.

Consumption of a meal for most adults requires a minimum of 15 to 20 minutes. However, sometimes dependent eaters are rushed to finish meals in 5 to 10 minutes (Saunders et al., 1992). Older adults generally have a slower reaction time than younger adults, so it is sensible to provide a slower, rather than faster, mealtime. A *pace* that is too rapid may lead to choking or refusal to eat. One solution is to feed people in a group setting (Hogstel and Robinson, 1989). Feeding several persons who eat at different rates simultaneously in a group maximizes the efficiency of caregiver time and enables a slower eating pace. Even regressed older adults may use mealtime as a social opportunity.

Most people have strong *food preferences*. Ignoring those preferences, especially with persons who are unable to feed themselves, is inhumane. The practice of combining all food on a plate is inappropriate. Few adults would choose to have their scrambled eggs and oatmeal combined. Caregivers need to recognize the importance of normalizing food intake. Failure to provide nourishment in a normal manner fosters undernutrition.

Performance of the activities of daily living consumes a great deal of time for dependent older adults. Feeding occurs three or more times each day. It is a major activity during which considerable communication may take place. Attention to *verbal and nonverbal aspects of communication* is important. Mealtime provides an opportunity to engage the older adult socially and to send messages that strengthen self-esteem. A depersonalized or threatening feeding environment discourages optimal food intake and minimizes self-worth.

ENTERAL NUTRITION. Enteral nutritional therapy is an option when the older adult is unable to meet nutritional needs orally but has normal gastrointestinal function. Enteral feeding may be used to supplement oral intake or to provide total nutrient requirements.

The most common sites used for enteral feeding are the stomach and jejunum. Placement of a feeding tube will depend on the

T A B L E   1 9 – 8
Complications of Enteral Tube Feeding

COMPLICATION	MANAGEMENT
Mechanical	
Nasopharyngeal irritation	Use small-bore pliable tube Provide nose and mouth care Monitor for nasopharyngeal bleeding and infection
Tube obstruction	Flush tube with 30–60 ml warm water after each feeding, every 4 hours with continuous feeding, and before and after medication administration Use liquid medications if available; crush tablets and dissolve in 10–15 ml water before administration; do not mix medications with formula Use infusion pump for high-viscosity formulas Switch to less calorie-dense formula
Aspiration	Keep head of bed elevated 30–45 degrees Check tube placement prior to feeding Check gastric residual volume prior to feeding; stop feeding and notify physician if residual is >100 ml or twice the hourly rate of continuous feeding Assess for abdominal distention, symptoms of gastric reflux, and bowel sounds Stop feeding if nausea or vomiting occurs Use small-bore pliable feeding tube to minimize gastroesophageal relaxation Reduce rate and/or concentration of formula
Tube migration	Stabilize tube position appropriately Mark tube at insertion site; check marking prior to feeding Check G-J tube insertion site for drainage Notify physician of signs of tube migration
Infection	Clean G-J tube insertion site daily Stabilize tube position appropriately Monitor for local signs of skin infection
Gastrointestinal	
Dry mouth	Provide mouth care
Distention	Check tube placement
Bloating	Assess bowel sounds; measure abdominal girth Keep tube clamped between intermittent feedings; remove air from delivery system before connecting to feeding tube Check gastric residual; stop feeding and notify physician if residual >100 ml or twice the hourly rate of continuous feeding Reduce rate and/or concentration, increase slowly Switch to continuous drip or different formula Encourage ambulation

older adult's medical condition and the anticipated length of time that enteral therapy will be used. Nasogastric and other transnasal tubes are used for short-term therapy. Feeding tubes placed in the stomach and jejunum either surgically or by percutaneous endoscopy are preferred for permanent or long-term enteral feeding. A jejunostomy tube is indicated for the older adult who has a diminished or absent gag reflex, to reduce the risk of aspiration.

A number of commercially prepared formulas are available. Selection depends on nutrient and fluid needs, the patient's ability to digest and absorb nutrients, and the type of feeding tube used. Standard formulas are available in isotonic and hypertonic forms.

Tube feedings can be delivered by continuous drip, intermittent infusion, and bolus administration. The method of delivery de-

pends on the location of the feeding tube, type of formula used, and tolerance for the feeding. Bolus administration is used only with nasogastric and gastrostomy tube feeding. Formula is given by gravity with a large barrel syringe over 15 to 30 minutes, four to six times a day. Bolus feeding is not well tolerated. Intermittent feeding by slow gravity drip or infusion pump over 30 to 60 minutes helps alleviate problems of intolerance encountered with bolus administration. The preferred method is continuous drip over 16 to 24 hours using an infusion pump to maintain consistent flow rate, thus minimizing feeding intolerance. Feedings delivered to the small intestine, duodenum, and jejunum require use of an infusion pump to prevent the dumping syndrome.

Isotonic formulas are started full strength

TABLE 19–8
Complications of Enteral Tube Feeding *Continued*

COMPLICATION	MANAGEMENT
Nausea, vomiting	Assess bowel sounds; check for distention and rigidity; measure abdominal girth Stop feeding and notify physician Check gastric residual
Diarrhea (>5 stools/24 hr)	Give formula at room temperature Use aseptic technique with formula preparation Do not hang formula longer than 6 hours Reduce rate and/or concentration of formula; increase slowly Use lactose-free formula or switch to different formula Check placement of gastric tube for migration to small intestine Assess medications for side effect of diarrhea Obtain diagnostic studies: stool culture, *Clostridium difficile* toxin Monitor intake and output
Constipation	Use fiber-enriched formula Add free water if intake is not greater than output by 500–1000 ml Encourage ambulation Monitor intake and output
Metabolic Hyperglycemia	Monitor for signs of hyperglycemia and infection Check blood glucose level and administer insulin as prescribed Use infusion pump to insure consistent flow rate Reduce flow rate; change formula to lower calorie content
Hypoglycemia	Monitor for signs of hypoglycemia Check blood glucose level; notify physician
Hypernatremia, dehydration	Monitor for signs of hypernatremia and dehydration Monitor serum sodium, BUN, hematocrit, urine specific gravity Monitor intake and output, weight Assess medications for effect on fluid and electrolyte balance Increase fluid intake Use formula with less protein
Hyponatremia, overhydration	Monitor for signs of hyponatremia and fluid overload Monitor intake and output, weight Assess medications for effect on fluid and electrolyte balance Use only 30–50 ml of water to flush feeding tube Change formula dilution; use calorie-dense formula

Data from Chernoff, R. Nutritional support in the elderly. *In* Chernoff, R. (ed.). *Geriatric Nutrition: The Health Professional's Handbook.* Gaithersburg, MD: Aspen Publishers, 1991, pp. 401–408; Young, C.K. and White, S. Tube feeding at home. *Am J Nurs* 92(4):46–53, 1992; Dudek, S.G. *Nutrition Handbook for Nursing Practice.* 2nd ed. Philadelphia: J.B. Lippincott, 1993, pp. 353–375; Sacks, G.S. and Brown, R.O. Drug-nutrient interactions in patients receiving nutritional support. *Drug Ther* 24(3):35–42, 1994; Shuster, M.H. and Mancino, J.M. Ensuring successful home tube feeding in the geriatric population. *Geriatr Nurs* 13(2):67–81, 1994.

at a rate of 25 to 50 ml per hr, increased by 25 ml per hr over 12 to 24 hours as tolerated and until the desired rate to meet nutrient needs is achieved. Hypertonic formulas should be diluted to isotonic strength when initiated. The concentration is increased every 8 to 12 hours as tolerated to full strength, then the rate is increased 25 ml per hr every 8 to 12 hours until the desired rate to meet nutrient needs is achieved. The rate and the concentration should never be advanced at the same time (Davis, 1991).

Complications of enteral therapy may be mechanical, gastrointestinal, or metabolic. These complications and related management measures are presented in Table 19–8.

TOTAL PARENTERAL NUTRITION.
Total parenteral nutrition (TPN) is indicated when oral intake or enteral feeding is inadequate to meet metabolic needs for more than 3 to 5 days. Other indicators for TPN include conditions in which bowel rest is desirable or the gastrointestinal tract is nonfunctioning. The solutions are administered through a catheter inserted into the superior vena cava via the subclavian or internal jugular vein, where a high rate of blood flow enables rapid dilution to avoid irritation of venous endothelium.

TPN solutions are prepared under aseptic conditions and individualized based on nutrient needs and laboratory tests. Nutrients provided include dextrose, amino acids, electrolytes, vitamins, minerals, and fat emulsions. Solutions are delivered at a continuous rate via an infusion pump to prevent metabolic complications. TPN infusion rates are gradually advanced to the desired caloric intake, allowing body adaption, and gradually decreased before discontinuing therapy to avoid rebound hypoglycemia.

Mechanical, metabolic, and sepsis complications can occur with TPN. These complications are mostly avoidable with proper care and well-defined protocols. Three potential complications of TPN and related preventive administration measures are presented in Table 19–9.

Home TPN is now a common mode of therapy for persons who do not need to be hospitalized but can benefit from continued nutritional support. With adequate instruction and supportive follow-up, an older adult and/or caregiver can successfully manage TPN at home.

T A B L E   1 9 – 9
Three Complications of Parenteral Nutrition and Preventive Measures

COMPLICATION	PREVENTIVE MEASURES
Infection	Refrigerate solution until 30 min before using
	Use new infusion set with each new bag of solution; change filters every 24 hr
	Maintain an aseptic delivery system
	Maintain sterile, dry occlusive dressing over catheter insertion site
	Perform dressing change and skin care at catheter insertion site using aseptic technique
	Monitor vital signs q 4 hr
Air Embolism	Use Valsalva maneuver when changing tubing
	Clamp catheter when changing tubing
	Remove air from tubing before connecting to catheter
	Maintain secure catheter and tubing connections
Hypoglycemia, Hyperglycemia	Observe for signs of hypo/hyperglycemia
	Monitor serum glucose and potassium
	Administer regular insulin as ordered
	Use an infusion pump to insure constant rate of solution delivery
	Gradually increase and decrease infusion rate when initiating and discontinuing TPN
	Monitor intake and output

Data from Davis, C. Nursing care of total parenteral and enteral nutrition. *In* Fischer, J.E. (ed.). *Total Parenteral Nutrition.* 2nd ed. Boston: Little, Brown, 1991, pp. 112–121; and Weinsier, R.L. and Morgan, S.L. *Fundamentals of Clinical Nutrition.* St. Louis: C.V. Mosby, 1993, pp. 158–159.

Impaired Swallowing/Dysphagia

Definition and Scope

Dysphagia refers to difficulty in swallowing. Concurrent xerostomia (dry mouth), fatigue or activity intolerance, and decreased chewing ability further complicate this problem. Persons with dysphagia are at risk for nutritional deficiency because of their inability to ingest sufficient amounts of essential nutrients.

Dysphagia may be divided into two types:

- Oropharyngeal or transfer dysphagia
- Esophageal dysphagia (Castell, 1990)

Trouble initiating a swallow or voluntary transfer of food or fluid from the mouth into the esophagus is termed *oropharyngeal* or *transfer dysphagia*. Other symptoms associated with transfer dysphagia are nasal regurgitation, coughing during swallowing, and dysarthria due to weakness of palatal muscles. Difficulty with food and/or fluid transport down the esophagus after swallowing is termed *esophageal dysphagia*. Characteristic of esophageal dysphagia is a sensation of food stopping or sticking after it has been swallowed.

Etiology

Dysphagia can result from a number of causes: esophageal motility disorders, stroke, Parkinson's disease, other degenerative neuromuscular disorders, and mechanical obstruction such as stricture or spasm. A complete evaluation to identify the cause of dysphagia is necessary for development of an effective treatment plan. Radiographic studies of swallowing or endoscopy or both usually are necessary.

Management

The goal of dysphagia management is to enhance swallowing ability to meet fluid, calorie, and other essential nutrient needs. Achievement of this goal requires a collaborative effort by the nurse, physician, speech therapist, and dietitian.

Management measures focus on the prevention of aspiration, use of specific feeding techniques, and diet modification (Donahue, 1990; Ferri, 1994). Dysphagia diet staging and feeding techniques and tips are presented in Table 19–10.

Health-Seeking Behaviors and Knowledge Deficit

The nursing diagnosis Health-Seeking Behaviors refers to individuals in stable health

T A B L E   1 9 – 1 0
Dysphagia Diet

Stage I —Dysphagia purée, no liquids	Stage IV —Dysphagia mechanical soft foods, no liquids
Stage II —Dysphagia purée plus thick liquids	Stage V —Dysphagia mechanical soft foods plus thick liquids
Stage III —Dysphagia purée plus thin liquids	Stage VI —Dysphagia mechanical soft foods plus thin liquids

STAGE I—DYSPHAGIA PURÉE, NO LIQUIDS

No liquids are provided unless specified by physician's order. Includes smooth, moist, and puréed foods that require little or no chewing but form a moist, cohesive bolus.

Food Group	Foods Allowed	Foods Avoided
Milk products	Pudding, custard, ice cream, plain or flavored yogurt (without fruit)	All others
Meat, poultry, and eggs	Puréed meat, chicken, fish; soufflés, soft cooked or poached eggs	All others
Vegetables and fruits	Puréed vegetables, fruits; applesauce, frozen fruit juices	All others
Breads and cereals	Thick cooked cereals, mashed potato	All others
Fats	Butter, margarine, sour cream	All others
Miscellaneous	Salt, pepper, ketchup, mustard, jelly, gelatin dessert	None

STAGE II—DYSPHAGIA PURÉE PLUS THICK LIQUIDS

Includes all foods allowed in stage I with the addition of the following *thick liquids.*

Food Group	Liquids Allowed	Liquids Avoided
Milk products	Thickened eggnog, Carnation Instant Breakfast, milk shakes	All others
Soups	Thick creamed soups	Broth
Fruits	Thinned puréed fruits, nectar, vegetable juice	All others

STAGE III—DYSPHAGIA PURÉE PLUS THIN LIQUIDS

Includes all foods allowed in stage II with the addition of the following *thin liquids.*

Food Group	Liquid Allowed	Liquids Avoided
Milk products	Eggnog, Carnation Instant Breakfast, milk	None
Soup	Thin creamed soups, broth	None
Beverages	Coffee, tea, soda, fruit juices	None

Note: Once a patient has mastered stage III, the diet can be either progressed in consistency (i.e., to stage V) or changed to purée.

STAGE IV—DYSPHAGIA MECHANICAL SOFT FOODS, NO LIQUIDS

No liquids are provided unless specified by physician's order. Includes minced and soft foods that require little or no chewing but form a soft, cohesive bolus.

Food Group	Liquids Allowed	Liquids Avoided
Milk products	Pudding, custard, ice cream, cream pies; plain, flavored, fruited yogurt	All others
Cheeses	Small-curd cottage cheese, ricotta cheese, American cheese, grated cheese	All others
Eggs	Soft scrambled eggs, crustless quiche, soufflés, egg salad	All others
Meat, fish, and poultry	Ground meat or poultry with gravy; chicken or tuna salad (without celery); meat loaf; hamburger; baked or broiled fish; salmon loaf; pasta casseroles	All others
Vegetables	Cooked and diced carrots, beets, chopped or creamed spinach, butternut or acorn squash	Raw vegetables, other cooked vegetables
Potatoes, rice, and noodles	Mashed or baked (without skin) potatoes, macaroni and cheese, egg noodles, spaghetti with gravy or sauce	Rice, coarse grain (kasha, buckwheat, bran)
Fruit	Mashed banana, canned or cooked fruits cut into small pieces	Fruits with pits, raisins; all others
Breads and cereals	Bread, soft rolls, muffins, soft French toast, pancakes, cooked cereal, dry cereals soaked in milk, cakes without nuts	Dry crackers, breads with seeds, raisins, nuts
Fats	Butter, margarine, sour cream, gravy, mayonnaise	Nuts, seeds

Table continued on following page

TABLE 19–10
Dysphagia Diet *Continued*

STAGE V—DYSPHAGIA MECHANICAL SOFT FOODS PLUS THICK LIQUIDS

Includes all food from stage IV with the addition of *thick liquids* as outlined in stage II.

STAGE VI—DYSPHAGIA MECHANICAL SOFT FOODS PLUS THIN LIQUIDS

Includes all food from stage IV with the addition of *thin liquids* as outlined in stage III.

Note: Once a patient has mastered stage VI, the diet can be either progressed in consistency (i.e., to regular) or changed to mechanical soft foods.

Patients at stages I and IV need to have fluid status monitored and fluid requirements met by alternate means.

Milk products may not be tolerated by individuals who are susceptible to increased mucus production probably secondary to casein, a milk protein. If this becomes a problem, substitutes should be found.

Suggestions for Dietitians:
1. A member of the medical or nursing staff or dysphagia team should be present at the bedside when a patient initially receives a dysphagia diet or advances to a higher stage, to evaluate the patient's tolerance of the stage.
2. The dietitian should work closely with medical and nursing staff for continued evaluation of the patient's diet tolerance and progression.

3. Calorie counts are indicated to evaluate adequacy of intake and to justify the need for supplementation or nutrition support.
4. The dietitian should work closely with the dysphagia team for physiological evaluation of the patient's ability to chew and swallow to select the correct diet stage.
5. The dietitian should encourage small, frequent meals, particularly in the first stages of the diet.
6. As a guide, the following list gives a progression of food consistencies in order of increasing swallowing difficulty:
   - stiff jelled consistency
   - standard jelled consistency
   - thick purées
   - applesauce consistency
   - thick soup consistency
   - nectar consistency
   - standard thin liquids
   - chunk consistency (ground or diced)

Eating Tips:
1. Food should be taken in small portions (1/2 tsp at a time).
2. The patient should sit upright with hips flexed at a 90° angle.
3. If possible, the neck should be at a 90° angle and flexed slightly forward.
4. The patient should sit up for 15 to 30 minutes both before and after meals.
5. Food should be placed on the unaffected side when possible.
6. Cold or hot foods may be better tolerated than foods at room temperature.

From Antiaspiration-dysphagia diet. *In* Diet manual. New York: Memorial Sloan-Kettering Cancer Center, 1989. Reprinted by permission; and Bloch, A.S. Nutrition Management of the Cancer Patient. Rockville, MD: Aspen Publishers, 1990. With permission.

---

who are actively seeking ways to achieve a higher level of health. The nursing diagnosis Knowledge Deficit refers to situations in which the individual lacks specific information to make informed decisions about health care. Both diagnoses are applicable to two important aspects of nursing care addressing nutritional needs: screening and education.

Nutrition Education

Providing learning experiences involves a needs assessment, development of objectives, identification of content, selection of learning activities, implementation of learning activities, and evaluation of learning. To be effective, planned learning experiences need to incorporate principles of adult learning as well as accommodate normal age-related physical changes. Older adults are most interested in information that is of immediate use, problem-centered, and based on their own identified learning needs (Knowles, 1970). To facilitate information processing,

teaching strategies need to compensate for reduced visual and auditory acuity, short-term memory, and attention span (Kicklighter, 1991; Weinrich and Boyd, 1992). Appropriate strategies include a nondistracting environment, small groups, shorter teaching sessions, presentation of one to three new ideas at a time, and uncluttered large print visuals.

A nutrition instruction model that has been effective in changing dietary behaviors in the elderly is one based on the principles of activated health education (Kupka-Schutt and Mitchell, 1992; Mitic, 1985). This model involves three phases of instruction. In the first phase, *nutrition skills experiences*, participants are shown how to evaluate their dietary intake. During the second phase, *cognitive nutrition instruction*, participants are provided nutrition information based on their needs and interests, using a variety of teaching strategies. In the final phase, *affective nutrition instruction*, participants set their own goals and develop a plan for making changes to improve their dietary intake.

DETERMINE YOUR NUTRITIONAL HEALTH

The Warning Signs of poor nutritional health are often overlooked. Use this checklist to find out if you or someone you know is at nutritional risk.

Read the statements below. Circle the number in the yes column for those that apply to you or someone you know. For each yes answer, score the number in the box. Total your nutritional score.

	YES
I have an illness or condition that made me change the kind and/or amount of food I eat.	2
I eat fewer than 2 meals per day.	3
I eat few fruits or vegetables, or milk products.	2
I have 3 or more drinks of beer, liquor or wine almost every day.	2
I have tooth or mouth problems that make it hard for me to eat.	2
I don't always have enough money to buy the food I need.	4
I eat alone most of the time.	1
I take 3 or more different prescribed or over-the-counter drugs a day.	1
Without wanting to, I have lost or gained 10 pounds in the last 6 months.	2
I am not always physically able to shop, cook and/or feed myself.	2
TOTAL	

Total Your Nutritional Score. If It's —

0-2 **Good!** Recheck your nutritional score in 6 months.

3-5 **You are at moderate nutritional risk.** See what can be done to improve your eating habits and lifestyle. Your office on aging, senior nutrition program, senior citizens center or health department can help. Recheck your nutritional score in 3 months.

6 or more **You are at high nutritional risk.** Bring this checklist the next time you see your doctor, dietitian or other qualified health or social service professional. Talk with them about any problems you may have. Ask for help to improve your nutritional health.

Implementing Nutrition Screening and Intervention Strategies

These materials developed and distributed by the Nutrition Screening Initiative, a project of:

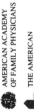 AMERICAN ACADEMY OF FAMILY PHYSICIANS

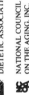 THE AMERICAN DIETETIC ASSOCIATION

NATIONAL COUNCIL ON THE AGING, INC.

Remember that warning signs suggest risk, but do not represent diagnosis of any condition. Turn the page to learn more about the Warning Signs of poor nutritional health.

The Nutrition Checklist is based on the Warning Signs described below. Use the word DETERMINE to remind you of the Warning Signs.

Disease
Any disease, illness or chronic condition which causes you to change the way you eat, or makes it hard for you to eat, puts your nutritional health at risk. Four out of five adults have chronic diseases that are affected by diet. Confusion or memory loss that keeps getting worse is estimated to affect one out of five or more of older adults. This can make it hard to remember what, when or if you've eaten. Feeling sad or depressed, which happens to about one in eight older adults, can cause big changes in appetite, digestion, energy level, and well-being.

Eating poorly
Eating too little and eating too much both lead to poor health. Eating the same foods day after day or not eating fruit, vegetables, and milk products daily will also cause poor nutritional health. One in five adults skip meals daily. Only 13% of adults eat the minimum amount of fruit and vegetables needed. One in four older adults drink too much alcohol. Many health problems become worse if you drink more than one or two alcoholic beverages per day.

Tooth loss/ mouth pain
A healthy mouth, teeth and gums are needed to eat. Missing, loose or rotten teeth or dentures which don't fit well or cause mouth sores make it hard to eat.

Economic hardship
As many as 40% of older Americans have incomes of less than $6,000 per year. Having less -- or choosing to spend less -- than $25-30 per week for food makes it very hard to get the foods you need to stay healthy.

Reduced social contact
One-third of all older people live alone. Being with people daily has a positive effect on morale, well-being and eating.

Multiple medicines
Many older Americans must take medicines for health problems. Almost half of older Americans take multiple medicines daily. Growing old may change the way we respond to drugs. The more medicines you take, the greater the chance for side effects such as increased or decreased appetite, change in taste, constipation, weakness, drowsiness, diarrhea, nausea, and others. Vitamins or minerals when taken in large doses act like drugs and can cause harm. Alert your doctor to everything you take.

Involuntary weight loss/gain
Losing or gaining a lot of weight when you are not trying to do so is an important warning sign that must not be ignored. Being overweight or underweight also increases your chance of poor health.

Needs assistance in self care
Although most older people are able to eat, one of every five have trouble walking, shopping, buying and cooking food, especially as they get older.

Elder years above age 80
Most older people lead full and productive lives. But as age increases, risk of frailty and health problems increase. Checking your nutritional health regularly makes good sense.

The Nutrition Screening Initiative, 1010 Wisconsin Avenue, NW, Suite 800, Washington, DC 20007
The Nutrition Screening Initiative is funded in part by a grant from Abbott Laboratories, a division of Abbott Laboratories

FIGURE 19-5

Nutrition checklist. (From Gallagher-Allred, C.R. Implementing Nutrition Screening and Intervention Strategies. Washington, D.C.: Nutrition Screening Initiative, 1993, pp. 89–90. Reprinted with permission by the Nutrition Screening Initiative, a project of the American Academy of Family Physicians, the American Dietetic Association and the National Council on the Aging, Inc., and funded in part by a grant from Ross Products Division, Abbott Laboratories.)

Level II Screen

Complete the following screen by interviewing the patient directly and/or by referring to the patient chart. If you do not routinely perform all of the described tests or ask all of the listed questions, please consider including them but do not be concerned if the entire screen is not completed. Please try to conduct a minimal screen on as many older patients as possible, and please try to collect serial measurements, which are extremely valuable in monitoring nutritional status. Please refer to the manual for additional information.

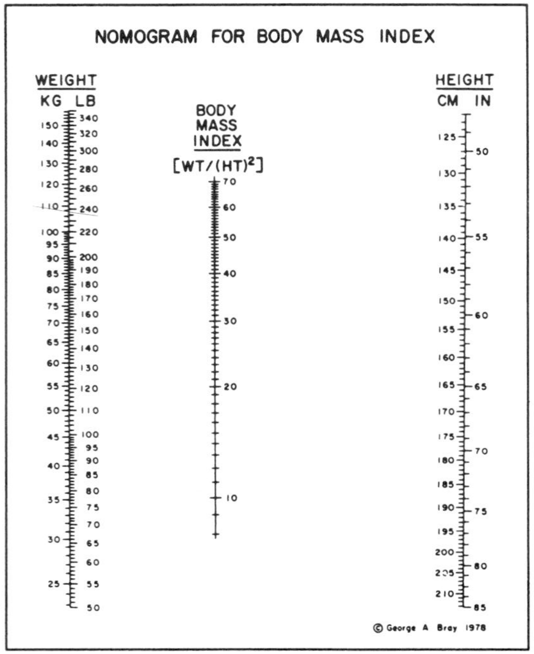

Anthropometrics

Measure height to the nearest inch and weight to the nearest pound. Record the values below and mark them on the Body Mass Index (BMI) scale to the right. Then use a straight edge (paper, ruler) to connect the two points and circle the spot where this straight line crosses the center line (body mass index). Record the number below; healthy older adults should have a BMI between 24 and 27; check the appropriate box to flag an abnormally high or low value.

NOMOGRAM FOR BODY MASS INDEX

© George A. Bray 1978

Height (in): _____
Weight (lbs): _____
Body Mass Index (weight/height²): _____

Please place a check by any statement regarding BMI and recent weight loss that is true for the patient.

☐ Body mass index <24
☐ Body mass index >27
☐ Has lost or gained 10 pounds (or more) of body weight in the past 6 months

Record the measurement of mid-arm circumference to the nearest 0.1 centimeter and of triceps skinfold to the nearest 2 millimeters.

Mid-Arm Circumference (cm): _____
Triceps Skinfold (mm): _____
Mid-Arm Muscle Circumference (cm): _____

Refer to the table and check any abnormal values:

☐ Mid-arm muscle circumference <10th percentile

Implementing Nutrition Screening and Intervention Strategies

☐ Triceps skinfold <10th percentile
☐ Triceps skinfold >95th percentile

Note: mid-arm circumference (cm) - (0.314 x triceps skinfold (mm)) = mid-arm *muscle* circumference (cm)

For the remaining sections, please place a check by any statements that are true for the patient.

Laboratory Data

☐ Serum albumin below 3.5 g/dl
☐ Serum cholesterol below 160 mg/dl
☐ Serum cholesterol above 240 mg/dl

Drug Use

☐ Three or more prescription drugs, OTC medications, and/or vitamin/mineral supplements daily

---

Clinical Features

Presence of (check each that apply):

☐ Problems with mouth, teeth, or gums
☐ Difficulty chewing
☐ Difficulty swallowing
☐ Angular stomatitis
☐ Glossitis
☐ History of bone pain
☐ History of bone fractures
☐ Skin changes (dry, loose, nonspecific lesions, edema)

Eating Habits

☐ Does not have enough food to eat each day
☐ Usually eats alone
☐ Does not eat anything on one or more days each month
☐ Has poor appetite
☐ Is on a special diet
☐ Eats vegetables two or fewer times daily
☐ Eats milk or milk products once or not at all daily
☐ Eats fruit or drinks fruit juice once or not at all daily
☐ Eats breads, cereals, pasta, rice, or other grains five or fewer times daily
☐ Has more than one alcoholic drink per day (if woman); more than two drinks per day (if man)

Living Environment

☐ Lives on an income of less than $6000 per year (per individual in the household)
☐ Lives alone
☐ Is housebound
☐ Is concerned about home security

☐ Lives in a home with inadequate heating or cooling
☐ Does not have a stove and/or refrigerator
☐ Is unable or prefers not to spend money on food (<$25-30 per person spent on food each week)

Functional Status

Usually or always needs assistance with (check each that apply):

☐ Bathing
☐ Dressing
☐ Grooming
☐ Toileting
☐ Eating
☐ Walking or moving about
☐ Traveling (outside the home)
☐ Preparing food
☐ Shopping for food or other necessities

Mental/Cognitive Status

☐ Clinical evidence of impairment, e.g. Folstein<26
☐ Clinical evidence of depressive illness, e.g. Beck Depression Inventory>15, Geriatric Depression Scale>5

Patients in whom you have identified one or more major indicator* of poor nutritional status require immediate medical attention; if minor indicators are found, ensure that they are known to a health professional or to the patient's own physician. Patients who display risk factors of poor nutritional status should be referred to the appropriate health care or social service professional (dietitian, nurse, dentist, case manager, etc.).

These materials developed by the Nutrition Screening Initiative.

*see Table 19-11.

	Men		Women	
Percentile	55-65 y	65-75 y	55-65 y	65-75 y
Arm circumference (cm)				
10th	27.3	26.3	25.7	25.2
50th	31.7	30.7	30.3	29.9
95th	36.9	35.5	38.5	37.3
Arm muscle circumference (cm)				
10th	24.5	23.5	19.6	19.5
50th	27.8	26.8	22.5	22.5
95th	32.0	30.6	28.0	27.9
Triceps skinfold (mm)				
10th	6	6	16	14
50th	11	11	25	24
95th	22	22	38	36

From: Frisancho AR. New norms of upper limb fat and muscle areas for assessment of nutritional status. Am J Clin Nutr 1981; 34:2540-2545. © 1981 American Society for Clinical Nutrition.

FIGURE 19-6

Screening tool for clinical settings. (From Gallagher-Allred, C.R. Implementing Nutrition Screening and Intervention Strategies. Washington, D.C.: Nutrition Screening Initiative, 1993, pp. 97-98. Reprinted with permission by the Nutrition Screening Initiative, a project of the American Academy of Family Physicians, the American Dietetic Association and the National Council on the Aging, Inc., and funded in part by a grant from Ross Products Division, Abbott Laboratories.)

TABLE 19-11

Nutrition Screening Initiative Risk Factors and Indicators of Poor Nutritional Status

RISK FACTORS
Inappropriate food intake
Poverty
Social isolation
Dependency/disability
Acute/chronic diseases or conditions
Chronic medication use
Advanced age (80+)

MAJOR AND MINOR INDICATORS

Major Indicators
Weight loss of 10 lbs. +
Underweight/overweight
Serum albumin below 3.5 gm/dl
Change in functional status
Inappropriate food intake
Midarm muscle circumference <10th percentile
Triceps skinfold <10th percentile or >95th percentile
Obesity
Nutrition-related disorders
Osteoporosis
Osteomalacia
Folate deficiency
B_{12} deficiency

Minor Indicators
Alcoholism
Cognitive impairment
Chronic renal insufficiency
Multiple concurrent medications
Malabsorption syndromes
Anorexia, nausea, dysphagia
Change in bowel habit
Fatigue, apathy, memory loss
Poor oral/dental status
Dehydration
Poorly healing wounds
Loss of subcutaneous fat or muscle mass
Fluid retention
Reduced iron, ascorbic acid, zinc

From The Nutrition Screening Initiative. *Report of Nutrition Screening I: Toward A Common View.* Washington, D.C.: 1991.

During this phase, the instructional climate is nonevaluative, encouraging expression of feelings about dietary change and fostering peer support.

Nutrition Screening

Based on recommendations from the 1988 Surgeon General's Workshop on Health Promotion and Aging and the U.S. Department of Health and Human Services Report *Healthy People 2000*, the Nutrition Screening Initiative (NSI) was formed in 1990 as a 5-year project to promote improved nutritional care for older adults. This project is sponsored by the American Academy of Family Physicians, the American Dietetic Associa-tion, and the National Council on Aging, Inc. A multidisciplinary Blue Ribbon Advisory Committee and Technical Review Committee provide expert advice and support for the project.

NSI has created an interdisciplinary, community-based model for nutrition screening and intervention that encourages use of existing programs and resources. Tools developed through this project enable a tiered approach to nutrition screening. The *DETERMINE Your Nutritional Health Checklist* (Fig. 19-5) is a self-test checklist designed to increase the awareness of older adults or their caregivers of warning signs of poor nutrition. The *LEVEL I SCREEN* and *LEVEL II SCREEN* (Fig. 19-6) are designed for use by health care professionals. Interventions delineated by NSI for risks and problems identified from these screening tools address social services, oral health, mental health, medication use, nutrition education and counseling, and nutrition support. The NSI model for nutrition screening and intervention has been successfully incorporated into community meal programs, senior centers, adult day care centers, home services programs, ambulatory health care facilities, hospitals, and long-term care facilities under the leadership of nurses and other professional health care providers.*

SUMMARY

Nurses have many opportunities to promote health in older adults. A growing body of knowledge about the impact of nutritional alterations in later life, along with increased and sophisticated methods of assessment and treatment, has expanded nutritional therapy into a truly multidisciplinary endeavor. To serve older persons best, nurses in all care settings should routinely conduct nutritional assessments and intervene when possible to promote optimal nutritional status.

REFERENCES

Ausman, L.M. and Russell, R.M. Nutrition in the elderly. *In* Shils, M.E., Olson, J.A. and Shike, M. (eds.). *Modern Nutrition in Health and Disease.* Vol. 1, 8th ed. Philadelphia: Lea & Febiger, 1994, pp. 770–780.

*For copies of NSI screening tools, implementation manuals, and other publications, write to Nutrition Screening Initiative, 2626 Pennsylvania Avenue, Washington, D.C. 20073.

Bonnel, W.B. The nursing home group dining room: Managing the work of eating. *J Nutr Elderly* 13(1):1–10, 1993.

Bowman, B.A., Rosenberg, I.H. and Johnson, M.A. Gastrointestinal function in the elderly. *In* Munro, H.I. and Schlierf, G. (eds.). *Nutrition of the Elderly*. New York: Raven Press, 1991, pp. 43–50.

Bray, G.A. and Gray, D.S. Obesity. Part I—Pathogenesis. *West J Med* 149:429–441, 1988a.

Bray, G.A. and Gray, D.S. Obesity. Part II—Treatment. *West J Med* 149:555–571, 1988b.

Campillo, B., Bories, P.N., Devanlay, M. et al. Aging, energy expenditure and nutritional status: Evidence for denutrition-related hypermetabolism. *Ann Nutr Metab* 36:265–272, 1992.

Castell, D.O. Eating and swallowing disorders. *In* Hazzard, W.R., Andres, R., Bierman, E.L. and Blass, J.P. (eds.). *Principles of Geriatric Medicine and Gerontology*. 2nd. ed. New York: McGraw-Hill, 1990, pp. 1115–1160.

Chernoff, R. Nutritional support in the elderly. *In* Chernoff, R. (ed.). *Geriatric Nutrition: The Health Professional's Handbook*. Gaithersburg, MD: Aspen Publishers, 1991, pp. 397–413.

Chumlea, W.C. Anthropometric assessment of nutritional status in the elderly. *In* Himes, J.H. (ed.). *Anthropometric Assessment of Nutritional Status*. New York: Wiley-Liss, 1991, pp. 399–418.

Chumlea, W.C., Roche, H.F. and Steinbaugh, M.L. Estimating stature from knee height for persons 60 to 90 years of age. *J Am Geriatr Soc* 33(2):116–120, 1985.

Committee on Diet and Health. *Diet and Health: Implications for Reducing Chronic Disease Risk*. Washington, D.C.: National Academy Press, 1989.

Davis, C.L. Nursing care of total parenteral and enteral nutrition. *In* Fischer, J.E. (ed.). *Total Parenteral Nutrition*. 2nd ed. Boston: Little, Brown, 1991, pp. 111–126.

Dolan, T., Monopole, M.P., Kaurick, M.J. and Rubenstein, L.Z. Geriatric grand rounds: Oral disease in older adults. *J Am Geriatr Soc* 38:1239–1250, 1990.

Donahue, P.A. When it's hard to swallow: Feeding techniques for dysphagia management. *J Gerontol Nurs* 16(4):6–9, 1990.

Drugay, M. Nutritional evaluation: Who needs it? *J Gerontol Nurs* 12(4):14–18, 1986.

Dudek, S.G. *Nutrition Handbook for Nursing Practice*. 2nd ed. Philadelphia: J.B. Lippincott, 1993.

Dwyer, J.T., Gallo, J.J. and Reichel, W. Assessing nutritional status in elderly patients. *Am Family Phys* 47(3): 613–620, 1993.

Eaton, M., Mitchell-Bonair, I.L. and Friedman, E. The effect of touch on nutritional intake of chronic organic brain syndrome patients. *J Gerontol* 41(5):611–616, 1986.

Ferri, R.S. *Care Planning for the Older Adult: Nursing Diagnoses in Long-Term Care*. Philadelphia: W.B. Saunders, 1994.

Fischer, J. and Johnson, M.A. Low body weight and weight loss in the aged. *J Am Diet Assoc* 90(12):1697–1706, 1990.

Graham, K.M., Pecoraro, D.A., Ventura, M. and Meyer, C.C. Reducing the incidence of stomatitis using a quality assessment and improvement approach. *Cancer Nurs* 16(2):117–122, 1993.

Grant, J.P. *Handbook of Total Parenteral Nutrition*. 2nd ed. Philadelphia: W.B. Saunders, 1992.

Hall, G.R. Chronic dementia: Challenges in feeding a patient. *J Gerontol Nurs* 20(4):21–30, 1994.

Ham, R.J. Indicators of poor nutritional status. *Am Family Phys* 45(1):219–228, 1992.

Hogstel, M.O. and Robinson, N.B. Feeding the frail elderly. *J Gerontol Nurs* 15(3):16–20, 1989.

Horwath, C.C. Nutrition goals for older adults: A review. *Gerontologists*, 31(6):811–821, 1991.

Keller, H.H. Malnutrition in institutionalized elderly: How and why? *J Am Geriatr Soc* 41(11):1212–1218, 1993.

Kenny, S.A. Effect of two oral care protocols on the incidence of stomatitis in hematology patients. *Cancer Nurs* 13(6):345–353, 1990.

Kicklighter, J.R. Characteristics of older adult learners: A guide for dietetics practitioners. *J Am Diet Assoc* 91(11):1418–1422, 1991.

Knowles, M. *The Modern Practice of Adult Education: Andragogy Versus Pedagogy*. New York: Association Press, 1970.

Kupka-Schutt, L. and Mitchell, M.E. Positive effect of a nutrition instruction model on the dietary behavior of a selected group of elderly. *J Nutr Elderly* 12(2):29–53, 1992.

Lange-Alberts, M.E. and Shott, S. Nutritional intake: Use of touch and verbal cueing. *J Gerontol Nurs* 20(2): 36–40, 1994.

Lee, C.J., Warren, A.P., Godwin, S. et al. Impact of special diets on the nutrient intakes of southern rural elderly. *J Am Diet Assoc* 93(2):186–188, 1993.

Lipschitz, D.A. Nutrition and aging. *In* Evans, J.G. and Williams, T.F. (eds.). *Oxford Textbook of Geriatric Medicine*. Oxford: Oxford University Press, 1992, pp. 119–127.

Lohman, J., Martorell, R. and Roche, A.F. (eds.). *Anthropometric Standardization Reference Manual*. Champaign, IL: Human Kinetics Books, 1988.

Lutz, C.A. and Przytulski, K.R. *Nutrition and Diet Therapy*. Philadelphia: F.A. Davis, 1994.

Mahan, L.K. and Arlin, M. *Krause's Food, Nutrition and Diet Therapy*. Philadelphia: W.B. Saunders, 1992.

Martin, W.E. Oral health in the elderly. *In* Chernoff, R. (ed.). *Geriatric Nutrition*. Gaithersburg, MD: Aspen Publishers, 1991, pp. 107–181.

Mitic, W. Nutrition education for older adults: Implementation of a nutrition instruction program. *Health Educ* 16:7–9, 1985.

Morley, J.E. Appetite regulation by gut peptides. *Annu Rev Nutr* 10:383–395, 1990.

Morley, J.E. and Silver, A.J. Anorexia in the elderly. *Neurobiol Aging* 9:9–16, 1988.

Murphy, C. Nutrition and chemosensory perception in the elderly. *Crit Rev Food Sci Nutr* 33:3–15, 1993.

Opheim, C. and Wesselman, J. Optimal dietary prescribing in the nursing home. *Geriatrics* 45(7):66–71, 1990.

Osborn, C.L. and Marshall, M.J. Self-feeding performance in nursing home residents. *J Gerontol Nurs* 19(3): 7–14, 1993.

Phillips, P.A., Rolls, B.J., Ledingham, J.G.G. et al. Reduced thirst after water deprivation in healthy elderly men. *N Engl J Med* 311(12):753–759, 1984.

Pi-Sunyer, F.X. Obesity. *In* Shils, M.E., Olson, J.A. and Shike, M. (eds.). *Modern Nutrition in Health and Disease*. 8th ed. Philadelphia: Lea & Febiger, 1994, pp. 984–1006.

Powers, J.S. and Folk, C. Nutritional concerns in the elderly. *South Med J* 85(11):1107–1112, 1992.

Robinson, C.H., Weigley, E.S. and Mueller, D.H. *Basic Nutrition and Diet Therapy*. 7th ed. New York: Macmillan, 1993.

Roe, D.A. *Geriatric Nutrition*. Englewood Cliffs, NJ: Prentice-Hall, 1983.

Roe, D.A. Drug-nutrient interactions in the elderly. *Geriatrics* 41(3):57–74, 1986.

Rogers, J.C. and Snow, T. An assessment of the feeding behaviors of the institutionalized elderly. *Am J Occup Ther* 36(6):375–380, 1982.

Rolls, B.J. Regulation of food and fluid intake in the elderly. *Ann N Y Acad Sci* 561:217–225, 1989.

Rudman, D. and Cohan, M.E. Nutrition in the elderly. *In* Calkins, E., Ford, A.B. and Katz, P.R. (eds.). *Practice of Geriatrics.* 2nd ed. Philadelphia: W.B. Saunders, 1992, pp. 19–32.

Rudman, D. and Feller, A.G. Protein-calorie undernutrition in the nursing home. *J Am Geriatr Soc* 37(2):173–183, 1989.

Russell, R.M. and Suter, P.M. Vitamin requirements of elderly people: An update. *Am J Clin Nutr* 58:4–14, 1993.

Saunders, H.N., Hoffman, S.B. and Lund, C.A. Feeding strategy for dependent eaters. *J Am Diet Assoc* 92(11): 1389–1390, 1992.

Schiffman, S.S. and Warwick, Z.S. Effect of flavor enhancement of foods for the elderly on nutritional status: Food intake, biochemical indices, and anthropometric measures. *Physiol Behav* 53:395–402, 1993.

Shaw-Stiffel, T.A., Zarny, L.A., Pleban, W.E. et al. Effect of nutrition status and other factors on length of hospital stay after major gastrointestinal surgery. *Nutrition* 9(2):140–145, 1993.

Silver, A.J. Aging and risks for dehydration. *Cleveland Clin J Med* 57(4):341–344, 1990.

Silver, A.J. The malnourished older patient: When and how to intervene. *Geriatrics* 48(7):70–74, 1993.

Sullivan, D.H. Risk factors for early hospital readmission in a select population of geriatric rehabilitation patients: The significance of nutritional status. *J Am Geriatr Soc* 40(8):792–798, 1992.

Sullivan, D.H., Patch, G.A., Walls, R.C. and Lipschitz, D.A. Impact of nutrition status on morbidity and mortality in a selected population of geriatric rehabilitation patients. *Am J Clin Nutr* 51:749–758, 1990.

Suski, N.S. and Nielsen, C.C. Factors affecting food intake of women with Alzheimer's type dementia in long-term care. *J Am Diet Assoc* 89:1770–1773, 1989.

Walker, D. and Beauchene, R.E. The relationship of loneliness, social isolation, and physical health to dietary adequacy of independently living elderly. *J Am Diet Assoc* 91(3):300–304, 1991.

Weinrich, S.P. and Boyd, M. Education in the elderly: Adapting and evaluating teaching tools. *J Gerontol Nurs* 18(1):15–20, 1992.

Weinsier, R.L. and Morgan, S. *Fundamentals of Clinical Nutrition.* St. Louis: C.V. Mosby, 1993.

Welch, P.K., Dowson, M. and Endres, J.M. The effect of nutrient supplements on high-risk long-term care residents receiving puréed diets. *J Nutr Elderly* 10(3):49–62, 1991.

Welnetz, K. Maintaining adequate nutrition and hydration in the dysphagic ALS patient. *Can Nurse* 93(3):30–35, 1983.

White, J.V. Risk factors for poor nutritional status in older Americans. *Am Family Phys* 44(6):2087–2097, 1991.

Care Settings

5

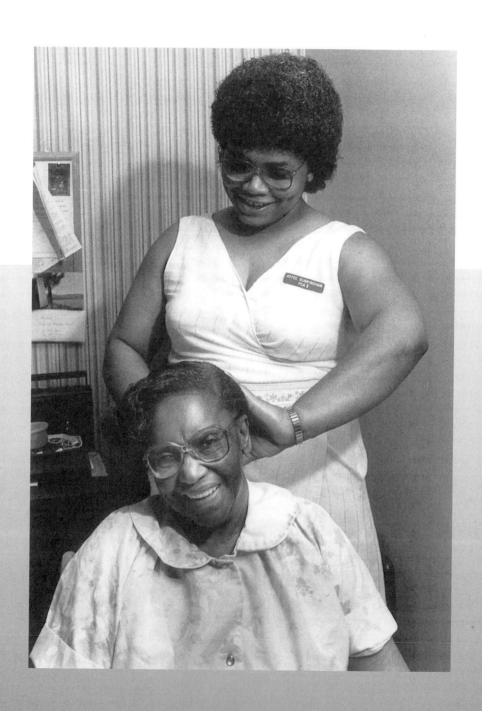

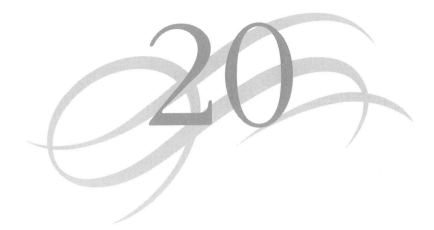

Context of Services—
Network of Care

SUSAN J. BARNES

OBJECTIVES

Define long-term care in the broad context of the health care continuum.

❖

Identify and describe health services available in the community that are appropriately used by older people.

❖

Discuss hospital usage, the Medicare Prospective Payment System and DRGs (diagnosis-related groups), hospital services related to the elderly, and managed care.

❖

Relate the current system of nursing home care to issues such as reimbursement, patient classification and health policy, and service and ownership patterns.

❖

Apply concepts of health promotion to long-term care of the elderly.

❖

Discuss practice and educational and political initiatives in long-term care.

are as important as the services provided in understanding its impact on the health of older people.

Prior to 1932, the elderly were not singled out as a discrete group of adults in the medical care or health care system. Infectious diseases were still the leading cause of death, and little attention was paid to the problems of those with chronic diseases. Care of older people took place in either the home with untrained family members as caregivers or almshouses for those who had no family. People paid what they could afford for their care; there was no health insurance (Dolan, 1983).

Today, chronic illness is the leading cause of death and disability in the United States, and increasing numbers of people are living into older age. Significant changes have occurred in health care financing and delivery since the days of the almshouse. Major federal legislation since 1932 (Table 20–1) has spawned a broad array of services, so that care of the elderly has moved from being a fairly small, unsophisticated endeavor to a large-scale, bureaucratic, expensive enterprise. Development of the current system of care has been tainted by special interest groups and the economic welfare of professionals, sometimes at the expense of the

Nursing interventions for the elderly are carried out in the context of the health care system. The *history, philosophy, economics,* and *interrelationships of* the system components

TABLE 20–1
Historical Events Affecting the Health Care System

TIME	EVENT	IMPACT ON CARE OF THE ELDERLY
1932	Social Security Act	Increased financial security for the elderly
1940s	Widespread use of antibiotics	Increased life expectancy; chronic diseases now major causes of death rather than infectious diseases
1950s	Amendments to Social Security Act	Vendor payments to nursing homes caring for the elderly allowed
1951	First White House Conference on Aging	Brought visibility to problems of the aged; began process of national level–policy making to address problems of the aged. White House Conferences on Aging have been held each decade since this time
1965	Medicare (Title XVIII of the Social Security Act)	National medical insurance for all older adults; federal government involved in setting standards for institutions providing care for the aged for the first time
	Medicaid (Title XIX of the Social Security Act)	Acute illness care widely available to people regardless of their ability to pay; increased federal regulation of hospitals, nursing homes; proliferation of nursing homes
	Title XX of the Social Security Act	In-home services for medically indigent elderly more widely available through social services agencies
1965	Older Americans Act	Established aging networks throughout the states, introduced the concept of a "focal point" for services to the aged, funded noninstitutional health services external to the social services agencies
1972	Medicare reform legislation and changes in regulations	Established intermediate care facilities as a new type of reimbursed nursing home care
1981	Omnibus Reconciliation Act	Medicare reform: waived three-day prior hospitalization requirement for extended care benefits, removed limit on number of home health visits allowed
1982	Tax Equity & Fiscal Responsibility Act (TEFRA)	Introduced prospective reimbursement for hospitals under Medicare; also initiated promulgation of regulations for hospice to allow reimbursement for hospice care under Medicare and Medicaid
1993	Health Care Reform	Concept of universal coverage. Full impact on availability of services not yet known; however, many private companies are merging to form managed care corporations

well-being of the older persons for whom the system was created. The health care reform effort begun in 1993 is an attempt in one sense to deal with these difficulties. New trends toward managed care may hold promise in better coordinating care for the elderly.

The current state of health care for the elderly is complex, controversial, and, at times, unsatisfactory. The complexity of the health care system for the elderly is not a new phenomenon, nor is it necessarily the result of governmental intervention in health services. Thomas (1969, quoting Boas, 1933) described the health care system in New York City in 1933 as follows:

Thus we find a very confused picture—patients at home who should be in hospitals, patients in hospitals who should be in less complex institutions, patients in homes for the aged that are not prepared to minister to their needs, patients in convalescent homes occupying beds needed for another purpose. A mad confusion of patients and institutions . . . It is really a scene of the greatest disorder that presents itself as the report unfolds the many types of agency that contribute to the care of the chronic sick: public and private hospitals, homes for the aged, convalescent homes, nursing and visiting doctor services, aftercare agencies for sheltered work, medical social service departments, and family service agencies.

Sixty years later, similar confusion exists. Care of the aged has never occupied a place of distinction in the American health care system. There were cries for reform as early as the early 1900s (Crane, 1907), when it was noted that the majority of those in almshouses were aged and infirm and treated not according to their health needs but according to their social status (Butler, 1975). However, apathy has surrounded policy development until recently (Vladeck, 1980). The 1993 Health Care Reform initiatives are the most recent attempt to deal with the discrepancies in care for the American population, especially the elderly. Despite the difficulties encountered in legislative reform, practice reform can be seen in movements toward a system of managed care (Kane, 1995).

LONG-TERM CARE

In 1988, approximately 6.9 million older people needed long-term care. By the year 2000, the number is expected to increase to 9 million (U.S. Senate Special Committee on Aging, 1991). Long-term care (LTC) is generally defined as

. . . a range of services that addresses the health, personal care, and social needs of individuals who lack some capacity for self-care. Services may be continuous or intermittent, but are delivered for a sustained period to individuals who have a demonstrated need, usually measured by some index of functional dependency (Kane and Kane, 1982).

Long-term care in its broadest definition implies both a range of services and a concept of care. The various types of care and services encompassed in the LTC continuum include both community-based services,

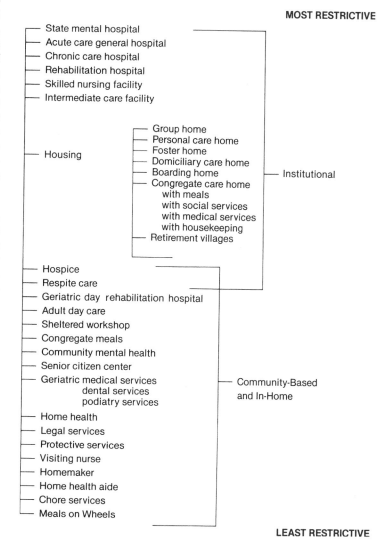

MOST RESTRICTIVE

- State mental hospital
- Acute care general hospital
- Chronic care hospital
- Rehabilitation hospital
- Skilled nursing facility
- Intermediate care facility

- Housing
  - Group home
  - Personal care home
  - Foster home
  - Domiciliary care home
  - Boarding home
  - Congregate care home
    with meals
    with social services
    with medical services
    with housekeeping
  - Retirement villages

— Institutional

- Hospice
- Respite care
- Geriatric day rehabilitation hospital
- Adult day care
- Sheltered workshop
- Congregate meals
- Community mental health
- Senior citizen center
- Geriatric medical services
    dental services
    podiatry services
- Home health
- Legal services
- Protective services
- Visiting nurse
- Homemaker
- Home health aide
- Chore services
- Meals on Wheels

— Community-Based and In-Home

LEAST RESTRICTIVE

FIGURE 20–1

Continuum of care for the elderly. (From Brody, S.J., Masciocchi, C. Data for long-term care planning by health systems agencies. *Am J Public Health* 10: 11, 1980.)

Service Needs of the Chronically Impaired Elderly	Medicaid (Title XIX of the Social Security Act)	Medicare (Title XVIII of the Social Security Act)	Social Services (Title XX of the Social Security Act)	Supplemental Security Income (Title XVI of the Social Security Act)	Administration on Aging	Veterans Administration
Medical services	X	X				X
Home nursing services	X	X				
Home health aide	X	X	X		X	X
Homemaker services			X		X	
Personal care	X		X			X
Chore/home repair services			X		X	
Home-delivered meals			X		X	
Shopping assistance			X		X	
Transportation			X		X	
Adult day care			X			
Housing assistance						
Congregate housing/domiciliary homes/adult foster care			X	X		
Respite care			X			
Congregate meals			X		X	X
Day hospital services	X					
Social/recreational services					X	
Legal and financial counseling			X		X	
Mental health services		X	X			
Information and referral			X		X	X

FIGURE 20–2

Major federal programs funding community services for the elderly.

such as home health care and nutrition programs, and institution-based services, such as boarding homes, chronic care hospitals, and nursing homes. Traditionally, LTC has been defined primarily as those services that were provided in an institutional setting over an extended period of time. Individuals needing continuous care often had few, if any, options for home-based care; however, in recent times, individuals often have been able to remain in their homes if needed health and social services were regularly provided. Figure 20–1 presents an example of a typical continuum of services now available in many communities.

The availability and specific nature and quality of services vary among and within each locale, presenting problems for the elderly, their caregivers, and policy makers alike. The late congressional representative Claude Pepper, who chaired the U.S. Bipartisan Commission on Comprehensive Health Care and for whom the commission was renamed, stated:

When an older person has a need for a particular service, for example in-home health services, where can he turn for help? The answer, unfortunately, is, "It all depends." Home health and supportive services are provided under Medicare, Medicaid, the social services program under Title XX of the Social Security Act, home health demonstration grants under the Public Health Services Act, two different titles of the Older Americans Act, the Senior Companion and RSVP volunteer programs under ACTION, the Older Americans Community Service Employment Program, Senior Opportunities and Services under the Community Services Act, and other statutes. All of this adds up to a bewildering maze of programs and regulations that is a nightmare for the elderly person trying to find his or her way through it (Pepper in the U.S. House, 1977, quoted in Estes, 1979).

Figure 20–2 lists the various funding sources that help support this continuum of services.

In summary, the following generalizations apply to the systems of health care for the elderly.

1. There are many components to the health care system for the elderly.
2. The components of the system vary considerably from one locale to another.
3. There are institutional and noninstitutional providers of services, and the institutional providers of care dominate the system.
4. There is a lack of well-trained geriatric experts available, and most older people receive their care from generalist health care providers or from specialists in fields other than geriatrics or gerontology. These professionals have little or no formal training in the special needs of the elderly and tend to deliver services in a fragmented manner rather than in a coordinated or team mode.
5. There is a considerable amount of governmental involvement in health care of the elderly, particularly in the areas of financing of medical care as well as financing and standard setting for long-term care.
6. There are few formal linkages between various components of the health care system. This is a by-product of the political process that brought about funding

for the system, which sought to preserve the professionals' sense of autonomy from the federal government.

The functioning of the system of health services to the elderly can be best described as disorganized, inefficient, and expensive. Confusion is generated for providers and consumers alike as they attempt to determine appropriateness of the eligibility for services. Despite the years of attempting to coordinate and coherently plan services, there is all too often the familiar story of the aged individual who just "fell through the cracks." In the system of health and long-term care, this generally means that the older person does not fit into any pre-established bureaucratic category and therefore will have to make do without needed help because of regulatory constraints or lack of availability of a needed service (Korn et al., 1989). The human costs of such disorganization in care are brought to life in the two examples that follow.

CASE STUDY. At Home

Mr. Smithy is an 85-year-old retired farmer who has "never been sick a day in his life." His daughter, hearing an advertisement for a "health fair," decides to take him along with her and they both have their blood pressures checked. Mr. Smithy's reading is 190/90. The screener suggests that Mr. Smithy see his doctor to recheck his blood pressure.

As Mr. Smithy has no regular doctor, he goes to the local hospital's ambulatory care clinic. Another reason he chooses the clinic is that he is afraid he may not be able to afford a private doctor. He has no insurance, and Social Security is his only source of income.

The clinic doctor examines him and prescribes hydrochlorothiazide, 25 mg per day. The medicine and its purpose are explained to Mr. Smithy, and he is told to return to the clinic in one week.

The prescription is filled on the way home, and the next morning Mr. Smithy, after experiencing some difficulty removing the childproof cap on the medicine bottle, takes one tablet with breakfast, as instructed.

Later that day he feels dizzy when he gets up from a chair and assumes that it is because of the new medicine. He decides not to take any more.

The following week his daughter takes him back to the clinic, where this time he sees a different doctor. His blood pressure reading is 192/94. The doctor tells Mr. Smithy to take two hydrochlorothiazide tablets each morning and return to the clinic in one week.

- Outreach mechanism—no primary care provider

- No explanation of side effects

- Poor continuity of care

- Poor assessment for compliance influenced by decreased continuity

continued on following page

CASE STUDY. At Home

continued

Mr. Smithy decides to follow the doctor's advice this time but is now unable to remove the lid from the medicine bottle. Embarrassed at not following the directions before and not wanting to be a bother to his daughter, he does not take the pills. The following week he returns to the clinic, his blood pressure reading unchanged. He sees a third doctor this time, who decides that he is refractory to diuretics and prescribes methyldopa (Aldomet). Again, the prescription is filled on the way home. This time Mr. Smithy asks his daughter to remove the cap before she leaves. He takes the drug as prescribed, and his blood pressure at the next clinic visit is 140/70. He now feels less energetic and does fewer things around the house. The following clinic visit he is told that he will not need to return to the clinic for a month. Mr. Smithy gradually becomes less and less able to care for himself, and his daughter becomes worried.

At the next clinic visit Mr. Smithy's daughter voices her concerns to the doctor. He notes the patient's complaints of decreased energy and appetite and new onset of constipation and decides, given the patient's age, to admit him to the hospital for a work-up of an occult malignancy. At this hospital, the clinic physicians do not attend patients in the hospital, so Mr. Smithy comes into the hospital under the care of a new doctor, a general internist.

- Further fragmentation of care

IN THE HOSPITAL

Mr. Smithy is admitted that day and prepared for upper and lower GI series. The second night in the hospital, unused to the environment and suffering from mild dehydration and electrolyte imbalance (undetected by nurse or physician staff), he experiences some confusion. He gets out of bed, despite the side rails, to go to the toilet, becomes dizzy because of his hypovolemia and decreased blood pressure, falls to the floor, and sustains a fractured left hip.

- Inadequate assessment by physicians or nurses

After an orthopedist confirms the diagnosis of hip fracture, he is scheduled for surgery the following day. He is then transferred to the orthopedic floor, and his medical care is assumed by the orthopedist. After Mr. Smithy has received physical therapy for 10 days, the surgeon decides that he

CASE STUDY. At Home

continued

has reached maximum benefit from his hospitalization, so arrangements are made for him to be transferred to a nursing home to receive further physical therapy. The hope is that he will eventually return home. (No one mentions to the patient or his daughter the possibility of receiving physical therapy from a home health agency.) After several days of waiting for a nursing home bed to become available, Mr. Smithy is placed in a nursing home 75 miles from his daughter's home. During his hospitalization his daughter visited him daily.

Prior to the nursing home placement, Mr. Smithy had remained alert and oriented but had shown variable motivation in physical therapy. Upon hearing of his pending transfer to the nursing home, he becomes more withdrawn. He fears that he will never return home again. Ten years before, his wife had entered a nursing home after suffering a stroke, and he swore then that he would rather die than go to a nursing home.

He is too tired and lethargic to stop his transfer to the nursing home, and so he enters, some 3 weeks after admission to the hospital. At this point his medical care is transferred to yet another physician, because he will be so far away and because none of his previous physicians sees patients in nursing homes.

IN THE NURSING HOME

At the nursing home he receives exemplary nursing care and physical therapy and slowly regains his ability to walk and do for himself. One of the staff recognizes that his blood pressure is low for his age, and he is taken off of all blood pressure medications. His daughter is able to visit weekly and is encouraged by his progress. Mr. Smithy is encouraged by the difference in the staff in this nursing home compared with the nursing home his wife had died in.

One month after admission, Mr. Smithy's daughter receives notification that Mr. Smithy no longer qualifies for skilled nursing care. This means that either the family must pay for his nursing home care privately (at a rate of $_____ per month) or Mr. Smithy must leave the facility.

- Poor care coordination/discharge planning

- Poor preparation for adjustment (transfer) to nursing home

- Further fragmentation of medical care

- Astute nursing assessment

- Reimbursement issues often control type of care received

continued on following page

CASE STUDY. At Home

continued

The social worker in the nursing home explains to Mr. Smithy's daughter that there is a possibility that home health services could be reimbursed under Medicare, meaning that he could continue to have physical therapy and a home health aide to assist with his personal care. Under these circumstances, Mr. Smithy's daughter feels that she could care for him in her home. The decision is made to discharge Mr. Smithy to his daughter's home.

- Care coordination—counseling about care options

BACK AT HOME

Once at home, Mr. Smithy's progress is even more rapid. Within 2 weeks, the home health agency notifies the patient's daughter that because he has reached his rehabilitation goals, he no longer qualifies for either physical therapy or home health aide services under Medicare.

Mr. Smithy voices his desire to return to his own home. Despite some misgivings, his daughter supports his decision, and he returns home to live independently, with somewhat more help with housekeeping and grocery shopping from his daughter than in the past.

- More care decisions influenced by reimbursement

CASE STUDY.

Miss Able is a 76-year-old retired bookkeeper. Her only living relative, a niece named Ms. Helpful, noticed during a recent visit that Miss Able's house was not well kept, which was unusual for her fastidious aunt. She further observed that there were several past-due bills in evidence. Knowing that Miss Able had always been frugal, the niece had difficulty believing that lack of money was a problem. Further investigation revealed that Miss Able had not recorded any checks for several months, again something most out of character.

Miss Able's niece had recently been to a program in her community on Alzheimer's disease and decided to have her aunt medically and psychiatrically evaluated. She took her aunt to the local university hospital, and after extensive outpatient evaluation, the diagnosis of senile dementia of the Alzheimer's type was made. The following information pertains to Miss Able's functional status at this time.

- Outreach function performed by family

CASE STUDY.

continued

MENTAL ABILITIES Awake, alert, oriented to place and person, unable to perform simple calculations, easily distractable and unable to concentrate on a task for longer than three minutes, able to perform only single-stage commands. Remembers birth date but not age; long-term memory intact, but short-term and recent memory totally unreliable.

- Substantial cognitive impairment

PHYSICAL ABILITIES Able to ambulate without assistance, able to wash face and hands and brush teeth if materials are set up and supervision given, able to toilet self independently, able to feed herself independently, unable to perform any instrumental activities of daily living.

- Mild functional impairment

SOCIAL SUPPORT No close friends or living relatives other than Ms. Helpful and her next-door neighbor, Mr. Nice. Retired for 11 years, he lives in the apartment building where she has resided for the past 35 years. No consistent participation in church or civic activities.

- Limited social supports

MEDICAL PROBLEMS None documented except for mild osteoarthritis in right hip; physical examination unremarkable except for unkempt appearance and mild obesity. Laboratory data, including SMA-12, CBC, thyroid panel, and B_{12} and folate levels, all within normal limits.

MEDICATIONS Occasional aspirin for hip pain, occasional Ex-Lax for constipation.

Miss Able and her niece were referred to the evaluation team's social worker and gerontological nurse for assistance in designing an appropriate long-term care plan. Their recommendations included the following.

- Comprehensive assessment and care planning received

LEGAL/FINANCIAL Obtain power-of-attorney for Miss Able and determine her assets available for use in obtaining long-term care.

CARE Encourage Miss Able to continue to perform those tasks that she is able to perform, assist Ms. Helpful with those tasks that she can safely assist with, and obtain help in the home or regular involvement in an adult day care program to assist with supervision of Miss Able and to prevent "burnout" of Ms. Helpful. They also counseled Ms. Helpful on how to structure activities so they would be less frustrating for Miss Able to maximize her functional capacity.

continued on following page

CASE STUDY.

continued

No specific recommendations for treatment, but a recommendation that Miss Able be seen at least semiannually by an internist or family practice physician so that a medical practitioner would be familiar with her baseline medical status, against which any changes in mental or functional status would be evaluated.

A home visit was made to evaluate the adequacy of Miss Able's home environment and to make recommendations for environmental modifications that would enhance Miss Able's functioning. The recommendations included placing a nightlight in Miss Able's bedroom and bathroom, placing grab rails next to the toilet, obtaining a raised toilet seat, and reducing the number of utensils and appliances in the kitchen.

Miss Able's niece decided to move Miss Able down to her home, where she knew the community resources best. She also decided that she would keep Miss Able in her home as long as possible.

Following the move to Ms. Helpful's home, Miss Able's symptoms worsened considerably. Miss Able began to be extremely restless in the evening but showed little interest in helping her niece with even the simplest of chores. She also became incontinent at night and spent progressively more time during the day in the easy chair. Previously a very docile individual, she seemed to withdraw more and more. She sometimes accused Ms. Helpful of stealing her money.

• Change in patient's location results in functional decline

Ms. Helpful voiced these concerns to Miss Able's physician but received little help. The physician believed that there was nothing more that he could do for Miss Able because of the irreversible nature of her disease and could not understand why the niece was so insistent that her aunt be reevaluated. The physician did agree to sign a referral and treatment plan form so that visiting nurses could go out and visit.

• Coordination with new service provider achieved

The home health nurse made an assessment visit, where it was clear to her that the niece was only marginally coping with the situation. The niece, although somewhat sophisticated about the nature of the patient's illness, had difficulty adjusting to her new role as full-time caregiver. The nurse suggested that the niece try to find some kind of help in the home to relieve the stress on her.

• Lack of necessary supportive care in community or adequate reimbursement for chronic dependency

The nurse informed the niece that, under Medicare regulations, she could not continue

CASE STUDY.

continued

to see Miss Able because she had no need for skilled nursing care. Admittedly, Miss Able required a great deal of care, including 24-hour supervision, assistance with bathing, dressing, and meal preparation, and reminders to eat and drink fluids properly, but none of this constitutes skilled nursing care according to the Medicare definitions. The other agencies in the community providing companion or home health aide–type services already had extensive waiting lists, so Miss Able's niece's only option was to try to find someone on a private pay basis. The average rate for this service was $6.50 per hour. At this rate, Miss Able's niece would spend three fourths of her paycheck for care while she was at work and would not be able to keep up with other household payments. Miss Able's bank account and Social Security income would only pay for a fraction of the cost. The only other alternative offered to Ms. Helpful was nursing home placement. There, once Miss Able had applied for Medicaid, Miss Able's savings would be used to pay for the nursing home care until that money ran out. Under Medicaid, the cost of the nursing home not covered by Miss Able's Social Security check would be supplemented by Medicaid.

Ms. Helpful felt that her aunt did not belong in a nursing home, since she could still do things for herself, and so, despite some misgivings, she decided to leave Miss Able by herself while she was at work. She locked the door when she left, called to check on her during the day, and prayed that no harm would come to her aunt. Eventually, Miss Able was admitted to the hospital because she had become extremely lethargic and had stopped eating.

In the hospital she improved dramatically with IV hydration. The niece was advised to place the patient in a nursing home, but the niece refused. The niece also refused to take the patient home from the hospital, because she felt she could not properly care for her aunt. Eventually, because of threat of legal action over the unpaid hospital bill, the niece agreed to nursing home placement. Because of bed shortages in the county of residence, Miss Able was placed in a nursing home several hundred miles from her niece.

Miss Able died in this nursing home 3 years later, a Medicaid recipient and ward of the state.

- Importance of adequate financial resources

- Suboptimal compensation for inadequate resources precipitates acute illness and hospitalization

- Nursing home bed shortages coupled with inadequate home care resources precipitate family breakup

PATTERNS OF HEALTH CARE UTILIZATION

Older people have a greater prevalence of chronic conditions than the population at large and are the primary users of health care services. Although they constitute only 12 per cent of the population, they account for 31 per cent of all hospital discharges and one third of the country's personal health care expenditures. Health care utilization is also greatest among the *old-old* and in the last year of life. People over 85 are three times more likely to lose their independence, seven times more likely to enter a nursing home, and two and a half times more likely to die compared with persons 65 to 74 years of age. The elderly use medical personnel and facilities more frequently than the young, they are hospitalized approximately twice as often, stay twice as long, and use twice as many prescription drugs (U.S. Senate Special Committee on Aging, 1991).

Community Health Services

"Informal supports" provide the majority of community services to older adults who have disabling health problems but live outside institutions. Relatives represent 84 per cent of all caregivers for males and 79 per cent for females. More wives than husbands provide care to disabled spouses, reflecting the fact that women outlive men by an average of seven years. More than one third of all elderly disabled men living in the community are cared for by a wife, whereas only one tenth of all elderly disabled women are cared for by a husband (Manton and Liu, 1984).

The goal of community-based services is to promote the independence of the elderly and to provide an alternative to institutional care. The focus is generally on all individuals aged 60 and older. Community services are provided in physicians' offices, clinics, HMOs, nurse-managed centers, nutrition sites and/or senior centers, mental health clinics, day hospitals and outpatient surgery clinics, rest homes, and day care centers. Other services are provided through home health agencies, homemaker/chore service programs, hospice, health education programs, wellness programs, home-delivered meals, respite care, case management, and transportation services (Igou et al., 1989; Bremer, 1989).

Physician Services

Utilization of physician services increases with age (Table 20–2). In 1989, people aged 65 to 74 years averaged 8.2 physician contacts whereas those aged 45 to 64 averaged 6.1 physician contacts. Additionally, since the enactment of Medicare, the average number of physician contacts and the percentages of persons 65 and over reporting that they had seen a physician in the last year have increased significantly, especially for people with low incomes (U.S. Senate Special Committee on Aging, 1991).

Physicians in private practice provide the

TABLE 20 – 2
Number of Physician Contacts and Interval Since Last Physician Contact, by Age: 1989

AGE GROUPS	CONTACTS			PER CENT DISTRIBUTION OF PEOPLE BY INTERVAL SINCE LAST CONTACT			
	Number (thousands)	Per Cent Distribution	Average Number per Person, per Year	Less Than 1 year	1 to Less Than 2 Years	2 to Less Than 5 Years	5 Years or More
All ages	1,322,890	100.0	5.4	77.4	10.2	8.7	3.8
Under 5 years	126,309	9.5	6.7	93.3	5.0	1.2	0.4
5 to 17 years......	157,698	11.9	3.5	76.3	13.4	8.1	2.3
18 to 24 years	98,233	7.4	3.9	72.2	13.0	11.2	3.6
25 to 44 years	398,368	30.1	5.1	72.8	11.3	11.2	4.7
45 to 64 years	283,351	21.4	6.1	76.5	9.2	9.0	5.3
65 to 74 years	145,949	11.0	8.2	85.1	5.3	5.6	4.0
75+	112,982	8.5	9.9	89.1	4.0	4.0	2.9
65+	258,931	19.6	8.9	85.9	4.7	4.9	3.5

Note: Data include office visits, telephone consultations, hospital contacts (including emergency room and outpatient visits but excluding inpatient visits), and other modes of contact. Data exclude people in institutions.

From National Center for Health Statistics. Current estimates from the National Health Interview Survey, 1989. *Vital and Health Statistics* Series 10, No. 176, October 1990.

majority of medical care for the elderly. Their goal is to diagnose and treat diseases. There is considerable diversity among the types of physicians who care for older patients. They may be generalists or specialists, but few have specialized training or interest in the care of the elderly (Kane, 1980). Most of the specialists are in the field of internal medicine. Practice patterns are diverse and include both group and solo practitioners. Some physicians view patients holistically and serve as counselors, teachers, and coordinators of care. The primary focus of most, however, is on diagnosis and treatment of diseases.

Fragmentation of medical care is a problem for many older persons. The trend toward specialization in medical care, coupled with the prevalence of multiple organ system dysfunction associated with aging, results in some older adults *literally having a specialist for each disease*. Coordination among the physicians can be as large a dilemma as coordination among providers of the other health services. Older people frequently complain of depersonalized care, because despite the "special" care for each organ system, *no one treats the whole individual*. Current efforts at health care reform are expected to incorporate the use of case managers to assist individuals in locating and receiving appropriate care.

Physicians also serve as gatekeepers to other services within the continuum of care for elderly people, including hospitals, nursing homes, laboratory services, rehabilitation services, nursing services, and pharmaceutical services. Some physicians practice within a team approach to medical care, meaning that they routinely consult with members of other disciplines in assessing the needs of older patients and in planning their care. Some share office space with members of other disciplines such as nurses, psychologists, and nutritionists. The norm in private practice, however, is for physicians to provide medical care in their offices and refer to other practitioners without a great deal of interaction or joint planning with the other care providers.

Historically, individuals have looked to physicians for help in solving a wide range of human problems. This is particularly true of the current cohort of aged individuals, who remember the days of the general practitioner who made housecalls and was a community figure as well as a technical expert. Currently few physicians are able to fulfill expectations of those who desire help with the broad array of health problems that elderly people encounter because of time constraints, financial constraints, and the complexities of the helping network.

Outpatient Clinics

These may be associated with community or teaching hospitals, or with community service agencies. Their focus is generally on patients with chronic disease problems, such as diabetes and hypertension, but patients with any medical or surgical problem, acute or chronic, can be seen. The goal is to diagnose and treat the presenting illness.

Many services are offered through an outpatient clinic, including physician services, nursing services, rehabilitative services, and laboratory and diagnostic services. In large hospitals, the clinics are usually organized along medical subspecialty lines. This can be problematic for the elderly, who frequently have multiple chronic diseases and thus may be cared for in several clinics, rather than receiving coordinated medical and health care in one central place.

Roles that nurses fulfill in this setting include assessor, triage officer, coordinator of care, teacher, and case manager. When nurses work as case managers in these settings, they fulfill two roles, one as patient advocate and one as gatekeeper. Tension can develop as the nurse strives to balance the two roles (Kane, 1992).

Traditionally, through doctors and hospitals, outpatient clinics provided medical care for the indigent on a charity basis. With the advent of Medicare and Medicaid, physicians now have a source of reimbursement for their services, so the clinics no longer operate on a strictly charitable basis. However, there is still a need for indigent care, which these clinics often fill. In addition, some private practice physicians do not accept Medicaid patients, and many do not accept assignment for Medicare services (meaning that the patient still is left with between 20 and 50 per cent of the professional service charges to pay out of pocket), so that a demand remains for outpatient clinic services.

Community Mental Health Centers

Established by the Community Mental Health Act of 1962, these centers were the focal point of deinstitutionalization of the mental hospital population. The purpose of these centers was to prevent psychiatric hospitalization. In some communities, they have developed into a focal point for the receipt of outpatient psychotherapy services. In other communities, they serve as a screening point for people referred for psychiatric hospitalization and provide only limited aftercare services for those discharged from mental hospitals. Funding difficulties have reduced their potential for impact in the preventive realm.

The range of services available varies among communities but may encompass outpatient psychotherapy, including individual, group, and family therapy; partial hospitalization (or day hospital) services; psychotropic medication prescription and ongoing evaluation for side effects of medication; consultation and education services to the community; drug and alcohol treatment programs; sheltered workshops; and services to those with mental retardation. Typically these centers are staffed by a multidisciplinary group of professionals, including psychiatrists, psychologists, nurses, social workers, recreational therapists, and paraprofessional staff. Nurses fulfill the roles of psychotherapist, teacher, case manager, consultant, and manager.

Medicare and Medicaid reimbursement exists for outpatient psychotherapy, but increasing limits have been placed on the amount of service an individual can receive (Morgenlander and Greenwald, 1985). Most centers have some form of sliding-scale fee schedule. The 1990s have brought cutbacks in federal funding for staff in these programs, so their continued success and the range of services provided are often dictated by local political and social considerations.

Certain expectations of patients, based on a psychotherapy model developed for younger individuals, may inhibit the use of these centers by elderly people. For example, many centers do not provide services in peoples' homes, expecting that if patients are "motivated" they will come in to the clinic to seek help. This is clearly impractical for some dependent older persons who are in need of psychotherapeutic services.

Historically, mental health centers have been underutilized by elderly people, mainly because of a combination of factors, including reluctance on the part of elderly people to use mental health services, "gerontophobic" mental health clinicians, and difficulties in physical access to these centers (Butler, 1975). However, mental health clinics do remain a potential, if grossly underutilized, resource for the mental health needs of elderly folks.

Home Health Care

In the past several decades, the focus of health care services has been concentrated on institutional care, particularly on acute care hospital settings. Although home health services have been provided by visiting nurse associations, public health and social services, home health agencies, families, and volunteers, the percentage of total public health care funding for home care has been relatively small. Data from the National Center for Health Statistics have shown that little more than 10 per cent of Medicare, Medicaid, and other public funds was allocated for home care in 1991 (National Center for Health Statistics, 1992). Although home health services still account for a relatively small share (7.8 per cent) of Medicaid expenditures for elderly people, it is the most rapidly growing category, increasing tenfold between 1975 and 1989 (Thomas et al., 1989).

The current prospective payment policy for Medicare is having an impact on home health agencies through changes in hospital admission policies and redirection of caregiving resources. Hospital discharge planners, nurses, physicians, hospital social workers, and allied health personnel must work closely with home health care providers to ensure a smooth transition from the hospital to the home. Home care represents one cog in a wheel of emerging health care networks that compete for the traditional acute care patient.

In conjunction with high-technology services, markets for health promotion/maintenance/prevention services will continue to expand. According to Senator Bill Bradley (1984), long-range planning for health care services should emphasize health maintenance and illness prevention to promote a health care system based on prospective payment rather than cost reimbursement. Even more emphasis can be expected on this as systems of managed care emerge with the current health care reform. This would shift the emphasis from illness care to maintenance of health and prevention of illness. Strategies for prevention would include incentives to maintain healthy lifestyles, such as proper diet and exercise, and discourage such habits as smoking and alcohol consumption. Long-term care should also be fully integrated into the total health care system and eventually integrated into capitated health systems, such as Health Maintenance Organizations. The goal of capitated services is to provide the most cost-effective services possible.

Definition of Home Health

The most useful and complete definition of home care is that presented by the group of five national organizations involved in promoting quality home care: the Assembly of Outpatient and Home Care Institutions, American Hospital Association; the National Association of Home Health Agencies; the National Home Caring Council; the Council of Home Health Agencies and Community Health Service; and the National League for Nursing. Their definition states

Home health service is that component of comprehensive health care whereby services are provided to individuals and families in their places of residence for the purpose of promoting, maintaining or restoring health or minimizing the effects of illness and disability. Services appropriate to the needs of the individual patient and family are planned, coordinated and made available by an agency or institution, organized for the delivery of health care through the use of employed staff, contractual arrangements, or a combination of administrative patterns. These services are provided under a plan of care which includes appropriate service components such as, but not limited to, medical care, dental care, nursing, physical therapy, speech therapy, occupational therapy, social work, nutrition, homemaker, home health aide, transportation, laboratory services, medical equipment, and supplies (McNamara, 1982).

Overview/History of Home Health

The Boston Dispensary created the first home care program around 1800. A founding principle established by the Boston Dispensary related to the home care issue: "The sick, without being pained by separation from their families, may be attended and relieved at home" (Irwin, 1978). During this time period the poor and homeless received care in the hospital, whereas the wealthy patients were treated at home. In the late 1800s lay persons organized and offered home nursing services. Voluntary agencies began providing home nursing care around this time, and these later became visiting nurse associations. Around 1900, graduate nurses began to provide home nursing care. With advancing technology and improving sanitation and living conditions, health care needs shifted from communicable diseases to long-term illnesses. Hospitals became overcrowded and attempted to alleviate this problem by developing home care for discharged hospital patients. By the mid 1940s, home health care providers included government agencies, voluntary health associates, private insurance companies, and hospital-based programs. The passage of Medicare in 1965 had great impact on the expansion of home care during the next two decades, with federal regulations for home care agencies requiring them to provide nursing and one additional service. In recent years, cost-containment efforts, owing to the rising cost of health care, have increased the focus on home health care (Greene et al., 1993).

Types of Home Health Agencies

Home health care is provided by hospitals, private profit and nonprofit agencies, and public agencies, such as public health and social service departments.

HOSPITAL-BASED HOME HEALTH AGENCIES. Hospitals establish their own home health agencies to maintain control of these services. Hospital-based home health agencies can be beneficial; however, many hospitals lack the administrative expertise or necessary resources to operate a home health agency (Pyles, 1984). The advantages of hospital-based home health agencies are threefold: financial, organizational, and community. Financial benefits include providing an additional source of revenue and retaining patients within the hospital system. Organizational benefits include the use of available health staff, management, and support services and increased control of health care services. Services can also be provided where there is a gap in existing home health services. Advantages to the community include ensuring continuity of care between the hospital and the community, providing integration of health programs and services, and using the community as a hospital referral source.

Since hospitals are focusing attention on reduced length of stay, it is important for them to be able to refer patients easily to home health agencies and skilled nursing facilities. Hospitals may provide posthospitalization services directly or arrange referral of patients to existing home health agencies. These arrangements assure prompt hospital discharge and ready referral to home health agencies. Home health agencies that have good referral arrangements with hospitals can ensure growth and stability in patient referral networks. Thus patient referral becomes increasingly important with increased competition in home health care and as the possibility of a prospective system for home health care is explored by the government (Tillman, 1984).

When there is a good relationship between a hospital and a home health agency, the hospital can identify specific diagnosis-related groups (DRGs) where home health can help to reduce the length of stay and to monitor screening and discharge procedures. Hospitals can also monitor physician referrals to home health and how these contribute to control of inpatient costs. The use of home care as an alternative or supplement to inpatient care can be facilitated by in-hospital training and education of hospital staff and physicians regarding the effectiveness of home health care (Pyles, 1984).

PROFIT/NONPROFIT/PUBLIC HOME HEALTH AGENCIES. Profit making or proprietary home care companies are licensed by individual states for governmental reimbursement. Nonprofit home care agencies frequently oppose this licensing, and few states allow proprietary agencies to participate. Profit making companies often bypass the licensing requirement and contract with certified agencies, supplying home care services for them to people covered by the federal programs. Many proprietary agencies belong to the Home Health Services and Staffing Association, composed of 11 investor-owned and tax-paying organizations. Members of this association, including Manpower Health Care Services, Medical Personnel Pool, and Upjohn Health Care Services, Inc., provide professional nursing care; physical, occupational, and speech therapy; medical and social services; home health aid; and medical supplies and equipment.

Nonprofit agencies provide essentially the same services as for-profit agencies; however, each agency is autonomously run by members of local communities. They are governed by a Board of Directors, made up of community members from various areas of expertise pertaining to the running of the agency, such as registered nurses, physicians, allied health care providers, business people, and community leaders. Agencies are funded by reimbursement from federal, state, and private insurance (Medicare, Medicaid, Blue Cross), direct payment from the patient, and contributions.

Public agencies that provide home care are the Health Departments and the Departments of Social Services. Health Departments generally have a range of services, such as nursing, home health aid, and physical and occupational therapy. Social Services may provide "chore" services for homebound elderly who need help with household chores such as cooking, cleaning, and personal care. Medicare and Medicaid fund the bulk of these services.

Concerns about the increasing role of proprietary interests in health care generally are widespread (Institute of Medicine Commit-

tee, 1986a). These concerns are particularly pertinent to the home health sector, as the ownership structure of home health has changed radically during the 1980s. The Omnibus Reconciliation Act of 1980 changed the ownership patterns of home health agencies in two ways: (1) by removing the restriction barring certification of proprietary home health agencies in states without home licensure laws, and (2) by liberalizing the conditions under which Medicare would reimburse home care. The result was an eight-fold increase in the number of proprietary home health agencies between 1980 and 1984 (from 186 to 1569), compared with less than a twofold increase for hospital-based and not-for-profit home health agencies, compared with no growth for governmental and visiting nurse association home health agencies (Institute of Medicine Committee, 1986b, citing Health Care Financing Administration [HCFA] data). The majority of Medicare-certified home health agencies are now owned by for-profit organizations.

The Institute of Medicine's Committee on Implications of For-Profit Enterprise in Health Care (1986a,b) identifies two major themes in the debate over the potential effects of proprietary interests in health care and suggests that both views oversimplify the complex issues involved. The two major themes can be summarized as follows:

1. For-profit health care organizations are antithetical to the traditional values of health care institutions and threaten the autonomy and ideals of the health care professions.
2. For-profit health care organizations provide new impetus for innovation, are more responsive to the needs of patients and care providers, and provide more efficient management and new sources of capital for the provision of health care.

The report further characterizes some powerful stereotypes held of the various ownership models in health care, which can be summarized as follows: (1) governmental: last resort, inefficient but equitable; (2) not-for-profit: volunteerism, charity, community; (3) for-profit: efficient, innovative but self-interested. The Committee report contends that these notions, although popular and powerful in shaping opinions, may be out-moded distinctions. Distinctions commonly made between proprietary and not-for-profit organizations are summarized in Table 20–3. However, the distinctions between these two forms of organization have become blurred for a variety of reasons, including, among others:

- The increasing dependence of both types of organizations on fee-for-service revenues;

- The trend in not-for-profits to expand to take advantage of economies of scale;

- The reality that not-for-profits can and do make surplus over revenues (a euphemism for profit) that is generally used as working capital to improve or expand services; and

- The tendency for development of not-for-profit subsidiaries of proprietary organizations as well as proprietary branches of not-for-profit organizations.

Although it is useful to understand some of the distinctions between proprietary and nonproprietary providers, many questions about the influence of ownership remain unanswered. The Committee concludes that in acute hospital care, there is little evidence to support the notion that proprietary ownership has had a negative effect on the quality of care (Gaumer, 1986). However, in long-term care institutions, which have been owned predominantly by proprietary interests, there are data to suggest that quality of care may suffer when profits are put first. To quote:

The preponderance of evidence from the relatively few studies that systematically address quality of care and ownership differences suggests the superiority of nonprofits—particularly of the church-related nonprofits. The data from the state surveys strongly support this finding. Studies using a variety of quality measures—resource inputs, licensure violations, complaints, and outcome-oriented measures of quality—are fairly uniform in finding nonprofit facilities superior in quality to for-profit nursing homes (Hawes and Phillips, 1986, pp. 520–521).

To summarize, studies on acute care show few adverse effects of proprietary interests on quality, whereas the data on long-term care suggest the reverse. It may be that the natural history of proprietary interests in health care is an erosion of quality, or this may be a trend unique to long-term care institutions. Gerontological nurses should be intensely interested in how quality in home care is affected by the changing patterns of ownership and work diligently to protect high standards of care.

Rules and Regulations

FEDERAL REGULATIONS. Federal regulations for home health agencies are described by HCFA, Title 42, Public Health, entitled "Conditions of Participation; Home

TABLE 20-3

Common Distinctions Between For-Profit and Not-for-Profit Organizations

FOR-PROFIT	NOT-FOR-PROFIT
Corporations owned by investors	Corporations without owners or owned by "members"
Can distribute some proportion of profits (net revenues less expenses) to owners	Cannot distribute surplus (net revenues less expenses) to those who control the organization
Pay property, sales, income taxes	Generally exempt from taxes
Sources of capital include a. Equity capital from investors b. Debt c. Retained earnings (including depreciation and deferred taxes) d. Return-on-equity payments from third-party payers (e.g., Medicare)	Sources of capital include a. Charitable contributions b. Debt c. Retained earnings (including depreciation) d. Governmental grants
Management ultimately accountable to stockholders	Management accountable to voluntary, often self-perpetuating boards
Purpose: Has legal obligation to enhance the wealth of shareholders within the boundaries of law; does so by providing services	*Purpose:* Has legal obligation to fulfill a stated mission (provide services, teaching, research, etc.); must maintain economic viability to do so
Revenues derived from sale of services	Revenues derived from sale of services and from charitable contributions
Mission: Usually stated in terms of growth, efficiency, and quality	*Mission:* Often stated in terms of charity, quality, and community service, but may also pursue growth
Mission and structure can result in more streamlined decision making and implementation of major decisions	Mission and diverse constituencies often complicate decision making and implementation

From Gray, B.H. Profits and health care: An introduction to the issues. In Gray, B.H. (ed.). *For-Profit Enterprise in Health Care.* Washington, D.C.: National Academy Press, 1986.

Health Agencies," in Chapter IV—Health Care Financing Administration. To participate as a home health agency in the health insurance program for the aged (Medicare), an institution must be a "home health agency" within the meaning of section 1861(o) of the Social Security Act:

The term "home health agency" means a public agency or private organization, or a subdivision of such an agency or organization, which

1. Is primarily engaged in providing skilled nursing services and other therapeutic services;

2. Has policies, established by a group of professional personnel (associated with the agency or organization), including one or more physicians and one or more registered professional nurses, to govern the services (referred to in paragraph 1) which it provides, and provides for supervision of such services by a physician or registered professional nurse;

3. Maintains clinical records on all patients;

4. In the case of an agency or organization in any State in which State or applicable local law

provides for the licensing of agencies or organizations of this nature, (A) is licensed pursuant to such law, or (B) is approved, by the agency of such State or locality responsible for licensing agencies or organizations of this nature, as meeting the standards established for such licensing;

5. Has in effect an overall plan and budget that meet the requirements of subsection (z); and

6. Meets such other conditions of participation as the Secretary may find necessary in the interest of the health and safety of individuals who are furnished services by such agency or organization. . . .

STATE REGULATIONS. State regulations for the establishment and operation of home health agencies vary from state to state. They are patterned after the federal regulations in regard to administrative policies, financial and statistical records, personnel, and policy making. Service requirements, in addition to skilled nursing service, include the provision of at least one other therapeutic service, e.g., physical, speech, or occupational therapy; medical social services; or home health aide services.

Hospital Discharge Planning

The hospital discharge planner helps to facilitate the transition from hospital to home care. This includes preadmission planning for elective admissions, assessment of referral and discharge needs, setting up actual discharges and referrals, follow up of discharged patients who have been referred to home health care, and education of patients who may require home health services in the future. Close involvement with hospital social workers is necessary to identify referral and discharge needs. The hospital discharge planner may also be in a position to evaluate which patients exceed DRG length-of-stay requirements to provide data for DRG re-evaluation. Since DRGs have been instituted, patients tend to be more acutely ill and are discharged earlier and sicker, requiring increased home health services. This necessitates home health nurses with a higher degree of expertise and the ability to maintain good communication between the discharge planner and the home health agencies.

Patients are expected to be able to care for themselves during the time that agency staff are not present. For people with significant functional disabilities, this may require the presence and active support of family and/or friends. Without such support, individuals are unlikely to receive substantial benefit from home health services. In theory, there is no distinction between the functional level of recipients of skilled nursing care in a nursing home and the functional level of those receiving skilled nursing care at home. In practice, the key difference seems to be the level of family support available to the individual.

Roles that nurses play in this setting include direct care provider, case manager, supervisor of paraprofessionals, and community care coordinator. In contrast to the nursing home setting, there is more opportunity for professional nurses in this setting to provide direct care to patients. A key role that the nurse plays is that of care coordinator, because for patients at home, failure to coordinate services often means that the patient does without needed services.

There is little direct physician involvement in care once the initial referral has been written, except for routine renewal of orders and telephone consultation. Very few physicians deliver services in the home. The activity of rehabilitative staff may be quite extensive, depending upon their availability and the philosophy of the agency.

Hospice

Hospice is defined as a concept of care for dying patients that emphasizes family-centered care, sophisticated pain and symptom management in terminal illness, and care of the bereaved. The focus of care is on terminally ill patients and their families, with the expressed goal of helping them to live as fully as possible until death occurs. Services included in such a program of care vary according to the nature of the particular hospice. Some are based in hospitals, but the vast majority in the United States are home-based. Most provide round-the-clock professional nurse availability, chaplain service, medical services, and a strong volunteer service. Patients are expected to be aware of their prognosis and to have a life expectancy of six months or less. Because most hospices are not institutionally based, they usually require that a family member or close friend be involved.

Hospice is a relative newcomer to the spectrum of services for the aged in the United States. The movement was inspired by hospice programs in the United Kingdom, most notably by the work of Dr. Cicely Saunders, a nurse and physician and the founder and director of St. Christopher's Hospice in London. Hospice in the United States began in the mid-1970s as a voluntary effort, and reimbursement for such services under Medicare began in 1984. Controversy currently exists about the nature of governmental involvement, for there is concern that the reimbursement levels set by government are too low to enable the delivery of the high quality of care for which hospices have become known (Hays, 1986).

Rest Homes

The general category of rest homes includes domiciliary homes, board and care homes, family care homes, and group homes. The goal is to provide room, board, and personal care for those individuals who cannot provide this service for themselves. The focus is generally on those dependent elderly who do not require regular nursing intervention or observation but who cannot live independently or on younger individuals who have mental illness or mental retardation. Reimbursement for rest home care comes from private dollars or from state and county funds for indigent persons.

The advantage of rest homes is that a less institutional atmosphere may prevail because the residents are generally less impaired than those in intermediate care facilities (ICFs) or skilled nursing facilities (SNFs). However, it is far from a certainty that domiciliary homes will be "home-like." The atmosphere in domiciliary homes is highly variable, being a product of many factors, including the values, philosophy, and expertise of the owners and operators as well as the local health and social regulations governing the operation of domiciliary homes.

Residents of rest home facilities are expected to conform to house rules, and they must be transferred to another type of facility, either a hospital or nursing home, if they require significant medical or nursing attention. (The exception is the availability of home health service delivery in cooperation with the rest home staff. With the growth of home health services, this is becoming less of an exception, but the majority of rest homes do not care for individuals requiring significant medical or skilled nursing intervention.)

The role of nurses and other health professionals in these facilities is quite limited. Licensure is generally required to operate rest homes, but in many states there is no requirement for significant health professional input. Because home health services may be available to residents, there is potential for nurses and other health professionals to provide direct services. In addition, some homes obtain consultation and staff training from health professionals. Historically, these facilities are closest to the almshouses and homes for the aged as they existed prior to Medicare. Concerns have been raised about

the quality of care in these settings and the risk that residents who require greater care than can be provided are not transferred in a timely manner.

Nutrition Sites/Senior Centers

Older people who are in need of socialization and a good meal may participate in senior center programs. The programs are supported by Title XX funds, and participants pay a small fee for their lunch, often on a sliding-scale basis. In addition to recreational activities, such as singing, card playing, and arts and crafts, some centers serve a linkage function, providing easier accessibility to other community services. Health-related assessments and learning experiences are provided in such areas as blood pressure and oral cancer screening, nutrition counselling, and exercise. Transportation is usually provided to the centers.

Case Management, Home Care, and Day Care Services

Services arranged by many of the previously mentioned agencies include case management, home-delivered meals, and day care, provided by chore workers, home health aides, and homemaker/home health aides. *Case managers* identify, negotiate, and coordinate a package of services for individual clients. This service package is designed to reduce some of the difficulties of negotiating a complex health care service system (Leath and Thatcher, 1991). *Chore workers* and *homemaker/health aides* assist with household chores such as meal preparation, housework, and grocery shopping and may provide companionship. In some agencies, they are allowed to assist with simple personal care tasks. This is highly variable from locale to locale and generally depends on local interpretation of Title XX guidelines. *Home health aides* provide personal care under the supervision of registered nurses. Reimbursement is through Medicare, Medicaid, and private insurance or private pay.

Home-delivered meals, also known as Meals-on-Wheels, offers one hot meal per day to homebound individuals who are unable to prepare a meal for themselves. There are often provisions for special diets, and some programs deliver meals on weekends and holidays. Volunteers usually deliver the meals; however, general program funding may be public or private.

Day care is a program of structured activity designed to provide socialization and meaningful activity for aged persons with mental or physical infirmity. Day care is usually a term reserved for use with "social model" programs, whereas the term day hospital is reserved for programs organized according to a medical model. Either program may have various types of health professionals coming in to provide service or consultation.

In most localities, there is a greater need for some services, such as homemakers, home health aides, and meals-on-wheels, than is available. Most services are provided on a sliding-scale fee basis or without charge to the target population. Typically, there is no means test, meaning that, regardless of income level, any older person is eligible to receive services. Service recipients constitute a varied population, ranging from those who merely require the security of a daily telephone call to those who require multiple services, without which they would require institutional care. Clients are expected to be able to make alternative arrangements on weekends and holidays and to be fairly self-sufficient or to have family who can assist.

Roles for nurses and other health professionals in this service network also vary. Usually the services operate on a social model rather than a medical or health model, so that social workers and paraprofessional workers predominate. When nurses and other health professionals are used, it is generally in the role of teacher, consultant, assessor, and, sometimes, coordinator of care.

Many of these services are funded through the Older Americans Act, which was originally passed in 1965 with a broad mandate to help older Americans. The goals of the Older Americans Act are (Butler, 1975, p. 329)

1. An adequate income
2. The best possible physical and mental health
3. Suitable housing
4. Full restorative services
5. Opportunity for employment without age discrimination
6. Retirement in health, honor, and dignity
7. Pursuit of meaningful activity
8. Efficient community services when needed
9. Immediate benefit from proven research knowledge
10. Freedom, independence, and the free exercise of individual initiative

However, most localities use many sources of funding to support a specific service, as funding from Older Americans Act monies is often inadequate to meet the need. The demonstration projects and training that have been funded have resulted in the development of the services listed previously, along with agencies to help deliver the services. Such agencies are generally known as Councils on Aging or Departments on Aging. Needs assessment and service coordination take place on a regional level, through statewide Area Agencies on Aging.

Hospital-Based Services

Hospitals are major providers of health and related services to older adults; of all persons aged 65 and older, one in five is admitted to the hospital each year. Older individuals also make 2.5 million visits each year to hospital emergency rooms. In 1991, people over age 65, who represented 12 per cent of the population, accounted for 35 per cent of the discharges and 45 per cent of the days of hospital care (Graves, 1993).

Hospital Usage

Short-stay hospital admissions for the elderly have decreased slightly in the last few years. However, hospital use increased between 1965, the year Medicare was enacted, and 1983 by more than 50 per cent. In 1987, people over age 65 years (12 per cent of the population) accounted for 31 per cent of all hospital discharges and 42 per cent of all short-stay hospital days of care. The population aged 75 years and older (5 per cent) accounted for 16 per cent of all hospital discharges and 23 per cent of all hospital days (Table 20–4). The average hospital stay for people aged 65 to 74 years was about 8 days in 1987 compared with about 9 days for the 85 and over group (Fig. 20–3). Most hospital admissions of older people are for acute episodes of a chronic condition. The most common principal diagnoses of the elderly are diseases of the circulatory system (32 per cent), heart disease (21 per cent), digestive diseases (12 per cent), respiratory diseases (10 per cent), and neoplasms (10 per cent) (National Center for Health Statistics, 1989).

Despite the large numbers of elderly patients in acute care hospitals, most of these institutions have no comprehensive geriatric program geared to the long-term medical, rehabilitative, and social needs associated with acute illness. Hospitals are acute care oriented, with a major focus on diagnosis and treatment of acute illness.

Within the hospital setting, patients should conform to sick role behavior. Once they have achieved maximum medical benefit from the hospitalization, they should be discharged elsewhere (regardless of the availability or desirability of aftercare ser-

TABLE 20 – 4
Utilization of Short-Stay Hospitals for Selected Age Groups: 1987

| | DISCHARGED PATIENTS | | | DAYS OF CARE | | | |
AGE GROUPS	Number in Thousands	Per Cent Distribution	Rate per Thousand	Number in Thousands	Per Cent Distribution	Rate per Thousand	Average Length of Stay
All ages	33,387	100.0	138.2	214,942	100.0	889.4	6.4
45 to 64	7,099	21.3	156.9	48,360	22.5	1,068.6	6.8
65 to 74	4,963	14.9	280.9	40,534	18.9	2,294.4	8.2
75 to 84	3,968	11.9	426.6	35,403	16.5	3,806.3	8.9
85+	1,528	4.6	532.9	14,459	6.7	5,043.4	9.5
65+	10,459	31.3	350.5	90,397	42.1	3,029.9	8.6

From National Center for Health Statistics. National Hospital Discharge Survey: Annual Summary, 1987. *Vital and Health Statistics* Series 13, No. 99, April 1989.

vices). Roles of nurses in the hospital setting include bedside caregiver, teacher, discharge planner, administrator, utilization review co-ordinator, clinical specialist, and manager. Clinical specialists in gerontological nursing appear to be relatively rare in a hospital setting.

The 20th century has seen the development of the hospital as the cornerstone of modern medical practice. The organizational development of the hospital system can be traced from its beginnings in a church-based model to a charity-based model, through the community hospital movement to the increasingly prevalent corporate structure of today's hospitals. It is worth noting that many still regard the hospital as a charitable or community institution, whereas the predominant thinking of the administration may be corporate in style and not focused on charitable or community goals.

Prospective Payment/DRGs

The predominant source of payment for hospital services to the aged is Medicare and third-party insurers, such as Blue Cross/ Blue Shield. The Medicare prospective payment system for inpatient hospital services was signed into law in April, 1983. Research conducted by Yale University and results of the DRG system in New Jersey and a modified DRG system in Maryland in large part form the basis for the national prospective payment system. It is based on a set of DRGs that classifies patients according to diagnosis. Under the DRG system, hospitals receive a fixed payment per case based on the patient's diagnosis or DRG category placement (Overview, 1984).

The HCFA is responsible for determining DRG rates utilizing historical cost data. DRG classifications are recalibrated at least once every 4 years (Johnson, 1985). DRG payment methodology is adjusted according to local wage variations and urban and rural locales. In 1987, a phase-in program was completed so that all DRG-based payments are based on national rates. Adjustments will be made for atypical cases with extended lengths of stay (outliers). Institutions and services that were originally excluded from the DRG prospective payment system are being re-examined for inclusion. These include psychiatric hospitals, rehabilitation hospitals, and home-based rehabilitation.

To reduce costs, hospitals and physicians discharge patients as early as possible, increasing the number of admissions to skilled nursing facilities and home health agencies (Lorenz, 1984). Discharged patients are not as fully recovered as those with longer hos-

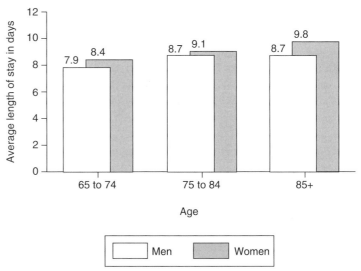

FIGURE 20 – 3

Duration of stay by the elderly in short-stay nonfederal hospitals by age: 1987. (From National Center for Health Statistics. "National Hospital Discharge Survey: Annual Summary, 1987." *Vital and Health Statistics* Series 13, No. 99, April 1989.)

pital stays, so they require higher levels of care in these settings. High-technology services traditionally provided in the acute care hospital setting, such as intravenous hydration, antibiotic therapy, chemotherapy, enteral and parenteral nutrition, ventilator care, apnea monitoring, insulin therapy, and kidney dialysis, are now included in home health care services (Coleman and Smith, 1984). A Lackawanna County, Pennsylvania, study (Frayne, 1985) showed that the majority of the 39 physicians surveyed confirmed the predictions in the literature regarding the increase in the number of referrals to home health agencies and skilled nursing facilities due to DRGs.

Hospital Services to the Aged

The elderly are receiving increased attention by hospital administrators. Changes in Medicare reimbursement have provided powerful incentives to seek the most cost-effective ways of caring for older patients. Direct involvement by the hospital in home health care, nursing home care, and a variety of other, less intense, support services may be on the increase in the next decade. According to Campion and associates (1983), hospitals must make a commitment to long-term care for chronically ill older patients; however, fundamental changes in the hospital environment and in reimbursements would be required. Provisions such as congregate meals, demedicalization of patients, geriatric training for staff, long-term care units, and case management to ease transitions from home care to acute care would greatly improve hospital care for the aged.

Apparently, many hospitals are beginning to offer a more varied array of services for the elderly. A survey conducted by the American Hospital Association in 1981 showed that many hospitals offered services specifically for older people. Services most frequently offered included discharge planning, information and referral, patient/family education, skilled nursing facilities, and psychosocial counseling. Other services included intermediate care facilities, home-delivered meals, and home health care (Evashwick et al., 1985).

Nursing Home–Based Services

Only about 5 per cent of all older adults are in nursing homes at any given time; however, 25 per cent will need long-term care assistance during their later years. In 1985, approximately 1.5 million older adults resided in nursing homes (U.S. Senate Spe-

cial Committee on Aging, 1991). About 2 per cent were aged 65 to 74, 7 per cent were aged 75 to 84, and about 16 per cent were over the age of 85 (Fig. 20–4). The rate of nursing home use by the elderly has almost doubled since the introduction of Medicare and Medicaid in 1966, from 2.5 to 5 per cent of the over-65 population.

Nearly 68 per cent of all nursing home residents are without a spouse, as compared with just over 40 per cent of the noninstitutionalized elderly. According to the Senate Subcommittee on Aging (1985–86),

Such statistics, along with those which show that nursing home residents tend to have health problems which significantly restrict their ability to care for themselves, suggest that the absence of a spouse or other family member who can provide informal support for health and maintenance requirements is the most critical factor in the institutionalization of an older person. It is likely that the nursing home population will continue to grow rapidly, partly because of the growth in the size of the very old population, and partly because of the increasing gap in life expectancy between husbands and wives.

Projections compiled by demographers Manton and Liu predict that between 1985 and 2000, the nursing home population will increase by 47 per cent from 1.5 to 2.1 million, and, by 2040, it will more than double to 4.4 million. Nursing home residents are disproportionately very old, female, white, and currently unmarried.

Although there are three times more nursing home beds than hospital beds, it is recognized that nursing homes by tradition are isolated from the mainstream of modern medicine. "The majority [of nursing homes] have no formal links to other health providers and are physically isolated from community hospitals, physicians' offices and other community health care resources" (Aiken et al., 1985). Many members in the helping professions—nursing, medicine, social work, physical therapy—receive little or no education specific to the care of the elderly. Few professional students have opportunities to care for older persons in nonhospital settings. Many of the health problems that result in admission to nursing homes are poorly understood because of the disinterest of researchers and clinicians.

Historical Development of the Nursing Home

In the 1930s, the development of welfare, loan, housing, and rent programs, as well as the Social Security Administration, created a new concept of income maintenance for the elderly. Although the income support helped older people to be more self-sufficient, it did not encourage families to provide care for the elders in their homes, as was the intent. Instead, privately owned boarding homes sprang up to care for displaced elderly. As these facilities added nurses to their staff, the name "nursing home" emerged (Moss and Halamandaras, 1977).

Legislation authorizing grants and loans for building long-term care institutions activated a surge of growth in the industry. In 1939, there were 1200 facilities in the United States with 25,000 beds; in 1976, there were over 23,000 facilities with over 1.3 million beds. The greatest rate of increase in the number of both nursing homes and nursing home beds occurred from 1961 to 1965 because of the availability of guaranteed loans authorized by the Federal Housing Administration for new construction (Jones, 1982). The passage of Title XVIII (Medicare) in 1965 and Title XXIX (Medicaid) in 1967 also contributed to the expansion of the nursing home industry.

The rapid and unchecked growth of the nursing home industry combined with new funding sources provided opportunities for investors to succeed financially without maintaining adequate standards of care for the nursing home residents. Many nursing home operators had little knowledge of or interest in the special needs of residents. In addition, lax enforcement standards provided few incentives to correct the deficiencies and abuses that occurred. Investigations in the 1970s uncovered a wide variety of criminal activities including finance and reimbursement fraud, vendor kickbacks, embezzlement of residents' assets, and extortion from residents' families. These scandals undermined public confidence in nursing homes and led to demands for coercive government regulation. At the federal level, conditions for participation and standards of care were established to qualify a nursing home for Medicare and Medicaid reimbursement; at the state level, licensure laws were enacted (Rango, 1982).

Stringent regulations, new reporting mechanisms, and more strictly enforced standards led to decreased growth of the nursing home industry. Many states restricted the number of nursing home beds to control health care expenditures (Rango, 1982). Restrained growth was accompanied by an increasing demand as the aging population needing long-term care increased. Thus, long waiting lists and lengthy delays became

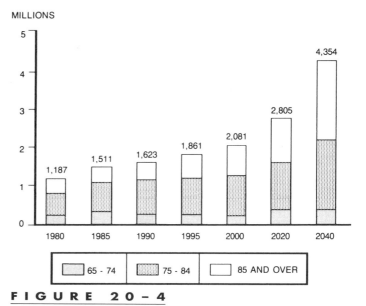

MILLIONS

FIGURE 20 – 4

Nursing home population projections: Persons 65 years and older by age group, 1980–2040. (From Manton, K. and Liu, K. The future growth of the long-term care population: Projections based on the 1977 National Nursing Home Survey and the 1982 Long-Term Care Survey. Presented at the Third National Leadership Conference on Long-Term Care Issues: "The Future World of Long-Term Care." Washington, D.C., March 7–9, 1984.)

common and contributed to the imbalance that exists today between the supply and demand of nursing home services.

The Nursing Home

The term "nursing home" is used to describe institutions that serve individuals with chronic illnesses and physical impairments. The focus of care is on those who do not require hospitalization but are unable to care for themselves. Although there are two types of nursing homes—*skilled nursing facilities* (SNF) and *intermediate care facilities* (ICF)—the term nursing home is often loosely applied to residential care homes that deliver personal care and other non–health care services.

Nineteen per cent of nursing homes are certified for skilled care (Medicare), 31 per cent are certified for intermediate care (Medicaid), and approximately 24 per cent are certified for both skilled and intermediate care. Twenty five per cent of all nursing homes are not certified by either Medicare or Medicaid and thus are not required to comply with the standards that allow for participation in these programs (Jonas, 1981). In some states (such as California), skilled nursing facilities dominate the nursing home industry, whereas in other states (such as Texas), intermediate care facilities dominate.

The term extended care facility (ECF) is chiefly of historical interest. The ECF was conceived as being attached to and operated by a hospital, utilized primarily in the recovery from acute illness, and was not intended for the care of individuals with chronic illness. Reimbursement for extended care through the Medicare program was a logical extension of Medicare's focus on care for acute medical problems. The ECFs were later renamed skilled nursing facilities (SNFs).

The SNF is designed to provide rehabilitative care for individuals who have the potential to regain function. Services include physician care; professional nursing and rehabilitative services; physical and occupational therapy; pharmacy, dietary, and social services; laboratory and radiological services; dental care; and activities. SNF residents may be in need of technical care requiring the skills of a registered nurse. Operationally, this care has come to be defined as provision of one or more of the following: observation during an acute or unstable phase of an illness, administration of enteral feedings or intravenous fluids, bowel and bladder retraining (for a limited period of time), administration of intramuscular or intravenous medications, and changing of sterile dressings. Persons not fitting into any of these categories are deemed to be in need of custodial care and thus are ineligible for skilled nursing care benefits under any third-party reimbursement source.

Requirements for professional nurse staffing in an SNF vary from state to state; the federal government only requires that there be "sufficient staff to meet the needs of the patients" (Code of Federal Regulations, 1986). Usually, however, there is an R.N. or L.P.N. on staff, and 50 per cent or more of the patients receive nursing care. All care is to be provided under the guidance of an individualized multidisciplinary plan of care. The professional nursing staff generally function in a supervisory capacity over nursing assistants, who provide most of the "hands on" care.

Requirements for training of nursing assistants vary from state to state. Federal requirements specify that nursing assistants receive in-service training and that personnel not be assigned tasks beyond their level of training and ability. Such standards, although certainly appropriate, have proven to be notoriously difficult to monitor (Vladeck, 1980).

ICFs are health-related facilities designed to provide custodial care for individuals unable to care for themselves because of mental or physical infirmity. They are not considered by the government to be medical facilities and thus receive no reimbursement under Medicare. They do, however, receive the bulk of their financing under Medicaid. As with the SNFs, staffing requirements vary from state to state. However, federal regulations require a registered nurse to serve as director of nursing and a licensed nurse to be on duty at least 8 hours per day.

Health care professionals involved in nursing homes include physical, occupational, and recreational therapists, social workers, dietitians, and physicians. The degree of involvement of these other workers is highly variable. Physicians frequently have been criticized for not being sufficiently involved in nursing home care. They are required to visit monthly (SNF) or bimonthly (ICF) and as the patient's condition warrants. However, much of the physician involvement in nursing homes takes place over the telephone. Allied health professionals are often involved only on a part-time contractural basis or as consultants to paraprofessionals. The exception is physical therapy; in SNFs, there is usually a regular staff member providing physical therapy services.

Expectations for nursing home residents vary from facility to facility. Generally, however, the residents are not acutely ill, but they may have significant physical and/or mental disabilities. They are expected to "do as much for themselves as they can" within the limits of staff patience and time constraints; however, the residents' independence is often sacrificed in the interests of time. Aberrant behavior is generally accepted, up to the limits of violence toward other residents or staff. There is no requirement for family involvement, and the institution may, for those individuals without family, take over responsibilities traditionally reserved for family, such as handling of financial affairs.

Roles of professional nurses in nursing homes include manager, coordinator of nursing care plans, supervisor of paraprofessional staff, staff development coordinator, and direct caregiver. Many nurses feel frustrated about their inability to give direct care in these settings because of the low nurse-patient ratio and the burden of administrative duties. Nurses who have been able to provide direct care to patients cite the increased autonomy associated with nursing home care as a source of job satisfaction. They assume a large amount of responsibility and require sophisticated skills to carry out their tasks.

Reimbursement

Medicare, Title XVIII of the Social Security Act, is the major health program for financing acute care for the elderly, with a focus on hospital care. Medicare currently prohibits payment for most long-term or custodial care and accounts for only 1 per cent of nursing home funds (Waldo et al., 1989). For nursing home care to be covered, stringent requirements for "skilled care" must be met, and the reimbursement period is limited to 100 days per year. Few private insurers offer long-term care benefits, so even if farsighted individuals wished to obtain private insurance including these benefits, it would be difficult or prohibitively expensive.

Medicaid, Title XIX, is operated jointly by federal and state governments. This program provides health services to low income persons of all ages, the blind and permanently disabled, the medically needy, and the aged. The major payer of nursing home costs, Medicaid accounted for 43 per cent of nursing home funds in 1989. To be eligible for Medicaid, the person must demonstrate financial need. For the elderly needing nursing home care and lacking sufficient private funds to pay for care over an indefinite period of time, Medicaid is the only option. Unfortunately, this requires that people divest themselves of personal assets (home, car, savings) to become eligible for enrollment. This process, known as the "spend down" requirement, is extremely traumatic to families (Lazenby and Letsch, 1989). Not wanting to impoverish both spouse and family, prospective nursing home residents may resort to concealing assets or transferring them to other family members or may even seek a legal divorce as a way of limiting personal financial liability.

The importance of Medicare and Medicaid to institutional long-term care is underscored by cost data. In 1989, the cost of long-term care was estimated at $32 billion, and about two thirds of this, $21 billion, went for nursing home care, the fastest growing segment of the health care industry (Lazenby and Letsch, 1989). By 1990, nursing home costs were over $48 billion and of this, almost half came from public funds. The Medicaid and Medicare programs contribute 51 per cent of nursing home funds, with private pay accounting for 43 per cent and 6 per cent coming from other sources.

It has been noted that almost one third of the nursing home patients who eventually become Medicaid certified enter as private pay patients, and as many as two thirds of the group entering as private pay convert to Medicaid status during their stay. Therefore, it is not surprising that patients receiving Medicaid occupy 80 per cent of nursing home beds (Campion et al., 1983).

It is unfortunate that many elderly incorrectly assume that, should the need arise, nursing home care after hospitalization would be covered automatically by Medicare. And although Medicare can provide up to 100 days of benefits provided minor requirements are met, a "rude awakening awaits most nursing home applicants when they learn they have been declared ineligible" (Loeser et al., 1983, p. 353). The Medicare statute requires that the individual need "skilled" nursing care and specifically excludes custodial care. Furthermore, the distinctions between skilled and custodial care can vary from state to state. Insurance carriers who administer the program variously interpret the law, and decisions related to benefits are often arbitrary and unpredictable. Appeals go to the same carrier instead of an impartial regulatory body (Loeser et al., 1983). Thus, posthospitalization payments for nursing home care are denied to a portion of elderly, leaving few alternatives for payment short of bankrupting their financial resources and assets.

Under the current federal system of patient classification, reimbursement is based on the care providers and the medical technologies employed rather than on individual patient needs. The American Nurses' Association (ANA) Committee on Skilled Nursing Care (1975) delivered testimony to the Senate Subcommittee on Long-Term Care on the problems of providing "skilled nursing" as it is presently defined by Medicare and Medicaid. The committee strongly recommended the deletion of the term skilled nursing from the federal regulations and that the corresponding level of care concept be changed to reflect patient needs.

The present classification of intermediate and skilled nursing care facilities overlooks personal needs, resulting in undesirable restrictions on care for patients needing varying levels of attention and medical services. It is only through a flexible classification of patients and a system of matching services to needs that an acceptable delivery of health care for the elderly can be provided (American Nurses' Association, 1975, p. 4).

Although individual needs should be the common denominator in determining the kind and intensity of care the resident requires, there should also be some mechanism for continuous evaluation.

The long-term needs of the individual, constantly affected by his changing state, can be seen only on a continuum. His status may reflect variances in his ability to ambulate, the degree or extent of disability, his ability to communicate, his mental alertness, or his level of orientation. Nursing services in long-term care must be flexible in responding to the constantly fluctuating needs of those individuals who are receiving care. Focusing upon the individual's needs is in direct contrast to the present vertical hierarchy of levels of care, which is based on the numbers and/or kinds of isolated, individual procedures required. The kind, complexity, frequency, and duration of nursing care needed by an individual patient within any given time may vary considerably (American Nurses' Association, 1975, pp. 5–6).

The ANA Committee further challenged the logic of the current level of care, which distinguishes skilled from intermediate care on several grounds. First, the distinctions of these two categories for reimbursement are artificial and the term skilled care is a misnomer. For example, when is "unskilled" care an appropriate health care service? Arguments supporting the contributions of professional nursing center on the differences between therapeutic and custodial care. When applying a therapeutic focus, nursing goals address the effects of chronicity, the developmental stages of the life cycle, and the effects of institutionalization upon a person. In meeting these goals, professional nursing is accountable for health assessment, health maintenance, and restorative nursing care. Differentiating care and reimbursement should begin with patient needs.

Second, the committee proposed that regulations should recognize the different competencies of personnel providing care to the elderly and that effective round-the-clock nursing care involves an appropriate combination of personnel depending on the care needs of the residents (American Nurses' Association, 1975, p. 19). Professional nurses are underrepresented in staffing patterns and seriously underutilized as well, spending little time in direct patient care. Licensed nursing staffing patterns in nursing homes are often guided by government regulations only, which set minimum standards for "safe" care and again focus on restrictive functions of the licensed staff (such as performing medical treatments and administering medications). The ANA Committee concluded that serious attention must be given to the problem of the unclear and mislabeled levels of care and the severe under-utilization of professional nursing in the nursing home. The crisis associated with cost of care has caused several proposals to emerge regarding the problem and future options. Most involve the federal government (Mitty, 1988; Polich, 1989; Rantz, 1990).

Patient Classification and Health Policy in Long-Term Care

Gerontologists have pointed out the inadequacy of the current patient classification system for reimbursement. Kane, Bell, and associates (1983) have proposed a system of nursing home reimbursement based on patient outcomes. Reform of the current system, they feel, should address these goals:

1. Provision of an incentive for high-quality care defined in broad terms to include social and psychological as well as physical health.
2. Discouragement of market skimming whereby certain patients (usually those needing the least care in a category) are admitted whereas others with greater care needs are not.
3. Overcoming the general tendency toward assuming that more is necessarily better and, especially, the perverse incentive of cost reimbursement that rewards the development of increased dependency.
4. Minimization of the negative aspects of regulation (i.e., to avoid both the record keeping burden and the constraints on creativity).
5. Use of the free market as much as possible to encourage the expansion of good homes and the closure of poor ones (Kane, Bell, et al., 1983, p. 200).

The key feature of the proposed reform is that payment for care is linked to the outcome of care. So, rather than awarding a fixed payment determined by the existence of medical diagnoses and treatments, which is currently the case, the payment is based on the predicted clinical prognosis for the patient and the amount depends on whether the patient "gets better, stays the same, or gets worse." Under the current system, the focus is on levels of care, not on progress or outcome; and good and bad care are reimbursed equally.

The National Long-Term Care Facility Plan, conducted by the Department of Health, Education, and Welfare, developed a patient appraisal mechanism that identifies physical, psychological, and social needs and determines whether services are being rendered to patients according to those needs (Abdellah et al., 1979). The result of this effort was the PACE instrument: Patient Appraisal, Care Planning, and Evaluation. Derived from a health model rather than a medical model, PACE includes information about resident characteristics, functional capacity, plans for individual goals, and whether those goals have been met (Abdellah et al., 1979). The PACE tool allows the recording of an amalgamation of information systematically contributed from different disciplines.

Effective use of a patient care management system facilitates comprehensive patient care evaluation, systematic monitoring of changes in patient health status, and formulation of a baseline for developing or modifying standards of care. Original work was conducted by four universities (Case Western Reserve University Medical School, Harvard University, Johns Hopkins University School of Hygiene and Public Health, and Syracuse University Research Corporation) during the early 1970s. From this effort the Patient Classification Form (PCF) was developed to serve several purposes: management of individual patients, administration of long-term care within the institution and the community, policy making, epidemiological research, and education (Kane et al., 1992). Abdellah and coworkers noted that the patient's status can be reviewed, quality of care monitored, resources allocated appropriately, and patient care planning decisions made (Abdellah et al., 1979).

A subsequent version of the PACE system has evolved from the PCF, known as PACE II or Patient Care Management (PCM). The original PCF was criticized for its underrepresentation of psychosocial components. The basic components of the PCM build on those of the PCF with several additions, particularly in the area of psychosocial factors. One section records the need for nursing procedures, special procedures, rehabilitative and restorative care, and teaching and psychosocial therapies; other sections record medication use (type and frequency, side effects, drug interactions, and drug dependence) and medical conditions.

Although the PCF was designed to be used in all long-term care sites, it was tested primarily in nursing homes. Nurses have found the classification record useful in caring for patients, since organization of information ensures that no observation about the patient is omitted and that the same information is available to all caregivers.

The final model of the Program for All-Inclusive Care for the Elderly capitated acute and chronic care for older patients in need of long-term care. Community involvement is stressed in lieu of institutional care. Currently, the model has been replicated at eight sites around the country (Kane et al., 1992).

Using data from the application of a comprehensive classification tool, Cavaiola and Young (1980) developed an "integrated procedure that would link the assessment process to a classification process and subsequently the performance time data to a nursing staff allocation model responsive to the requirements of a mix of patients classified as to their levels of care" (p. 285). The approach is based on three interrelated processes:

- Formal assessment of a variety of key functioning status items, behavioral status indicators, and medically defined conditions;

- Development of a practical post-assessment level of care classification method that can be used to determine patient placement within the long-term care system and to indicate particular nursing care activities called for; and

- Use of mathematical programming techniques to evaluate alternative nursing staff allocations and their costs within a long-term care facility.

This approach has many practical uses and is unlike earlier developments of classification methods in its mathematical linkage to calculate nursing staff numbers and ratios. For example, Cavaiola and Young (1980) point out that the Katz Index of Independence in Activities of Daily Living (ADL), a commonly used measure of physical function, does not infer or specify nursing resources required. They conclude that this model would be useful for costing out various ratios and mixes of professional and nonprofessional nursing staff according to the intensity of nursing care required by the resident. However, this classification model appears somewhat restrictive in its focus on tasks (such as bed making, bathing, oral hygiene, catheterization, and so on) and its exclusion of skills such as teaching, pain management, bereavement counseling, psychological support, and care of the dying patient. Perhaps inconsistencies in practice and inadequate documentation prohibit the generalization that these are expected nursing functions in long-term care.

Efforts to formulate a national policy on long-term care have thus far been unsuccessful. The elderly and chronically ill or disabled face limited care options and confusing financing mechanisms for long-term care. Many elderly who need long-term care confront a financial crisis as there is no unified program available that offers comprehensive services and rational payment schemes. A few private insurers are experimenting with long-term care insurance, but coverage may still be somewhat limited and costs expensive. However, increasing interest in and support of long-term care insurance options by groups such as the American Association of Retired Persons should stimulate greater development.

Changing Conditions in the Nursing Home Industry

Service Patterns

Promotional advertisement of nursing home services reflects the intent of nursing home operators to improve the negative image of the nursing home and to market the excellent services that are available to the community. The nursing home as a service agency is changing from a relatively closed system, that is, providing services primarily for its own residents, to an open system, providing a multitude of services to community residents. Among these services are day care and rehabilitation programs, respite care, nutrition services, and outpatient diagnostic and evaluation services. Nursing homes are also extending their services by developing linkages with teaching institutions so that students in the health professions have opportunities to learn about the elderly in nursing homes through direct care and research.

While providing a valuable community service, institutions stand to gain from the influx of new people. Maximal use of resources increases the efficiency of an organization. The input of community residents, educators, students, family members, and others serves as a quality control mechanism. Nursing homes are also interfacing with hospitals and community agencies to facilitate discharge planning so that individuals receive the most appropriate kinds of services.

Ownership Patterns

Almost 80 per cent of the nursing homes in the United States are proprietary and managed by either individual operators or corporate chains. A minority are nonprofit and operated by churches, civic groups, and the government: state, county, or the federal Veterans Administration. For independent proprietary operators, high operating costs, tightening governmental controls, and low reimbursement payments make nursing

home management extremely complex and perhaps not very profitable. Failure of small nursing homes due to increasing health care costs and the trend in the health care market toward corporate growth have created a new profile of the nursing home industry. Big corporate chains are buying out independently owned nursing homes or smaller chains, and the proportion of chain-operated nursing homes is increasing. About half of the country's 1.3 million nursing home beds are controlled by proprietary corporations operating at least five homes, and the top 20 chains run one third of the industry.

Beverly Enterprises is an example of the corporate growth in the nursing home industry. Wohl (1984) reports that Beverly Enterprises, the nation's largest operator of skilled and intermediate care facilities, owns 700 nursing homes totalling 80,000 beds. In addition, he notes that 20 per cent of its stock is owned by the Hospital Corporation of America (HCA), the largest operator of acute care facilities; as of 1982, HCA owned or managed hospitals totalling almost 51,000 beds. In a joint venture with Upjohn Health Care Services, a subsidiary of Upjohn Pharmaceutical Company, Beverly Enterprises delivers in-home health services. Upjohn, one of the world's largest manufacturers of drugs and pharmaceuticals, also has a vested interest in the elderly, who, as a group, consume the largest amount of drugs of any group in the United States. National Medical Enterprise, the fifth largest acute care chain, owns Hillhaven, the second largest nursing home chain with 32,000 beds. National Medical Enterprise also owns hemodialysis stations, home health agencies, Medi$ave Pharmacies, and a variety of other medical product and service businesses. Other corporations may also own other services, such as emergency centers and hotel services (linen, laundry), needed in the nursing home, further capturing a market on health-related services.

The profit motive of many corporations has been criticized regarding several issues. One issue centers on the fairness of corporate profits being made at the public's expense. Over half of corporate revenues come from federal and state funds through Medicare and Medicaid. Another issue considers ethical questions that arise from relationships among hospitals, nursing homes, home health agencies, drug companies, and businesses and services. Some corporations exercise control over such a broad network of services needed by the elderly that they virtually monopolize the market. And finally, the primary focus of profit-oriented business on the "bottom line" does not ensure that compromises in patient care will not be made.

Whether high-quality health care can be delivered while turning a profit is still to be reconciled. Advocates of corporate growth argue that greater management efficiency and economies of scale can be achieved as resources are pooled and shared and goods and supplies purchased in bulk at greater discounts. As a result, profit stems from better management and not necessarily at the expense of quality of patient care.

There is no doubt that the economics, politics, and ethics of long-term care affect the delivery of nursing care to nursing home residents. Directors of nursing and administrators are faced with these issues and must make management decisions within a complex management environment. Gerontological nurses must become informed of the political and corporate issues that influence patient care. Strong nursing leadership is crucial to the attainment of resources and services essential for high-quality care.

Because of the skyrocketing costs associated with long-term care, many institutions and agencies are moving in the direction of managed care. Health care reform efforts have served to accelerate this move (Dee-Kelly et al., 1994). Managed care has promise not only for controlling costs but also for preventing some of the scenarios described in the case studies in this chapter. Managed care is defined by different agencies in specific ways, but a broad definition is the provision of supervision for care provided to an individual in order to better utilize and coordinate resources to both control costs and maximize benefit to the client. Various professionals such as social workers may fulfill the role of case manager. However, the role can be seen as an extension of the historical role of the public health nurse. The role requires setting goals for restoration or rehabilitation, coordination and referral of required services, and termination of services when full benefit has been achieved. Services that can be called into play include skilled nursing services, home health aide services, physical therapy, occupational therapy, speech therapy, social services, and physician intervention. The goal of managed care is to use available resources in the most efficient way possible.

Health maintenance organizations, preferred provider organizations, competitive medical plans, and public health departments are those currently leading the way in utilization of managed care. Home care agencies and institutional settings will most likely view managed care as an opportunity (Dee-Kelly et al., 1994).

HEALTH PROMOTION IN THE CONTEXT OF LONG-TERM CARE

Given the increasingly older population and the heavy utilization of health care services among elderly people, the question arises as to the efficacy of health promotion as a means of solving some of the burdensome problems related to these issues. There are three major issues in regard to the elderly and health promotion:

- Demographics of the older population
- Focus of health promotion
- Approaches to health promotion

Demographics

One of the most important demographic facts affecting health care is the aging of the U.S. population. The number of people aged 65 years or older is growing more rapidly than any other segment of the population. Not only are there more older people in the United States today, but they are living longer. By the year 2020, the number of people over 65 years should reach 50 million, or 17 per cent of the population. By the year 2030, the proportion of the population over 65 years of age will be 22 per cent. In addition, the death rate has decreased from 5600 per 100,000 in 1900 to 3100 per 100,000 in 1977 for those aged 65 to 74 years (U.S. Senate Special Committee on Aging, 1991).

The population of older Americans is a richly diverse group with a heterogeneous economic and health status. The "young old," aged 60 to 74 years, are vastly different in activity level and health status from the "old old," aged 75 years and over. It is the very old who are at greater risk for severe illnesses that often persist as chronic illnesses or disabilities (Self/Health/Care, 1982).

Elderly persons are much more likely to suffer from multiple chronic and disabling illnesses than the young. Eighty per cent of older Americans have one or more chronic conditions, and, as a result, approximately 40 per cent are limited in at least one activity of daily living. The elderly use a disproportionately higher number of health services than other age groups and account for one third of the health care expenditures in the United States. The leading causes of death among the elderly are heart disease, cancer, and stroke (U.S. Senate Special Committee on Aging, 1991).

Focus of Health Promotion

Given these figures, the focus for health promotion programs and their goals for the elderly are necessarily different from those for the young. Older people are at risk for chronic disease, hospitalization, dependency, and institutionalization. In many cases, we must deal with already existing chronic diseases rather than their prevention. Primary, secondary, and tertiary prevention are terms that take on new meanings when applied to older persons with impairments, disabilities, or handicaps associated with chronic disease. According to Kane and colleagues (1985),

the distinctions between primary, secondary, and tertiary prevention fit poorly into the language of chronic disease. A condition may be simultaneously a preventable disease (and thus a problem in its own right) and a precursor (or risk factor) for another condition that could subsequently ensue. For example, . . . hypertension is a problem itself and a risk factor for stroke and heart disease. Thus one can attempt primary prevention of hypertension (through diet modification, for example), whereas control of hypertension (tertiary prevention) becomes primary prevention for stroke.

The issue is where health promotion programs should be focused and what realistically is most effective for the older age group.

Although the majority of programs for the elderly have been tertiary care, disease oriented, and targeted to the sick elderly, increasing attention recently has been devoted to primary activities, such as physical exercise and diet modification, to maximize wellness and reduce risk factors for the well elderly (Kane, R.L., et al., 1983; Fries et al., 1989; Fries, 1992). These are especially appropriate for the "young old." Thus the foci of health promotion programs can range from disease-specific self-management goals to general health promotion goals and can include individual and group efforts related to spiritual, emotional, and psychological as well as physical health concerns (Woomert and Leonard, 1984).

Approaches to Health Promotion

The approach to health promotion programs for the elderly should be wide ranging and should consider basic developmental and psychosocial needs in addition to physical needs. According to Maddox (1985),

interventions should focus on three areas: (1) those that are macroscopic and focus on changing environments (societal); (2) those that concentrate on modifying the immediate environment; and (3) those that concentrate on individuals. Most conventional health promotion programs in the United States have tended to exclude the elderly as a group, first because their focus is on categorical disease prevention more appropriate to the young, and second because the health problems of the elderly seem more like social and economic problems than the categories of problems usually encountered by health care organizations. Basically, two broad strategies for programming appear appropriate for the elderly population:

1. Enhancing the capability of individuals to function independently in the activities of daily living, and
2. Making the environment as supportive as possible (Toward a Strategy, 1982).

The special problems of reaching the elderly through health promotion programs are mainly related to attitudes, beliefs, and knowledge. Many health care providers and the older people themselves have the attitude that the symptoms and problems they are facing are merely normal occurrences associated with aging. They tend to minimize the problems, and often there is no attempt to treat or prevent them. There is often a devaluing of older people, and because they are at the end of the life span, attempts at health promotion do not seem worth the effort. Health professionals may also think that older people are incapable of learning new behaviors or changing old ones.

Leigh and Fries (1992) have demonstrated that health habits in elderly people are related to consequent health care costs, so that health promotion is economically justified. Fries and colleagues (1989) have also shown the need for successful aging programs to focus on health promotion in the older population.

Beliefs about health also may interfere with attempts toward health promotion in the elderly. The Health Belief Model (Rosenstock, 1966; Becker, 1974) shows that people are more likely to take health actions when they are motivated, when they perceive an impending illness to be severe, when they perceive themselves to be susceptible to an illness, when they perceive health actions to be efficacious, and when barriers to health actions are not too great. Older people who already have chronic illness may not feel that preventive actions would be useful (motivation) and worth the effort to change behavior and lifestyle (barriers). If they have become increasingly dependent, they may believe that they have little control over their health and may not perceive that the health behavior is efficacious. Finally, they may believe that, regardless of the severity of the illness or their susceptibility, it is too late to do anything anyway.

Lack of knowledge about health and health care services may also prevent older persons from seeking health promotion interventions. Older people may not be aware that there are primary, secondary, and tertiary prevention strategies that would benefit them. They may also equate health care with sickness-oriented medical care and be reluctant to spend the time, money, and energy on health promotion programs.

Six desired outcomes of health promotion programs are (1) cost containment; (2) survivorship or decreased mortality; (3) decreased morbidity, including impairment; (4) better quality of life; (5) behavior change; and (6) increased productivity. However, since the major health issue of older people is maximizing functional independence and minimizing dependency associated with chronic illness and disability, the criteria for evaluation of health promotion programs probably should focus more narrowly on functional independence and quality of life.

The "compression of morbidity" is an important concept in health and wellness promotion for older adults. The purpose is to delay the onset of the first major disease, infirmity, or disability. This increases the length of "quality" life and decreases the time spent with debilitating illness in a lifetime (Fries et al., 1989; Fries, 1992).

One more issue related to outcomes is whether the cost of health promotion programs for the elderly is worth the effort. Is increased quality of life or increased functional independence measurable in terms of cost effectiveness? Are we willing to use money for quality of life issues? More research must be carried out to attempt to answer these questions.

REHABILITATION IN THE CONTEXT OF LONG-TERM CARE

The overlap among primary, secondary, and tertiary prevention in the elderly points to the need for a strong rehabilitation component in long-term care. Rehabilitative measures cannot be separated easily from health promotion and disease prevention measures in the face of multiple, concurrent chronic illnesses. Therefore the concept of rehabilitation for older persons may be considered in terms of primary, secondary, and tertiary prevention, depending on the level of functioning.

The aim of rehabilitation is either to restore individuals to their former level of functioning or to maintain or maximize remaining function (Williams, 1984; Brummel-Smith, 1993). Prevention of secondary complications, such as muscle contractures, decubitus ulcers, disuse atrophy, and psychological problems, is also of utmost importance. Rehabilitation can and should be carried out in all health care settings by a variety of health care professionals with active involvement of the patients and their families. The location of the rehabilitation environment depends on the needs of the patients and their social and formal support systems.

The Rehabilitation Team

Because of the wide-ranging needs of older patients as a result of the combined effects of environment, significant others, and their general condition, teamwork is vitally important. The rehabilitation team is made up of the patient, family, nurse, physical therapist, occupational therapist, speech therapist, social worker, recreation therapist, and physician. The team can function in all rehabilitation settings, but the make up varies according to the needs of the patient and the availability of particular health care professionals.

The role of the nurse on the rehabilitation team is to coordinate care, provide patient and family teaching, and promote the functional independence of the patient. The nurse also helps to prevent secondary complications by providing patient care, either directly or indirectly, with special attention to elimination, mobility, nutrition, and emotional support. The nurse is in the best position to observe for changes in function and small accomplishments, which should be shared frequently with the older patients, their families, and the team members.

The Rehabilitation Environment

Community

The home environment is frequently the best setting for rehabilitation of the elderly. Older people can have the emotional security of familiar people and personal possessions, fewer inconveniences, and lower costs. The restorative results are usually equal or superior to those in more formal environments. Difficulties associated with rehabilitation in the home environment are overprotection and overindulgence by well-meaning family members, tendency to backslide on the prescribed regimen owing to the absence of an established routine, unavailability of special equipment, and physical obstacles in the home. Assessment of the home environment for appropriateness of rehabilitation should include all of the positive and negative factors, including physical and social supports, the structure of the environment, family interactions, and availability of equipment.

Hospital

The inpatient rehabilitative setting may be located in either a unit in a general hospital or a single-purpose rehabilitation institute. Older people who are best served in a formal hospital setting include those who do not have expert medical care elsewhere, who lack a supportive rehabilitative environment at home, and who need a structured setting for motivation and independence. Additional advantages include the availability of staff and facilities to care for acute problems and comprehensive evaluation and treatments by a multidisciplinary team.

Sometimes the patients' limited restorative potential may not warrant the structured environment of the hospital. However, health care professionals must take care to avoid negative stereotyping of the aged during the decision-making process regarding placement. Older people frequently benefit from formal rehabilitation programs and should not be ruled out solely because of age. In some cases, older patients may adjust poorly to the hospital environment; in other cases, the hospital environment may provide enough security that the older patients do not want to leave.

Nursing Home

Patients who need rehabilitation after hospitalization may be discharged to a nursing home for a period of time. Rehabilitative services in nursing homes vary according to the facility, the type of payment schedules (i.e., Medicare, Medicaid, or private pay), location, and staff. Some nursing homes provide mainly custodial care, so that discharge planning should include an investigation into the type and quality of rehabilitation services offered. Older people frequently dread the possibility of nursing home placement and all its connotations. The nurse must work with the patients and families to allay fears, concerns, and guilt associated

with nursing home placement and should emphasize the rehabilitation potential of the facility and the possibility of returning home if it is realistic.

INITIATIVES IN LONG-TERM CARE

Practice Initiatives

As health care providers recognize the growing proportion of older people in our society and the market potential they represent, increasing numbers of health care providers may identify themselves as geriatric experts. Additionally, service providers, such as hospitals, nursing homes, and community-based agencies, have begun to explore new ways of configuring service to better serve this important sector of the health marketplace. For example, it is no longer uncommon for hospitals to own health agencies; nursing homes are beginning to offer day care services, along with their traditional services; and home health agencies are providing highly technological services (such as intravenous therapy and enteral nutrition programs), which formerly were simply unavailable at home (Huey, 1985). Such innovation has the potential for providing more options in care for elderly people, including better coordination of services and less fragmentation.

Educational Initiatives

Pressure has been placed on the institutions training health care professionals to do more to prepare their graduates to provide good health care for the elderly. Such pressure has stimulated some academic settings to try alternative models of health professional education involving new patterns of student rotation and health services. Examples include the teaching nursing home and some nurse-run clinics, designed to provide health promotion services to the elderly while teaching nursing students about health in elderly people. It is hoped that these efforts will combine with forces in the marketplace to increase the number of properly prepared gerontological health care practitioners.

Political Initiatives

Other promising signs that system change is in the offing include increasingly popular and political support for home-based long-term care. This is demonstrated by the support for federal reimbursement for home health and hospice care and state and local support for community-based long-term care demonstration projects. These are designed to address some of the problems of coordination of care and inefficiency that currently plague noninstitutional services in the "continuum of care," and there is hope that such community-based services will prove to be more cost effective than the institutional alternative (although this has yet to be proven). Should this eventually prove to be true, there would be more sound rationales for reimbursement of services on a chronic disease model rather than only on a medical model.

The federal government, with enactment of the Tax Equity and Fiscal Responsibility Act of 1983, began implementation of a prospective reimbursement system for hospital care under Medicare. It is believed that this will be a powerful tool for containing health care costs. Such a change in financing health care costs for the elderly has already had a profound effect on the manner in which services are delivered (American College of Hospital Administrators, 1984). The total nature of the impact is relatively unclear. However, it is expected that the prospective reimbursement will likely spread to other sectors of the health care system, including other reimbursors and other subunits within the health care system.

SUMMARY

Funding of various demonstration projects during the 1970s fostered development of "alternatives" to nursing home care, such as expanded in-home services and adult day care, among others. Despite the piloting of many new types of services, few of these have found their way into the mainstream of the health care system. Many of these programs, such as adult day care and senior centers, have foundered on the shoals of inadequate funding and reimbursement mechanisms. Other services, such as home-delivered meals and hospice, seem more likely to be incorporated into the mainstream of health services for the aged.

The 1980s were a period of heightened awareness and concern about rapidly rising costs and a shift in focus from federal to state and local governments in both the regulation and finance of health care. Changes in health care financing for the elderly in the 1960s and 1970s spearheaded the development of nursing homes as we know them today. Many believe that the health care reform currently being developed will shape health care delivery to old people in the future and will establish the standard for the

manner in which older people receive their health care for the next several decades.

Although an in-depth analysis of the impact of such changes in the health care system for the elderly is beyond the scope of this book, it should be appreciated that powerful forces for change exist, affording some hope that a system that is based on the principle of targeting specific services to shifting individual needs in a coordinated fashion may someday emerge. It seems clear that during the next several years, owing to the pressures of cost, demographics, and dissatisfaction with the status quo, there will be some consolidation of the aging services network. It is possible that the effective services developed during the demonstration projects of the 1970s and 1980s will become a part of the mainstream of care and that those that are not shown to be effective will be eliminated from the scene, thus reducing some of the confusion surrounding care of elderly people. However, because of the history of service development for the elderly, clinical leaders must be alert for loss of services that are effective but not politically attractive or that may be portrayed as too costly when the evaluation period for cost is too short. The current wave of cost consciousness may bring some rationality to a very complex service delivery system, but there is, at the same time, risk of losing some worthwhile, innovative services.

REFERENCES

Abdellah, F.G., Foerst, H.V. and Chow, R.K. PACE: An approach to improving the care of the elderly. *Am J Nurs* 79:1109–1110, 1979.

Aiken, L.H., Mezey, M.D., Lynaugh, J.E. et al. Teaching nursing homes: Prospect for improving long-term care. *J Am Geriatr Soc* 33:196–201, 1985.

Allen, J.E. *Key Federal Requirements for Nursing Facilities.* New York: Springer Publishing Company, 1992.

American College of Hospital Administrators. *Health Care in the 1990's: Trends and Strategies.* Chicago: Arthur Anderson & Company, 1984.

American Nurses' Association. Nursing and Long-Term Care: Toward Quality Care for the Aged. ANA Publication #GE4 3M, April 1975.

Becker, M.H. *The Health Belief Model and Personal Health Behavior.* San Francisco: Society for Public Health Education, 1974.

Boas, E. Foreword. *In* Jarret, M.C. *The Problem of Chronic Illness.* Vol. 1: *Chronic Illness in New York City.* New York: Columbia University Press, 1933, p. xiii.

Bradley, B. DRGs—An alternative to medicare cuts. *Caring* 3:41–42, 1984.

Bremer, A. A description of community health nursing practice with the community-based elderly. *J Commun Health Nurs* 6(3):173–184, 1989.

Brummel-Smith, K. Research in rehabilitation. *Clin Geriatr Med* 9:895–904, 1993.

Butler, R.N. *Why Survive: Being Old in America.* New York: Harper & Row, 1975.

Campion, E., Bang, A. and May, M. Why acute-care

hospitals must undertake long-term care. *N Engl J Med* 308:71–75, 1983.

Cavaiola, L.J. and Young, J.P. An integrated system for patient assessment and classification and nurse staff allocation for long-term care facilities. *Health Serv Res* 15:281–306, 1980.

Code of Federal Regulations. *Public Health.* Parts 400–429 (rev.). Washington, D.C.: U.S. Government Printing Office, 1986.

Coleman, J.R. and Smith, D.S. DRGs and the growth of home health care. *Nurs Econ* 2:391–395, 1984.

Crane, C.B. Almshouse nursing: The human need; The professional opportunity. *Am J Nurs* 7:872–877, 1907.

Dee-Kelly, P.A., Heller, S. and Sibley, M. Managed care. An opportunity for home care agencies. *Nurs Clin North Am* 29(3):471–481, 1994.

Dolan, J. *Nursing in Society: A Historical Perspective.* Philadelphia: W.B. Saunders, 1983.

Estes, C.L. *The Aging Enterprise.* San Francisco: Jossey Bass, 1979.

Evashwick, C.J., Rundall, T. and Goldiamond, B. Hospital services for older adults. *Gerontologist* 25:631–637, 1985.

Frankfather, D., Smith, M. and Caro, F. *Family Care of the Elderly.* Lexington, MA: D.C. Heath Company, 1981.

Frayne, L.J. DRGs—The impact on physician home health referrals. *Caring* 4:60–63, 1985.

Fries, J.F. Strategies for reduction of morbidity. *Am J Clin Nutr* 55(6 Suppl):1257S–1262S, 1992.

Fries, J.F., Green, L.W. and Levine, S. Health promotion and the compression of morbidity. *Lancet* 1(8636):481–483, 1989.

Gaumer, G. Medicare patient outcomes and hospital organization mission. In Gray, B.H. (ed.). *For-Profit Enterprise in Health Care.* Washington, D.C.: National Academy Press, 1986, pp. 354–374.

Graves, E.J. National Hospital Discharge Survey: Annual Summary, 1991. National Center for Health Statistics. Vital and Health Stat 13(114), 1993.

Greene, V.L., Lovely, M.E. and Ondrich, J.I. The cost-effectiveness of community services in a frail elderly population. *Gerontologist* 33(2):177–189, 1993.

Hawes, C. and Phillips, C.D. The changing structure of the nursing home industry and the impact of ownership on quality, cost and access. In Gray, B.H. (ed.). *For-Profit Enterprise in Health Care.* Washington, D.C.: National Academy Press, 1986, pp. 492–541.

Hays, J.C. Hospice policy and patterns of care. *Image* 18:92–97, 1986.

Hazzard, W.R., Andres, R., Bierman, E.L. and Blass, J.P. *Principles of Geriatric Medicine and Gerontology.* 2nd ed. New York: McGraw-Hill, 1990.

Huey, F. What teaching nursing homes are teaching us. *Am J Nurs* 85:678–683, 1985.

Igou, J.F., Hawkins, J.W., Johnson, E.E. and Utley, Q.E. Nurse-managed approach to care. *Geriatr Nurs* 10(1):32–34, 1989.

Institute of Medicine Committee on Implications of For-Profit Enterprise in Health Care. Profits and health care: An introduction to the issues. In Gray, B.H. (ed.). *For-Profit Enterprise in Health Care.* Washington, D.C.: National Academy Press, 1986a, pp. 3–18.

Institute of Medicine Committee on Implications of For-Profit Enterprise in Health Care. Changes in the ownership, control and configuration of health care services. In Gray, B.H. (ed.). *For-Profit Enterprise in Health Care.* Washington, D.C.: National Academy Press, 1986b, pp. 24–46.

Irwin, T. *Home Health Care: When a Patient Leaves the Hospital.* New York: Public Affairs Committee, 1978.

Johnson, K.A. Exploring home health care opportunities as a result of the Prospective Payment System. *Caring* 4:54–60, 1985.

Jonas, S. *Health Care Delivery in the United States.* New York: Springer Publishing Company, 1981.

Jones, C. *Caring for the Aged.* Chicago: Nelson-Hall, 1982.

Kane, R.A. Case management in long-term care: It can be ethical and efficacious. *J Case Manage* 1(3):76–81, 1992.

Kane, R.L. *Geriatrics in the United States: Manpower Projections and Training Considerations.* Santa Monica, CA: Rand Corporation, 1980.

Kane, R.L. Improving the quality of long-term care. *JAMA* 273(17):1376–1380, 1995.

Kane, R.L., Bell, R.M. et al. *Outcome-Based Reimbursement for Nursing Home Care.* Santa Monica, CA: Rand Corporation, 1983.

Kane, R.L., Illston, L.H. and Miller, N.A. Qualitative analysis of the program of all-inclusive care for the elderly (PACE). *Gerontologist* 32(6):771–780, 1992.

Kane, R.L. and Kane, R.A. (eds.). *Values and Long-Term Care.* Lexington, MA: Lexington Books, D.C. Heath and Company, 1982.

Korn, K., Iverson, L.H. and Pastor, B. The need to reform the long-term care system. *Caring* 8(8):42–48, 1989.

Lazenby, H.C. and Letsch, S.W. National health expenditures, 1989. *Health Care Financ Rev* 12(2), 1989.

Leath, C. and Thatcher, R.M. Team-managed care for older adults. A clinical demonstration of a community model. *J Gerontol Nurs* 17(7):25–28, 1991.

Leigh, J.P. and Fries, J.F. Health habits, health care use and costs in a sample of retirees. *Inquiry* 229(1):44–54, 1992.

Loeser, W., Dickstein, E. and Schiavone, L. Medicare coverage in nursing homes—a broken promise. *N Engl J Med* 304:353–355, 1983.

Lorenz, B.R. Prospective reimbursement in health care and related problems and opportunities for home health agencies. *Caring* 3:27–28, 1984.

Maddox, G.L. Intervention strategies to enhance well-being in later life: The status and prospect of guided change. *Health Serv Res* 19(Part II):1007–1032, 1985.

Manton, K. and Liu, K. *The Future Growth of the Long-Term Care Population: Projections Based on the 1977 National Nursing Home Survey and the 1982 Long-Term Care Survey.* Presented at the Third National Leadership Conference on Long-Term Care Issues: "The Future World of Long-Term Care." Washington, D.C., March 7–9, 1984.

McNamara, E. Hospitals rediscover comprehensive home care. *Hospitals* 56:60–66, 1982.

Mitty, E.L. Resource utilization groups: DRGs move to long-term care. *Nurs Clin North Am* 23(3):539–557, 1988.

Morgenlander, K.H. and Greenwald, D.E. Psychiatric DRGs: The legal and ethical impact. *Qual Rev Bull* 11(6):175–179, 1985.

Moss, F. and Halamandaras, V. *Too Old, Too Sick, Too Bad: Nursing Homes in America.* Germantown, MD: Aspen Systems Corporation, 1977.

National Center for Health Statistics. *Tabulations.* Reported in U.S. Senate Special Committee on Aging. Developments in Aging: 1984, Vol. 1.

National Center for Health Statistics. National hospital discharge survey: Annual summary. *Vital and Health Statistics* 13(99), 1989.

National Center for Health Statistics: *Health United States, 1992.* Data from the Office of National Health Statistics, Health Care Financing Administration: National health expenditures, 1991. *Health Care Financing Review* 14(2). HCFA Pub. 03335. Washington, D.C.: U.S. Government Printing Office, 1992.

Overview of the Medicare DRG system. *Caring* 3:15–19, 1984.

Polich, C.L. Financing long-term care: The role of

the federal government. *Caring* 8(4):16–19, 22–23, 1989.

Pyles, J.C. Referral arrangements between hospitals and home health agencies. *Caring* 2:54–56, 1984.

Rango, N. Nursing-home care in the United States: Prevailing conditions and policy implications. *N Engl J Med* 307:883–889, 1982.

Rantz, M.J. Inadequate reimbursement for long-term care: The impact since hospital DRGs. *Nurs Health Care* 11(9):470–472, 1990.

Rosenstock, I. Why people use health services. *Milbank Mem Fund Q* 44:94–127, 1966.

Self/Health/Care and Older People. New York, World Health Organization, 1982.

Thomas, W.C., Jr. *Nursing Homes and Public Policy: Drift and Decision in New York State.* Ithaca, N.Y.: Cornell University Press, 1969.

Thomas, W.R., Clauser, S.B., and Baugh, D.K. Trends in Medicaid payments and utilization, 1975–1989. *Health Care Financ Rev* 1990 Supplement, 1989.

Tillman, E. The Medicare prospective payment system: New problems and opportunities. *Caring* 2:24–26, 1984.

Toward a Strategy for Health Promotion Among the Elderly: A Background Paper. Special Report prepared for the W.K. Kellogg Foundation. Chapel Hill, NC: UNC–CH Health Services Research Center, 1982.

United States Department of Health and Human Services. *Health Care Financing: Program Statistics.* Bethesda, MD: HCFA Publication No. 03270, U.S. Department of Health and Human Services, 1983.

United States Department of Health and Human Services. *Personnel for Health Needs of the Elderly Through the Year 2020.* Bethesda, MD: National Institute on Aging, Public Health Service, Department of Health and Human Services, Pub. No. 87-2950, 1988, p. 199.

United States Department of Health and Human Services. *Special Report on Aging 1990.* Washington, D.C.: National Institute on Aging, 1990.

United States Department of Health and Human Services. *The Use of Formal and Informal Home Care by the Disabled Elderly.* Agency for Health Care Policy and Research Pub. No. 93-0004, 1992.

United States Department of Health, Education and Welfare, Public Health Service. *A Guide to Medical Self-Care and Self-Help Groups for the Elderly.* Washington, D.C.: U.S. Government Printing Office, 1979.

United States Senate Special Committee on Aging. *Aging America: Trends and Projections.* Washington, D.C.: U.S. Department of Health and Human Services.

Vladeck, B.C. *Unloving Care.* New York: Basic Books, Inc., 1980.

Waldo, D.R., Sonnefeld, S.T., McKusick, D.R., and Ross, H.A. Health expenditures by age group, 1977 to 1987. *Health Care Financ Rev* 10(4), 1989.

Williams, T.F. (ed.). *Rehabilitation in the Aging.* New York: Raven Press, 1984.

Wohl, S. *The Medical-Industrial Complex.* New York: Harmony Books, 1984.

Woomert, A. and Leonard, A. An overview of health education programs for the elderly: Current directions in health promotion and disease prevention. Paper presented at the American Public Health Association, 112th Annual Meeting, Anaheim, CA, November 11–15, 1984.

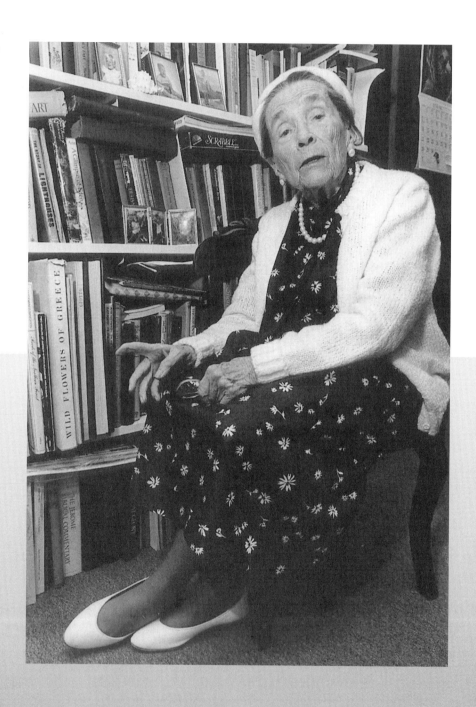

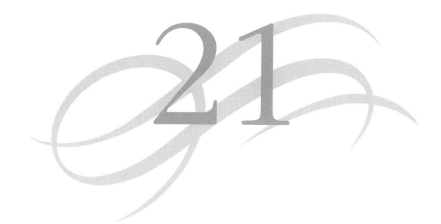

Nursing Diagnoses Influenced by Setting of Care

SUSAN ANN RUZICKA

OBJECTIVES

Identify nursing diagnoses that are influenced by various care settings.

❖

Discuss the definition and scope of the problem, theoretical issues, and contributing factors for each, nursing diagnosis as they relate specifically to the elderly.

❖

Conduct a nursing assessment on an older client related to each nursing diagnosis.

❖

Formulate a plan of care and nursing interventions for older clients for each nursing diagnosis.

❖

Evaluate the plan of care and nursing interventions for older clients for each nursing diagnosis.

The process of nursing care is influenced by the setting in which the nurse and patient are located. Certain diagnoses are subject to the influence of the care setting. Both the institutional standards of care and the policies influence the selection and the use of particular nursing diagnoses. The use of a particular nursing diagnosis also depends on the availability of resources to effectively manage the defined need of a patient. For example, long-term care facilities have a larger percentage of residents with disruptive behaviors that increase risk of injury, potential nonadherence to therapy, and overall impaired health maintenance. Lack of resources to maintain the individual in the community often prompts the change in care setting to a long-term care facility that provides the patient with more effective management.

The common thread among the diagnostic categories discussed in this chapter is that assessment or treatment in each category is influenced by setting of care.

DIVERSIONAL ACTIVITY DEFICIT

Definition

Diversional activity deficit is ". . . the state in which an individual experiences a decreased stimulation from or interest or engagement in recreational or leisure activities [Note: Internal/external factors may or may not be beyond the individual's control]" (Doenges and Moorhouse, 1993, p. 163). Defining characteristics of this deficit currently accepted by the North American Nursing Diagnosis Association (NANDA) include a patient's statements of boredom, desire for something to do, and inability to pursue usual hobbies because of illness or physical or environmental limitations (Doenges and Moorhouse, 1993).

Theoretical Issues

Time Utilization

People use time in one of four ways: work, rest, leisure, and self-care. Achieving a balance among all these activities is a self-care requirement.

Cultural group identification influences the meaning and values attached to the use of time. For example, the Protestant work ethic focuses on productivity and work, placing less value on leisure pursuits. Eastern cultures and religions place a higher value on contemplative activities than do Western cultures.

Industrialization and increase in life expectancy have influenced the roles of work and leisure in people's lives. The transformation from an agrarian society to an industrialized society has dramatically reduced the percentage of time spent working. The trend of early retirement also reflects on the increased time spent in leisure activities as people age. Fewer than 15 per cent of Americans aged sixty-five years and older are in the work force (Dychtwald and Flower, 1989).

Many of these retirees have guided their lives by the Protestant work ethic, which values work much more than leisure. Surveys performed by the American Association of Retired Persons and the National Council on Aging found 40 per cent of retired people would rather be working. Fulfillment, control over their own lives, and a sense of usefulness to society are some of the reasons for this interest in working.

Developing a new view of leisure can be challenging. Leisure makes up the majority of time for elders. Strategies that allow a sense of fulfillment and control of self within the framework of leisure are essential.

AGING-RELATED CHANGES AFFECTING TIME UTILIZATION. Restructuring the use of time as one ages is necessary because of factors such as age-related changes, disease-associated changes, and socially defined limitations and demands.

Age-related changes in the body have been identified throughout this text. The process of aging slows functioning to some degree but has minimal impact on ability of overall performance. The patterns of function may change, but the overall outcome is minimally altered. For example, as people age, their patterns of sleep change. With age, sleep is less deep, and their patterns of sleep and rest change. The overall outcome of feeling rested after uninterrupted sleep, however, does not change.

As discussed in Chapter 2 of this text, most of the elderly have one or more chronic diseases. The pathophysiological changes and the effects of medications taken to manage disease greatly affect the elderly's use of time.

Pathological processes and states often place additional burdens on the older person that dramatically affect time use. The demands to spend additional time in self-care activities stem from four sources:

1. Self-monitoring response to disease
2. Carrying out of therapeutic regimens
3. Compensating for function lost to illness
4. Seeking of professional assistance for treatment of the disease

The time to accomplish these tasks must be taken from work, leisure, or rest activities.

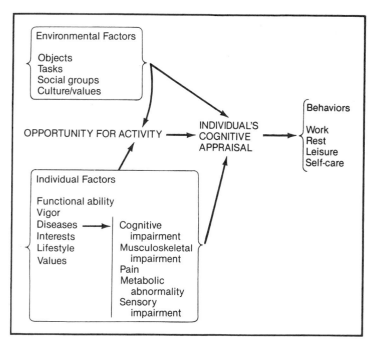

FIGURE 21-1

Contributing factors to diversional activity deficit.

Social factors also affect the use of time. An example of this is the increasing trend of grandparents' caring for their grandchildren. Dual-income families, single parenthood, and divorce have affected this trend. Loss of societal partners and spouses influences the use of time.

Nurses should consider the various dimensions of time use in older adults because processes associated with aging result in slowed task performance and changes in roles. For many, the changes are complementary. As time required for performance increases, the number of roles and task demands decreases, and a new and satisfactory equilibrium is reached. For others, an imbalance occurs, either because of role loss preceding lost capabilities or because roles are not relinquished despite disability. Imbalances between activity and ability may result in maladaptive responses by the older person, such as boredom, loss of self-confidence, fear, and arrested development (Kreidler et al., 1994; Windriver, 1993; Dychtwald and Flower, 1989).

Contributing Factors

Diversional activity deficit is most likely to occur in persons who lose meaningful roles. Factors contributing to diversional activity deficit are shown in Figure 21–1.

Examples of contributing factors would be the following:

An elderly man played cards weekly with friends. Within a few years, his card playing companions either died, were institutionalized, or relocated nearer to their children's homes. The elderly man lost his social group of many years in a brief period of 24 months.

An elderly woman cared for her husband for 71 years in a variety of ways. This role became increasingly consumed with basic care tasks. Her husband needed assistance ambulating, toileting, grooming, and dressing. She derived meaning and satisfaction from this role. Her husband's death placed a huge void in her life.

LIFESTYLE AND HEALTH STATUS. The relationship between lifestyle and health status is significant. Research shows that a lifelong diversity of interests and activities supports successful adaptation (Somers and Fabian, 1981; Dychtwald and Flower, 1989). Lifestyle choices reflect types of activities that are important to each individual. Knowledge of those activities guide the nurse in identifying what is meaningful to the individual. Walker et al. (1988) studied six health-promoting lifestyles: self-actualization, health responsibility, exercise, nutrition, interpersonal support, and stress management. They found that encouragement and facilitation of healthy lifestyles reduces the likelihood of premature death and enhances the quality of life (Lorenson, 1992). There is continuity throughout the lifespan regarding activities and interests. Individuals with diverse interests are thought to be at less risk of diversional activity deficit than those with only one or two interests.

ENVIRONMENTAL INFLUENCES. Both the physical and the social environments are powerful shapers of activity patterns. The concept of environmental layers—objects, tasks, social group, and culture and values—provides a useful framework for analysis of the influence of environment on activity pattern (Barris et al., 1985).

Objects of only one type are not conducive to a variety of behaviors. For example, if a person lives in one room where the only objects are related to rest or self-care, such as a hospital or nursing home room, he or she is unlikely to engage in work or leisure activities. The individual would need to leave the room to engage in other pursuits. Those with mobility impairments would have a particularly difficult time. Conversely, if there are no suitable rest or self-care objects in a senior center or health clinic, attending such places is less attractive for those who have greater-than-average personal care requirements.

The *task demands* of the environment may also shape the types of activity for the older person. If toileting requires excessive time because of the physical layout of the environment (e.g., shared bathrooms, long distances), then increased time must be devoted to self-care, which generally is taken from leisure time or work time. The task demands of work may exceed the older person's capabilities. For example, holding down a volunteer job may require reliable transportation, thus eliminating a potential activity in the work domain for the older person without access to good transportation.

Social groups to which the individual belongs also influence the diversity of activities available. Some social groups, such as churches, fraternal organizations, and some community voluntary organizations, afford a wide range of activities. The older person who is physically isolated from interacting with such groups through inadequate transportation, physical illness, or psychological illness is at high risk for diversional activity deficit.

As noted, the cultural group to which a person belongs affects the structure of time use. Individuals who must lie in an environment with a different *culture or set of values* than their own are at high risk for diversional activity deficit (Smith et al., 1986). For example, the old man who has worked all his life and defines his self-worth in terms of work-related accomplishments and productivity is at great risk for adjustment problems if he is institutionalized in an environment in which the activities are all leisure- or self-care oriented.

Assessment

Detailed assessment of someone suspected of having diversional activity deficits builds on the data gathered in the screening psychosocial assessment (see Chapter 16). The response to the request "Describe what you did yesterday," followed by clarification that yesterday was a typical or an unusual day, should be analyzed to determine the percentage of time the individual spends in self-care activities, work, rest, and leisure. Although specific age norms have not been validated, a total lack of work or leisure activities suggests diversional activity deficit.

Table 21–1 details a few assessment maneuvers and their rationale. The nurse should determine the client's satisfaction with the prevailing level and variety of activities. The nurse should ask whether cer-

TABLE 21-1
Assessment Maneuvers for Diversional Activity Deficit

QUESTION/MANEUVER	RATIONALE
1. Describe what you did yesterday. Was this a typical day for you?	Screens for deficit
2. Are there things that you wish you could do but are not now doing?	Probe for satisfaction with current activity level and diversity
3. When you want to have a really good time, what do you do?	Taps pleasurable, enjoyable activities
4. Prior to—(retirement, this hospitalization, this illness, coming to the nursing home), how did you spend your time?	Screens for recent changes in work/rest/play/self-care time utilization

tain types of activities are missing from the person's life. An impaired health status, the perception of leisure as inappropriate for adults, or other factors may interfere with the variety of activity. The nurse should assess the individual's perception of his or her present activity level. Knowledge of past activity patterns are helpful in the planning of effective care. Desired activities, frequency of those activities, and presence of barriers to those activities are essential to the assessment. The nurses should ask what the individual does for pleasure or enjoyment. Absence of a positive response suggests diversional activity deficit and possibly depression and deserves an in-depth investigation. Interest inventories are sometimes used by recreational or occupational therapists to facilitate planning and to stimulate the older person to consider a wider range of activity options.

Planning

The interdisciplinary approach to the management of diversional activity deficit is beneficial to the individual. Inclusion of family, significant others, and the individual enhances the process. If a change in activity pattern is indicated, the individual's response may vary. Some may feel great relief and may welcome change, whereas others may feel very threatened and insecure regarding the change in routine. A team approach with the individual and the support person being involved in the recognition and management of the deficit increases the probability for its success. Restructuring routine habits, whether they are pleasurable or not, can be a stressful experience. An understanding of the individual's response and

perception of these proposed changes is critical. This knowledge guides the choice of strategies and how those strategies are implemented.

Individuals who are involved in the identification of the diversional activity deficit and who agree that it is a problem are more likely to be involved in the implementation of strategies to eliminate the deficit. Individuals with a lifestyle of solitary pursuits require a strategy much different than those engaged in group activities. A caveat applies: if one type of activity has been lost through health status or environmental changes, the substitute activity should be of a similar type. For example, the college professor who is forced to retire should be counseled to turn to activities that replace the lost gratification of the job. If the professor most enjoyed interacting with students, activities that allow continuing a mentoring role are most appropriate.

Another individual who most enjoyed making grandfather clocks found enjoyment piecing together interwoven wooden baskets. Individuality in the planning phase is of great importance. Lack of attention to this area could lead to other problems, such as lack of self-esteem and identity (Kenny, 1990).

Interventions

Orem's (1980) taxonomy of helping methods provides a useful organizing framework for discussing interventions for diversional activity deficit.

DOING FOR THE CLIENT. Nurses seldom provide recreational pursuits for patients, although the nurse may elect to do something entertaining or diverting on a short-term basis to raise the client's awareness that diversional pursuits are worthwhile. Guiding the client through referral to other professionals is a common intervention for the individual with diversional activity deficit. The client may not be aware of the various counseling services available: vocational rehabilitation, recreational therapy, and occupational therapy. The nurse is more often involved in the evaluation of the effectiveness of the specific interventions and shares this information with other health care professionals.

SUPPORTING ANOTHER (PHYSICALLY OR PSYCHOLOGICALLY). The older person may require considerable support to engage in a new diversional activity. There are many disincentives to older persons' participating fully in adult life. For example, individuals with a series of personal losses of friends, spouses, or both, may be more hesitant in expending energy toward new social experiences. Encouragement or assistance in compensating for physical limitations may make the difference between successful intervention and failure.

PROVIDING AN ENVIRONMENT THAT PROMOTES DEVELOPMENT. Several elements in the older person's environment may not be conducive to diversional activity. The necessary privacy or solitude for contemplative pursuits may be missing in an institution or a busy household. Simple modifications, such as "do not disturb" signs or enforced quiet hours, may transform the situation into one that permits the desired activity. Physical features like lighting or background noise may require modification, too. Insufficient lighting intensity will render needlework or crocheting nearly impossible for those with visual impairment. In a similar manner, proper control of background noise may make dining an enjoyable experience. Methods that can promote successful activities include networking individuals with similar interests and matching needs of individuals. For example, an individual who enjoys gardening but cannot participate in that activity because of physical limitations may be paired with someone who knows little about gardening but enjoys tasks and following directions in accomplishing projects. Together, they may serve each other in creating a beautiful garden, thereby enhancing one another's quality of life.

It is important to be cautious in networking to avoid a sense of burden or obligation.

TEACHING. This is a commonly used intervention for diversional activity deficit. The nurse may provide information about other resources that can help resolve the personal or environmental lack—Talking Books, transportation, adaptive equipment, and the senior center.

Evaluation of Nursing Care

Criteria for evaluation of nursing care for the person with diversional activity deficit are as follows:

1. The person verbalizes or demonstrates satisfaction with his or her present activity level and use of time.
2. The individual is happily integrated into social groups and/or is involved in solitary pursuits that are stimulating.
3. The individual verbalizes or demonstrates sufficient time to engage in desired activities.

4. The person exhibits or verbalizes a decreased sense of burden.

HEALTH MAINTENANCE ALTERATION

Definition and Scope of Problem

Health maintenance alteration is defined by NANDA as the "inability to identify, manage, and/or seek out help to maintain health" (Doenges & Moorhouse, 1993, p. 225). NANDA further states that this diagnosis ". . . contains components of other nursing diagnoses. We recommend subsuming health maintenance interventions under the 'basic' nursing diagnosis when a single causative factor is identified (e.g., Knowledge Deficit, Communication, Impaired; Verbal, Thought Processes, Altered; Individual/Family Coping, Ineffective)" (Doenges and Moorhouse, 1993, p. 225).

Theoretical Issues

Many issues influence health maintenance in the elderly population, including increased percentage of the total population, increased health costs, use of national health care resources, increased numbers of economically poor elderly, and changes in family structure (Somers and Fabian, 1981). The family is more mobile today, and children are often far away and unable to care for their frail elders. The traditional informal caregiver, the eldest daughter, may be working full time, financially supporting her post–college-aged children and managing a family without a spouse.

No universal definition of health exists. It is multidimensional and varies depending on the culture, the institution, and the setting in society.

Setting of Care

The practice of health maintenance management varies considerably from one setting to another. Resources to maintain elderly persons at this most independent level vary greatly. Rural communities far from well-established metropolitan medical centers have less access to programs that could enhance the quality of life of their elderly. Physical and economic limitations also restrict access to health care providers. Continuing care and easing the transition from the acute care setting to the less acute community setting are becoming increasingly important services.

Most individuals discharged from the hospital to their home are dependent on themselves for management of their medical regimens. Often, this is a time of great anxiety and vulnerability, predisposing the elderly person to the ill effects of stress (Zarle, 1989). Individuals who have limited capacity for health maintenance management often end up in institutions, where they are more dependent on facility staff to assist in health maintenance.

Individuals in the community are at risk for altered health maintenance for a variety of reasons, many of which are listed earlier. Altered cognition, altered sensation, changes in mobility, lack of resources or access to resources, and inability to perform instrumental activities of daily living (IADLs) or basic activities of daily living (ADLs) are some of the factors that increase the individual's risk for altered health maintenance.

Individuals in long-term care facilities are prone to relocation stress, acute confusion, decreased self-esteem, decreased locus of control, and excess functional disability. Altered Health Maintenance is a helpful diagnosis in identifying a general area of concern, while continued assessment and identification of the specific etiology are being performed.

Recommendations for Health Maintenance in the Aged

Despite the controversies surrounding definitions of health and the efficacy of health maintenance programs, certain recommendations regarding health maintenance activities are widely accepted. The recommendations of the Canadian Task Force on the Periodic Health Examination for health maintenance procedures for the elderly are summarized in Table 21–2.

Contributing Factors

Individual Factors

IMPAIRED COMMUNICATION. Impaired communication skills affect maintenance of health in several ways. Hearing loss may result in older individuals' having inadequate information about their disease process, leading to ignorance about special care required because of the disorder or treatment regimen. Reading disabilities, whether due to visual disturbance or illiteracy, may have a similar effect. The inability to communicate verbally because of aphasia or cognitive impairment makes it difficult to report symptoms or historical aspects of an

TABLE 21–2
Healthy People 2000: Recommendations for Older Adults

PHYSICAL ACTIVITIES	BENEFITS
Participation in leisure time physical activity on a regular basis	Reduced risk of coronary heart disease, hypertension, non–insulin-dependent diabetes mellitus, colon cancer, depression, and anxiety Increased bone mineral content, reduced risk of osteoporotic fracture Enhanced maintenance of body weight Increased longevity and maintenance of functional independence
Regular contact with a primary health care provider ● Screening mammography ● Breast examination ● Papanicolaou test ● Prostate examination ● Pneumococcal immunization ● Influenza vaccination ● Review of prescribed and over-the-counter medications, dosage, and use ● Screen for etiology of reversible dementia, incontinence, depression	Prevention of disabling and life-threatening diseases and conditions
Participation in formal and/or informal social networks on a regular basis	Decreased risk of social isolation as a result of loss of spouse, retirement, or changes in social role Decreased risk of depression

Adapted from *Healthy People 2000: National Health Promotion and Disease Prevention Objectives.* United States Department of Health and Human Services, Public Health Service, DHHS Publication No. (PHS) 91-50213, Washington, D.C., 1990.

illness; thus, accurate diagnosis becomes more difficult. Disorders common among the elderly that lead to communication difficulties include cerebrovascular accident, dementia, delirium, depression, macular degeneration, and presbycusis. People with these disorders should be considered at risk for health maintenance alteration.

COGNITIVE IMPAIRMENT. Cognitive impairment contributes to health maintenance alteration because memory and judgment are affected. For example, the individual with coronary artery disease may forget to report episodes of chest pain or lack the problem-solving ability to use rest periods or nitroglycerin to relieve symptoms of angina. Dementia, delirium, and depression all may affect judgment, problem-solving ability, and memory.

ACTIVITY INTOLERANCE. Extreme activity intolerance may affect health maintenance by reducing the energy available to the individual to engage in health-maintaining behaviors. People who are chronically fatigued may omit their usual oral hygiene routines because it is simply too tiring. In a similar manner, it may be too energy-consuming to travel to appointments, necessitating some form of home care or arrangement for a rest area at the clinic.

MOBILITY IMPAIRMENT. Types of altered physical mobility that potentially contribute to altered health maintenance include diminished hand strength, impairments in fine motor coordination, and impaired ability to transfer and ambulate. Diminished hand strength and dexterity affect the ability to self-administer medications, both oral and injectable. Difficulties in transfer ability increase the complexity of visits to primary care providers and professionals who use specialized chairs and equipment, such as dental hygienists.

INEFFECTIVE COPING. Alterations in health maintenance that result from ineffective individual coping may become manifest as self-neglect or denial of problems. Coping difficulties also may interfere with problem-solving abilities and judgment.

CHRONIC DISEASES. Specific disease states influence the activities required to maintain health (Orem, 1980). Diseases like chronic obstructive pulmonary disease, diabetes mellitus, hypertension, and peripheral vascular disease require new self-care behaviors to maintain health. For example, individuals with diabetes mellitus must learn, among other things, to inspect their feet on a regular basis because of the high morbidity associated with foot ulcers in diabetics. In most people, minor foot trauma is a trivial occurrence. Older people with multiple chronic diseases must learn many new tasks to manage their health problems optimally and are therefore at high risk for alterations in health maintenance management.

Social Factors

FAMILY DYNAMICS. Ineffective family coping may also contribute to altered health maintenance, particularly for elderly individuals who require the assistance of a caregiver. In the simplest case, the older person relies on family only for simple forms of assistance, such as transportation to medical appointments. In more complex instances, a family member may be the older person's primary caregiver. When difficulties arise in the family unit, the reliability of the caregiver may suffer. Families also may experience conflict over priorities in health care for the elderly member. Individual members may disagree over how money is to be allocated for care, or they may disagree about

the extent of medical intervention desired. Unless there is a mechanism for the older person's wishes to be considered, psychological and spiritual health may be compromised.

ECONOMIC FACTORS. Economic factors influence access to health maintenance services. Medicare does not pay for preventive care, and many prosthetic devices that would also allow greater independence in function (such as dentures, arm slings, and shower chairs) are considered "luxury items" by insurance carriers and therefore are not reimbursed. Old people in poverty thus have more limited access to health-maintaining services and equipment.

ATTITUDES. Attitudes of health care providers also may limit access to health-maintaining services or equipment. Some professionals consider it inappropriate to refer old people for psychotherapy, on the grounds that the personality is relatively fixed in old age. Such a stance ignores the growing body of literature revealing that old people can benefit from psychotherapy. A similar problem exists with rehabilitative services.

RELIGIOUS BELIEFS. Religious beliefs also can affect health maintenance in the aged. Certain religions—for example, Jehovah's Witnesses and Christian Scientists—eschew some but not all types of medical intervention. Some members of these groups fear losing control over decisions about their care to the medical institution and avoid traditional forms of health care completely.

Environmental Factors

In the community, the accessibility of health care providers is influenced by the availability of public transportation, the presence of ramps for wheelchairs, and the ease of negotiating the office or clinic surroundings. In hospitals and nursing homes, accessibility of care is governed by institutional policies, the services rendered in the institution, and the "gatekeepers" for those services. In both settings, the physician is designated the official gatekeeper, but nurses have tremendous influence over decisions about access to care. Nurses make decisions about when to give *pro re nata* medications and when the patient has a new health problem requiring evaluation or intervention by other health team members.

Assessment

Assessment of individuals or groups for health maintenance alterations is guided by the defining characteristics listed by Doenges and Moorhouse (1993, p. 225):

- Demonstrated lack of knowledge regarding basic health practices
- Demonstrated lack of adaptive behaviors to internal and/or external environmental changes
- Reported or observed inability to take responsibility for meeting basic health practices in any or all functional pattern areas
- History of lack of health-seeking behavior
- Expressed interest in improving health behaviors
- Reported or observed lack of equipment and financial aid/or other resources
- Reported or observed impairment of personal support systems

High-risk groups include people living in institutions, homebound people, those who have difficulty performing activities of daily living, those with cognitive impairments, and those with severe sensory impairments.

Interview

The individual suspected of having altered health maintenance management should be interviewed to understand his or her perspective on the following:

- Personal definition of health
- Self-perception of health status
- Satisfaction with current health status
- Personal health goals
- Usual mode of obtaining health information
- Self-care, health, and illness behaviors, including last immunizations, health examination
- Access to various health care providers
- Beliefs about aggressiveness of medical care

Some individuals are unable to articulate their health goals and practices or no longer carry primary responsibility for self-care activities. People with moderate-to-severe dementia and those with severe physical impairment are in this category. In such situations, health maintenance practices are assessed as just outlined, but the primary caregiver is the informant. The older person still should be included in the assessment so that the older person participates to the full-

est extent possible. Although judgment or ability to carry out an activity may be impaired, the individual may have strong feelings about health care that deserve full expression. Jewel and Peters (1989) developed an assessment guide to organize assessment data in a useful way. Nine areas were addressed:

1. Ability to act independently.
2. Habits, customs, values, and beliefs. The nurse should look for behaviors that are valued by the groups, such as respect for elders, privacy, courtesy, humor, pride, cleanliness, public image, and others. The nurse should determine attitudes toward birth, death, illness, sex roles, aging, and others and should determine personal habits, such as alcohol intake, drug use, smoking, personal hygiene, sleeping patterns, and exercise habits.
3. Health and illness beliefs and practices. The nurse should elicit the patient's theories of health and illness—what do they believe makes them sick or keeps them well? Examples are heat or cold, yin-yang (a belief predominant in Eastern cultures), germs, supernatural visitations, and "hard work and right living." The nurse should look for preventive practices and should also determine the patient's healing systems, such as folk healers, scientific healers, and religious healers. Does the person use home remedies, drug stores, herbal shops, health food stores or others?
4. Nutritional practices and beliefs, including food preparation, availability of food, shopping practices, excesses and deprivations, and cultural variations in food preferences.
5. Utilization of health care services and attitude toward health care—understanding of scientific health care and when and how to enter the system.
6. Experiences with the professional health care system—has the bureaucracy prevented the patient from receiving humane care when needed? Has the patient received preventive care that he or she can use?
7. Cultural and social class responses to stress, illness, and disability—what does the person do when he or she gets sick?
8. Medication use—understanding of side effects, self-medication.
9. Preventive health measures.

Observation

In addition to using interview techniques, the nurse should observe the individual's performance of selected self-care maneuvers, such as medication administration, foot care, and meal planning. Inquiring about hypothetical situations allows the clinician to assess the individual's understanding of appropriate symptom reporting and management of therapeutic regimens. An example is "If you were making the bed and began to experience tightness in your chest, what would you do?"

Considerations in Home Care

Nurses in home health settings have a unique opportunity to assess family approaches to health maintenance. When family members become primary caregivers for a dependent older person, issues of family health maintenance influence the health maintenance of the elderly. The nurse should identify the caregivers' perceptions of their own health problems and self-care practices. Failure to do so represents a lost opportunity to help prevent caregiver burnout. Especially for a spouse or an only child providing care, the burden of caregiving may demand new strategies for self-care that are unknown to the family member. Techniques of stress management, body mechanics, and transfer skills or opportunities for respite care are samples of the new health maintenance skills a family caregiver may need to develop.

Planning

Individual Considerations

When working with people to establish a plan for health maintenance, it is important to know whether the person has the capacity to make decisions about health maintenance and the ability to carry out those decisions. Orem's (1980) distinctions between supportive-educative, partly compensatory, and wholly compensatory modes of nursing intervention provide a useful means of categorizing patients (see Chapter 1). Some clients require only information about resources for health maintenance or recommendations regarding the type or frequency of health maintenance activities. Others require varying degrees of assistance in developing and implementing a health maintenance program, ranging from formulating goals and strategies to relying on institutional policy for all health maintenance care.

Nurses may have to work with a family in planning a health maintenance program for patients with partly or wholly compensatory nursing care systems. The process increases in complexity with more individuals involved because a greater variety of beliefs and values must be considered. Techniques useful in planning include values clarification exercises, assignment of specific responsibilities within the family or kin network, and development of explicit guidelines for communication. Focusing on the values and beliefs of the individual being assisted or cared for gives all persons involved in planning the individual's care a common point of reference and more appropriate guidelines. If the individual is cognitively impaired, this process is more challenging.

Community Considerations

At the group level of organization, planning for health maintenance becomes quite complex. Activities such as control of nosocomial infection, development of fall-related injury prevention programs, establishment of do-not-resuscitate policies, and ascertainment of new community health problems are all examples of health maintenance planning at the small group or community level. The large-scale health maintenance plan may be the responsibility of quality assurance departments, infection control departments, or clinical nurse specialists. It should be guided by the philosophy or mission statement of the institution and should be derived from scientifically based assessment data.

Interventions

Etiologic factors and settings of care influence interventions for health maintenance alterations. Table 21–3 provides examples of interventions possible in the particular locations of care, according to diagnosis.

Evident is the generalist approach. The plan of care is modified to best meet the individual goals through implementation of the intervention and evaluation of individual's responses to the intervention. The nursing priorities are threefold: (1) further assessment of causative or contributing factors, (2) assistance in maintaining and managing desired health practices, and (3) promotion of wellness through teaching and discharge considerations (Doenges and Moorhouse, 1993; Miller et al., 1987; Kenney, 1990; Schank, 1990).

Further Assessment of Causative and Contributing Factors

Assessment of functional abilities is an important aspect of health maintenance. Focusing on functional abilities is critical for

TABLE 21 – 3
Sample Interventions for Altered Health Maintenance

DIAGNOSIS	EXPECTED OUTCOME	INTERVENTION
Nursing Home Alteration in health maintenance, related to impaired ability in communication and dysfunctional grieving	Client will identify two effective methods in grieving within the next thirty days and use these methods with verbal cuing from staff	Assist client in identification of appropriate grieving methods Identify etiology of impaired communication Establish routine times to actively listen to client Use positive verbal praise when appropriate grieving methods are used
Hospital Alteration in health maintenance, related to lack of knowledge of available resources and impaired motor skills secondary to recent CVA	Client will have established resources to assist in completion of activities of daily living by (set date for accomplishment)	Assist in identifying formal and informal resources in the community Use positive reinforcement when client practices new strategies learned in PT/OT Use fellow health disciplines in promoting health maintenance, e.g., social work, physical therapy
Community Alteration in health maintenance, related to cognitive impairment and ineffective family coping	Client will safely perform activity of daily living with verbal cuing and nonverbal gestures by family/caregiver by (set date for accomplishment) Client and caregiver will use respite services appropriately by (set date for accomplishment)	Assist client and caregiver in recommended health practices Inform client and caregiver of available respite services and adult daycare services Use positive verbal praise when recommended health practices are implemented and used appropriately

CVA = cerebrovascular accident; OT = occupational therapy; PT = physical therapy.

promoting optimal performance and independence. Assessment of ADLs and IADLs helps to determine a realistic level of functional ability. Assessing at different times of the day is important, especially in the home setting. Individuals may fear institutionalization and may make appearances that they can effectively manage independently when the reality is otherwise. Using one's senses in this assessment is helpful. For example, odors of poor hygiene, rotten food, or unkempt pets are clues regarding inadequate health maintenance. Visually noting empty pantries or refrigerators, poor personal grooming, or safety hazards, such as unsafe pathways or poor lighting, are additional clues.

Use of adaptive equipment and behaviors; utilization of formal (e.g., medical center programs) and informal (e.g., neighbors) resources; use of communication skills and resources; and presence and/or use of alcohol, narcotics, over-the-counter remedies, or home practices (e.g., baking soda after each meal, butter on wounds) are important and need to be documented. Recent changes in lifestyle, recent personal losses, recent

changes in motivation or participation in activities, and recent changes in health or perception of health are also important to document. Documentation of these assessment cues provides the opportunity to further define the cause of the person's inability to effectively manage his or her health. The cues may together form a cluster that defines more appropriate, tailored nursing diagnoses.

Assistance in Maintaining and Managing Desired Health Practice

The focus at this level of intervention is heavily dependent on effective communication. The first step in effective communication is listening. The nurse should listen to the elderly person's concerns, perceptions, and routines, and should listen to the pace and tone of the elderly person's speech. Most communication is nonverbal. The nurse should observe the expressions, eye contact, and musculature of the face and body movements. This information identifies the issues that are important to the individual, which will be used in mutual goal setting. Health care providers should communicate their roles and the reason for their presence.

Communication of identified self-care deficits, availability of resources, use of resources, and identified strengths of the individual are necessary. Actual networking with health care or community resources to meet the individual's needs is a critical step. Monitoring effectiveness of resource utilization is helpful in maintaining and managing desired health practices.

Promotion of Wellness Through Teaching and Discharge Planning

Effective discharge planning enhances the quality of life for the elderly and reduces readmissions and the overall cost of health care. Interventions helpful for the nurse to implement include assisting the individual in the development of realistic strategies. For example, in the acute care setting, elderly people are often discharged with multiple problems, such as wound care, recommendations for changes in lifestyle, decreased energy, inability to independently perform ADLs and IADLs, and new medications. Hospitalization is a stressor, but being sent home with the aforementioned challenges can be overwhelming to the individual.

The nurse is an advocate for the client. Communication and clarification among the health team, the individual and the family, and the services to be utilized are important. The elderly person's or guardian's understanding of referral services is necessary in arranging referrals. The elderly individual may be more reassured if he or she is given a contact person who serves as a liaison to be contacted by the individual in times of need.

Acute care settings may relocate the individual to a floor that focuses on rehabilitation as a stepping stone to the home. Others may use long-term care settings as an intermediate step. Rehabilitation and long-term care facilities often allow their residents a trial period before discharging them. They send the individual home for the weekend to see what concerns may arise and how well prepared the individual is in the home setting.

The role of the nurse in the management of altered health maintenance is essential to the positive outcome for the elderly patient.

Evaluation

Criteria for evaluation of successful management are specific to the strategies and the type of interventions used.

Individual Care

At the individual level, criteria include the following:

- Health status is congruent with the goals mutually set by the client and the provider.
- Health habits are consistent with accepted recommendations for health maintenance.

Group Care

At the group level of organization, the following criteria apply:

- A health maintenance program is in place that is consistent with accepted recommendations for health maintenance in the elderly.
- How often do preventable problems (such as pressure sores, contractures, infections) occur?
- Exacerbations of chronic disease or acute illness episodes are identified promptly.
- Difficulties in obtaining needed resources for clients—for example, adaptive equipment, prostheses, dental care—are resolved.

No specific recommendations about the timing of evaluation of health maintenance activities for the elderly can be made, but tradition suggests an annual cycle of review. Most primary care providers schedule an annual health review, and review of health maintenance practices is appropriately included in this activity. Periodic review allows an opportunity to review health maintenance practices in light of the changes in medication regimen or health status that may have occurred at another point during the year, when the focus of care was episodic. Institutionally, policies and departmental goals are often formulated on an annual basis. It is appropriate that policies affecting health maintenance be considered at the same time.

IMPAIRED HOME MAINTENANCE MANAGEMENT

Definition and Scope of Problem

Impaired home maintenance management is defined as "inability to independently maintain a safe, growth-promoting immediate environment" (Doenges and Moorhouse, 1993, p. 232). This nursing diagnosis appropriately focuses on both the individuals and their caregivers. For example, if a spouse caring for an individual falls and breaks a hip and home maintenance cannot be maintained, this diagnosis would be properly used.

ACCEPTABLE ENVIRONMENTS FOR THE AGED. A safe, growth-promoting immediate environment implies one in which basic physiological and psychological needs can be met. This environment has two parts: the physical environment and the social or interpersonal environment. Essential aspects of the physical environment include a room temperature of between 65° and 80°F; freedom from disease-carrying pests; access to clean drinking water, toilet facilities, and cooking and refrigeration facilities; and adequate space for sleeping. Essential aspects of the social and interpersonal environment include the presence of individuals who can provide support, stimulation, and feedback about behavior. Such personal contacts do not need to live with the elderly individual. Access to these individuals must be realistic, acknowledging the elderly persons cognitive and physical limits. Failure to diagnose and manage this problem leaves an older adult at high risk for frequent reinstitutionalization, injury, or death. Those who cannot maintain a safe and clean household are more vulnerable to physiological and psychological injury as a result of lack of support processes basic to human adaptation (e.g., adequate nutrition and social interaction). A minor cut of the foot in this environment could, through inattention, lead to sepsis. Trauma from a fall, left undetected, could lead to catastrophic consequences. The section on social isolation in Chapter 17 contains a detailed discussion of the impact of lack of interpersonal and social supports.

MEANING OF HOME. Verwoerdt (1976, p. 229) defines home as "a place where one belongs and where one has one's belongings . . . where a family lives." Independent living has been the norm for adults in Western society, although in the last decade there has been a growing trend for young to middle-aged adults to reside with their parents. Most elderly persons were most probably comfortable living independently. The loss of independent living is frightening and has the potential to affect an elderly person's self-esteem. In addition, a marked change in the perception of role can be noted. To transition from an independent to a somewhat dependent role is difficult under the best of situations. Critical assessment before such transitions is essential. The social elements of home—a sense of security, unconditional love, and acceptance—are important dynamics that have an influence on whether the transition is a positive or negative experience. Involving the elderly person in the decision-making processes that affect their lives is helpful and allows re-evaluation and renegotiation of role expectations. Research also shows that existence of basic shared values and belief systems among intergenerational families is beneficial in solidarity (Somers and Fabian, 1981). Support for the formal or informal caregiver is equally important.

Contributing Factors

Many factors related to impaired home maintenance management may be found in the elderly individual's social system. The demographic characteristics of the elderly, described in Chapter 15, highlight the heightened risk status of the elderly. Advanced age is associated with increased prevalence of chronic disease, functional impairment, diminished economic resources, and diminished numbers of readily available relatives and friends. These characteristics have direct implications for the older person's ability to maintain a home.

Persons who are at high risk for impaired home maintenance management include those who *live alone*, those who have experienced *recent change in lifestyle or role*, those with *diseases* that are likely to result in diminished physical or mental function (such as metastatic cancer or newly diagnosed Alzheimer's disease), those with an active *alcohol abuse* problem or recent history of alcoholism, and those who live with a *spouse who is in poor health*. The nurse who cares for an elderly individual in the hospital, in a skilled nursing facility, or in the community should be alert to these risk factors and, if the factors are present, should assess critically to confirm or rule out this diagnosis. Individuals with impaired home maintenance management require particularly careful discharge planning from institutions. Formal support services from community-based agencies are frequently required to prevent or delay institutionalization.

Studies have shown that elderly persons who do not have a caregiver present in the community and are not adherent to the prescribed plan of care are more likely to be placed in an institution. Key elements to assess in detail are caregiver ability, follow-up care, and client adherence to prescribed plan of care (Weaver and Bryant, 1990).

In sum, the ability to perform home maintenance management may be expressed as follows:

$$\text{Home Maintenance Management} = \begin{cases} + \text{Client Abilities} \\ - \text{Environmental Demands} \\ + \text{Client Coping Resources} \\ + \text{Social Support} \end{cases}$$

Assessment

To make the diagnosis of impaired home maintenance management, information must be collected about the individual's lifestyle, household arrangements, requirements for self-care, and presence or absence of support persons from the kin network or neighborhood. A home visit, preferably by the nurse who will be responsible for the client's ongoing care, is extremely helpful. If this is not possible, the next best information can be obtained by validating the patient's perceptions of the home situation with that of a family member or close friend who has been in the home recently. The informant can be interviewed about the physical environment and the social supports readily available to the client. The client and home environmental factors detailed in Table 21–4 should be assessed.

It is not possible nor desirable to collect all the information cited in Table 21–4 on every patient during the initial assessment. The starred items are useful screening questions. Answers to these questions that suggest that the client has heightened needs for assistance or has an unusually meager support network merit further assessment. Once this information has been collected, the nurse should consider the client's self-care and home maintenance requirements, along with identified supports available to assist the client. If there is a significant gap between available resources and the client's desired lifestyle, then the diagnosis of Impaired Home Maintenance Management is justified. The remainder of the assessment process should be devoted to determining the contributing factors to the impairment in the individual case.

Planning

Once the diagnosis Impaired Home Maintenance has been established, coordination of plans for intervention is essential. Because the pattern of funding for services to the elderly is fragmented, arriving at the appropriate mix of services for the older client may be problematic. It is helpful during assessment to contact community agencies, family, and neighbors previously involved in the client's care. This provides an important foundation for joint home management planning. Regardless of the setting from which the care planning is conducted, it is worthwhile to appoint a group leader who is responsible for seeing that all parties are included and that a written plan for home maintenance management is developed, with a timetable for implementation. Someone should be appointed to be responsible for day-to-day monitoring of the effectiveness of the plan. This person may be the client, a family member, a neighborhood helper, or a professional caregiver. Ideas for contingency plans, or what to do if the proposed plan is not successful, should be discussed. Critical thinking, using creativity within the framework of nursing science, and involving elderly persons in the planning stage are essential. Especially for cognitively impaired elderly persons, it is important to focus on safety, comfort, and security and to let the person being cared for share the sense that the nurse is focused on their safety, comfort, and security.

Considerations for Institutionalized Clients

If the client is in an institution (hospital, rehabilitation center, or nursing home), a target discharge date and level of function should be established as soon as possible. This allows the caregivers in the community (family, neighborhood helpers, and community agency personnel) as much time as possible to arrange for the necessary home supports, which may include making structural modifications to the home, obtaining equipment and supplies, and arranging for caregivers prior to discharge. Such targeting also promotes realistic planning by the caregivers, who may otherwise operate under the erroneous assumption that the client will not be discharged until a return to baseline function has been achieved. For those clients going from a hospital to a nursing home, the nurse should try to give the nursing home as much advance notice as possible, so that the necessary preparations are carried out before the transfer.

Considerations for Clients at Home

If the client is already in the community, it may be more challenging to bring together

T A B L E   2 1 – 4
Nursing Assessment for Impaired Home Maintenance Management

ASSESSMENT PARAMETER	RATIONALE
Client Considerations	
What is the lifestyle of the client—feelings regarding household cleanliness, food preparation, desire to remain in current household?	Need this information to determine gap between preferred lifestyle and current client capabilities and supports
How long has the client lived in this current residence?	Gives information about potential impact on individual of change in home environment
*How does the client currently carry out the instrumental activities of daily living (IADLs), such as meal preparation, housekeeping, grocery shopping, laundry, transportation to and from medical appointments, social engagements?	Data about functional abilities and degree of social support currently available
Who lives with the client (if anyone)?	Identifies source of social support
Who does the client identify as the person(s) he/she would turn to for help on a short-term basis? on a long-term basis?	Identifies source of social support
*What is the impact of the client's current diseases on: Requirements for self-care? Ability to carry out IADLs? Ability to continue to live in the home environment?	Specifies need for supportive services Specifies need for lifestyle change
What modifications in lifestyle are likely to be required in order to optimally convalesce from or adapt to the client's diseases?	Identifies and helps specify potential for home modification if needed
Physical Environment	
Is the home rented or owned? If rented, how much is the monthly rent?	Quantifies degree of environmental demand on client at home.
What type of plumbing and toilet is currently in use?	Helpful in determining whether environment is compatible with client's limitations
What types of heating and cooling systems are in use?	
What type of refrigeration system?	
*What physical barriers to accessing vital areas of the house exist? (One-story versus multistory dwelling, stairs to enter the home, presence/absence of ramps, handrails, doorways or areas too small for wheelchairs?)	Points toward need for modification of home environment
*Is there evidence of inability to maintain sanitation? (Moldy food in refrigerator, presence of roaches, ants, flies, etc.)	Pathognomonic of diagnosis
Social Environment	
*Is there someone who can care for the client if necessary: On a short-term, drop-in each day basis? On a short-term, live-in basis? On a long-term, drop-in basis? On a long-term, live-in basis?	Quantifies degree of social support available
Who are these people? (names, relationship to client, physical proximity to client, telephone numbers)	Additional validation of amount of social support available; information needed for planning
What additional roles do these individuals fulfill? What will they have to give up (if anything) to assume these care/support responsibilities?	Partially predictive of stability of support network
What nonfamily informal supports are available in the client's neighborhood? (e.g., grocery stores and pharmacies that deliver, church or fraternal groups that assist with instrumental tasks on a dependable basis)	Further specification of supports available
What formal supports exist in the client's community? Home health agency Voluntary agencies that provide services to the elderly Units of government that provide services to the elderly, such as social service departments and councils on aging	

* Particularly useful screening questions.

the various parties involved in continuing the home maintenance plan. In some communities, there is an established mechanism for achieving interagency and caregiver input into a plan for home maintenance management. Where such mechanisms exist, they are very helpful in preventing duplication of effort, waste of scarce resources, and fragmentation of care. Sometimes, the various caregiving agencies involved have competing priorities and may be accustomed to responding only to crises. In this instance, the nurse should provide leadership in convening and coordinating a planning group.

Interventions

The interventions chosen for resolution of impaired home maintenance management depend largely on the contributing factors and the resources available to the client. Because most older adults have a strong desire to remain in their homes despite significant functional impairment, various strategies for coping with impaired home maintenance management exist.

To best meet individuals' needs through nursing intervention, the nurse must set priorities. The priorities used are the same as those used in altered health maintenance: (1) further assessment of causative and contributing factors, (2) assistance in maintaining and managing desired home environment, and (3) promotion of wellness through teaching and discharge considerations (Doenges and Moorhouse, 1993).

Further Assessment of Causative and Contributing Factors

An in-depth assessment of the individual's disability and intact abilities is helpful. The etiology for the disability and the degree of functional ability guide the health care team in successful management of the patient's problem. Assessment of the elderly person's knowledge base and information provides cues. The person could be functioning based on misinformation or lack of information. Other areas to assess in more detail are the environment, the support systems, and the financial resources. These areas need to be intact so that the elderly person is ensured a safe home situation. In-depth assessment is the first step in intervention.

Assistance in Maintaining and Managing Desired Home Environment

A home visit is the optimal starting point for this intervention. As in altered health maintenance, the focus is on avoiding promotion of dependence. Coordination with other services, formal and informal, in meeting the objective of a safe, nurturing environment is necessary. Such areas for intervention include adaptive equipment in the bathroom, household repair and maintenance, opportunities of social engagement, and/or respite care for caregivers.

Promotion of Wellness Through Teaching and Discharge Planning

As previously mentioned, effective individualized discharge planning enhances the quality of life for the elderly, reduces readmissions, and lowers the overall cost of health care. Actively assisting older adults and/or caregivers in the identification of environmental hazards is appropriate. For example, many elderly persons are at high risk for hyperthermia, resulting in death during hot summer months. Identifying the ill effects of heat and teaching the steps in identifying increased temperature and the actions to take when it occurs are helpful. A check system (in which someone calls daily to check the elderly person, use of cool compresses, increased fluid intake, and adequate ventilation systems all are active interventions. It is necessary to go beyond identifying environmental hazards to provide information, resources, and positive reinforcement for behaviors that enhance a healthy environment.

Once again, communication among the resources—health care providers, caregivers, and the elderly individual—must be clarified. Documentation and follow-up are helpful in minimizing miscommunication and increasing the likelihood for success. Long-term planning should be discussed once a trusting rapport is established.

Evaluation

Criteria for evaluating the effectiveness of a plan to resolve impaired home maintenance management are based on the criteria outlined in the mutually set goals and objectives.

1. Is the client living according to preferred lifestyle? If not, have all the acceptable alternatives been explored? Is the current arrangement the most acceptable one available? The ultimate goal is to allow individuals to pursue preferred lifestyles. The stability of the plan is related to the money available, the number of individuals involved, and the restrictiveness of the plan.

2. Is the client free from undue risk to health in the current living situation? If the answer is no, does the client understand and accept the level of risk to health? If the client is unable to understand the risks involved, does a responsible other person (family, friend, or guardian) understand these risks and

judge them to be in accordance with risks the client would accept if he or she were able to understand them?

No life situation is risk-free—chronic disease often increases risk. Professionals have a responsibility to share information about risks inherent in life situations because of disease, and the client has the responsibility of making a decision about acceptability of risks.

3. Is someone responsible for the ongoing monitoring of the adequacy of the home maintenance plan?

4. Do plans exist for reassessment or alternative arrangements if the current plan becomes inadequate to meet the client's home maintenance management needs? Complex plans have an increased potential for breakdown. Failure of a plan does not relieve the professional of responsibility for developing a safe alternative plan.

To evaluate care effectively, the clinician should know the individual's preferred lifestyle, the risks to health status, and the presence of another to monitor adequacy of the care plan, based on previously obtained psychosocial assessment data.

HIGH RISK FOR INJURY

Definition and Scope of Problem

High risk for injury is defined as a state in which the individual is at risk for injury as a result of environmental conditions that interact with the individual's adaptive and defensive resources (Doenges and Moorhouse, 1993, p. 274). Older persons are at high risk for injury because of diminished homeostatic reserves, which results from aging changes and the increased prevalence of chronic diseases that impair healing processes and predispose to functional impairments. However, potential for injury is by definition an environmentally dependent diagnosis. Therefore, the hazards and supportiveness of an environment will vary with the setting of care. Likewise, the range of interventions available to prevent injury in older people vary considerably from one setting to the next.

The consequences of injury are often more severe in older persons. Injury accounts for one of every eight hospital admissions, resulting in a greater burden on society than any single disease (Ryan et al., 1993; Rice et al., 1989). Adults aged 75 years and older have three times the risk of that of all other ages combined to suffer an injury-related hospitalization and death (Rice et al., 1989). Ryan et al. (1993) noted, "Falls are the most common nonfatal injury and the second leading cause of death from unintentional injury." Moss (1992) noted that in the elderly, only patients with malignancies have longer hospitalizations. The National Committee for Injury Prevention (Rice et al., 1989) documented that almost half the fatal falls in those aged 65 years and older occurred in the home.

Selected defining characteristics of potential for injury (Doenges and Moorhouse, 1993) include

- Biochemical and regulator alteration: sensory impairment, integrative and effector dysfunction, tissue hypoxia, immune and/or autoimmune dysfunction, malnutrition, abnormal blood profile (leukocytosis and/or leukopenia, altered clotting factors, thrombocytopenia, sickle cell, thalassemia, decreased hemoglobin level), and orthostatic changes in blood pressure

- Physical alteration: altered skin integrity (bruising, skin tears, burns), altered mobility (unsteady gait, loss of limb, reduced muscle mass and function), vision impairment, hearing deficits, effects from disease and medication, and history of falls

- Psychological alteration: affective disorders, changes in orientation, changes in cognition (especially judgment)

- External biochemical alteration: immunization level of community pollutants, poisons, drugs, and nutrients (vitamins, food types)

- External physical alteration: design, structure, and arrangement of community, building, and/or equipment (e.g., steep stairs, poor lighting, scattered rugs, new unfamiliar adaptive equipment, new unfamiliar floor plan, lack of telephone), and impairment in mode of transport or transportation

- People/provider: presence of communicable disease, lack of support system or systems, and non-nurturing behavior

Theoretical Issues

ECOLOGICAL MODEL OF ACCIDENTAL INJURY. Accidental injury in the elderly has been conceptualized by Hogue

(1982) as the mismatch between environmental demand and individual competence. Donley (1985/1986) noted that ". . . the physical and social environment of care are untapped resources in caring for the elderly." Factors related to mobility enhancement can also be viewed as factors that influence injury in the elderly. Theoretically, the more one does to promote competence in older people, the less likely the older people are to experience injury or its adverse sequelae. The ecological approach to injury prevention in older people greatly simplifies interpretation of the voluminous literature on injury and injury prevention in the aged because nurses can consider the studies on personal competence enhancement and environmental simplification in the development of strategies to prevent injury, rather than memorizing lists of risk factors. Social environmental factors and functional health have a positive impact on the well-being of the elderly (Gould, 1992).

INJURY PREVENTION. Haddon (1968) and Waller (1980) developed the concept of phases of injury to guide prevention efforts. The model presupposes that the agent of all injuries is unintentional energy exchange, rather than stairs, rugs, stoves, or automobiles. They describe three phases: the preinjury phase, including all the events that lead to the unintended exchange of energy; the injury phase, in which the energy acts on human tissue; and the postinjury phase, in which emergency services and follow-up care may affect patient outcomes from the injury (Hogue, 1982). Consideration of the various phases of injury prevention allows for broader perspectives on injury prevention strategies. Broadening the concept of injury prevention to include postinjury events provides a basis from which reduction in fall-related injuries that results from excellent emergency and rehabilitation services can be explained.

RISK. Humans do not normally exist in a risk-free environment. A tenuous balance exists between an environment that is sufficiently challenging to promote growth and skill development and one that is potentially hazardous. Institutional providers of health care are increasingly concerned about preventing injury because of the possibility of being considered liable for the injury. However, injury can result from overprotectiveness as well. Individuals who are restrained in wheelchairs because of ataxic gait or impaired judgment, "to prevent a fall," are placed at a new type of risk for injury related to disuse atrophy (Bortz, 1982). As the individual's activity is restricted, his or her limited competence becomes further compromised, so that a fall is now more likely to occur, and, if it does, the possibility of injury from the fall is enhanced. For example, older people living in the community who fall are sometimes institutionalized so that they will have closer supervision. The intent to prevent injury is admirable, but such an intervention is misguided. The individual becomes more likely to fall because the new environment presents unfamiliar challenges. Although the individual will be found more quickly if a fall occurs, and emergency help will be obtained more promptly, the questions of cost and benefit to the individual must be raised. Is the price of the added protection worth it? It depends on the people involved and their individual values. Injury prevention, like drug therapy, must be tailored to the individual. It seldom involves interventions with no adverse side effects (Donius and Rader, 1994; Kayser-Jones, 1992).

Contributing Factors

Major contributors to injury in the elderly include falls, poisoning, trauma to lower extremities, burns, altered host defense mechanisms, and adverse drug reactions. The prevalence and nature of adverse drug reactions are well described in Chapter 18 and are not repeated here. Individual and environmental factors that predispose older persons to falls, poisoning, trauma, burns, and infection are reviewed next.

PERSONAL COMPETENCE. Factors contributing to accidental injury in old people from poisoning, falls, trauma, and burns are numerous and interactive and include sensory impairment, cognitive impairment, affective disorder, osteoporosis, muscle weakness, decreased endurance, balance problems, anxiety, and polypharmacy.

ENVIRONMENTAL CONTRIBUTORS. Any environment is potentially hazardous if there is a mismatch between the individual's personal competence and the degree of challenge, or stress, in the environment. For example, environmental contributors to falls include poor lighting, many stairs, poor household repair, equipment in poor repair, clutter, chairs that are too low, beds on rollers that cannot be stabilized before transfer, and personnel untrained in transfer techniques.

Environmental contributors to poisoning include poor lighting, unsafe storage of toxic chemicals, poverty, lack of opportunity to learn about medications and their toxic effects, and unclear dosage instructions from health care providers.

Assessment

Determination of potential for injury requires assessment of person-environment fit, and lifestyle. Successful injury prevention efforts require knowledge of measures that are realistic to apply in the preinjury, injury, and postinjury phases of tissue damage. Therefore, information is required about the older person, the physical environment, and the interpersonal environment. Because the likelihood of accidental injury is a function of person-environment fit, major changes in either health status or living situation should prompt assessment for potential for injury.

INDIVIDUAL ASSESSMENT. Individuals at highest risk of potential for injury of all types are those with cognitive impairments, particularly when judgment is impaired (Tinetti et al., 1988). When mental status testing reveals impaired judgment, the diagnosis of potential for injury can be made on the basis of this finding alone. Steps should be taken immediately to remove toxins from the environment, and an injury surveillance system should be established. This involves development of an early warning system for injury, such as periodic checks throughout the day for the person at risk for falls or regular assessment for minor trauma that may go unreported.

Another high-risk group for injury are those with severe sensory impairments. Vision loss and diminished tactile sensation are primary contributors, although patients with impaired balance are also at risk. Careful assessment of visual acuity, including peripheral fields; hearing; balance; and sensitivity of extremities to temperature, light touch, pinprick, and proprioception is necessary. Those with moderate-to-severe impairments deserve intervention. Spilker and Semonin-Holleran (1987) reported on the successful adaptation of the Cincinnati Stroke Scale to identify individuals with potential for injury related to sensory or motor deficits. Their adaptation rates the extent of facial and gaze palsy, ability to hold arms and legs against gravity, visual field defects, decreased sensation, and unilateral neglect. The nursing literature does not provide useful guidance beyond these general maneuvers as to useful assessment protocols to identify individuals at particular risk for motor vehicle accidents, poisoning, or thermal injury. The role of the nurse's critical thinking is of great significance. Thorough

assessment of the individual's physical ability, the caregiver's ability, the required follow-up, and the client's adherence to the prescribed plan of care is critical.

A specific guide for assessment of those at risk of fall-related injury is found in Table 21–5. The assessment tool focuses on preinjury factors that may be manipulated.

ENVIRONMENTAL ASSESSMENT. The United States Consumer Product Safety Commission publishes a "Home Safety Checklist" that provides a useful guide to prevent accidental injury in the home. It may be used to guide the nurse's assessment of the home environment. For older people who are motivated to enhance the safety of their homes, the checklist is also suitable as a self-assessment tool.

In institutional settings, the primary cause of injury is falls. Environmental assessment to prevent falls includes bed and toilet seat height, average chair height, night lights, distance to the nearest bathroom, clutter in the hallways, and use of signs to clearly label rooms and hallways.

Planning

The setting of care greatly influences planning for injury prevention. Many institutions have formal assessment tools identifying individuals at high risk for injury, accompanied by safety protocols that can be tailored to the individual's needs. Reducing the threat from the strange and challenging environment should be emphasized. In the community, it may be more difficult to assess the physical environment, unless home visits by nurses are ordered. The focus is often on monitoring functional status changes that may precipitate injury. Protocols for general personal competence enhancement are often indicated, as well as careful evaluation of the risk/benefit ratio of drugs thought to predispose one to falls, such as those with hypotensive effects and central nervous system depressants.

Changes in cardiovascular (orthostatic hypotension, cardiovascular disease), neurological (visual and auditory changes, decreased proprioception, pathologies—transient ischemic attacks, Parkinson's disease, cerebrovascular accidents, peripheral neuropathies, dementia), musculoskeletal (decreased strength and tone, gait changes, loss of bone mass), and urological (incontinence, nocturia) activity and changes in sleep patterns all need to be assessed because they place the elderly person at higher risk for fall (Moss, 1992). Careful review of medications and history of falls should be assessed and documented.

T A B L E 2 1 – 5
Assessment Protocol for Fall-Related Injury

Goals of Assessment:
1. Determine the individual's likelihood of falling
2. Determine the individual's likelihood of sustaining serious injury in a fall
3. Determine the individual's ability to secure appropriate and timely assessment and emergency care in the event of a fall

SPECIFIC ASSESSMENT MANEUVER	RATIONALE
History Taking Previous falls Predisposing medical conditions Drugs currently taken, especially diuretics and sedatives and tranquilizers Presence of neurological symptoms, such as dizziness, vertigo, diplopia, weakness, or numbness; or cardiac symptoms such as palpitations Patient's perception of competence in own environment Ask if someone lives with client or drops by daily. If not, is client connected to a Lifeline system, telephone reassurance system, or some other network?	People who fall, fall again Certain medical conditions have been associated with falls, particularly heart disease, stroke, vertigo, or with increased injury from falls, such as osteoporosis Diuretics and sedatives have been associated with increased incidence of falls in the community Neurological symptoms are associated with increased incidence of falls Cardiac arrhythmias associated with falls Anxiety may lead to reduced mobility, which may lead to disuse atrophy, which may lead to increased potential for falls Many old people live alone. This helps determine whether individual requires counseling regarding telephone reassurance systems, or other means of regular, periodic checking to ensure access to appropriate postfall assistance
Physical and Functional Assessment Apical pulse—rate and rhythm Blood pressures in lying and standing position Observe degree of postural sway with eyes open and closed Observe gait and note type of shoe Observe ADL capability and endurance Rapid, rhythmic alternating movements, or finger-to-nose pointing Mental status examination such as the FROMAJE Visual acuity: distance and peripheral fields	Cardiac arrhythmias may precipitate falls Orthostatic hypotension may contribute to falls Increased postural sway may predispose to falls by reducing ability to compensate if off balance Abnormal gait and use of assistive devices are associated with increased risk of falling. Improper footwear may contribute to falls ADL abnormalities are associated with increased risk of falling. Also, fatigue may predispose to injury Cerebellar dysfunction predisposes to falls Depression may lead to inattentiveness, which may predispose to falling. Cognitive impairment is associated with increased incidence of falls. Results help determine whether patient teaching strategy needs modification Vision is necessary to see and avoid obstacles. Visual perception abnormalities are associated with increased incidence of falls

Environmental Assessment
Where possible, do a home visit and evaluate home environment. If this is not possible, send a visiting nurse. If this is not an option, inquire of patient and or family regarding:
  Presence of hazards: throw rugs, clutter, inadequate lighting, stairs in poor repair or without visibility strips or handrails
  Presence of factors that might help prevent a fall or reduce injury, such as grab rails in bathroom, nonskid mats in bathtub or on sink, raised toilet seat, suitable chairs, carpeting properly secured
	Environmental factors can often be modified to allow the individual to function more safely and independently. Specific interventions need to be tailored to the individual patient situation
	These have been associated with increased incidence of falls
	
	Such prudence deserves recognition and reward. Also provides opportunity regarding the need for these environmental supports if relocation occurs

It should be evident from this protocol that the adequacy of the environment is related to the functional competence of the individual. It is thus difficult to list attributes of the home environment that are in and of themselves hazardous. What may appear hazardous to one individual may serve an important purpose to the person living in the home.

When possible, passive interventions such as environmental modification are preferable to interventions that require individual behavior change (Moss, 1992: Kayser-Jones, 1992; Gould, 1992; Taft et al., 1993; Rader, 1991).

Interventions

PREINJURY PHASE. Two categories of intervention are available: environmental modification and intervention with the individual. The importance of enhancing individual competence in preventing injury cannot be overemphasized. Treatment of sensory dysfunction, mobility disorders, and cognitive dysfunction has tremendous potential benefit for the elderly. Environmental modifications must be tailored to the individual's level of impairment. Safety proofing the environment for an individual with cognitive impairment includes locking up toxic substances, including medications, and providing a safe, but limited, area in which to wander that includes barriers to stairwells and automobile traffic. Stoves can be turned off, and only the most necessary electrical appliances need be left in the living area. Matches should be removed.

Unfortunately, in institutional settings, the predominant form of injury prevention is physical restraint, in the form of side rails, "gerichairs," and cloth restraints. The use of restraints in accidental injury prevention should be extremely limited because of the many associated adverse effects. Individuals who have little or no control of posture require some form of passive restraint, unless there is a constant attendant. Individuals with equivocal body control may best be treated with careful supervision by staff and family or friends.

The hazards of restraints cannot be overemphasized. First, there is a problem of false security. Restrained patients actually require even *more* supervision than those who are unrestrained because there is risk of injury on the restraint itself as a result of improper positioning or patient agitation. Many have encountered patients who, restrained in a wheelchair, fall and pull the entire piece of equipment on top of them. Second, restraints are dehumanizing. Patients complain of being tied-up, and a clear message is sent that the patient is "not in his or her right mind." Finally, use of a restraint may actually increase the older person's predisposition for injury by increasing muscle atrophy and decreasing skill in getting around. For all these reasons, restraints should be regarded as a temporary measure only.

Creative alternatives to restraining patients in institutional settings are emerging. They include high-technology devices, such as audible warning signals for patients who have gotten out of bed unassisted, to low-technology solutions, such as family and staff education about the risks and benefits of restraints in preventing fall-related injury. Many institutions have implemented "wandering gardens" to allow individuals to avoid the hazards associated with restraints. The gardens prevent a person from wandering in an unsafe manner by providing a protective environment (Rader, 1991; Taft et al., 1993; Donius and Rader, 1994; Kayser-Jones, 1992).

INJURY PHASE. Placing carpet on hardwood or slate floors and removing sharp objects from the living area may help reduce the amount of impact experienced in a fall, thereby reducing the extent of injury.

To reduce the amount of injury from poisoning, the amount of toxic substances in the house can be limited at one time if it is not possible to lock up all toxins.

Thermal injuries may be reduced by turning down the hot water heater. The Consumer Product Safety Commission recommends that the maximum temperature for hot water be 120°F, which results in a full-thickness burn after 10 minutes of exposure (Hogue, 1982).

POSTINJURY PHASE. Ideally, accidental injuries should be prevented, but in some instances, this simply is not possible. Therefore, nurses should attend to optimizing postinjury prevention efforts, to minimize the long-range effects of an injury. Many communities have emergency call systems, such as "Lifeline," that allow older people at risk of falling ready access to postfall assistance. The systems work by activating a central emergency call board (such as in an emergency room) when the client pushes a button. These buttons are generally small and may be worn on light clothing. Other alternatives include daily checking systems, in which neighbors, friends, or family members telephone the older person each day.

An example of a fall-related injury prevention protocol developed for a nursing home is shown in Table 21–5. It includes both preinjury and postinjury interventions to reduce injury.

Evaluation

The following are criteria for evaluation of nursing care for those with potential for injury:

1. What is the incidence of injury in the target client population? How does it compare with national averages?

2. What is the incidence of functional impairment attributable to injury in the client population?

3. Are the patients assessed for potential for specific injuries: fall-related injury, other trauma, burns, poisoning?

4. Are steps taken to reduce the at-risk individual's likelihood of sustaining injury?

5. Is the client's lifestyle adversely affected by the injury prevention program?

6. What is the cost of the injury preven-

TABLE 21-6
Harmful Health Practices, Effects on Health in the Later Years, and Preventive Measures

HARMFUL HEALTH PRACTICE	POSSIBLE EFFECT ON HEALTH	PREVENTIVE MEASURES
Lack of physical activity and fitness	Diabetes, osteoporosis, heart disease, stroke, colon cancer, obesity, depression	Increase moderate daily physical activity and reduce sedentary lifestyle
Obesity	Heart disease, hypertension, atherosclerosis, cancer, stroke non-insulin-dependent diabetes mellitus	Maintain ideal body weight Maintain low-cholesterol, low-fat ($<30\%$), nutritious diet with plenty of vegetables, fruits, and grain products
Cigarette smoking	Heart disease; cancers of the lung, larynx, pharynx, oral cavity, esophagus, pancreas, and bladder; chronic bronchitis and emphysema	Stop smoking or do not start smoking
Alcohol and drug abuse	Malnutrition, cirrhosis of the liver, brain damage, mental status changes, homicides, suicides, and motor vehicle fatalities	Limit alcohol intake and stop using drugs or do not start Participate in 12-step program for rehabilitation
Stress	Stress-related conditions, such as hypertension and heart disease	Recognize and modify stressors Use a stress management program, such as exercise or biofeedback

Adapted from *Healthy People 2000: National Health Promotion and Disease Prevention Objectives.* United States Department of Health and Human Services, Public Health Service, DHHS Publication No. (PHS) 91-50213, Washington, D.C., 1990.

tion program to the individual, family, and facility or agency?

NONCOMPLIANCE

Definition and Scope of Problem

Noncompliance is ". . . a person's informed decision not to adhere to a therapeutic recommendation" (Doenges and Moorhouse, 1993, p. 283). Doenges and Moorhouse (1993) further explain, "Noncompliance is a term that may create a negative situation for patient and caregiver that may foster difficulties in resolving the causative factors. Since patients have a right to refuse therapy, we see this as a situation in which the professional need is to accept the patient's point of view/behavior/choice(s) and

work together to find alternate means to meet original and/or revised goals."

Theoretical Issues

Some find the concept of compliance objectionable because it implies that the client is passive in the therapeutic relationship, and it connotes an unbalanced power relationship between nurse and client (DiMatteo and DiNicola, 1982; Edel, 1985). The idea that clients should unquestioningly accept whatever prescriptions the health care professional offers is not consistent with models of practice that seek to promote independence and self-reliance. In a client-professional relationship characterized by mutuality—that is, the professional has special expertise about health matters but serves as a *consultant* to the client, who has the responsibility to decide whether a treatment plan is acceptable—the notion of compliance has limited usefulness except as an indicator of client-professional miscommunication. To remove the connotations of power and dependency inherent in the term compliance, other terms have been developed, such as adherence, cooperation, collaboration, therapeutic alliance, and concordance. They are often used interchangeably with compliance (Morris and Schulz, 1992; Fahlberg et al., 1991; Kenny, 1990; Walker et al., 1988; Hurd and Butkovich, 1986).

Despite many limitations, the term compliance is used by health professionals and is an accepted nursing diagnosis by NANDA; therefore, it is included in this discussion.

Consequences of Noncompliance

The consequences of noncompliance vary from trivial to life threatening (Table 21-6). If an older person elects not to follow an exercise regimen as prescribed, his or her quality of life may be reduced along with endurance and ability to withstand injury, but the immediate effects of these problems are not life threatening. In contrast, serious illness and death may ensue in individuals with congestive heart failure who take their diuretics and digitalis erratically. Because the elderly tend to have multisystem disease and be quite vulnerable to adverse side effects of drugs, it is important to determine to what extent prescriptions are being followed. Failure to do so may result in misdiagnosis and inappropriate alterations in medication type or dosage, which ultimately contribute to the disability of the older person.

The consequences of the patient being labeled as "noncompliant" are not trivial. The term noncompliance is sometimes used simply because the person does not cooperate with a clinician's wishes. If the label of noncompliance is applied without sufficient supporting data and investigation into the contributors, an individual may be denied appropriate treatment because another clinician feels the prescriptions would not be carried out. When there is frequent turnover in primary caregivers, such labels may follow a client for a long time, presenting a serious barrier to good care.

Models of Causation

Morris and Schulz (1992) viewed compliance as a process and as an outcome. They noted the lack of a consistent measure in determining compliance, which makes it difficult to apply to health practice. Fahlberg et al. (1991) acknowledged the concept of empowerment in enhancing health practices. The intent of empowerment is ". . . to enable people to increase their capacity to enhance their own health as they define it, both individually and collectively" (Fahlberg et al., 1991). Assumptions basic to empowerment philosophy are that

1. People are part of a reality that includes physical, biological, spiritual, psychological, historical, cultural, social, economic, and political perspective.
2. People know their own realities better than anyone else.
3. People have greater potential to both grow and transform their world when basic needs are met and social-structural barriers are removed.
4. Empowerment involves increasing people's "power to" rather than people's "power over."
5. Empowerment is a process begun and experienced by an individual or group; it is not something one bestows on another.
6. Empowerment increases the capacity to grow and truly change the social reality.
7. It is essential that people participate in any plan affecting their health and lives.

Application of this concept to health education allows for greater trust by participants, increased sense of self-worth, and better utilization of resources.

A strong focus on the individual's perception and the development of a trusting collaborative relationship between the individual and nurse can facilitate mutual goal setting and create success for the individual. Often through institutional routines, elderly people are encouraged to become more dependent. For example, when an elderly person is admitted to a hospital, the nurse often assumes many of the tasks the individual previously performed such as cutting up food, dressing, and getting medication ready (Kenny, 1990). The nurse may be more effective in overseeing the individual who prepares his or her own medications than in actually administering the medication and fostering dependence of the individual. In this way, the nurse may identify the specific areas in which the individual needs help to maintain adherence to the mutually set plan of care.

For instance, Hurd and Butkovich (1986) found that functional limitations were a significant source of problems of compliance in taking medication. They found some elderly persons had difficulty removing the safety caps and that others could not differentiate between the blue and green colors of medications. Some elderly persons could not read the small type on the medication label. The errors made were related to physical limitations. Walker et al. (1988) reported that elderly people scored higher overall in health-promoting lifestyles than both young and middle-aged adults. They found that older adults are definitely a heterogeneous population with a wide variety of needs for health promotion. Health promotion is appropriate for the older as well as for the younger population.

Contributing Factors

Doenges and Moorhouse (1993) suggested three nursing priorities for effective intervention. The first nursing priority is to determine the reason for nonadherence to the prescribed plan of care. It is important to seek the individual's perception and understanding of the situation. Cultural values, health and spiritual beliefs, and developmental issues are all relevant to effective care planning and need to be explored by the nurse. Review of the present treatment and of past health care management is helpful. It is important to actively listen to the elderly person's comments and descriptions and to assess the social characteristics, demographic factors, educational factors, and personality of the individual or group. This information helps in the development of effective teaching strategies and the proper use of resources. Equally important are the

BOX 21-1
Assessment for Etiology of Nonadherence to Prescribed Plan of Care

Individual's Perception of Prescribed Plan of Care
- Self-perceived health status
- Personality
- Developmental issues
- Education level
- Self-esteem
- Locus of control
- Sense of safety and hope

Cultural and Social Milieu
- Cultural values
- Social groups
- Social roles
- Primary native language
- Length of illness
- Anticipation of needs before change of health care settings

individuals' native language and his or her ability to read. Assessment of the individual's or group's self-esteem, level of anxiety, locus of control, sense of safety, hopefulness, and security may offer insight in determining the reason for nonadherence to a mutually set plan of care. The length of illness can often be a factor. A long-term chronic disease can challenge one's sense of independence. Also significant are the self-assessment of the health professional's values and the role these values play in the care, communication, and relationship with the elderly person.

The second nursing priority is to assist elderly people to develop strategies for effective management. A therapeutic relationship between elderly patients and nurses is essential. Involvement in the goal setting, planning, and implementation by elderly patients in the plan of care is critical. This involvement encourages the role of health care as it is most helpful, as facilitator or collaborator. Use of the strengths of the elderly individual, knowledge of his or her limitations, and use of resources to best meet his or her needs assist the elderly person to develop effective strategies. Establishing small goals that build on each other and planning celebrations when those goals are met promote self-esteem and adherence to the plan of care.

A critical area of assisting individuals is appropriate discharge planning. Transitions in health care delivery—for example, dis-charge from hospital to home care—often are stressful. The importance of communication between services and anticipation of true needs cannot be underestimated. Providing information on how to access and utilize the resources is an appropriate nursing intervention. It is important that the nurse have elderly patients verbalize this information in their own words or demonstrate an understanding of it. The nurse needs to be realistic in the delivery of such information. Overwhelming the individual accomplishes nothing. It is best to give information in small amounts and to build on that information once the person has integrated it.

The third priority is health promotion. The more tailored and individualized the health promotion, the more likely it will be implemented. As Walker et al. (1988) noted in their study, the older population is a heterogeneous group with a variety of health care needs. The nurses' role is one of facilitating the successful meshing of healthy lifestyle practice with the elderly person's present lifestyle and health needs. Creativity, as well as a holistic understanding of individuals and of the nursing science of the elderly, are needed. The nurse using these three elements can be successful in health promotion of the elderly.

REFERENCES

Barris, R., Kielhofner, G., Levine, R. et al. Occupation as interaction with the environment. *In* Kielhofner, G. (ed.). *A Model of Human Occupation.* Baltimore: Williams & Wilkins, 1985.

Bortz, W. Disuse and aging. *JAMA* 248:1203–1208, 1982.

DiMatteo, M.R. and DiNicola, D.D. *Achieving Patient Compliance: The Psychology of the Medical Practitioner's Role.* New York: Pergamon press, 1982.

Doenges, M. and Moorhouse, M. *Nurse's Pocket Guide: Nursing Diagnoses with Interventions.* Philadelphia: F.A. Davis, 1993.

Donius, M. and Rader, J. Use of side rails: Rethinking a standard of practice. *J Gerontol Nurs* 20(11):23–27, 1994.

Donley, R., Sr. The teaching nursing home project. *Gerontol Geriatr Educ* 6(2):76–80, 1985/1986.

Dychtwald, K. and Flower, J. *Age Wave: The Challenges and Opportunities of an Aging American.* Los Angeles: Tarcher, 1989.

Edel, M.K. Noncompliance: An appropriate nursing diagnosis? *Nurs Outlook* 33:183–185, 1985.

Fahlberg, L., Poulin, A., Girdana, D. and Dusek, D. Empowerment as an emerging approach in health education. *J Health Educ* 22(3):185–193, 1991.

Gould, M.T. Nursing home elderly: Social-environmental factors. *J Gerontol Nurs* 18(8):13–20, 1992.

Haddon, W., Jr. The changing approach to the epidemiology, prevention and amelioration of trauma: The transition to approaches etiologically rather than descriptively based. *Am J Public Health* 58:1431, 1968.

Hanson, M., Kennedy, F., Dougherty, L. and Baumann,

L. Education in nursing diagnosis: Evaluating clinical outcomes. *J Contin Educ Nurs* 21(2):79–85.

Hogue, C.C. Injury in late life: Part I. Epidemiology. *J Am Geriatr Soc* 30(3):183–190, 1982.

Hoskins, L., McFarlane, E., Rubenfeld, M. et al. Nursing diagnosis in the chronically ill: Methodology for clinical validation. *Adv Nurs Sci* 17(5):256–262, 1986.

Hurd, P. and Butkovich, S. Compliance problems and the older patient: Assessing functional limitations. *Drug Intell Clin Pharm* 20:228–231, 1986.

Jewel, M. and Peters, D. An assessment guide for community health nurses. *Home Healthcare Nurse* 7(5):32–36, 1989.

Jirovec, M. and Maxwell, B. Nursing home residents: Functional ability and perceptions of choice. *J Gerontol Nurs* 19(5):13–20, 1993.

Kayser-Jones, J. Culture, environment, and restraints: A conceptual model for research and practice. *J Gerontol Nurs* 18(11):13–20, 1992.

Kenny, T. Erosion of individuality in care of elderly people in hospital—an alternative approach. *J Adv Nurs* 15:571–576, 1990.

Kreidler, M., Campbell, J., Lanik, G. et al. Community elderly: A nursing center's use of change theory as a model. *J Gerontol Nurs* 20(1):25–30, 1994.

Kriegler, N. and Harton, M. Community health assessment tool: A patterns approach to date collection and diagnosis. *J Community Health Nurs* 9(4):229–234, 1992.

Lorensen, M. Health and social support of elderly families in developed countries. *J Gerontol Nurs* 18(6):25–32, 1992.

McMurray, A. Expertise in community health nursing. *J Community Health Nurs* 9(2):65–75, 1992.

Miller, J., Steele, K. and Boisen, A. The impact of nursing diagnoses in a long-term care setting. *Nurs Clin North Am* 22(4):905–911, 1987.

Morris, L. and Schulz, R. Patient compliance—an overview. *J Clin Pharm Ther* 17:283–295, 1992.

Moss, A. Are the elderly safe at home? *J Community Health Nurs* 9(1):13–19, 1992.

Oberst, M. Perspectives on research in patient teaching. *Nurs Clin North Am* 24(3):621–627, 1989.

Orem, D. *Nursing Concepts of Practice.* New York: Mc-Graw-Hill, 1980.

Rader, J. Modifying the environment to decrease use of restraints. *J Gerontol Nurs* 17(2):9–13, 1991.

Rice, D.P. et al. Cost of injury in the United States: A report to Congress. San Francisco Institute of Health and Aging University of California, San Francisco; and Baltimore: Injury Prevention Center, Johns Hopkins University, 1989.

Roberts, B. and Wykle, M. Pilot study results: Falls among institutionalized elderly. *J Gerontol Nurs* 19(5):13–20, 1993.

Ryan, J.W., Dinkel, J.L. and Petrucci, K. Near falls incidence: A study of elder adults in the community. *J Gerontol Nurs* 19(12):23–28, 1993.

Sawin, K. and Heard, L. Nursing diagnoses used most frequently in rehabilitation nursing practice. *Rehabil Nurs* 17(5):256–262, 1992.

Schank, M. Wanted: Nurses with critical thinking skills. *J Contin Educ Nurs* 21(2):86–89, 1990.

Smith, N.R., Kielhofner, G. and Watts, J.H. The relationships between volition, activity pattern, and life satisfaction in the elderly. *Am J Occup Ther* 40:278–283, 1986.

Somers, A. and Fabian, D. *The Geriatric Imperative: An Introduction to Gerontology and Clinical Geriatrics.* New York: Appleton-Century-Crofts, 1981.

Spilker, J.A. and Semonin-Holleran, R. Injury, potential for related to sensory or motor deficits: Using the stroke scale to validate defining characteristics of this nursing diagnosis. *In* McLane, A. (ed.). *Classification of Nursing Diagnoses: Proceedings of the Seventh Conference.* St. Louis: C.V. Mosby, 1987.

Taft, L., Delaney, K., Seman, D. and Stansell, J. Dementia care: Creating a therapeutic milieu. *J Gerontol Nurs* 19(10):30–39, 1993.

Taival, A. and Raatikainen, R. Finnish nursing homes: Client well being and staff development. *J Gerontol Nurs* 19(2):19–24, 1993.

Tinetti, M.E., Speechly, M. and Ginter, S.F. Risk factors for falls among elderly persons living in the community. *N Engl J Med* 319:1701–1707, 1988.

Verwoerdt, A. *Clinical Geropsychiatry.* Baltimore: Williams & Wilkins, 1976, p. 229.

Walker, S., Volkan, K., Sechrist, K. and Pender, N. Health-promoting life styles of older adults, correlates and patterns. *Adv Nurs* 11(1):76–90, 1988.

Waller, J.A. Injury as a public health problem. *In* Last, J.M. (ed.). *Rosenau's Preventive Medicine and Public Health.* New York: Appleton-Century-Crofts, 1980.

Weaver, F. and Bryant, F. An analysis of decision making in discharge planning. *Eval Health Professions* 13(1):121–142, 1990.

Windriver, W. Social isolation: Unit based activities for impaired elders. *J Gerontol Nurs* 19(3):15–21, 1993.

Woolley, N. Nursing diagnosis: Exploring the factors which may influence the reasoning process. *J Adv Nurs* 15:110–117, 1990.

Zarle, N. Continuity of care: Balancing care of elders between health care settings. *Nurs Clin North Am* 24(3):697–705, 1989.

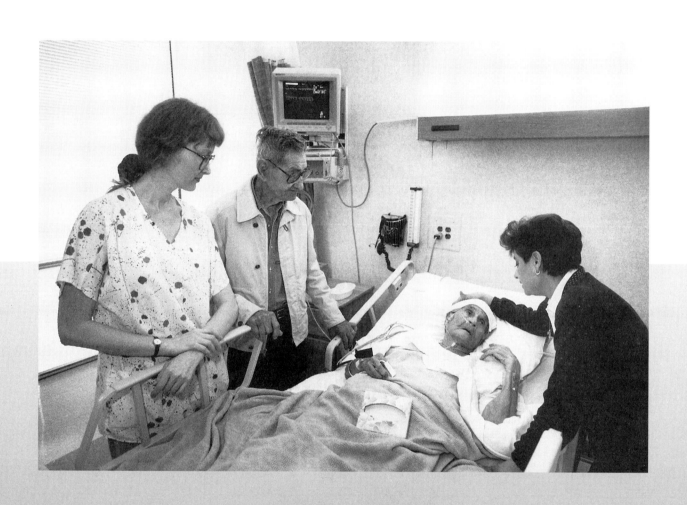

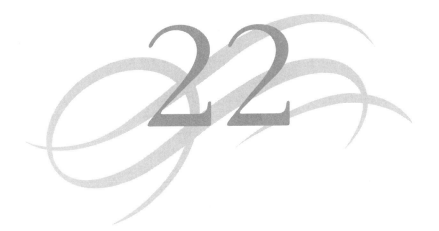

Gerontological Nursing in Acute Care Settings

NANCY J. GIRARD

OBJECTIVES

Describe the hospitalized elderly, including the frequency and outcome of hospitalization, the impact of hospitalization, and the functional status of the patient.

❖

Discuss the importance of discharge planning and its problems and difficulties.

❖

Analyze concepts in the care of hospitalized elderly in relation to altered homeostasis, the impact of the hospital environment, ethical conflicts, and time use.

❖

Demonstrate the workings of the geriatric multidisciplinary team in the hospital.

❖

Differentiate four types of care in an acute care setting: medical, surgical, psychiatric, and rehabilitative.

❖

Analyze the rehabilitation needs of older adults in the acute care setting.

❖

Explain common gerontological nursing problems in the hospital, particularly delirium, urinary incontinence, immobility, and falls.

The purpose of acute care is to stabilize patients with life-threatening disorders. An acute illness, by definition, is one that is "characterized by symptoms that are of relatively short duration, are usually severe, and affect the functioning of the patient in all dimensions" (Potter and Perry, 1993). Hospitals, therefore, are tertiary care centers for these short-term, serious illnesses. Hospitalization typically occurs when procedures required to diagnose, monitor, or treat patients' conditions require 24-hour care by a multidisciplinary team of health professionals. When the illness is stabilized, it is time to discharge the patient from the hospital.

Hospitals also have served as places of last resort, where people with diseases and disabilities too complex for outpatient, community, or nursing home care are taken. For many older adults, hospitals represent a place where people go to die, and hospitalization is met with dread and fear. Although hospitals traditionally have been the setting in which most acute care has been offered, recent concerns about the high cost of hospi-

talization have brought about some changes in the approach to the provision of acute care. Conditions that once were treated only in the hospital, such as respiratory failure requiring ventilator support, are now managed in long-term acute care facilities and in specialty nursing homes (Zuckerman et al., 1993). Factors affecting the decision to discharge the patient from an acute care institution are complex. The dual role of the hospital, as the provider of acute care and the provider of last resort, is at the center of the dilemma regarding timing of discharge.

The focus of this chapter is on the unique responses and needs of hospitalized older patients, with an emphasis on discharge planning and coordination.

PROFILE OF HOSPITALIZED ELDERLY PATIENTS

Older people are admitted to hospitals from the community or from nursing homes; many come into the hospital via the emergency department because they are seriously ill. Past assumptions and generalizations of the older adults' use of emergency departments as a primary care center for nontraumatic and nonacute problems are inaccurate. Rather, most elderly patients are sicker and are much more likely to use ambulance transportation, to require more testing and observation in the emergency department (Singal et al., 1992), and to be admitted to intensive care beds (Strange et al., 1992) than are younger patients.

Hospitalization of the elderly today usually represents an acute situation in which intensive care is needed. Elderly persons are hospitalized about twice as often as younger persons, and they stay in the hospital twice as long. Further, the introduction of prospective payment systems and managed care is affecting the delivery of health care to this population (Fillit, 1994).

The elderly report that they come to the emergency department because they feel too sick to wait for a clinical appointment with their physician. They are self-referred or are referred by the physician or other health care provider. The elderly are not frequent attenders in the emergency department. Contrary to common perceptions, their emergency department visits are appropriate and are not used for extraneous factors, such as loneliness and neglect (Eagle et al., 1993). Strange et al. (1992) reported on data compiled for 1,193,743 patient visits to the emergency department in 1990. They found that 32 per cent of the elderly seen in the emergency department were admitted to hospitals, versus 7.5 per cent of the younger patients. Admission did not depend on whether the patient came from the community or a nursing home. The most common diagnostic-related group (DRG) categories on admission from the emergency department were cardiovascular problems, fractures and dislocations, neurological problems, respiratory problems, and gastrointestinal problems (Strange et al., 1992; Eagle et al., 1993).

Keating (1992) investigated surgical procedures performed on 57 female and 17 male nursing home residents with a median age of 86. The types of procedures were fractured hip repair (n = 42), amputation (n = 10), general and abdominal surgery (n = 14), genitourinary surgery (n = 6), and other (n = 8). Eighty per cent were classified as American Association of Anesthesiologists (ASA) classification of III or above, and 63 per cent of the cases were emergencies. The mean hospital stay was 13 days. Major complications were seen more often in ASA class IV patients, in patients who underwent emergency procedures, and in those who underwent general anesthesia. All deaths occurred in emergency procedures with ASA class IV patients. The overall mortality rate was 3.8 per cent. This rate is comparable to or better than general elderly population surgical rates.

This difference in the course and outcome of hospitalization between patients is due to the presence of comorbidity or health complications. There appears to be a distinction in the treatment course and outcomes of hospitalization between patients who come with a rehabilitation classification of their diagnosis and those with a medical or surgical diagnosis. Miller et al. (1994) compared the DRG classification with the geriatric assessment unit in a community hospital with a rehabilitation facility. One hundred fifty-five subjects with a mean age of 78 years were followed up for 1 year. Outcomes measured were mortality, nursing home use, activities of daily living, and charges for follow-up or additional medical services. The patients who were admitted with a medical or surgical diagnosis were in the hospital almost 3 weeks before a geriatric consultation was received. Mortality was lower in the rehabilitation group, and more patients in the rehabilitation group were able to maintain a residence in the community. In addition, those with cognitive impairment were two times as likely to remain hospitalized for 6 or more days (Weiler et al., 1991).

In summary, older adults admitted to the hospital tend to be older, tend to be sicker with more illnesses, tend to have fewer social supports, may have mental impairment, and have a higher mortality than younger patients.

Functional Status

Aging physiology and chronic conditions in the elderly often result in functional impairments. Older people who are hospitalized are more likely to experience changes in functional status and ability than are younger people. A systematic approach to establishing baseline data related to function enables identification of changes from that baseline and promotes timely interventions for minimizing disability and maximizing independence.

Attending to the functional status of older people in the acute care setting is important for several reasons. First, older people fear the prospect of dependency, and therefore an essential health outcome is the maintenance of remaining functional ability. Second, care for dependent people is often more costly because it is labor intensive. The promotion of independent function, therefore, influences cost containment efforts by reducing length of stay and need for labor-intensive services, such as personal care assistance. Finally, people with functional impairments need more individualized social service and nursing interventions to promote their remaining capabilities and to arrange for needed support services after they are discharged from the hospital.

Older adults frequently still are not given the rehabilitation opportunities readily available to the young. Many health care professionals believe that older adults do not have the potential or reasons for rehabilitation or for being maintained at their present level of functioning. The belief that dependency and dying are synonymous with old age must change if a model of care that includes rehabilitation of functional skills is to be developed. Older patients must also be permitted to take responsibility for their own needs. Nurses must allow patients to determine the amount and degree of risk patients are willing to take to improve function. In an effort to combat prejudices toward the elderly, many nursing schools are including attitudinal content in their curriculum. Rehabilitation issues are also now clearly defined and identified in nursing standards, and the scope of nursing practice has been defined by the American Nurses' Association and the Association of Rehabilitation Nurses (Butler, 1991).

In addition to functional problems, older adults often have multisystem problems, altered homeostasis, normal aging sensory changes, and multiple therapeutic regimens that are further affected by the hospital environment. The traditional problem-oriented approach to care can lead to the development of a formidable list of problems that, when taken collectively, may discourage both the caregiver and the patient. In contrast, nursing care that focuses on supportive, outcome-oriented care helps increase the level of functioning in daily activities and decreases dependency.

Functional outcome-oriented care (Mitchell, 1993) involves the same assessment, data collection, planning, and evaluation of any nursing care plan. However, in functional outcome-oriented care, the patient has a stronger role in working with the caregiver to determine what their goals will be and how they will be accomplished. Thus, data collection is effective if it is focused on the functional health patterns approach (Iyer, 1994).

The functional data collection includes health perceptions and beliefs of the patient, nutrition, elimination patterns, activity levels, sleep patterns, cognitive status, self-health perceptions, sexuality, coping levels and abilities, values and religion, and physical abilities (Iyer, 1994). Nursing care based on goals developed with a functional assessment focuses on the strengths and remaining abilities of the patients. This approach enables the patient to return to his or her desired lifestyle rather than attempting to treat all of the nursing diagnoses or problems individually.

Impact of Hospitalization

Hospital admission may be the final event that upsets the delicate balance maintained in the frail, impaired elderly person (Guyatt et al., 1993). Older people with a multitude of chronic illnesses who have been in a community or nursing home setting show a functional decline in spite of successful treatment of the condition for which they were admitted (Creditor, 1993). In some cases, diagnostic and treatment procedures meant to cure can trigger negative reactions that become additional conditions needing care. Hospitalization can provoke a vicious cycle of dependency and permanent impairment. Some studies have shown that negative effects of hospitalization begin by the second day after admission (Hirsch et al., 1990).

Complications, such as adverse drug reactions, confusion, bladder and respiratory infections, falls, and incontinence, increase with age in hospitalized patients. Even if the complication is rectified during hospitalization, many elderly patients are no longer independent on discharge (Creditor, 1993) (Fig. 22–1).

Nosocomial Infection and Iatrogenesis

A nosocomial infection is one that is acquired in a health care institution (Potter and Perry, 1993) and was not present when the patient was originally admitted. The acute care settings are very likely places for these situations to occur because of the extremely ill populations and the virulent microorganisms that may also be resistant to antibiotics and bactericidal drugs. A common example is methicillin-resistant *Staphylococcus aureus*. Enterococcus has also been found to become resistant to vancomycin, which makes it virtually untreatable. This microorganism causes many of the diseases to which the elderly are especially susceptible, such as blood, wound, and urinary tract infections (Martin, 1994). In addition to resistant strains of microorganisms, the elderly are very vulnerable to opportunistic microorganisms, which invade the elderly more often because of their decreased immune response. Nosocomial infections can come from the patient (endogenous) or from another person (exogenous) (Girard, 1995).

An iatrogenic infection is a nosocomial infection that results from a diagnostic or therapeutic procedure. For example, the insertion of and infrequent care for an indwelling urinary bladder catheter is a major cause of bladder infection. Other causes of iatrogenic problems are overuse or misuse of drugs (Gravely and Oseasohn, 1991), prolonged immobilization, and malnutrition or dehydration related to withholding of, or inability to take, food or fluids.

Age-related physiological changes contribute to infections in susceptible patients. The changes most often are in the urinary and respiratory tracts. The bladder has decreased ability and sphincter tone, contributing to urine retention. The lungs have reduced ciliary action, which inhibits removal of mucus. There is an accompanying decline in muscle mass and a stiffening in the thoracic cage, further decreasing respiratory ability (Stanley, 1992).

Emotional Reactions

Emotional reactions to hospitalization are significant in all age groups but may be more intense in the elderly. Anxiety, depression, agitation, and disorientation are emotional or psychological reactions that can re-

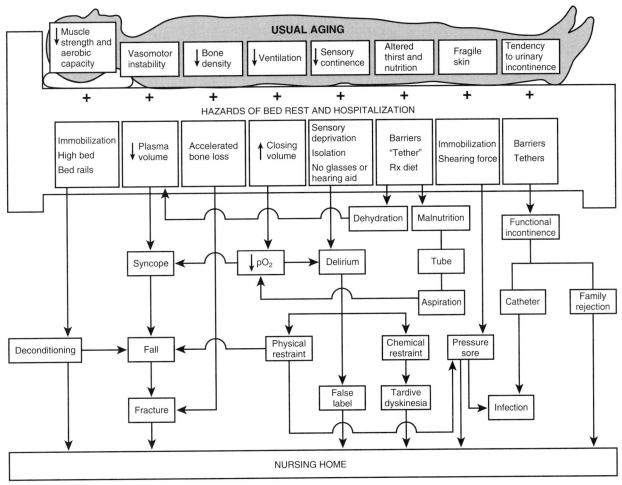

FIGURE 22-1

Hazards of hospitalization for elderly patients. (From Creditor, M.C. Hazards of hospitalization of the elderly. *Ann Intern Med* 118(3):219–223, 1993.)

sult from fears of hospitalization, diagnostic testing, treatment, or hospital routines. For many older people, admission to a hospital signals impending death, and this fear is heightened by the daily routines of the hospital, such as blood drawing, specimen collecting, or nursing care.

The hospital can induce feelings of helplessness, role loss, dependency, and isolation. Meaningful relationships may be jeopardized by limited visiting hours, and this kind of deprivation emphasizes the essentially alienating process inherent in hospitalization. Older patients who are left alone for long periods of time often complain of an ill-defined malaise, which can progress quickly to confusion.

Measures that nurses can take that are helpful in counteracting negative emotional reactions to hospitalization include the following:

1. Visit the patient frequently, especially in the beginning of the hospitalization. Provide a supportive environment.

2. Orient the patient to hospital routines immediately on admission.

3. Explain the diagnostic tests and treatments. Explain the rationale for the various procedures.

4. Use drugs appropriately and judiciously for the treatment of anxiety, agitation, and insomnia.

5. Anticipate common problems, such as nocturnal falls, incontinence, missed meals, or lack of sleep. Take appropriate prophylactic measures.

6. Begin discharge planning on the day of admission (Blaylock and Cason, 1992).

DISCHARGE PLANNING AND CONTINUITY OF CARE

Older patients benefit from discharge planning because they have more complicated and multiple illnesses. Nursing and regulatory standards (such as the Joint Commission on the Accreditation of Health Care Organizations) stress the importance of such coordinated multidisciplinary planning.

With the advent of the Medicare prospective payment plan based on DRGs, hospital stays for the elderly have shortened significantly. The general consensus among health care providers is that all patients are now being discharged "quicker and sicker." Therefore, discharge planning must begin immediately on admission. Older patients, their families, and all the members of the health care team should be involved in the planning and continuity of care.

Discharge planning is an ongoing process that involves collaboration and communication between individuals and agencies to facilitate the passage of a patient as smoothly as possible from one environment to another. The process of discharge planning involves assessing the abilities and limitations of patients during hospitalization, planning for continuity of health care on discharge, and coordinating individual, family, hospital, and community resources needed to implement the discharge plan. This planning is frequently incorporated as a component of case management or managed care (Madrid, 1994; McNabb, 1994).

Criteria for outcomes of patient care must be developed for effective discharge planning. These criteria include the following:

1. Patient and family knowledge of the medical diagnosis and treatment, self-care or assistive needs, functional abilities, and directions for follow-up care and physician and/or clinic visits (Potter and Perry, 1993)

2. Coordination of community, rehabilitation, and resource support systems needed to provide continuing care

3. Arrangements for relocation of the patient to another health care institution or facility if needed, including financial, physical, and emotional considerations

Because discharge planning begins on admission, an accurate assessment must be completed, which includes the physical, cognitive, and emotional abilities of the patient. Effective assessment of the elderly should include age, functional status, mental abilities, social support, living situation, behavior patterns, mobility, sensory deficits, medications, and number of past readmissions to an acute care facility. A risk assessment tool is provided in Figure 22–2 (Blaylock and Cason, 1992).

Most health care institutions today have developed their own patient discharge information forms. Often, one form must be completed as near as possible to admission for high-risk patients, and another form must be completed at discharge that includes instructions the patients take home.

The early discharge planning team includes nurses, social service personnel, and physicians. Families are also involved when appropriate. This planning fulfills criteria of the Healthcare Financing Administration (HCFA), which requires concrete, documented evidence of multidisciplinary planning. These forms contain plans that are revised throughout the patient's hospitalization so that he or she is ready for discharge in a timely manner.

The patient discharge information form summarizes the patient education that has taken place throughout hospitalization and the care needs that are still present at discharge, and it is usually completed by the nurse. It should include directions on skills such as dressing changes or catheter care and the patient's ability to perform that self-care. Discharge information can include the need for family involvement and the resources and/or equipment needed after discharge (Fig. 22–3). Regulatory requirements for documenting must be met for home care financial reimbursement to be received. This documentation should include

1. Continuing problems stemming from the diagnosis, such as a diabetic's inability to self-administer insulin or difficulty ambulating after hip replacement

2. Continuing need of skilled care, such as wound or ostomy care

3. Record of objective data, such as pain, blood pressure, and nutritional intake, that reflect continuing problems at the time of discharge (Potter and Perry, 1993)

Problems and Difficulties

Acute care nursing hospital beds are often occupied by patients who do not require acute medical or surgical nursing care. Many of these patients are older adults who are not able to function independently after discharge for physical or cognitive reasons, and they require placement in a nursing home or an extended care facility. The longer they remain in the hospital, the less likely they are to use the services that the acute care hospitals provide. A major problem is the posthospitalization placement. This is due to the limited availability of intermediate and extended acute care facility

Blaylock Discharge Planning Risk Assessment Screen

Circle all that apply and total. Refer to the Risk Factor Index.*

Age
    0 = 55 years or less
    1 = 56 to 64 years
    2 = 65 to 79 years
    3 = 80+ years

Living situation/social support
    0 = Lives only with spouse
    1 = Lives with family
    2 = Lives alone with family support
    3 = Lives alone with friends' support
    4 = Lives alone with no support
    5 = Nursing home/residential care

Functional status
    0 = Independent in activities of daily living
          and instrumental activities of daily living
    Dependent in:
    1 = Eating/feeding
    1 = Bathing/grooming
    1 = Toileting
    1 = Transferring
    1 = Incontinent of bowel function
    1 = Incontinent of bladder function
    1 = Meal preparation
    1 = Responsible for own medication adminis-
          tration
    1 = Handling own finances
    1 = Grocery shopping
    1 = Transportation

Cognition
    0 = Oriented
    1 = Disoriented to some spheres† some of the
          time
    2 = Disoriented to some spheres all of the time
    3 = Disoriented to all spheres some of the time
    4 = Disoriented to all spheres all of the time
    5 = Comatose

Behavior pattern
    0 = Appropriate
    1 = Wandering
    1 = Agitated
    1 = Confused
    1 = Other

Mobility
    0 = Ambulatory
    1 = Ambulatory with mechanical assistance
    2 = Ambulatory with human assistance
    3 = Nonambulatory

Sensory deficits
    0 = None
    1 = Visual or hearing deficits
    2 = Visual and hearing deficits

Number of previous admissions/emergency room visits
    0 = None in the last 3 months
    1 = One in the last 3 months
    2 = Two in the last 3 months
    3 = More than two in the last 3 months

Number of active medical problems
    0 = Three medical problems
    1 = Three to five medical problems
    2 = More than five medical problems

Number of drugs
    0 = Fewer than three drugs
    1 = Three to five drugs
    2 = More than five drugs

Total score:

*Risk Factor Index: Score of 10 = at risk for home care resources; score of 11 to 19 = at risk for extended discharge planning; score greater than 20 = at risk for placement other than home. If the patient's score is 10 or greater, refer the patient to the discharge planning coordinator or discharge planning team.
† Spheres = person, place, time, and self.

FIGURE 22-2

Blaylock Discharge Planning Risk Assessment Screen. (From Blaylock, A. and Cason, C. Discharge planning: Predicting patients' needs. *J Gerontol Nurs* 18(7):5–10, 1992. Copyright 1991, Ann Blaylock.)

GOOD CARE HOSPITAL
PATIENT DISCHARGE INFORMATION SUMMARY

| (Patient name plate) | Date __12-20-94__   Time ___11:30 am___ |

DISCHARGED VIA: [ ] Ambulatory   [x] Wheelchair   [ ] Stretcher
DISCHARGED TO: [x] Home   [ ] Home with home health care
                   [ ] Skilled nursing facility   [ ] Rehabilitation unit
                   [ ] Other _____
DISCHARGE STATUS: BP__122/74__ PULSE __76__ RESP __18__
        WOUND _Clean, dry, Ø discharge, sutures intact_
        MOBILITY _Able to walk unassisted_
        SELF CARE ABILITY _Able to care for self_
        KNOWLEDGE   [x] can repeat all information given below
                    [x] returned demonstration correctly
                    [x] can perform skill with assistance _(dressing change)_
                    [x] family or significant other can perform skill and
                        repeat information
        OTHER _Wife present for discharge instruction_

DISCHARGE INFORMATION

PHYSICIAN/CLINIC VISIT APPOINTMENT: Date ___12-27-94___   Time __1:30 pm__
        Place _University clinic, 3rd floor, room 211_
        Physician _Kancut_   Phone _211-1227_

INSTRUCTIONS:

        Activity: _As tolerated. Do not lift weights over 5lbs. or drive car without physician consent._

        Medications: _Tylenol tab. ī or īī every 3–4 hours if needed for discomfort. Call physician if
                      discomfort greatly increases._
        Diet: _Resume pre-hospital diabetic diet. Try to keep blood glucose around 120–160
               to promote healing._
        Wound care: _Clean twice a day with warm water and mild soap. Apply one 4X4 gauze dressing_

        Other: _Watch for signs of infection (redness, tenderness, pain, discharge, swelling). Notify
                doctor immediately._

RESOURCES GIVEN: _1 box 4X4's, 1 box tape, Tylenol._
SPECIAL INSTRUCTIONS: _Keep clinic appointment and bring glucose chart._

[ ] Valuables from cashier   [x] Meds from pharmacy
[x] Discharge supplies   [x] Release forms signed

My discharge instructions have been explained and a copy has been given to me.

(Patient)/significant other ___Joe Patient___   Relation _____
Nurse ___N. Nurse RN___

FIGURE 22–3

Sample discharge form.

beds in the community, conflicts among placement and funding agencies, confusing policies and procedures for placement, family considerations and concerns, delays in obtaining legal status such as guardianships, and communication lapses. Thus, the barriers to expeditious rehabilitation and discharge of hospitalized elderly patients can be summarized into four categories:

1. Patient care issues
2. Structural and administrative issues
3. Community-related issues
4. Financial and legal issues

Patient care issues include focusing care only on the acute problem, without consideration of the long-term implications and rehabilitation needs. They can also include failure of the staff to recognize problems outside the physical needs of the patient; for example, psychological (fear of body loss, fear of dying), cognitive (confusion, inability to recall information), or emotional problems (depression).

Structural and administrative issues include communication problems between health providers, lack of coordination between departments and institutions, inadequate financial coverage for rehabilitative services, and unavailability of the services or equipment. In spite of the degree of severe illness in most older adults, the trend is to discharge them rapidly, often before optimal health can be achieved in the hospital environment. Lack of acute extended care facilities and rehabilitation and follow-up services and poor liaison among facilities outside the hospital have been identified as problems in the discharge process.

Community-related issues center on poor coordination between inpatient and community services and lack of services in the community. The small number of long-term facilities that can accept patients with ongoing acute problems also hinders discharge. For example, patients who have stabilized physiologically but still have intravenous lines or needs related to ventilator care must be placed in long-term facilities that are licensed to care for such patients.

Lastly are financial and legal issues, which involve the third-party reimbursement system and the impact of managed care allotments on those resource distributions.

For all of these reasons, multidisciplinary case management is proving to be an acceptable model of health care delivery. It reduces fragmentation, promotes a higher quality of care, and is more cost effective (Trella, 1993). Possible reasons for readmission to the acute care hospitals are inadequate medical management, patient noncompliance, exacerbation of an acute condition, and emergency situations. Many of these readmissions might have been prevented if appropriate planning and interventions had occurred.

Inappropriate placement is another problem after hospitalization. If discharge planning does not begin early in the hospitalization, older patients may be inappropriately placed in a nursing home or may otherwise be readmitted to a hospital. Routine assessment of functioning may help to facilitate planning by predicting the level of care that will be required after discharge. An ongoing functional assessment would not only help to ensure appropriate placement, it would also result in a reduced length of hospital stay.

Discharge to the Community

Many elderly persons today are benefiting from a multidisciplinary case management–managed care approach (Propotnik et al., 1993). This method of care delivery ensures a better continuity of care through collaborative efforts and timely discharge planning (Connors, 1992). Hospitalized elderly patients can be categorized in terms of their discharge plans: (1) those who have steady support in the community, usually from a spouse or family member, and are likely to resume their lives as they existed previously and (2) those for whom the hospital stay offers an opportunity to introduce a definite change in living arrangement.

When older patients are discharged from the hospital to their home, psychological, physiological, social, economic, and functional factors must be considered. The family situation, including pre-existing physical problems and chronic illness, should be determined, and the layout of the home, need for assistive devices, prescription and nonprescription medications, affordability of special diets and medications, and need for services need to be considered.

Patients who return to their homes have a much higher incidence of acute care nursing needs today that must be coordinated before their discharge from the hospital. For example, patients may go home with respiratory equipment, which can range from oxygen supplements to ventilator assistance. Medical equipment needed after discharge also requires careful planning before discharge. These technologies can include special beds, monitoring devices, pain relief devices, and fluid administration equipment. Plans must also include supplies for needs such as wound care, diabetes care, and ostomy care (Zastocki, 1994). Thus, patient and family discharge teaching and information are essential to ensure knowledgeable care and prevention of complications that would lead to readmission.

Medication noncompliance has been a concern for decades and is more so today, with increasing numbers of patients receiving multiple-medication regimens. In one study, 76 per cent of the subjects were noncompliant when many drugs were prescribed, even when adequate teaching was provided. This was a primary factor for readmission to the hospital. Reasons for noncompliance were multiple (Gravely and Oseasohn, 1991), indicating further rationale for case management.

Discharge planning should include an assessment of the amount of professional intervention needed in the community, and the availability of the following supports should be assessed: a supportive physical and social environment, a mutually caring personal relationship with one or more persons, and a mutually caring professional relationship with one or more health providers. A discharge planning and assessment form should be completed by a multidisciplinary team, using patient and family input.

Discharge to a Nursing Home

Long-term care needs have greatly increased. The presence or absence of social support may determine the likelihood of being discharged from a hospital to a nursing home. An estimated 2.7 million elderly need functional assistance, either in their own home or in extended care facilities (Rice, 1989). The American Academy of Orthopedic Surgeons estimated that 40 per cent of the more than 280,000 older adults with hip fractures annually will be discharged to long-term care facilities (Zuckerman et al., 1993). Placement to a nursing home or another institutional care facility can often be difficult. Many hospital patients are occupying acute care hospital beds only because nursing home beds are not available.

Some hospitals, especially those with excess bed capacity, located in rural areas lacking community and nursing home services, are solving the problem by developing "swing beds." The term *swing bed* is used because the patient may swing between acute and skilled or intermediate care as his

or her needs require (Sloane et al., 1981). The swing bed model has been found to be a potentially cost-effective way to meet the need for long-term care services close to the patient's home without new nursing home construction. Because of the effectiveness of this care delivery system, the Omnibus Reconciliation Act of 1980 authorized rural hospitals with fewer than 50 beds to be reimbursed for providing skilled nursing services to Medicare or Medicaid beneficiaries and for providing intermediate care to Medicaid beneficiaries.

KEY CONCEPTS IN CARE OF ELDERLY PATIENTS IN THE HOSPITAL

Altered Homeostasis

Homeostasis is achieved by complex regulatory mechanisms that keep the individual within a narrow range of normal physiological function. With aging, adaptive reserves are reduced, and homeostatic mechanisms are impaired, leading to increased vulnerability to physiological and psychological disruption. The health care provider should know the parameters of normal age-related physiological changes. For example, there are normal changes in laboratory values with older adults (Table 22–1).

The normal physiological changes of aging must also be considered in planning for quality acute care of the older adult. These changes occur in the cardiovascular, respiratory, renal, and immune systems.

Hospitalized old people typically have one or more decompensated diseases, making homeostasis even more difficult to maintain. Nurses, therefore, should continually consider the diminished homeostatic response of the aged when planning and implementing care.

For example, an 87-year-old woman was hospitalized for treatment of a septic left knee. She experienced hypovolemia as a result of the sepsis and subsequently developed congestive heart failure as a result of overzealous intravenous fluid support. The patient was then put on bedrest to await definitive diagnosis of her knee pathology and to minimize her pain. She was given narcotic analgesics to ease her pain. She subsequently developed a sacral pressure sore, atelectasis, and delirium. Overzealous treatment of the initial symptoms without sufficient thought given to the impact of advanced age on homeostatic mechanisms,

TABLE 22-1
Laboratory Values for Older Adults

TEST	UNCHANGED/SAME AS YOUNGER REFERENCE	DECREASE WITH OLDER SUBJECTS	INCREASE WITH OLDER SUBJECTS
CBC			
RBC	Unchanged	or Slight decrease	
Hgb	Unchanged	or Slight decrease	
Hct	Unchanged	or Slight decrease	
RBC indices	Unchanged		
WBC count	Unchanged		
Differential			
Basophils	Unchanged		
Eosinophils	Unchanged		
Myelocytes	Unchanged		
Bands	Unchanged		
Monocytes	Unchanged		
Lymphocytes	Unchanged	or Slight decrease	
Platelets	Unchanged		
ESR			Slight increase
B_{12}		Decrease	
Folate/folic acid		Decrease	
TIBC/transferrin	Unchanged		
Serum Fe	Unchanged		
Blood chemistry			
Electrolytes			
Na	Unchanged	or Slight decrease	
K	Unchanged		or Slight increase
Cl	Unchanged		
Ca	Unchanged	or Slight decrease	
P	Unchanged		
Mg		Decrease	
Glucose			
FBS	Unchanged		or Slight increase
PPBS			Increase
OGTT			Increase
HgA_{1c}			Increase
End products of metabolism			
BUN	Unchanged		or Slight increase
Creatinine	Unchanged		or Slight increase
Creatinine clearance		Decrease	
Bilirubin	Unchanged		
Uric acid			Slight increase
Liver function tests			
ALAT (SGPT)	Unchanged		
AST (SGOT)	Unchanged		
LDH	Unchanged		or Slight increase
Alkaline phosphatase			Gradual increase
Total Protein	Unchanged	or Slight decrease	
Albumin		Decrease	
Globulin	Unchanged		
Lipoproteins			
Total cholesterol			Gradual increase
LDL			Increase
HDL	Unchanged	or Slight decrease in women	or Slight increase in men
Triglycerides			Increase
Thyroid function tests			
T_4	Unchanged	or Slight decrease	
T_3		Decrease	
TSH			Slight increase

Reproduced with permission from the article "Interpretation of Laboratory Values in Older Adults" by K.D. Mellillo, from the July, 1993 issue of *The Nurse Practitioner,* © Springhouse Corporation.
CBC = complete blood count; RBC = red blood cell; WBC = white blood cell; Hgb = hemoglobin; Hct = hematocrit; ESR = erythrocyte sedimentation rate; TIBC = total iron-binding capacity; FBS = fasting blood sugar; PPBS = postprandial blood sugar; OGTT = oral glucose tolerance test; HgA_{1c} = hemoglobin A_{1c}; BUN = blood urea nitrogen; ALAT (SGPT) = alanine aminotransferase (serum glutamic-pyruvic transaminase); AST (SGOT) = aspartate aminotransferase (serum glutamic-oxaloacetic transaminase); LDH = lactate dehydrogenase; LDL = low-density lipoprotein; HDL = high-density lipoprotein; T_4 = thyroxine; T_3 = tri-iodothyronine; TSH = thyroid-stimulating hormone.

such as cardiopulmonary, renal, and central nervous system function, led to further problems for this patient. Eventually, through gentle diuresis, gradual remobilization, good pulmonary toilet, an aggressive pressure sore prevention program, and in-depth discharge planning, she regained her self-care abilities.

Care in today's acute care hospital system is often organized according to specialty units that tend to treat one organ system aggressively without necessarily considering the potential adverse effects on other organ systems, or they do not consider the fact that older people may react differently to treatment because of the physiological changes of aging. For example, the optimal treatment for a particular infection may be administration of aminoglycoside antibiotics. But, if the potential for drug-drug interactions that increase the likelihood of ototoxicity or nephrotoxicity of these agents is ignored, severe functional impairments may result. Similar examples can be generated for nearly every organ system.

Impact of the Hospital Environment

The hospital environment is quite different from the home environment of most older people. The hospital environment is designed to facilitate the efficient delivery of acute nursing and medical care. In the physical environment, space is conserved to contain costs and to reduce the amount of time that health care professionals must spend moving from patient to patient. Beds are often left in a higher-than-normal position from the floor to reduce strain on nurses' backs. The physical layout of beds or rooms is often designed to maximize ability to supervise a large number of patients simultaneously. In certain instances, hospital architects have made compromises to promote patient privacy (for example, in constructing private rooms), but most environmental features are designed for the convenience of hospital staff. Environmental noise is dominated by a cacophony of alarms, beepers, pages, and housekeeping activities rather than by the sound of human voices. Odors in the hospital consist of urine, feces, and wound drainage, or antiseptics and deodorizers. Visual stimuli are predominantly pieces of highly technical medical equipment, such as intravenous lines and pumps, cardiac monitors, and oxygen and suction units.

The interpersonal aspects of the environment are also targeted to promote efficiency of medical care rather than normal physiological functioning. Calls for help are usually indicated by lights or intercom rather than by face-to-face communication. Hospital routines do not necessarily promote physiological sleep-wake patterns or nutritional habits, nor do they support the practice of individual health behaviors.

The net result of the design characteristics of most hospitals is an environment that is extremely supportive, even prosthetic, for health professionals but challenging and, in some cases, overwhelming for a functionally impaired elderly patient. Hospital nurses should therefore include an environmental assessment and should attempt to provide as therapeutic an environment as possible to enhance the older person's functional independence and control.

Ethical Conflicts

Many ethical conflicts may arise in the hospital setting (Fahey, 1989). One central dilemma is the conflict between the hospital, which is primed to provide every technological advantage and health care opportunity to the older patient, and the potential of that same technology to do harm. Most older people benefit from a judicious use of technology, but restrained or prudent use of technology by individuals who are trained to apply a specific technique or procedure is sometimes difficult to achieve. For example, when sudden death occurs in the hospital, an entire cascade of events is automatically brought into play unless a "do not resuscitate" (DNR) order has been written and properly communicated to the staff.

Patients can be admitted to the hospital with living wills or advanced directives already in place concerning heroic care. These must also be communicated to the health care team. Decisions regarding their care should be directed by the patient and/or family. However, consider the problem of the elderly patient and family who have none of these care directives in place, or who, after agreeing to a DNR order, feel that the health care team is no longer interested in the patient. They may feel that the patient does not belong in the hospital despite the fact that he or she has a remedial problem, such as dehydration, that negatively influences her or his functional status.

The Patient Determination Act of 1990 was passed to rectify some of the ethical dilemmas involving unwanted aggressive technological therapy for the elderly. The act defined advance directives, which include living wills, durable powers of attorney, and restriction of select and specific care, such as cardiopulmonary resuscitation (Schonwetter et al., 1993; Sachs, 1992).

Time Use

Hospital nurses have a tremendous number of responsibilities to the older patient and to other team members. Accomplishing these responsibilities competently and efficiently has become more difficult because of the increased complexity of patient care since 1981, under Medicare's prospective reimbursement system.

The average length of hospital stays has decreased, resulting in smaller numbers of patients who are well known to the hospital staff. From the nurse's perspective, the following question arises: When I have all these responsibilities and a limited amount of time, how are priorities best established? The major options for spending time in patient care include

- Prevention
- Treatment
- Collaborative roles in monitoring and treating clinical problems
- Independent responsibilities
- Patient teaching
- Working with families

Setting priorities for these functions depends on several factors, including the skill and availability of other health team members, the adequacy of posthospitalization resources for both long-term and short-term care, and the philosophy and skills of the nursing service and the individual nurse. In settings in which the physician staff is highly dependent on nurses to monitor clinical problems, failure to give functional care needs a high priority may be life threatening. However, if nurses do not place a high priority on independent nursing functions, such as promoting physiological activity, sleep or rest, elimination patterns, and adequate nutritional intake, the patient will suffer over the long term, and preventable diseases will ensue.

STRUCTURE OF CARE IN THE HOSPITAL

The Geriatric Multidisciplinary Team

Multidisciplinary teams are becoming increasingly popular as a means of providing holistic care to older patients in acute care settings. The reason is that care of the elderly is so complex that the expertise and input of several different disciplines are needed. One profession is severely limited in its ability to handle the multiplicity of problems encountered in elderly patients. The multidisciplinary team that uses a case management–managed care delivery model is especially effective with the elderly. In one case management implementation project (Trella, 1993), positive results included better coordinated care, earlier therapies and discharge planning, better clarification of ethical issues, less task-oriented care, and elimination of unnecessary treatments.

A multidisciplinary team is a small group whose members share common goals, possess the diversity of skills and professional orientations needed to achieve those goals, and coordinate their efforts to provide services to a patient or group of patients through systematic communication (Dugan and Mosel, 1992). Teams are usually made up of a core group consisting of a nurse, social worker, and physician with special training in geriatrics. Other members of the team may include an occupational therapist, a physical therapist, a psychologist, and a clinical pharmacist.

Complex geriatric patients are found through admission, chart review, or referrals from staff. Assessments are made by each member of the team that are pertinent to the team member's discipline. The team usually has an initial case conference after the assessments are made to develop a plan of care. Weekly conferences and rounds are made, with staff members providing care. Specific problems of care are discussed, including ethical dilemmas related to cardiopulmonary resuscitation, withholding of treatment, and use of limited resources after discharge. Discharge planning, follow-up, and continuity of care are emphasized.

The success of multidisciplinary geriatric team-managed care, particularly on a geriatric unit, has been encouraging. Improvements in placement location, functional status, diagnosis of treatable disorders, and drug management were seen in older patients admitted to a geriatric activity center (Zuckerman et al., 1993). Staff response was very positive, and members of the health care team became more sensitive to the needs of their elderly patients.

Care of the Older Medical Patient

Elderly patients who are occupying beds on medical floors reflect the trend of increased numbers of chronically ill in the acute care setting. The increase in chronically ill elderly, especially those with multiple chronic illnesses and functional disabilities, has given rise to many problems for both patients and staff in acute care hospitals, where care and services are organized around the disease-illness model. Medical services predominantly oriented toward acute care resulted in negative consequences for the chronically ill recovering from an acute illness and whose need was for rehabilitative and preventive measures. However, within this context of caring for "low-priority" patients, nurses have been able to derive satisfaction in their work through interacting with the patients and through seizing on opportunities to be innovative. Because the needs of these patients have been predominantly "nursing" rather than "medical," nurses have had the opportunity to experience relative independence and freedom to try new approaches, thus affirming their professional identity.

The Case for a Professional Nursing Model of Care for Older Medical Patients

Many nurses who care for older medical patients advocate professional care delivery models (Mayer et al., 1990), such as nursing case management (Cohen and Cesta, 1993). General case management has been defined as a "system of health assessment, planning, service procurement/delivery/coordination and monitoring to meet the multiple needs of clients" (Zander, 1990). Managed care, on the other hand, usually refers to organizational structure. It originally was designed for health maintenance organizations in the 1970s and operated with federal funding. The main element of managed care is control through ownership or contractual agreement and is associated with for-profit organizations, such as insurance companies, health care institutions, or independent medical practice arrangements (Zander, 1990).

The basic concepts of professional nursing care delivery include autonomy and accountability, promotion of cost-effective, high-quality patient outcomes, and a professional knowledge base (Mayer et al., 1990). There is direct communication between the nurse and other caregivers on the health care team. The nurse may act as a leader, communication facilitator, clinician, resource person, and quality control agent for the unit. Primary functions of a nurse case manager are multiple and are inter-related with all aspects of holistic care needs of the elderly (Bower, 1992):

- Coordinating care and services for identified patient population
- Performing case finding and screening
- Assessing the biopsychosocial needs of the patient and family
- Assessing patients' coping and adaptive abilities, their formal and informal support systems, and their self-care abilities
- Gathering all information and synthesizing interdisciplinary problem identification
- Acting as resource in identifying and linking the patient with most appropriate resource, person, or institution to solve the patient's problems in a timely manner
- Procuring services, making eligibility decisions, and authorizing hospitalization, rehabilitation, or home care needs
- Facilitating access to health care
- Acting as a problem solver and a decision maker
- Providing direct patient care when necessary
- Acting as a liaison and facilitating communication
- Educating
- Documenting
- Monitoring and evaluating client and program outcomes

Older medical patients can have multiple problems and may react in various ways to their hospitalization. Having a variety of caregivers can produce confusion, disorientation, misperception of signs and symptoms, and misinterpretation of clues to alterations in function. Professional nursing care can facilitate both an accurate baseline assessment and recognition of deviation from that baseline while the older person is in the hospital, and it can provide an anchor for the patient and the family. The nurse can also communicate any concerns and problems to the various hospital professionals involved in the team care of the patient.

Health care financing today has affected all patients, particularly older hospital patients. Because a complication can mean extended hospitalization, it is essential that nurses plan, coordinate, and provide patient care in order to detect early signs and symptoms of trouble. Nursing care must be carefully and effectively planned to maximize available time and also must be well coordinated. Ongoing team management is essential because of the short hospitalization time. Because patients are being discharged earlier, patient and family teaching assumes even greater importance, necessitating that discharge planning begin the day of admission.

Dependency and Functional Problems

Elderly medical patients are at special risk for losing control and regressing or becoming dependent. The need for control becomes increasingly varied with older age. In some cases, detrimental effects on health may occur as a result of control of activities, circumstances, or health restrictions; in other cases, greater control produces other negative consequences, such as stress, worry, and self-blame.

Conditions that tend to increase dependency in older patients result from changes in the internal and external environment, including medications, disease processes, aging processes, nurse-patient interactions, rigid schedules, and the hospital setting itself.

Miller (1985) found that different methods of nursing care had an impact on dependency in older patients. When care was provided in a "task-allocated" unit, the patients became more dependent than did those in an "individualized care" unit, generally because nurses and nonprofessional caregivers who were task oriented were more likely to be preoccupied with accomplishing certain tasks, such as bathing, feeding, and dressing, than with the rehabilitative care of an individual patient. In addition, the longer older patients were hospitalized, the more dependent they became.

It is important for nurses who are caring for older medical patients to make a special effort to increase independent functioning and to promote control beginning on the first day of hospitalization. Discharge planning, patient and family teaching, and other strategies for maximizing independence should be an integral part of the nursing care plan. This process can be difficult in an acute care unit that is poorly staffed because it often takes longer and requires more patience to encourage disabled, chronically ill elderly patients to care for themselves. However, in the long run, preventing decline (Inouye et al., 1993) and maintaining functional capacity and independence are more beneficial for patient and staff alike.

CASE 1.   Ms. A's Admission to a General Medical Ward

Ms. A is an 83-year-old white unmarried woman, a retired college professor of romance languages. She is hospitalized for left knee pain with effusion, hypotension, and fever of unknown etiology. Her other medical problems include hypertension and hypoalbuminemia.

Before the hospitalization, she was functionally independent, living alone with her pet dog on a farm where other relatives lived close by. By her sister-in-law's report, she regularly walked 1 mile per day. The patient had only one prior hospitalization, in France during the 1930s for appendicitis. During the hospitalization, she develops the following complications: a grade 2 sacral pressure sore, delirium, congestive heart failure, atelectasis, dependency in self-care, and learned helplessness. For a period of time, she requires supplemental feeding through a nasoduodenal tube. She is discharged to a nursing home to regain her lost self-care abilities and eventually returns home.

ANALYSIS OF NURSING CARE NEEDS
Universal Self-Care Requisites

1. Food. Monitor calorie and protein intake to ensure sufficient to alleviate protein malnutrition and to prevent caloric malnutrition.

2. Fluid. Minimal fluid requirement is 1800 ml per day.

3. Air. Supplemental oxygen is required sporadically.

4. Elimination. The patient's usual bowel pattern is once each day without the use of laxatives.

5. Safety. The patient is unable to stand or transfer unassisted because of pain in

continued on following page

CASE 1.   Ms. A's Admission to a General Medical Ward

continued

left knee. Requirement for pain medication increases the likelihood of clouded consciousness, necessitating side rails and more supervision.

6. Social interaction/solitude. The patient's usual pattern is living alone and inviting guests or visiting with family during her daily walk. During hospitalization, the patient has limited control over the timing of interactions with others.

7. Activity/rest. The patient is placed on bedrest because of sepsis and pain in knee. Requires in-bed exercise program, including passive range of motion to the left knee within pain tolerance; turning schedule, to prevent pressure sores and atelectasis; and isometric exercises to preserve strength in other muscle groups.

8. Sense of normalcy. The patient's normal state is disrupted by feeding tube requirements for assistance in personal care activity and by disruptions in social interaction patterns.

Developmental Self-Care Requisites

1. Altered homeostasis. The patient is at higher-than-average risk for adverse drug reactions, including superinfection from antibiotic therapy. She is at risk of overhydration from use of intravenous fluids and nasoduodenal tube. She is at high risk for pressure sore development because of her immobility and reduced nutritional status.

2. Loss. The patient admits to having no recent major life change or losses. Potential losses represented by this hospitalization include loss of sense of normalcy, loss of usual daily habits, and loss of independence.

3. Role change. No recent role changes before hospital admission are evident. The patient has not had to assume a sick role in more than 50 years.

4. Dependence/independence. The patient presents as an extremely self-reliant person with little experience in a dependent role. She is likely to need assistance in striking a healthy balance between appropriate dependence and independence.

Health Deviation Self-Care Requisites

1. Congestive heart failure. This condition results in sodium-restricted diet.

2. Knee sepsis. This condition results in increased use of pain medication and use of activity restriction.

3. Malnutrition. This condition results in use of feeding tube.

NURSING DIAGNOSES
(Ackley and Ladwig, 1993)

1. Nutrition, Altered: Less than Body Requirements, probably related to inadequate protein intake; manifested by hypoalbuminemia without other signs of nutrient deficiency

2. Skin Integrity, High Risk for Impairment, related to immobility, nutritional deficit; Norton score = 13

3. Mobility, Impaired Physical, related to pain and medical therapy for left knee sepsis; manifested by prescribed bedrest, inability to move in bed easily without pain

4. Self-Care Deficits, in bathing, hygiene, dressing, toileting, related to pain, bedrest; manifested by inability to perform these self-care activities without assistance

5. Comfort, Altered, related to inflammation in left knee joint, secondary to streptococcal infection

6. Thought Processes, Altered, related to atelectasis, drug side effects, reduced sensory inputs; manifested by illogical speech

7. Powerlessness, related to prolonged hospitalization, functional impairments, inexperience with health care system; manifested by limited participation in discharge planning process, passive acceptance of nursing home placement, refusal to acknowledge that eventual return to home is possible

8. Home Maintenance Management, Impaired. Meal preparation, related to reduced endurance secondary to prolonged period of dependency; manifested by inability to stand long enough to prepare a meal

9. Gas Exchange, Impaired, related to alve-

CASE 1.   Ms. A's Admission to a General Medical Ward

continued

olar collapse secondary to immobility; manifested by diminished breath sounds, dullness to percussion, and decreased PO_2

PREVENTABLE PROBLEMS AND THEIR IMPACT ON FUNCTIONAL COMPLICATIONS

PRESSURE SORES Pressure sores are predictable, preventable problems in most hospitalized older persons. In this instance, the patient had significant risk (Norton score = 13), yet no systematic pressure sore prevention efforts were initiated until a grade 2 pressure sore had appeared. Once the sore developed, an eggcrate mattress was installed, and a regular turning schedule was implemented. The sore healed before discharge from the hospital.

DELIRIUM Delirium in the geriatric patient is common in acute care situations and can affect as many as 80 per cent of those hospitalized (Foreman, 1991; Evans et al., 1993). Although the etiology of delirium is not precisely defined, several factors in this patient may have contributed, including the use of central nervous system depressant medications (narcotic analgesics), atelectasis, infection, sensory deprivation from prolonged bedrest, and congestive heart failure. The patient's delirium manifested with agitated behavior when she could not find a favorite television show. This patient was fortunate for several reasons:

1. She was not incorrectly diagnosed as demented. Instead, she received supplemental oxygen empirically on the basis of a prior diagnosis of atelectasis, and her delirium resolved.

2. Her delirium presented in an obvious, fairly benign pattern. Not all delirium is manifested by agitated behavior, and some observers believe that this situation is often overlooked by medical and nursing staff and may therefore go untreated.

3. Had her delirium been manifested by more serious behavioral disturbances, such as combativeness or wandering behavior, she may well have received another medication, which could have clouded the diagnosis and treatment picture.

CONGESTIVE HEART FAILURE This patient's

congestive heart failure was induced by overaggressive fluid replacement to correct her admission hypotension. According to Lipsitz et al. (1986), older individuals who do not have pre-existing cardiomegaly are less likely to develop congestive heart failure, even with volume overload. However, underlying heart disease should have been suspected in this patient because she had long-standing hypertension and possible endocarditis. Thus, a quiescent cardiac problem, coupled with decreased homeostatic reserve, precipitated a new medical problem. After diuresis for several days with furosemide, the patient required no further diuretic therapy or fluid restriction.

ATELECTASIS A common problem in surgical settings, atelectasis may also occur in medical settings in which the patient is relatively immobile and central nervous system depressant drugs are used. Both situations occurred in this case. There is controversy in the nursing literature about the relative effectiveness of treatments such as incentive spirometry and use of blow bottles or an intermittent positive-pressure breathing apparatus, compared with deep-breathing exercises in preventing atelectasis. For this patient, no one anticipated the likelihood of atelectasis, and so treatment with supplemental oxygen became necessary; incentive spirometry was added after the problem was diagnosed. Although low-flow, supplemental oxygen is a relatively benign intervention, it carries the risk of further immobilizing the patient as well as inducing dependency on the oxygen. Anticipation of the problem and institution of preventive measures earlier would have been preferred.

DEPENDENCE IN SELF-CARE The patient had been fully independent at home before this hospitalization. She had significant pain and immobility from the infection in her knee, and therefore some dependence in activities of daily living was to be expected. During the course of the hospitalization, she became completely dependent on staff for assistance in all activities of daily living. Nursing staff reacted with some frustration at what they perceived as her excess disability, but only late in the hospitalization did they set consistent expectations that she assume increasing responsibility for her self-care. Perform-

continued on following page

CASE 1. Ms. A's Admission to a General Medical Ward

continued

ing self-care tasks is one method of exercising and maintaining strength and skill during periods of restricted activity and mobility.

LEARNED HELPLESSNESS Learned helplessness is a situation in which individuals perceive that they have little influence over their lives and rely excessively on others. As time for discharge approached, the patient did not discuss or initiate any plans for discharge. The nurse discharge planner was struck by the disparity between the patient's functional status before admission and her ready acceptance of nursing home placement. There were sufficient informal and formal supports available to the patient to allow for her eventual return home if she was motivated and could see herself as functioning

independently once again. Team conferences, which were intended to work toward discharge and included the patient, sister-in-law, physical therapist, primary nurse, physician, and nurse discharge planner, were convened 2 weeks before discharge. The goals of the conferences were to help the patient and her family appreciate the extent of progress made during the hospitalization and to communicate clearly the goals to be attained before discharge home would be feasible. The conferences helped to empower the patient by allowing her to ask questions of the team and to participate in goal setting and decision making about her disposition. Had the team approach not been used, with the goal of fully involving the patient in disposition decisions, she would probably have remained in the nursing home permanently.

Care of the Older Surgical Patient

In 1988, 40 per cent of all geriatric patients admitted to acute care hospitals required surgery (Jackson, 1988). It is believed that this figure is higher in the 1990s. Surgical interventions for older adults have become more common and successful. Chronological age is no longer the primary means of assessing surgical risk or predicting morbidity and mortality; biological and psychological factors are also considered in the surgical decision-making process. Surgical goals for the elderly can be classified into the following categories: (1) complete restoration of health, (2) diminished disability, and (3) limited postponement of inevitable death. Nursing plans and interventions must take into account the effects of normal physiological aging (Dellasega and Burgunder, 1991) (Table 22–2). Quality of life must be considered in the decision to perform surgery, especially if the surgery is performed with the goal of postponing death. The perioperative period (preoperative, intraoperative, and postoperative) is one that is stressful, frightening, and lonely for the older patient.

Risk Factors

Surgical risk is the probability of morbidity and mortality that results from preopera-

tive preparation, anesthesia, surgery, and postoperative convalescence. Studies that have attempted to quantify mortality in elderly surgical patients have lacked consistency because they do not have a standardized system of reporting. For example, studies do not differentiate between nonviable and potentially viable patients, operative and nonoperative mortality, medical and surgical causes of postoperative mortality, and existence or nonexistence of residual malignancy. Patients older than 85 years are the fastest-growing surgical population (Arron et al., 1992). Studies generally have shown that surgical morbidity and mortality are higher in older than in younger patients, but outcomes for even the most difficult surgical procedures in the elderly are favorable if appropriate attention is given to all factors that affect the degree of operative risk (Nunnelee et al., 1993). Morbidity and mortality are generally associated with pathological changes rather than with normal aging changes, and emergency surgery carries a much higher risk than elective surgery.

Chronological age can serve as a rough index for consideration of the increased incidence of concurrent chronic diseases, which may have a profound effect on surgical outcome. Older people often have advanced primary disease, which increases surgical risk. Diseases that increase the risk of death

T A B L E   2 2 – 2
Selected Nursing Interventions for Elderly Surgical Clients

SYSTEM	AGE-RELATED CHANGE	NURSING INTERVENTION
General appearance	Change in height, weight, and fat distribution	Accurate assessment of physical parameters. Provide for warmth.
Integument	Diminished integrity 2° to loss of subcutaneous fat and decreased oil production, elasticity, and hydration	Avoid trauma, careful preoperative preparation. Use other means to assess oxygenation and hydration, such as evaluation of mucous membranes, laboratory studies, and urine output.
Sensory-perceptual	Decline in vision and hearing ability; dryness of mouth	Compensate for sensory deficits: speak low, not loud; minimize noise in environment; stay within patient's field of vision when speaking; encourage patient to wear hearing aid to the operating room. Moisture measures when NPO.
Respiratory	Decreased efficiency of cough reflex and decreased aeration of lung fields	Teach coughing and deep breathing exercises and remind patient to do them. Assess baseline parameters. Constant monitoring.
Cardiovascular	Less efficient, decreased adaptation to stress	Monitor for hypotension and shock. Assess for thrombosis formation. Assess for cardiac dysrhythmias.
Gastrointestinal	Decline in gastric motility	Encourage intake of nutritious meals, soft diet. Assist with feeding. Monitor bowel function.
Genitourinary	Decreased efficiency of kidney; loss of bladder control	Monitor intake and output, electrolyte levels. Assess for drug side effects. Assist with voiding as needed.
Musculoskeletal	Stiffness of joints; decrease in strength; bones become brittle	Careful positioning on operating room bed. Move carefully and gently. Prevent pressure sores.
Cognitive-psychosocial	Reaction time decreases; intellectual ability stable; prone to delirium and altered mental status while in hospital	Provide ample time for decisions. Implement safety measures. Talk to patient as an adult, not a child. Orient frequently.

Adapted from Dellasega, C. and Burgunder, C. Perioperative nursing care for the elderly surgical patient. *Today's OR Nurse* 13(6):15, 1991.
2° = secondary; NPO = nothing by mouth.

can be grouped into (1) those that occur to varying degrees in all aging individuals, (2) those that are not universally present but have an increased incidence with age, and (3) those that are not related to aging but have more serious consequences in older persons.

Specific factors associated with surgical risk are related to cardiac and pulmonary problems, nutritional status, and mental health. Most morbidity that occurs with surgery in the elderly is associated with cardiovascular and pulmonary complications. Ischemic heart disease is the most serious risk factor in older patients. The occurrence of a myocardial infarction within the 3 months preceding surgery is associated with either another myocardial infarction or cardiac death in 39 per cent of surgical patients. This figure decreases to 15 per cent if surgery occurs 3 to 6 months after a myocardial infarction and decreases further to a constant 5 per cent risk factor after the 6-month interval (Goldman, 1983). Congestive heart failure also presents a cardiac risk that should be treated before surgery.

Pulmonary risks include the common pulmonary complications (respiratory insufficiency, pneumonia, and atelectasis) that occur more frequently in the elderly as a result of surgery, especially in those with pre-existing chronic lung disease.

Nutritional status affects the success with which the older person withstands the stress of surgery. Many older people, especially those with cancer or those facing emergency surgery, are significantly malnourished. It is useful to improve the nutritional status of older patients before surgical procedures are carried out, if possible.

Mental health problems, such as dementia and depression, can affect surgical outcome. Demented patients do not respond well to instructions and can obstruct normal recovery in their confusion. Depressed older people may not have the will to recover and so may not respond well to the stress of the surgery.

A positive aspect related to surgical intervention in the elderly is the individual's longevity. Survival to advanced age in itself is predictive of more years of survival. These are the very people who have survived heart disease, cancer, and accidents. They have certainly demonstrated durability and resilience and are probably better surgical risks than are feeble, pessimistic younger patients.

Preoperative Care and Management

Preoperative assessment and management of the elderly patient are important phases of care. The perioperative nurse, anesthesia provider, and surgeon work as a team to provide optimal outcomes of the surgery and the anesthesia. A thorough assessment should include an identification of the presenting illness in the context of coexisting disease and age-related changes (Meckes, 1991).

A careful history and physical examination can reveal any medical or psychological problems that may complicate the operation and recovery. Of particular interest to the perioperative nurse are the decreased function in the cardiovascular system, reduced immune ability, slow metabolic rate, decreased skin thickness and muscle volume, decreased mobility, rigidity of limbs and joints, and decreased pressure and touch receptors (Horner, 1993). Awareness of present or past medical diagnoses can also help in planning high-quality perioperative care. Such diagnoses include arteriosclerotic cardiovascular disease; myocardial infarction; chronic obstructive pulmonary disease; hypertension; diabetes; renal, liver, gastrointestinal, and endocrine dysfunction; neurological abnormalities; and arthritis. Laboratory results should be carefully monitored. Parameters outside normal values should not be considered to be common to aging, but rather to be due to a disease process. For example, anemia is a pathological condition and is not a normal occurrence with aging (Melillo, 1993).

All medications should be noted, including over-the-counter drugs (Meeker and Rothrock, 1995). The patient should be asked about aspirin intake because many older patients take aspirin for arthritis but do not consider it a drug. Postoperative bleeding problems can occur because of the effects of aspirin on the clotting cascade. Mental status and attitude toward the surgery should also be noted. The patient's general mood is a valuable clue to how the older patient will withstand the surgical procedure. A hopeful outlook, controlled anxiety, and a will to live indicate a good surgical risk (Meeker and Rothrock, 1995).

During the preoperative period, older patients should be kept out of bed and as mobile as possible. This helps to maintain a positive nitrogen balance and prevents musculoskeletal atrophy due to disuse, sodium retention, respiratory and venous stasis, pressure sores, and bladder dysfunction (Girard, 1994b).

Nutritional rehabilitation should be carried out whenever possible to decrease the incidence of wound infection and wound dehiscence and to compensate for the catabolic effects of major surgery and feeding difficulties in the postoperative period. Because elderly patients are more apt to have nutritional deficits than are younger patients, they are more prone to postoperative complications. For example, if the patient is protein-calorie deprived because of age, he or she will have decreased albumin levels. Hypoalbuminemia has been related to delayed surgical wound healing and an increased potential for development of pressure sores (Johnson, 1993). An assessment of malnutrition risk factors should be conducted before surgery. Both enteral and parenteral feeding before and after surgery have had beneficial effects on postoperative morbidity and mortality.

Management of medical conditions preoperatively can improve operative risk. For example, patients with chronic obstructive pulmonary disease secondary to bronchitis or emphysema should be weaned from cigarette smoking, given expectorants and possibly bronchodilators, and treated with broad-spectrum antibiotics before surgery to decrease the quantity of purulent secretions (Van Buren, 1984). In some cases, drugs such as digoxin and nitroglycerin are discontinued during the perioperative period unless otherwise indicated. If an antiarrhythmic drug is needed, it may be given parenterally until oral ingestion is possible. Diuretics and antihypertensive drugs may be taken as needed but should not be used routinely in the postoperative period.

Diabetic patients are susceptible to many complicating conditions postoperatively. However, with metabolic control, even elderly patients can have a relatively normal recovery period. Withholding all insulin until the postoperative period is not recommended, because it places the patient in a catabolic state even before the surgical stress (Hammonds, 1991). Optimal methods of achieving glycemic control vary (Rosenberg, 1990); they include infusing insulin with an intravenous pump, giving boluses as needed, using a computerized biofeedback loop that continuously reads the blood glucose levels and delivers an appropriate dose of insulin, or giving insulin by subcutaneous injections (least favored method) (Gisler,

1994). Many physicians advocate partial dosing the day of surgery: administering ⅓ to ⅔ the usual dose of intermediate-acting insulin subcutaneously because exogenous insulin is needed even in the preoperative fasting state. Optimal fasting glucose levels are debated and range between 100 and 150 mg per dl to 150 and 200 mg per dl intraoperatively (Schwartz et al., 1990; Hammonds, 1991). Whatever the range desired, it is important to keep the levels consistent rather than fluctuating greatly anytime during the perioperative period.

Preoperative teaching is an extremely important part of the preparation for surgery in the elderly because it helps to allay fears and to elicit full cooperation during the postoperative course. Older people are as able to learn as younger people (Merriam and Caffarella, 1991). However, because of sensory deficits and changes in cognition, the learning process may take longer in older than in younger people. Sensory impairments and environmental influences, such as noise and distractions, must be considered in any preoperative teaching experience. A suggested teaching protocol can include the following (Girard, 1994b):

1. Sit close so that the patient can see your face and read your lips if needed.
2. Talk slower and pitch voice tone lower—do not raise your voice volume.
3. Minimize environmental background noises.
4. Show or draw pictures as well as present the surgical information verbally.
5. Give procedural information if the patient has a moderate amount of anxiety (what is going to happen, and when).
6. Give sensory information if the patient's anxiety level is high (what the patient will see, feel, and hear), rather than detailed procedural information.
7. Include family or significant other in the teaching.

Emphasis should placed on the need for mobility, aeration of the lungs, safety (e.g., prevention of falls), and adequate elimination.

Consent for Surgery

No surgery can be performed without the informed consent of the patient. Elements of informed consent include an explanation in lay terms of the nature and purpose of the surgery; disclosure of the attendant risks, inconvenience, hazards, and problems in recuperation; information about the risk of declining the procedure; explanation of alternative modes of treatment; knowledge of the identity of the person performing the operation; and guarantee that all questions will be answered. The physician has the legal duty to make certain that the patient understands the information that is relevant to his or her decision (Harris and Velligan, 1992).

Age does not preclude the elderly from having the right to informed consent if they are capable of making decisions. No one is authorized to give consent for any older person unless the older person has been declared incompetent and has been assigned a legal guardian (see Chapter 3). Older people have every right to determine what is done to their bodies.

It is important to be sure that consent is truly "informed" in elderly patients. The normal changes associated with older age (sensory changes in vision and hearing, slowed reaction time, slowed learning processes, decreased short-term memory) as well as the impact of various chronic illnesses can influence the person's perception and understanding of the explanation and teaching related to the consent form. In many cases, older patients are overwhelmed by the newness of the hospital environment and the number and variety of health care team members visiting either in groups during rounds or in and out during the day. They may feel intimidated and may hastily sign a consent form without fully understanding all of the implications of a surgical procedure. The nurse can aid in the consent process by being a stable and consistent health care provider, clarifying or giving further explanations, and listening attentively to any questions and anxieties raised.

Preoperative Medication

Preoperative medication is given to alleviate apprehension, reduce secretion of mucus in the upper respiratory tract, decrease stomach acidity, and facilitate the induction and maintenance of general anesthesia. The intensity and duration of the therapeutic effects of the drugs are usually increased in the elderly owing to age-related functional and pathological changes that may interfere with the absorption, binding, distribution, metabolism, and excretion of drugs (see Chapter 18 for a discussion of pharmacology in the aged).

Premedications that cause minimal circulatory and respiratory depression are generally chosen for older patients. Dosages may be reduced by a third to half the amount that would be given to a younger person of the same size. Narcotics are given for their analgesic and hypnotic effects, as well as for an anesthetic adjunct. Narcotics depress the respiratory center in the central nervous system. This is a particular problem in older patients because respiratory reserve decreases in old age, causing older people to compensate by increasing the respiratory rate. Because narcotics tend to depress elevated respiratory rates more than they do normal rates, they have a greater effect on respiratory exchange. Narcotics should be given preoperatively to older people only if they have pain (Duncalf and Kepes, 1986).

Barbiturates, used for sedation, can have an exaggerated depressant effect or, conversely, may produce excitement or various psychotomimetic symptoms in elderly patients. Drugs that are considered safe for preoperative use are diphenhydramine, paraldehyde, chloral hydrate, and glutethimide. Anticholinergic drugs, such as atropine and scopolamine, should be used sparingly, if at all, in the elderly. With today's balanced and controlled anesthesia, premedication of elderly patients with sedatives or anticholinergics is seldom warranted and, if used, may create more serious problems than preoperative anxiety or hypersalivation. Older persons are more sensitive to the central nervous system and ophthalmic effects of the drugs, especially elevated temperature, tachycardia, and glaucoma (Miller, 1994).

Intraoperative Care

During the intraoperative period, perioperative nurses, surgeons, and anesthesia providers monitor older patients closely and treat them carefully to prevent postoperative complications. Anesthesia is chosen in consideration of normal aging changes, which can cause diminished circulation to the heart and other vital organs. Physiologically, there is increased potential for hypovolemia, hypoxia, and lower-than-normal perfusion pressures. Major perioperative nursing considerations include ensuring safety, maintaining skin integument, monitoring homeostasis, creating and maintaining a sterile environment, and monitoring psychological status (Association of Operating Room Nurses, 1994).

Proper positioning on the operating table is vital to minimize injury or trauma to bones, joints, nerves, and blood vessels (Meeker and Rothrock, 1995; Atkinson, 1992). The spine and limbs are padded and supported to prevent fractures, muscle tears, pressure paralysis of the nerves, and damage to blood vessels. Awareness of a history of chronic conditions, such as osteoarthritis, wasted flaccid muscles, loss of adipose tissue, and hemiplegia, is important information that should be communicated to the perioperative nurse. For example, an older patient with atherosclerosis would be positioned to prevent ischemia to already compromised vessels, which would help prevent postoperative complications, such as venous thromboses.

Vital signs and temperature are monitored with all patients, but particular emphasis is placed on temperature monitoring with the elderly. Older people are prone to complications of hypothermia, so the following steps can be taken to maintain body normothermia (Atkinson, 1992):

1. Warm all fluids (both blood and crystalloid).
2. Maintain a reasonable operating room temperature when the surgical procedure does not contradict it.
3. Keep abdominal viscera covered with warm laparotomy pads.
4. Use warm saline lavage of the abdominal cavity when not contraindicated.
5. Minimize operating time.
6. Use appropriate warming blankets and head covers.

Hypothermia increases the risks of cardiovascular, respiratory, and renal complications (Burkle, 1988). The nurse must be aware of the potential for hypothermia as a result of the surgery both intraoperatively and immediately postoperatively.

Anesthesia

The two major types of anesthesia administration are regional and general. Regional anesthesia is the loss of sensation in a localized body area without the total loss of consciousness. It includes injections of a local anesthetic agent into the spine at the lumbar or sacral areas, which numbs all areas below the nerve juncture. Anesthetic agents can also be injected into regional nerve bundles (such as at the brachial plexus) or infiltrated locally to numb a small area. Local anesthesia is used for minor operations on the extremities, cataract surgery, and dental extractions. Techniques include infiltration, intravenous regional blockade, and peripheral neural blockade. These cause little systemic effect and are quite safe for the elderly (Miller, 1994).

Spinal anesthesia is a form of regional anesthesia that is useful for surgery of the lower body and extremities. Because of spinal arthritis, it may be difficult for the elderly patient to bend enough to have a needle inserted into the spinal canal. However, regional anesthesia is often preferred for the elderly because there is no direct central nervous system involvement (Meeker and Rothrock, 1995). An amnestic or analgesic agent is frequently given along with regional anesthesia. Spinal anesthesia is also especially suitable for elderly patients who may have cardiac or respiratory conditions. It is commonly used today for both inpatient and ambulatory surgeries for patients of all ages. There are no demonstrated differences in mortality or morbidity between general and regional anesthesias (Weitz, 1990).

An amnestic or analgesic agent is frequently given along with regional anesthesia. These new sedation drugs cause a temporary decline in elderly patients' ability to retrieve information, or remember (Girard, 1994a). This information should be shared with patients because they often believe they have permanent memory loss or, worse, had a stroke during the surgery.

General anesthesia acts on the central nervous system to produce deep unconsciousness. It is administered by inhalation or intravenous methods of delivery. The choice of general or regional anesthesia is made according to the needs of the anesthesia provider and surgeon, along with the preference of the patient. Some of the considerations used to make the choice include patient age, pre-existing medical illnesses, acuity of the immediate surgical problem, nature of the surgery to be performed, psychological status of the patient, and the patient's desires and past surgical and anesthesia history (Meeker and Rothrock, 1995). A form of balanced anesthesia is used today that usually includes the following (Meeker and Rothrock, 1995; Stoelting, 1993):

- A preoperative oral antacid to decrease the possibility of aspiration of stomach acid during surgery

- A fast-acting intravenous induction agent, which immediately causes loss of consciousness

- An intravenous muscle-paralyzing agent

- An inhalation agent administered via an endotracheal tube placed after the patient is asleep

During insertion of the endotracheal tube, the neck must be hyperextended. If the elderly patient has cervical arthritis, the anesthesiologist or nurse anesthetist should be informed, to prevent inadvertent damage during the procedure (Girard, 1994b).

Elimination time of general anesthesia may be decreased because of age-related lung, renal, and liver changes. Altered cardiac and tissue perfusion also decreases anesthesia clearance (Stoelting, 1993). A preoperative cognitive baseline assessment is necessary to identify postoperative ability accurately. Temporary confusion and decreased mental ability are common in the elderly after a surgical experience and should not be diagnosed as permanent elderly dementia (Girard, 1994b).

Hypotension and thrombus formation are the most serious potential side effects (Merli, 1990). They result from vasodilation and peripheral pooling of blood and decreased central venous return to the heart.

Local anesthesia with intravenous conscious sedation is frequently used today in minor surgical procedures. This procedure involves the use of a narcotic analgesic agent and an amnestic agent. Perioperative nurses are frequently the ones who administer and monitor intravenous conscious sedation. They must be educated to perform this skill according to regulations and standards within the institution and the profession (Association of Operating Room Nurses, 1994).

Postoperative Care

The major goal in postoperative care is to enable the older patient to return to normal functioning as soon as possible. Because aging body systems, especially the cardiovascular, pulmonary, and renal systems, have more difficulty coping with stress and because many concomitant chronic illnesses exist, recovery may take longer. Older people may take as long as 4 to 6 months to recover (return to baseline) from major surgery such as prostatectomy or hip replacement.

Older patients should be monitored carefully for complications. Frequent checks of vital signs and renal output during the immediate postoperative period can help identify any changes in condition. Mental status checks should be performed routinely to identify an acute confusional state.

Postoperative problems most frequently encountered in the elderly are hypotension, hypothermia, respiratory problems, thrombophlebitis and thromboembolism, acute renal failure, delirium, and alterations in fluid, electrolyte, and nutritional balance. In many cases, because older patients do not exhibit the classic symptoms of these complications, the complications may go unnoticed. The nurse is in the best position to carefully monitor, note, and report any changes in status so that early treatment can begin. In addition to knowing the normal physiology of the older adult, the nurse should be aware of changing laboratory values in the older adult (Melillo, 1993) (see Table 22–1).

An older postsurgical patient often requires more nursing care than a younger patient. Early mobilization and ambulation are of utmost importance to prevent pressure sores (which can develop in less than 24 hours), urinary incontinence, pulmonary complications, and other systemic effects of immobility. Pain management is as important for older patients as for younger ones. Regular doses rather than "whenever needed" administration of analgesics can decrease the rate of confusion and can allow the initiation of rehabilitation earlier in the postoperative course. Because older patients may respond differently to pain medication, lower doses of medication can be used to provide relief. Dose should be determined on an individual basis once an adequate amount of analgesia has been found.

Postoperative confusion, a difficult nursing care problem, may be manifested in different forms, such as disorientation, lethargy, anxiety, paranoia, aggressive behavior, and visual hallucinations (Evans et al., 1993). In some cases, "sundowning" may occur, meaning that the patient becomes confused and agitated only at night. During the postoperative phase of hospitalization, many factors may contribute to confusion, including environmental factors, sensory deprivation, untoward drug reactions, vascular problems, metabolic influences, and infection. Treatment is directed at recognizing and alleviating the underlying cause. Every effort should be made to enhance alertness through reality orientation, environmental cues, and personal interactions. It is helpful to have a family member stay with the patient as much as possible.

Discharge planning should begin as early as the first day of hospitalization (Zuckerman et al., 1993). In some cases, older people do not have support at home, so they must be discharged to a nursing home until they can function independently. Early identification of informal and formal support systems and community services can make discharge planning easier. Discharge planning can help to shorten the hospital stay and can ensure the elderly patient of a supportive environment either at home or in a nursing home.

CASE 2. Mr. B's Surgery

Mr. B is a 74-year-old black man admitted to the hospital for treatment of a nonhealing wound on his left ankle. He has had a medical history of insulin-dependent diabetes mellitus for 20 years, peripheral vascular disease, cerebrovascular disease with a mild left cerebral stroke 2 years ago, hypertension, and a right below-knee amputation 6 years ago. After 2 weeks of treating the ankle wound with wet-to-dry dressings and debridement in the whirlpool, there is no improvement. The patient undergoes surgery for a left below-knee amputation with general anesthesia; the operation is successful, and the stump wound begins to heal well.

Postoperatively, Mr. B receives the usual intravenous fluids and gradually progresses to an 1800-calorie American Dietetic Association (ADA) diet. His appetite is poor, and he frequently refuses to take medications. He voids poorly and is catheterized with a Foley catheter; several days later, he develops a urinary tract infection and is started on intravenous antibiotic therapy. Although his mental status was mildly impaired before admission (forgetting names and dates), it becomes worse in the hospital. Before surgery, he is disoriented to time and place and had visual hallucinations, as evidenced by his talking to people in his room when he is alone. After surgery, he is disoriented to time, place, and person and becomes agitated and combative at times (especially after trips to the x-ray department). Restraints are placed on his wrists to prevent him from pulling out his indwelling urinary catheter.

CASE 2. Mr. B's Surgery

continued

ANALYSIS OF NURSING CARE NEEDS
Universal Self-Care Requisites
1. Food. The patient is receiving an 1800-calorie ADA diet.
2. Fluid. Minimal fluid requirement is 2000 ml per day, and more is required postoperatively to replace blood lost during surgery and fluid lost from drainage.
3. Air. The patient is breathing room air. He is using a turning, coughing, and deep-breathing regimen to prevent atelectasis and pneumonia after general surgery.
4. Elimination. The patient eliminates at regular times; assistance is needed in getting onto commode to evacuate bowels. He may need a stool softener until bowel activity and peristalsis increase. His catheter bag requires emptying every 8 hours, possibly more often if the patient is getting ready to walk. The patient may need a leg bag to facilitate mobility.
5. Safety. The patient is at increased risk of falls secondary to loss of leg, disorientation, and change in environment.
6. Social interaction/solitude. No data are available.
7. Activity/rest. No data are available.
8. Sense of normalcy. No data are available.

Developmental Self-Care Requisites
1. Altered homeostasis. The patient is at risk for numerous problems secondary to altered homeostasis, including volume overload, pressure sores, malnutrition, and delirium.
2. Loss. Recent life changes are not noted. However, the patient has just experienced loss of the second lower extremity and will have to develop new means of transferring and ambulating. Limited information is available about his ability to cope with his previous amputation.
3. Role change. The patient has experienced a sick role for some time, given the extent of his nonhealing ulcer. His challenge now is to adapt to the new limitation in his mobility.
4. Dependence/independence. The patient has been self-reliant except for dressing changes before admission, with limited help from his wife. His return home will depend on his ability to resume his previous independent lifestyle.

Health Deviation Self-Care Requisites
1. Peripheral vascular disease. This condition requires regular inspection of stump site to note any early signs of skin breakdown. It also requires daily stump care, including emollients to prevent skin breakdown.
2. Indwelling catheter with infection. Fluid and nutritional intake should be monitored for adequacy in light of additional demands represented by infection. Long-term goals for elimination need to be established.

NURSING DIAGNOSES
(Ackley and Ladwig, 1993)
1. Altered Thought Processes, related to delirium and dementia; manifested by disorientation, memory loss
2. Infection, High Risk, related to indwelling catheter and surgical intervention
3. Skin Integrity, High Risk for Impairment, related to impaired microcirculation and immobility
4. Nutrition, High Risk for Alteration; Less than Body Requirements, related to delirium in hospital environment versus ineffective individual coping; manifested by decreased intake postoperatively
5. Mobility, Impaired Physical, related to inadequate rehabilitation after leg amputation; manifested by inability to transfer without maximal assistance
6. Urinary Elimination, Altered Patterns, related to side effects of drugs versus delirium; manifested by poor voiding postoperatively, placement of indwelling catheter
7. Constipation, High Risk for, related to immobility, side effects of drugs
8. Coping, Individual, At Risk for Ineffective Coping Strategies, related to loss of limb

continued on following page

CASE 2. Mr. B's Surgery

continued

9. Injury, High Risk for, related to decreased mobility and delirium

10. Self-Care Deficits, in Bathing, Dressing, Toileting, related to decreased mobility, delirium; manifested by inability to perform these tasks without assistance

11. Home Maintenance Management, High Risk for Impairment, related to self-care deficits and decreased physical mobility.

PREVENTABLE PROBLEMS AND THEIR IMPACT ON FUNCTIONAL STATUS

INDWELLING URINARY CATHETER Patients experience voiding difficulties postoperatively for one of several reasons:

- Side effects of anticholinergic medications result in hypertonic urinary sphincters.

- Dehydration occurs postoperatively.

- Delirium makes it difficult to follow through with instructions to void.

- The aging bladder changes.

Although initially it may be necessary to catheterize a patient, use of an indwelling catheter should be reserved for individuals who require careful monitoring of urinary output or for those who have anatomical obstructions of the urinary tract. Long-term use of an indwelling catheter invariably leads to urinary tract infection, which impedes mental function and rehabilitation from surgery.

POOR EATING The patient's failure to eat properly postoperatively could result from a variety of causes, including delirium; nausea from the anesthesia, analgesic agents, or antibiotics; not being accustomed to or not liking hospital food; dysphagia secondary to impaired oral-motor reflexes (exacerbation of

old stroke symptoms); new onset of strokes; and depression. Careful evaluation of the factors contributing to poor eating should be undertaken, and remedial action should be taken. Poor nutritional status is likely to compromise wound healing and resolution of the urinary tract infection. Nutritional deprivation may also contribute to delirium. Options for treatment depend on the etiological factors (see Chapter 19 for suggestions about detailed assessment and options for intervention for poor nutritional status).

DELIRIUM Sources of delirium include environmental dislocation; adverse drug reactions, including postanesthesia effects; urinary tract infection; malnutrition; hypoglycemia or hyperglycemia; and fluid and electrolyte disturbances. Treatment of delirium should include addressing all reversible physiological problems and providing for the patient's safety and self-care deficits in the interim. More careful attention to preoperative nutritional status and more conservative treatment of voiding problems may have prevented the delirium, as may have the use of a spinal rather than a general anesthetic.

RESTRAINTS Use of restraints is to be avoided whenever possible for several reasons: (1) the patient's autonomy is violated, and (2) restraints may precipitate or exacerbate agitation. If the patient had not been catheterized, restraints may not have been necessary. Options other than restraints to contain difficult or dangerous behavior include use of family or friends to remain with the patient at all times and removal of the offending agent (in this case, the indwelling catheter) (Stolley, 1995; United States Food and Drug Administration, 1992). Hospital routines should also be examined because they may contribute to patient agitation. See Chapter 24 for further discussion of restraint alternatives.

Care of the Older Psychiatric Patient

Older people with psychiatric problems may need institutionalization for therapy, stabilization, or maintenance. General and psychiatric hospitals are appropriate settings for emergency and short-term psychiatric care; state and mental hospitals are appropriately used for long-term care. Psychiatric home care is a growing service, with delivery of care by a psychiatric nurse practitioner or a psychiatric clinical nurse specialist (Blazek, 1993; Kozlak and Thobaben, 1992). Events that may precipitate admission to a psychiatric unit include the following:

1. Potentially harmful behavior, such as self-neglect or wandering
2. Harmful behavior, such as heavy drinking, fire setting, or violence
3. Environmental factors, such as depletion of funds, loss of a caretaker, or physician's recommendation
4. Depression, delusion, incoherence, or other disturbances of thought or feeling
5. Physical factors, such as strokes, falls, malnutrition, or feebleness

The criteria for psychiatric hospitalization of the elderly are outlined according to the appropriateness of the admission. Older people considered appropriate for admission include those with functional psychoses and without significant physical illness or disability for whom outpatient treatment is not feasible; those with depression; those with alcoholism and without significant physical illness or disability who need a period of inpatient treatment for their alcoholism after detoxification; and those with severe organic brain disorders who cannot be managed at home. It is important for the nurse to be able to differentiate among dementia, delirium, and depression (Table 22–3). Older people who are inappropriate for admission are those with delirium related to a physical illness that requires medical care, those who are moribund or comatose, those with major medical problems and minor mental symptoms, those who are mildly confused as a result of dementia and are better treated or managed at home, and those who need only adequate living accommodation and social supports (Kemp, 1993).

Voluntary admission to a psychiatric unit with both patient and family participating in decision making is always preferred. However, in some cases, involuntary commitment is necessary. Legal justification for commitment is based on imminent physical danger to self, imminent danger to others, and a clear and present need of immediate care or treatment. Commitment can be made only through a physician, preferably a psychiatrist, but often a family physician is involved in the handling of a psychiatric emergency. Prescreening admission teams, composed of a nurse, social worker, and psychiatrist, are effective in evaluating the need for psychiatric care and obtaining appropriate placement, whether it be in the hospital or the community.

Finding appropriate placement for an older person with psychiatric symptoms is difficult. In many cases, a decision must be made whether to place the patient in a medical unit or a psychiatric unit because so many elderly have a mix of medical and psychiatric problems. Some institutions are developing an alternate level of care unit for elderly patients who do not require extended acute care but are unable to find placement in extended care centers (Liukkonen, 1992). Consequences of misplacement include prolonged hospitalization; increased mortality; increased incontinence, restlessness, disorientation, or immobility; and reduced staff efficiency.

Frequently, older people come to the emergency department after a psychiatric or medical crisis. In many cases "emergency shelter" admission is required for evaluation and decision making. "Short-term hospitalization" usually refers to hospital stays lasting from a few days to 3 months. Diagnosis and treatment are especially successful for delirium and functional disorders. During short-term hospitalization, maintenance of orientation is especially important and can be achieved through the use of personal belongings, frequent family contacts, and unrestricted visiting hours. Families display a range of emotions during such hospitalization, including relief, guilt, failure, and grief. They may have been taking care of the older person for years, and the hospitalization may be the culmination of a long and trying ordeal. Geropsychiatric nurses should be supportive and nonjudgmental, especially if family members find it emotionally difficult to visit (Liukkonen, 1992).

The Environment

The physical environment should provide a setting for treatment that is both safe and therapeutic. The normal changes of aging as well as the consequences of multiple chronic illnesses should be considered in the design of the psychiatric unit. For confused and wandering older patients, color coding, the buddy system, and adequate staff can be used for orientation programs. Large signs on the doors of patients' rooms, such as "MRS. SMITH'S ROOM," are also helpful. Safety devices such as grab bars, call buttons, good illumination, and nonslip floors are essential.

Temperature control is important for older patients, who are especially prone to hypothermia and hyperthermia. Excessive heat can cause rapid development of dehydration or dangerously elevated body temperatures in older patients who are taking phenothiazines or anticholinergic drugs. Air tempera-

TABLE 22-3

Differentiating Dementia, Delirium, and Depression

	DEMENTIA	DELIRIUM	DEPRESSION
Orientation	Disoriented	Disoriented	Seems disoriented
Judgment, impairment	Focus on irrelevant	Yes or no	Appears to have poor judgment
Memory	Impaired, recent events; remote, intact	Impaired, recent events	Appears impaired, decreased ability to concentrate
Behavior	Agitation or apathy; unable to perform self-care	Agitation, changes in sleep, unable to perform self-care	Self-neglect, changes in appetite, agitation or apathy
Onset	Gradual, months to years	Rapid, hours to days	Rapid, but lasting at least weeks
Mood/affect	Labile, inappropriate	Varies	Hopeless, worried
Speech	Sparse, repetitive, does not complain of deficits; later does not attempt to conceal problems	May be incoherent, sparse, or fluent	Understandable; "I don't know," "I guess so"; complains of memory problems
Prognosis	No return to predemented state	Resolves with treatment of cause	Resolves with treatment of cause or with treatment of the depression, e.g., antidepressants

From Guin, P. and Freudenberger, K. The elderly neuroscience patient: Implications for the critical care nurse. *AACN* 3(1):102, 1992.

ture should be maintained between 68°F and 83°F with adequate control of humidity.

The social environment should provide stimulation (without overstimulation), independence, and rehabilitation. Generally, age integration is preferred over age segregation because older people on age-integrated units tend to function better than those on age-segregated units. Sexually integrated units also apparently promote acceptance and practice of realistic and appropriate sex roles and help to improve grooming and manners.

Violence is sometimes a concern on psychiatric units, especially among different age and sex groups. Depp (1981) found that younger and stronger patients were responsible for most assaults on psychogeriatric patients. Depp also found that the behavior of the victim may have precipitated the assault, and the victims were often described as unusually intrusive and meddlesome. Another study (Donat, 1986) found that assaults were second in frequency only to falls in incidents reported on a psychogeriatric unit. Most incidents involved aggressors described as having "problem behaviors," and victims were described as more cognitively impaired and less mobile than younger and stronger patients. In addition, victims were often wanderers who invaded the personal space of other patients. Most altercations occurred during periods of low staffing, and when staff was increased, the number of altercations decreased.

The use of restraints to prevent wandering should be discouraged and used only in emergency situations. Other methods of relieving anxiety and agitation, such as personal contact and touch, are preferred. Seclusion and restraint are still overused methods of control in many hospitals (Betemps et al., 1992). However, restraints or seclusion should never exceed 2 hours without review and rewriting of the order by a physician.

Treatment Modalities

MILIEU THERAPY. Institutional psychogeriatric care can promote a dependency role in older adults, resulting in deterioration of ego skills and regression. The purpose of milieu therapy is to design an environment that will encourage socialization and self-management. All elements of the environment are used as therapeutic agents, including the staff, the patients, the treatment program, and the setting. Patients are provided with opportunities to assume the normal social roles of friend, consumer, worker, and citizen. Levels of activities are broken down into steps that become increasingly complex as patients progress. Milieu therapy works best for patients who have been very regressed and socially deprived. Problems associated with milieu therapy in the elderly include lack of patient potential for change, rigid attitudes of staff members, chronic shortage of funds and personnel, and lack of desirable community alternatives to hospital care.

INDIVIDUAL PSYCHOTHERAPY. Although individual psychotherapy was once thought to be inappropriate for the elderly, many therapists now are achieving successful outcomes. When working with older patients, several modifications should be made in the approach to therapy. The therapist usually takes on a more active role, environmental manipulation is often beneficial, and some educational techniques may be used. In addition, resistance and transference are handled carefully and gently, and therapy is tapered but rarely terminated. Because older people experience so many losses, the loss of the therapist may not be bearable. If therapy must be terminated at some point, the patient must be prepared in advance to deal with the feelings involved.

GROUP THERAPY. Group therapy is an economical method of providing psychotherapeutic intervention for institutionalized elderly (Finkel, 1990). Generally, the purpose of group therapy is to help group members solve immediate problems rather than to promote insight or personality changes. The approach is more directive than that used with groups made up of younger patients, and group leaders should provide support, encouragement, and empathy because of the many losses that preoccupy older people (Saul and Saul, 1990). Group leaders must also be aware of, and compensate for, the physical problems associated with aging, such as sensory deficits, decreased energy levels, and problems associated with chronic illnesses.

Several modalities for group therapy are used with older patients, including reality orientation, validation therapy, remotivation therapy, reminiscing therapy, and group psychotherapy.

Reality Orientation. Reality orientation was developed by a nurse and a psychologist (Taulbee and Folsom, 1966) in an Alabama Veterans Administration hospital. It is designed to help reduce confusion and disorientation in people suffering from dementia. Although it is useful in orienting the patient, studies show that it has no significant effect on mental status, level of depression, or functional status (Scanland and Emershaw, 1993). Group meetings are held for about half an hour, Monday through Friday, and are usually led by a nursing assistant or activities coordinator. The size of the group should be limited to four members because of the high demands on the group leaders. Reality orientation is enforced throughout the 24-hour period by the entire staff and through use of environmental cues. Sign boards with the day of the week, date, next holiday, and next meal written on them are placed in view of the patients, and patients are reminded of who and where they are, the date, and the time. Misperceptions of the environment, which can occur frequently as a result of the aging process, are corrected. Two major problems with reality orientation are (1) lack of consistent enforcement over a 24-hour period and (2) not keeping the sign board up to date. Often, someone forgets to change the date or the next meal on the board, producing even more confusion.

Validation Therapy. Validation therapy is sometimes offered as an alternative to reality orientation in the confused and disoriented elderly. The primary goal is to give confused older persons a sense of identity, dignity, and self-worth. It can help maintain or improve aspects of cognitive or behavioral functioning in the confused older adult (Hitch, 1994). According to the originators of validation therapy, change in behavior is slow and fluctuates daily, but after a period of several years, improvements in continence, speech, affect, and awareness of the external environment can be noted.

The basic premises underlying validation therapy are (1) there is logic behind all behavior, and (2) there are different stages and levels of disorientation among elderly patients who are diagnosed with organic mental disorders. By establishing trust, a caregiver can explore the older person's free associations, body language, "nonsense syllables," and fantasies to find the meaning behind the person's bizarre behavior. The caregiver helps disoriented persons "make sense" by tying together their behavior with logical meaning. In the process, confused older persons gain a new sense of dignity and identity because the caregiver has "validated" their feelings. The caregiver becomes the link between past associations and present reality, which sometimes leads to an awareness of external reality. Group leaders are advised to use supportive behavior, develop skills in assessment, build trust, and develop a therapeutic environment for the confused elderly patient. Group sessions are limited to four to five patients and last for 15 to 45 minutes. Direct eye contact, exploration of feelings, and use of touch mimicking behaviors are therapeutic strategies that help the group leader to find logical meaning behind fantasies, rhyming, or repetitive body movements. The therapist may use statements such as the following: "Are you singing because it makes you feel better? Let's sing together." "Are you banging the chair because you are angry?" "You are making a fist—perhaps because you are angry?" The therapist looks for the underlying feeling for clues to "decode" the behavior. Validation therapy requires a large amount of energy and patience, and results come slowly. Therapists are advised to use outside sources for support and maintenance of adequate levels of energy.

Remotivation Therapy. The purposes of remotivation therapy are to resocialize regressed and apathetic patients and to reawaken their interest in the environment. It is important to discover ways to measure incentives for health promotion in the elderly and to understand their neglect in self-care (Pascucci, 1992). Group meetings, led by a specially trained nursing assistant for 10 to 15 patients, are usually held once or twice weekly. The meetings are highly structured and are located in a classroom setting in which props are used to stimulate discussion of a particular topic. Each session includes five basic steps (American Psychiatric Association, 1965):

1. Climate of acceptance, which consists of introductions and getting acquainted
2. Bridge to reality, which encourages individuals to participate in reading and discussing newspaper articles and poetry
3. Sharing of the experiences of the world, which provides development of topics for discussion
4. Appreciation of the work of the world, which prompts individuals to think about work in relation to themselves
5. Climate of appreciation, which is a time to express pleasure that the group has met and to plan the next meeting

Older people often have difficulty with steps 2 and 4 (reading aloud and considering the work world). The group also does not give the members the opportunity to explore feelings or to behave spontaneously because of its structured nature. However, it does offer the opportunity to increase the participants' sense of reality, practice healthy roles, and realize a more objective self-image.

Reminiscing Therapy. The purpose of reminiscing and life review (Haight and Burnside, 1993) is to share memories of the past, increase self-esteem, increase socialization, and increase awareness of the uniqueness of each participant (Ashton, 1993). The groups are usually made up of six or eight participants who meet once or twice a week for about 1 hour. Subjects for discussion include holidays, major events, birthdays, travel, and food.

Matteson (1984) found reminiscing groups to be a useful mode of alleviating depression in the institutionalized elderly. Reminiscence in the elderly is part of the normal life review process that takes place when a person approaches death and that can be used as a tool to resolve past conflicts, reintegrate them, and find new significance to one's life. The process of reorganization and reintegration provides a means by which older people can achieve a new sense of identity and a more positive self-concept, as well as promote health and coping abilities (Newbern, 1992; Moore, 1992).

Group Psychotherapy. Group psychotherapy provides a supportive mode of therapy for older patients and is at the same time a time-saving and economical method for the therapist (Finkel, 1990). Goals of group psychotherapy include alleviation of psychiatric symptoms, ability to interact successfully in a group, increase in self-esteem, and ability to make decisions and function more independently. The group experience helps to decrease the sense of isolation, facilitate development of new roles or re-establish familiar roles, provide information on a variety of topics for other group members, and provide group support for effecting change or enhancing self-esteem. Group therapy for the elderly differs from therapy for younger people in that there is more personal sharing of information by the therapist, physical contact, tolerance of silence, intergenerational conflict and struggle to adapt, and emphasis on reminiscence and life review. The leader should be a professional with a background in psychiatric theory and group dynamics. Group size may vary according to the goals, but a 6- to 12-member group usually works best. Desirable group characteristics include a relative homogeneity of problems, needs, and mental status; sexual integration; and regular times and places for meeting.

Outcomes of Institutional Treatment

Goals of institutionalization for the psychogeriatric patient are to provide the most effective treatment possible and the maximum potential rehabilitation or simply to slow the rate of disability, provide humane comfort and support, or achieve death with dignity. Outcomes of care are affected mainly by the type of presenting problem and the nature of the therapy. For example, patients with organic mental disorders or physical disease are less likely to be released than those with affective disorders. Excessive morbidity and mortality occur in older patients with physical illnesses who are admitted to psychiatric hospitals. Patients who are discharged within 3 months of admission have a better chance of successful return to the community than do those who are hospitalized longer.

CASE 3. Ms. X's Psychiatric Problem

Ms. X is a 67-year-old black woman admitted to the inpatient psychiatry service for diagnosis and treatment of bizarre, psychotic, and agitated behavior. Her behavior disorder includes an inability to sit still, picking at things in the air as if she were hallucinating, and a thought process that is completely disorganized, with her speech showing an extreme flight of ideas. She tries to undress the male psychiatrist during the screening examination. Two months before her admission, she underwent a right simple mastectomy for breast cancer. Her other medical problems include obesity and hypertension.

After careful psychiatric evaluation and a computed tomographic scan of her head, no brain metastasis is found, and the diagnosis of psychotic agitated depression is made. She is initially treated medically with thioridazine (Mellaril), 50 mg four times a day. After resolution of her florid symptoms of psychosis, she continues to exhibit a global mental impairment consistent with chronic dementia. Family history confirms that the patient has had a long, gradual history of decline in memory and self-care abilities.

ANALYSIS OF NURSING CARE NEEDS
Universal Self-Care Requisites
1. Food. The patient is receiving an 1800-calorie weight-reduction diet.

2. Fluid. Minimum requirement is 1800 ml of fluid per day.

3. Elimination. The patient needs a toileting schedule because she is currently incontinent of both urine and feces.

4. Social interaction/solitude. The patient swings between being withdrawn and hypomanic and is socially inappropriate.

5. Activity/rest. The patient has had a sedentary lifestyle; increased activity would promote faster weight loss and resolution of obesity.

6. Sense of normalcy. The patient has no breast prosthesis.

Developmental Self-Care Requisites
1. Altered homeostasis. The patient has decreased neuronal reserve and ability to cope with change in new environments owing to disease and drug effects.

2. Major loss. Two months before admission, the patient had a right simple mastectomy without breast prosthesis or implant; otherwise, no change has occurred in her lifestyle.

3. Role change. None has been identified.

4. Dependence/independence. The patient receives assistance with activities of daily living from daughter with whom she lives.

Health Deviation Self-Care Requisites
1. Psychosis/dementia. The patient needs supervision to prevent injury from wandering and bothering other patients and needs reminders to take medicine, eat, and not become overactive.

2. Depression. The patient needs assistance for resolving loss and for controlling psychotic behavior.

3. Obesity. The patient needs to decrease calorie intake.

NURSING DIAGNOSES
(Ackley and Ladwig, 1993)
1. Coping, Impaired, related to recent loss of breast, dementia

2. Nutrition, High Risk for Alteration; Greater than Body Requirements, related to excess calorie consumption relative to activity level

3. Self-Care Deficit, Total, related to psychosis

4. Thought Process, Altered, related to major depression

5. Body Image, Altered, related to surgical removal of breast

6. Injury, High Risk for, related to orthostatic hypotension as a side effect of medication

7. Mobility, Impaired Physical, related to extrapyramidal side effect of medication

COURSE OF TREATMENT AND ITS IMPACT ON FUNCTION
The two immediate goals for Ms. X were to ensure her safety and to obtain an accurate diagnosis of her underlying behavioral disturbance. Awareness of

continued on following page

CASE 3. Ms. X's Psychiatric Problem

continued

culturally appropriate care needs to be considered when planning goals (Reynolds, 1992). She was treated with thioridazine, 50 mg four times daily, which controlled her agitation. Nursing care consisted of creating the proper therapeutic milieu, monitoring the patient for development of physical complications of pharmacotherapy, and assisting with performing basic self-care needs. The ward norm was for individuals to be dressed in street clothes and to tidy their living space. The therapeutic milieu consisted of the judicious use of one-to-one guidance and supervision regarding self-care activities; encouragement to involve herself in group activities, such as a reminiscence group; and attendance in a low-intensity exercise group. Her nurse therapist advocated a breast prosthesis for her. Regular nursing

assessment was also required to monitor the patient's response to her medications and to be alert for oversedation, postural hypotension, or extrapyramidal symptoms.

After the first week in the hospital, the patient was able to engage in ward activities, such as dressing herself with prompting and tidying the area about her bed. Her medications were gradually decreased over the next 6 weeks, and she continued to show increased self-care ability to the extent that she could perform all basic activities of daily living independently, with verbal prompting. She was discharged to her home in her daughter's care because she continued to be unable to perform self-care activities as a result of her underlying dementia, which was diagnosed for the first time during this hospitalization.

REHABILITATION OF OLDER PATIENTS

Hospitalized elderly people may suffer from acute problems related to previously existing chronic illness, or they may be newly diagnosed with conditions such as stroke, heart disease, or diabetes. In any case, older people have the potential for rehabilitation and should not be excluded from rehabilitative programs simply because of their age (Tucker, 1993). Older patients, even the very old and mentally compromised, benefit from rehabilitation in hospital settings. Major benefits were related to increased independent functioning and return to the prehospital setting (Tucker, 1993).

Principles of Rehabilitation

Rehabilitation, or restorative nursing, is generally described as the restoration of the individual with a functional deficit to the fullest physical, mental, social, vocational, and economic usefulness of which he or she is capable. The aim of rehabilitation is "to restore individuals to their former functional and environmental status, or alternatively, to maintain or maximize remaining function." Standards and scope of practice have been defined to guide the evaluation and promotion of the restoration of function (Butler, 1991).

Other terms related to rehabilitation that are usefully defined and clarified are *impairment, handicap,* and *disability.* An impairment is an objective, quantifiable pathophysiological condition that does not always result in secondary disability. Handicap always follows impairment and is an extra burden that the individual must either overcome or circumvent to avoid significant reduction of a specific functional ability. Disability indicates a failure to function at a reasonably expected level for an individual; it does not refer to an anatomical defect.

Terms for three types of handicaps that have been used to describe patients with chronic psychiatric problems (Goldberg et al., 1985) can also be used to describe older patients with both physical and mental impairments:

1. *Primary handicaps,* consisting of the disabilities that are basically part of the illness

2. *Secondary handicaps,* consisting of non-adaptive reactions to the illness, together with negative attitudes on the part of important people in the patients' environment, such as relatives or members of the hospital staff

3. *Premorbid handicaps,* consisting of ways in which patients may be disadvantaged in terms of personality, low intelligence,

physical disabilities, and poor social skills before their illness

The degree to which these handicaps exist affects the degree of disability in an older patient and, in turn, the success of the rehabilitative program. For example, an older person who has a stroke is likely to have certain disabilities associated with the disease, such as hemiplegia, aphasia, and emotional lability (primary handicaps). The patient may have difficulty in working through the grieving process and in accepting the physical, social, and professional losses brought about by the infirmity.

The belief held by some health care professionals that older adults have little rehabilitation potential may also play a role in the inability of many older patients to accept their loss and maximize their remaining functional ability. The negative attitudes held by both patient and staff may produce secondary handicaps. Pre-existing chronic illnesses or lack of accomplishment of developmental tasks associated with later life can result in premorbid handicaps.

Primary, secondary, and premorbid handicaps can negatively affect motivation for rehabilitation and can interfere with the rehabilitative process. Older patients often appear unmotivated for rehabilitation, and "poor motivation" is frequently the reason given for excluding them from rehabilitation programs. However, adults learn new information that has meaning to them (Merriam and Caffarella, 1991), and past rehabilitation efforts may have been more what the care provider determined was needed, rather than what the patient determined he or she wanted. In addition, the traditional culture of a hospital that emphasizes cure rather than long-term management can subtly interfere with motivation for rehabilitative efforts in older patients and staff. Older rehabilitation patients should be assessed for levels of motivation, and the health professionals who are working with them should assess their own attitudes as well as the environment to determine whether or not the process is being facilitated.

Effect of Aging on Rehabilitation

Older people differ from younger people, not only physically but also psychologically, socially, and developmentally. The aging process causes a decreased capacity to adapt to stress and maintain homeostasis, and the high incidence of multiple chronic conditions aggravates an already disabling primary problem. There may be some cognitive slowing with aging and an increased potential for confusion and delirium associated with disease. Major depression or depressive symptoms are present in 20 to 40 per cent of people older than 60 years (Valente, 1994). Older people may have suffered many losses and may be living alone with few supports. Developmentally, older people are adjusting and adapting to the demands of older age. All of these factors alter the approach to rehabilitation in the aged.

Goals

Rehabilitation goals for older patients differ from those in younger patients. Whereas the goal for young people is to return to home, family, community, work, and previous lifestyle, this may not be realistic for older people. The traditional aim of rehabilitation programs has been to restore vocational potential with an emphasis on placement in jobs. For older people, maintenance of independence in activities of daily living and restoration to an acceptable quality of life may be the primary foci.

Long-range goals for an older patient include reasonable functional improvement, maintenance of existing abilities, retardation of deterioration, and prevention of secondary complications. The goals of treatment must be realistic, and the goal-setting process should involve the patient, family, and health care team. Sufficient time must be allowed to reach the goals set because it is expected that a longer time is needed for rehabilitation of the old than the young (Calvani and Douris, 1991). If older patients are returning to the care of family members, then personal self-care, even with supervision, may be an appropriate goal. However, if the older person lives alone, a greater degree of independence must be achieved.

Short-term goals and objectives can enhance the rehabilitative process for caregivers and patients alike. Small achievements help to mark progress that otherwise may be overlooked and can encourage the caregiver and patient to press on. Daily objectives should be developed according to individual needs. The atmosphere should be stimulating and should provide opportunities to overcome obstacles, such as frustration, lack of motivation, and poor self-image.

Strategies

Basic principles of rehabilitation for older adults include the following:

1. Control the underlying disease or impairment. Treat the underlying causes of delirium, control concurrent illnesses, and carefully evaluate pain and its management.

2. Develop functional abilities. Capitalize on existing abilities and focus on strengths rather than weaknesses. Balance exercise with rest. Encourage the patient to resume activities gradually.

3. Prevent secondary disabilities. Promote physical activity within the limits of the patient's capability to prevent complications of immobility. Provide a positive atmosphere for rehabilitation to increase motivation in the patient and the staff. Begin rehabilitative measures immediately, before complications and secondary disabilities develop.

4. Preserve the dignity of the individual. Promote self-esteem, self-respect, and self-confidence.

CASE 4. Ms. O's Rehabilitation

Ms. O is a 78-year-old white widow and retired bookkeeper. She has one son who lives in the same town. She suffered a right-sided cerebrovascular accident with left-sided flaccid hemiplegia and emotional lability but no speech impairment or swallowing difficulty. She is admitted to the rehabilitation unit in the hospital for treatment to restore independence in self-care abilities. During the course of the hospitalization, the health care team is able to prevent contractures, and Ms. O learns how to perform a pivot transfer and walk in the parallel bars. She develops independence in eating and becomes continent of stool. Because she develops shoulder-hand syndrome and is unable to achieve urinary continence, the indwelling catheter remains in place. She cannot propel a wheelchair independently, and she cannot shift her weight sufficiently while sitting to prevent pressure sores independently. Her behavioral problems do not abate, and she develops a more pronounced learned helplessness syndrome. Initially, she is discharged to home with daily caregivers, but within 2 weeks, she is admitted to an intermediate care facility in a town 50 miles away from her home.

ANALYSIS OF NURSING CARE NEEDS
Universal Self-Care Requisites

1. Food. The patient is receiving a regular diet. She requires assistance in setting up foods and utensils and needs to be reminded of food on her left side because of left-sided hemianopsia. The patient uses a plate guard. No calorie or salt restriction is necessary. The patient's height and weight are within normal limits. There is no evidence of malnutrition.

2. Fluid. Minimal requirement is 2000 ml per day.

3. Air. The patient is breathing room air and has no evidence of chronic lung disease.

4. Elimination. The indwelling catheter remains because of urinary incontinence. The patient senses the urge to defecate but is sometimes incontinent because of mobility problems.

5. Safety. The patient is unable to transfer independently but manages a one-person pivot transfer safely. The patient is tall but not obese. She tends to become anxious during transfers, increasing the likelihood of injury.

6. Social interaction/solitude. The patient hates to be left alone. She calls for help repeatedly if left alone for even short (5-minute) periods of time but is then apologetic; she says she wants to cooperate.

7. Activity/rest. The patient tolerates exercise programs poorly. She complains of heart racing and chest pain and becomes dyspneic. She is in chronic atrial fibrillation, but electrocardiograms during periods of chest pain reveal no changes from baseline. The patient complains bitterly of pain on the affected side, particularly in the upper extremity. The patient re-

CASE 4. Ms. O's Rehabilitation

continued

sists efforts to exercise passively her left upper extremity.

8. Sense of normalcy. The patient has had little experience with dependency. Her roles before the cerebrovascular accident centered around church activities, including volunteer work, Sunday school class, and worship service. She lived alone and maintained house with only limited assistance from her son for home maintenance chores.

Developmental Self-Care Requisites

1. Altered homeostasis. The patient is at high risk for pressure sores, infection, delirium, depression, deep vein thrombosis, and constipation.

2. Loss. The patient has suffered catastrophic loss of self-care abilities and potential loss of her home.

3. Role change. The patient is currently unable to carry out many accustomed roles. Friends from church visit regularly, but the patient is used to being the visitor, not the patient.

4. Dependence/independence. Historically, the patient has had little experience with the dependent role.

Health Deviation Self-Care Requisites

1. Atrial fibrillation. The patient requires periodic assessment for evidence of congestive heart failure.

2. Cerebrovascular accident. The patient requires a daily exercise program to prevent adverse consequences associated with hemiplegia.

NURSING DIAGNOSES
(Ackley and Ladwig, 1993)

1. Skin Integrity, High Risk for Impaired, related to immobility

2. Coping, Individual, High Risk for Alteration, related to unresolved losses; manifested by activity intolerance

3. Self-Care Deficit, Dressing, Ambulation, related to learned helplessness and decreased mobility

4. Mobility, Impaired Physical, related to hemiplegia

5. Urinary, Reflux Incontinence, related to detrusor instability

6. Thought Process, High Risk for Alteration, related to ineffective coping

7. Sensory Perceptual Alterations, Auditory and Tactile, Left Hemianopsia, and Left Hemiplegia, related to cerebrovascular accident

8. Comfort, Altered, related to shoulder-hand syndrome and indwelling catheter

---

PREVENTABLE PROBLEMS AND THEIR IMPACT ON FUNCTION By traditional standards of rehabilitation—that is, completely independent function—Ms. O's success in rehabilitation is partial. She is virtually independent in transfer, is continent of feces, and can self-propel her wheelchair, yet several problems remain. She is not sufficiently independent in self-care to allow her to return home. She retains an indwelling catheter and is at high risk for pressure sores. The success of her rehabilitation must be evaluated based on what is feasible given her premorbid personality, her other medical problems, and the length of time allowed for rehabilitation.

By her own report, premorbidly she had little experience with illness and a poor tolerance for pain. She has lived a sedentary life and has cardiac disease, both of which limit her endurance. The amount of time she spent in rehabilitation was brief, only 1 month. This is too short a period of time to fully accept the body image changes that accompany a dense hemiplegia and to become socialized into the impaired role. Therefore, she required additional time for rehabilitation after her discharge from the hospital. During this time, she completed a partial rehabilitation and became as independent in self-care as possible, given her impairment and emotional lability.

Ideally, the rehabilitation team considers postrehabilitation plans and communicates them to the next team of health professionals who will care for the patient. Unfortunately, in this case, good communication was lacking, and the home care helpers did not follow through on a care plan that promoted independence. After only 2 weeks at

continued on following page

CASE 4. Ms. O's Rehabilitation

continued

home, Ms. O required too much from the limited home care available to her. She then was placed in the intermediate care facility, where an occupational therapist and a gerontological nurse specialist reinstated a rehabilitative care approach.

This patient exemplifies two challenges of geriatric rehabilitation: (1) the need to extend rehabilitation over a lengthy time period and (2) the need to address premorbid personality traits. Because little progress would be made until the patient's learned helplessness was addressed, the occupational therapist and gerontological nurse developed a written schedule of exercises and posted it on the patient's door. When these were performed, a colorful check was marked in the appropriate box. The goal of the schedule was to reinforce the concept that the patient's behavior made a difference in her functioning level.

Gradually, Ms. O engaged in a daily exercise program. She did not develop flexion contractures, and she progressed to the point that discharge to a rest home was seen as possible. A properly placed grab rail was installed in her bathroom, and she was trained in its use in transferring onto the toilet. She regained independence in transfer to and from the toilet, which allowed removal of the indwelling catheter and resumption of urinary continence over the course of 2 months. She had experienced considerable discomfort from the indwelling catheter. Within several months, she was independent enough to be discharged to a rest home (a lower level of care).

The transfer had two advantages: (1) she was closer to her home community and could see old friends more regularly, and (2) fewer staff were available to reinforce dependency. Had Ms. O regressed further in her activities of daily living, she would have had to transfer to a facility farther away from her son. This was a powerful incentive for her to maintain her newly developed independence.

GERONTOLOGICAL NURSING PROBLEMS IN THE HOSPITAL

Delirium or Acute Confusional State

Delirium, or an acute confusional state, occurs in half to a third of all older patients at some point in their hospitalization and must be correctly addressed (Linderborn, 1988). Delirium is a disturbance of cerebral function with global cognitive impairment that has an abrupt onset, is brief in duration, and is characterized by evident concurrent disturbances in attention, sleep-wake cycle, and psychomotor behavior. (For a more detailed discussion of delirium, see Chapter 9.) Confusion is an important consideration in the treatment of older patients because in some cases it may be the only sign of serious disease in the elderly. van der Kooij (1993) believes that reality orientation and validation approaches are useful in distinguishing the needs of the disoriented elderly. There are four main types of behavior that may indicate the presence of confusion in hospitalized elderly:

1. Verbal or behavioral manifestations of disorientation to time or place

2. Inappropriate behaviors, such as pulling at tubes or dressings, getting out of bed when not indicated, and physical combativeness

3. Inappropriate communication, such as noncommunicativeness, verbal combativeness, and incoherent, nonsensical, or unintelligible speech

4. Visual or auditory hallucinations

Predisposing factors for confusion in hospitalized elderly are increasing age, baseline brain damage, drug or alcohol addiction, fatigue, social and psychological stressors, recent change in location, and sleep deprivation. The numerous causes of confusion include drugs, alcohol withdrawal, infections, metabolic disorders, cardiac disorders, cancer, trauma, and cerebrovascular disorders (Patterson, 1993). Confusion can also result from misperceptions of the environment caused by age-related sensory changes.

Reversal of an acute confusional state can be dramatic if the underlying cause is removed. The nurse can assist in the treatment of the confused patient by using a problem-solving process of assessment and intervention. Use of the steps of the nursing process (assess, plan, implement, and evaluate) facilitates a comprehensive plan of care. Comprehensive geriatric care can be planned for the high-risk problems that can affect cognition. These problems include fluid deficit, electrolyte imbalance (Antonelli et al., 1993), respiratory insufficiency, alterations in core body temperature, hyperglycemia or hypoglycemia, and drug toxicity. The cause of the confusion becomes apparent with sufficient and correct data, and thus the intervention can be determined. By directing nursing interventions toward the many behaviors associated with confusion, the nurse can help the older patient maintain or regain his or her level of cognitive function.

Urinary Incontinence

Incontinence is a prevalent problem in both surgical and medical elderly patients. Continence is achieved early in the life cycle and is associated with adulthood and dignity. Its absence is a key contributor to social isolation or institutionalization in the elderly (see Chapter 14 for further discussion of incontinence).

Urinary incontinence is usually brought about by a number of factors, many of which are treatable or reversible. The major causes of incontinence are atrophic vaginitis, medications, metabolic abnormalities, mental status changes, prostatic obstruction, fecal impaction, autonomic neuropathy, urinary tract infection, cystocele and rectocele, detrusor instability, psychological regression, immobility, and restraints. The consequences of incontinence are skin irritation and breakdown, worsening of pressure sores, institutionalization, social isolation, social breakdown syndrome, and decreased self-esteem.

Assessment should include a thorough history of patterns of incontinence, including its relationship to coughing, laughing, or straining; dribbling versus flooding; patterns suggestive of a behavioral component; and the onset and duration of the problem. A physical examination should be based on the possible contributors to incontinence, including a vaginal examination in women and a prostate examination in men, bladder distention, postvoiding residual capacity, impaired mobility, and impaired mentation. Laboratory tests should include a complete urinalysis and culture.

Treatment should be aimed at reversing any underlying causes. Examples of treatment are strengthening sphincters with Kegel exercises and biofeedback, treating infections, removing impactions, altering drug regimens, and treating delirium and depression. In the hospital setting, several environmental and behavioral techniques may be employed to enhance continence. Decreasing the distance to the toilet and removing obstacles in the way, initiating a schedule for toileting (night and day), and providing privacy for voiding may be helpful. For patients who have problems with mobility, having a bedside commode or keeping a bedpan within easy reach can eliminate some episodes of incontinence.

Patient teaching is often useful in helping the patient and family to be involved in the management of urinary elimination. The patient can be taught to maintain a schedule of voiding using environmental and behavioral cues, such as after meals, before bedtime, and before or after favorite television shows. Patients can enlist the aid of families as helpers to remind them to use the bathroom or commode. Patients and families can also be taught to keep records of voiding and incontinence patterns to manage their own continence and maintain a feeling of control and independence.

Immobility

There are very few reasons for immobilizing hospitalized elderly. Only acute catastrophic events, such as severe blood loss, fresh trauma, head injury or insult, burns, and hip fractures are legitimate reasons for immobilization. Factors that cause immobilization in the hospital that are not legitimate reasons include environmental barriers, such as bedrails, restraints, high beds, and lack of staff to help with mobility; cognitive impairment; central nervous system disorders; pain with movement; affective disorders; sensory changes; terminal illness; and acute episodes of illness. Common consequences of immobility are bowel and bladder incontinence, bedsores, emotional trauma, depression, weakness, sensory deprivation, sleep disorders, and potential electrolyte imbalances.

Conscious attempts at mobilization of hospitalized elderly should be made continually. Older patients should be moved frequently, and the frequency and desired movement should be specified. Examples of specified frequency of desired movement are "up in a chair for all meals," "weight-bearing transfers twice a day," and "walk to the toilet three times a day."

Exercises, whether range of motion,

stretching, or flexing, can be graded, performed without movement, and performed anywhere by even the most immobilized patient. For example, fracture patients can tighten and relax muscles in an immobilized extremity to improve recovery of function after removal of a cast or traction, or patients in pain can move slowly and smoothly while deeply breathing to ease pain and anxiety. Exercises that can be performed in bed are deep breathing, neck rolls, knee to chest movement, pelvic tilts, head raising in prone and supine positions, unilateral leg lifts, foot dorsiflexion, rolling, and prone lying. Exercises that can be performed in a chair are deep breathing, head rolls, knee to chest movement, head to knee movement, shoulder rolls and lifts, weight shift (hip to hip), leg lifts, ankle rotation and dorsiflexion, and ankle placement on the knee.

Falls

Hospitalized elderly are at special risk of falling. Not only do they experience varying degrees of physiological decline associated with the aging process, but they are also confronted with an acute illness superimposed on existing chronic disease. Older patients are commonly subjected to the effects of multiple medications, complex diagnostic and therapeutic procedures, and an unfamiliar environment—all contributors to the likelihood of falling. Other factors that are commonly implicated in falling episodes include new drug regimens, orthostatic hypotension, muscle weakness, deconditioning (periods of bedrest or other periods of inactivity), poor judgment (dementia, delirium, depression, denial of aging), changes in coordination, sensory changes, environmental hazards, and inadequate lighting.

In one study, 90 per cent of all accidents were falls, and most falls were in patients over the age of 60 (Goodwin and Westbrook, 1993). Although falls account for the greatest number of injuries in older patients in hospital settings, most falls produce no injury (62 per cent). They usually occur during periods of activity, especially during changes in position or posture. Falls from wheelchairs and beds are common, particularly during transfer.

Falls are frequently preventable. Ongoing assessment should be carried out to identify older patients at risk for falling during hospitalization and to determine the need for interventions. A careful history should include information on previous falls, presence of predisposing medical conditions, drug intake (especially new medications), complaints of neurological symptoms, reports of comfort and mobility in the patient's own environment, and validation of information with significant others. A physical and functional assessment should include pulse and blood pressure (lying, sitting, and standing); observation of postural sway; determination of the ability to transfer, ambulate, and use mobility aids and assistive devices; and a mental status evaluation. Environmental factors to be assessed include seat height, depth, and stability compared with patient height and agility; footwear and flooring compared with patient alertness and mobility; bed height and stability; lighting and clutter in the patient area; availability of safety equipment and patient's ability to use it; and condition and use of ambulatory equipment.

Interventions are based on the need for individualized care of high-risk patients to maintain mobility and functional status. A program of gait training, muscle-strengthening exercises, and movement therapy can increase mobility, coordination, dexterity, and balance. Careful monitoring of medications can help to avoid the effects of polypharmacy and unnecessary sedation. Possible drug effects that can cause falls are hypoglycemia; orthostatic hypotension in patients taking diuretics, antidepressants, vasodilators, beta blockers, antiagitants, or other antihypertensives; and ataxic gaits in patients taking phenytoin.

Older patients should be thoroughly oriented to their environment, and an ongoing evaluation of their adjustment to the unfamiliarity of the acute care setting should be carried out. The use of volunteers or a patient buddy system might be effectively implemented to assist new patients to adapt to the hospital and its routines. Additional recommendations for preventing falls include the use of low beds with half side rails, stabilization of movable furniture, provision of patient footwear with nonskid soles, proper use of walking aids, and availability of corrective devices for visual and hearing deficits. Environmental modifications to promote safety include adequate sources of lighting, particularly at night; clear walking surfaces made with adequate friction, a nonglare finish, and energy-absorbing material; raised toilet seats; horizontal as well as vertical handrails; well-designed furniture of the correct height; and wheelchairs with seat belts (McVey, 1985).

Nurses are often confronted with the dilemma of whether to encourage older patients to maintain their physical activity in spite of the possible danger of falls or to confine them and risk the consequences of immobilization. It is generally thought that the risks associated with immobility are greater than the risks of falls, and many gerontologists would rather encourage activity than immobility. Sometimes, restraints are used to prevent falls (Betemps et al., 1992); however, there is a lack of research to support the use of physical or chemical restraints as deterrents to fall-related injuries. In fact, restraints in some cases may encourage falls (Stolley, 1995; United States Food and Drug Administration, 1992). Therefore, nurses should think carefully before advocating a restraint system. The need for restraints should be reviewed every 24 hours, and restraints should be removed for remobilization of patients every 30 to 45 minutes.

Alternative approaches to restraints may include using the presence of family members, assisting with mobility, and reorienting the patient.

REFERENCES

Ackley, B. and Ladwig, G. *Nursing Diagnosis Handbook: A Guide to Planning Care.* St. Louis: C.V. Mosby, 1993.

American Psychiatric Association. Remotivation Kit. Washington, D.C.: American Psychiatric Association, 1965.

Antonelli, I.R., Gemma, A., Capparella, O. et al. Postoperative electrolyte imbalance: Its incidence and prognostic implications for elderly orthopedic patients. *Aging* 22(5):325–331, 1993.

Arron, M., Martin, G. and Webster, J. Perioperative care of the elderly. *Compr Ther* 128:4–10, 1992.

Ashton, D. Therapeutic use of reminiscence with the elderly. *Br J Nurs* 2(18):894, 896–898, 1993.

Association of Operating Room Nurses. *Standards and Recommended Practices for Perioperative Nursing.* Denver: AORN, Inc, 1994.

Atchinson, D. Restorative nursing: A concept whose time has come. *Nurs Homes* 41(1):8–12, 1992.

Atkinson, L.J. *Berry and Kohn's Operating Room Technique.* 7th ed. St. Louis: Mosby-Year Book, 1992, p. 70.

Bandman, E.L. Tough calls: Making ethical decisions in the care of older patients. *Geriatrics* 49(12):46–49, 51–53, 1994.

Beck, L.H. Perioperative renal, fluid, and electrolyte management. *Clin Geriatr Med* 6(3):557–567, 1990.

Betemps, E.J., Buncher, C.R. and Oden, M. Length of time spent in seclusion and restraint by patients at 82 VA Medical Centers. *Hosp Community Psychiatry* 43(9):912–914, 1992.

Blaylock, A. and Cason, C. Discharge planning. Predicting patients' needs. *J Gerontol Nurs* 18(7):5–10, 1992.

Blazek, L.A. Development of a psychiatric home care program and the role of the CNS in the delivery of care. *Clin Nurse Specialist* 7(4):164–168, 1993.

Bower, K. *Case Management by Nurses.* American Nurses' Association. Kansas City: American Nurses' Association, N-32. 4-5, 1992.

Burgin, A. and Schuetz, M.P. Establishing an alternate level of care unit. *J Nurs Adm* 22(9):62–65, 1992.

Burkle, N.L. Inadvertent hypothermia. *J Gerontol Nurs* 14(6):26–30, 1988.

Butler, M. Geriatric rehabilitation nursing. *Rehabil Nurs* 16(6):318–321, 1991.

Calvani, D.L. and Douris, K.R. Functional assessment: A holistic approach to rehabilitation of the geriatric client. *Rehabil Nurs* 16(6):330–336, 1991.

Cohen, E. and Cesta, T. *Nursing Case Management: From Concept to Evaluation.* St. Louis: C.V. Mosby, 1993, pp. 36–42.

Connors, H.R. Case management: Within and beyond the walls: Nursing assessment and management of the frail elderly (NAMFE) program—eight learning modules. *In Perspectives in Nursing, 1991–1993.* NLN Publications 41-2472:113–120, 1992.

Cornoni-Huntley, J., Blazer, D.G., Lafferty, M.E. et al. *Established Populations for Epidemiologic Studies of the Elderly.* Vol. II. National Institute on Aging, United States Department of Health and Human Services, Washington, D.C., NIH Publ. No. 90-495, 1990.

Creditor, M.C. Hazards of hospitalization of the elderly. *Ann Intern Med* 118(3):219–223, 1993.

Dellasega, C. and Burgunder, C. Perioperative nursing care for the elderly surgical patient. *Todays OR Nurse* 13(6):12–17, 1991.

Depp, F.C. Preventing injuries inflicted on elderly psychiatric patients by other patients. *Issues Ment Health Nurs* 3:353–363, 1981.

DesHarnais, S.I., Chesney, J.D. and Fleming, S.T. Should DRG assignment be based on age? *Med Care* 26(2):124–131, 1988.

Donat, D.C. Altercations among institutionalized psychogeriatric patients. *Gerontologist* 26:227–228, 1986.

Dugan, J. and Mosel, L. Patients in acute care settings. Which health care services are provided. *J Gerontol Nurs* July:31–35, 1992.

Duncalf, D. and Kepes, E.R. Geriatric anesthesia. *In* Rossman, I. (ed.). *Clinical Geriatrics.* 3rd ed. Philadelphia: J.B. Lippincott, 1986, pp. 494–510.

Eagle, D.J., Rideout, E., Price, P. et al. Misuse of the emergency department by the elderly population: Myth or reality? *J Emerg Nurs* 19(3):212–218, 1993.

Evans, C.A., Kenny, P.J. and Rizzuto, C. Caring for the confused geriatric surgical patient. *Geriatr Nurs* 14(5):237–241, 1993.

Fahey, C.J. Ethics and aging. *Gerontologist* 29(1):6–7, 1989.

Fillit, H. Challenges for acute care geriatric inpatient units under the present Medicare Prospective Payment System. *J Am Geriatr Soc* 42:553–558, 1994.

Finkel, S.I. Group psychotherapy with older people. *Hosp Community Psychiatry* 41(11):1189–1191, 1990.

Foreman, M.D. The cognitive and behavioral nature of acute confusional states. *Schol Inquiry Nurs Pract* 5(2):3–26, 1991.

Girard, N. Anesthesia and learning: The mind-body connection. *Semin Periop Nurs* 3(3):121–132, 1994a.

Girard, N. Asepsis. *In* Gruendemann, B.J. and Fernsebner, B. (eds.). *Perioperative Nursing.* Boston: Jones and Bartlett, 1995.

Girard, N.J. Geriatric surgery. *In* Phippen, M.L. and Wells, M.P. (eds.). *Perioperative Nursing Practice.* Philadelphia: W.B. Saunders, 1994b, pp. 817–842.

Gisler, J. Surgical wound healing and diabetes mellitus. University of Texas Health Science Center at San Antonio, San Antonio, TX, 1994 (unpublished paper).

Goldberg, E.L., Van Natta, P. and Comstock, G.W. Depressive symptoms, social networks and social support of elderly women. *Am J Epidemiol* 121(3):448–456, 1985.

Goldman, L. Cardiac risks and complications of noncardiac surgery. *Ann Surg* 198:780, 1983.

Goodwin, M.B. and Westbrook, J.I. An analysis of patient accidents in hospital. *Aust Clin Rev* 13(3):141–149, 1993.

Gravely, E.A. and Oseasohn, C.S. Multiple drug regimens: Medication compliance among veterans 65 years and older. *Res Nurs Health* 14:51–58, 1991.

Guin, P. and Freudenberger, K. The elderly neuroscience patient: Implications for the critical care nurse. *AACN* 3(1):98–105, 1992.

Guyatt, G.H., Eagle, D.J., Sackett, B. et al. Measuring quality of life in the frail elderly. *J Clin Epidemiol* 46(12):1433–1434, 1993.

Haight, B.K. and Burnside, I. Reminiscence and life review: Explaining the differences. *Arch Psychiatr Nurs* 7(2):91–98, 1993.

Hammonds, W. Anesthesia for the diabetic patient. *In* Davidson, J.K. (ed.). *Clinical Diabetes Mellitus: A Problem Oriented Approach.* 2nd ed. New York: Thieme, 1991, pp. 648–654.

Harris, D. and Velligan, T. *Texas Statutes Affecting Nursing Practice.* 5th ed. Eau Claire, WI: Professional Education Systems, 1992.

Hirsch, C.H., Sommers, L., Olsen, A. et al. The natural history of functional morbidity in hospitalized older patients. *J Am Geriatr Soc* 38:1296–1303, 1990.

Hitch, S. Cognitive therapy as a tool for caring for the elderly confused person. *J Clin Nurs* 3(1):49–55, 1994.

Horner, J. The aging client: A perioperative approach. *Semin Periop Nurs* 2(4):226–230, 1993.

Inouye, S.K., Acampora, D., Miller, R.L. et al. The Yale Geriatric Care Program: A model of care to prevent functional decline in hospitalized elderly patients. *J Am Geriatr Soc* 41(12):1345–1352, 1993.

Iyer, P.W. The nursing process: The basis for nursing care. *In* Bolander, V.B. (ed.). *Sorensen and Luckmann's Basic Nursing. A Psychophysiologic Approach.* 3rd ed. Philadelphia: W.B. Saunders, 1994, p. 109.

Jackson, M.F. High risk surgical patients. *J Gerontol Nurs* 14(1):8–15, 1988.

Johnson, L.J. Nutrition and wound healing. *Semin Periop Nurs* 2(4):238–242, 1993.

Keating, H.J., III. Major surgery in nursing home patients: Procedures, morbidity, and mortality in the frailest of the frail elderly. *J Am Geriatr Soc* 40(1):8–11, 1992.

Kemp, B.J. Psychological care of the older rehabilitation patient. *Clin Geriatr Med* 9(4):841–857, 1993.

Kozlak, J. and Thobaben, M. Treating the elderly mentally ill at home. *Perspect Psychiatr Care* 28(2):31–35, 1992.

Linderborn, K.M. The need to assess dementia. *J Gerontol Nurs* 14(1):35–39, 1988.

Lipsitz, L.A., Pluchina, F.C., Wei, J.Y., Minaker, K.L. and Rowe, J.W. Cardiovascular and norepinephrine responses after meal consumption in elderly (older than 75 years) persons with postprandial hypotension and syncope. *Am J Cardiol* 58:810–815, 1986.

Liukkonen, A. The nurse's decision-making process and the implementation of psychogeriatric nursing in a mental hospital. *J Adv Nurs* 17(3):356–361, 1992.

Madrid, C. Orthopedic case management in a collaborative practice. *Semin Periop Nurs* 3(1):16–21, 1994.

Martin, M.A. Methicillin resistant *Staphylococcus aureus*: The persistent resistant nosocomial pathogen. *Curr Clin Top Infect Dis* 14:170–191, 1994.

Mayer, G.G., Madden, M.J. and Lawrenze, E. *Patient Care Delivery Models.* Rockville, MD: Aspen Publishers, 1990.

Matteson, M.A. Group reminiscing for the depressed institutionalized elderly. *In* Burnside, I. (ed.). *Working with the Elderly: Group Processes and Techniques.* Monterey, CA: Wadsworth Health Sciences Division, 1984.

Matteson, M.A. and McConnell, E. *Gerontological Nursing: Concepts and Practice.* Philadelphia: W.B. Saunders, 1988.

McNabb, M.S. HMO case management and the surgical patient. *Semin Periop Nurs* 3(1):22–26, 1994.

McVey, L.J. Falls in the acute care setting. Paper presented at the International Congress of Gerontology, New York, July 1985.

Meckes, P.F. Geriatric surgery. *In* Meeker, M. and Rothrock, J. (eds.). *Alexander's Care of the Patient in Surgery.* 9th ed. St. Louis: Mosby-Year Book, 1991, pp. 1004–1017.

Meeker, M. and Rothrock, J. *Alexander's Care of the Patient in Surgery.* 10th ed. St. Louis: Mosby-Year Book, 1995.

Mellillo, K.D. Interpretation of laboratory values in older adults. *Nurse Pract* 18(7):59–66, 1993.

Merli, G.J. Prophylaxis for deep vein thrombosis and pulmonary embolism in the geriatric patient undergoing surgery. *Clin Geriatr Med* 6(3):531–541, 1990.

Merriam, S.M. and Caffarella, R.S. *Learning in Adulthood.* San Francisco, CA: Jossey-Bass Publishers, 1991.

Miller, A. A study of the dependency of elderly patients in wards using different methods of nursing care. *Age Ageing* 14:132–138, 1985.

Miller, R.D. (ed.). *Anesthesia.* Vol. 1, 4th ed. New York: Churchill Livingstone, 1994.

Miller, S.T., Applegate, W.B., Elam, J.T. and Graney, M.J. Influence of diagnostic classification on outcomes and charges in geriatric assessment and rehabilitation. *J Am Geriatr Soc* 42:11–15, 1994.

Mitchell, P. Perspectives on outcome-oriented care systems. *Nurs Adm Q* Spring:1–7, 1993.

Moore, B.G. Reminiscing therapy: A CNS intervention. *Clin Nurse Specialist* 6(3):170–173, 1992.

Newbern, V.B. Sharing the memories: The value of reminiscence as a research tool. *J Gerontol Nurs* 18(5):13–18, 1992.

Nunnelee, J.D., Kurgan, A. and Auer, A.I. Distal bypasses in patients over age 75. *Geriatr Nurs* 14(5):252–254, 1993.

Pascucci, M.A. Measuring incentives to health promotion in older adults. Understanding neglecting health promotion in older adults. *J Gerontol Nurs* 18(3):16–23, 1992.

Patterson, B.J. Comprehensive care for the elderly. *Can Fam Physician Med Fam Can* 39:1380–1391, 1993.

Phippen, M. and Wells, M.A. (eds.). *Perioperative Nursing Care.* Philadelphia: W.B. Saunders, 1993.

Potter, P. and Perry, A. *Fundamentals of Nursing.* 3rd ed. St. Louis: Mosby-Year Book, 1993, pp. 720–723.

Propotnik, T., Schaffner, A. and LaLonde, J. Providing acute geriatric care. *Nurs Management* 24(10):61, 1993.

Reynolds, C. An administrative program to facilitate culturally appropriate care for the elderly. *Holistic Nurs Pract* 6(3):43–42, 1992.

Rice, D. The characteristics and health of the elderly. *In* Eisdorfer, C., Kessler, D. and Spector, A. (eds.). *Caring for the Elderly.* Baltimore: Johns Hopkins University Press, 1989, pp. 3–25.

Rodin, J. Aging and health: Effects of sense of control. *Science* 233:1271–1276, 1986.

Rosenberg, C. Wound healing in the patient with diabetes mellitus. *Nurs Clin North Am* 25(1):247–261, 1990.

Sachs, G.A. Caring for older cancer patient: Practical decision-making guidelines with a focus on advance directives. *Oncology* 6(2 suppl):131–135, 1992.

Saul, S. and Saul, S.R. The application of joy in group

psychotherapy for the elderly. *Int J Group Psychother* 40(3):353–363, 1990.

Scanland, S.G. and Emershaw, L.E. Reality orientation and validation therapy. Dementia, depression, and functional status. *J Gerontol Nurs* 19(6):7–11, 1993.

Schick, F.L. *Statistical Handbook on Aging Americans.* Phoenix, AZ: Oryx Press, 1986.

Schonwetter, R.S., Walker, R.M., Kramer, D.R. and Robinson, B.E. Resuscitation decision making in the elderly: The value of outcome data. *J Gen Intern Med* 8(6): 295–300, 1993.

Schrier, R.W. *Geriatric Medicine.* Philadelphia: W.B. Saunders, 1990.

Schwartz, J.G., Phillips, W.T. and Aghebat-Khairy, B. Revision of the oral glucose tolerance test: A pilot study. *Clin Chem* 36(1):125–128, 1990.

Singal, B.M., Hedges, J.R., Rousseau, E.W. et al. Geriatric patient emergency visits: Part 1. Comparison of visits by geriatric and younger patients. *Ann Emerg Med* 21:802–807, 1992.

Sloane, P.D., Redding, R. and Wittlin, L. Longest-term placement problems in an acute care hospital. *J Chron Dis* 34:285, 1981.

Stanley, M. Elderly patient in critical care: An overview. *AACN Clinical Issues in Critical Care Nursing* 3(1):120–128, 1992.

Stoelting, R.K. (ed.). *Anesthesia and Co-existing Disease.* 3rd ed. New York: Churchill Livingstone, 1993.

Stolley, J.M. Freeing your patients from restraints. *Am J Nurs* February: pp 27–31, 1995.

Strange, G.R., Chen, E.H. and Sanders, A.B. Use of emergency department by elderly patients: Projections from a multicenter data base. *Ann Emerg Med* 21(7): 818–824, 1992.

Taulbee, L. and Folsom, J. Reality orientation for geriatric patients. *Hosp Community Psychiatry* 175:133–135, 1966.

Trella, R. Multidisciplinary approach to case management of frail, hospitalized older adults. *J Nurs Adm* 23(2):20–26, 1993.

Tucker, N.J. Geriatric rehabilitation: Nursing challenge of the '90s. *Rehab Nurs* 18(2):114–146, 1993.

United States Food and Drug Administration. *Food and Drug Administration Safety Alert: Potential Hazards with Restraint Devices.* Rockville, MD: United States Department of Health and Human Services, 1992.

Valente, S. Recognizing depression in elderly patients. *Am J Nurs* 94(12):18–25, 1994.

Van Buren, C.T. Surgery in the older patient. *In* Levenson, A.J. and Porter, D.M. (eds.). *An Introduction to Gerontology and Geriatrics: A Multidisciplinary Approach.* Springfield, IL: Charles C. Thomas, 1984, pp. 341–355.

van der Kooij, C. Reality orientation, validation and the reality of the disoriented old old. *Vard Nord Utveckl Forsk* 13(4):4–8, 1993.

Weiler, P.G., Lubben, J.E. and Chi, I. Cognitive impairment and hospital use. *Am J Public Health* 81(9):1153–1162, 1991.

Weitz, H. Noncardiac surgery in the elderly patient with cardiovascular disease. *Clin Geriatr Med* 6(3):511–527, 1990.

Zander, K. Second generation primary nursing: A new agenda. *J Nurs Adm* 15(3):18–24, 1985.

Zander, K. Managed care and nursing case management. *In* Mayer, G.G., Madden, M.J. and Lawrenz, E. (eds.). *Patient Care Delivery Models.* Gaithersburg, MD: Aspen Publishers, 1990, p. 37.

Zastocki, D.K. Home care nursing. *In* Bolander, V.B. (ed.). *Sorensen and Luckman's Basic Nursing. A Psychophysiologic Approach.* 3rd ed. Philadelphia: W.B. Saunders, 1994, p. 399.

Zuckerman, J.D., Fabian, D.R., Aharanoff, G. et al. Enhancing independence in the older hip fracture patient. *Geriatrics* 48(5):76–81, 1993.

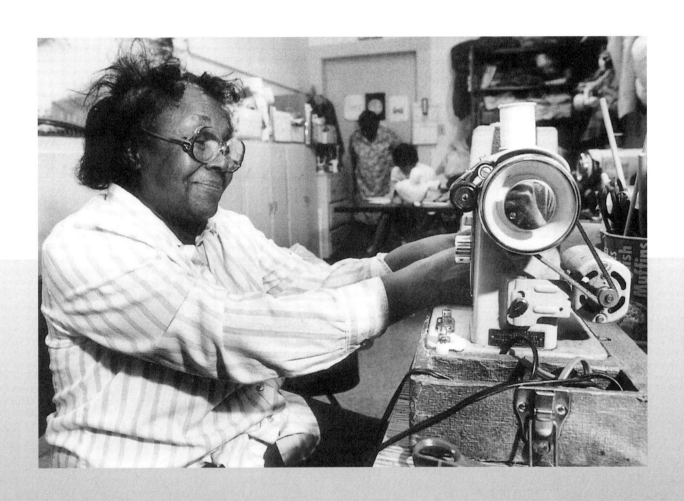

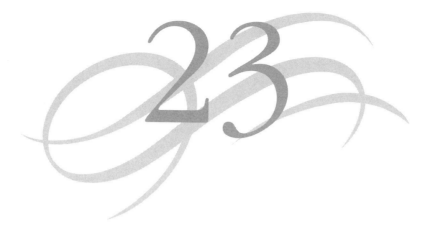

Gerontological Care in Community Care Settings

S U S A N   J .   B A R N E S

OBJECTIVES

Define the concept of community and discuss the relationship of the community to health and the elderly.

❖

Discuss the history of community health nursing and the role of the community health nurse.

❖

Conduct a community assessment with a focus on aging and formulate a plan for nursing intervention with the community as the client.

❖

Conduct an assessment of an older individual in the community and formulate a plan for nursing intervention with the individual and family as clients.

IMPORTANCE OF COMMUNITY

Communities are where people live and from where people derive the social meaning in their lives. Gerontological nursing should therefore always be concerned with the communities of older clients.

Definition

The idea of community has many definitions. One way of viewing community is as

a consciously identified population with common needs and interests, which may include occupation of common physical space, which is organized and engages in common activity including differentiation of functions and adaptation to its environment in order to meet the common needs. Its components include the individuals, groups, families, and organizations within its population and the institutions it forms to meet its needs. Its environment is the society within which it exists and to which it adapts, and other communities and organizations outside itself that impinge on its functioning (Anderson and Carter, 1974, p. 47).

Communities, Health, and Aging

Communities have informally and formally provided for the health of their members for all recorded history. Western civilization has made formal efforts to provide health services to the community since the late 19th century (Clemen-Stone, et al., 1991). Nurses have been key professionals in re-solving community health problems. Problems associated with aging represent a community health challenge for a number of reasons:

1. Many of the problems associated with aging are preventable through lifestyle modifications (Koop, 1991).

2. Older people are the most frequent consumers of primary health care services of any age group in the country (United States Senate Special Committee on Aging, 1991).

3. Older people are most likely to require long-term, supportive services to maintain independence in the community (Bremer, 1989; Johnson, 1990).

Nurses working in community health settings, such as public health agencies, nurse-managed health centers, ambulatory care clinics, home health agencies, and other community-based agencies, have a tremendous opportunity to influence the health of aging people at both community and individual levels of care.

Community care is influenced by family attitudes and behaviors in several ways. Family and cultural values shape and reinforce lifestyles, which in turn influence health status. To help people alter their lifestyles, an attempt should be made to understand the purposes served by the individual's current lifestyle (Hinds et al., 1992). Families are also the mainstay of long-term caregiving. Provision of services from a health or social service agency is usually only an adjunct to ongoing family care. Therefore, careful assessment of family strengths, limitations, and goals is essential in providing appropriate supportive services to meet the goals of both the individual and the family.

To find solutions to problems associated with aging in the community care setting, goals should be formulated to guide the problem solving. For the *community*, the goal is to recognize, prioritize, and mobilize to bring about a healthy community. The community should recognize the problems associated with aging, prioritize the problems that are most pressing, and mobilize the community itself to solve the problems. For the *family*, the goal is to help older people meet their needs in a personally desirable way within the family context. The older person's values should predominate, but collaboration with family members should also take place, so that needs are met and the family network remains intact. For *older individuals*, the goal is to stay as functionally independent as long as possible according to their lifestyles. Therefore, their wishes and preferences must be respected as they are assisted in maintaining their independence.

COMMUNITY AS CLIENT

Solutions to community health needs must first involve the community that is experiencing the problems. John Dewey (quoted in Citizens Board of Inquiry into Health Services for Americans, 1972) expressed this philosophy quite aptly:

No matter how ignorant any person is, there is one thing he knows better than anybody else, and that is where the shoes pinch his own feet, and that is because it is the individual that knows his own trouble, even if he is not literate or sophisticated in other respects. The idea of democracy as opposed to aristocracy is that every individual must be consulted in such a way actively, not passively, that he himself becomes part of the process of authority, of the process of social control, that his needs and wants have a chance to be registered where they count in determining social policy.

Community health needs can best be addressed by nurses who are knowledgeable and interested in the health of the whole community. It is essential that the community health nurse work as an ally of consumers, both to increase their participation and to help empower the elderly and their families to effect positive changes in health care programs. Community health nurses must be knowledgeable about public policy and must use their influence to support the community they serve (Stewart and O'Rawe Amenta, 1993).

Community Health Nursing

History

The concept of community health nursing originated with the activities of public health nurses, who have been seen as social reformers as well as caregivers for the sick since the formation of district nursing associations (Brainard, 1985). Many years ago, Wald identified the *community* as the focus of public health nursing and emphasized the nurse's responsibility in collaborating with others in the community to promote health.

Our basic idea was that the nurse's peculiar introduction to the patient and her organic relationship with the neighborhood should constitute the starting point for universal service to the region. Our purpose was in no sense to establish an isolated undertaking. We planned to utilize, as well as to be implemented by, all agencies and groups of whatever creed which were working for social betterment, private as well as municipal. Our scheme was to be motivated by a vital sense of the interrelation of all these forces. For this reason, we considered ourselves best described by the term "public health nurses" (Wald, in Anderson, 1983).

Harmer (see Skrovan et al., 1974) saw nursing as "linked with every social agency which strives for . . . the preservation of health . . . and is . . . not only concerned with the care of the individual, but with the health of a people." In the 1960s, the American Nurses' Association Public Health Nurses' Section (1964) recognized that public health nursing had responsibility in "diagnosis, planning and treatment of *community* ills—those of the body politic. . . ."

Role of Community Health Nurse

A role for the community nurse practitioner, who sees the *community* rather than the individual or family unit as the client, has evolved. The practitioner, in collaboration with the community, defines what its health problems are and assists in defining the community's priorities, resources, and an acceptable approach to the problems. Community nurse practitioners are taught skills of community development, needs assessment, and evaluation. To establish trust and rapport with the community as well as to act as an effective facilitator, community nurse practitioners should be active participants in community groups, such as churches, schools, and clinics and community centers. Sources of assessment data may include census records, police reports, clinic records, and vital statistics (Anderson and McFarlane, 1988; Clark, 1992).

The community health nurse must first work with the community to define what it sees as its health problems and possible resources and solutions. The following process is adapted from a World Health Organization (WHO) paper on development of successful health education programs:

1. Analyzing people's values, interests, and needs as they relate to health, especially within the perspective of other perceived priorities
2. Determining customary practices
3. Defining specific objectives
4. Identifying positive and negative factors that affect health practices
5. Determining existing and needed resources
6. Intervening based on the above information

7. Evaluating the influence of the intervention(s) on health-related behavior, and modifying the intervention as necessary (WHO, 1978).

Community Assessment: Focus on Aging

Numerous community assessment guides exist in the community health nursing literature; one focuses explicitly on the aging population as a community (Mezey et al., 1993). Assessment of the aging population in a community should provide a basis for the development of programs to achieve primary, secondary, and tertiary prevention of the common problems afflicting older people and their families. Definition of aging as a lifelong process allows the community health nurse to consider people of *all* ages as potential recipients of prevention services. The focus on prevention of problems associated with advanced age is an important focus for the community health nurse.

The continued evolution of the community health nurse is evidenced in the emergence of positions-titled case managers in managed care settings. The nurse is the professional who has the breadth of education and experience to be able to assist a client in the community to make use of the most appropriate services in the most timely manner (Zander, 1988). Currently, professional organizations representing nursing are working on establishing these roles as nursing roles. In the end, the role of case manager may go to a variety of individuals including nurses and social workers. An accurate and useful community assessment begins with observation and vital statistics information. The nurse interested in the geriatric portion of the population can focus on that aggregate only after assessing the community as a whole. For example, if the community is experiencing problems with gang activity, the effect on the elderly may be profound. Those who would normally perform shopping and yard work independently may, out of fear, delay venturing outdoors and voluntarily become housebound. The individual suffers from lack of activity and social contact. Consequently, mental and physical health may decline. Hogue (1977) suggested the following questions as a guide for community assessment:

1. What is the health of the group served?
2. What factors seem to be associated with this health status?
3. What can be done about the health status?

4. How well are interventions designed to affect health status being performed?

Research regarding public health and wellness strategies for the older population and the compression of morbidity is progressing (Hubert et al., 1993; Leigh and Fries, 1992–1993; Fries, 1992). Specific community assessment efforts made by nurses concerned with prevention of age-associated disability and premature mortality should include evaluation of the

- Prevalence of risk factors for age-related problems
- Existing programs for lifestyle modification
- Functional status of older people
- Existing programs for screening the health assessment of older people
- Existing programs for long-term care

Each element of community assessment is described more fully in the paragraphs that follow.

Risk Factors for Aging-Related Problems

It is interesting that in general the elderly take better care of their health than do the nonelderly (United States Senate Special Committee on Aging, 1991). Even so, most problems experienced by the elderly have a behavioral component that can be altered (Fries et al., 1993). The list of age-related problems and associated risk factors contained in Table 23–1 is generated from national statistics on age-related disability and mortality, the gerontology and geriatrics literature, and the author's experience in common problems associated with aging. Estimation of prevalence rates of many of these disorders can often be obtained from regional or state planning offices, universities, or direct care providers.

When prevalence rates for a specific community or aggregate are not available on a disease or disability of interest, it is possible to design methods to evaluate the prevalence of the problem using community survey methods or key informant methods. For more detailed assistance with these methods, see Anderson and McFarlane (1988). Estimation of the prevalence of a problem is often necessary to justify allocating resources to a specific program. When the prevalence rate of a specific disorder in a given community greatly exceeds national or state averages, special programming may be indicated.

Lifestyle Modification Programs

Development of healthy lifestyles in people of all ages is likely to reduce age-related disability and premature death (Leigh and Fries, 1992–1993). Many of the diseases that plague older people, including heart disease, cancer, diabetes, stroke, chronic lung disease, and substance abuse, are partially amenable to prevention through lifestyle modification. Modifiable lifestyle factors implicated in these disorders include

- Diets that are too high in calories, cholesterol, fat, or sodium
- Lack of regular aerobic exercise
- Cigarette smoking
- Inadequate coping resources and stress-reduction skills

Because the adverse effects of lifestyle are often not experienced until middle age or old age, it is important for younger people to become more knowledgeable about the aging process so that they understand the rationale for modifying their lifestyles in young adulthood.

Wellness-type programs that help promote healthy lifestyles include both educational offerings and facilities and programs that promote or support the desired behavior. For example, educational programs in secondary schools about the hazards of smoking may be beneficial, but smoking cessation groups exemplify programs that help to support a change in lifestyle. Similarly, health education about the benefits of regular exercise may help to persuade some people to begin a personal exercise program, but the development of high-quality facilities for exercise, such as those available at Young Men's Christian Associations (YMCAs) or provided by some employers, is also a useful element of a lifestyle modification effort.

INVENTORY. The community assessment should include an inventory of the existing wellness programs as well as programs that have been tried and found unsuccessful in the past. Because there are no generally accepted standards for minimum community efforts for promoting wellness, the community assessor must consider the priorities of the community and the prevalence of specific problems in the community to make decisions about the adequacy of the range of existing programs.

QUALITY AND ACCESSIBILITY. Once the existing programs have been catalogued, determining the quality and accessibility of the programs is worthwhile. Quality is most

T A B L E   2 3 – 1

Major Age-Related Health Problems and Associated Risk Factors

MAJOR AGE-RELATED PROBLEMS	ASSOCIATED RISK FACTORS
Stroke	Smoking
	Sedentary lifestyle
	Cardiovascular disease
	Hypertension
Cancer	Environmental exposure to carcinogens
	Tobacco use (both smoking and smokeless tobacco)
	Family history of cancer
	Presence of "premalignant lesions"
	Diet
Cardiovascular disease (including congestive heart failure and peripheral vascular disease)	Smoking
	Sedentary lifestyle
	Diet high in cholesterol
	High serum triglycerides
	Family history of cardiovascular disease
Chronic lung disease	Smoking
	Exposure to environmental toxins, such as coal dust, cotton dust, asbestos
Dementing disorders	Hypertension, as in Binswanger's dementia or multi-infarct dementia
	Social isolation
	Sensory deprivation
Depression	Multiple losses
	Family history
	Social isolation
	Multiple drug use (as adverse side effect of drug therapy)
Adult-onset diabetes mellitus	Obesity
	Sedentary lifestyle
	Family history
Digestive disorders	Diet
Substance abuse	Family history
	Limited coping resources
	Social isolation
Hip fracture	Osteoporosis
	Frequent falls
	Depression
	Dementia
	Reduced physical agility
Inappropriate institutionalization	Shortage of community-based supportive services
	Lack of geriatric multidimensional assessment services
	Lack of preinstitutionalization screening program
Elderly neglect or abuse	Inadequate family resources for long-term care
	Inadequate community-based services for long-term care
Poverty	Inadequate planning for postretirement income
	Catastrophic medical illness with inadequate insurance coverage
Family caregiver burnout	Insufficient knowledge of difference between normal aging process and results of disease
	Insufficient information about techniques of care
	Inadequate community support services
	Inadequate access to rehabilitatively oriented care
	Inadequate emotional support

difficult to assess because the field of health and wellness promotion is so young. However, standards for the establishment of fitness programs are emerging. Accessibility is somewhat easier to estimate. For example, evaluation of the accessibility of a fitness program might include some of the following questions: Are most of the fitness programs developed by employers for current employees and thus not accessible to retirees or unemployed persons? Or are the programs developed by the government but underfunded so that they operate only on Monday through Friday during usual working hours, thus excluding access by most employed persons? Are the waiting lists prohibitively long? Finally, is access to the fitness program restricted by finances? What is the enrollment fee for most programs? The same types of questions can be applied to other health promotion activities, such as weight reduction support groups, classes on "You and Your Aging Parent," and preretirement planning groups. Table 23–2 summarizes some examples of community-based wellness programs that are likely to affect health positively in old age (Leigh and Fries, 1992–1993). Programs that are entirely missing from or inaccessible to large segments of the community suggest a need for further program development. Program development must always proceed according to the jointly derived priorities of the assessor and the community. Priorities in health promotion programming are particularly susceptible to influence from individuals in the community because there is a relative lack of evidence about the efficacy of strategies for lifestyle modification relative to cost, which might outweigh individual opinion.

Functional Status of Elderly People

Knowledge of the proportion of older people in the community who suffer from disabilities should underlie the development of assessment and support services for elderly individuals, so that secondary and tertiary prevention services can be most effectively developed and targeted (Hubert et al., 1993). As is the case with determining the prevalence of selected conditions that commonly affect older people, much of the necessary information can be derived from existing surveys of the community, which are available from local, regional, or state agencies. When the information is not available, several approaches can be used to ascertain the extent of functional disability in the aged. Methods such as the Older Americans Resources and Services (OARS) instrument have been applied to large community samples using trained interviewers rather than professional assessments (Pfeiffer, 1975; see also Chapter 2). Other assessments include the Hebrew Rehabilitation and Care for the Aged (HRCA) Vulnerability Index (Morris et al., 1984). The HRCA combines self-report or proxy report of performance and capability on key instrumental and personal activities of daily living (ADLs), orientation, and activity level. In addition, screening assessment tools that allow estimation of the prevalence of specific age-associated disabilities, such as musculoskeletal impairment, and that are appropriate for large population studies are beginning to appear in the literature (Jette and Branch, 1984).

If the prevalence of a functional disability in the older population of a community is much greater than the national average, existing support services should be scrutinized. The use of a more scientific epidemiological method to study aging has developed over the past 15 years, and progress has been made in its application (Davies, 1988). Maintenance of autonomy is the goal for the elderly, so loss of autonomy is the focal point of the epidemiological study of elderly persons. Great care should be taken when extrapolated data are used because the unique attributes of the community will not be taken into account.

Screening and Assessment Programs

Secondary prevention of disease is based on the ability to identify disease as early as possible, so that the disease can be more readily treated or managed and adverse sequelae prevented. Early detection of disease in the elderly is hampered by the current system of Medicare reimbursement, which specifically denies reimbursement for disease detection in the absence of a specific diagnosis. The controversy over both Medicare and private insurance payment for preventive health care has long been raging. With current health care reforms, it is expected that a more significant emphasis will be placed on screening and preventive health measures.

Some practitioners carefully circumvent the reimbursement obstacle by providing disease screening services as part of other disease-related care, but individuals who do not receive medical care for chronic diseases must pay for disease detection privately. Some public health agencies have provided multiphasic screening clinics to screen for common treatable diseases such as anemia, hypertension, tuberculosis, glaucoma, diabetes, and certain malignancies. Other commu-

T A B L E   2 3 – 2

Examples of Community-Based Wellness Programs Designed to Promote Healthy Aging

TARGET AGGREGATE	PROGRAM DESCRIPTION	RATIONALE

Young people, unselected for risk factors	1. Educational programs on:
	  Aging as a normal, lifelong process, influenced by lifestyle choices
	  Exercise as a key element of healthy aging and disease prevention
	
	  Nutrition as a key element of healthy aging and disease prevention
	
	  Substance abuse: alcohol, drugs, and cigarettes as major problems in our society that adversely affect health
	
	  Stress reduction and management
	2. Facilities for:
	  Access to recreational pursuits
	  Access to examples of high-quality nutrition (e.g., in school cafeteria)
	  Exposure to role models who exemplify successful stress reduction techniques rather than turning to substance abuse
		Increase understanding and coping skills for dealing with aging-related changes
		Sedentary lifestyle implicated in much age-related pathology (e.g., hypertension, cardiovascular disease, diabetes, obesity, depression)
		Poor nutrition implicated in much age-related pathology (e.g., hypertension, cardiovascular disease, obesity, cancer)
		Much morbidity and early mortality associated with substance abuse (e.g., organic brain disease, liver disease, chronic lung disease)
		Increased coping skills may decrease reliance on drugs as escape
		Reinforce educational programming. Actions speak louder than words. Build healthy lifestyle habits early

Employment-age adults, unselected for risk factors	1. Educational programs on:
	  Exercise and health protection
	  Nutrition and disease prevention
	  Stress management techniques
	  Aging process and its impact on emotional health, family relationships
	  Availability of community resources to care for dependent older family members
	2. Facilities to promote and reinforce healthy lifestyles:
	  Work safety program to identify and control health hazards in the workplace
	  Access to exercise places and equipment (in the workplace or in the community)
	  Cafeterias and other eating places that promote and reinforce good nutrition
	  Access to support groups for developmental and health-related life crises (e.g., unemployment and job finding skills, new parenthood, caring for dependent adult relatives, and disease-specific conditions)
		Same as for school-aged children. Provide opportunity for adults to learn what they did not learn as children. Lifestyle modification still possible and useful in adulthood

Older adults (postretirement age)	1. Educational programs in:
	  Difference between normal aging process and disease
	  Importance of *exercise* in maintaining health despite disease
	  Importance of proper *nutrition* in maintaining normal body function
	  Importance of maintaining and developing *social ties* as buffer against losses associated with aging
	  Availability of resources for exercise, nutrition, and socialization
	  Availability of resources to care for dependent older family members or friends
	  Availability of home maintenance and repair programs
	2. Programs that provide:
	  Age-appropriate exercise classes
	  Educational opportunities in retirement
	  Transportation to exercise and social opportunities
		Know when to seek professional help for disease symptoms. As for younger age groups, lifestyle modification is still possible and potentially effective in staving off end-stage disability

Not age specific	Air pollution controls Water pollution controls Hazardous waste disposal	Needed to prevent morbidity and premature mortality from lung disease and malignancies

nities accomplish the same goal through the use of community health and wellness fairs, in which professionals volunteer their time on a periodic basis to provide screening services. Where screening programs exist, it is important to evaluate the effectiveness of follow-up from the screening tests because if a potential disease is identified but appropriate evaluation and treatment are not carried out, then the screening has not accomplished the goal of secondary prevention (see related case history, Chapter 20).

Another issue in secondary prevention programs for the elderly is identification of the full range of assessment and screening that should be applied to older people. For example, multiphasic screening approaches have traditionally focused on *diseases* that first manifest themselves in middle age rather than on *disabilities* that manifest themselves in late life. The question of whether screening maneuvers specific to the elderly, such as the detection of mobility problems, should be undertaken with the goal of preventing disability in advanced old age remains to be answered. The focus of secondary prevention efforts has been disease specific and is based on the medical model of care. In the elderly, secondary prevention should have a multidisciplinary focus that emphasizes prevention of disabilities (Hogue, 1982a and 1982b). A growing number of studies are demonstrating the efficacy of home-based, nurse-run screening programs in the prevention of mortality and morbidity in the aged (Leath and Thatcher, 1991; Hendricksen et al., 1984; Vetter et al., 1984).

Examples of useful screening maneuvers specific to the elderly can be gleaned from clinical anecdotes. For example, one astute clinician has noticed that many older people, because of reduced joint mobility and lower extremity muscle weakness, tend to fall down into chairs rather than transferring gently, possibly predisposing to compression fractures and increased musculoskeletal pain. If screening programs included assessment of transfer abilities, specific exercises could be prescribed to remedy the incorrect transfer technique, perhaps preventing further musculoskeletal impairment. Another example pertains to drug screening. Adverse drug reactions increase with the number of medications taken. Many older people consult more than one primary care provider, who has little or no knowledge of what the other practitioner is prescribing. Periodic drug regimen review by a qualified professional is a screening maneuver that can prevent adverse drug reactions or interactions.

Yet another example of screening, which was developed after clinical observation, is that regarding falls and fall-related injury prevention. Falls are not just accidents and often can be prevented with appropriate interventions. Assessing the individual for relevant risk factors frequently associated with falling is critical. These factors can include medications that contribute to postural hypotension or vertigo, muscular and/or skeletal impairment, confusion, and decreased sensorial functioning. Environmental factors in the home should also be examined and include the presence of unanchored scatter rugs, crumbling flooring or sidewalks, slick floors, and inadequate handrailing (Kippenbrock and Soja, 1993; Edwards et al., 1993).

The community assessor has the responsibility to consider the availability of screening and assessment services to the elderly in the community and whether the services are adequate to prevent common problems confronting the aged. This aspect of community assessment is particularly difficult because most screening and assessment services for the aged are not segregated and clearly identified but are included in other primary health care. Thus, the assessor must become knowledgeable about the nature of the services provided to the elderly in primary care settings as well as the services provided in senior centers, rest homes, adult day programs, public health departments, and pharmacies.

Programs for Care of Dependent Older People

Tertiary prevention is concerned with promotion of independent function and prevention of further disease-related deterioration. The purpose of many community-based, long-term care services is to promote independence in the community without compromising the health of younger family members. The hazards of institutionalization are well described in the literature and include increased mortality, decreased social opportunity, and learned helplessness.

IDENTIFICATION OF GAPS IN SERVICE NETWORK. Communities differ greatly in the extent and depth of the community support services that are available. The full range of possibilities currently reported in the literature is described in Chapter 20. The community assessor should identify gaps in the network of services as well as the accessibility of the services. Barriers to obtaining services include financial, bureaucratic, and transportation or personal mobility barriers. Extensive waiting lists, limited service hours, and highly centralized locations of services are all signals that service delivery may not be matched to service need. Waiting lists generally indicate either that there is insufficient service for all who need it or that services are inappropriately targeted. One North Carolina survey showed that a high percentage of people receiving chore services had no documented functional impairment (Nelson, 1986), yet there were large numbers of functionally impaired people on the waiting list.

ASSESSMENT OF QUALITY OF SERVICES. Another element in evaluation of existing programs for dependent older people includes an assessment of the quality of the service. Selective interviews with care recipients and their family members as well as with the personnel delivering the service are indicated. Anecdotal reports sometimes indicate that problems exist with caregivers. Notation of this in the community assessment and development of a strategy to address the problem are important tasks for the community health nurse interested in high-quality long-term care in the home. Monitoring the quality of care in highly decentralized care systems such as home care is recognized to be difficult. More and more agencies are employing a managed care approach.

DETERMINING HOME HEALTH CARE NEEDS. One model for determining home health care needs in a local community lists three components to be assessed:

1. Need for services
2. Services already provided
3. Implications for nursing education, service, and research

Information acquired to determine need for service should include an overview of both the health care system, especially its organization, payment systems, and health care providers, and the types of health care needs of the consumers. Services provided should be described in terms of the existing relationships among the various components of the long-term care continuum (primary care, hospital, long-term care institutions, home care), discharge planning, and availability of professional services. Implications for nursing education, service, and research are directly related to provision of care in the home health setting. Nurses must be educated to provide services to homebound clients, and they should be conducting research to enhance their assessment practices (see Fig. 23–1, Box 23–1, and Table 23–3).

Planning and Intervention

Planning at the community level is an extremely complex activity that requires knowledge of the community power structure as well as knowledge of the needs of the community. Factors other than simply the assessed needs of the community may dictate the types of community health programming in a specific community. In programming for aging individuals, this situation is further complicated by the fact that problems of older persons typically transcend a number of service agency boundaries. For example, older people may simultaneously receive services from a home health agency, a community mental health center, a social services agency, voluntary organizations, and an ambulatory care clinic. Achieving consensus on the priorities for preventive services for the elderly among the various community agencies may be difficult indeed, particularly when the needed services may have to compete for funding with more familiar and popular services, such as day care for children. The specific techniques and subtleties of planning at the community level for the elderly are beyond the scope of this book. Interested readers should consult the community health planning, community health nursing, and community organization literature for specific information on this topic (Spradley, 1985). The case examples in this chapter provide some insights into the complexity of planning for the needs of older people at the community level. The paragraphs that follow provide an overview of the kinds of programs that might be stimulated by a community nursing professional interested in prevention of aging-related problems.

Prevention Programming

The nurse's specific role in the community usually influences the opportunities chosen to develop various preventive programs. For example, public health nurses whose responsibilities include serving in an outpatient clinic as well as providing home health services have the opportunity to use their knowledge about preventable musculoskeletal disabilities seen in the home to enhance musculoskeletal screening and intervention in the outpatient clinic. Occupational health nurses may identify the need in middle-aged workers for information about changes with aging and services for older family members and may then develop an educational series in collaboration with a local home health care provider. Nurses in an ambulatory care clinic, noting the high prevalence of obesity and hypertension, may stimulate the development of a weight-reduction support group in their community.

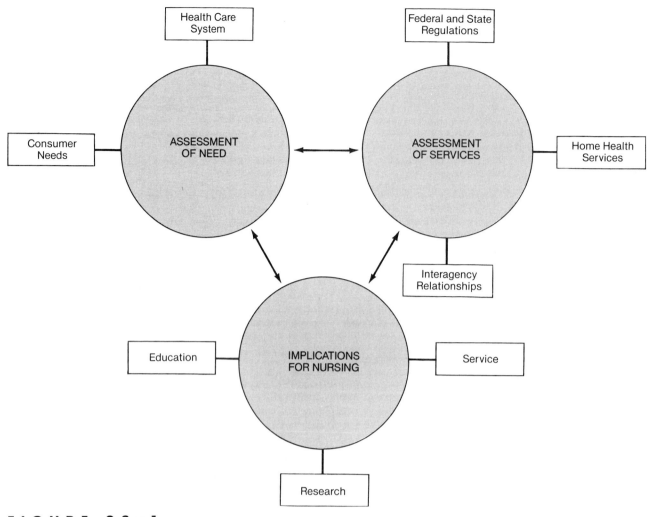

FIGURE 23-1

Assessment model for home health care.

Development of Needed Services

At the tertiary level of prevention, the case management approach has been advocated both as a way to coordinate a complex array of services and as a means of systematizing needs assessment for long-term care services. Case managers, who assess complex cases and design care plans with comprehensive needs of the patients and their families in mind, have a special opportunity to document the lack of needed services because of the comprehensiveness of the service they provide (Zander, 1988; Lajeunesse, 1990; Brockopp et al., 1992). If the administration of the case management service is attuned to presenting data about the gaps in services to community decision makers, then case management serves an important function in the community as well as for individual patients. Unfortunately, there is seldom a systematic means of assessing when the range of services is inadequate to serve the long-term needs of the elderly. Generally, new services are developed in response to some perceived crisis or as a response to a funding initiative.

Evaluation

Four criteria can be applied to the effectiveness of the nursing process at the community level: (1) the cost of care, (2) the care being delivered in the least restrictive environment, (3) the prevalence of selected disorders generally considered preventable, and (4) the quality of care.

Few guidelines specify the definition of a "reasonable sum of money" to be expended on community health for the elderly. A great deal depends on the community's values concerning the importance of caring for the elderly and its beliefs about the efficacy of preventive services. Because various eth-

BOX 23-1
Independent Living Assessment

1. RESIDENT'S WISHES
Desired living site ⎯⎯⎯⎯⎯⎯⎯⎯⎯⎯⎯⎯⎯⎯
Ambivalence ⎯⎯⎯⎯⎯⎯⎯⎯⎯⎯⎯⎯⎯⎯⎯⎯
Plans to manage at site successfully ⎯⎯⎯⎯⎯⎯

2. FAMILY CONCERNS
Informant ⎯⎯⎯⎯⎯⎯⎯⎯⎯⎯⎯⎯⎯⎯⎯⎯
Relationship ⎯⎯⎯⎯⎯⎯⎯⎯⎯⎯⎯⎯⎯⎯
Ambivalence ⎯⎯⎯⎯⎯⎯⎯⎯⎯⎯⎯⎯⎯⎯
Support needs seen ⎯⎯⎯⎯⎯⎯⎯⎯⎯⎯⎯⎯
Plans to get support needs met ⎯⎯⎯⎯⎯⎯⎯

3. INDEPENDENCE OF RESIDENT IN ACTIVITIES OF DAILY LIVING

	INDEPENDENT	WITH HELP	SPECIFY KIND OF HELP AND BY WHOM
Mobility in apartment			
Walks to meals			
Gets own mail			
Feeds self			
Bathes			
Dresses			
Takes medications			
Maintains personal hygiene			

4. RESIDENT'S SAFETY

	ADEQUATE	DEFICIENT	SPECIFY HOW
Overall mental status			
Appropriate in relationships			
Hearing			
Mobility			
Vision			
Communication			
Ability to make decisions			

5. FINANCIAL/LEGAL CONSIDERATIONS
Financial constraints ⎯⎯⎯⎯⎯⎯⎯⎯⎯⎯⎯⎯
Power of attorney ⎯⎯⎯⎯⎯⎯⎯⎯⎯⎯⎯⎯⎯
Helper with business affairs ⎯⎯⎯⎯⎯⎯⎯⎯

Summary of recommendations:

Date ⎯⎯⎯⎯⎯⎯ Signature ⎯⎯⎯⎯⎯⎯⎯⎯⎯⎯⎯⎯

T A B L E 2 3 – 3
Assessment Model for Home Health Care

I. Assessment of need
  A. Overview of health care system
    1. Organization
    2. Payment systems
    3. Health care providers
  B. Needs of health care consumers
    1. Medical diagnoses
    2. Nursing diagnoses and nursing needs
    3. How needs best met
II. Assessment of services
  A. Federal and state regulations
  B. Home health services
    1. Number
    2. Location
    3. Type
    4. Services provided
  C. Interagency relationships
    1. Hospital discharge planning
    2. Coordination of care
    3. Communication among health care professionals
III. Implications for nursing
  A. Education
  B. Service
  C. Research

nic groups and communities differ in their willingness to institutionalize dependent elderly persons, the community health budget cannot be evaluated without considering the values and health care expenditures of the community as a whole. Communities differ in the degree to which they expect families to shoulder the burden of dependent care and the degree to which they expect support from government or industry.

Cost of community care must also be evaluated according to the outcomes obtained. Unfortunately, many cost studies on alternatives to long-term care have neglected to include adequate measures of effectiveness. For example, community-based alternatives to long-term care have been criticized as not being cost-effective compared with nursing home care because the average longevity of the client is greater in the community than in the nursing home (Weissert, 1985). If the goal is to care for dependent older people until they die, then the nursing home seems to be the more cost-effective alternative. If, however, the goal is to promote health and prevent premature mortality, the nursing home, although less costly, is not the most effective alternative.

Delivering care in the least restrictive environment means that institutionalization is forestalled whenever possible, and maximum autonomy is promoted. Access to the full range of community health and support services must be available for this goal to be achieved.

The prevalence of selected disorders in the community is an index of the effectiveness of certain prevention programs. Communities with accessible, well-developed fitness programs may over time demonstrate lower-than-average rates of cardiovascular disease. Care must be taken in selecting target disabilities to allow an appropriate length of time to see the effects of the preventive effort. For example, in 1964, over half of the adult American population smoked. After the initiation of broad-based prevention programming, the number was down to 33 per cent in 1981. Education and awareness efforts were continued, and by 1984, the number was down to 26 per cent. This success is tempered by the fact that smoking remains one of the primary public health problems, causing 175,000 "excess" deaths (35 per cent of all cancer deaths) per year (Koop, 1991).

Likewise, the impact of a hypertension screening program on the prevalence of stroke-related disabilities may take 20 years or more to assess.

The impact of reinforcing healthy lifestyles in school-aged children and in the workplace may take even longer to evaluate. However, the impact of an educational program on body mechanics for family caregivers of older people may be evaluated by comparing the incidence of back strain complaints in the specific age range served in the clinic where the course was offered before and after the course offering. Community health nurses should remember that significant decreases in such disorders may take a generation or more to achieve, and the time frame for evaluation of health promotion strategies should be modified to account for the long-range nature of the effects of these interventions.

Starfield (1974) suggested a set of criteria to evaluate quality of care based on a continuum of levels of well-being with a focus on individual functional levels. The categories are listed according to complexity of measurement, beginning with the best-defined categories:

1. Longevity and prognosis: normal versus premature death
2. Activity: functional versus disabled
3. Comfort: comfortable versus distressed
4. Satisfaction: acceptance of one's health status or health care
5. Disease/morbidity: not detectable versus permanent
6. Achievement or level of accomplishment: achieving versus not achieving

7. Resilience (the ability to cope with adversity, including resisting a health threat and responding to stress): resilient versus vulnerable

Care is evaluated in terms of how well a provider helps a client move toward the positive end of the continuum. Evaluation of prevention-oriented programming is difficult but should be incorporated in planning to provide feedback to community planners about which programs increase well-being among the elderly.

Development of Community Health Services

In the late 1970s, the federal government mandated that Community Mental Health Centers (CMHCs) offer specialized services to the elderly. The mandate stemmed in part from national service utilization data showing that only 4 per cent of community mental health center clients were over age 65, although they represented 10 per cent of the population as a whole and were thought to have a larger-than-average prevalence of emotional and cognitive disorders.

Let us suppose that a gerontological nurse specialist with expertise in psychiatric/mental health nursing was hired to direct the services of a community mental health center in a rural southeastern community. The charge was to see a caseload of elderly outpatient psychotherapy clients and to develop preventive, educational, and therapeutic programs according to the needs of the community. This example describes the steps of the nursing process used by the nurse specialist.

Assessment

A general systems model guided the community assessment. The goals of the assessment were to

1. Identify factors in the community that contribute to or detract from the *emotional well-being* of older people and their families.
2. Describe the *range of services* available to older persons and their families.

The nurse specialist collected data over a 6-month period and organized it into the following categories: *contextual data, inputs, process,* and *products.*

Contextual Data

The major employers in this rural, conservative, southeastern community are two textile mills and one large defense contractor. The people have strong church affiliations, and the churches are active in community affairs and problems. There is a history of coordinated community action to address local problems. The CMHC has a reputation for implementing innovative prevention and treatment programs and fostering interagency working relationships. The goal of the CMHC is to increase the number of elderly persons served by the center.

Inputs

The community assessment revealed that funding sources for mental health programs came from several sources: federal and state grants, county funding, fee-for-service arrangements, insurance (including Medicare and Medicaid), United Way agencies, and other charitable contributions. A statewide Title XX needs assessment discovered that loneliness and poverty were widespread for elderly people in the area, and there were only 250 nursing home beds.

Three important considerations would influence the development of a mental health program:

- National estimates suggest that *50 to 80 per cent* of the elderly may require some type of mental health service.
- Family members' inability to cope with relatives suffering from *dementia* is a common outpatient problem.
- *Depression and adjustment reaction to late life* is a commonly diagnosed problem in outpatient therapy populations.

The nurse specialist grouped the inputs under three headings: governmental human services agencies, nongovernmental agencies, and informal groups.

INPUTS FROM GOVERNMENTAL HUMAN SERVICES AGENCIES. The Public Health Department was the *only* provider of home health services. The Department of Social Services operated a small-chore worker program and supervised rest home operators. The CMHC had a strong consultation and education component, liaison with industry and area businesses through employee assistance programs, adult outpatient service clinicians involved with an adult day hospital program, a substance abuse program, and a long history of providing high-quality consultation and preventive services. A Community Action Agency sponsored five congregate nutrition sites throughout the county. The housing authority ran two congregate housing projects for senior citizens, with social workers based at each project. The recreation department runs the only senior center in the county and provides staff support for the council on aging, a senior volunteer program, and a senior transportation program; the department also convenes a forum of presidents of senior citizens clubs throughout the county. The community college runs a licensed practical nurse program and has a broad array of adult education and noncurricular programs.

INPUTS FROM NONGOVERNMENTAL AGENCIES. Meals on Wheels, a private non-profit organization, does friendly visiting in addition to delivering meals; it is interested in writing a proposal for funding a homemaker–home health aide program. Several Protestant church ministers are concerned about the problems of and ministry to the aged; some senior citizens clubs operate through the churches. There are two hospitals in the county, one with an inpatient psychiatric unit and a skilled nursing facility attached. Two intermediate care nursing homes besides the hospital facility are in the area. Several small domiciliary homes are operated throughout the county; the larger rest home, with about 60 beds, has a large census of chronic psychiatric patients.

INPUTS FROM INFORMAL GROUPS. A loose confederation of clergy is concerned about community problems. The community council is composed of members from key county and nonprofit agencies as well as charitable organizations; it discusses community problems and new programs for development. An interagency luncheon group of people from governmental human services meets monthly to facilitate communication between county agencies.

Process

INTRA-AGENCY COMMUNICATIONS. The community assessment identified three sources of intra-agency communications: regular staff meeting, biweekly grand rounds, and the lunchroom.

INTERAGENCY COMMUNICATIONS. On the individual client level, many workers believed that CMHC employees do not readily share client information, which impedes service delivery. Others believed that criteria for being screened at the mental health center were unduly restrictive. On the program level, openness was expressed about joint ventures, such as collaboration on training, patient evaluation, family conferences, and grant development. On the community service planning level, informal exchanges usually preceded a formal presentation at the community council or interagency groups.

DAY-TO-DAY INTERACTIONS. The CMHC had to improve certain aspects of its current programs for the elderly and their families. Patients may be reluctant to come into the mental health center to be served,

and the staff is not trained to recognize normal aging changes and their impact on the function of the aged. On the other hand, about a third of the staff in adult services are particularly interested in working with the elderly.

The senior center and congregate meal sites provide accessible, pleasant environments that are conducive to socialization but cannot serve persons with severe functional or cognitive impairments.

The housing authority has people on its social work/outreach staff who are very concerned about maintaining the independence of marginally functional individuals as much as possible. The staff is attentive to subtle changes in clients' behavior. The agency is limited, though, because it can only provide direct services to clients who live independently.

Products

Specific mental health services to the elderly include family counseling, inpatient psychiatric services, sheltered workshop (old people have low priority because of their limited remaining worklife), a day hospital program (most clients are younger adults), and substance abuse counseling.

There are also three specialized geriatric services available: outpatient psychotherapy, preventive group work, and case-oriented and program-oriented consultation to rest homes and nursing homes regarding behavioral problems in the elderly.

Gaps in the service delivery network for old people include no adult day care service, no respite services, and few home health aide providers. In addition, *many family members have unresolved problems in caring for relatives suffering from dementia or depression.*

Conducting the Assessment

The nurse specialist used a variety of means to collect the assessment data. Key members of the community, including workers in all relevant human services agencies, were interviewed to ascertain their view of the community's approach to the problems of older people and their families. Specific questions were asked about the adequacy of services, unmet needs, and barriers to increasing services to older people. Each element in the service delivery network was assessed in terms of how it approached services to older people and how its mission to older people was conceived.

Diagnostic Summary

Strengths of the community include the following:

- Good mental health center commitment to preventive as well as treatment services
- Many possible funding sources to support service expansion
- Good working relationships between formal and informal service providers
- Most elements of a continuum of long-term care services are already in place
- Strong lifespan approach to preventive community mental health
- Orderly interagency communications processes and community problem-solving processes

Problems with providing mental health service to the elderly and their families include

- Gaps in services (no homemaker–home health aide service, no adult day care, no family-centered prevention, and limited department of social services interest in the aged)
- No ongoing consultation or direct service provision in rest homes or nursing homes
- Difficult access to outpatient mental health services by debilitated older people
- Space in mental health center too small to permit program expansion; not barrier-free for physically handicapped
- Mental health center staff not perceived as good team players by other agency staff
- Lack of training in aging by all community human service professionals
- Lack of awareness of special problems of the aged in obtaining human services from bureaucracies

Planning

The many strengths of the community in human services delivery suggested that much could be accomplished to strengthen the network of services to the elderly and their families. The nurse specialist elected to work toward several goals simultaneously for two reasons: (1) progress was likely to be slow on some fronts, and (2) success in achieving some goals would increase her credibility and in turn her ability to achieve more complex goals.

The highest priority for services in the community was lack of an *adult day care* program, but development of this would also be the most difficult to achieve because

it required new space, start-up funding, and new staff. Other high priorities included

- Development of preventive services for family members of dependent older people
- Development of ongoing consultation and direct services to nursing homes and rest homes
- Education of other human service professionals in the community in aging process and addressing the special needs of the elderly
- Increasing access to mental health services for dependent older persons

Areas in which special opportunities existed but were of lesser urgency included developing support groups for individuals with specific aging-related problems, such as widowhood, sensory loss, or chronic diseases, and fostering the development of preretirement counseling in the community through a liaison with industry or the community college's adult education program.

Interventions

To build on existing strengths in the mental health center, the nurse specialist first moved to affirm the efforts of the mental health center staff who had been working with the elderly prior to her arrival. She negotiated with two other adult services therapists to continue the weekly "sharing" group they had begun in a senior nutrition site as a preventive and outreach service while expanding the service to two other nutrition sites. She acquired new psychotherapy patients by referral only from the existing outpatient therapists and was available for consultation on problems of the aged for individual, family, and group psychotherapy sessions.

Next, the nurse specialist got to know the other agency personnel in the community. No educational or speaking engagement was turned down during the first 6 months. Such invitations offered opportunities to foster trust with other community members while increasing the visibility of the mental health center's commitment to geriatric care. In addition, community consciousness was raised, and people became aware of the special needs of the elderly and their families.

In the community at large, the nurse specialist affirmed some of the concerns voiced about access to the mental health center for dependent elderly people and pledged to work diligently to improve access. She scheduled joint home visits with some of the nurses at the public health department and social workers at other community agencies to provide mental health consultation and to foster enhanced interdisciplinary communication.

Finally, an advisory, or "steering" committee for program development of geriatric services was formed consisting of the *nurse specialist*, the heads of *consultation and education* and *adult services*, the *program evaluator* for the mental health center, adult services *therapists* with expressed interest in working with the aged, the head of the *substance abuse prevention program*, the *director of nursing* in the public health department, the chair of the *senior citizens club coalition*, the head of the *home-delivered meals agency*, and one of the *active ministers* in town. It is important to note that this steering committee was an *informal* group. The nurse specialist frequently consulted these key people for advice on program development but never convened the entire group for a meeting. The rationale behind not having the committee as a whole meet was to avoid the slowness of a highly bureaucratized group and to avoid the group process impeding the development of fresh ideas and programs. Subgroups met as needed to enhance efficiency, or when it was desirable to brainstorm in small groups, or when programmatic decisions would affect some segment of the larger group.

The community assessment outlined was shared with the advisory committee, along with a preliminary plan for addressing the prioritized needs. The advisory committee's ideas were particularly helpful in developing approaches for new services. For example, the advisors encouraged work on all goals simultaneously and facilitated introductions to key members of the community, such as the fiscal officer of the mental health center and members of the community council. They also suggested that an attempt to revitalize the Council on Aging would be an excellent move to increase visibility and to provide a ready forum for receiving feedback about program development ideas.

The progress of program development then became opportunistic. As opportunities for collaborative work with other individuals or agencies were presented that were consistent with the overall plan of development, such projects were taken on. For example, the agency in charge of home-delivered meals prepared a proposal to develop a homemaker–home health aide service. The nurse specialist wrote letters of support for the proposal and, once it was funded, assisted in part of the curriculum development and training for the new workers that emphasized helping skills and teaching about the normal aging process. When the substance abuse division chief wanted to develop a grant proposal to enhance prevention services directed toward women, the nurse specialist successfully lobbied to focus the proposal on women in transition throughout the life cycle, thus beginning work on preventive mental health services for women in times of transition, such as retirement, widowhood, and assuming a caregiver role for dependent older family members.

A program of regular, case-oriented consultation was established with all three nursing homes and one rest home in the area. This increased the accessibility of both direct psychotherapy services to dependent older people and education to staff regarding techniques that foster positive adjustment to institutional life.

Education about the benefits of an adult day care program targeted toward the needs of dependent older people and their families was directed at diverse groups in the community, including the clergy, the mental health center staff, and other human services agencies.

A family education and support group was led with another mental health center clinician as co-therapist. It was a close-ended, weekly group of six sessions, designed to enhance the knowledge base of family members about the normal aging process and human responses to various chronic diseases. Selected other members of the community were called on to assist with some of the teaching. At the first group of sessions, many of the participants were agency personnel (for example, public health nurses), who came both because they had to help the elderly and their families professionally and because they wanted help with personal situations.

Evaluation

The nurse specialist left the mental health center before the full impact of the program development efforts could be assessed. The major accomplishments of the geriatric program development in the community 3 years later included

- Two geriatric day care centers in the county: one run by the mental health center and one privately run, but both receiving extensive community support

- Increased willingness on the part of mental health center staff to consult with staffs of rest homes and nursing homes

- Continued support for a geriatric mental health specialist

- Increased numbers of older people receiving outpatient psychotherapy services
- Increased availability of prevention services to older people and their families
- Increased knowledge of the special problems of older people by human service workers in the county

Multidisciplinary Team Assessment of Long-Term Care Services

A nurse responsible for management of human services in a mixed urban/rural county in the southeast was able to identify difficulties in the long-term care services delivery system for the elderly in her county. Indications that the system was in trouble included

- Long waiting lists for some in-home services
- Significant numbers of patients in the county hospital remaining longer than medically necessary because no nursing home beds were available
- Fragmented community service system
- Discontent in the professional community about the comprehensiveness of home care services offered

The nurse contracted with a university-based, multidisciplinary team to assess the long-term care service delivery system in the county. They were also asked to develop and implement a case management program for the elderly in need of long-term care. The team was composed of a health care administrator with expertise in adult education and a pastoral care background, an occupational therapist with extensive experience working with severely handicapped individuals, a gerontological nurse specialist, a medical social worker with training in counseling psychology, and an internist interested in problems of the aged.

Assessment

A community assessment similar to the one in the previous example was conducted using a general systems framework. The three assessment goals were to

1. Identify the status of long-term care in the community
2. Identify barriers to optimal long-term care for the elderly
3. Identify the components of the long-term care system

Contextual Data

There was increased concern about containing hospital costs both nationally and lo-

cally, a state limitation on construction of new nursing home beds, and heightened awareness of the problems of older persons in long-term care.

Inputs

Inputs were from old people with functional impairments, families trying to care for old people, governmental agencies (e.g., the public health department, Department of Social Services, and community mental health centers), and private sector agencies (proprietary home health care agencies, six proprietary nursing homes, several proprietary domiciliary homes, and one proprietary hospital). The voluntary sector was represented by two hospitals, the Council on Aging, a hospice, and Meals on Wheels. Reimbursors included Medicare, Medicaid, and private insurers. The new Medicaid waiver project reimbursed chore services, Meals on Wheels, case management, adult day care, increased professional nursing care, and rehabilitative therapies.

Process

Interagency communications were hindered by several factors. There was little joint program planning, except between the Council on Aging and the public health department. Multiple assessments were performed by different agencies, and little information was shared. There were multiple points of entry into the long-term care system and long waiting lists. Clinicians did not have specialized training in geriatrics, which resulted in decreased sensitivity to the special needs of older people, barriers to receiving care, and inadequate time frames for rehabilitation. The various agencies adopted narrow concepts of coordinated care within a highly bureaucratized system of care.

Products

Limited competition and minimal teamwork among agencies resulted in fewer service options for old people and their families. Patients were poorly served because of regulations, fiefdoms created by various funding sources, and restricted social work practice in the hospital.

Conducting the Assessment

The multidisciplinary team identified key agencies that provided long-term care services in the community. Heads of agencies as well as individual clinicians were interviewed to determine

- Their ideas about how care for the aged was carried out

- The criteria for admission and discharge to and from various service programs
- How eligibility for services was assessed
- How services were delivered
- How agencies interacted with each other
- What gaps in service were perceived

These data were combined with statistical information available from the county manager's office and the state Department of Human Resources concerning the amount and sources of funding expended for long-term care in the county. Individual older people and their families as well as physicians in private practice in the community were interviewed regarding unmet but needed services and the availability of existing services.

Diagnoses

1. Elderly persons and their families have difficulty obtaining continuous reliable care because of fragmented delivery of long-term care related to diverse funding sources and unduly restrictive sets of services being offered by single agencies.

2. Patient and family choices of care providers are limited owing to unfair restraint of private agencies' growth by county agency dominance of referral patterns and caseloads.

3. Service options for older people and their families are limited.

4. Bias exists toward institutional care for dependent older people.

Planning and Intervention

Based on the community assessment data, the community nurse gave the multidisciplinary assessment team sanction to lead a series of interventions designed to improve the coordination and quality of community-based, long-term care services to the elderly and their families. Two goals of the project were: (1) better coordination of care in order to provide comprehensive care options for patients and their families at the lowest possible cost, and (2) lobbying to change existing barriers to better coordination of care.

First, a plan for implementation of a Medicaid Section 2176 community-based, long-term care waiver project was developed, using a centralized, hospital-based case management approach. Plans were also developed for expanding the service to community-based sites pending evaluation of the effectiveness of the hospital-based program. The rationale for beginning with a hospital-based program was that patients in the hospital were most vulnerable to inappropriate institutionalization because of three factors: (1) the pressures to discharge patients from the hospital to the first available setting, regardless of its appropriateness, (2) the vulnerability of the elderly to functional decline while in the hospital environment, and (3) the county's concern about wasting scarce hospital resources on patients who no longer required acute care, even though there was no long-term care facility available.

The team formed and staffed a community long-term care provider forum for the purpose of facilitating communications. The assessment team also recommended that a community long-term care advisory board be formed to begin to address some of the financial and administrative barriers to efficient, comprehensive, readily accessible, community-based long-term care. A policy board was formed that included members of the state legislature, advisory board members of each of the key human services agencies in the county, and a consumer representative. The case-management project actively sought, assessed, and then presented to the board for their consideration cases that exemplified some of the systemic dilemmas in long-term care. Examples of cases brought before the board included the following:

- A case highlighting the need for less cumbersome guardianship procedures as well as the need for a public guardian other than the social services agency

- A case highlighting the bias toward institutionalization by Medicaid eligibility determinations because institutions have a higher nonmedical care cost of living allowance and have greatly streamlined eligibility recertification procedures

- Cases demonstrating how limited Medicare reimbursement adversely affects clinical decisions about need for rehabilitative services, despite the presence of alternative sources of funding

- Cases demonstrating the adverse effects of the virtual monopoly on services held by one of the home health agencies in the county.

Evaluation

The project was operational for 18 months. During this time, the following objectives were accomplished:

1. Three hundred three patients qualifying for institutional long-term care were served in the community at an average cost that

was 40 per cent of the current nursing home reimbursement rate.

2. Legislators and other community leaders gained increased understanding of the barriers to expanded community-based long-term care services, including different Medicaid eligibility rules for institutional and community populations that favor institutionalized residents, and the fragmentation of services among various agencies.

3. A uniform assessment tool for long-term care services was developed and accepted for state-wide use but was not adopted by all local agencies for intake assessment.

According to the criteria for evaluation of community care presented earlier, the nursing service to the community was successful at delivering care in a high-quality, cost-effective manner in the least restrictive environment possible to 303 elderly persons in need of long-term care. No data were collected that allow comparison of the incidence or prevalence rates of preventable disorders in this population with those in institutional settings or in those receiving traditional community long-term services.

The intervention was not successful in sustaining itself. The other community agencies lobbied successfully with the county commissioners to terminate the project on the grounds that it duplicated existing services in the community. Thus, although an intervention or new service may be successful according to objective criteria, it may be politically unsupportable.

Proper Placement of Residents in a Retirement Community

A private, nonprofit life care community has 320 older persons living independently in their own apartments. There is a 60-bed inpatient facility with 30 skilled nursing beds and 30 domiciliary home beds to accommodate residents with acute, chronic, rehabilitative, or terminal care needs. Primary care services are delivered on site by a geriatric nurse practitioner and a part-time clinic physician as well as by community physicians in their offices. There is a home health nurse/wellness coordinator who sees residents in their apartments for acute and chronic problems. Inpatient care is delivered by nursing staff led clinically by another nurse practitioner who specializes in care of the elderly.

The level of care committee is an interdisciplinary group that meets every 2 weeks to discuss proper placement for residents who have borderline functional ability or those in transition from one level of care to another.

Community Health Problems

Although the health care system was designed to allow residents with functional dependencies to transfer to the inpatient facility, many residents prefer to stay in their apartments as long as possible despite chronic illness and functional disabilities.

General Needs of the Borderline Residents

Residents who have borderline function have the following general needs:

- Supervision of health care conditions, including multiple medical disorders
- Supervision of medication regimens
- Varying amounts of help with activities of daily living (ADLs)
- Varying amounts of help with instrumental ADLs
- Social support
- Coordination of caregiving activities
- Regular evaluation of their functional status
- Regular evaluation of their safety within their own environment
- Respect for the wishes of clients to be as autonomous as possible
- Varying amounts of help from family members
- Freedom from caregiving of more frail residents by neighbors

System Constraints

The health care system in this particular community operates under a number of constraints. First, it is committed to maintaining an environment of independent living and wellness to attract other active, independent retirees as new residents; in addition, the socialized payment system must be fair so that the very dependent residents do not consume more than their share of health care resources. Limited home health services are available because Medicare does not fund home health services provided by the community staff, since the facility is not licensed as a home health agency. (A certificate of need would not be extended for this license, because home health services would be provided only to a very small number of persons, and there is already an operational home health agency in the area.) The facility is reluctant to use the local home health agency because of the need for close coordination of care, and many of the needs are not for reimbursable "skilled nursing."

Among the residents, a great need is for custodial care, but there is a reluctance to use multiple privately hired nursing assistants who require supervision and coordination in the independent living units. On the other hand, 24-hour per day qualified nursing care is provided in the inpatient unit, where nursing needs can be met more efficiently by the staff than in the community at large.

Assessment

In view of the preceding needs and constraints, the need is for development of a plan to honor the residents' desire for independent living in the least restrictive environment while not taxing the socialized system of health care for the general community and destroying the norm of independent living for the retirement community.

Planning

1. Evaluate the needs of individual residents in terms of the general needs listed earlier. See the assessment form in Box 23–1 (p. 907).
2. Develop a specific care plan for each resident that the home health nurse will administer and coordinate.
3. Help residents and their families hire needed private aides for necessary help with activities of daily living and instrumental activities of daily living and supervise these caregivers.
4. Discuss the care plan at the level of care meeting so that an interdisciplinary team, including an administrator, may have input about the appropriateness of the use of health care resources.
5. Incorporate the families and residents' physicians in planning and supporting the individualized care plans.
6. Allow residents to come to the health center for short stays as necessary to decrease resistance to possible institutionalization and to acclimate the resident to the supportive environment.
7. Schedule regular outpatient visits to the clinic as residents are able to obtain health care services independently.
8. Allow input from independent living residents about the proper solution to the appropriate level of care problem through the residents' association.
9. Hire a private aide to work with the home health nurse to increase services and decrease supervisory needs but require that

residents pay an additional charge for this service.
10. Require that residents wear street clothes in public areas.

Evaluation

The foregoing plan has worked well, with the decision making and evaluation taking place at the semimonthly level of care meeting. At that time, caregivers present individualized care plans and hear other relevant information from the administration, the residents, and the director of nursing regarding the availability of inpatient beds. When a resident's functional status is quite limited, the group acts as a forum for an objective critique of the care plan and the appropriateness of placement. The committee thus evaluates whether the care plan is adequate and the resident seems sufficiently functional to remain in the apartment without unduly taxing the community's health care resources. A system of checks and balances at level of care meetings works well to individualize patient care and preserve the autonomy of residents in keeping with the facility's concern for overall fairness and emphasis on promoting functional independence.

INDIVIDUAL AS CLIENT

Most elderly persons prefer to stay in their own homes in familiar communities for as long as possible. As people get older, they often fear that they may have to leave home for health reasons. Their fear is realistic because acute and chronic health problems associated with aging often dictate at least temporary changes in environment, leading the elderly to reside in places they would prefer not to. Their desire to stay at home challenges the health care system to study their special needs and devise solutions that will accommodate them in the most acceptable way. Nurses working in the community who focus on care for individual clients use different specific approaches in the nursing process. The goals of prevention of excess disability and promotion of health apply at both the community and the individual client levels.

Assessment

Nurses in primary care settings have the most interaction with older individuals. As health promotion activities gain greater acceptance among the elderly, it can be expected that the sophistication of this aspect of assessment will increase. If in current health care reform, reimbursement systems change to prepaid models, the emphasis on health promotion and disease prevention should become more pronounced.

Home health nurses have already experienced changes in the nature of their client population owing to the advent of prospective payment for hospitals under Medicare. There is now an increased demand for technologically oriented care and an increased level of acute care for patients in the home, necessitating certain clinical skills in home health nurses previously required only in the hospital setting (Haddad, 1987). Although the focus of nursing care in home and clinic settings is changing to include more acutely ill patients, nurses must remain attentive to the preventive and rehabilitative aspects of care if older people are to be well served.

Primary Care Settings

In primary care, the purposes of assessment are to identify the risk factors for functional impairment, to assist in early detection of treatable disease, and to develop a database for providing continuous care. Primary care providers generally have the advantage of ample opportunity to gather assessment data over an extended period of time rather than being under pressure to perform a comprehensive assessment on the first visit. Although the older person's and family members' concerns should be conscientiously assessed on each visit, other parameters should also be routinely assessed, including

1. Activities of daily living: walking, transfer, bathing, dressing, continence, eating
2. Instrumental ADLs: telephoning; household chores, including meal preparation; transportation and shopping; and administering one's own medication
3. Mental status
4. Lifestyle, including exercise, diet, use of social drugs
5. Nutrition
6. Social support network
7. Family support
8. Recent life changes
9. Review of desires in regard to a living will, aggressiveness of care
10. Sensory impairments: hearing, vision, peripheral sensation
11. Immunizations
12. Cancer detection protocol: breast, colorectal, prostate, cervical, oral

13. Fall-related injuries
14. Review of medications for possible adverse reactions

More in-depth assessment of these domains is required in selected cases, depending on the individual situation. For more detailed discussion of assessment maneuvers, see Chapter 2.

Individuals without functional impairment should receive an assessment that is focused on health maintenance and health promotion, with in-depth assessment of health problems guided by findings on the history, review of systems, and physical examination. Baseline measures of basic and instrumental ADLs, cognitive status, and social support should be obtained but in less detail than in the multiply impaired individual.

Home Care Settings

People seen in home care settings often have complex problems and suffer from multiple impairments. A comprehensive, multidimensional assessment is therefore indicated and should be obtained as soon as possible following admission to the home care service. An example of a multidimensional assessment format used successfully in a community-based long-term care project appears in the Appendix. It is an efficient means for recording a rather extensive database. This type of assessment is also appropriate for a subset of ambulatory care patients—that is, those who have multiple functional impairments. Domains to be assessed include

1. Environment
2. Activities of daily living
3. Instrumental ADLs
4. Mental status
5. Lifestyle
6. Social support network
7. Family history
8. Recent life change screening
9. Review of desires in regard to living will, aggressiveness of care
10. Sensory impairment
11. Fall-related injury potential
12. Review of medications for possible adverse reactions
13. Physical assessment to document baseline pathological findings
14. Pressure sore risk
15. Need and adequacy of care given by others.

The conduct of the assessment is highly individualized according to the needs of the patient and the family and according to the style of the nurse. The end point of the assessment process should be a comprehensive database from which changes can be observed, along with a concise listing of nursing diagnoses.

Planning and Intervention

Two issues in community-based care of the elderly are pervasive: (1) determining the most appropriate location of care for older people with multiple impairments and (2) obtaining adequate support for families of individuals with multiple impairments.

Disposition Determination

Determining the ultimate disposition or living situation for an older person can be particularly difficult. Often, elderly people want to remain independent at home, but there may be questions about the wisdom of such a decision. A person's mental or physical health may have a direct impact on where that person can safely live. Use of practical guidelines for making realistic determinations is possible.

Three fundamental questions must be addressed in determining the disposition of an older person who wants to live alone but is at risk for some untoward event: (1) What does the older person want? (2) Can the basic care needs of the person be met at home? (3) Is the older person basically safe at home alone? These three questions have been expanded into an assessment form that can guide the deliberations of an interdisciplinary team that decides with the client and the family where the older person will live (see Independent Living Assessment earlier in this chapter and the case example "The Retirement Community Resident" later in this chapter).

CLIENT DESIRES. Asking older adults what they want to do sounds rather obvious; however, health care providers often listen more attentively to the opinions of the older person's children than to the older person. The feelings and desires of the older person cannot be ignored, because to do so violates that person's basic human rights. Legally, older people cannot be forced to do something against their will unless they have been declared incompetent (see Chapter 3). The reasons for the older person's choice should be explored thoroughly. The nurse should find out why individuals want to live at home—specifically, what problems or advantages do they foresee, and what difficulties are anticipated in living in another place. Parnell (1982) noted that the costs of keeping a frail person at home come in two forms: (1) financial expense to pay for needed services in the home and (2) emotional expense of family concern over the risky situation.

FUNCTIONAL STATUS. Evaluation of a client's ability to get basic needs met at home involves assessment of the capacity in ADLs as well as ability to perform instrumental ADLs, such as food preparation, telephone use, medication administration, laundry, and housekeeping. These requirements may be met in many ways, such as through the use of home-delivered meals and in-home help for part of the day (United States Department of Health and Human Services, 1992). Family, neighbors, or privately paid helpers may enable an older adult to stay at home longer (Wilson et al., 1989). Although assessments are imprecise, the primary provider can monitor whether needs are being met adequately by watching the client's weight at regular intervals, observing for evidence of falls, and observing the home for cleanliness and orderliness.

SAFETY CONSIDERATIONS. Assessing safety in the home is also important. Does the individual know how to summon emergency help? Are home adaptations made to compensate for decreased mobility and dexterity? Cognitive impairments often present a more serious threat to safety than does physical impairment. Judgment and insight should be assessed. For example, people who know they are having problems are likely to call for help and remain safely in the home until help arrives. Individuals with impaired judgment may present a hazard to themselves as well as to their neighbors, as when an older person forgets to turn off the stove. In isolated instances, a choice may be made to preserve the older person's autonomy at the risk of serious injury; however, few would agree that the impaired older person has a right to put others at risk of serious injury. In such cases, interventions such as disconnecting the stove and bringing meals in from outside may be a reasonable compromise.

Medication use is another important factor to consider when evaluating whether or not an older person can safely remain at home alone. Sometimes, the deciding factor in whether or not a cognitively impaired individual can remain at home alone is the nature of the medication regimen. Some individuals do not require medications or can do without drugs such as calcium supplements if necessary, whereas others must have medication regularly to maintain health. There are various systems to help forgetful persons take their medicines (see examples in Chapter 18). Preparing and labeling medications for each day is one strategy for simplifying medication administration. Medication calendars, which show each type of pill with its time of administration and have a space for marking when the pill is taken, are useful to individuals with early memory impairment.

Functionally impaired individuals who want to stay at home but require assistance or supervision with ADLs are often helped by paraprofessional personnel (see Chapter 20). Some controversy exists about the amount of training and supervision necessary for paraprofessionals to function effectively in a helping role with the elderly, and requirements vary from state to state. A number of curricula and training guides have been developed, although none is universally accepted. The National Homecaring Council's *Accreditation Manual* specifies 60 hours of generic classroom training, augmented by frequent supervision in the practice setting. A minimum of 40 hours of basic training is required before a nurse's aide can give personal care to patients, and a total of 8 hours of in-service training annually is required (National Homecaring Council, 1982).

Family Caregivers

It is impossible to discuss care of the functionally impaired at home without discussing the role of *family caregivers* and their need for support. Families can be a natural support network, but tasks and responsibilities must be clearly delineated, and family members must be willing and able to share in accomplishing these tasks. Needs that a family member cannot meet must be identified and help sought through community agencies, volunteers, friends, or privately paid helpers.

POTENTIAL STRESSORS. Most family members are concerned and involved with their elders. Caring for elderly family members presents many *potential stressors* on the family unit because of altered role relationships, value conflicts between younger adults and older people, the need to confront one's own aging and mortality, financial burdens, and the difficulty of obtaining needed resources and services from the long-term care and health care systems. However, there is a potential for mutual benefit in a caregiving relationship that ranges from financial benefits to deepening of satisfying emotional relationships (see Chapter 15). Nurses should be skilled at assessing family support and signs of caregiver strain. Chapters 16 and 17 include instruments that can be used to assess family structure, functioning, and indices of caregiver burden.

TECHNIQUES TO ENHANCE FAMILY FUNCTION. The community-based gerontological nurse's repertoire should include techniques to enhance family function and reduce caregiver burden. Factors associated with positive relationships between the elderly and their family members include shared decision making and shared values (Stuart and Snope, 1981), a history of open communication and discussion of conflicts and feelings as they occur, physical proximity, a well-developed sense of self and one's priorities, an ability to have fun together, an ability to set limits without guilt, mutual expression of support and affection, and regular communication. When the older person is supported by a large extended family, it is worthwhile determining how equitably the workload is distributed. If only one or two family members are providing the bulk of support, consider in what ways the others might contribute, such as through financial assistance or provision of nonpersonal care services, such as occasional meal preparation, assistance with yard work, or shopping. When family stress is high, it is important to consider temporary care alternatives outside the family, such as respite care services.

SUPPORT GROUPS. Another useful method of supporting caregiving family members is the formation of *support groups* (Russell et al., 1989; Kernich and Robb, 1988; Pesznecker and Zahlis, 1986). Hartford and Parsons (1982) identified the following problems while working with caregivers of aged relatives and friends:

- Difficulty in deciding about relocation of an elder
- Acting on a decision to relocate an elderly person
- Deciding when it is appropriate to make decisions for the elderly person
- Involvement with other caregivers who offer either too much or too little help
- Coping with feelings of entrapment, frustration, and guilt
- Dealing with the elderly person's fear of loss of control or fear of being a burden

Knowledge of strategies for managing these difficult issues facilitates coping with the stressors inherent in caring for an impaired relative. Nurses can foster the development of family support groups to meet this goal.

Coordination of Services

The role of the gerontological nurse in the primary health care setting depends on the nurse's job as negotiated with the employer. Increasingly, nurses in primary care settings are responsible for counseling in health promotion, coordination of needed in-home services and referrals to other providers, monitoring of response to chronic diseases, and teaching about self-care practices for disease-related conditions. Nurses with geriatric nurse practitioner preparation offer the additional services of diagnosis and management of acute and chronic problems, including prescribing medication, as allowed in some states. Nurses in home health settings have greater interaction with family members than do nurses in primary care settings. The nurse may be the primary support person and teacher of caregiving techniques, and the nurse is often the primary resource person when the patient's condition changes. The nurse has first-hand data about the home environment and its effects on patient and family coping and should take responsibility for communicating this information to other caregivers as indicated. Finally, home health nurses are often responsible for supervising home health aides and other paraprofessionals in the home.

Managed Care and the Elderly

Most elderly people receive funding for health care through the Medicare/Medicaid system. However, many are enrolled in health maintenance organizations (HMOs) or other prospective payment organizations, which are managed care–based systems. Even those in community agencies may find that they have a case manager whose job is to coordinate appropriate services relevant to their needs. This trend has been necessitated by the rising cost of health care and the disorganization surrounding provision of varying services.

The goal of HMO coverage is to provide access to medical care while containing costs. This goal is to be accomplished by using the most cost-efficient methods of treatment and eliminating unnecessary care. However, the cost incentive involved causes the HMO to increase volume of services. There is concern that the elderly do not benefit from enrollment in a managed care system as opposed to remaining in a fee-for-service situation. Both health care providers and recipients are concerned about the impact of cost containment on the quality of care (Boland, 1993).

At the same time, organizations that employ a kind of community-based managed care that uses the services of a case manager show promising outcomes. This team approach is not necessarily new but is appropriate in the current health care environment, which has so many unrelated services that can be of benefit to the elderly who wish to remain independent as long as possible. A demonstration project has been undertaken in Arkansas. The North Little Rock Community Seniors Health Services project has a goal to assist older adults to manage their own health care, maintain or improve their health, and continue living in their own homes (Leath and Thatcher, 1991). Each client who enrolls is given a comprehensive assessment of all health and social needs. Team members include a clinical nurse specialist as team coordinator, a gerontological nurse practitioner, a clinical pharmacist, a clinical nutritionist, a geriatrician who works with the client's private physician, and a social worker. After the initial evaluation, the agency then provides direct service delivery, health promotion services, and disease prevention services; coordinates resource referrals; and monitors clients' health status as long as they wish. The preliminary reports of the success of this project are very positive (Leath and Thatcher, 1991).

Evaluation

No matter who the primary provider of care for the older person is, the essentials of caring for the elderly consist of competence, comprehensiveness, continuity, and coordination. *Competence* means that the care is based on scientific principles of gerontological care, drawing from research in the nursing, biomedical, pharmacological, nutritional, psychosocial, and rehabilitation literature. Satisfactory care is delivered only when care providers understand their limitations as well as their strengths and refer to other providers appropriately to maximize the functional potential of their clients.

Comprehensiveness means that the approach to the client is holistic. Every need the client perceives is related to health—be it physical, emotional, social, or spiritual. Distress is felt by the older adult in many ways, and one system may affect another. In other words, psychological or spiritual distress may manifest itself through the body in the form of a headache, abdominal cramping in an irritable colon, or an ulcer. Effective care must deal with the source of the problem as well as its physical manifestations. (For specific ideas about psychosocial care, see Chapters 16 and 17.) Comprehensiveness also means that the patient's environment is important and must be included in assessing and managing a client's problem. Death of a spouse, a move to another house or community, or a lack of access to transportation all affects a person's health and must be dealt with in a comprehensive health program. Comprehensive care means that the nurse must view elderly clients from many perspectives, including health habits and lifestyle characteristics.

Continuity means that persons are cared for whatever their location. Because their care extends over time, their history and caretaking are relevant to any immediate problem. It is essential to gather baseline data on every elderly client. Only then can a provider know whether an arrhythmia is an old or a new finding or whether a blood pressure reading is abnormal. Follow-up is also essential for both acute and chronic problems. Ideally, every time an older client leaves an encounter with a primary care clinician, a follow-up appointment should be made. Patients should know that if a problem is not improving, they should not hesitate to call. Many older people need to know that some problems are not curable but can be controlled. Accurate, complete documentation is essential for continuity of care. Elderly clients often have long problem lists, the contents of which should be addressed individually over time and at regular intervals. Acute or chronic problems should be easily traced, and their status should be quite clear from review of the chart. For example, the presence of chronic bibasilar rales is important in assessing or monitoring a client with cardiopulmonary problems.

Coordination is another essential ingredient in geriatric care that involves many providers, disciplines, and agencies. The nurse can provide the link among all the helping professionals who may not know what the others are doing. One specialist physician may be prescribing a drug that is essentially the same as that prescribed by another physician or is contraindicated given the long list of other medications prescribed for various chronic illnesses. None of the providers may be aware of all the over-the-counter medications an older person is taking. As health care reform is implemented, the use of case managers may improve overall coordination.

A paramount goal of all primary care is to help clients be as functional and independent as possible within their preferred lifestyle. Nearly all older people dread becoming dependent. Achieving the aims cited above within a complex, fragmented health care delivery system requires scrupulous attention to the four hallmarks of high-quality care in the elderly: competence, comprehensiveness, continuity, and coordination.

The following examples describe some of the complexities of care for individuals in the community setting. The first case focuses on an ambulatory care patient with multiple chronic problems. The second involves a terminally ill client, estranged from his family, who wants to remain at home as long as possible and requires sophisticated and well-coordinated care. The last example concerns an elderly woman living in a retirement community who is struggling to maintain her independent living status despite substantial functional impairments.

CASE 1.   The Ambulatory Care Patient

Ms. E.B. is a 67-year-old black woman seen in a general medical clinic for the following problems: adult-onset diabetes mellitus, congestive heart failure, obesity, and polymyalgia rheumatica. She lives with some of her children and works full-time as a housekeeper in the hospital.

CONDUCTING THE ASSESSMENT The assessment was conducted during the course of several vists to the clinic and included one home visit. Orem's (1995) self-care deficit framework was used as a nursing "review of systems," and the framework outlined earlier in the section on primary care was used to collect the remainder of the assessment information.

ASSESSMENT DATA
Universal Self-Care Demands
1. Air. No difficulties
2. Fluid. Takes diuretic to control congestive heart failure
3. Food. Takes in more calories than needed for activity level
4. Elimination. No problems
5. Rest activity. Experiences dizziness while working; often fatigued after work
6. Solitude/social interaction. Feels that she has to help with babysitting family members, even when she would rather be alone
7. Injury prevention. Engages in regular foot care regimen; has evidence of peripheral neuropathy
8. Normalcy. Continues employment despite being older than retirement age and despite multiple chronic diseases. Has leadership role in extended family network

Health-Deviation Self-Care Demands
1. Diabetes mellitus: does not understand relationship between activity, diet, and insulin. Has no regular system for monitoring blood glucose, is frequently hyperglycemic when seen in clinic, and has symptoms attributable to poor blood glucose control (dizziness, fatigue).
2. Congestive heart failure: adheres to medication regimen but has poor understanding of heart failure and relationship between exercise, diet, and medication requirements.
3. Polymyalgia rheumatica: well controlled on low doses of steroids.

Developmental Self-Care Requisites
1. Acceptance of chronic disease
2. Adjustment to role changes accompanying aging

Aging-Specific Assessment Parameters
1. Activities of daily living status. Independent in all basic ADLs and all instrumental ADLs except driving.
2. Mental status. No evidence of cognitive impairment.
3. Nutritional status. Obese: 20 per cent over ideal body weight; hematological indices normal, hyperglycemic.
4. Social support. Lives with three children (of six), who provide transportation and assist with grocery shopping. Patient provides assistance with grocery shopping, contributes financially to the household. Patient does not identify a confidante. Is active in local church and neighborhood activities, has many friends in the workplace, and is referred to by many as "Mama."
5. Family assessment. Family communications not completely open, although children do communicate with each other about patient's health status and needs.
6. Recent life changes. None identified.
7. Review of desires regarding living will, aggressiveness of care. Deferred because of other priorities in assessment and care.
8. Sensory impairment screening. No hearing impairment evident on "whispered word" test. Able to read small print with glasses, distance visual acuity = 20/40 by Snellen chart. Decreased sensitivity to light touch and pinprick in lower extremities to calf.
9. Immunization status. Tetanus, influenza, and Pneumovax up to date.
10. Cancer detection status. Does not perform breast self-examination, has had Papanicolaou smear within the past year, stools for occult blood negative. Mammogram 1 year ago negative.

CASE 1. The Ambulatory Care Patient

continued

11. Fall-related injury assessment. Risk factors include dizziness, cluttered home environment.

12. Medications. Insulin, NPH, 30 units every morning; methyldopa (Aldomet), 250 mg twice a day; furosemide (Lasix), 80 mg every morning; potassium chloride, 20 mEq every morning; digoxin (Lanoxin), 0.125 mg every day.

DIAGNOSTIC FORMULATION

1. Noncompliance with diabetic diet as related to negative side effects of prescribed treatment

2. High Risk for Injury as related to neuropathy and dizziness secondary to diabetes mellitus and cluttered home environment

3. Ineffective Individual Coping as related to unsatisfactory support systems

PLANNING AND INTERVENTIONS The primary goal set with the patient was to better understand the relationship between her symptoms of dizziness, blood glucose level, diet, and activity. She declined offers to teach her how to monitor her blood glucose level at home for 2 months. At this time, she was hospitalized in a hyperosmolar state. The primary care nurse visited her in the hospital to assess the nature of the diabetic teaching being provided and to determine whether the patient's readiness to learn had changed.

Both the patient and one daughter had become highly motivated to learn about home glucose monitoring and how to improve dietary control over diabetes. Home health referral was made for teaching home blood glucose monitoring during convalescence from the hospitalization. The clinic nurse and home health nurse were in close communication about the pacing of instruction and about the patient's recording her activity and diet information along with blood glucose levels. The patient was able to master the skill of blood glucose monitoring and used the information to understand the effect of diet and exercise on glucose levels and symptoms.

EVALUATION Ms. B's activity level improved as a result of losing approximately 30 pounds and because she was no longer dizzy. Her comfort level increased because she no longer experienced daily episodes of dizziness and fatigue. Through mastery of a new skill, she was able to achieve better control over a chronic disease and make active choices about lifestyle modifications rather than blindly following a behavior pattern that contributed to poor control of her chronic diseases.

CASE 2. The Terminally Ill Client

Mr. W.H. is a 70-year-old retired black man referred to home health for terminal care after discharge from the hospital. His diagnoses include metastatic brain cancer, seizure disorder, bilateral pleural effusions, and a history of alcoholism. He lives alone in a subsidized housing project.

UNIVERSAL SELF-CARE REQUISITES

1. Air. Becomes short of breath with moderate activity.

2. Fluid. No difficulties.

3. Food. Is unable to shop for groceries or prepare meals independently but can eat independently.

4. Elimination. No problems.

5. Activity/rest. Lethargic at times, denies sleep disorder.

6. Solitude/social interaction. Unable to interact with friends at local convenience store because "they wouldn't want to see me like this."

continued on following page

CASE 2.   The Terminally Ill Client

continued

7. Safety. At high risk for fall-related injury.

8. Normalcy. In terminal stage of illness but is adamant about not going to a nursing home until "I can't make it on my own any more." Does not believe that time is now.

HEALTH-DEVIATION SELF-CARE REQUISITES

1. Requires twice-daily dexamethasone (Decadron) to control cerebral edema; has history of steroid psychosis in the past because of improper dosing

2. Requires twice-daily phenobarbital to control seizure disorder (not able to tolerate phenytoin)

3. Requires assistance with activities of daily living because of weakness related to cerebral edema, pleural effusions, cognitive impairment

DEVELOPMENTAL SELF-CARE REQUISITES

1. Acceptance of one's own mortality

2. Completion of unfinished business

ASSESSMENT PARAMETERS FOR HOME-BASED CARE

1. Environmental assessment. Lives alone in a two-story subsidized housing project apartment, where bedroom and toilet are upstairs. He sleeps on the sofa and has a bedside commode.

2. Activities of daily living status. Requires assistance with meal preparation, grocery shopping, medication administration, dressing, and bathing. Can eat, transfer, ambulate, and toilet self independently using bedside commode but cannot empty bedside commode alone.

3. Mental status. Has focal defects, including poor short-term memory, poor judgment, and limited reasoning ability. However, states a strong desire to remain at home as long as possible despite admittedly limited reserve. Can verbalize risks of staying at home alone.

4. Lifestyle assessment. He lived a "drifter's life" for many years. Is used to making his own decisions, managing his own affairs. Has alienated most of his family, although his sister, who lives fairly close by, expresses sporadic interest in his care. Recreational activities prior to present illness included playing checkers at neighborhood store daily.

5. Social support status. One neighbor across terrace looks out for him in a friendly way—checks to see that he gets up each morning, fixes occasional meals. Sister willing to assist with finances, but patient resists this. Formal agencies involved include home health agency, Council on Aging, social services. Hospice not involved because patient has not identified a primary caregiver.

6. Family status. No children. Only relatives close by are a sister who is inconsistently involved. She feels he should be in a nursing home or living with her, which he refuses to do. He would prefer to go to a nursing home first.

7. Recent life changes. None other than onset of cancer and its resultant functional limitations.

8. Desires regarding aggressiveness of care: does not want heroic measures taken. Has been through course of palliative radiation therapy. Says he will agree to go to nursing home when he can no longer care for self. Understands that he has cancer, and that it is not curable.

9. Sensory impairment. Hemiparesis (left-sided), although he has only weakness, not true paralysis, decreased sensation to pinprick and light touch. Vision and hearing intact.

10. Fall-related injury risk. At high risk, secondary to environmental problems (e.g., steep stairs) and intrinsic factors such as hemiparesis, weakness, poor judgment, lethargy from medications, and seizure disorder.

11. Medications include dexamethasone and phenobarbital.

12. Baseline pathological findings include left-sided hemiparesis, bilateral pleural effusions, dysarthria, dependence in activities of daily living.

13. Risk of pressure sore development at present. Mild, with a Norton score of 16, based on his relative functional in-

CASE 2.   The Terminally Ill Client

continued

dependence (ability to ambulate, continence).

DIAGNOSTIC FORMULATION

1. Impaired Home Maintenance Management as related to chronic debiliting disease (cancer) and impaired mental status
2. Self-Care Deficit: Bathing/Hygiene, Dressing/Grooming, Instrumental (medication administration) as related to cognitive and physical deficits
3. Ineffective Individual Coping as related to terminal illness
4. Spiritual Distress as related to crisis of illness and lack of support network
5. High Risk for Injury as related to altered cerebral function, environmental hazards, and alcoholism
6. Activity Intolerance as related to pleural effusion

PLANNING AND INTERVENTION The health care team, including the home health nurse, physician, and case manager, agreed to support the patient's goal of staying at home as long as possible. To assist with instrumental ADLs and to supervise one time slot of medication administration, homemaker services were obtained. This individual was assigned to do light housekeeping, meal preparation, and grocery shopping, and to empty the bedside commode, as well as to provide some social stimulation. She came for 3 hours each day in the afternoon, 7 days per week. The presence of the homemaker, combined with daily home health aide visits, allowed for a twice-daily checking on the patient and the ability to call for help if the patient had fallen. A home health aide visited 7 days per week in the morning to assist with personal care, fix a hot breakfast, and supervise morning medication administration. She was supervised by the home health nurse, who also provided some limited counseling services to the patient. The home health nurse organized the medication administration schedule, so that it

was as simple as possible for the patient and helpers to understand. A medication calendar was used, with administration times set at breakfast and at bedtime. The home health agency was on call on a 24-hour per day basis to the patient and family, as well as to the paraprofessional helpers. The nurse–case manager was responsible for coordinating the overall plan of care, ensuring that accurate financial records were kept to continue Medicaid coverage for services, and communicating with the patient's sister. The case manager was also responsible for calling in adult protective services if the patient's situation became blatantly unsafe, so that nursing home placement could be arranged. The case manager provided assistance in life review and acceptance of dying, and counseling about what to do when more assistance than could be obtained in the home would be needed.

In less than 1 week, the patient became too weak to be able to care for himself adequately during the times when there was no help available. His increasing lethargy caused him to be admitted to the hospital emergency room pending identification of a nursing home bed. His total time in hospital was less than 24 hours. He died within 1 week of admission to the nursing home.

EVALUATION The care provided for the patient was less expensive than institutionalizing him directly from the hospital. It also conformed to the patient's wishes. He was cared for in the least restrictive environment possible. The patient's death was not hastened by the plan of care implemented; he functioned at a more autonomous level than if he had been institutionalized during the entire illness; and his level of comfort about admission to the nursing home was much greater because he had had the opportunity to try to make it on his own at home. His acceptance of the nursing home placement was greater than it would have been if placement had been effected from the hospital.

CASE 3.   The Retirement Community Resident

Mrs. N.C. is a 78-year-old white woman who has been discharged from the retirement community health center to her apartment where she lives alone. She has the following medical problems: (1) seizure disorder and (2) three cerebrovascular accidents resulting in gait instability, inability to talk intelligibly, drooling and swallowing difficulties, and slight right hemiparesis. The major problem is whether this woman is capable of living at home safely and performing her ADLs.

CONDUCTING THE ASSESSMENT The assessment was conducted during the course of several visits to the apartment by various care providers including the home health nurse, physical therapist, speech therapist, and geriatric nurse practitioner. Orem's (1995) self-care framework was used to assess this patient and her environment.

ASSESSMENT DATA
Universal Self-Care Demands
1. Air. No difficulties
2. Fluid. Has slight dependent edema
3. Food. Has to eat puréed food and cannot shop or prepare own food
4. Elimination. No problems
5. Rest/activity. Walks very slowly with some gait instability with her walker in the apartment. Does some exercises to strengthen her arms and legs. Is fatigued by some effort. Sleeps with no problems
6. Solitude, social interaction. Has a regular friend who sees her two or three times a day. Daughter who lives in nearby town visits every day or two. Has daily private aide whom she likes
7. Safety. At some risk for falls; minimal risk for aspiration
8. Normality. Is very motivated to stay in her own apartment. Feels move to nursing home will herald her death

Health-Deviation Self-Care Requisites
1. Seizure disorder. Takes phenytoin, 300 mg a day, and has been seizure-free for years.
2. Post cerebrovascular accident. Requires puréed food to be brought to her but can feed herself. Cannot communicate verbally. Walks unsteadily with walker.

Developmental Self-Care Requisites
1. Acceptance of chronic disease and state of dependency
2. Acceptance of worsening functional state with every subsequent cerebrovascular accident
3. Acceptance of possible death or permanent debility with next cerebrovascular accident

Assessment Parameters for Home-Based Care
1. Environmental assessment. Lives alone in small apartment where she can get to bathroom, bedroom, kitchen, and living room with a walker. This apartment is located very close to main administrative building and is easily accessible for helpers stopping in.
2. Activities of daily living status. Requires assistance with meal delivery, grocery shopping, medication administration, dressing, and bathing. Can eat, ambulate, and toilet self independently.
3. Mental status. Although the patient is quite intelligent and motivated, she shows some evidence of rigidity in dealing with care issues. She understands risks of staying at home alone. Does not seem cognitively impaired, but this needs to be tested.
4. Lifestyle assessment. This woman is extremely independent despite her disabilities and has shown her determination and resilience in overcoming past deficits after strokes. She enjoys being alone and prefers little interaction with others except for her friend, daughter, and caregivers.
5. Nutritional status. Thin. Her weight is stable at about 95 pounds.
6. Social support. Boyfriend visits two to three times a day. Daughter visits every day or two. Next door neighbor is very friendly and willing to be "on call" for problems. Caregivers have formed close relationships with her.

CASE 3. The Retirement Community Resident

continued

7. Family assessment. One daughter who lives in nearby town is very involved in supporting her and helping to arrange care. She supports her attempt to live independently because this obviously means so much to her mother. She shops for her.

8. Recent life changes. Only the cerebrovascular accident which has necessitated puréed diet, caused gait instability, and worsened her speech.

9. Desires regarding aggressiveness of care. Has living will but wants to live as long as she can remain independent. When she is no longer able to live independently, she has little interest in living in an institution.

10. Sensory impairment. Right slight hemiparesis with sensation intact. Vision and hearing intact. Able to tolerate puréed diet without difficulty.

11. Immunization status. Tetanus, influenza, and Pneumovax up to date. Tuberculosis test within past 2 years.

12. Cancer detection status. Performs breast self-examination. Had Papanicolaou smear 1 year ago. Stools for occult blood negative. Has never had mammogram.

13. Fall-related injury assessment. Risk factors include gait instability with right-sided hemiparesis; small apartment, impossibility of communicating verbally (e.g., using the phone).

14. Medications. Phenytoin, aspirin, dipyridamole (Persantine), propantheline bromide (Probanthine), Metamucil, Peri-Colace, multivitamins.

DIAGNOSTIC FORMULATION

1. Impaired Communication as related to effects of aphasia and manifested by difficulty calling for help

2. High Risk for Injury as related to altered cerebral function and altered mobility

3. Impaired Home Maintenance Management as related to cerebral vascular accident

4. Self-Care Deficit Syndrome as related to pathophysiological and maturational factors

PLANNING AND INTERVENTION The primary goal was to arrange care for this woman in her apartment to support her living as independently as possible. Because her illness was quite stable, plans needed to focus on helping her make arrangements to meet her needs for performing ADLs and instrumental ADLs and making her environment safe.

To ensure that her basic care needs were met on a daily basis and that someone would check on her to make sure she had not fallen, arrangements were made for a private aide to come for 4 hours every morning. She would bring her breakfast from the dining room and fix her lunch before she left about noon. She would help her bathe and dress and do exercises. Another aide would bring her dinner and be sure she was set for this meal. After dinner, her boyfriend would come over for a visit and help her get ready for bed. She was responsible for being sure she used her walker at all times to get around the apartment. One goal was to increase her ambulation to the point where she could eventually go to the dining room occasionally for a meal.

To facilitate communication in the event she needed help, the following code was set up: she would pull the emergency cord in the bathroom or living room if she fell. When the health center responded to the call she would not answer the phone, and therefore the health personnel would come immediately. If she needed health center personnel but not for an emergency, she would pull the emergency cord, and when the health center personnel called she would answer the phone and make a noise that would let them know this was not an emergency. They would come at the earliest convenience. Another resource for getting help was to call her boyfriend or her neighbor, and when they answered she would make a guttural sound that would let them know she needed something. She uses good judgment in not abusing these privileges. When people visit her apartment, she is able to communicate by writing or using her alphabet board to spell out words.

To maintain her motivation, short-term goals such as going to the dining room for a meal will be set. Plans are being made to

continued on following page

CASE 3. The Retirement Community Resident

continued

have her come to the physical therapy room each morning with her aide to do her regular exercises with the rehabilitation aide. Her daughter and caregivers will continue to support her zest for independent living but will talk with her about the eventuality of care in the health center when the time comes. As the opportunity arises, she can participate in some life review discussions and think about what she wants regarding aggressiveness of care.

To monitor the patient's progress, the home health nurse will visit weekly, and the geriatric nurse practitioner will visit monthly.

EVALUATION This patient has been able to stay at home in her own familiar surroundings, maintaining as much independence as possible. At the same time, her care needs have been met to provide protection, safety, and basic ADLs. She has maintained her social support and self-respect as she slowly accepts the reality of her impairments, but she thrives on her sense of mastery in a difficult situation.

SUMMARY

The challenges for gerontological nurses practicing in community care settings are tremendously varied, ranging from community-wide assessment and intervention to large-scale prevention of the many problems accompanying old age and providing highly focused individualized care to a complex older person and family. The gerontological nurse practicing in the community must be self-directed and capable of practicing with a widely scattered multidisciplinary team to be most effective.

A community health model has been presented as one way of addressing problems associated with aging from a preventive stance. Care of individuals in the community has been discussed, emphasizing assessment and respect for individual autonomy. Recent concerns about burgeoning health care costs suggest that noninstitutional options for care will expand; thus, community care for the elderly is likely to become even more important in the coming decades. Payment systems must become more progressive to allow maximum utilization of new specialized providers, such as geriatric nurse practitioners and gerontological nurse specialists. Expanded reimbursement systems and prepaid health plans are two examples of providing the elderly with the skills of nurses specially prepared to meet their needs without imposing undue financial burdens. Gerontological nurses have an important opportunity to exercise leadership in the development of high-quality long-term care and health promotion for the elderly in the community.

REFERENCES

American Nurses' Association. Ad Hoc Committee. Public Health Nurses' Section. *Nature of Public Health Nursing.* New York: American Nurses' Association, 1964.

Anderson, E. Community focus in public health nursing: Whose responsibility? *Nurs Outlook* 31:44–48, 1983.

Anderson, E.T. and McFarlane, J.M. *Community as Client: Application of the Nursing Process.* Philadelphia: J.B. Lippincott, 1988.

Anderson, R.E. and Carter, I.E. *Human Behavior in the Social Environment: A Social Systems Approach.* Chicago: Aldine, 1974, p. 47.

Bayer, R. Ethical challenges in the movement for home care. *Generations* 9:44–47, 1986–1987.

Boland, P. *Making Managed Health Care Work: A Practical Guide to Strategies and Solutions.* Gaithersburg, MD: Aspen Publishing, 1993.

Brainard, A.M. *The Evolution of Public Health Nursing.* New York: Garland Publishing, 1985.

Bremer, A. A description of community health nursing practice with the community-based elderly. *J Community Health Nurs* 6(3):173–184, 1989.

Brockopp, D.Y., Porter, M., Kinnaird, S. and Silberman, S. Fiscal and clinical evaluation of patient care: A case management model for the future. *Journal of Nursing Administration* 22(9):23–27, 1992.

Citizens Board of Inquiry into Health Services for Americans. *Health Your Self.* Washington, D.C.: American Public Health Association, 1972.

Clark, M.J. *Nursing in the Community.* Norwalk, CT: Appleton & Lange, 1992.

Clemen-Stone, S., Eigsti, D.G. and McGuire, S.L. *Comprehensive Family and Community Health Nursing.* 3rd ed. St. Louis: Mosby-Year Book, 1991.

Davies, A.M. Epidemiology and services for the aged. *Public Health Rep* 103(5):516–520, 1988.

Edwards, N., Cere, M. and Leblond, D. A community-based intervention to prevent falls among seniors. *Fam Community Health* 15(4):57–65, 1993.

Fries, J.F. Strategies for reduction of morbidity. *Am J Clin Nutr* 55(6 suppl):1257S–1262S, 1992.

Fries, J.F., Koop, C.E., Beadle, C.E. et al. Reducing health care costs by reducing the need and demand for medical services. The Health Project Consortium. *N Engl J Med* 329(5):321–325, 1993.

Funk, S.G., Tornquist, E.M., Champagne, M.T. and Wiese, R.A. *Key Aspects of Elder Care: Managing Falls, Incontinence, and Cognitive Impairment.* New York: Springer Publishing, 1992.

Haddad, A.M. *High Tech Home Care: A Practical Guide.* Rockville, MD: Aspen, 1987.

Hartford, M. and Parsons, R. Groups with relatives of dependent adults. *Gerontologist* 22(3):394–398, 1982.

Hendricksen, C., Lund, E. and Stromgard, E. Consequences of assessment and intervention among elderly people: A three year randomized controlled trial. *BMJ* 289:1522–1524, 1984.

Hinds, P.S., Chaves, D.E. and Cypess, S.M. Context as a source of meaning and understanding (originally appeared *In* Hinds, P.S., Chaves, D.E. and Cypess, S.M. *Qualitative Health Research.* 1992, Vol. 2, Issue 1 (pp. 61–74)). *In* Morse, J.M. *Qualitative Health Research.* Newbury Park, CA: Sage Publishing, 1992, pp. 31–42.

Hogue, C.C. Epidemiology for distributive nursing practice. *In* Hall, J. and Weaver, B.R. (eds.). *Distributive Nursing Practice: A Systems Approach to Community Health Nursing.* Philadelphia: J.B. Lippincott, 1977, pp. 193–210.

Hogue, C.C. Injury in late life: Part I. Epidemiology. *Am Geriatr Soc* 30:183–190, 1982a.

Hogue, C.C. Injury in late life: Part II. Prevention. *Am Geriatr Soc* 30:276–280, 1982b.

Hubert, H.B., Bloch, D.A. and Fries, J.F. Risk factors for physical disability in an aging cohort: The NHANES I Epidemiologic Followup Study. *J Rheumatol* 20(3):480–488, 1993.

Jette, A. and Branch, L. Musculoskeletal impairment among the non-institutionalized aged. *Int Rehabil Med* 6(4):158, 1984.

Johnson, M.A. Growing old in America: Health care for the elderly. *In* Wold, S.J. (ed.). *Community Health Nursing: Issues and Topics.* Norwalk, CT: Appleton & Lange, 1990.

Kernich, C.A. and Robb, G. Development of a stroke family support and education program. *J Neurosci Nurs* 20(3):193–197, 1988.

Kippenbrock, T. and Soja, M.D. Preventing falls in the elderly: interviewing patients who have fallen. *Geriatric Nursing* 14(4):205–209, 1993.

Koop, C.E. *Koop: The Memoirs of America's Family Doctor.* New York: Random House, 1991.

Lajeunesse, D.A. Case management: A primary nursing approach. *Caring Magazine,* August: 13–16, 1990.

Leath, C. and Thatcher, R.M. Team-managed care for older adults: A clinical demonstration of a community model. *J Gerontol Nurs* 17(7):25–28, 1991.

Leigh, J.P. and Fries, J.F. Associations among healthy habits, age, gender, and education in a sample of retirees. *Int J Aging Hum Dev* 36(2):139–155, 1992–1993.

Mezey, M.D., Rauckhorst, L.H. and Stokes, S.A. *Health Assessment of the Older Individual.* 2nd ed. New York: Springer Publishing, 1993, p. 246.

Morris, J.N., Sherwood, S. and Mor, V. An assessment tool for use in identifying functionally vulnerable persons in the community. *Gerontologist* 24:373–379, 1984.

National Homecaring Council. *Homemaker–Home Health Aide Services Self Study Manual.* New York: National Homecaring Council, 1982.

Nelson, G.M. Functional assessment of elderly subjects in four public welfare settings. Working paper, Durham County Department of Social Services, Community Alternatives Program, Durham, NC, 1986.

Orem, D. *Nursing: Concepts and Practice,* 5th ed. St. Louis: Mosby-Year Book, 1995.

Parnell, J. Clinical comment. *Nursing Mirror,* p. 46, Sept 22, 1982.

Pesznecker, B.L. and Zahlis, E. Establishing mutual-help groups for family-member care givers: A new role for community health nurses. *Public Health Nurs* 3(1):29–37, 1986.

Pfeiffer, E. *Multidimensional Functional Assessment: The OARS Methodology.* Durham, NC: Duke University Center for the Study of Aging and Human Development, 1975.

Russell, V., Proctor, L. and Moniz, E. The influence of a relative support group on carers' emotional distress. *J Adv Nurs* 14(10):863–867, 1989.

Skrovan, C., Anderson, E. and Gottchalk, J. Community nurse practitioner: An emerging role. *Am J Public Health* 64:847–853, 1974.

Spradley, B.W. The community: Assessment and planning. *In* Spradley, B.W. (ed.). *Community Health Nursing: Concepts and Practice.* 2nd ed. Boston: Little, Brown, 1985.

Starfield, B. Measurement of outcome. *Milbank Memorial Fund Q* Winter: 39–50, 1974.

Stewart, R. and O'Rawe Amenta, M. Policy, politics, legislation, and public health nursing. *In* Swanson, J. and Albrecht M. (eds.). *Community Health Nursing: Promoting the Health of Aggregates.* Philadelphia: W.B. Saunders, 1993.

Stuart, M. and Snope, F. Family structure, family dynamics, and the elderly. *In* Somers, A.A. (ed.). *The Geriatric Imperative.* New York: Appleton-Century-Crofts, 1981.

United States Department of Health and Human Services. *The Use of Formal and Informal Home Care by the Disabled Elderly.* Washington, DC: U.S. Government Printing Office, October 1992.

United States Senate Special Committee on Aging, the American Association of Retired Persons, the Federal Council on the Aging, and The United States Administration on Aging. *Aging America: Trends and Projections.* Washington, DC: U.S. Government Printing Office, 1991.

Vetter, N.J., Jones, D.A. and Victor, C.R. Effect of health visitors working with elderly patients in general practice: A randomized controlled trial. *BMJ* 289:369–372, 1984.

Weissert, W.G. Seven reasons why it is so difficult to make community-based long-term care cost effective. *Health Serv Res* 20(4):423–433, 1985.

Wilson, R.W., Patterson, M.A. and Alford, D.M. Services for maintaining independence. *J Gerontol Nurs* 15(6):31–37, 1989.

World Health Organization, Regional Office for the Eastern Mediterranean. Health education with a special reference to the primary care approach. *Int J Health Educ* April/June (suppl), 1978.

Zander, K. Nursing case management: Resolving the DRG paradox. *Nurs Clin North Am* 23(3):503–520, 1988.

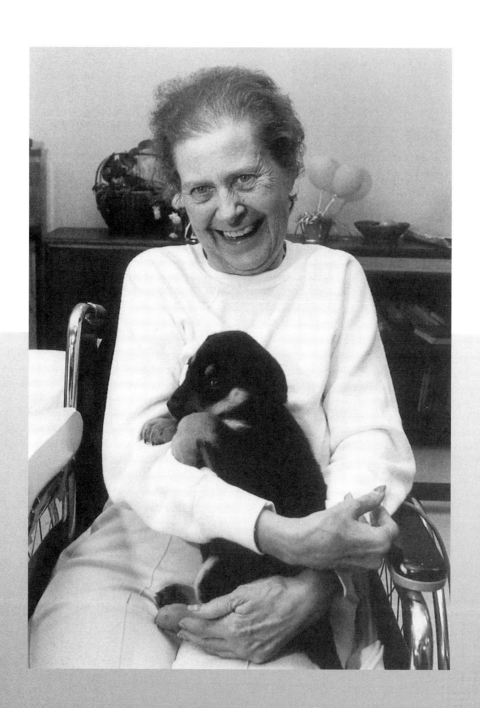

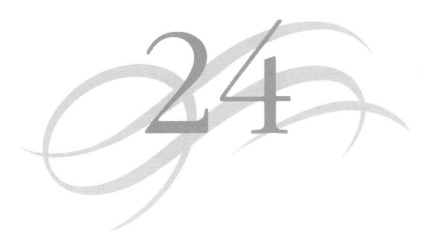

Gerontological Nursing in Long-Term Care Facilities

DEBORAH LEKAN-RUTLEDGE

OBJECTIVES

Describe the long-term care nursing facility, the nursing home resident, and relocation and transition to the long-term care nursing facility.

❖

Discuss the social and physical environment of the long-term care nursing facility and measures for its enhancement.

❖

Compare staff roles and interdisciplinary team responsibilities in the long-term care nursing facility.

❖

Interpret the need and implementation of advocacy and rights for long-term care nursing facility residents.

❖

Formulate a nursing model for long-term institutional care of the elderly.

THE LONG-TERM CARE NURSING FACILITY

Admission to a long-term care nursing facility is a significant event in the lives of older persons and their families. Although only about 5 per cent of the elderly population resides in a long-term care nursing facility, it is estimated that more than half of all older persons will be admitted to such a facility at some point in their life. Transition to the nursing facility may be anticipated by the individual with both optimism and reluctance. Many older persons prefer to "age in place," that is, to remain in their own familiar and secure environment, even as their ability to safely do so may be questioned. A transition of this magnitude may be feared because of the disruption and uncertainty that this change may bring. For many, continuing care in a long-term care nursing facility offers security, stability, needed care and services, and safety. In this most challenging setting, nurses have an enormous opportunity to provide creative, innovative care in working with residents, their families, and other health professionals. The complexity of both the service delivery within the nursing facility organization and the unique needs of the residents demands nurses' leadership and management expertise as well as their clinical expertise.

The long-term care nursing facility is a health care institution with a rich history in social, demographic, and legislative change. During the 19th century, religious orders and benevolent citizens established almshouses and poor farms to care for dependent, chronically ill patients. At the turn of the century, as the number of hospitals grew and hospital stays grew shorter, almshouses and poor farms were gradually replaced by private charitable homes, board and care homes, and rest homes. As medical and technological advances led to prevention of communicable diseases, quicker recovery from illness, and increased survival, the population of elderly and disabled persons increased, as did the need for institutional long-term care. A number of legislative initiatives helped establish the nursing home industry as a dominant provider of long-term care. The Social Security Act passed in 1935, creating a source of funds that individuals could use to pay for their own health services. Because payment with these funds to public facilities was restricted, the growth of for-profit facilities began. The Medicare and Medicaid amendments to the Social Security Act, which passed in 1965, created payment systems for the elderly and the poor while fostering the growth of long-term care in the private sector. Hospitals concentrated on acute care because they had little incentive to develop long-term acute care services (Tellis-Nayak, 1988). The need for long-term care beds grew in the 1960s, when the mentally ill population were discharged from institutions with few community-based alternatives available, and in the 1980s, when the Medicare prospective payment system was imposed on hospitals, resulting in a higher rate of discharge from the hospital of elderly persons who were still acutely ill. Social changes since the 1960s raised society's awareness of the non-therapeutic conditions under which many residents received care in nursing homes, creating growing consensus about patients' rights and quality of care. The Omnibus Reconciliation Act (OBRA), passed by Congress in 1987, introduced substantial reform in residents' rights, the facility survey process, nurse staffing and training standards, and quality monitoring in the nursing facility. As standards for excellence and quality in long-term care have evolved, long-term care nursing facilities have increasingly developed and implemented innovations that enrich the quality of life of residents and provide a challenging and stimulating practice environment for nurses.

There are more than twice the number of nursing facility beds as hospital beds in the United States. In 1939, there were 1200 nursing facilities (Burke and Donley, 1987). Currently, approximately 2.3 million elderly persons reside in over 19,000 nursing facilities in this country at an annual cost per resident of $20,000 to $36,000. One in five elderly over age 65 will spend time in a nursing facility, and for those over 85, this number is one in three (Mezey et al., 1989). Reflecting the shift in the delivery of long-term care services from custodial to prevention of acute exacerbation of illness and improved management of chronic diseases, the long-term care nursing facility is challenged to meet community standards for quality of care.

The Contemporary Long-Term Care Nursing Facility

Gerontological nursing in the long-term care nursing facility is not easily defined or categorized in terms of resident population, services, and nursing roles. The long-term care nursing facility offers continuing care for chronically ill, disabled, and medically frail persons, promoting the highest practicable level of functioning for all residents. The population characteristics and the service delivery in the long-term care nursing facility create a paradoxical view. For example, the long-term care nursing facility is both a home to many residents and a health care institution offering a number of health services. Many long-term care nursing facilities offer a full range of rehabilitation and specialized services that facilitate discharge to the home. Residents have more functional impairments with greater acuity in long-term care, yet approximately half stay less than 3 months (Spence and Weiner, 1990). Although the nursing facility is commonly associated with the care of the elderly, a small percentage of residents are chronically or terminally ill infants, children or young adults, patients with acquired immunodeficiency syndrome, and those with spinal cord injuries. The intensity of care is often perceived as long term, nonemergency, or custodial; however, this setting in fact may often resemble acute care with high acuity levels, high prevalence of acute episodic illnesses, and the availability of nursing and medical resources and various laboratory and diagnostic technologies. In one study, it was reported that over a 3-month period, 89 per cent of residents in a nursing facility experienced between one and eight "adverse clinical events," defined as any acute or subacute change in the resident's health status detected from specific signs, symptoms, and/or laboratory findings that suggest acute or subacute illness (Bernardini et al., 1993). In close to one quarter of these events, complex care management was needed.

It is also a paradox that although the name "nursing facility" or "nursing home" connotes that the primary service in this setting is professional nursing, most nursing facilities are staffed with few positions for professional registered nurses (RNs). By regulation, only one RN is required to be on duty 8 hours per day 7 days per week, compared with hospital staffing in which higher RN staffing ratios are the norm, and RNs are on staff 24 hours per day. According to the American Nurses' Association (ANA), there is one nurse per 100 residents in long-term care, in contrast to hospitals, which average one nurse per 4.5 patients (ANA, 1986). Although advanced technologies and health professional resources may not predominate in most nursing facilities, these resources are increasingly available and appropriately used to improve resident care outcomes.

Comparisons can be drawn between the long-term care nursing facility and the critical care unit. In each setting, there is recognition of the complex and dynamic patient conditions and the nurse's autonomy and independence in preventing, identifying, reporting, and intervening in acute medical problems (Foyt, 1991). Like in the critical care unit, resolution of many episodic acute problems in the nursing facility is accomplished because key resources, such as advanced practice clinical nurse specialists and nurse practitioners, are available. Early recognition of acute illness results in more timely intervention that may avert the need for costly hospital transfers. The opportunity to pursue nontraditional nursing roles, experience challenging and diverse work situations, and exercise a high level of autonomy in patient care often attracts nurses to the long-term care nursing facility (Bandriet, 1992; Robertson and Cummings, 1991; Rountree and Deckard, 1986).

THE NURSING HOME RESIDENT

Prospective nursing home residents typically need intense care before their nursing home placement. Such care may include physical care as well as help with other social and instrumental activities, such as meal preparation, housekeeping, shopping, managing finances, and transportation to appointments. When sufficient numbers and types of resources, including family, friends, community programs, and formal services, are coordinated and used by the older person, remaining in the home is often feasible and preferable for the older person. When the need and demands for care exceed the abilities of the family or the availability and accessibility of long-term care services, then institution-based long-term care options are sought. Smallegan (1985) noted that a decision to enter a nursing home is always a result of inadequacy—finances, health, social supports, emotional strength, or other ability to cope. Interviews with decision makers for newly admitted nursing home residents about problems preceding admission revealed that the residents were receiving substantial care from family members and friends before admission. Multiple functional impairments and complex medical and social circumstances interact to produce excessive caregiving burdens. The study findings substantiated that families do make significant contributions in caring for their elderly members and usually do not inappropriately or prematurely admit them to institutions. When the burden of managing care exceeds the family's ability to provide such care, nursing home placement becomes an important option.

Social changes occurring after World War II introduced trends toward the dissolution of family caregiving networks. Many adult children left their home communities to seek career opportunities in distant locations. As parents aged, fewer family members were available to provide assistance. Friends and community-based services became increasingly important in meeting instrumental and caregiving needs. In spite of this trend, approximately 80 per cent of services rendered to the elderly in the community are still provided by families. A significant number of nursing facility residents have no extended care networks, and nursing facilities are disproportionately occupied by the unmarried,

widowed, or childless (Sloane and Gwyther, 1980; United States Department of Health and Human Services, 1991).

Residence in a nursing facility offers numerous benefits. Access to professional nursing services and other health professionals; health monitoring; timely evaluation and treatment of illness; the convenience of having available basic services, such as meals, laundry, housekeeping, and personal assistance; and the stability of being in a safe setting of care make this setting attractive. Many individuals can function at a higher level when the appropriate services are available. Special environmental design features in the nursing home can enhance physical mobility and social interaction. For the person needing round-the-clock personal assistance and care, the nursing home may be the most economical and practical solution (Sloane and Gwyther, 1980). Smith and Bengtson (1979) reported on the positive effect of nursing facility placement on family relationships. More than two thirds of family members of nursing home residents interviewed indicated that they experienced a renewed closeness and strengthening of family ties, a discovery of new love and affection or a continuation of closeness. In only 10 per cent were there negative patterns, and there was no evidence that the resident had been abandoned. Family relationships seemed to be renewed or strengthened at least in part because of the release of the family from the strain of caregiving.

Nursing home residents are older and more medically frail than elderly persons residing in the community. The median age of nursing home residents is 81 years, whereas the median age of the general population over 65 is about 72 years. The nursing facility population is predominantly white (93 per cent); only 6 per cent of the residents are black, and fewer than 1 per cent are Hispanic, compared with 11.7 per cent and 6.5 per cent of the total United States population, respectively. Residents tend to be single: 83 per cent are widowed or never married, compared with 44 per cent single persons in noninstitutionalized elderly (Schick and Schick, 1994).

In areas where there may be limited access to long-term care services, such as in rural communities, there may be a greater number of highly impaired older persons residing in the home (Kane and Kane, 1981). Families provide most long-term care services in our country, directly by providing care, and indirectly by coordinating the delivery of both formal and informal services for the individual. Approximately 9 million people of all ages who need long-term care live in the community, compared with fewer than 2 million persons, primarily older persons, who live in institutional settings (Heine and Bahr, 1993). The limited availability of nursing facility beds available to older persons without formal or informal social networks means that many older persons attempt to manage without needed services. Rural elderly are especially isolated from communities and may have difficulty securing services.

Relocation and Transition to the Long-Term Care Nursing Facility

Abrupt change in the living situation challenges the older person's coping abilities, putting the individual at high risk for loss of physical or psychological function. Unfamiliar environments are particularly stressful because there is a loss of personal control and routines. Transition from the home or hospital to the nursing facility, whether temporary or permanent, is a stressful event for the older person. The degree to which the person exercises control over the environment and participates in the decision-making process can positively influence the transition. Preadmission visits should be encouraged, and prospective residents should be given opportunities to express concerns and realistically appraise the options. Rosswurm (1983) noted that the predictability of the move, the reason for the move, and the degree of control the elderly person has in the decision-making process and in other events surrounding the move all affect the relocation. Planned preparation for transition to the nursing facility is widely acknowledged to be essential to successful transition.

Numerous studies on the negative consequences of relocation to new environments, including mental hospitals and nursing facilities, concluded that mortality was high during the first month and during the first year (Camargo and Preston, 1945; Whittier and Williams, 1956). These studies helped generalize the opinion that relocation itself was hazardous, even life threatening, apart from conditions associated with the move (Coffman, 1981). Terms such as *transplantation shock, transfer trauma, relocation trauma,* and *relocation effect* described the perceived dangers of relocation. Subsequent review of these studies have determined that methodological flaws in the studies made those conclusions questionable and probably overrated (Borup, 1981; Coffman, 1981; Borup, 1983). Although the effect of relocation on

mortality in later studies was shown to be insignificant, it is believed that certain factors mediate relocation, including the degree of environmental change, the type or quality of environmental change, the degree of preparation for the change, and whether the relocation was voluntary or involuntary (Mirotznik and Ruskin, 1984).

Studies on adverse behavioral and health effects of relocation suggest that residents may become passive, having less involvement in social interactions and organized activities (Bourestom and Tars, 1974). Patnaik et al. (1974) studied resident and staff behavior patterns before and after involuntary relocation and found that given the marginal adaptive reserves characteristic of elderly people, more residents were observed to restrict themselves to their bedrooms, fewer were observed in the lounge, and more passive behavior was exhibited (more staff were noted to be performing tasks for the resident). This behavior was interpreted as an appropriate way for residents with diminished competence to orient themselves to a new environment; however, longitudinal measurements of these behaviors that would note permanent declines in behavior patterns were not taken (Patnaik et al., 1974). Brody et al. (1974) reported that personality variables, including depression, aggression, resistance, anger, demandingness, neurosis, and anxiety, all increased after relocation, especially anxiety and depression, but returned to baseline status after 2 weeks.

Physical health may be affected by relocation. Changes in appetite, physical activity, mood, and cognitive function leading to acute confusion or delirium are signs of distress. New environments can be overwhelming, disorienting, and exhausting to the new resident. Individuals with cognitive and sensory deficits who are physically frail are the most vulnerable and have the most serious adverse relocation effects. Engle and Graney (1993) reported on a large prospective study investigating the stability of residents' mental status, function, and mood during the first and second week after nursing home admission. These findings documented improvement in hygiene, grooming, dressing, and transferring, whereas feeding, ambulation, urination, and defecation were stable. Tired and depressed moods improved, and other affective states, such as anger, loneliness, fear, and cheerfulness, remained stable. This study provided data suggesting that negative aspects of nursing home admission may be less than anticipated.

A study attempting to determine the effectiveness of planning and preparing to move

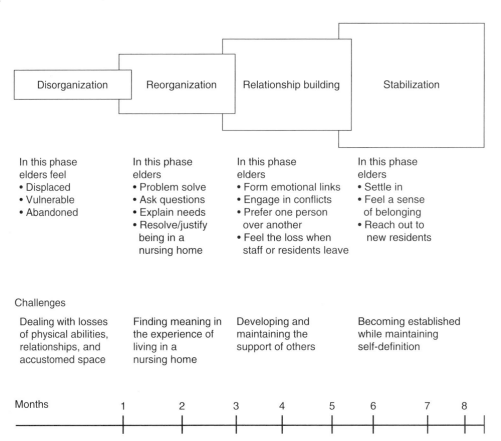

FIGURE 24–1

The process of adjusting to a nursing home. (From Brooke, V. Your helping hand: How to tailor your approach in each phase of adjustment. *J Gerontol Nurs* 10(3): 126–128, 1989.)

Disorganization	Reorganization	Relationship building	Stabilization
In this phase elders feel • Displaced • Vulnerable • Abandoned	In this phase elders • Problem solve • Ask questions • Explain needs • Resolve/justify being in a nursing home	In this phase elders • Form emotional links • Engage in conflicts • Prefer one person over another • Feel the loss when staff or residents leave	In this phase elders • Settle in • Feel a sense of belonging • Reach out to new residents

Challenges

Dealing with losses of physical abilities, relationships, and accustomed space	Finding meaning in the experience of living in a nursing home	Developing and maintaining the support of others	Becoming established while maintaining self-definition

Months 1 2 3 4 5 6 7 8

a group of elderly veterans to a new facility showed that the group that received preparation interventions experienced fewer illnesses, such as fever, pneumonia, and urinary and respiratory infection and fewer transfers to the hospital, than did a control group who did not receive the interventions (Petrou and Obenchain, 1987). In the intervention group, several months were devoted to preparation, which included frequently discussing key aspects of the move, selecting one's roommate, seeing photos of the new location, and conducting site visits to the new location. The time spent building familiarity with the new facility and presenting opportunities for individual decision making facilitated the residents' acceptance of the move and eased the transition.

Adaptation to the nursing facility environment can be seen as a socialization continuum. Brooke (1989) discussed four phases that most residents progress through while adjusting to a nursing facility (Fig. 24–1): disorganization, reorganization, relationship building, and stabilization. In the disorganization phase, the resident may feel a pervasive sense of loss and grieving about his or her health status and new environment. The resident may also feel overwhelmed by the

challenge of learning about a new living situation. In the reorganization phase, the resident attempts to understand the environment and to find meaning and autonomy in daily experiences. The resident may attempt to justify and resolve being in a nursing facility and may see personal benefit. During the relationship-building phase, the resident forms emotional links with other residents and staff and may experience conflict or frustration in these attachments. When the stabilization phase is reached, the resident's roles and routines are established, but he or she may still have fears and anxieties about the future.

Specific nursing approaches proposed by Brooke (1989) focus on learning the resident's perceptions, goals, and feelings regarding the new living situation. Frequent one-on-one contacts orient the resident to new routines; determine the resident's preferences and habits, which may be incorporated into the care plan; and acknowledge and understand the emotional state of the resident. Reminiscence therapy may help residents examine and accept losses and separate past from present events. Obtaining a list of important dates, such as anniversaries and birthdays, can stimulate discussion about fond memories. Problem solving in difficult situations should involve the resident and ask that he or she take initiative in identifying needs, previous coping mechanisms, and choices possible for that situation.

Orientation to the facility, staff, and routines should be carried out at a self-paced speed to avoid overwhelming the resident (Wolanin, 1978). Paying extra attention to rest and comfort needs and maintaining previous routines (meals, therapy, elimination, ADL, and recreational activities) can help the resident adjust. The resident should be encouraged to personalize his or her living space with special belongings.

Societal norms for transition to, and living in, the nursing facility are lacking. Aside from the personal distress that may be caused by other losses encountered in nursing home admission—perhaps one's home, belongings, social network, health status, and finances—the resident may feel a lack of social context within which health-directed and goal-directed behavior can occur. As a result, passive, dependent behavior may prevail, along with feelings of loss of control and helplessness.

Learned helplessness (Seligman, 1975) is the situation in which the individual perceives that the outcome of an event is independent of any voluntary response. As such, any attempt by the individual to influence the outcome is perceived as futile. The effects of learned helplessness are manifested in apathy, depression, decreased cognitive function, and increased emotionality and fear (Decker and Kinzel, 1985). Long-term care institutions tend to foster dependency because of inflexible daily routines, rigid policies and procedures, and lack of choice in all but a few matters. Promoting resident autonomy in making choices, even if the choices seem insignificant, can help increase a sense of independence, personal decision making, and control.

CREATING A THERAPEUTIC SOCIAL AND PHYSICAL ENVIRONMENT

The dynamic interaction between the individual and the environment (physical and social) is a powerful influence that can foster independence and competence as well as create and perpetuate unnecessary dependency. Thus, certain features of the physical and social environment reinforce dependent behavior or fail to reward and reinforce in-

dependent behavior. Likewise, a therapeutic environment enables and sustains higher levels of function to the extent that higher function is attainable.

Social Environment

The social environment provides a context in which behavior can be adaptive or maladaptive. Studies indicate that the social environment influences autonomy and participation in self-care. Evans (1979) stated that man is a social being who has a continuing need for human interaction to develop and maintain social relatedness and personal validation and to meet others' needs. For the elderly, the natural support system of the family and other social groups dwindles, and many social ties may no longer be available. Nursing staff become significant participants in the resident's social network. As such, nursing staff play a vital role in helping the resident adjust to this new living environment.

The therapeutic social environment should provide a humane and caring milieu in which older persons receive confirmation of who they were and who they are now. The milieu should help residents "reconnect" with themselves, their lives, and their situations by integrating meaningful rituals and routines into daily activities (Kastenbaum, 1983). A positive supportive environment should foster self-confidence and hopefulness and enhance expectations. The essential features of the milieu include an atmosphere of acceptance, trust, and positive expectations. Positive expectations are conveyed through touch, words of encouragement, and articulation of choices to be made by the resident. Involving the residents in decision making improves activity levels and psychological outlook. Even if the choices are limited, the actual perception held by residents that they have the right to choose is a powerful force that counteracts feelings of hopelessness (Mercer and Kane, 1979).

Storlie (1982) proposed that less emphasis be placed on protection and control and that staff make allowances for increased independence and choice whenever possible. Strict adherence to rules and overprotection of residents from the "hazards of exertion" often dehumanize residents by depriving them of any mastery over their situation (Kahana, 1973).

Extra attention to the new resident's social needs is necessary during the first several weeks after admission. Frequent visits from family and friends can buffer the overwhelming effects of being moved to a strange new environment. For individuals without family or friends, a few selected staff members and residents can be designated to assist and support the resident. Ascertaining the residents' previous socialization patterns is crucial to avoid imposing unrealistic demands and expectations. Older persons who have lived alone for a long time may find group living situations very stressful. For many older persons, one confiding and trusting relationship can have a greater positive effect than multiple, superficial contacts.

As a measure of quality of care, nursing routines and practices should be examined to determine if such practices either discourage or deny residents opportunities for performing self-care or for engaging in personal decision making. Many nursing personnel are unaware of the extent to which even small choices are not offered to residents when it would be important to do so.

Physical Environment

Functional impairment and sensory deficits are prevalent among nursing facility residents. The design and structure of the nursing home must take this characteristic into consideration. Interventions to modify the environment make tasks easier for the elderly. The physical environment should encourage the elderly to move about and pursue interests independently without fear of overexertion or of getting lost or injured. Structural and design measures to simplify the environment promote resident function and mobility.

Color discrimination decreases with age. Studies have shown that red-orange tones are easier to distinguish than are the cooler blue-green tones. Color selection for walls, floors, and furnishings may reflect the preference of administration or interior designers more than choices to enhance color contrast. Neutral colors, such as buff, white, gray, and pale blue and green, are the colors most frequently seen in institutions (Andreasen, 1985). Furniture, carpet, drapes, and other fixtures blend together, making it difficult for residents to distinguish the boundaries of chairs, pathways, and other objects. This may inhibit residents from moving about freely without feeling cautious. Bright colors and different textures should be used in the design of the environment. Walls and doors painted in contrasting colors to identify bathrooms, social spaces, and exits provide visual markers for room recognition. Lettering on doorways and signs should be large and clearly marked.

Glare is an important consideration in nursing homes. Tiled floors and light-colored walls reflect light, which may blur the resident's field of vision. Glare can be painful for the person with cataracts. Lighting decisions should take into consideration the increased illumination needed by the elderly and the hazards posed by both glare and shadows. Lighting should be indirect and should come from natural sources if possible. Louvered window shades can divert the bright rays of the sun and still allow natural light to enter.

Hallways should be wide to allow for easy passage of wheelchairs and other carts and equipment. Recessed spaces should be designed to accommodate food, linen, and medication and housekeeping carts. Recessed spaces could also accommodate several chairs for residents who need a rest when walking or who just like to "people watch."

Furniture should be selected with consideration of the physical characteristics of the residents. Chairs with low seats and without arms can be difficult for elderly people to get in and out of. Chair selection should take into account the height, width, and depth of the chair and the elevation of the arms; the chairs should also be stable. Upholstery should be firm, to provide support and to prevent the person from sinking too deeply into the seat.

Carpeted floors are desirable because they buffer noise, reduce the abrasive impact of falls, and appeal to residents who might leave their rooms more frequently because carpeting provides steadier footing and eliminates slipping (Andreasen, 1985). Carpeting may influence behavior: one study demonstrated that patients were more careful about spillage, neater in personal appearance, more willing to help others to the bathroom, and more eager to show visitors around the unit if it was carpeted. Carpeting also helps create a homelike atmosphere.

Wheelchair-bound residents should be able to reach light switches, sinks, mirrors, shelves, desks, windows, and other utilities. Wall pictures and news items posted on bulletin boards should be at eye level. Andreason (1985, p. 21) noted: "Special considerations must be made for these individuals whose living space has shrunk to the size of a chair . . . nursing staff must be sensitive to the way the chair isolates a resident from the physical environment . . . and provide enriching experiences . . . to keep them in contact with the environment."

Residents should be encouraged to personalize their rooms by having familiar objects in view to promote a sense of familiarity and comfort. All residents need some territory or space to call their own, a place to be physically separated from others (Roosa, 1982). Nurses should always be sensitive about personal boundaries and private space. Personal mementos serve as a reminder of important events from the resident's life history. They also stimulate interest and conversation in staff, other residents, and visitors.

STAFF ROLES

In the long-term care nursing facility, the nursing staff, medical director, and other interdisciplinary team members make significant contributions to the care of the resident.

Nursing Staff

Professional nurse staffing in the nursing facility consists of three groups: administrative nurses (nurse administrators and directors of nursing), staff nurses (RNs and licensed practical nurses [LPNs]), and nurses with advanced clinical preparation in the care of the elderly (including nurse practitioners and clinical nurse specialists).

Nurse staffing in the nursing facility can be viewed as a pyramid structure, with licensed nursing staff (RNs and LPNs) at the top of the pyramid, denoting their lesser number, and certified nursing assistants forming the base of the pyramid, denoting their greater number. Certified nursing assistants have the most frequent contact with residents: they make up 71 per cent of full-time nursing staff and provide between 80 and 100 per cent of personal care (National Center for Health Statistics, 1989; Diamond, 1986). LPNs represent 17 per cent of the nursing staff; RNs represent only 12 per cent of the nursing staff (National Center for Health Statistics, 1989). Labor costs account for approximately 60 per cent of costs in the nursing facility. The minimal use of RNs in long-term care is attributed to cost-control mechanisms. The primary service in the nursing facility is nursing care, which is need based rather than disease based. Nursing care is also low technology, which is somewhat "invisible" given its human relations focus, rather than high technology,

which is more visible. Unfortunately, minimum standards determined by state regulations and reimbursement systems foster the use of the least expensive resources for most care. Minimum staffing standards defined by each state are in part driven by the cost of long-term care borne by each state through the Medicaid program. Increasing patient care acuity levels of residents combined with a therapeutic focus in care mandated by OBRA regulations has renewed attention on the role of the RN. The RN has increased authority and autonomy in the coordination of resident care from assessment, intervention, evaluation, and ongoing quality monitoring of resident outcomes.

Nurse administrators and directors of nursing form the core of administrative personnel in the nursing facility, retaining 24-hour accountability for residents and staff, in contrast to acute care, in which managerial and clinical responsibilities are shared by a bureaucracy of nursing, medical, and administrative staff. Larger nursing facilities may have additional nursing positions for assistant director of nursing and staff development and quality assurance personnel. In many facilities, these responsibilities are carried out by the same person, but in smaller facilities, the director of nursing would also be responsible for these duties. Roles and responsibilities of the nurse administrator and director of nursing have been described to broadly encompass organizational management (including establishing goals, policies, procedures, budget, and quality assurance), human resources management (recruiting and retaining staff, scheduling, and creating work climate), nursing and health service management (developing philosophy, goals, objectives for nursing, implementing and evaluating nursing, and ensuring residents' rights), and professional nursing and long-term care leadership (creating linkages with community resources, affecting public policy, and continuing professional growth) (Lodge, 1987) (Fig. 24–2).

Registered nurses have responsibility for resident assessment and careplanning, supervising and evaluating the implementation of resident care plans, supervising and directing the care given by nursing assistants, and administering direct care, treatments, medications, and other procedures. In charge nurse roles, RNs or LPNs assume responsibility for a caseload of residents for assessment and treatment and for monitoring the care provided by nursing assistants. Nurses in the nursing facility not only assume major responsibility for the residents'

ASSUMPTIONS

Long-term care is where professional nursing will have a major impact.

The health care delivery system of the future will be different from the present system.

The aging population is increasing and requiring additional and different kinds of health care services.

The national movement toward self-care and personal responsibility for health has direct implications for nursing services.

Better educated, more articulate consumers have higher expectations of the quality of nursing services they will receive.

Changing family structures and relationships influence nursing services for the elderly.

The frail elderly population increasingly comprises a greater percentage of institutionalized persons and requires more complex nursing care.

The nurse administrators/directors of nursing are responsible for the management and improvement of nursing care delivery.

The compensations of nurse administrators/directors of nursing will be commensurate with their role, responsibilities, and qualifications.

The complexity of the role requires that the nurse administrators/directors of nursing place increased emphasis on administrative responsibilities.

There is a common core of knowledge for nurse administrators/directors of nursing.

Knowledge about aging is also essential for the nurse administrator/director of nursing in long-term care.

The standards developed by nursing organizations as they relate to nursing administration are criteria for quality nursing services and education.

Increasing competition in the health care industry requires a marketing orientation by nurse administrators/directors of nursing.

Cost containment is and will continue to be a major issue in health care.

Quality long-term care requires collaboration among individuals and professional organizations.

ROLES AND RESPONSIBILITIES

The nurse administrator in long-term care has four major roles with related responsibilities: organizational management (member of management team), human resources management, nursing/health services management, and professional nursing and long-term care leadership.

Organizational Management

As a member of the management team, the nurse administrator/director of nursing in long-term care

- Serves as a member of the executive staff of the organization and develops effective working relationships with the chief executive officer and the medical director
- Participates in development of institutional policies
- Shares in development of long-range plans for the institution
- Participates in development and administration of an evaluation plan for the institution based on institutional goals and objectives and on nursing standards
- Works in establishing and facilitating effective employer-employee relations
- Minimizes legal risks
- Participates in establishing and maintaining management information systems to facilitate administration of the institution's nursing department
- Designs and implements organizational structure for the nursing department
- Formulates and administers policies and procedures for the nursing department
- Implements federal, state, and local regulations pertaining to nursing service
- Develops long-range plans for the nursing department
- Formulates and administers the departmental budget based on nursing department goals and projected revenue
- Participates in establishing a competitive wage, salary, and benefit plan for nursing services staff
- Operates the department in a cost-effective manner
- Designs and implements a quality assurance program for nursing care
- Formulates and administers an evaluation plan for nursing services in relation to the department's established goals, objectives, and standards
- Raises consciousness, educates, and participates in formulating policy relative to bioethical issues
- Initiates research projects that address problems and issues specific to the nursing department

Human Resources Management in Nursing

As the person responsible for nursing personnel, the nurse administrator/director of nursing in long-term care
- Recruits, selects, and retains qualified nursing staff
- Develops and implements a master staffing plan based on client needs and nursing service goals and standards
- Initiates and approves position descriptions for nursing personnel
- Promotes a scheduling system that balances employee and client needs
- Formulates, implements, and evaluates a departmental plan for orientation and staff development
- Assists individual staff members in development of career plans
- Designs and implements a performance appraisal system for nursing
- Promotes resolution of conflicts
- Promotes and implements personnel policies
- Creates a work climate that promotes a high-quality work life

Nursing/Health Service Management

As the person ultimately responsible for the quality of nursing care, the nurse administrator/director of nursing in long-term care
- Develops philosophy, goals, and objectives for the department of nursing
- Assesses the implementation of effective strategies and methods for delivery of nursing services
- Implements actions to meet and maintain nursing care standards
- Cooperates in developing and implementing a process for an interdisciplinary approach to health care services
- Facilitates creative use of community resources
- Ensures that clients' rights are protected
- Encourages independence of clients through use of self-care and rehabilitation concepts
- Initiates formal or informal testing of nursing interventions
- Evaluates the organization of nursing care
- Evaluates plans of nursing care

Professional Nursing and Long-Term Care Leadership

As the professional nurse and leader in long-term care, the nurse administrator/director of nursing in long-term care
- Plans for future health and nursing care actions based on social, economic, political, and technological changes
- Promotes changes in community health care systems based on social, economic, political, and technological changes
- Encourages innovative methods for delivery of long-term care
- Encourages entrepreneurial activities associated with development of nursing models for health care delivery focusing on health promotion, health education, and direct services
- Establishes linkages with existing community resources
- Influences public policy affecting long-term care and nursing
- Establishes relationships with colleges and universities to promote formal educational opportunities for nursing staff, faculty practice, student learning experiences, and research
- Promotes a positive image of long-term care and long-term care institutions
- Seeks opportunities for personal and professional growth

In addition, curriculum implications for each role and responsibility were suggested for graduate programs in nursing.

The following qualifications were recommended for the nurse administrator in long-term care:

1. 1982: baccalaureate in nursing.
2. 1992: master's degree in nursing with specialized preparation in administration. Experience in nursing practice required, with middle-management and long-term care nursing experience desirable.
3. Certification in nursing administration for long-term care highly desirable.

Lodge, M.P. Professional Education and Practice of Nurse Administrators/Directors of Nursing in Long-Term Care. *Executive Summary. Kansas City, MO: American Nurses' Foundation, 1987.*

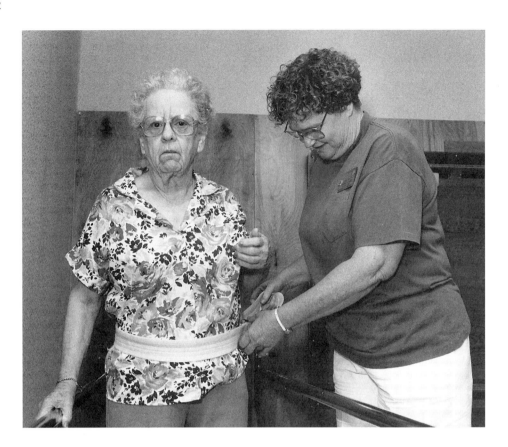

FIGURE 24 – 2

Adjusting to the nursing home.

health care but they also function as unit managers with day-to-day responsibility for management of staff issues. LPNs fulfill a wider range of resident care and managerial responsibilities in the nursing facility than in other settings of care. Management and leadership skills are as critical as clinical expertise to ensuring quality care.

The role of the nurse practitioner in the nursing facility has also evolved as an approach to providing primary care to nursing facility residents. Early studies suggest that nurse practitioners are cost-effective providers and have a positive impact on quality indicators, such as reducing hospitalization and improving functional status in residents (Kane et al., 1991; Kane et al., 1989b). When asked about their perceptions of their impact on resident status, geriatric nurse practitioners in one study reported they had a positive effect in reducing hospitalization; improving physical, cognitive, and social functioning and comfort of residents; and improving relationships with physicians (Kane et al., 1989a). The evaluation of the Robert Wood Johnson Teaching Nursing Home project, which used nurse practitioners in a more comprehensive capacity, showed that geriatric nurse practitioners had a positive impact on numerous quality measures (Mezey and Scanlon, 1989; Kane et al.,

1989a). The use of nurse practitioners promotes closer monitoring and early identification and intervention for acute and chronic illness and fosters health promotion and restorative care. Nurse practitioners are valuable resources to nursing staff for continuing education and training. In general, nurse practitioners "enhance the facility's capability of managing patients with increased levels of complexity" (Mezey and Scanlon, 1989, p. 66). The presence of nurse practitioners alone cannot guarantee improvement in quality; the practice environment is a critical variable in determining the degree to which positive change may take place. Conditions in the immediate practice environment, such as organizational policies, procedures, management directives, and regulatory constraints, can either thwart or facilitate potential contributions of the nurse practitioner (Kane et al., 1989a). The expanding role of the nurse includes mechanisms for independent reimbursement, thus allowing for full utilization of this role. Nurse practitioners and clinical nurse specialists in rural areas may be reimbursed for services in Medicare- and Medicaid-approved nursing facilities. National efforts to remove barriers to reimbursement for advanced-practice nurses in nonrural areas continue.

The use of nursing staffing ratios as a

measure of quality of resident care in nursing homes is a subject of intense interest in all settings of care. In general, research on quality of care has focused on organizational variables, such as organization ownership (for profit, not for profit, government owned, or religious affiliated), organization size, organizational expenditures, administrative practices, staff characteristics, and resident satisfaction (Sheridan et al., 1992). Few studies have examined this issue in the long-term care nursing facility. An important study by Linn et al. (1977) found that higher numbers of RN hours per patient were associated with improved functional status, survival, and discharge to the community. Braun (1991) reported on the relationship between measures of nursing home quality and patient outcomes on mortality, rehospitalization, and discharge in elderly veterans. The study found improved prediction of mortality associated with the number of RN hours per patient, thus further substantiating the link between quality of care outcomes and professional nursing staff. The low number of budgeted RN positions in the long-term care nursing facility continues to be a concern, particularly in light of increasing resident care acuity levels and complexity of care and treatment. A federally funded research and demonstration project under the auspices of the Health Care Financing Administration entitled the Multi-State Nursing Home Case-Mix Payment Demonstration is studying the relationship between resident characteristics and resource utilization as measured by nursing and other staff who provide care to residents. The results of this study will provide data about appropriate staffing levels based on case mix.

Nursing staff turnover in the nursing facility continues to be a significant problem. The nursing facility industry has one of the highest turnover rates in the health care field. Vacancy rates are highest in nursing facilities, although this figure represents only 10 per cent of the work force across settings of care (Hassanein, 1991). There is a persistent shortage of nursing staff in many nursing homes, and turnover among all levels of staff (RNs, LPNs, and nursing assistants) also affects staffing. High turnover of nurses and insufficient staffing contribute to more negative outcomes in nursing facility residents, whereas higher staffing levels and low RN turnover are related to functional improvement (Spector and Takada, 1991). In addition to adverse effects on residents, turnover has negative consequences on staff morale, task efficiency, and satisfaction.

Studies of turnover have measured variables on staff characteristics (age, education, sex, ethnicity, attitudes, knowledge about elderly), facility characteristics (ownership, physical environment, staff patterns, turnover and absenteeism, salary and benefits, management patterns), and resident characteristics (age, acuity, functional impairments). Tellis-Nayak asserts that turnover is not the real problem of nursing homes, that turnover is ". . . merely a symptom of an underlying unwholesome malaise" emanating from an unmotivating, uncaring environment (1988, p. 139). Nursing facilities with low turnover rates demonstrate attributes of a moral and cultural environment that is committed to service and caring. Caring for and about employees is as important as caring for residents. In outstanding nursing facilities, a pervasive philosophy is communicated to the employees that is based on mutual respect, trust, expectations, pride, and recognition for the employees' work. There is open two-way communication and commitment to solving problems as a team. In addition to a positive organizational culture, specific rewards to motivate staff, including job mobility, educational advancement, good salary and benefits, and bonuses, can be effective in increasing staff retention. Tellis-Nayak notes that it is misguided to blame employees when care lags in the nursing facility. Staff members have ongoing needs to belong, be loyal, take pride in their work, and feel a sense of satisfaction and achievement. On the importance of systematically valuing nursing aides, Tellis-Nayak notes:

The unsuccessful homes have somehow not tapped that reservoir of goodwill and generosity that reside inside them. They may have, in fact, turned them off, or even alienated them. But the successful homes all follow a simple path to success, a sure-fire strategy. They act as if their aides are their most precious resource, and so they cultivate them with care and concern. It is positively edifying to see how they transform their caregivers into caring caregivers (1988, p. 146).

Medical Director

The medical director is a physician, ideally board certified in geriatrics, who assumes responsibility for establishing administrative and clinical practice standards within the nursing facility. The position of medical director was created in the 1970s as a means of improving physician participation and improving the medical care in the nursing facility. Now, federal regulations require all nursing facilities to have a medical director (Elon, 1993). Medical directors have both administrative and clinical responsibilities. Usually, medical directors follow a caseload of residents for whom they are the primary physicians. In general, the medical director is accountable for the following (Zimmer et al., 1993, p. 130):

- Develop and revise policies and standards
- Communicate with attending physicians about policies, standards, and patient problems
- Assist in in-service training
- Arrange for medical coverage when necessary
- Help ensure that emergency care is available
- Participate in comprehensive care planning
- Help identify and correct problems in quality of care by serving on committees (utilization review, quality assurance, infection control)

Employee health activities, such as pre-employment screening and annual physical examinations, may also be a responsibility of the medical director, although it has been noted that the use of nonphysicians, such as nurse practitioners, may be more cost-effective (Elon, 1993). Surveys report that medical directors spend less than 1 to 2 hours per week fulfilling their responsibilities (Zimmer et al., 1993). Given the scope of their responsibilities, it is questionable whether this is enough time to allow for meaningful contributions. Although participation may be limited by the level of reimbursement currently available for such activities, it is likely that the role of the medical director will increase or that models for practice will change to more fully utilize advanced-practice nurses in collaborative relationships with physicians.

Social Worker

The full-time social worker is required in Medicare-approved nursing facilities with more than 120 beds. The social worker is often used in the admission process to ascertain admission status and billing and to help families resolve considerations associated with the resident's transition to the nursing facility. The social worker is also involved in obtaining the social history and in partici-

pating in the comprehensive care plan. Social workers interact with residents and families to facilitate admission to the nursing facility as well as to help plan discharge activities and coordinate the use of community resources. Social workers may also conduct group activities as part of the activities program as well as conducting one-on-one counseling sessions.

Pharmacist

Pharmacists have an active role in monitoring medication regimens to assist in reducing polypharmacy, drug-drug interactions, adverse side effects, suboptimal dosage, and long-term complications. Pharmacists periodically review medication to evaluate efficacy, and they document any problems the resident may be experiencing as a result of the medication regimen. For some medications, such as psychotropic drugs, adverse signs and symptoms related to the drug are documented on a flow sheet and reviewed by the pharmacist. Based on periodic medication review, recommendations for changes in the drug, dosage, and schedule may be made, as may suggestions for a drug holiday or discontinuation of drug therapy.

A number of studies on medication administration in the nursing facility showed inappropriately high use of antipsychotic and antianxiety drugs. OBRA guidelines stipulate that antipsychotic drugs may be used only when the resident demonstrates psychotic symptoms, such as delusions, paranoia, and hallucinations, but they may not be used when "problem behaviors," such as wandering, pacing, and calling out, are the only symptoms (JCAHO, 1992). The facility must document the drug and dosage and the resident's behavior, as well as the effectiveness of the drug in reducing the frequency and intensity of the behavior (JCAHO, 1992). A pharmacist consultant can greatly enhance drug surveillance.

Dietitian

The registered dietitian assesses, supervises, and evaluates the diets provided to residents. Residents receiving special diets, such as low-salt or diabetic diets, are provided with tasteful food choices that are consistent with specified dietary guidelines. On a regular basis, residents are assessed, using nutritional indicators to determine the adequacy of nutritional intake and to ascertain any changing needs that may warrant a change in diet. Monthly weight, food intake patterns, and other nutritional data, such as laboratory values for glucose, albumin, and protein levels, are evaluated. Abnormal changes in weight and intake patterns trigger in-depth assessment and follow-up. Registered dietitians must be very creative in providing tasteful food choices to large numbers of residents with widely varying food preferences. The dietary department can be extremely helpful in the implementation of programs that address fluid hydration in underhydrated residents, fiber supplementation in residents with chronic constipation, and restorative feeding programs in residents advancing from tube feeding to a pureed or semisolid diet.

Activities Director

The activities director is responsible for providing a schedule of daily activities that foster an environment that is interesting, stimulating, and meaningful. An active volunteer force is helpful in providing for programs that occur in groups as well as singly. General group activities may include current events discussions, organized singing, cards and games, book clubs or book readings, ice cream socials, and religious services. Pet therapy, music therapy, art therapy, exercise, and horticulture therapy are among the more specialized activity programs. In addition to social activities, the activities director also facilitates meetings of the residents' council. Nursing facilities judged as being of high quality demonstrate high rates of resident participation and involvement in activities programs offered in groups or singly (Tellis-Nayak, 1988).

Other Interdisciplinary Team Members

Interdisciplinary team members may also include rehabilitation specialists (physical, occupational, and speech therapists), a podiatrist, a psychiatrist, a psychologist, a geropsychiatric nurse clinical specialist, an audiologist, and a dentist. Family members and friends of the resident should also be involved in interdisciplinary team meetings when appropriate.

Interdisciplinary Team Responsibilities

The role of the interdisciplinary team has been long recognized as an essential component in geriatric care. Geriatric problems commonly require complex systems of care

that involve numerous services and therapies that cut across professional domains. Of paramount importance is that all team members see themselves as part of a unified approach to the care of the resident; no single therapist's approach should be considered in isolation from other disciplines. Interdisciplinary team meetings are held regularly to review each resident's care and to communicate each discipline's plan of care and its effectiveness. The resident should be involved in team meetings whenever feasible, and family members and significant others should be included as well.

The gerontological nurse is essential in providing a leadership role—nursing represents the vital link in development and implementation of the plan of care 24 hours a day. The gerontological nurse integrates treatment recommendations into a coherent plan of care and is in frequent contact with the resident and family to evaluate its effects. Using nursing theory and nursing diagnosis as the framework for interdisciplinary team communication and careplanning, Wright (1993) described how this model was implemented in a 240-bed nursing facility. Using a nursing theory model facilitated team communication once team members were educated about the nursing process and nursing theory. The rationale for adopting this model for the interdisciplinary team and committing time and resources to accomplish this process was based on the nature of the problems most often encountered by residents and the need to find a common ground to name those problems for which resident-centered goals may be established. The success of this initiative warrants further application and study.

The involvement and role of the nursing assistant is key in the implementation of the care plan. Nursing assistants provide the majority of direct physical care to residents, yet they are typically underused as key participants in careplanning. Dawes (1981) described the difficult role of the nursing assistant who may not feel a part of the interdisciplinary team. The aide may have daily interchanges with other team members, but relationships with professionals depend on "accidents of personality or personal initiative" (p. 269) rather than on the formal organizational structure. Systematic mechanisms for involving nursing assistants in interdisciplinary team meetings affirm their important role in implementation of the care plan and ongoing observation of the resident's status and response to care. This also ensures that the caregiver responsible

946 CHAPTER TWENTY-FOUR

for most of the direct care fully understands the goals of the care plan and individual role responsibilities.

Multi-State Nursing Home Case-Mix and Quality Demonstration

The Health Care Financing Administration (HCFA) funded a research and demonstration project to test a resident information system and resident classification system for equitable payment and for quality monitoring of process and outcomes relative to case mix. An expanded version of the Minimum Data Set (MDS) called the MDS+ is being used in this project. The MDS+ contains additional information about rehabilitation and special nursing procedures that more closely reflects the intensity of nursing care. To develop the classification system, HCFA collected detailed data in approximately 200 nursing facilities in six states about resident status and staff time measurements of all care provided by nursing, ancillary staff, and consultants. The demonstration states were Texas, New York, Kansas, Maine, South Dakota, and Mississippi. Resident characteristics and resource use were analyzed to differentiate residents, resulting in a 44-group classification system. Subsequent implementation of the classification tool was conducted in the demonstration states in 1991. The resulting Medicare and Medicaid reimbursement model using the classification systems is under development. This initiative is one effort to establish appropriate nursing staffing and reimbursement guidelines for nursing facilities. The results of this effort will radically change the way in which nursing homes are reimbursed for the services they deliver.

QUALITY OF CARE

The implementation of The Nursing Home Reform Act (PL 100-203) of the OBRA 1987 heralded a new era in the quest for quality of care and residents' rights in the long-term care nursing facility. The achievement of nursing home reform comes after years of consumer activism, health professional advocacy, and legislative initiatives on behalf of nursing facility residents. In 1986, the National Citizens' Coalition for Nursing Home Reform reported on a project entitled "A Consumer Perspective on Quality Care: The Resident's Point of View." This project developed recommendations for nursing home reform based on interviews with over 450

residents across the country. Quality of care components cited in resident group interviews across the country are listed in Table 24-1. The variable of quality identified as most important was staff characteristics and services, particularly that staff had good attitudes toward the resident, that they promptly attended to their needs, and that they provided good care. The other variables of quality are as pertinent today as they were when the study was completed. Findings from this report strongly influenced OBRA legislation by articulating resident/consumer expectations for care. The Institute of Medicine (1986) released a report on a 2.5-year study entitled *Improving the Quality of Care in Nursing Homes,* which contained more than 400 pages of analysis and recommendations that focused on regulatory changes addressing a number of issues, including quality of care, residents' rights, staffing and training, and survey and certification processes. The outstanding panel of experts that participated in the development of this document strongly supported major change in the long-term care nursing facility.

At the core of the OBRA legislation is the recognition of the need to define and articulate quality in long-term care and to hold the long-term care nursing facility accountable for meeting high-quality standards. OBRA states that the purpose of the long-term care nursing facility is to bring each resident to the highest practicable level of mental, physical, and psychosocial well-being in an environment that emphasizes residents' rights. This is achieved by focusing on quality of life as well as on quality of care.

OBRA law includes new regulatory requirements that must be met by nursing facilities as conditions of participation in the Medicare and Medicaid programs and thus be eligible for reimbursement. The methodology for evaluating the quality of care in the nursing facility changed from an emphasis on documentation of policies and procedures and structural characteristics (termed *paper compliance*) to an emphasis on outcomes of care and services as evidenced by direct observation of, and interaction with, residents. The outcome-oriented survey process shifted the focus to measuring the effectiveness of resident care. The MDS for resident assessment provided the mechanisms for ongoing outcome evaluation.

A summary of the major provisions of OBRA follows (Gerontology Institute, 1991, pp. 7–9):

TABLE 24-1
Quality of Care Components

1. Staff
   Good attitudes and feelings
   Prompt attention to needs of residents
   Good care (general) by staff
   Adequate numbers of staff
   Qualified, good staff
   Staff selection and training
   Continuity of staff
   Staff supervision
   24-hour-a-day staffing by nurses
2. Environmental
   A private room
   Larger rooms
   Security
   Temperature controls
   Privacy
   Quiet
   Call light visible, responded to
   Safety
   Better lights
3. Food
   Variety
   Choice
   Proper preparation
   Served hot
   Pleasant, proper service
   Evening snacks
   Resident input
4. Activities
   Broad range available
5. Medical care
   Quality care
   Physicians responding when needed
   Opportunity to see a physician privately
6. Cleanliness of the environment
7. Administration
   Good strong administration
   Supervision of administrators
   Access to administrator
   Enforcement of rules
8. Religion
9. Resident council and residents' rights and participation in community activities
10. Transportation provided by van or bus for residents

Recommendations to Promote Quality Care in Nursing Homes

1. Have open lines of communication at all levels, among residents and health care providers.
2. Mandate preservice and in-service training for all workers and improve conditions for workers.
3. Elevate residents' rights to a condition of participation and mandate opportunities for residents' involvement in personal and institutional decision making.
4. Give residents regular opportunities to participate in inspections and to offer their views on public policy related to nursing homes.
5. The community should take a more active role in nursing home life, and nursing homes should promote community involvement.

Adapted from National Citizens Coalition for Nursing Home Reform. *A Consumer Perspective on Quality Care: The Resident's Point of View.* 1986.
* Based on open-ended discussions with groups of nursing home residents across the country.

1. *Requirements for care.* Comprehensive assessment using a uniform resident assessment tool of every resident and a written plan of care describing the medical, nursing, and psychosocial needs of the resident and how those needs will be met.

   Annual comprehensive assessment of activities of daily living and periodic assessment when acute medical or functional changes occur.

   Preadmission screening and annual resident reviews to detect mental illness or mental retardation. Nursing facility placement of these individuals is inappropriate unless they also need nursing care or have been a resident of the facility for at least 30 months.

2. *Resident rights.* When admitted to the nursing home, residents are to be informed of their rights verbally and in writing, which include the right to

   Choose one's own physician and be consulted on a plan of care, including the right to refuse treatment

   Be free from chemical and physical restraints

   Enjoy privacy and confidentiality of personal and medical records and protection of personal funds

   Voice grievances without fear of reprisal and gain prompt attention to, and resolution of, those grievances

   Organize and participate in residents' groups with family members able to meet in family groups

   Have access to federal or state surveys of the facility and to a local or state long-term care ombudsman

   Receive services with reasonable accommodations of individual needs and preferences

3. *Staffing and training.* Facilities must have at least one RN on duty 8 hours a day, 7 days a week, and an LPN (licensed practical nurse) on duty 24 hours a day, 7 days a week.

   Nurses' aides or nursing assistants must undergo at least 75 hours of approved training and pass a competency evaluation. States must develop and maintain registries of those aides who have satisfied the requirements and any aides who have been found to have abused or neglected residents.

4. *Survey and certification.* States must conduct unannounced standard surveys of nursing facilities at least once a year, but no less often than every 15 months. An extended survey is to be carried out at any facility found to be providing substandard care.

Surveys are to include an audit of a sample of resident assessments and interviews with residents to determine the quality of care being provided.

States must set up procedures to investigate complaints about violations of standards.

5. *Enforcement and sanctions.* A state or the federal government can immediately appoint a temporary manager or end a facility's participation in Medicare or Medicaid if a facility is found to be out of compliance with OBRA provisions.

Intermediate sanctions can be applied to facilities that are out of compliance, including denial of payment for new Medicare or Medicaid admissions, civil penalties of $10,000 per day for each day the facility is out of compliance, and appointment of a temporary manager.

Denial of payment for new admissions will be automatic if a nursing facility is found to be out of compliance for 3 consecutive months.

Ensuring Quality

The ultimate goal of the OBRA Nursing Home Reform Act is to ensure better quality of care and service in long-term care nursing facilities. OBRA targets the most important elements of the residents' care and quality of life. Successfully meeting these requirements is facilitated by having an effective quality improvement program (JCAHO, 1992). OBRA regulations stipulate that nursing facilities must have a quality assessment and assurance committee that meets at least quarterly. This committee would consist of the director of nursing services, a physician, and at least three other members of the facility's staff (JCAHO, 1992). The goal of the committee is to develop ongoing quality assessment and assurance activities necessary to monitor quality indicators and to develop appropriate plans of actions to correct identified quality deficiencies.

Quality improvement mechanisms are being adopted throughout the health services and business world. Three features that describe quality improvement are (JCAHO, 1992, p. 8)

1. Creation of a supportive, customer-focused, and quality-driven internal environment fueled by leadership commitment
2. Systematic identification of the processes that are critical to meeting customer needs and expectations
3. Use of statistical tools to describe, measure, and continuously improve the efficiency and effectiveness of these key processes

The process of quality improvement is ongoing, comprehensive, and interdisciplinary, and the nature of problem solving is built on a belief of shared accountability and responsibility for identifying problems and their solutions. The methods of quality improvement go beyond the quality assurance activities common in health care organizations. Although quality assurance methodology relied heavily on data collection and on performance indicators, the approach to solving problems often focused blame on individuals (Tellis-Nayak and Snyderman, 1992). Quality improvement emphasizes that processes determine outcomes, and that problems associated with quality are usually multifactorial and symptomatic of more widespread implementation problems, which often involve personnel from many departments and from management. To address these issues, the quality improvement approach involves the following: a commitment to make ongoing improvements; hands-on involvement of management; use of interdepartmental teams to analyze problems, organize data collection, and develop solutions; and inclusion of all levels of employees in the process (Tellis-Nayak and Snyderman, 1992).

Describing what constitutes quality of care and how it should be measured is at once broad and complex. Quality of care generally encompasses the resident's satisfaction with care, the efficacy of care, the technical proficiency and performance of providers, the accessibility and continuity of care, and the cost-effectiveness of care (McElroy and Herbelin, 1989).

The OBRA regulations require that at least annually, the quality assessment and assurance committee addresses each of the following (McElroy and Herbelin, 1989, p. 9):

1. Prevention and occurrence of infectious diseases
2. Promotion of behavioral, cognitive, and social functioning
3. Preservation of quality of life
4. Use of medications, including a review of each resident's drug regimen
5. Use of chemical and physical restraints

6. Suitability, adequacy, and implementation of nursing care plans

7. Frequency and seriousness of accident and incident reports, and preventive measures

8. Frequency and resolution of residents' grievances and complaints about quality of care

The quality assessment and assurance committee develops systematic, ongoing procedures for monitoring process and outcome for these and other areas of concern related to individual residents as well as groups of residents. For the individual resident, steps aimed at both prevention and early identification should be evidenced in resident assessment and careplanning. The goal of a quality improvement program is to identify problems early when they are minor and to initiate timely intervention. On a facility-wide basis, the problems would be monitored in terms of prevalence, severity, intervention, and resolution. Individual resident problems of special concern that are high risk and have serious consequences (such as pressure ulcers, malnutrition, and urinary incontinence) warrant quality improvement activities.

Quality of Care Indicators

Indicators, by definition, "are measures of performance that can be used to monitor care or service; the measures can be related to either the process or the outcome of care" (JCAHO, 1992, p. 41). Processes are the activities carried out by staff, such as bathing, feeding, and ambulating, and the activities that facilitate resident care, such as staff education. Outcomes are the products of one or more processes and may include pressure ulcers, weight loss, and falls (JCAHO, 1992). Many aspects of care may be seen as both processes and outcomes; however, the indicator must be measurable in objective terms.

A number of quality of care indicators are evaluated as evidence of substandard care. Monitoring specific quality of care indicators should be part of an ongoing quality improvement plan in the nursing facility. A high prevalence of problems associated with quality indicators suggests systemic problems with care. Table 24–2 lists a number of important quality indicators. State surveyors evaluate these quality indicators during their review of care to determine whether the nursing facility would be charged with deficiency penalties.

The residents' viewpoint about the quality of care is an important mechanism for en-

T A B L E   2 4 – 2
Quality of Care Outcomes in Nursing Facility Residents

- Maintenance or improvement of functional abilities in performing activities of daily living
- Psychosocial status, including activities and social services assessment and care planning
- Pressure sore prevention
- Nutritional status and hydration
- Maintenance or improvement of range of motion
- Maintenance of urinary continence or implementation of effective bowel and bladder retraining programs
- Accident prevention, principally preventing falls
- Drug use, including the use of psychoactive drugs
- Potential or actual abuse or neglect
- Prevention and management of infectious disease

Adapted from Joint Commission on Accreditation of Healthcare Organizations (JCAHO). *Quality Improvement in Long Term Care.* Oakbrook Terrace, IL: JCAHO, 1992, p. 66. © JCAHO 1992. Reprinted with permission.

suring quality. In a study that developed a quality of care survey instrument based on the National Citizens' Coalition for Nursing Home Reform project, 17 variables were rated on a five-point scale in terms of importance and frequency of occurrence in the facility (Bliesmor and Earle, 1993). Most of the residents interviewed considered the 17 quality indicators to be important aspects of their care. The authors recommended that on admission and periodically thereafter, residents be asked to rank quality indicators as part of an ongoing quality monitoring effort. Consistent with quality improvement philosophy, the nursing staff and administration and other employees would also be involved in monitoring quality indicators.

Special Resident Care Issues

A primary goal in resident care is that each resident reaches his or her highest level of well-being and functioning that is attainable. Common functional impairments that require systematic measures for prevention, early identification, and treatment include urinary incontinence, falls and fall-related injuries, physical and chemical restraints, dysmobility, pressure ulcers, and pain.

Urinary Incontinence

Urinary incontinence, which affects over half of all nursing home residents, is a distressing, costly, and time-consuming problem. Inadequate assessment of urinary incontinence may result from the belief that very little can be done about this problem. Thorough assessment to identify treatable factors and underlying contributing factors results in timely appropriate treatment that can potentially reverse the incontinence. Incontinence can be reversed in almost half of the elderly patients who develop it, and in the remainder, it can be cured or improved in as many as two thirds (Resnick and Yalla, 1985). Treating causative and contributing factors such as urinary tract infections, deliriums, vaginitis, urethritis, and constipation can result in improvement or cure of urinary symptoms and urinary incontinence.

Toileting programs have long been a mainstay of systematic approaches to treating or managing incontinence. Scheduled toileting, prompted voiding, bladder training, habit training, and patterned urge response toileting offer various individualized approaches to meeting toileting needs in residents. In particular, prompted voiding and patterned urge response toileting have been shown to significantly improve or reverse incontinence in approximately 35 per cent of incontinent residents (Schnelle, 1990; Colling et al., 1992). Staff management and statistical quality control measures facilitate long-term staff implementation of prompted voiding and provide mechanisms for feedback on staff performance and resident outcomes. In addition to a successful toileting program, other measures to enhance bladder function include fluid hydration, urge control exercises, pelvic muscle exercises, bowel management with diet and fiber supplementation, and skin care protocols.

Urinary tract infections require protocols for prevention and treatment. A high prevalence of urinary tract infection may be associated with poor care practices, such as underhydration of residents, improper handling of urinals and bedpans, and inadequate bathing techniques and perineal care. Urinary tract infections can be prevented by measures that prevent cross-contamination of residents (using handwashing and good hygiene, never sharing urinals and bedpans, and providing private bathrooms for individuals with an infection) and increase the resident's resistance to bacterial proliferation (good nutrition, hydration, mobility, prevention of overdistention of the bladder and fecal impaction) (McConnell, 1984).

Judicious and infrequent use of urethral catheters is imperative because of the adverse consequences of infection, sepsis, discomfort, and psychological distress. Urinary incontinence can be successfully managed without long-term use of indwelling urinary catheters in most incontinent residents. The estimated prevalence of urethral catheter use in the nursing facility is between 2 and 28 per cent, but only 2 to 4 per cent of residents may actually require catheterization (Urinary Incontinence Guideline Panel, 1992). Excessive use of urethral catheters is considered to be an indicator of poor care.

Quality improvement measures should address assessment and treatment procedures, toileting and fluid hydration procedures, catheter and other assistive device protocols, bowel management procedures, and a monitoring system to evaluate treatment effectiveness and resident outcomes.

Falls and Fall-Related Injuries

Falls are of particular concern in the elderly because of their serious immediate and long-term consequences. Falls occur with greater frequency in the elderly, and the mortality, morbidity, disability, and need for medical services are greater in this age group than in any other. Tinetti et al. (1986) emphasized the importance of recognizing falls as preventable, not inevitable, events.

In a prospective study of falls in three large intermediate care facilities, Tinetti et al. (1986) assessed residents with a fall risk index that is composed of scales for mental status, physical health, balance, gait and mobility, self-perceived health and mobility problems, and hearing and vision. The assessment focuses on the actual performance of certain maneuvers (such as walking at a normal and an accelerated pace, withstanding sternal pressure, turning the head, bending down, rising from a sitting position) rather than on extensive physical examination and diagnostic studies. This is primarily because in the elderly, there is no consistent relationship between anatomic or biochemical abnormalities (or physical signs) and function (Tinetti, 1986).

In this study, Tinetti et al. found that as the number of disabilities increased, the percentage of residents who had recurrent falls increased. No resident with three or fewer abnormalities fell more than once, whereas every resident with seven or more did. In addition, one third of those who had recurrent falls fell during an acute illness. The environment appears to have played a minor role in fall causation, with only a few falls being related to extrinsic factors (such as missing a chair while sitting down). Different classes of drugs often implicated in fall causation (such as diuretics, antihypertensives, and neuroleptics) were not clearly related to falls, with the exception being that antidepressant, phenothiazine, and sleeping medication use was more common in those who fell. Although 20 per cent of those who fell sustained injury, including fractures, other outcomes—such as fear of falling and decreased mobility and independence—are also important sequelae. In later studies, Tinetti et al. (1991, 1992) compared the occurrence of falls and injuries in nursing home residents who were and those who were not physically restrained in a study in 12 nursing facilities. The investigators reported that in 349 falls by 122 residents who were restrained (usually as a measure to decrease falls), serious injury was significantly associated with restraint use after adjustment for multiple variables believed to be associated with falling or with serious fall-related injury.

Fall risk assessment and fall prevention are important initiatives in the nursing facility. Systematic, facility-wide measures for fall prevention combined with individual-focused measures toward risk reduction may reduce the occurrence of falls and fall-related injury. Environmental measures to increase safety include increased lighting, carpeting in high-traffic areas, nonskid floor surfaces, clutter-free walkways, and bed stabilizers. Increased observation by staff may warrant a reorganization of staffing patterns or assignments. Individual measures to increase mobility include exercises for gait stability, balance, and endurance. Range-of-motion exercises, foot care, and appropriately fitted walking aids are also helpful. Minimizing sensory deficits and medication side effects can enhance overall functioning. These measures help increase the overall competence of the individual to meet environmental demands, meet mobility needs, and reduce the risk of injury. Although multiple individual, organizational, and environmental approaches could be implemented, an individualized approach, with particular vigilance being placed on the resident at high risk for injury, may offer a high degree of efficacy while being sensitive to the cost of some interventions (Ginter and Mion, 1992). Neufeld et al. (1991) described the implementation of a multidisciplinary falls consultation service that was made up of medical, nursing, rehabilitation, and administration staff in a nursing facility to gather data, evaluate falls, and provide mechanisms to intervene. General approaches such as purchasing and designing new beds and chairs were implemented, as were individual interventions, such as reducing medication and restraint use.

Physical and Chemical Restraints

One of the most important outcomes of the OBRA regulation is the limitation in the use of chemical and physical restraints. The restraint reform of OBRA mandates that the rights of nursing home residents to humane care and alternatives to restraints must be upheld. Although restraints have been used to protect the resident from injury, there is evidence suggesting that restraints not only do not prevent injury but may be hazardous and may increase the risk of injury and death (Evans and Strumpf, 1990; Stolley, 1995; Tinetti et al., 1991; Tinetti et al., 1992; United States Food and Drug Administration, 1992). The national movement toward restraint-free care, combined with residents' rights, has significantly fostered restraint reduction in nursing facilities.

A 3-year statewide demonstration project to reduce restraints in Oregon, funded by the Robert Wood Johnson Foundation, was undertaken in cooperation with the state Senior and Disabled Services Division and the support of state nursing home associations (Rader et al., 1992). The project aims included the following:

1. Develop criteria and guidelines for the use of providers and regulators for restraint reduction.
2. Provide training, protocols, and consultation for providers, regulators, and advocates to facilitate implementation of the guidelines.
3. Resolve problems that arise among consumers, providers, and regulators during implementation.

The overall goal was to develop a model program for restraint reduction that would facilitate adoption of these approaches across the country. Although the program is still under way, evidence suggests that restraint use is declining. In another project, Strumpf et al. (1992) described the components of an educational program on restraint reduction and how to manage the change within organizations. Staff response to the program was enthusiastic, although the staff also reported frustration in determining alternative care practices for difficult resident behaviors. The educational program consists of 10 modules, which are each 30 minutes long. In addition, a companion manual was developed for the program to facilitate dissemination (Strumpf et al., 1992).

Systematic efforts toward restraint reduction and elimination require significant commitment from administration, stability in nursing leadership, and recognition of nursing staff who are involved in day-to-day implementation. Practical methods for managing mobility and behavioral issues must be articulated for problems that in the past would have resulted in the use of restraints. Frequent dialogue with the resident's family and significant others and the interdisciplinary team is important in the decision-making process to eliminate restraints so that risks and benefits may be articulated and weighed.

In some nursing facilities, restraints have been completely eliminated. Proponents of restraint elimination emphasize that if the option to restrain, even under certain conditions, exists, then efforts at restraint elimination are diluted because there is an implication that a small group of people exists for whom restraints are appropriate (Kane et al., 1993). Debate also continues about what constitutes a restraint, what may be substituted for a restraint, and what is an acceptable level of risk accepted by the nursing facility balanced against protection of the resident from injury. Terminology used by advertisers to describe products used for restraints, such as "safety devices," "postural supports," and "patient aids," obscures the issue by promoting the benign nature of this practice. Restraints constructed to look like clothing promote acceptance by health professionals and patients by "disguising" the intended function of the garment.

Often, restraints are used to provide a mechanism to keep the resident from falling out of the bed or chair as a result of trunk instability, muscle atrophy and weakness, or hemiplegia. Johnson (1991) described five alternatives to restraints that serve to position the resident. For the resident who slides out of the wheelchair, a zippered pillowcase was filled with foam beans or peanuts (used in mailing) and/or beans from a beanbag chair, sealed, and then positioned on the seat of the wheelchair under the knees, thereby providing resistance to the trunk and helping to prevent it from sliding downward. Another alternative used for the resident with hemiplegia involved the purchase of a large foam square cut to fit over the arm of the wheelchair. This square is covered with a pillowcase to prevent soiling. The foam stabilizes and provides trunk and arm support. For residents who attempt removal of intravenous or feeding tubes, a soft foam football is placed in the hand, which is then covered with a stockinette. When alternatives such as these are used, they should be implemented based on an individualized assessment of the resident and used not as a substitution of one restraint for another but to facilitate positioning, comfort, and mobility.

Unfortunately, the use of restraints may continue to be justified in specified situations. Staff may often feel compelled to use restraints for legal liability reasons (Evans and Strumpf, 1989), and the use of restraints may be associated with poor staffing (Sloane and Mathew, 1991). Restraint use must be accompanied by frequent nursing observation, documentation, and repositioning. Any restraint policy should emphasize that a restraint is always an unusual and temporary measure and should be considered a last resort.

Special care units have evolved in response to the identified needs of residents with cognitive impairment in an effort to group residents and provide targeted therapeutic services to promote adaptive behavior and social interaction (Sloane and Mathew, 1991). A high degree of variability among special care units has been documented, and the efficacy of this approach to care has not been established (Sloane and Mathew, 1991). Special care units offer a controlled, low-stimulus environment and a staff that is skilled in the principles of creating and implementing a therapeutic milieu. Reminiscence therapy, activity therapy, and validation fantasy may be used extensively. The use of psychotropic drugs is typically limited, and the use of restraints is avoided. Sloane et al. (1991), in a case-control study of 31 special care units and 32 traditional units, found that physical restraints were used in 18.1 per cent of patients with dementia versus 51.6 per cent of patients on traditional units. Ongoing activity programs provide a healthy outlet for stress and an opportunity to participate in meaningful and entertaining activities. Balancing physical activity and rest helps the cognitively impaired person avoid overexertion and excess weight loss. Environmental awareness is increased through the use of environmental cues (calendars, clocks, and reality orientation boards) and gentle reminders by staff to describe and explain daily routines and events. The therapeutic environment of the special care unit should provide a setting in which the resident may become more socially adjusted and less agitated, wander less, be free of restraints, receive fewer drugs, and achieve a balance of physical activity and rest. Staff should receive specialized training on the care of residents with cognitive impairment.

Quality monitoring of restraint use should focus on prevalence; duration of use; alternative modes of managing behavior; indications for use and type of restraint used; family and resident's input; and documentation of restraint use protocols, including repositioning, range of motion, orientation, skin care, resident's response while in restraints, and any complications associated with the use of restraints, such as injury or falls.

Dysmobility

Promoting mobility is a major focus of nursing care in the nursing facility. The consequences of immobility are well established and are largely preventable (Miller, 1975). Body movement and exercise can retain flexibility and strength that may otherwise decrease or be lost with disuse. Mobility strategies balance activity and rest to prevent fatigue. Fatigue can lead to weakness and a decreased level of performance.

Efforts to promote mobility are directed toward planning and coordinating mobility-enhancement programs for groups as well as maximizing opportunities in everyday routines for physical activity (Bassett et al., 1982; Paillard and Nowak, 1985). Van Oteghen (1987) described an exercise program for persons with Parkinson's disease that includes stretching exercises and short workouts on exercise bicycles and rowing machines. The exercises help improve posture, balance, flexibility, and strength. Even frail elderly persons may benefit from structured, guided, individualized exercise programs.

Mobility-enhancing strategies can be implemented during everyday activities, such as bathing, dressing, transferring, sitting in a chair, and eating a meal. Exercises to promote flexibility, strength, and range of motion can be performed during normal care in very little time. These are critically important in chairbound and bedbound residents to prevent contractures, muscle wasting, and muscle weakness. Systematic measurement of ability and progress toward goals is imperative to document the impact of preventive and restorative care.

Some residents benefit from a group exercise program that is tailored to their needs. For residents who are more frail, an individualized program conducted one on one at the patient's bedside may be more appropriate and effective. Positioning, passive and active range-of-motion exercises, and assisted participation in activities of daily living become priorities.

Quality monitoring should address targeted needs of residents, enrollment and participation in various group and one-on-one exercises, and mobility-enhancement programs. Measurement of outcomes, such as distance walked, endurance, transfer skill, activity of daily living skills, and range of motion, should be included in program evaluation and quality monitoring.

Pressure Ulcers

Many residents in the nursing facility with impaired mobility, cognition, nutritional status, and incontinence would be deemed to be at high risk for the development of pressure ulcers. The prevalence of pressure ulcers in the nursing facility is estimated to be about 10 per cent. Their high cost in terms of medical and nursing treatment, disability, and pain and discomfort warrants aggressive efforts toward their prevention, early identification, and treatment. Early identification and aggressive intervention that focuses on increasing the resident's biological competence through nutritional management, and interventions to enhance mobility and pressure relief and reduction, should be systematically implemented and documented. Using the wound, ostomy, and continence nurse consultant may be extremely helpful in difficult wound healing situations as well as providing consultation on new technologies such as skin care products and devices.

Quality monitoring should include policies that address frequency of skin assessment and ulcer measurement and staging, treatment protocols for wound healing and nutritional approaches, and methods for mobilization, pressure relief, and reduction.

Pain

The prevalence of pain in nursing facility residents is estimated to be greater than 70 per cent (Ferrell et al., 1990). This is not surprising, because the prevalence of chronic diseases that are associated with pain, such as arthritis, is very high in the elderly. For many persons, there may be more than one source of pain. Also, one must also consider pain that may be associated with immobility and muscle atropy and weakening. The impact of pain in all spheres of function can lead to adverse consequences: decline in physical performance, psychological stress, and disrupted social patterns. Elderly persons have lifelong experience with pain of different types and therefore have a unique perception of pain. Pain may be interpreted as a sign of progressing disease, and fears surrounding increasing pain levels may intensify.

Pain assessment in the nursing facility resident poses unique problems. Pain perception in the elderly may be different than in younger persons, such that symptoms may be blunted or atypical. Pain assessment in the cognitively impaired is limited, and nurses must rely on behavioral changes, such as increased agitation, rather than on objective measures. Nursing approaches should first include a pain history, a pain record (over the course of 24 to 48 hours) using a visual analogue scale, and a pain coping inventory. Treatment should be individualized and should include both pharmacological and behavioral interventions and physical agents, such as hot or cold applications.

Quality monitoring should address policies directing when and how pain is assessed, the use and effectiveness of pharmacological and nonpharmacological therapy, and the resident's quality of life as a result of therapy.

The Survey Process in the Long-Term Care Nursing Facility

Long-term care nursing facilities undergo intense surveys to obtain licensure, certification, and accreditation. The survey process evaluates different aspects of the care delivery system to determine whether the facility meets standards of care as required by federal OBRA regulations. OBRA surveyors perform 12 tasks during a survey (JCAHO, 1992, p. 59):

1. Off-site survey preparation	Surveyors collect information about recent surveys, abuse reports, ombudsman reports about complaints, and minutes of residents' council meeting.
2. Entrance conference	Surveyors interview the facility administrator about detailed information about the facility, residents, staff, and daily routines.
3. Orientation tour	Surveyors tour the facility to observe the environment, identify potential residents to be interviewed, and identify possible patterns of poor care, as evidenced by such problems as pressure ulcers, poor grooming of residents, lack of water at bedside, and high use of restraints.
4. Resident sampling	Surveyors select a case-mix stratified sampling of residents to include four categories: physically independent and interviewable, physically dependent and interviewable, physically independent and noninterviewable, and noninterviewable who do not require total staff assistance. Interviews address quality of care and residents' rights.
5. Environmental quality assessment	Surveyors observe the impact of the environment on the residents' quality of life, freedom of choice, health, and safety. For cognitively impaired residents, surveyors observe for methods for memory stimulation and social support.
6. Quality of care assessment	Surveyors examine the resident assessment and care plan for the sampling of residents as it relates to improvement, maintenance, or decline of function. Special attention is given to negative outcomes, such as pressure ulcers, infection, undernutrition, dehydration, and infectious diseases.
7. Resident rights interviews	Surveyors interview resident and family members about their satisfaction with care and their ability to exercise rights and choice in everyday life.
8. Dietary services system assessment	Surveyors examine food preparation procedures, sanitation, nutritiousness, dining experience, and distribution.
9. Medication pass	Survey team nurse or pharmacist observes at least two nurses administering medication and calculates medication administration error rate. Also evaluates appropriateness of medication regimen.

10. Closed-record review (transfers, discharges) — Surveyors assess appropriateness of transfers, notification procedures, and quality of discharge planning. Examine reasons for transfer to the hospital to determine if clinical indicators of poor care were present.

11. Formation of a deficiency statement — Survey team reviews and analyzes observations and findings to determine whether facility has severe and frequent problems warranting a deficiency rating.

12. Exit conference — Survey team presents its findings to facility personnel. If deficiency ratings are lodged, the facility may provide additional information to clarify or explain, and the findings are re-evaluated. Residents and ombudsman may be present at the meeting. When deficiencies are noted, plans for correction are discussed. Severe deficiencies may result in fines and denial of participation in Medicare and Medicaid.

Preparing for a site visit is the culmination of the year's activities toward quality improvement. Although the survey process is stressful and intense, it provides a good opportunity to carefully examine facility-wide and resident-focused practices. Quality improvement is not a steady state of perfection but an operational system that continuously examines how well problems are identified, monitored, and managed.

Evaluating and Choosing a Long-Term Care Nursing Facility

Once the decision is made about transition to a long-term care nursing facility, the difficult task of selecting a facility lies ahead. First, available nursing facilities should be identified. Names of nursing facilities may be obtained from local councils on aging, the department of social services, the state department of human resources, and the nursing facility association.

Evaluating and choosing a long-term care nursing facility are affected by subjective opinions and first impressions that may or may not reflect usual practices. A systematic evaluation of structure, process, and outcome variables can be accomplished by using various sources of information. State surveys of the nursing facility are mandated by law to be accessible to the public. Information about deficiencies and citations may be obtained from state agencies responsible for surveying nursing facilities. When visiting a facility, it is important to carefully interview the administrators of the nursing facility with regard to the philosophy of care; the resources available to meet the prospective resident's needs; the availability of RNs, advanced practice nurses, and physicians to meet ongoing and episodic needs of residents; nurse staffing patterns; and conditions under which residents may be transferred out of the facility. Clarify financial details concerning what is and is not covered in the daily rate or by insurance carriers. It is also important to observe care being delivered to residents at different times of the day and to observe staff communication patterns. A guide to evaluating and choosing a nursing home is found in Table 24–3.

INNOVATIONS

The long-term care nursing facility is recognized as an important site for advanced nursing practice and nursing education. Innovations in the nursing facility have affected the quality of care provided to residents and the formal education of nursing students. Mechanisms to establish formal linkages and clinical partnerships between the nursing facility and schools of nursing have contributed to advancements in clinical practice, education, and research. The teaching nursing home innovation exemplifies the collaboration between nursing facilities and schools of nursing.

The Teaching Nursing Home

The teaching nursing home concept is modeled after the university-affiliated teaching hospital. The concept was developed as a systematic approach to close the gaps between long-term care and academic medical centers. The teaching nursing home is the result of several public and private programs that have supported the joining of the academic community with long-term care fa-

T A B L E   2 4 – 3
Checklist for Evaluating a Long-Term Care Nursing Facility

CHECKLIST	QUESTIONS AND OBSERVATIONS	FACILITY 1	FACILITY 2	FACILITY 3
Location	Is location convenient for family and friends to visit? Is it close to public transportation if visitors use this form of transportation? Is it located in a safe neighborhood?			
Telephone contact	Is telephone contact courteous and friendly? Do staff seem interested and helpful? Are you often put on hold for lengthy periods of time?			
Size and ownership	How many beds are certified for skilled care, intermediate care, assisted living, rest home, or home for the elderly? What level of care will the applicant need? Is ownership not for profit, government, proprietary (for profit); is it owned by a corporate chain? Has the facility earned accreditation with JCAHO?			
Administration	Do administrator and director of nursing seem knowledgeable about resident physical and psychosocial needs, have a positive attitude about restorative and rehabilitative care, and demonstrate a commitment to individualized care, dignity, and resident rights? What are their qualifications, and how long have they held their positions? Do they interact openly with staff and residents? Are facility policies clearly presented? Ask to see the most recent state inspection report (Statement of Deficiencies and Plan for Correction), which by law is a public document that must be posted. Ask to see the written policy on quality of life and ask how it is implemented.			
Nursing services	Do staff interact positively with residents? Are staff professional, well groomed, courteous? Is the staff/patient ratio adequate to meet resident needs? How many RNs are on site daily in addition to the director of nursing? What is CNA/resident ratio for skilled and intermediate residents for the day and evening shifts? What is the state minimum for staff ratios? What is the turnover rate in the past year? Talk with staff members to find out about their educational preparation, workload, job enjoyment, turnover, absenteeism, overtime, and teamwork/relationships with other staff members. Are any RNs certified in gerontological nursing? Observe staff providing care to residents. Interact with residents and ask about their satisfaction with care.			
Facility tour	Is the facility neat, clean, free of odors, uncluttered, and cheerful? Is the background noise a low hum, or do hallways and public areas sound noisy, do sounds bounce off walls and floors, and are televisions or radios played loudly? How do staff members address each other? Do resident calls for assistance seem to go unanswered by staff? Do public areas look welcoming and comfortable for visiting? Are rooms personalized with belongings from home? Can residents bring favorite pieces of furniture and pictures for hanging? Is there adequate space for storing clothing and belongings? Will the bathroom accommodate a wheelchair and additional helpers comfortably? Is the bathroom equipped with a shower, if that is important to the applicant? Does the sink accommodate someone in a wheelchair? Visit during mealtime to observe the food service: does the food look and smell appealing; is it served in a timely manner? What kind of assistance is provided to resi-			

cilities (Schneider, 1985) in an endeavor to expand the knowledge of geriatric problems and geriatric care.

Modeling the long tradition in acute care between hospitals and medical schools, formal affiliations between nursing homes and academic centers have been forged to accelerate faculty participation in research, education, and clinical practice in the nursing home. Some models promote basic biomedical research in geriatric problems, whereas other models emphasize faculty practice, education of students, intervention studies for clinical problems, and exploration of care delivery models. Interdisciplinary team collaboration is emphasized in most teaching nursing home projects.

Sponsorship of teaching nursing home programs has been provided by a variety of organizations: the Robert Wood Johnson

T A B L E   2 4 – 3

Checklist for Evaluating a Long-Term Care Nursing Facility   *Continued*

CHECKLIST	QUESTIONS AND OBSERVATIONS	FACILITY 1	FACILITY 2	FACILITY 3
	dents who need help with feeding? Are there safety features, such as handrails, good lighting, even surfaces, and nonskid floors? Is there an outdoor, enclosed, shaded, public space for gardening, visiting, and walking?			
Special needs	How equipped is the facility in meeting special needs of the applicant? Are physical, occupation, and speech therapies available? Are there special programs developed for residents with Alzheimer's disease or for residents dependent on ventilators or enteral feeding, wound care, AIDS care, or hospice care? Do staff members have appropriate training? Is the medical director board certified as a geriatrician? Are advanced-practice nurses available on site for monitoring of health problems?			
Fees	Does facility accept patients with Medicare and Medicaid funding? When private pay resources are expended, will Medicaid funding be accepted for qualified residents or will the patient need to secure other funds or be discharged? What costs and services are covered in the daily rate? Do supplies such as absorbant products, medical supplies, and pharmaceuticals lead to additional charges? Are charges and billing procedures clearly explained?			
References	Talk with knowledgeable health professionals, such as nurses, social workers, therapists, and physicians, who have had contact with the facility. Clergy or volunteers who regularly visit can also provide information. Contact community advisory groups, such as Friends of Nursing Home Residents or the long-term care ombudsman. Talk with residents about their feelings about living in the facility and about nursing staff competence, interest, and responsiveness to needs, privacy, quality of food, laundry services, and social and religious activities. Note recurrent complaints from residents.			
Family and community issues	Are there restricted visiting hours? Are there ongoing family programs, including support groups and educational programs. Are families invited to participate in daily activities and special events? Does the facility affiliate with community groups, associations, or schools of nursing, social work, or medicine?			
New admission procedure	Is a planned program for the orientation and adjustment provided for the new admission? How is the family involved? How are room assignments and roommate compatibility issues handled?			
General impression	Is your initial impression about the ambience of the facility positive or guarded? What "red flags" concern you the most? What positive things stand out? Would you rate the facility as excellent, good, questionable, or poor?			
Return visit	If you feel that the facility tour was inconclusive or that you need additional exposure to normal daily activities, a return visit should be planned, preferably at a different time of day than that visited previously.			

JCAHO = Joint Commission on Accreditation of Healthcare Organizations; RN = registered nurse; CNA = certified nursing assistant; AIDS = acquired immundeficiency syndrome.

Foundation in conjunction with the American Academy of Nursing, the W. K. Kellogg Foundation Community College–Nursing Home Partnership, the National Institute on Aging, and Beverly Enterprises. As a result of the widespread success of many teaching nursing home models, many academic centers, particularly schools of nursing, negotiate formal relationships for ongoing clinical teaching experiences for students. These relationships ideally focus on building a long-term relationship to foster the meeting of mutual goals so that both the nursing facility and the school of nursing perceive significant benefit.

The Robert Wood Johnson program with the cosponsorship of the American Academy of Nursing supported a 5-year demonstration project that ended in 1987 that linked 11 university schools of nursing with 12 nursing homes. The project funded between 1.5 and 2.0 full-time equivalent new positions in the 12 homes. The major objective was to change the nature of care in nursing homes by implementing a nursing model for practice to improve patient outcomes in a cost-effective manner. The main objectives of the project included improving the quality of care; advancing clinical nursing research; advancing the educational preparation of geriatric nurses; implementing programs for the prevention, identification, and management of common health problems encountered in the nursing home; enhancing recruitment of nurses into long-term care; and maximizing opportunities for faculty and students in education, research, and clinical practice (Aiken, 1985).

In a formal analysis of longitudinal and cross-sectional data in six of the teaching nursing homes, it was shown that quality of care improved, hospitalization rates decreased, staff turnover decreased, and critical indicators, such as urinary incontinence, bowel continence, functional status, and use of restraints decreased. Table 24–4 docu-

ments outcomes in the demonstration teaching nursing homes in comparison with a control group of nursing homes. It was further documented that the added cost associated with hiring a nurse clinician was offset by reducing the use of hospital services. The lasting impact of the Robert Wood Johnson teaching nursing home project is evident in the magnitude and the importance of the nursing research that was generated, the validation of a nursing model for practice, and the influence these data had on the passing of legislation for Medicare reimbursement of nurse practitioners for services in the nursing home (Mezey and Lynaugh, 1991).

The W. K. Kellogg Foundation Community College–Nursing Home Partnership project has, since 1986, sponsored a variety of activities at six demonstration sites in six states (Tagliareni et al., 1993). Nursing students participate in planned experiences with both well and frail elderly persons in nursing facilities. Community college nursing education programs, which are widely dispersed in both urban and rural areas, prepare more than 60 per cent of newly licensed RNs each year, thus helping to meet the needs of local communities. The three major goals of the project were (1) to develop nursing potential in long-term care settings through education, (2) to influence the redirection of associate degree nursing education to include active preparation for nursing roles in long-term care settings, and (3) to disseminate lessons learned through the establishment of regional resource centers (Sherman, 1993). The nursing facility teaching experience was designed to maximize opportunities to focus on assessment skills, chronic disease management and health maintenance, rehabilitation, leadership and staff management, and interpersonal relationships with staff. Students, faculty, nursing home staff, and interdisciplinary team members collaborate and provide care within a nursing model. One outcome of the project was the production of a videotape, *Time to Care: The Nursing Home Clinical,* and a handbook entitled *Teaching Gerontology: The Curriculum Imperative* (National League for Nursing). These resources are important and useful adjuncts to the clinical teaching experience in the nursing facility.

The National Institute on Aging of the National Institutes of Health conducts research with funding allocated by the United States Congress. The National Institute on Aging promotes biomedical, social, and behavioral research and training related to the aging process and the diseases and special

T A B L E   2 4 – 4
The Robert Wood Johnson Teaching Nursing Home Program Outcomes

	NURSING HOMES (%)	
	Teaching	Comparison
Hospitalization Rate Within 3 Months of Admission		
Before	19	13*
After	12	18*
Patient Status		
Bowel continence improved	55	33†
Dressing/transfer stabilized	54	47‡
Episodes of incontinence avoided with timed voidings	36	25‡
No restraints used on confused residents	41	32§
Restraints on confused residents checked every 30 minutes	44	31‖
Who Participated in Planning Care		
Nurse clinician	28	1*
Nurses' aide	55	29*
Physical therapist	61	68‡
Resident	12	17¶

Adapted from Mezey, M.D. and Lynaugh, J. Teaching nursing home program: A lesson in quality. *Geriatr Nurs* 11:76–77, 1991.
* Difference significant at a level of <0.001.
† Difference significant at a level of 0.004.
‡ Difference significant at a level of 0.01.
§ Difference significant at a level of 0.005.
‖ Difference significant at a level of 0.007.
¶ Difference significant at a level of 0.02.

problems of the elderly. Most of the research funded by the National Institute on Aging focuses on differentiating normal aging from disease and medical conditions associated with aging. The study of dementia, urinary function, sleep apnea, arthritis, respiratory function, falls, stroke, nutrition, exercise, and risk factors for institutionalization are among the funded projects (List et al., 1985).

Beverly Enterprises has used the teaching nursing home model for developing innovations and improvements in the delivery, financing, and quality of long-term care. Beverly Enterprises supports affiliations between corporate nursing homes and schools of medicine, nursing, and pharmacology. The programs conducted in the nursing homes are diverse: postdoctoral training programs in geriatric medicine, long-term care administration training and research programs, family medicine teaching rounds, and geriatric nurse practitioner and physician's assistant training (Pipes, 1985).

The teaching nursing home initiative has had a positive impact on the quality of care. McCracken Knights (1984) listed several valuable outcomes of the teaching nursing home program. Foremost is a major change in the way nursing problems are approached. The infusion of faculty and researchers into the clinical setting stimulates careful review of clinical problems and efficacy of treatment and management approaches. The direct impact on patient care has resulted in the development of effective strategies for common problems such as incontinence, confusion, skin impairment, feeding problems, and falls. Increased nursing responsibility for early identification, treatment, and management of episodic illness using defined protocols facilitates timely and appropriate care. With an everexpanding research base on significant clinical problems and the efficacy of specific interventions, the challenge to incorporate these approaches into practice presents ongoing challenges to nurses in the nursing facility.

Clinical Teaching in the Nursing Facility

The use of the long-term care nursing facility as a clinical teaching site for nursing students has been a long-debated academic topic in schools of nursing. Disadvantages in the use of this setting are often cited. However, the proliferation of literature documenting the unique advantages of this setting strongly supports the inclusion of long-term care nursing facility experience for all nursing students (Heine, 1993; Burke and Sherman, 1993).

The clinical teaching experience in the long-term care nursing facility should be recognized as an environment that is quite different from acute care, where most clinical teaching in many schools of nursing occur. The long-term care nursing facility is a setting that requires a shift in thinking about what would constitute a rich learning experience for the student. In many ways, the long-term care nursing facility is an ideal context for the student to assimilate the full scope of the nursing process in a resident-centered environment (Tagliareni, 1993). The long-term care nursing facility clinical experience offers numerous opportunities:

1. To focus on the resident as a unique individual, working with well elderly persons as well as with those who are acutely and chronically ill

2. To focus on health promotion, health maintenance, chronic disease management, and acute, episodic illness management under conditions that emphasize resident-centered continuity of care

3. To develop an appreciation for the aging experience by interacting with the nursing facility resident over an extended period of time

4. To learn and master advanced assessment skills and comprehensive functional assessment techniques and strategies

5. To experience the implementation of a nursing model that emphasizes function, individual choice, self-care, and teaching and learning

6. To experience the full richness of interdisciplinary team function and collaboration in the implementation of resident-focused care

7. To develop and participate in organized activities and groups for special needs or interests among residents

8. To articulate and come to value the purpose and significance of the role of the gerontological nurse in contributing to quality of care in the nursing facility

9. To implement managerial leadership skills with nursing staff and interdisciplinary team members

10. To understand the impact of public policy on the quality of care for residents and on nursing practice, particularly OBRA regulations and the role of quality improvement in long-term care

11. To cultivate sensitivity in working with the elderly and to consider future opportunities for working in long-term care nursing facilities

12. To differentiate the organizational culture and management practices of the long-term care nursing facility from those of other settings of care

Development of a clinical partnership between academic institutions and long-term care nursing facilities signifies an investment in the quality care of the resident. The reciprocal relationship between long-term care practice settings and academic institutions offers innovative solutions to challenges faced in both domains. For long-term care nursing facilities, keeping abreast of state-of-the-art innovations in care is stimulated by nursing faculty and students who have expertise, opportunity, and technical resources to explore in-depth special resident care problems. For nursing students, developing and mastering skills that will prepare them to be competent nurses in the care of the well, acutely ill, and frail elderly occur in a well-planned long-term care clinical experience. The teaching nursing home innovations have laid the groundwork for the design of successful clinical partnerships and clinical teaching experiences. Widespread adoption of the lessons learned in the teaching nursing home projects about designing long-term care nursing, facility-based experiences with the elderly is crucial to nursing's future in the care of the elderly.

PROFESSIONAL PRACTICE FOR NURSE ADMINISTRATORS/DIRECTORS OF NURSING IN LONG-TERM CARE

Nursing administrators and directors influence the quality of life of institutionalized elderly when they improve the delivery and the effectiveness of nursing care. The scope of influence and authority of this position significantly affects the quality and the effectiveness of the work environment and organizational climate. The Institute of Medicine (1986) affirmed that the delivery of high-quality care depends on effective administrative practices and nursing leadership. Achieving an effective organizational climate is dependent on knowledgeable, effective nursing leaders.

Sheridan et al. (1992) studied the organizational climate and nursing staff members' job attitudes, opinions toward elderly residents, and perceptions of the organizational climate in 25 nursing facilities, including facilities that failed to meet resident care standards required for state certification. Organizational climate was defined along four dimensions: human relations (administration has an interest in staff well-being); task orientation (staff job responsibilities and expectations are clear, and feedback and rewards are based on accomplishments); laissez-faire (administrative practices fail to state clear objectives, and reward policies lack incentives for doing a good job); and status orientation (administrative practices emphasize status differences between staff, which causes conflict). The study concluded that administration's human resource management policies, practices, and procedures are the underlying factors contributing to poor care in some nursing homes. Nursing administrators and directors of nursing have tremendous responsibility to translate organizational values and philosophical principles, policies, and procedures into clinical practice and care of residents.

Until 1983, the status of nurse administrators and directors of nursing in long-term care was largely unknown. Qualifications, roles, and responsibilities likely vary widely from state to state and from institution to institution. Typically, the primary mechanism for learning the skills needed to be successful in administrative positions was on-the-job training. Underpreparedness for administrative roles and responsibilities may contribute to the high turnover rate of nurses in this position. The American Nurses' Foundation and the Foundation of the American College of Health Care Administrators, with grant support from the W. K. Kellogg Foundation, addressed the status and learning needs of this professional group. A national survey of nurse administrators and directors in nursing homes provided information on biographical characteristics, employment characteristics, perceptions of roles and responsibilities, and continuing education preferences. Survey results of 1234 respondents formed a representative sample showing that the typical nurse administrator or director is a white (98 per cent) female (98 per cent) who is 45 years of age, has a nursing diploma, and has "risen through the ranks." About 11 per cent are licensed by the state in nursing home administration, and only 2 per cent are certified as nurse administrators or gerontological nurses (Lodge, 1987).

In the second phase, a comprehensive statement about the roles, responsibilities, and qualifications of the nursing administrator/director of nursing in long-term care was formulated. In this statement, four major roles with related responsibilities were identified: organizational management, human resource management, nursing/health service management, and professional nursing and long-term care leadership (Abedzadeh and Heine, 1992). This statement formally recognized the extensive areas of involvement of nurse executives.

The third phase developed a continuing education program, which included self-assessment, career counseling, and self-instructional curriculum modules. Six university schools of nursing became involved in the presentation of the curriculum clusters or modules. Topics included quality assurance, the budget process, nursing care standards, collection of patient care statistics, and nursing care plans (Lodge, 1987). This endeavor represents a significant step in strengthening the competencies of nurse administrators/directors in long-term care.

In a study to validate the statement of roles, responsibilities, and qualifications, a sample of nurse administrators in long-term care in one state was surveyed using a questionnaire based on the roles, responsibilities, and qualifications of the nursing administrator/director of nursing in long-term care (Abedzadeh and Heine, 1992). Forty-nine nurse administrators completed the questionnaire. All respondents were female, the average age was 45 years, and the majority (61 per cent) had a diploma or an associate's degree. The results indicated that the respondents rated the four role subscales as important and as relevant to their daily role performance. Activities related to daily role performance include developing long-range plans, philosophies, and goals for the nursing department; encouraging innovative methods of nursing care; and assessing the implementation of strategies for the delivery of nursing services. A few role responsibilities rated low for both importance and for participation include initiating research projects that address problems and issues specific to the nursing department, initiating formal or informal testing of nursing interventions, and influencing public policy affecting long-term care and nursing. Overall, there were high ratings for congruence between ratings of activities seen as important and role responsibilities and activities that the nursing administrator in long-term care actually performed. In general, those few role responsibilities that showed incongruency between importance and participa-

tion or performance may be related to the rater's educational background, the availability of human and fiscal resources, and corporate ownership of the facility.

Vaughan-Wrobel and Tygart (1993) documented the management education needs of nurse administrators in long-term care in one state-wide survey. Findings suggest that almost half (45 per cent) of the nursing administrators had been in their position 1 year or less, and half of this group, six months or less. Most (83 per cent) had diploma or associate nursing degrees; 9 per cent had bachelor's degrees in nursing. Most indicated that this was their first time in the position as nurse administrator. Although 71 per cent reported that they had the necessary management skills, 94 per cent indicated that they would participate in a guided self-learning management education program. High-priority areas for education as reported by the nurse administrators included the nurse as manager, human relations skills, and staffing and scheduling.

Recognition of the need for advanced education in long-term care nurse administration has implications for nursing education institutions, at the undergraduate as well as master's and continuing education levels. The statement of the roles, responsibilities, and qualifications of the nurse administrator in long-term care recommended that by 1992, a master's degree in nursing with specialized preparation in administration should be required for nurses in management positions. Until educational opportunities become more accessible and feasible to nurses practicing in, or aspiring to, these administrative roles, accomplishing this recommendation will be difficult. The specialized skills required by the nurse administrator, which historically have been learned on the job, form a growing and unique body of knowledge and skill, thus warranting advanced preparation and credentialing.

Professional Associations for Gerontological Nurses in Long-Term Care

The American Nurses' Association offers membership in the Council of Gerontological Nursing. The Council addresses policy and practice issues of concern at the state and national levels. The Council serves as a national network linking nursing education with nursing practice through the adoption of standards of practice, recommendations for nursing curriculums, and publication of a newsletter and other publications, and it provides opportunity for national certification. Professional certification through the American Nurses' Association is available for the following positions: gerontological nurse, gerontological clinical nurse specialist, geriatric nurse practitioner, and nursing administration.

The National Association for Gerontological Nursing also offers membership, continuing education through regional and national conferences, and network for communication. The Long Term Care Nurses' Association, which is affiliated with American Health Care Association, the trade organization representing proprietary nursing care facilities in the United States, addresses issues concerning nurses who work in the nursing facility exclusively. Membership in this organization provides access to conferences and workshops nationwide.

The National Association of Directors of Nursing Administration/Long Term Care is a nursing association established in 1987 to serve as a forum for the formulation, inquisition, publication, and dissemination of principles concerning the acceptable efforts and practices in long-term care nursing administration (Warden, 1993). The association has adopted a code of ethics and standards of practice that delineate guidelines for the profession. The association also offers educational scholarships and awards for innovative ideas in long-term care. A certification program is offered to members annually, as are a wide range of educational opportunities, including seminars, workshops, and national conferences. A mentor program is also under development in five regions of the country. Mentors provide assistance by telephone, mail, or on site. With a membership of 3000 and growing, this organization provides a professional network for directors of nursing administration in long-term care. News events and special articles are published in the journal *Geriatric Nursing*.

SUMMARY

Gerontological nursing in the long-term care nursing facility offers opportunities for professional growth in clinical practice, managerial leadership, research, and public policy. Nurses practice in this setting for the rewarding caregiving experiences and the opportunity to lend their professional nursing expertise to make a significant difference in the lives of residents. The field of nursing's expertise, power, and influence are critical to facilitating change to meet new challenges, foster innovation, and sustain high standards of nursing practice.

REFERENCES

American Nurses' Association, Council on Gerontological Nursing, and Council on Nursing Administration. Statements on training/staffing in nursing homes. *Oasis* 3(2):2–3, 1986.

Abedzadeh, C.B. and Heine, C. Roles, responsibilities, and qualifications of nurse administrators in long-term care facilities. *Geriatr Nurs* Nov/Dec, 13(6):325–328, 1992.

Aiken, L.H., Mezey, M.D., Lynaugh, J.E. and Buck, C.R. Teaching nursing homes: Prospects for improving long-term care. *J Am Geriatr Soc* 33:196–201, 1985.

Andreasen, M.E. Make a safe environment by design. *J Gerontol Nurs* 11:18–22, 1985.

Baltes, M.M. and Zerbe, M.B. Independence training in nursing home residents. *Gerontologist* 16:428–431, 1976.

Bandriet, L.M. Gerontological research. Evaluating the process. *J Gerontol Nurs* 19(9):33–38, 1993.

Barber, H., Jelinek, D., Barbe, M. et al. Helping the rural elderly. *J Gerontol Nurs* 10:105–109, 1984.

Bassett, C., McClamrock, E. and Schmelzer, M. A 10-week exercise program for senior citizens. *Geriatr Nurs* 3:103–105, 1982.

Bernardini, B., Meinecke, C., Zacarini, C. et al. Adverse clinical events in dependent long-term nursing home patients. *J Am Geriatr Soc* 41:105–111, 1993.

Bliesmor, M. and Earle, P. Research considerations: Nursing home quality perceptions. *J Gerontol Nurs* 19(6):27–34, 1993.

Borup, J.H. Relocation: Attitudes, information network and problems encountered. *Gerontologist* 21(5):501–511, 1981.

Borup, J.H. Relocation mortality research: Assessment, reply, and the need to refocus on the issues. *Gerontologist* 23:234–242, 1983.

Bourestom, N. and Tars, S. Alterations in life patterns following nursing home relocation. *Gerontologist* 14:506–510, 1974.

Braun, B. The effect of nursing home quality on patient outcome. *J Am Geriatr Soc* 39:329–338, 1991.

Brody, E. Long-term care of the aged. *Health Social Work* 2:30–59, 1977.

Brody, E., Kleban, M. and Moss, M. Measuring the impact of change. *Gerontologist* 14:299–305, 1974.

Brody, J.A. and Foley, D.J. Epidemiologic considerations. *In* Schneider, E.L., Wendland, C.J. and Zimmer, A.W. (eds.). *The Teaching-Nursing Home*. New York: Raven Press, The Beverly Foundation, 1985, pp. 9–26.

Brooke, V. Your helping hand: How to tailor your approach in each phase of adjustment. *J Gerontol Nurs* 10(3):126–128, 1989.

Burke, B. and Sherman, S. (eds.). *Gerontological Nursing: Issues and Opportunities for the Twenty-First Century*. New York: National League for Nursing Press, 1993.

Burke, M. and Donley, S.R. The educational experiment: A teaching nursing home. *J Gerontol Nurs* 13(1):36–40, 1987.

Camargo, O. and Presston, G.H. What happens to patients who are hospitalized for the first time when over 65? *Am J Psychiatry* 102:168–173, 1945.

Campion, E., Bang, A. and May, M. Why acute-care hospitals must undertake long-term care. *N Engl J Med* 308:71, 1983.

Chappell, N.L. and Novak, M. The role of support in alleviating stress among nursing assistants. *Gerontologist* 32(3):351–359, 1992.

Coffman, T.L. Relocation and survival of institutionalized aged: A re-examination of the evidence. *Gerontologist* 21:483–500, 1981.

Coffman, T.L. Toward an understanding of geriatric relocation. *Gerontologist* 23:453–458, 1983.

Colling, J., Hadley, B.J., Eisch, J. et al. Patterned urge response toileting for urinary incontinence: A clinical trial. *In* Funk, S.G., Tornquist, E.M., Champagne, M.T. and Wiese, R.A. (eds.). *Key Aspects of Elder Care: Managing Falls, Incontinence, and Cognitive Impairment.* New York: Springer Publishing, 1992, pp. 169–186.

Collopy, B., Boyle, P. and Jennings, B. New directions in nursing home ethics. *In* Mitty, E.L. (ed.). *Quality Imperatives in Long-Term Care: The Illusive Agenda.* New York: National League for Nursing, Pub. No. 41-2440, 1992, pp. 71–104.

Copp, L.A. Pain coping model and typology. *Image* 17(3):69–71, 1985.

Dawes, P.L. The nurse's aide and the team approach in the nursing home. *J Geriatr Psychiatry Neurol* 14(2):265–276, 1981.

Decker, S.D. and Kinzel, S.L. Learned helplessness and decreased social interaction in elderly disabled persons. *Rehabil Nurs* Mar/Apr:31–32, 1985.

Diamond, T. Social policy and everyday life in nursing homes: A critical ethnography. *Soc Sci Med* 23:1287–1295, 1986.

Elon, R. The nursing home medical director role in transition. *J Am Geriatr Soc* 41:131–135, 1993.

Engle, V.F. and Graney, M.J. Stability and improvement of health after nursing home admission. *J Gerontol* 48(1):S17–S23, 1993.

Evans, L.K. Maintaining social interaction as health promotion in the elderly. *J Gerontol Nurs* 5(2):19–21, 1979.

Evans, L.K., and Strumpf, N.E. Myths about elder restraint. *Image J Nurs Scholarship* 22(2):124–128, 1990.

Evans, L.K. and Strumpf, N.E. Tying down the elderly: A review of the literature on physical restraint. *J Am Geriatr Soc* 37:65–74, 1989.

Ferrell, B.A., Feffell, B.R. and Osterweil, D. Pain in the nursing home. *J Am Geriatr Soc* 38(4):409–414, 1990.

Foyt, M.M. No place for a critical care nurse? *Am J Nurs* 91(10):20, 1991.

Gerontology Institute. *The Nursing Home Reform Act of 1987: Provisions, Policies, Prospects.* Boston: The Gerontology Institute, University of Massachusetts, 1991.

Ginter, S.F. and Mion, L.C. Falls in the nursing home: Preventable or inevitable? *J Gerontol Nurs* 18(11):43–48, 57–58, 1992.

Hassanein, S.A. On the shortage of registered nurses: An economic analysis of the RN market. *Nurs Health Care* 12(3):152–156, 1991.

Heine, C. (ed.). *Determining the Future of Gerontological Nursing Education: Partnerships between Nursing Education and Practice.* New York: National League for Nursing Press, 1993.

Heine, C. and Bahr, S.R. New practice models in long-term care. *In* Burke, M. and Sherman, S. (eds.). *Gerontological Nursing: Issues and Opportunities for the Twenty-First Century.* New York: National League for Nursing Press, Publ. No. 14-2510, 1993, pp. 27–36.

Horowitz, M.J. and Schulz, R. The relocation controversy: Criticism and commentary on five recent studies. *Gerontologist* 23:229–234, 1983.

Institute of Medicine. *Improving the Quality of Care in Nursing Homes.* Washington, D.C.: National Academy Press, 1986.

Johnson, D. Make your own chairbound alternatives. *Geriatric Nurs* 11:18–19, 1991.

Johnson, M.A. and Werner, C. "We had no choice": A study in familial guilt feelings surrounding nursing home care. *J Gerontol Nurs* 8:641–645, 654, 1982.

Joint Commission on Accreditation of Healthcare Organizations. *Quality Improvement in Long Term Care: How Quality Improvement Can Help Fulfill OBRA '87 Requirements.* Oakbrook Terrace, IL: Joint Commission on Accreditation of Healthcare Organizations, 1992.

Jonas, S. *Health Care Delivery in the United States.* New York: Springer Publishing Company, 1981.

Jones, C. *Caring for the Aged.* Chicago: Nelson-Hall, 1982.

Kahana, E. The humane treatment of old people in institutions. *Gerontologist* 13:282–289, 1973.

Kane, R.A. and Kane, R.L. *Assessing the Elderly: A Practical Guide to Measurement.* Lexington, MA.: Lexington Books, 1981.

Kane, R.L., Garrard, J., Buchanan, J. et al. Assessing the effectiveness of geriatric nurse practitioners. *In* Mezey, M.D., Lynaugh, J.E. and Cartier, M.M. (eds.). *Nursing Homes and Nursing Care: Lessons from the Teaching Nursing Homes.* New York: Springer Publishing Company, 1989a.

Kane, R.L., Garrard, J., Buchanan, J.L. et al. Improving primary care in nursing homes. *J Am Geriatr Soc* 89:359–367, 1991.

Kane, R.L., Garrard, J., Skay, C.L. et al. Effects of a geriatric nurse practitioner on process and outcome of nursing home care. *Am J Public Health* 79(9):1271–1277, 1989b.

Kane, R.L., Williams, C.C., Williams, T.F. and Kane R.A. Restraining restraints. Changes in a standard of care. *Annu Rev Publ Health* 14:545–584, 1993.

Kastenbaum, R. Can the clinical milieu be therapeutic? *In* Rowles, G.D. and Ohta, R.J. (eds.). *Aging and Milieu: Environmental Perspectives on Growing Old.* New York: Academic Press, 1983.

Lester, P.B. and Baltes, N.M. Functional interdependence of the social environment and the behavior of the institutionalized aged. *J Gerontol Nurs* 4:23–27, 1978.

Lieberman, M. Instutionalization of the aged: Effects on behavior. *J Gerontol* 24:330–340, 1969.

Linn, M.W., Gurel, L. and Linn, B.S. Patient outcomes as a measure of quality in nursing home care. *Am J Public Health* 67(4):337–344, 1977.

List, N.D., Ory, M.G. and Hadley, E.C. The NIA teaching nursing home award program: A national program of research on geriatrics and long-term care. *In* Schneider, E.L., Wendland, C.J. and Zimmer, A.W. et al. (eds.). *The Teaching Nursing Home.* New York: Raven Press, 1985, pp. 89–98.

Lodge, M.P. *Professional Education and Practice of Nurse Administrators/Directors of Nursing in Long-Term Care.* Executive Summary. Kansas City, MO: American Nurses' Foundation, 1987.

McConnell, J. Preventing urinary tract infections. *Geriatr Nurs* 5(6):361–362, 1984.

McCracken Knights, A. Teaching nursing homes. A project update. *J Gerontol Nurs* 10(6):14–17, 1984.

McDonald, M.L. and Butler, A.K. Reversal of helplessness: Producing walk behavior in nursing home wheelchair residents using behavior modification procedures. *J Gerontol* 29:97–101, 1974.

McElroy, D. and Herbelin, K. Assuring quality of care in long-term care facilities. *J Gerontol Nurs* 15(7):8–10, 1989.

Mercer, S. and Kane, R.A. Helplessness and hopelessness among the institutionalized aged: An experiment. *Health Social Work* 4:91–116, 1979.

Mezey, M.D. and Lynaugh, J.E. Teaching nursing home program: A lesson in quality. *Geriatr Nurs* 11:76–77, 1991.

Mezey, M.D., Lynaugh, J.E. and Aiken, L.H. The Robert Wood Johnson Foundation. *In* Schneider, E.L., Wendland, C.J., Zimmer, A.W. et al. (eds.). *The Teaching Nursing Home.* New York: Raven Press, 1985, pp. 79–87.

Mezey, M.D., Lynaugh, J.E. and Cartier, M.M. Reordering values: The teaching nursing home program. *In* Mezey, M.D., Lynaugh, J.E. and Cartier, M.M. (eds). *Nursing Homes and Nursing Care. Lessons from the Teaching Nursing Homes.* New York: Springer Publishing, 1989, pp. 1–11.

Mezey, M.D. and Scanlon, W. Reimbursement options for encouraging geriatric nurse practitioner services. *In* Mezey, M.D., Lynaugh, J.E. and Cartier, M.M. (eds). *Nursing Care and Nursing Homes.* New York: Springer Publishing Company, 1989, pp. 62–74.

Miller, M.B. Iatrogenic and nurisgenic effects of prolonged immobility of the ill aged. *J Am Geriatr Soc* 23: 360–369, 1975.

Mirotznik, J. and Ruskin, A.P. Inter-institutional relocation and its effects on health. *Gerontologist* 24:286–291, 1984.

National Center for Health Statistics. The 1985 National Nursing Home Study. Washington, D.C.: United States Government Printing Office, DHHS PHS 89-1758, 1989.

National League for Nursing. *Time to Care: The Nursing Home Clinical* (video) and *Teaching Gerontology: The Curriculum Imperative* (companion book). 1991. Battle Creek, MI:. W.K. Kellogg; New York: National League for Nursing (distributor).

Neufeld, R.R., Tideiksaar, R, Yew, E. et al. A multidisciplinary falls consultation service in a nursing home. *Gerontologist* 31(1):120–123, 1991.

Ouslander, J.G., Kane, R.L. and Abrass, I.B. Urinary incontinence in elderly nursing home patients. *JAMA* 248(10):1194–1198, 1982.

Paillard, M. and Nowak, K.B. Use exercise to help older adults: Clients in acute care benefit from exercise and relaxation plan. *J Gerontol Nurs* 11(7):36–39, 1985.

Patnaik, B., Lawton, M.P., Kieban, M.H. et al. Behavioral adaptation to the change in institutional residence. *Gerontologist* 14:305–307, 1974.

Petrou, M.F. and Obenchain, J.V. Reducing incidence of illness post-transfer. *Geriatr Nurs* 8(5):264–266, 1987.

Pipes, L.J. The Beverly Enterprises teaching nursing home program. *In* Schneider, E.L., Wendland, C.J., Zimmer, A.W. et al. (eds.). *The Teaching Nursing Home.* New York: Raven Press, The Beverly Foundation, 1985.

Rader, J., Semradek, J., McKenzie, D. and McMahon, J. Restraint strategies: Reducing restraints in Oregon's long term care facilities. *J Gerontol Nurs* 18(11):49–56, 1992.

Resnick, N.M. and Yalla, S.V. Management of urinary incontinence in the elderly. *N Engl J Med* 313(13):800–804, 1985.

Robertson, J.F. and Cummings, C.C. What makes long-term care nursing attractive? *Am J Nurs* 91(11):41–46, 1991.

Roosa, W.M. Territory and privacy: Resident's views: Findings of a survey. *Geriatr Nurs* Jul/Aug:241–243, 1982.

Rosswurm, M.A. Relocation and the elderly. *J Gerontol Nurs* 9:632–637, 1983.

Schick, F.L. and Schick, R.S. *Statistical Handbook on Aging Americans.* Phoenix, AZ: Onyx Press, 1994.

Rountree, B.H. and Deckard, G.J. Nursing in long term care: Dispelling a myth. *J Long Term Care Adm* Fall:15–19, 1986.

Schafer, S. Modifying the environment. *Geriatr Nurs* May/Jun:157–159, 1985.

Schneider, E.L. Teaching nursing homes. *N Engl J Med* 308:336–337, 1985.

Schnelle, J.F. Treatment of urinary incontinence in nursing home patients by prompted voiding. *J Am Geriatr Soc* 38(3):356–360, 1990.

Schwab, M. Nursing care in nursing homes. *Am J Nurs* 75(10):181–185, 1975.

Seligman, M. *On Depression, Development and Death.* San Francisco: W.H. Freeman, 1975.

Sheridan, J.E., White, J. and Fairchild, T.J. Ineffective staff, ineffective supervision, or ineffective administration? Why some nursing homes fail to provide adequate care. *Gerontologist* 32(3):334–341, 1992.

Sherman, S.E. The Community College-Nursing Home Partnership. *In* Heine, C. (ed.). *Determining the Future of Gerontological Nursing Education. Partnerships between Education and Practice.* New York: National League for Nursing Press. Publ. No. 14-2508, 1993.

Sloane, P. and Gwyther, L. Nursing homes. *JAMA* 244: 1840–1841, 1980.

Sloane, P. and Mathew, L. (eds.). *Dementia Units in Long-Term Care.* Baltimore: Johns Hopkins University Press, 1991.

Sloane, P.D., Mathew, L.J., Scarborough, M. et al. Physical and pharmacologic restraint of nursing home patients with dementia: Impact of specialized units. *JAMA* 265(10):1278–1283, 1991.

Smallegan, M. There was nothing else to do: Need for care before nursing home admission. *Gerontologist* 25(4):364–369, 1985.

Smith, K.F. and Bengtson, V.L. Positive consequences of institutionalization: Solidarity between elderly parents and their middle-aged children. *Gerontologist.* 19(5, part 1):438–447, 1979.

Spector, W.D. and Takada, H.A. Characteristics of nursing homes that affect resident outcomes. *J Aging Health* 30(4):427–454, 1991.

Spence, D.A. and Weiner, J.M. Nursing home length of stay patterns: Results from the 1985 National Nursing Home Survey. *Gerontologist* 30:16–22, 1990.

Staats, D.O. Physical environments. *In* Cassel, C. and Walsh, J. (eds.). *Geriatric Medicine.* Vol. 2. New York: Springer-Verlag, 1984.

Stolley, J.M. Freeing your patients from restraints. *Am J Nurs,* Feb: 27–31, 1995.

Storlie, F.J. The reshaping of the old. *J Gerontol Nurs* 8: 555–559, 1982.

Strumpf, N.E., Evans, J.K., Wagner, J. and Patterson, J. Reducing physical restraints: Developing an educational program. *J Gerontol Nurs* 18(11):21–27, 1992.

Tagliareni, M.E. The nursing home clinical: New horizons for capitalizing on a caring experience. *In* Burke, M. and Susan Sherman, S. (eds.). *Gerontological Nursing: Issues and Opportunities for the Twenty-First Century.* New York: National League for Nursing Press, Publ. No. 14-2510, 1993, pp. 37–44.

Tagliareni, M.E., Carignan, A. and Austin, M. The community college–nursing home partnership: Improving care through education. *In* Heine, C. (ed.). *Determining the Future of Gerontological Nursing Education: Partnerships Between Education and Practice.* New York: National League for Nursing Press, 1993, p. 72.

Talbot, D.M. Assessing the needs of the rural elderly. *J Gerontol Nurs* 11:39–43, 1985.

Tellis-Nayak, M. and Snyderman, G. Quality improvement: The view from JCAHO. *Nurs Homes* Sept/Oct: 2022, 1992.

Tellis-Nayak, V. *Nursing Home Exemplars of Quality: Their Paths to Excellence.* Springfield, IL: Charles C. Thomas Publisher, 1988.

Tinetti, M.E. Performance-oriented assessment of mobility problems in elderly patients. *J Am Geriatr Soc* 34(2): 119–126, 1986.

Tinetti, M.E., Liu, W.L. and Ginter, S.F. Mechanical restraint use and fall-related injuries among residents of skilled nursing facilities. *Ann Intern Med* 1992, (6):369–374, 1992.

Tinetti, M.E., Liu, W.L., Marottoli, R.A. and Ginter, S.F.

Mechanical restraint use among residents of skilled nursing facilities: Prevalence, patterns, and predictors. *JAMA* 265:468–471, 1991.

Tinetti, M.E., Williams, T.F. and Mayewski, R. Fall risk index for elderly patients based on number of chronic disabilities. *Am J Med* 80(3):429–434, 1986.

United States Department of Health and Human Services. *Aging America: Trends and Projections.* Washington, D.C., Publ. No. (FCoA) 91-28001, 1994.

United States Food and Drug Administration. *FDA Safety Alert: Potential Hazards with Restraint Devices.* Rockville, MD: United States Department of Health and Human Services, 1992.

Urinary Incontinence Guideline Panel. *Urinary Incontinence in Adults: Quick Reference Guide for Clinicians.* AHCPR Pub. No. 92-0041. Rockville, MD: Agency for Health Care Policy and Research, Public Health Service, U.S. Department of Health and Human Services, March 1992.

Van Oteghen, S.L. An exercise program for those with Parkinson's disease. *Geriatr Nurs* 8(4):183–184, 1987.

Vaughan-Wrobel, B.C. and Tygart, M.W. Management education needs of nurse administrators in long-term care. *J Gerontol Nurs* 19(3):33–38, 1993.

Vincente, L., Wiley, J. and Carrington, R. The risk of institutionalization before death. *Gerontologist* 19:361–370, 1979.

Walsh, M.B. and Wilhere, S.P.G. The future of teaching nursing homes. *Geriatr Nurs* (9):354–356, 1988.

Warden, J.C. Professionalization, education, and commitment. *Geriatr Nurs* 14(1):6, 1993.

Whittier, J.R. and Williams, D. The coincidence in constancy of mortality figures for aged psychotic patients admitted to state hospitals. *Nerv Ment Dis* 124:618–620, 1956.

Wolanin, M.O. Relocation of the elderly. *J Gerontol Nurs* 4(3):47–50, 1978.

Wolanin, M.O. and Phillips, L.R. *Confusion: Prevention and Care.* St. Louis, MO: C.V. Mosby, 1981.

Wright, B.A. Behavior diagnoses by a multidisciplinary team. *Geriatr Nurs* Jan/Feb: 30–35, 1993.

Zimmer, J.G., Watson, N.M. and Levenson, S.A. Nursing home medical directors: Ideals and realities. *J Am Geriatr Soc* 41:127–130, 1993.

Zweig, J. and Csank, J. Effects of relocation on chronically ill geriatric patients on a medical unit: Mortality rates. *J Am Geriatr Soc* 23:286–291, 1975.

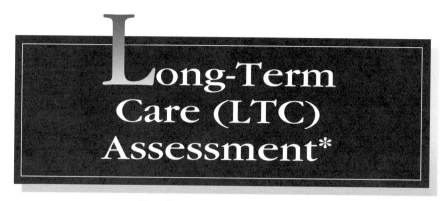

Long-Term Care (LTC) Assessment*

*See discussion on page 913.

Appendix

LTC ASSESSMENT—FACE SHEET

1. Target Population

( ) SNF/Medicaid eligible or pending

( ) ICF/Medicaid eligible or pending

( ) Voluntary private pay

( ) Potential Medicaid, if institutionalized

( ) Domiciliary

( ) Elderly/disabled applicant for LTC services

2. Basic Data

Name _____

Social Security Number _____

Address _____

_____ County _____

Phone. No. _____

Date of Birth _____

Sex ( ) Male ( ) Female

Race _____

Marital Status _____

Living Arrangement _____

3. Other Client Information

Physician _____

Emergency Contact _____

Medicaid Number _____

Medicare Number _____

Health Insurance (Company & Policy Numbers)

_____

_____

_____

_____

_____

Address _____ Phone No. _____

_____

Address _____ Phone No. _____

_____

F12 Prior Approval No. _____

F12 Date of Approval _____

CAP Eligibility Date _____

Veteran Status _____

Educational Status _____

Employment Status _____

Legal Status _____

Eligibility Category for SIS _____

4. Referral Information

Referral Source ( ) Self ( ) Family ( ) Friend ( ) Physician

( ) DSS ( ) Health agency ( ) Aging agency ( ) Other _____

Circumstances of Referral _____

Date of Referral _____

LTC ASSESSMENT *(Continued)*

5. Current Formal Service Provision

Agency	Services

PHYSICAL HEALTH

1. Health Problems   Client Name:

Health Problem	Date of Onset	Comments (Severity, Prognosis)

Senses	Good	Fair	Poor	None	Activity level	Active	Nonactive
Vision					Severely impaired		
Hearing					Somewhat impaired		
Speech					Unimpaired		

LTC ASSESSMENT *(Continued)*

2. Medications

Self-Administration ( ) Able to take medication in right doses at right time ( ) Can prepare and take medication with reminder ( ) Can take medication, needs assistance with preparation ( ) Unable to take medication without assistance		Comments	
Medication	Dosage/Frequency	Route	Note Any Compliance Problems

3. Health Treatment

Treatment Activity	Frequency	Done by	Additional Treatment Needed

New Treatment Needed	Frequency	

4. Describe General Physical Condition

5. Assistive Devices

	Needs	*Has*	*Uses*
Glasses/contacts			
Hearing aid			
Dentures			
Prosthesis			
Mobility aids			
Communication aids			

MENTAL HEALTH

1. FROMAJE Test

Client Name:

Date:

Areas

F = Function	A = Arithmetic
R = Reason	J = Judgment
O = Orientation	E = Emotion
M = Memory	

Ratings

1 = Normal, unimpaired performance
2 = Slightly impaired performance
3 = Totally impaired, cannot perform

	F	R	O	M	A	J	E	Total
Assessor Rating								
Family Rating (optional)								

2. Set Test Date:

Categories (0–10)

Animals _____

Colors _____

Vegetables _____

Cities _____

Total (0–40) _____

3. Narrative Description of Mental Status

4. Comments and Notes

LTC ASSESSMENT *(Continued)*

ECONOMIC STATUS

1. Available Income and Resources

Client Name:

(Check if client has income/resource. Enter amount if known.)	Spouse or other household member's income (enter if income resources affect client eligibility)

Client's income   Amount

( ) Social Security   _____
( ) SSI   _____
( ) Retirement   _____
( ) Salary   _____
( ) Other   _____
      TOTAL   _____

Resources

( ) Bank accounts   _____
( ) Life insurance   _____
( ) Stocks and bonds   _____
( ) Owns home   _____
( ) Other   _____
      TOTAL   _____

( ) Other financial assistance

   _____   _____

   _____   _____

Income   Amount

( ) Social Security   _____
( ) SSI   _____
( ) Retirement   _____
( ) Salary   _____
( ) Other   _____
      TOTAL   _____

Resources

( ) Bank accounts   _____
( ) Life insurance   _____
( ) Stocks and bonds   _____
( ) Owns home   _____
( ) Other   _____
      TOTAL   _____

( ) Other financial assistance

   _____   _____

   _____   _____

2. Average Monthly Expenses (Work Sheet)

3. Financial Affairs

Financial affairs are managed by
( ) Self _____
( ) Other _____
    Relationship _____
Are there financial assistance programs for which the client is potentially eligible? ( ) yes ( ) no
Identify _____
_____
_____
_____

4. Needs

Check if client experiences financial problems in meeting basic needs in the following areas:

             Comment
( ) Health services _____
( ) Medicines _____
( ) Food _____
( ) Clothing _____
( ) Fuel _____
( ) Housing _____
( ) Other _____

LTC ASSESSMENT *(Continued)*

5. Comments and Notes

ACTIVITIES OF DAILY LIVING

1. ADLs   Client Name:

	Dependency			Need Met by					Is Need Met Completely?	
	Independent	Partially Dependent	Totally Dependent	Family	Friend	Agency	Equipment	Type of Help/Frequency	Yes	No
Eating										
Dressing										
Bathing										
Toileting										
Urinary continence										
Bowel continence										
Ambulation										
Wheelchair use										
Transfers: Bed to chair										
In/out bath										
In/out car										
Communication system used										

2. IADLs

Meal preparation										
Shopping										
Money management										
Transportation										
Telephone use										
Equipment use										
Laundry										
Social participation										

LTC ASSESSMENT *(Continued)*

3. Family/Client Ratings

Describe any differences in ratings of client, family and interviewer

4. Additional Services Needed

Service	Frequency

5. Comments and Notes

HOME ENVIRONMENT

1. General Information

Client Name:

Location: ( ) Urban	Type of home: ( ) Apartment
( ) Rural	( ) Duplex
( ) Other	( ) House
Ownership ( ) Owns	( ) Single-story
of home: ( ) Rents	( ) Two-story
( ) Lives with relative	( ) Ground floor
( ) Government-subsidized	( ) Isolated
( ) Other _____	( ) Other _____

2. Problem Areas

Area	Safety	Adequacy	Accessibility	Comment
	(Check If a Problem)			
Heating				
Cooling				
Hot water				
Cold water				
Structural				
Electrical system				
Entrance(s)				
Windows				
Sleeping area				
Living area				

LTC ASSESSMENT *(Continued)*

2. Problem Areas *(Continued)*

Area	Safety	Adequacy	Accessibility	Comment
		(Check If a Problem)		
Eating area				
Bathing area				
Cooking area				
Phone system				
Telephone alert				
Washer				
Dryer				
Refrigeration				
Other				

3. Comments and Notes

SOCIAL SUPPORT

1. Usual Household Composition   Client Name:

Name	Age	Relationship to Client	Tasks Performed for Client	Days/Hours Available

2. Informal Care Providers (Other Than Household)

Name	Location	Phone	Tasks Performed	Days/Hours Available

LTC ASSESSMENT *(Continued)*

3. Family/Social Support System

Identify any concerns of family/significant others regarding clients being cared for at home:
Identify services family/social support system feels are needed for the client to stay at home:
Identify any concerns of the client regarding the adequacy of social support or being cared for at home:
Identify services the client feels are needed for the client to stay at home:

PLAN OF CARE

1. Identifying Information

Client's Name: _____   ( ) Initial Assessment

Social Security Number: _____   ( ) Reassessment

Date of Last Care Plan: _____   ( ) Plan Revision

LTC ASSESSMENT *(Continued)*

2. Assessment Summary (Check Each Area)

Area	Unimpaired	Mildly Impaired	Moderately Impaired	Severely Impaired
Physical health				
Mental health				
Economic status				
Activities of daily living				
Home environment				
Social support				

Assessor: _____   Assessor: _____

Agency: _____   Agency: _____

Phone No.: _____   Phone No.: _____

3. Plan of Care

List goals first, then describe the Action Plan, including relationships between formal and informal supports.

4. Equipment Justification (Durable Medical Equipment)

Include equipment specifications, costs, need for equipment, length of need, and recommendation for rental or purchase.

LTC ASSESSMENT *(Continued)*

CARE PLAN AGREEMENTS

1. Family/Social Support Responsibilities

Name	Relationship	Tasks to Be Performed	Days/Hours Available

Family/social support will assist with:

( ) Activities of daily living   ( ) Financial support

( ) Instrumental activities of daily living   ( ) Companion/oversight

( ) Emotional support   ( ) Other _____

2. Institutional Care

Have institutional options been discussed with the client?   ( ) yes   ( ) no

Comment on appropriateness of institutional care _____

_____

3. Agreements

The following persons have reviewed the Care Plan and agree to:

( ) Participate in the Care Plan as described

( ) Seek home care independently

    Identify reasons (if given) _____

    _____

( ) Participate in Care Plan pending placement in ICF/SNF or domiciliary home

( ) Seek placement directly into ICF/SNF or domiciliary home

( ) Other _____

Signature:	*Title/Relationship:*	*Date:*	*Verified by Case Manager:*
_____	Client	_____	_____
_____	Case Manager	_____	_____
_____	Physician	_____	_____
_____	Other _____	_____	_____
_____	_____	_____	_____

Source: North Carolina Department of Human Resources, Raleigh, NC, DHR647, 1984.

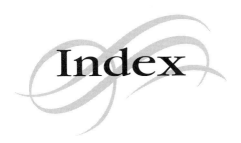

Index

Note: Page numbers in *italics* refer to illustrations; those followed by t refer to tables, and those followed by b refer to boxed material.

AARP (American Association of Retired Persons), 576
Abducens nerve, function of, 312t
Absolute threshold, in sensory systems, 356
Absorption, of drugs, 742
Abstraction, deficits in, 529
Abuse, definition of, 626–627
  of elderly. See *Elder abuse.*
  substance. See *Substance abuse.*
Accessibility, of lifestyle modification programs, 901–902, 903t
Accidental hypothermia, 418. See also *Hypothermia.*
Accidental injury, ecological model of, 845–846
Accommodation, of eye, 357–358
ACE (angiotensin-converting enzyme) inhibitors, cost comparisons of, 755t
  for hypertension, 230t
Acini, pancreatic, 362–363
Acoustic nerve, function of, 312t
Acquired immunodeficiency syndrome (AIDS). See *Human immunodeficiency virus (HIV) infection.*
Acral lentiginous melanoma, 188
Acrochordon (skin tag), 181
Actinic keratoses, 186, *186*
Actinic lentigo, senile (liver spots), *181*
Activities director, in long-term care facility, 945
Activities of daily living (ADL), assessment of, for community dwellers, 11, *11–13*
  dependence in, 487. See also *Self-care deficits.*
  dependency and, 621, *622*
  difficulties with, in elderly population, 562–563, 563t
  instrumental, 83–84, 86t
    dependency and, 621
    difficulties with, in elderly population, 562–563, 563t
  Katz Index of, 82t, 83
Activity, 409
  assessment of, 103t, 107
  physical. See also *Exercise(s).*
    contraindications to, 228t
    habitual, effects of, 227t
    requiring mild, moderate, and severe energy expenditure, 414t
Activity deficit, diversional, 830–834
  assessment of, 832–833, 833t
  definition of, 830
  evaluation of, 834
  factor(s) contributing to, *831*, 831–832
    environmental influences as, 832
    lifestyle and health status as, 832
  intervention in, 833–834
  planning and, 833
  theoretical issues in, 830–831

Activity deficit *(Continued)*
    time utilization in, 830–831
  health maintenance alteration and, 835–836
Activity intolerance, 409–417
  assessment of, 412–413, 413t, 414t
  definition of, 409
  evaluation of, 416–417
  factor(s) contributing to, 410–412
    age-related, 410
    cardiovascular and respiratory disorders as, 410
    hepatic and renal disorders as, 412
    neurological and musculoskeletal impairments as, 410–412, 411t
    nutritional, 412
    psychological influences as, 412
  planning and intervention in, 413–417
    age considerations and, 413–414
    energy conservation techniques and, 416
    exercise programs and, 415–416
    optimizing disease management and, 414–415
  scope of, *409*, 409–410
  self-care deficits and, 488–489
Activity theory, on aging, 592–593
Activity tolerance, assessment of, 413t
  impact of chronic diseases on, 411t
Acuity, visual, age-related changes in, 358, *359*
Acute care setting(s), gerontological nursing in, 855–893. See also *Hospital(s).*
Acute myocardial infarction, 234–235
  percutaneous transluminal coronary angioplasty for, 235
  thrombolytic therapy for, 234–235, 235t
Acute renal failure, 342–343
  treatment of, 343
Acute respiratory failure, as complication of COPD, 267
Acyclovir (Zovirax), for shingles, 189
Adaptation, ineffective coping and, 671–672
Adaptation, to stress, 19–20
Adaptive strategy(ies), to aging, 592
Adjustment disorder, with depressed mood, 639
ADL. See *Activities of daily living (ADL).*
Administrative issues, in discharge planning, 863
Adrenal cortex, age-related changes in, 358
ADRs (adverse drug reactions). See *Drug reaction(s), adverse.*
Adult day care, in social isolation, 723
Adulthood Isolation Index, 722t
Adverse drug reactions (ADRs). See *Drug reaction(s), adverse.*
Affect, changes of, in dementia of Alzheimer's type, 298

Affection, within families, 585
Affective needs, of family, 682
Affective status, unidimensional instruments for, 85–90, 89t, 90t, *91–92*, 93b–94b, 94–95, 95t, 96t
Age, chronological approach to, 6
  consideration of, activity intolerance and, 413–414
  functional approach to, 6–7
  median, of population, 557, *557*
  old. See also *Elderly.*
    definitions of, 6–7
Age differentiation, ageism and, 609, *609*
Age grading, 573–575
  effects of, on attitudes and behaviors, 574
    on intergenerational relationships, 574–575
    on transitions between age and categories, 575
Aged. See *Elderly.*
Ageism, 605–610
  age differentiation and, 609, *609*
  age integration and, 609, *609*
  consequences of, 608–609
  contributor(s) to, 606–608
    attitudes as, 605, 606
    beliefs as, 605, 606
    cultural factors as, 607–608
    labeling as, 607
    stereotyping as, 606–607
    values as, 606
  definition of, 605
  influence of, on health outcomes, 609
  nursing care and, 609–610
  scope of, 605–606
  social breakdown syndrome and, 608–609
  sociocultural factors and, 741
Agency for Health Care Policy and Research (AHCPR), 36
Age-specific reference values, for weight, 773t
Aggression. See also *Violence.*
  causation of, model of, *728*
Aggressiveness of care, ethical conflict over, for depressed patient, 151–154, *154*
Aging, 7–8
  accelerated, diabetes mellitus as state of, 365t
  adaptive tasks associated with, 591
  and family structure, 580
  Baltimore Longitudinal Study on, 226
  biological programming and, 166, 166t
  biological theories of, 159–170
    aging process and, 169, *169*
    at cellular level, 166–168, *167*
    at organ level, *168*, 169
    at tissue level, 168–169
    early, 162